PHYSIOLOGY IN CHILDBEARING

with anatomy and related biosciences

Dot Stables MSc BA(Hons) MTD DN RM RN

Formerly lecturer in applied biology, St Bartholomews, College of Nursing and Midwifery, City University, London, UK

With **Barbara Novak** MSc BEd(Hons) RN RSCN RM
Lecturer in applied biological sciences, City University, London, UK
(Chapters 2 and 48–53)

Foreword by:
Rosaline Steele MA BA MTD ADM RM RN
Director of Education and Practice Development,
The Royal College of Midwives Trust, London, UK

Baillière Tindall
Edinburgh London New York Philadelphia St Louis Sydney Toronto 1999

Baillière Tindall
An imprint of Harcourt Brace and Company Limited

First published 1999

ISBN 0 702 021350

British Library Cataloguing in Publication Data
A catalogue record for this book is available from the British Library.

Library of Congress Cataloging in Publication Data
A catalog record for this book is available from the Library of Congress

Note
Medical knowledge is constantly changing. As new information becomes available, changes in treatment, procedures, equipment and the use of drugs become necessary. The editors, contributors and the publishers have, as far as it is possible, taken care to ensure that the information given in this text is accurate and up to date. However, readers are strongly advised to confirm that the information, especially with regard to drug usage, complies with latest legislation and standards of practice.

Printed in China

PHYSIOLOGY IN CHILDBEARING

This book is dedicated to
the wonderful people who provide care
for mothers and babies throughout the world.

For Baillière Tindall

Publishing Manager: Inta Ozols
Project Manager: Karen Gilmour

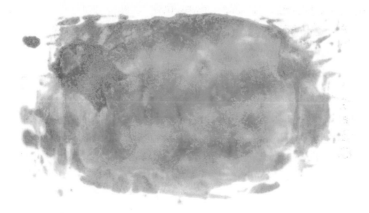

Contents

Foreword

It is an honour and a pleasure to be invited to write the foreword to *Physiology in Childbearing*; a book that will be warmly welcomed by student midwives and midwives already in practice, for the sound knowledge base it offers and the clarity of its contents.

Pregnancy, childbirth and parenting are activities normally overlooked by society as a whole until there is a real or perceived problem. However, midwives are very conscious of the need to support women and their families during this important period in their lives. *Physiology in Childbearing* provides midwives with a sound evidence base on which decisions for their practice can be made. As midwives we are proud to be part of a wonderful, challenging, and rewarding profession, which demands that a midwife has the knowledge and skills to practise with empathy and has the ability to support women and their families throughout pregnancy, labour and the postnatal period. As a midwife and a teacher of midwifery, I welcome the availability of a book on physiology, which is written in such an accessible format and which is a ready reference on all aspects of pregnancy and childbearing. There are a number of midwifery and medical texts available, which devote short sections to the physiology associated with childbearing. However, for the first time there is now a single text of quality and authority, written by a midwife, to which I can refer with ease and confidence.

The preparation and presentation of this book are not a complete surprise to those of us who are contemporaries of Dot Stables. Dot has always been keen to ensure that students at pre-registration and postgraduate level develop an accurate knowledge of the physiological process of pregnancy and childbirth, and through this book she has accomplished just that.

London, 1999 — Rosaline Steele

Introduction

As research and information increase, general textbooks for midwives have valiantly attempted to cover all aspects of midwifery theory and practice. However, even when written by multiple authors, they are increasingly unable to cover each subject in appropriate depth. Although they provide an excellent foundation on all aspects of pregnancy, labour and postnatal and neonatal care, it is essential that the student midwife, midwife practitioner and others caring for women during childbearing have access to more detailed knowledge on which to base their practice.

There have been many well-written books on the psychological and social implications of childbearing and there are many good textbooks of human anatomy and physiology for nurses. However, few that have been written specifically with the midwife in mind have approached sufficient depth of biology. Although the American textbook *Maternal, Fetal and Neonatal Physiology*, written by Susan Tucker Blackburn and Donna Lee Loper (1992), has much good information it does not cover labour and delivery and is therefore not sufficient for the practising midwife.

In my career as a teacher of midwifery to midwifery students and biology to all nursing and midwifery students, I am aware of the increasing need for appropriate books to deepen understanding. It is important for the reader to be aware that this book is about the biological sciences, in particular physiology, applied to human childbearing including the mother, fetus and baby. It is dedicated to introducing a wider appreciation of the biological sciences to those with little previous formal involvement in their study. The psychological and social status of the woman are of equal importance and the student is advised to read relevant texts.

It is important to remember that it is not sufficient to have knowledge of the reproductive organs only, as pregnancy, labour and the puerperium bring about major changes in each system of the woman's body. Also, an understanding of the development of the systems in the embryo and fetus and neonate, as well as problems affecting them, requires a detailed knowledge of their functions. For this reason a systems approach is used throughout the text. Allied biosciences have been integrated into the book where deemed necessary, including evolution, ecology, anatomy, biochemistry, genetics, embryology, microbiology, pharmacology, behavioural biology and any relevant pathophysiology.

Wherever possible, the application of theory to practice is discussed to demonstrate how knowledge of the biological sciences can enhance the care given to mothers and their babies. I remember being told by my nurse tutor, 'It is as important to make your patient safe as it is to attend to her emotional, spiritual and cognitive needs'. Surely the same tenet must be applied to the woman and her baby.

Therefore, the aims of the book are:

1 to enable an understanding of physiology and other sciences applied to childbearing to ensure safe and efficient practice;
2 to foster an integrated knowledge of applied biosciences and their importance to the understanding of humanity's place in nature;
3 to provide a biology textbook for basic and postbasic curricula students and practitioners of normal and abnormal midwifery;
4 to ensure the safety of mothers and babies both in the developed world and in those countries where care is less than adequate.

The book is divided into four sections. Section 1 covers preconception aspects of childbearing and includes the anatomy and physiology of the female and male reproductive system, fertility control, infertility and preconception care. The chapter on preconception care is presented at the widest level with environmental and lifestyle issues so that the practitioner is able to select appropriate advice both for the general public and for the couple seeking specific information.

Section 2 is divided into three parts. Section 2A is concerned with the development and growth of the fetus, its placenta and membranes. Embryology is presented in some detail but, it is hoped, in an easy-to-follow style. Problems of fetal health, growth and normality are covered. Section 2B is about the physiological adaptation of the woman's body to pregnancy. Each system is described in the non-pregnant state and, the alterations brought about by pregnancy and their significance to health are then discussed. Section 2C discusses pathophysiological states relevant to the pregnant woman. Again, a systems approach is taken and each disorder is discussed in depth with its management in terms of diagnosis and physical treatment outlined.

Section 3 is divided into two parts. Section 3A is about normal labour and includes management that arises from the knowledge of physiology. The onset and maintenance of labour are discussed. There is a chapter dedicated to each of the three stages of labour and one specifically to consider pain pathways and pain relief. Section 3B is concerned with abnormal labour. The effects of the powers, passenger and passages on the progress of labour are discussed.

Section 4 considers the mother and her baby in the puerperium. It is divided into two parts. Section 4A consists of six chapters written by Barbara Novak, a specialist in paediatric nursing and a midwife. These examine neonatal physiological adaptation to birth, the health of the neonate and some commonly encountered serious disorders. Section 4B examines the physiology of the breast and includes infant feeding. There is a chapter on the other physiological changes in the puerperium and the pathological conditions affecting the woman. The last chapter considers the development of mother–infant relationships in terms of biology although the student should not lose sight of the integration of biology, psychology and sociology in behavioural sciences.

Each chapter follows a similar format: there is a brief overview of the chapter contents, then the contents themselves and a summary of the main points. The latter is an aid to memory for revision and it should not be assumed that sufficient knowledge for practice can be gained by restricting reading to that information only. At the end of each chapter are the references followed by a list of recommended readings, some new, some highlighted from the reference list, which the author believes will further understanding of essential points.

We hope that you will find the content as fascinating as we do and that your care of mothers and babies within their families will be enhanced by this knowledge.

Dot Stables and Barbara Novak
1999

Acknowledgements

This book has had a prolonged gestation period and has developed to maturity in various units and schools of midwifery and, as time passed, schools of nursing. In particular, without the support of my friends and colleagues in the Department of Applied Biological Sciences at St Bartholomew's School of Nursing and Midwifery, City University, I would not have developed a knowledge base sufficient to support this project. Special thanks are due to Janet Vickers for her faith in my ability to teach biology to our students on many courses and to Clare Winter and Anna Hands for their early support of the project. Special thanks go to my colleague Barbara Novak for her helpful suggestions in the design of the book and her dedication to accuracy in those chapters under her development.

I owe a huge debt of gratitude to those midwives working in Ilford and Barking maternity hospitals who provided my experience and practice of midwifery and encouraged me to become a teacher. I would like to thank my tutors and colleagues for fostering my love of biological sciences, especially my tutor, colleague and friend, Florence Stephenson for first demonstrating so clearly the application of these sciences to the safety and well-being of mothers and babies.

The commitment and courage to undertake such an immense task was provided by Sheila Wood, former Head of Midwifery at St Bartholomew's School of Nursing and Midwifery, whose support and wisdom pointed me in the direction of academic writing.

Thanks are also due to the staff of Baillière Tindall, present and past, especially Sarah James who first contacted me about this book and to Inta Ozols and Karen Gilmour who have taken the project forwards.

Last but never least, I would like to pay tribute to the patient support of my husband Gordon Stables with whom I have shared an office during the two years of labour involved in writing this book. He has participated in the inevitable tribulations and joys and has provided guidance and information as required. Most of all, he has believed in me and provided encouragement.

Section

1

PRECONCEPTION

Section contents

One of the aims of this book is to enable an understanding of physiology and other biosciences applied to childbearing to ensure safe and efficient practice. This first section of the book provides basic knowledge to help understanding of the rest of the content. Chapter 1 introduces basic biochemistry for those who have no previous knowledge of the subject but the content will act also as a reference for those who have prior knowledge of the subject. Chapter 2 examines the nature of the cell and its interactions with other cells and systems. The role of the organelles, including the nucleus and cell division is explored. Before exploring the physiology of childbearing chapters 3 and 4 present the anatomy and physiology of the female and male reproductive systems. Chapters 5 and 6 examine fertility control and infertility. Chapter 7 is about preconception care and explores wide issues such as environment and lifestyle so that the practitioner is able to select appropriate advice both for the general public and for the couple seeking specific information.

Chapter

1 Basic biochemistry

In this chapter

INTRODUCTION

The study of the chemical basis for life enables a deeper understanding of physiology. The following information is given to enable an understanding of metabolic processes. It examines the basic chemical nature of the human body.

THE CHEMISTRY OF LIVING ORGANISMS

Atoms

Living organisms are made up of the same chemical elements found in all matter and elements are the smallest components of matter that cannot be broken down further. Over 100 elements are known and each has its own symbol. Elements consist of particles called atoms which are the smallest indivisible part of an element that still retains its chemical and physical properties. The study of physics has demonstrated that atoms are constructed from three subatomic particles called neutrons, protons and electrons (Davis 1996). The atom has a nucleus made up of neutrons and protons and the very small electrons are arranged in orbital shells surrounding the central nucleus (Fig. 1.1).

The formation within the atom is maintained by minute electrical charges. The neutrons of the nucleus carry no charge, the protons carry a positive charge and the electrons of the outer shells carry a negative charge. Electrons are the basis of electricity as they move along a conductor like a piece of wire. The number of protons is equal to the number of electrons so that most atoms are uncharged. Each element has a different number of electrons and protons and this is the basis for its atomic number.

Neutrons are heavy particles and contribute to the mass of the element. The number of neutrons and protons together give the element its mass number. This determines the atomic mass (atomic weight) of an element. Table 1.1 gives values for the six most common elements which make up 99% of living matter.

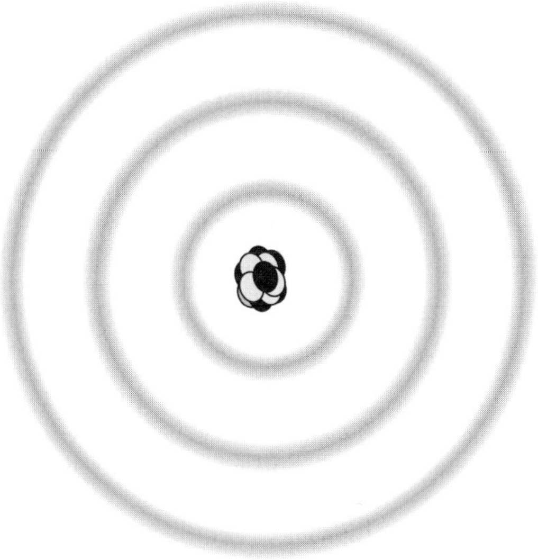

Figure 1.1 *Diagrammatic representation of the structure of an atom showing the nucleus surrounded by electron orbital shells (from Hinchliff SM, Montague SE, Watson R, 1996, with permission).*

Radioactive atoms

Variation in the number of neutrons in an atom leads to different forms of the element, called **isotopes**, with different mass numbers. In some isotopes the presence of extra neutrons causes them to be unstable. They will transform into a more stable configuration (break down or decay) during which they radiate energy and atomic particles. This is **radioactivity** and the

Table 1.1 *Values for the 6 most common elements which make up 99% of living matter.*

Element	*Atomic number*	*Number of protons*	*Number of neutrons*	*Mass number*	*Atomic mass*
Hydrogen	1	1	0	1	1
Carbon	6	6	6	12	12
Nitrogen	7	7	7	14	14
Oxygen	8	8	8	16	16
Phosphorus	15	15	16	31	31
Calcium	20	20	20	40	40

Table 1.2 *Examples of molecules*

<table>
<tr><th>Atomic element</th><th>Valency</th><th>Compound</th><th>Molecular formula</th><th>Molecular structure</th><th>Bond type</th></tr>
<tr><td>H</td><td>1</td><td>Hydrogen gas</td><td>H_2</td><td>H – H</td><td>Single</td></tr>
<tr><td>O</td><td>2</td><td>Oxygen gas</td><td>O_2</td><td>0 = 0</td><td>Double</td></tr>
<tr><td>O</td><td>2</td><td>Water</td><td>H_2O</td><td>H H
\ /
O</td><td>Single</td></tr>
<tr><td>N</td><td>3</td><td>Nitrogen gas</td><td>N_2</td><td>N ≡ N</td><td>Triple</td></tr>
<tr><td>N</td><td>3</td><td>Ammonia</td><td>NH_3</td><td>H
/
H – N
\
H</td><td>Single</td></tr>
<tr><td>C</td><td>4</td><td>Carbon dioxide</td><td>CO_2</td><td>O = C = O</td><td>Double</td></tr>
<tr><td>C</td><td>4</td><td>Methane</td><td>CH_4</td><td>H H
\ /
C
/ \
H H</td><td>Single</td></tr>
<tr><td>P</td><td>5</td><td>Phosphoric acid</td><td>H_3PO_4</td><td>OH
|
HO – P = O
|
OH</td><td>Single and double</td></tr>
</table>

Table 1.3 *The molecular masses of some common chemicals*

Molecular	*Calculation*	*Molecular*
Formula	N	Mass
H_2	1 + 1	2
O_2	16 + 16	32
H_2O	2 + 16	18
N_2	14 + 14	28
NH_3	1 + 1 + 1 + 14	17
CO_2	12 + 16 + 16	44
C_2H_5OH (ethanol)	12 + 12 + 1 + 1 + 1 1 + 1 + 16 + 1	46
$C_6H_{12}O_6$ (glucose)	(12 × 6) + (1 × 12) + (16 × 6)	180

isotopes are radioactive. Radioactive and stable isotopes have been used successfully in medical diagnosis and treatment (Cooper 1992).

Molecules

Atoms join together to form compounds by using chemical bonds. There are two kinds of chemical bond – the strong, stable covalent bond, which is hard to disrupt, and the weaker, less stable non-covalent bonds. The making and breaking of these chemical bonds is associated with energy changes; the more stable the bond, the greater the thermal (heat) energy needed to disrupt it. These bonds are formed by the electrons in the outer shell of the atom. Electrons may be donated, received or shared by atoms. One bond is formed by one electron but some atoms have more than one electron free to form bonds. The number of available electrons is called the atom's **valency**.

Covalent bonds – the sharing of electrons

When two or more atoms are joined together by the sharing of electrons a **molecule** is formed and the bonds are called covalent bonds. Some atoms require more than one electron to form a bond with another atom. Bonds may be single, as is seen in a molecule of hydrogen gas, or double, as in a molecule of oxygen gas. Some atoms require more than one electron to form a bond with another atom. Complex molecules can be built up by linkage of different atoms, depending on their valencies. Molecules can be represented as a molecular formula or a molecular structure, depending on how the information on their atomic structure is being used. Some examples are given in Table 1.2.

Carbon is essential for forming organic compounds – hence, the Star Trek carbon-based life forms!

Molecular mass (weight)

An immensely useful unit for measuring the concentration of a substance is the **mole**. This is the molecular mass expressed in grams. The molecular mass of a substance can be calculated by adding together the mass numbers of its component atoms. Some examples are shown in Table 1.3.

Non-covalent bonds

Non-covalent bonds are very important in stabilising the three-dimensional structure of biological molecules. There are four main types: the ionic bond, the hydrogen bond, the van de Waals interaction and the hydrophobic bond.

Ionic bonds (electrovalent bonds)

Ionic bonds are another way of forming compounds. Electrons are not shared by atoms but are donated from one atom to another, forming an electrovalent or ionic bond. The number of ionic bonds that can be formed is, as with covalent bonds, dictated by the valency. Atoms of metallic elements such as sodium, calcium and iron lose electrons readily. The loss or gain of an electron is called **ionisation** and the atom or group of atoms becomes an **ion**.

Electrons carry a negative charge so that atoms that lose an electron become positively charged and are known as **cations**. Sodium is such an element and the status of cation is shown by the addition of a plus sign – Na^+. The atom that receives an electron becomes negatively charged and is known as an **anion**. The status is shown by the addition of a minus sign, such as chlorine Cl^-. An atom or molecule that has lost or gained an electron in this way is said to have been **polarised**.

Salts

Cations are attracted to anions, giving rise to compounds called salts. The two elements mentioned above can be used to demonstrate the formation of a very well-known salt – sodium chloride. This chemical change occurs when sodium donates an electron to chlorine:

$$Na^+ + Cl^- \rightarrow NaCl$$

In this form the salt is crystalline and consists of a rigid lattice structure but if the salt is dissolved in water it dissociates into free ions which disperse in the solution.

Hydrogen bonding

Besides covalent and ionic bonds, a weak type of bond can occur between molecules. Molecules containing hydrogen atoms are attracted to each other by the weak positive charge left on the hydrogen atom when the only electron it contains is drawn towards the other element it is associating with. The association of oxygen and hydrogen to form water is a good example of this. These partial charges are represented by the Greek letter delta (δ) so that water can be represented as:

$$\begin{array}{c} \delta + H \backslash \\ O\delta - \\ \delta + H / \end{array}$$

Although there is no actual negative or positive charge, the water molecule has become polar. The two ends of the charge differ slightly from each other and are said to be **dipolar**. This ability of hydrogen to create weak bonds is essential for the formation of helical structures such as are found in proteins and in the double helix of DNA.

The van de Waals interaction

When two atoms approach closely to each other a weak attractive force called a van de Waals interaction is produced (Darnell et al 1990). Transient dipoles are created and the transient dipole of one atom disturbs the electron cloud of the other atom, creating a transient dipole in the other atom. There is then a weak attraction between the two dipoles.

Table 1.4 *Elements found in the human body*

Element	*Atomic symbol*	*Approximate weight (%)*
Oxygen	O	65
Carbon	C	18
Hydrogen	H	10
Nitrogen	N	3
Calcium	Ca	2
Phosphorus	P	1
		TOTAL = 99%
Potassium	K	0.35
Sulphur	S	0.25
Sodium	Na	0.15
Chlorine	Cl	0.15
		TOTAL = 0.9%
Magnesium	Mg	trace
Iron	Fe	trace
Zinc	Zn	trace
Copper	Cu	trace
Iodine	I	trace
Manganese	Mn	trace
Chromium	Cr	trace
Molybdenum	Mo	trace
Cobalt	Co	trace
Selenium	Se	trace
		TOTAL = 0.1%

Hydrophobic interactions

Non-polar molecules contain neither ions nor dipolar bonds. They are insoluble in water and are called hydrophobic which means 'water fearing'. A hydrophobic interaction is not a separate type of bonding force. It results from the energy needed to insert a non-polar molecule into water. The non-polar molecule cannot form hydrogen bonds and distorts the structure of water to make a cage around it. Non-polar molecules bind together comfortably using the van de Waals interaction. The hydrocarbons are the most common type of biological molecule and are virtually insoluble in water.

Table 1.5 *Types of chemical reaction occurring during metabolism*

Type	*Reaction*	*Typical processes*
Condensation	Combining molecules with the elimination of water	Formation of glycoside, ester and peptide bonds
Hydrolysis	Splitting a molecule with the addition of water	Digestion of carbohydrates, triglycerides and proteins
Dehydration	Removal of water from a molecule	Carbohydrate and fatty acid metabolism
Hydration	Incorporation of water into a molecule	Carbohydrate and fatty acid metabolism
Oxidation	Removal of hydrogen (or electrons)	Conversion of alcohols to aldehydes
Reduction	Addition of hydrogen (or electrons)	Biosynthesis of fatty acids
Carboxylation	Incorporation of carbon dioxide	Carbohydrate synthesis
Decarboxylation	Elimination of carbon dioxide	Fermentation, amine formation
Amination	Incorporation of amino group ($-NH_3$)	Amino acid biosynthesis
Deamination	Elimination of ammonia	Amino acid degradation
Methylation	Incorporation of methyl group ($-CH_3$)	Synthesis of DNA and adrenaline
Demethylation	Removal of methyl group	Amino acid degradation

COMPOSITION OF THE HUMAN BODY

The human body is made up of about two-thirds water. The other third is composed of six main elements and traces of other elements (Table 1.4).

Bonds and reactions

The types of non-covalent bonds that stabilise large biological molecules have been discussed. These bonds are not as stable as the covalent bond and that feature is essential to the working of the body to allow the compounds to change during chemical reactions without the need for large amounts of energy. Most chemical reactions in the body require the use of enzymes and their associated cofactors to act as catalysts. The types of chemical reaction found during the processes of metabolism are summarised in Table 1.5.

Summary of main points

- The study of the chemical basis for life enables a deeper understanding of physiology. The following information is given to enable an understanding of metabolic processes. It examines the basic chemical nature of the human body.
- Living organisms are made up of the same chemical elements found in all matter and elements are the smallest components of matter that cannot be broken down further. Over 100 elements are known and each has its own symbol. Elements consist of particles called atoms which are the smallest indivisible part of an element that still retains its chemical and physical properties.
- The formation within the atom is maintained by minute electrical charges. The neutrons of the nucleus carry no charge, the protons carry a positive charge and the electrons of the outer shells carry a negative charge. Electrons are the basis of electricity as they move along a conductor like a piece of wire. The number of protons is equal to the number of electrons so that most atoms are uncharged.
- Neutrons are heavy particles and contribute to the mass of the element. The number of neutrons and protons together give the element its mass number. This determines the atomic mass (atomic weight) of an element. Variation in the number of neutrons in an atom leads to different forms of the element called isotopes. In some isotopes the presence of extra neutrons causes them to be unstable. They will transform into a more stable configuration and radiate energy and atomic particles. Radioactive and stable isotopes are used successfully in medical diagnosis and treatment.
- Atoms join together to form compounds by using chemical bonds. There are two kinds of chemical bond – the strong, stable covalent bond, which is hard to disrupt, and the weaker, less stable non-covalent bond. The making and breaking of these chemical bonds is associated with energy changes; the more stable the bond, the greater the thermal energy needed to disrupt it.
- These bonds are formed by the electrons in the outer shell of the atom. Electrons may be donated, received or shared by atoms. One bond is formed by one electron but some atoms have more than one electron free to form bonds. The number of available electrons is called the atom's valency.
- When two or more atoms are joined together by the sharing of electrons a molecule is formed and the bonds are called covalent bonds. Complex molecules can be built up by linkage of different atoms, depending on their valencies. Molecules can be represented as a molecular formula or a molecular structure, depending on how the information on their atomic structure is being used.
- An immensely useful unit for measuring the concentration of a substance is the mole. This is the molecular mass expressed in grams. The molecular mass of a substance can be calculated by adding together the mass numbers of its component atoms.
- Ionic bonds are another way of forming compounds. Electrons are not shared by atoms but are donated from one atom to another, forming an electrovalent or ionic bond. The number of ionic bonds that can be formed is dictated by the valency. Atoms of metallic elements such as sodium, calcium and iron lose electrons readily. The loss or gain of an electron is called ionisation and the atom or group of atoms becomes an ion. Electrons carry a negative charge so that atoms that lose an electron become positively charged and are known as cations. Sodium is such an element, shown by the addition of a plus sign – Na^+.
- The atom that receives an electron becomes negatively charged and is known as an anion. The status is shown by the addition of a minus sign, such as chlorine Cl^-. An atom or molecule that has lost or gained an electron in this way is said to have been polarised.
- Cations are attracted to anions, giving rise to compounds called salts. The two elements mentioned above can be used to demonstrate the formation of a very well-known salt – sodium chloride. This chemical change occurs when sodium donates an electron to chlorine.
- Molecules containing hydrogen atoms are attracted to each other by the weak positive charge left on the hydrogen atom when the only electron it contains is drawn towards the other element it is associating with. The association of oxygen and hydrogen to form water is a good example. Although there is no actual negative or positive charge, the water molecule has become polar. The two ends of the charge differ slightly from each other and are said to be dipolar. This ability of hydrogen to create weak bonds is essential for the formation of helical structures such as are found in proteins and in the double helix of DNA.
- When two atoms approach closely to each other a weak attractive force called a van de Waals interaction is produced. Transient dipoles are created and the transient dipole of one atom disturbs the electron cloud of the other atom, creating a transient dipole in the other atom. There is a weak attraction between the two dipoles.
- Non-polar molecules contain neither ions nor dipolar bonds. They are insoluble in water and are called hydrophobic which means 'water fearing'. The non-polar molecule cannot form hydrogen bonds and distorts the structure of water to make a cage around it.
- The human body is made up of about two-thirds water. The other third is composed of six main elements – carbon, oxygen, hydrogen, nitrogen, phosphorus, calcium – and traces of other elements.
- Most chemical reactions in the body require the use of enzymes and their associated cofactors to act as catalysts.

References

Cooper GM 1992 Elements of Human Cancer. Jones and Bartlett, Boston.

Darnell J, Lodish H, Baltimore D 1990 Molecular Cell Biology, 2nd edn. Scientific American Books, New York.

Davis MG 1996 The chemistry of living matter, in Hinchliff ASM, Montague SE, Watson R (eds) Physiology for Nursing Practice, 2nd edn. Baillière Tindall, London.

Hinchliff SM, Montague SE, Watson R 1996 Physiology for Nursing Practice, 2nd edn. Baillière Tindall, London.

Recommended reading

Campbell MK 1995 Biochemistry, 2nd edn. WB Saunders, Philadelphia.

Cohen N (ed) 1991 Cell Structure, Function and Metabolism. Hodder and Stoughton, London.

Masterton WL, Hurley CN 1993 Chemistry: Principles and Reactions, 2nd edn. WB Saunders, Philadelphia.

Rose S 1991 The Chemistry of Life, 3rd edn. Penguin, Harmondsworth.

Sackheim GI, Lehman DD 1994 Chemistry for the Health Sciences, 7th edn. Macmillan, New York.

Wood EJ, Myers A 1991 Essential Chemistry for Biochemistry, 2nd edn. Biochemical Society, London.

Chapter 2

The cell – its structures and functions

In this chapter

PHYSICAL CHARACTERISTICS OF MAMMALIAN CELLS

The mammalian cell may be defined as the most fundamental, functional unit of the body. The complex genetic information contained within the nucleus governs its specific morphological features and explicit functional roles. Although there are over 200 different types of cells in the human body, they are assembled into a variety of tissue types such as the epithelia, the connective tissue, the muscle, the conducting neural tissue and non-conducting neuroglia. Most body tissue consists of an assembly of different cell types functioning in harmony.

According to Alberts et al (1994) mammalian cells average 5–50 μm in diameter. Their complex microstructure cannot be determined by using a light microscope at its normal limit of resolution, 0.2 μm. However, the electron microscope, with its resolution down towards 1 nm, has enabled us to reveal many complex cellular ultrastructures but in life these ultrastructures and their many microconstituents are not static but adapt as necessary. There is evidence to suggest that they are maintained by a continual assimilation of desirable matter from the extracellular environment in order to preserve the structural and functional integrity of the cell type.

CELL SIZE AND SHAPE

Although cells differentiate and modify their form and activities during their development and functional maturation, a common pattern of organisation can be determined in their final structure and functions in relation to a specific organ, system or the body as a whole. Knowledge of the 'size' of the cell is important. For instance, resting **lymphocytes** are amongst the smallest of cells, their average diameter being 6 μm, whereas **erythrocytes** are approximately 7.5 μm and columnar epithelial cells are 20 μm tall and 10 μm wide. Bannister et al (1995) argue that some mammalian cells are significantly larger than this. The **megakaryocytes** of the bone marrow may be over 200 μm in diameter and mature ova may be over 80 μm in diameter. Neurones and skeletal muscle cells are relatively large in size, but this may be due to their highly attenuated structural forms.

The dimensions of a cell may be partly determined by its metabolic requirements and corresponding biochemical circumstances concerning the rate of substrate diffusion across its highly selective plasma membrane (Guyton 1994). One of the major physical advantages of a particular cell may be its capacity to permit selective but rapid **diffusion of substrates** over short distances of up to 50 μm. This biophysical phenomenon appears to ensure that the metabolic needs of the active cells can be easily sustained. However, as cells increase in size, their increase in mass outstrips their surface area unless their shape changes to form an irregular or elongated surface structure. As many physiological processes, such as diffusion of gases, diffusion of ions and transport of nutrients, depend on the surface area of the cell, an increase in cell mass may contribute to an increasing difficulty of a given cell type to maintain efficient metabolic processes.

Furthermore, the larger the cell, the greater the distance of the cell periphery from the nucleus, so that exertion of nuclear control on the cytoplasm may become problematic. In larger cells such physiological and biochemical challenges appear to be overcome to some extent by a significant increase in the cells' relative surface area, either by folding the plasma membrane and forming microvilli or other surface protrusions or flattening the entire body of the cell. In both instances the cells generate a large surface area for efficient transport and diffusion of the necessary substrates.

Finally, the nuclear control in the larger cells can be enhanced by creating more nuclei in each cell, either by fusion of mononuclear cells, as in the skeletal muscle, or, more rarely, by the multiplication of nuclei without corresponding cytoplasmic division, as found in some epithelial cells. Bannister et al (1995) argue that to some extent cell surfaces adapt in order to perform their explicit functional roles effectively and efficiently. Given

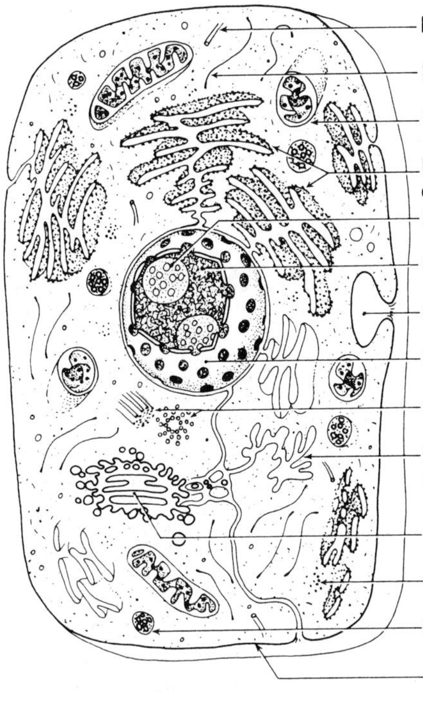

Figure 2.1 *Diagram of the ultrastructure of a cell (from Hinchliff SM, Montague SE, 1990, with permission).*

these circumstances, the external appearance of a cell type will vary widely depending on its specific functions, the need to interact with other cells and the external environment, as well as the characteristic nature of the internal structure which masterminds the activities of the individual cell.

CELL MOTILITY

Preston (1990) and Stossel (1994) argue that characteristics of cell motility are displayed by most cells. Generally, this involves the movement of the cytoplasm or specific **organelles** from one part of the cell to another. Cell motility can be influenced and, indeed, is dominated by various environmental factors, for example the migration of phagocytic white blood cells to a site of tissue injury or infection. However, humans are multicellular complex organisms and permissible cellular motility is likely to take place within a carefully defined biochemical and micro-anatomic world. Internal environmental factors will modulate the speed and direction of cell locomotion.

The uptake of materials from the extracellular environment, as in **endocytosis** and **phagocytosis**, and the reciprocal passage of large molecular compounds out of the cell by **exocytosis** demonstrate the need for cells to adapt in their functional roles as well as their anatomic positions. A further example of cell migration can be seen in fibroblasts during embryonic development. These become involved in an elaborate process known as **histiogenesis** contributing to the organisation of the neural crest and muscle fibre (Chapter 9) although their primary function is not cell locomotion but secretion of collagen essential to the extracellular matrix. Fibroblasts interact with collagen by means of adhesion plaques, through which they are able to exert traction on the matrix which, amongst other functions, plays a key role in the process of wound tissue healing.

THE EPITHELIAL CELLS

Bannister et al (1995) and Alberts et al (1994) hold that embryonically, epithelial cells are derived from the three germ layers, providing an internal and external covering for body surfaces. Thus, ectoderm, endoderm and mesoderm each contribute to the formation and development of some form of epithelium. The embryonic ectoderm contributes to the development of the epidermis, breast glandular tissue, cornea and the junctional zones of the buccal cavity and anal canal. The endoderm forms the epithelial lining of the alimentary canal and its glands, most of the respiratory tract and the distal tract of the urogenital tract. Finally, the mesoderm gives rise to the epithelium-like cells lining internal cavities such as the pericardium, pleural and peritoneal cavities, the lining of the blood vessels and lymph vessels and the proximal parts of the urogenital tract (see Chapter 8 for detail).

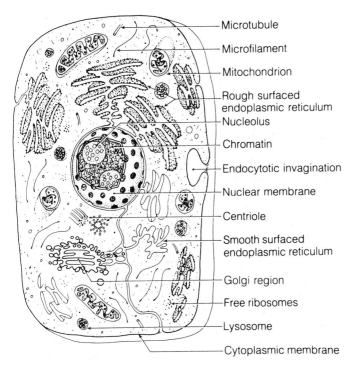

Given that the general function of the epithelia is to provide a covering for the body and its internal organs, it may be assumed that they also serve as selective barriers, facilitating or preventing substrates traversing the surfaces which they cover. Thus, some epithelia protect underlying tissue from dehydration, chemical or mechanical injury. Conversely, other epithelia function as sensory surfaces and many features of the neural tissue can be regarded as those of a modified epithelium.

Common classification of the epithelia

According to Bannister et al (1995), the polygonal, diverse shape of the epithelial cells appears to be partly determined by their cytoplasmic contents and partly by pressure and functional demands of the surrounding tissue. It is usual to classify the widely diverse epithelia into groups according to their structural and functional characteristics. Consequently, the following epithelial classifications are commonly used.

Simple epithelia

Simple epithelia are formed by single layers of cells resting on a basal lamina which consists of filamentous proteins and proteoglycans. These epithelia may be further subdivided according to the shape of their cells, which may be columnar, cuboidal, pseudostratifed and squamous types. The shape of the cell is largely related to cell volume, a point well illustrated by the squamous and low cuboidal epithelia. Where cells are small the volume of cytoplasm is relatively low, denoting few organelles and low metabolic activity. Conversely, the highly metabolically active epithelial cells such as the secretory forms contain abundant mitochondria and endoplasmic reticulum and are typically tall cuboidal or columnar. Simple epithelia are also capable of manifesting special functions and can be found forming cilia, microvilli, secretory vacuoles or sensory features.

Stratified or squamous epithelia

Stratified or squamous epithelia consist of superficial cells which are constantly replaced by their regenerating basal layers. Characteristically, these epithelia are composed of flattened, interlocking, polygonal cells. The cytoplasm of these cells may in some instances not exceed 0.1 nm thickness so that their nucleus may bulge into the overlying space. As squamous epithelium is so thin it appears to be ideally suited to facilitating efficient diffusion of gases and water. However, squamous epithelia also engage in active transport, a role indicated by their numerous endocytic vesicles. The most critical positions for squamous epithelia are in the lining of the lung alveoli (Chapter 18), the construction of the glomeruli and the thin segments of the loop of Henle (Chapter 19).

Cuboidal and columnar epithelia

Cuboidal and columnar epithelia consist of regular rows of cylindrical cells. Cuboidal cells are typically square whereas columnar cells are significantly taller in comparison to their diameter. Commonly, the free surfaces of columnar cells have microvilli, which are particularly suited to the absorptive role of the small intestine as they significantly enhance the surface area for absorption of water and nutrients (Chapter 21).

By contrast, the columnar epithelium of the gallbladder displays a characteristic brush border, essential to its concentration and storage of bile (Chapter 22). Ciliated columnar epithelium is found in much of the respiratory tract, the lining of fallopian tubes and uterine cervix. The proximal and distal convoluted segments of nephrons consist of large cuboidal cells with an extensive brush border capable of selective reabsorption of substances from the filtrate (Chapter 19).

Transitional epithelium

The characteristic feature of transitional epithelium is its thickness which is formed by an extended arrangement of 4–6 cells held together in a specific pattern by numerous **desmosomes** (filamentous structures). In stretching, these cells flatten without altering their position relative to each other. Most epithelial cells are attached to their basal lamina by slender processes, contributing to their characteristic organisation into a basal structure where they appear cuboidal and uninucleate when relaxed. At the surface of this multilayered epithelium, cells progressively fuse to form larger, at times binucleate but polyploid cells with a plasma membrane covered by **glycoprotein** particles.

This characteristic arrangement of epithelial cells has two distinctive roles. First, it facilitates expansion and contraction, stretching considerably without losing its structural integrity, and second, it provides an impermeable lining for organs that hold liquid containing some toxic metabolic end-products such as urea. Therefore, transitional epithelium is invaluable in forming an impermeable lining in the genitourinary tract.

Complex structures derived from epithelium

Complex organ structures which are largely derived from epithelia frequently retain highly familiar cellular characteristics. The capacity of the liver or the placenta to absorb, secrete and transport substrates illustrates the complex physiological roles some epithelial cells are capable of. Similarly, the complex and diverse forms of neural tissue are functional modifications of epithelia. Most of our neural tissue is highly differentiated in order to provide the body with a sophisticated network for processing and managing information.

THE CELL AND ITS PLASMA MEMBRANE

According to Alberts et al (1994) and Evans & Graham (1991), the cell membrane, also known as the plasma membrane, is the most common feature of all forms of epithelia and other cell types. Indeed, the existence of an appropriate plasma membrane is crucial to the functional integrity and survival of the cell. This specialised plasma membrane encloses the cellular content, defines its boundary and maintains the essential differences between the cytosol and the extracellular environment.

The lipid bilayer

In common with all biological membranes, the plasma membrane has a general structure consisting of a very thin lipid bilayer containing protein molecules (Bray et al 1994, Schmidt & Thews 1987). This complex arrangement of lipid and specialised proteins is held together predominantly by non-covalent interactions. However, plasma membranes are dynamic fluid structures capable of considerable adaptation because of the ability of most of their molecules to move about within the plane of the membranes.

One of the most characteristic features of plasma membranes is the arrangement of lipid molecules in a continuous double layer of about 5–7 nm thickness (Alberts et al 1994, Devlin 1990, Sherwood 1993). Although this lipid bilayer provides the basic structure of the membrane and serves as a relatively impermeable barrier to the passage of most water-soluble molecules, its suspended protein molecules also mediate many of the selective functions of the plasma membrane.

Functions of membrane proteins

The protein functions include the selective transportation of specific molecules across the plasma membrane and catalysing membrane-associated reactions. Some proteins serve as structural links connecting the plasma membrane to the cytoskeleton or to either the extracellular matrix or the adjacent cells as appropriate. Other proteins serve as specialised receptors for detection and transduction of chemical signals found in the cell's environment.

The complex role of the plasma membranes is partly attributable to their asymmetrical construction (Alberts et al 1994, Guyton 1994). This is best illustrated by the molecular lipid and protein compositions found on the outer and the inner surfaces of the membrane. For functional purposes the lipid–protein arrangements differ from one another, reflecting their different functions at the two distinctive surfaces of the membrane.

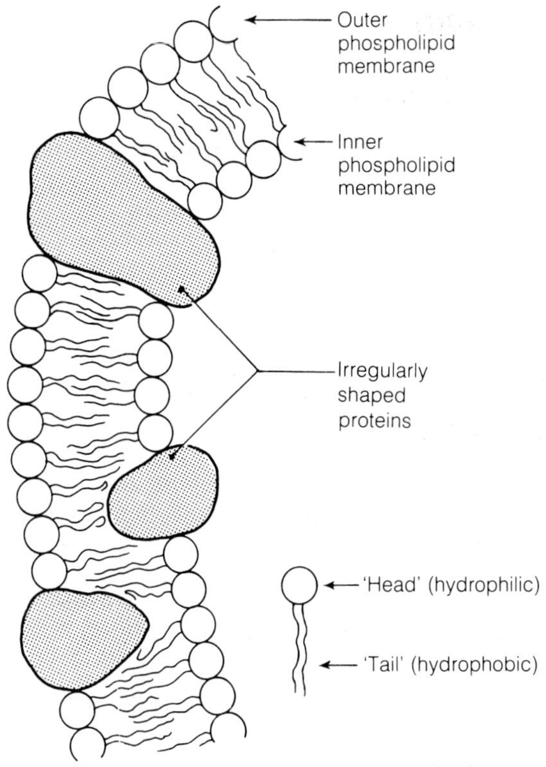

Figure 2.2 *Diagram of the fluid mosaic model of cell membrane structure (from Hinchliff SM, Montague SE, 1990, with permission).*

The phospholipid bilayer

The lipid bilayer provides the universal basis for the construction of the cell membrane (Alberts et al 1994, Bray et al 1994). The nature of this construction is probably attributable to the special properties of the lipid molecules, allowing them to assemble spontaneously into bilayers. This phenomenon is illustrated by the behaviour of the lipid molecules in certain physiological environments, as they are insoluble in water but dissolve readily in organic solvents.

The current understanding of the molecular phospholipid bilayer confirms that the membrane-forming lipid molecules consist of a hydrophilic polar head and a hydrophobic non-polar tail. The most abundant forms of lipid are the **phospholipids** which have a polar head group and two hydrophobic hydrocarbon tails which usually consist of fatty acids and differ in length. These characteristic differences in the length and saturation of the fatty acid tails are important because they influence the scope of the phospholipid molecules to pack against one another and construct the 'fluid' framework of a competent plasma membrane.

Thus, the shape and nature of the lipid molecules result in the spontaneous formation of these distinguished bilayers in aqueous solutions. When lipid molecules are surrounded on all sides by water they tend to aggregate so that their hydrophobic tails are buried in the dry, water-free interior and their hydrophilic heads are exposed to water. Furthermore, these lipid bilayers tend to close on themselves, forming sealed compartments, thereby eliminating any free spaces where the hydrophilic tails would be in contact with water. Damaged plasma membranes tend to reseal rapidly in order to avoid the exposure of the fatty acid tails to water.

The precise fluidity of the plasma membrane is, of course, biologically important to the survival of the cellular infrastructure and maintenance of efficient transport processes and enzyme activities. However, the lipid bilayer of many cell membranes is not exclusively composed of phospholipids and often contains cholesterol, glycolipids and glycoproteins. The cholesterol molecules make the lipid bilayer more stable and less deformable and decrease its permeability to small water-soluble molecules. A second significant role for the cholesterol molecules is to prevent the hydrocarbon chains from coming together, crystallising and so damaging the functional integrity of the plasma membrane. The role of the glycolipids and glycoproteins is to act as receptors for extracellular biochemical products.

The membrane proteins

Although the lipid bilayer provides the basic structure of biological membranes, most of the specific functions of the plasma membrane are carried out by the membrane proteins (Alberts et al 1994, Bray et al 1994). Therefore the quantities and types of proteins in a plasma membrane vary greatly, depending to a large extent on the overall functions of a cell. For instance, the neural myeline membrane serves mainly as an electrical insulation for nerve cells axons so that less than 25% of the membrane mass is protein. Conversely, membranes involved in energy transduction, such as the internal membranes of the mitochondria, are composed of approximately 75% protein.

The average content of protein in plasma membranes is about 50% of its total mass (Alberts et al 1994). However, because lipid molecules are considerably smaller in comparison to protein molecules, there are always many more lipid molecules in a plasma membrane than protein molecules; for example, there may be 50 lipid molecules for each protein molecule in a membrane that is 50% protein by mass.

Considerable evidence supports the current understanding that different membrane proteins are associated with the plasma membrane in different ways. A significant number of membrane proteins extend through the lipid bilayer with a small part of their mass on either side and are known as transmembrane proteins. They have distinctive regions that are hydrophobic and other specialised regions which are hydrophilic. Other membrane proteins are located entirely in the cytosol and are associated with the bilayer only by means of various types of lipid chains.

The transmembrane proteins

According to Guyton (1994) and Schmidt & Thews (1987), transmembrane proteins always appear to have a unique orientation in the plasma membrane which reflects the asymmetrical manner in which the protein may be synthesised in the endoplasmic reticulum and inserted into the lipid bilayer. Rather like the membrane lipids, membrane proteins do not flop across the lipid bilayers of the plasma membrane but do rotate about an axis which is perpendicular to the plane of the lipid bilayer, facilitating the process of **rotational diffusion**.

In addition, many membrane proteins are able to move laterally within the membrane, aiding the process of **lateral diffusion**. But cells can also confine proteins to specific domains within a plasma membrane. For example, in epithelial cells such as those lining the intestinal tract, some plasma membrane transport proteins are confined to the apical surface of the cells whereas others are confined to the basal and lateral surfaces. This asymmetrical distribution of membrane proteins is thought to be essential for the function of the epithelia. The lipid distribution of these two membrane domains also differs, demonstrating that epithelial cells control the diffusion of lipids as well as protein molecules.

The selective permeability of the plasma membrane facilitates free passage of some gases and water but restricts the movement of larger ions such as sodium, potassium, calcium, chloride and bicarbonate to their specific protein channels, which can be opened or closed in order to regulate transmembrane traffic. The selective passage of many of the other substances of large molecular weight such as glucose and amino acids is also limited to such protein channels. In most instances the protein channels are ion or substrate specific, allowing only one species of ion or substrate to diffuse through their apertures. Some lipid-soluble substances are permitted to pass directly through the lipid portion of the plasma membranes. A typical example of this form of diffusion is the entry of steroid hormones into the cytoplasm without passing through any form of protein channel.

By contrast, the uptake of larger molecules into the cell involves the invagination of a small segment of the plasma membrane which then forms small vacuoles or endocytic vesicles, which in turn take up the large molecules and aid their transportation to other regions within the cell. Similarly, the extrusion of organic molecules is achieved by exocytic vesicles, which fuse with the plasma membrane and release their content to the exterior.

THE CYTOPLASM AND ITS ORGANELLES

Every single living cell, in order to sustain its microstructures and functional competence, must communicate with its immediate environment. In prokaryotic cells (non-nucleated single cell organisms such as bacteria) the entire communication takes place across the plasma membrane. By contrast, eukaryotic (nucleated) cells have developed an elaborate internal membrane machinery that allows them to take up macromolecules by a process of endocytosis and eject molecular substrates as required by exocytosis. This elaborate internal membrane machinery is constructed by the complex arrangements of the cellular organelles which are cell specific and contained within the cytoplasm (Bannister et al 1995, Devlin 1990, Guyton 1994).

Cytoplasm

Cytoplasm makes up approximately half the cell volume (Alberts et al 1994). Due to its high protein content (20% by weight), it appears more like a gel than an aqueous solution which allows it to act as an effective framework for the suspension of small molecular structures, large particles and organelles. Organic and inorganic ions are dissolved in the aqueous phase of the cytoplasm and exchanged between the cell and the surrounding extracellular environment. Also dispersed in the cytoplasm are fat globules, glycogen granules, ribosomes and secretory granules.

The most important organelles contained within the cytoplasm are the endoplasmic reticulum, the Golgi apparatus, the lysosomes, the peroxisomes and the mitochondria. These organelles are cell specific and variations in densities may be found in different cells. However, their functional roles are unchanged across the different cell types.

The endoplasmic reticulum

Generally, the endoplasmic reticulum takes the shape of a specialised membranous structure organised into a network of tubular and flat vesicular sacs (Fig. 2.3). The tubules and the vesicular sacs are thought to interconnect so that the entire endoplasmic reticulum forms a continuous framework within the internal cellular space. The endoplasmic reticular membrane also forms a barrier between the cytosol and the reticular lumen and mediates the selective transport of molecules between these two compartments. The endoplasmic reticulum plays a central role in lipid and protein biosynthesis and is the site of

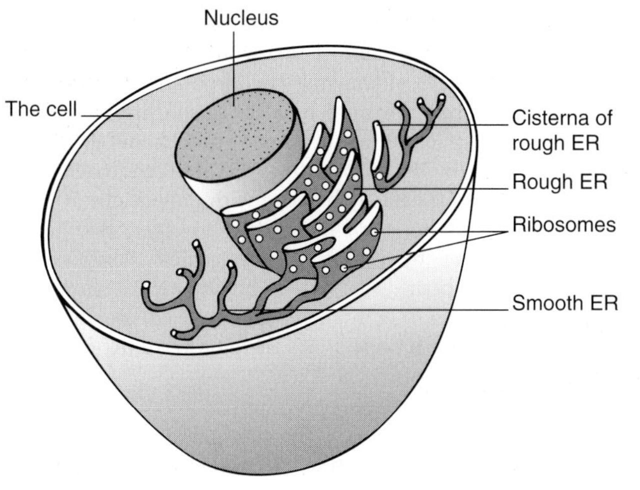

Figure 2.3 *The endoplasmic reticulum. The rough endoplasmic reticulum and smooth endoplasmic reticulum with their connections are illustrated.*

production of all the transmembrane lipids and proteins used in the ongoing construction of the cell's organelle, including itself!

There are two distinctive membrane types: the rough endoplasmic reticulum which displays a rich, characteristic arrangement of membrane-bound ribosomes and the smooth endoplasmic reticulum which lacks this arrangement of ribosomes. The role of the rough endoplasmic reticulum is to capture selected proteins from the cytosol as they are synthesised. These proteins are of two distinctive types, the transmembrane proteins and the water-soluble proteins, which are completely translocated across the membrane to be released into the endoplasmic reticular lumen.

Ribosomes

Ribosomes are particles or granules of no more than 25 nm in diameter, consisting of two-thirds ribonucleic acid and one-third protein. Each ribosome is made up of a large (60S) and a small (40S) subunit which play a critical role in protein synthesis. All ribosomes are produced in the nucleus of the cell under the direction of deoxyribonucleic acid (DNA). Each ribosome is 'programmed' to facilitate the synthesis of only one specific protein needed by that particular cell. Though free and attached ribosomes have the same structure, the types of protein they synthesise in the two locations are different.

In general, protein synthesised by ribosomes which are free in the cytoplasm are used for activities within the cell, such as cytoplasmic filament formation, whereas proteins synthesised by ribosomes which are attached to the endoplasmic reticulum enter the cisternae, then travel to the Golgi apparatus. These proteins are destined for secretion and use in the development or construction of intra- and extracellular substrates. Evidence presented by Alberts et al (1994) suggests that protein translocation into the cisternae occurs by virtue of specific protein-conducting channels in the membrane whose opening appears to be governed by signal peptides.

The smooth endoplasmic reticulum, though directly continuous with the rough endoplasmic reticulum, has a completely different form and function. It consists of a ribosome-free network of fine tubules. The distinctive biochemical reactions of the smooth endoplasmic reticula membranes are diverse, ranging from the synthesis of steroid hormones to detoxification of drugs (Schmidt & Thews 1987).

Golgi apparatus

Proteins synthesised by the rough endoplasmic reticulum are sequestered in transport vesicles and travel to the Golgi, where they are structurally modified and sorted according to their destination. Each Golgi apparatus is related to the endoplasmic reticulum and its membrane is similar in appearance to smooth endoplasmic reticulum. The apparatus itself consists of four or more stacked thin, flat vesicles lying very near the nucleus. The entire Golgi apparatus functions in close association with the endoplasmic reticulum and proteins from the endoplasmic reticulum are processed or 'fine-tuned' in the Golgi apparatus to form lysosomes, secretory vesicles or other cytoplasmic components (Fig. 2.4).

The lysosomes

Lysosomes are vesicular organelles formed by the Golgi apparatus and dispersed throughout the cytoplasm. In essence, the lysosomes form the digestive system of the cell and are capable of digesting and processing materials entering the cells from the extracellular environment prior to their release into the cytoplasm. They remove unwanted intracellular substances, damaged structures and foreign particles such as bacteria. The differentiation of lysosomes is cell dependent, but their usual microscopic appearance is confined to 250–750 nm in diameter. They are surrounded by a membranous lipid bilayer and are filled with large numbers of small granules 5–8 nm in diameter.

The granules are protein aggregates of hydrolytic, digestive enzymes. These hydrolytic enzymes are capable of splitting an organic compound into two or more parts by combining hydrogen derived from a water molecule with part of the compound and by combining the hydroxyl portion of the water

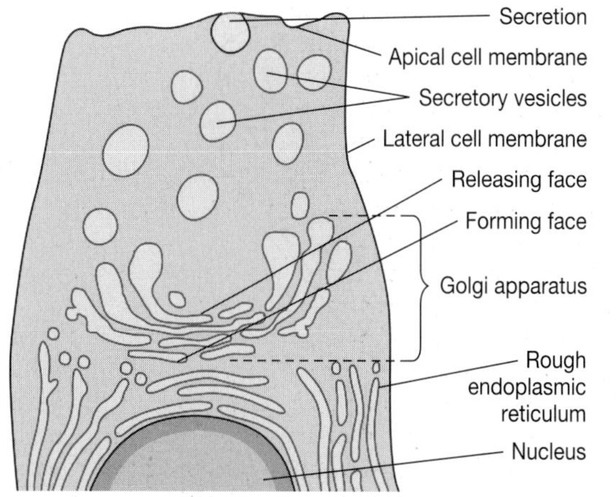

Figure 2.4 *Exocytosis of secretory proteins from the Golgi apparatus (from Hinchliff SM, Montague SF, Watson R, 1996, with permission).*

molecule with other parts of the compound. Proteins are hydrolysed to form amino acids and glycogen is hydrolysed to form glycose.

In conclusion, simple lysosomes are a group of membrane-bound organelles capable of breaking down polymers of all types. The low pH (<5) required for the hydrolysing activities is maintained by a membrane (ATP)-dependent hydrogen ion pump.

The peroxisomes

The peroxisomes are specialised vesicles believed to be formed by budding off from the smooth endoplasmic reticulum. They contain oxidases capable of catalysing many diverse reactions, including the oxidation of long chain saturated fatty acids not handled well by the mitochondria. Several of the oxidases are capable of combining oxygen with hydrogen ions from different intracellular chemicals to form hydrogen peroxide. This is also a highly oxidising substance which, in association with catalase, oxidises many substances that could be toxic to the cell. Therefore peroxisomes are particularly abundant in the hepatocytes of the liver where they are involved in cholesterol metabolism and gluconeogenesis. However, in other cell types peroxisomes contain different enzymes, such as in the myelin of the central nervous system where they express a capacity for the synthesis of plasmalogens and phospholipids.

The mitochondria

The mitochondria (Fig. 2.5) are the power centres of the cell, providing cells with energy in the form of adenosine triphosphate (ATP). Evidence suggests that without mitochondria, cells would be unable to extract energy from nutrients and oxygen and all cellular functions would cease (Alberts et al 1994, McKee & McKee 1996). The total number of mitochondria in various cell types differs, although it also depends on the energy requirement of the individual cell. Furthermore, mitochondria are concentrated in those parts of the cell most responsible for the major share of energy metabolism.

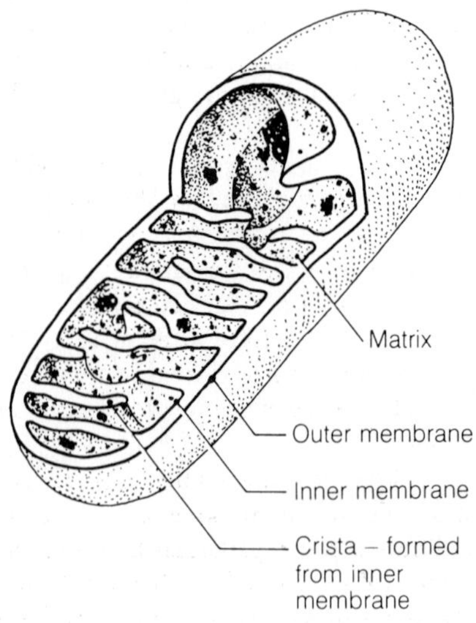

Figure 2.5 *Diagram of a mitochondrion (from Hinchliff SM, Montague SE, 1990, with permission).*

The size and shape of the mitochondria vary considerably; even within one cell the mitochondria divide, move, change shape and fuse. Consequently, some mitochondria appear globular and no more than a few hundred nanometres in diameter, whereas others may be large with dimensions of 1 μm in diameter and up to 7 μm in length. However, the fundamental structures of the mitochondria are chiefly composed of two limiting membranes, an outer and an inner. Numerous foldings of the inner membrane form the well-known mitochondrial cristae, which project into the interior of the organelle (Fig. 2.5).

Cristae

Cristae may be shelflike or tubular in structure onto which oxidative enzymes are attached. The innermost cavity of the mitochondrion is filled with a matrix containing large quantities of dissolved enzymes, necessary for extraction of energy from nutrients. These enzymes function in close association with the oxidative enzymes and enzyme partnerships within the mitochondria provide the critical mechanism for oxidation of nutrients with liberation of energy and formation of carbon dioxide and water. The liberated energy is used to synthesise the high-energy ATP. When necessary, the ATP is transported out of the mitochondria into the cytoplasm where it diffuses and releases its energy to support cellular activities.

Mitochondrial replication

Mitochondria are self-replicating. This replication appears to be induced partly by increased ATP requirements of the cell. Mitochondria contain their own genome and each mitochondrion usually contains multiple copies of its genome, which is double-stranded and read from opposing directions during transcription (Alberts et al 1994). In comparison to the nuclear genome, the mitochondrial genome is very small. In humans it consists of 16 569 nucleotide pairs in length and is extremely compact with almost no **intronic sequences**, or untranslated regions, between the coding genes. Because of the asymmetric distribution of guanines and cytosines between the two strands, one strand is heavier due to its guanine content and the opposing strand is lighter due to its cytosine content.

However, the majority of the proteins found in the mitochondria are encoded by the nuclear genome, translated into the cytoplasm of the cell and imported into the mitochondria by special amino acids. Receptors on the outer membrane of the mitochondria recognise and bind the protein and transport it to the import apparatus. A few proteins bypass this import system and integrate directly into the outer membrane without undergoing processing. The mitochondrial genome replicates independently of the nuclear genome but the complex process of energy production requires a high level of interdependence and communication between the two genomes.

THE CYTOSKELETON

The complex network of protein filaments that extends throughout the cytoplasm is known as the cytoskeleton. This is a highly dynamic structure that reorganises continuously as the cell changes shape, divides and responds to its environment (Schmidt & Thews 1987). It is directly responsible for much of the cellular movement such as the crawling of the cell, muscle contraction and the many changes in the shape of the developing vertebrate embryo. The cytoskeleton also provides the machinery for intracellular movement, such as the transport of organelles from one place to another within the cytoplasm, and the segregation of chromosomes at mitosis. The highly diverse activities of the cytoskeleton depend on three types of protein filaments: actin filaments, microtubules and the intermediate filaments.

THE NUCLEUS

Laskey (1987) suggests that the nucleus has long been considered the ultimate control centre of the cell. As the largest structure of the cell, it measures approximately 2–10 µm in diameter. Its position and number may vary with each cell type. Although mainly centrally situated, it is found in the periphery of adipocytes, at the base of epithelial and secretory cells and within the cell body of neurones. Most cells have only one nucleus but skeletal muscle cells and osteoclasts are examples of multinucleated cells.

Nuclei contain large quantities of DNA which holds the genetic blueprint. The nuclear genome determines the characteristics of proteins and enzymes contained in the cytoplasm of a specific cell type and controls the cytoplasmic activities and cellular reproduction (Alberts et al 1994, Cross & Mercer 1993, McKee & McKee 1996). In addition to the DNA, several other structures are essential to the normal functioning of the nucleus, namely the gel-like **nucleoplasm** and the **nucleoli**. The latter are the site of **ribosomal ribonucleic acid** (rRNA) synthesis.

The genetic material consisting chiefly of DNA is found in a thread-like mass known as **chromatin**. Prior to cellular reproduction the chromatin shortens and coils into rod-like bodies forming recognisable **chromosomes**. At the first stage of the DNA packing, it combines with proteins, known as **histones**. However, the entire DNA molecule is ultimately composed of several simple chemical compounds bound together in a regular pattern. The basic building blocks of the DNA molecule are **phosphoric acid**, a sugar called **deoxyribose** and four nitrogenous bases: two purines (**adenine** and **guanine**) and two pyrimidines (**thymine** and **cytosine**) identified by the single letters A, D, T and C.

The outermost part of the nucleus is formed by a complex nuclear membrane which is composed of two lipid bilayers approximately 20–40 nm apart from each other, enclosing the **perinuclear cisternae**. The outer nuclear membrane is continuous with the cell's endoplasmic reticulum. The intramembranous space of 20–40 nm is also continuous with the internal compartments of the endoplasmic reticulum. The entire nuclear envelope is penetrated by several thousand nuclear pores, making it permeable to substances of low molecular weight.

Large complex protein molecules surround these nuclear pores, leaving central smaller pores no larger than 9 nm in diameter but large enough to permit some molecules of up to 44 000 molecular weight to pass through with relative ease. Molecules of molecular weight less than 15 000 pass through the nuclear pores extremely rapidly. Warren (1987) suggests that the relative porosity of the nuclear membrane permits the necessary movement of messenger ribonucleic acid to the cytoplasm and entry of enzymes and histones into the nucleus during DNA replication.

Finally, the nucleolus, unlike most of the other organelles, appears not to have a limiting membrane. However, it usually contains large quantities of RNA and proteins similar to those found in the ribosomes. The nucleolus seems to become considerably enlarged when a cell is actively involved in protein synthesis when it also increases the size and enhances the shape of the nucleus. The nucleolus disappears during mitosis and is reassembled again in the daughter cells.

PLASMA MEMBRANE EXCITABILITY AND ION TRANSPORT

The hydrophobic interior of the plasma membranes acts as a barrier to the passage of most polar molecules. This barrier is crucially important to the overall function of a specific cell (Alberts et al 1994). It allows the cell to maintain concentrations of solutes in its cytoplasm that differ from those in the extracellular fluid and in each of the intracellular membrane-bound organelles. To maintain this barrier, cells have competent mechanisms for transferring specific water-soluble molecules across their membranes to obtain essential nutrients, excrete metabolic waste products and regulate intracellular ion concentrations. Transport of inorganic ions and small water-soluble organic molecules across the lipid bilayer is achieved by specialised transmembrane proteins, each responsible for the transfer of a specific ion or molecule or a group of closely related ions or molecules.

The two main classes of membrane proteins that mediate the transfer of small water-soluble molecules are called transport proteins. These are either **carrier proteins**, which shift specific molecules across the membrane, or **channel proteins**, which form a narrow hydrophilic pore allowing the passive movement of small inorganic ions across the lipid bilayer. Carrier proteins can be coupled to a source of energy which facilitates active transport.

This combination of selective passive permeability and active transport creates large differences in the composition of the cytosol compared with extracellular fluid or the fluid within membrane-bound organelles. By generating ionic concentration differences across the lipid bilayer, cell membranes are able to store potential energy in the form of **electrochemical gradients** which are used to drive various transport processes, convey electric signals in **electrically excitable cells** and generate ATP in the mitochondria.

Simple biochemistry experiments have demonstrated that the smaller the molecule and more soluble it is in oil, the more rapidly it will diffuse across a particular lipid bilayer (Alberts et al 1994, Guyton 1994, Schmidt & Thews 1987). Similarly, small non-polar molecules such as oxygen and carbon dioxide readily dissolve in lipid bilayers and diffuse rapidly across them. Uncharged polar molecules also diffuse rapidly across a bilayer if they are small enough. Thus water and urea cross rapidly while glycerol, a larger molecule, diffuses less rapidly and the more complex glucose diffuses hardly at all.

By contrast, the lipid bilayers are highly impermeable to charged molecules (ions), no matter how small they are. It would appear that the charge and the high degree of hydration of such molecules prevent them from entering the hydrocarbon phase of the bilayer. Therefore, to facilitate efficient transfer of ions, channel proteins consisting of highly selective pores form a continuous pathway across the plasma membrane to enable the specific hydrophilic solutes to cross the membrane without coming into direct contact with the hydrophobic interior of the lipid bilayer. Most channel proteins are species specific, permitting specific solutes to cross the membrane by passive diffusion.

Most channel proteins contained in the plasma membrane connect with the cytoplasm as well as the cell exterior. As these proteins are specifically concerned with the transport of inorganic ions, they are referred to as **ion channels**. These channel proteins have an advantage over the carrier proteins in that more than 1 million ions can pass through an open channel each second, which is a rate of 1000 times greater than the rate of transport of any known carrier protein.

Two important properties distinguish ion channels from single aqueous pores (Alberts et al 1994, Bray et al 1994). First, they show ion selectivity, permitting some inorganic ions to pass but not others. The second important distinction is that ion channels are not continuously open. Instead they have 'gates' which open briefly, usually in response to a specific stimulus, and then close again. The main types of stimuli known to cause ion channels to open are a change in the voltage across the membrane (voltage-gated channels), mechanical stress (mechanically gated channels) or the binding of a **ligand** (ligand-gated channels). The ligand can be either an extracellular mediator, a neurotransmitter or an intracellular mediator such as an ion or a nucleotide.

Although ion channels are responsible for the electrical excitability of muscle cells and mediation of electrical signalling in neurones, they are not restricted to electrically excitable cells. They are present in all cell membranes facilitating diffusion of their specific ion species. Perhaps the most common forms of ion channels are those that are permeable mainly to potassium ions. This makes the plasma membrane much more permeable to potassium ions than to any other ions and maintains a critical membrane potential or a significant voltage difference across all plasma membranes.

In contrast, carrier proteins, which are responsible for selective transport of substrates across the plasma membrane, bind the specific solute to be transported and undergo a series of conformational changes in order to transfer the solute across the membrane. Each of the carrier proteins has one or more binding sites for its substrate. The specialised transport process involves full saturation of the carrier sites. When all the binding sites are occupied, the rate of transport across the plasma membrane is maximal. However, the binding of a solute can be blocked by competitive inhibitors, which compete for the same binding sites and may or may not be transported by the carrier, or by non-competitive inhibitors which bind elsewhere and alter the structure of the carrier protein.

Carrier proteins are classified according to their functional capacity. Some carrier proteins are **uniporters** while other more complex proteins are **coupled transporters** where the transport of one solute depends on the simultaneous transfer of a second solute. This may be in the same direction (**symport**) or in the opposite direction (**antiport**). Examples include the take-up of glucose. Glucose is moved from the extracellular fluid, where its concentration is high relative to that in the cytosol, which is achieved by passive transport through glucose carriers operating as uniporters.

By contrast, the intestinal and kidney epithelial cells take up glucose from the lumen of the intestine and the lumen of the nephron respectively, where the concentration of glucose is low. In both these instances the epithelial cells are required to transport glucose actively across their plasma membrane along with sodium. Similarly, carrier proteins found in the plasma membrane of the human red blood cell are anion carriers that operate as an antiporter to exchange chloride for bicarbonate.

THE SODIUM–POTASSIUM PUMP

The concentration of potassium ions is typically 10–20 times higher in the cytoplasm than in the extracellular fluid, whilst the reverse is true of sodium. These significant ionic concentration differences are maintained by sodium–potassium pumps found in the plasma membrane of virtually all mammalian cells (Fig. 2.6). These appear to operate as antiporters, actively pumping sodium out of the cell against its steep **electrochemical gradient** found in the extracellular fluid and pumping potassium into the cell again against its steep electrochemical gradient. The sodium gradient produced by these pumps also regulates cell volume through its osmotic effects and is exploited to transport sugars and amino acids into the cells.

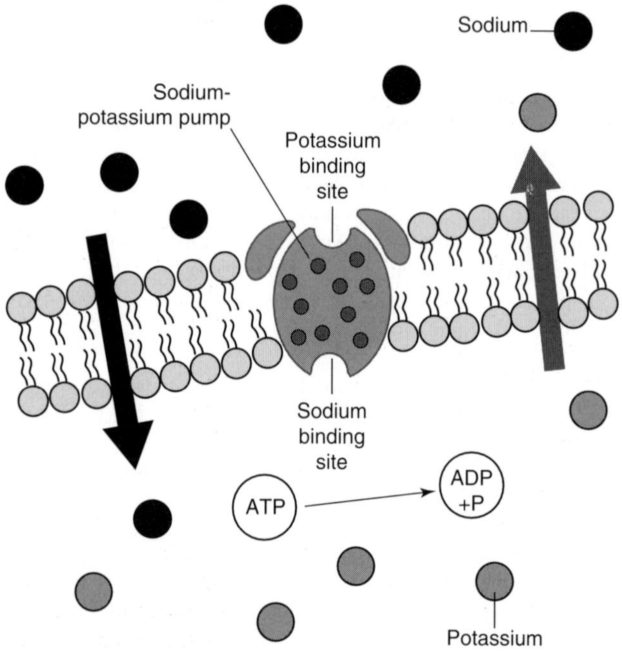

Figure 2.6 *Operation of the sodium–potassium pump. Three sodium ions are moved out of the cell and two potassium ions are moved into the cell. The energy is provided by hydrolysis of one molecule of ATP.*

Almost one-third of the energy of the cell is consumed in fuelling the sodium–potassium pumps. However, in electrically active nerve cells which are repeatedly gaining small amounts of sodium and losing small amounts of potassium during the propagation of nerve impulses, the pump energy requirements may increase to two-thirds. There is compelling evidence that ATP supplies the energy for pumping the sodium and potassium ions across the plasma membrane.

An enzyme, sodium–potassium ATPase, has been found, consisting of a large, multipass subunit approximately 1000 amino acids long and an associated smaller, single-pass glycoprotein. The former has binding sites for sodium and ATP on its cytoplasmic surface and a binding site for potassium on its external surface and is reversibly phosphorylated and dephosphorylated during the pumping cycle. The function of the glycoprotein is uncertain, except that it is required for the intracellular transport of the large subunit to the plasma membrane. Since the sodium–potassium ATPase drives three positively charged ions out of the cell for every two it pumps in, it creates an electrical potential with the inside surface of the plasma membrane negative to the outside surface. This effect seldom contributes more than 10% to the membrane potential.

The sodium–potassium ATPase does have a further function in regulating the volume of the cell. By controlling the solute concentration inside the cell it regulates the osmotic forces that influence cell expansion and dehydration. Cells usually contain a high concentration of solutes, including numerous negatively charged organic molecules (**fixed anions**) that are confined to the inside of the cell. The specific cations, such as sodium and potassium, are required for charge balance and create a large osmotic gradient that tends to 'pull' water into the cell. This is counteracted by an opposite osmotic gradient due to a high concentration of inorganic ions, mainly sodium and chloride, in the extracellular fluid so that the movement of sodium contributes to acceptable intracellular hydration.

CELL DIVISION

Mitosis

Controlled cell division is vital to human reproduction, tissue growth and repair, efficient immune defence mechanisms and countless other processes (Murray & Kirschner 1991). The cycle of cell division is the most critical and fundamental process by which all multicellular species replace cells damaged by wear and tear or lost as a consequence of programmed cell death. The body of a mature adult human being must be capable of programmed synthesis of millions of new cells simply to maintain its physical and physiological status quo (Alberts et al 1994).

Where natural cell division is halted, as for instance in exposure to a large dose of ionising radiation, the individual is likely to die within a few days because of rapid cell destruction. While the details of the cell cycle may vary, certain behavioural requirements of all cells are universal. In the first instance, cells have to coordinate various events in the cycle. They must, for example, avoid entering mitosis or meiosis until the chromosomes have been replicated. According to Mueller & Young (1995), failure to comply with this requirement can result in cells that lack a particular chromosome, an aberration which may give rise to cancer at a later stage.

Replication of deoxyribonucleic acid

In order to produce a pair of genetically identical daughter cells, the nuclear DNA must be precisely replicated and the replicated chromosomes must be separated into two genetically identical cells. Furthermore, the vast majority of cells also double their mass and duplicate all their cytoplasmic organelles in each cell cycle. Therefore, each cell which is genetically capable of division must be capable of coordinating a complex set of cytoplasmic and nuclear processes with one another during the actual cycle.

The duration of the cell cycle varies greatly from one cell type to another (Alberts et al 1994, Guyton 1994). However, a common standard does exist and the cell cycle for all dividing cells follows a template consisting of several distinct phases, namely **interphase**, **mitosis** and **cytokinesis**. Of these phases, mitosis, the critical process of nuclear division, is the most dramatic. Because cells require time to grow before they can divide, the standard cell cycle is fairly long, extending to approximately 12 hours or more in fast-growing mammalian tissue. In most cells the entire mitotic phase takes approximately an hour, which is only a very small fraction of the total cell cycle time.

- **Interphase** facilitates DNA replication. The vast amount of time that elapses between one mitotic phase and the next is taken up by the interphase, which consists of three distinctive phases: the **G1** or **gap1** phase, the **S** or **synthesis** phase and the **G2** or **gap2** phase. During the G1 phase the cells monitor their internal environment and their own size so that when the time is appropriate, decisive steps are taken that commit the cells to DNA replication which occurs in the S or synthesis phase of the cell cycle. The subsequent G2 phase appears to provide a safety gap, allowing the cell to ensure that DNA replication is complete before it enters into mitosis.
- During **mitosis** the nuclear membrane breaks down and the contents of the nucleus condense, forming visible chromosomes. The cell's microtubules reorganise to establish the mitotic spindle that will eventually separate the chromosomes. The cell seems to pause briefly in a state called **metaphase** as the duplicated chromosomes align on the mitotic spindle, in preparation for segregation. This segregation of the duplicated chromosomes marks the beginning of the **anaphase**, during which the chromosomes move to the pole of the spindle where they decondense and reestablish new intact nuclei.
- Only at this point is the cell pinched and gradually divided by a process of **cytokinesis** which is the critical point of the mitotic phase which terminates the end of the cell cycle.

Although the lengths of all phases of the cell cycle are variable to some extent, the greatest variation by far appears to occur in the duration of the G1 phase. One of the reasons for this variability is thought to be the cell's natural need to replicate. Thus, cells in G1, if not already committed to DNA replication, can pause in the progress around the cycle and enter a specialised resting state often referred to as the **G0 phase**.

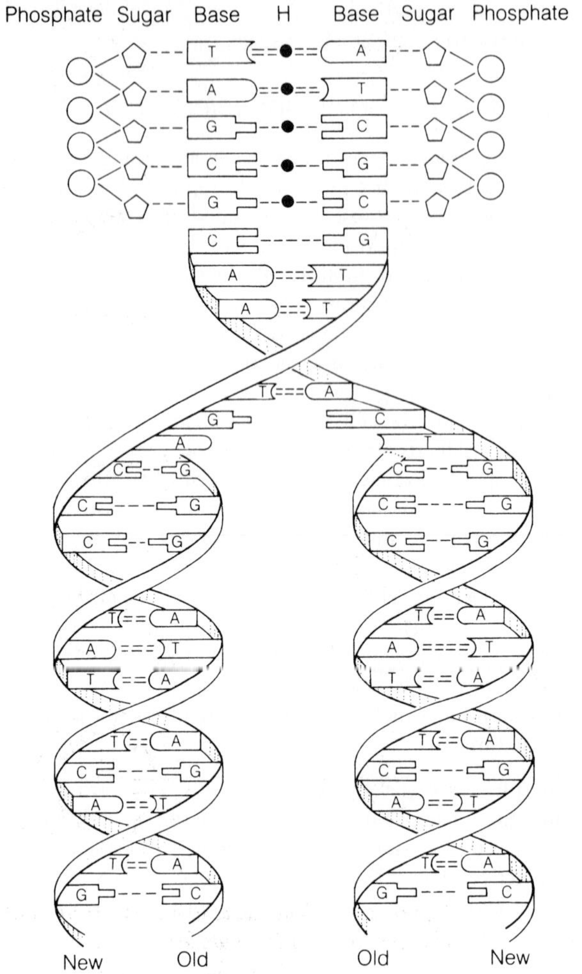

Figure 2.7 *The replication of DNA showing the unwinding of the double helix and the formation of new strands with complementary base pairs (from Hinchliff SM, Montague SE, 1990, with permission).*

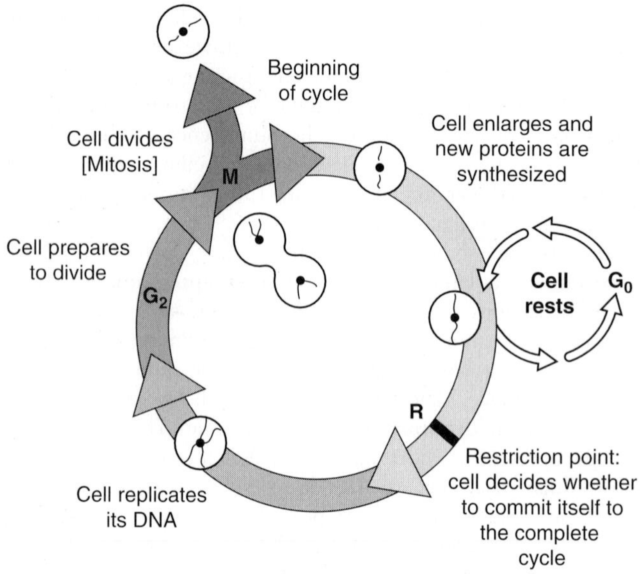

Figure 2.8 *Stages of the cell cycle (reproduced with kind permission of Barbara Novak).*

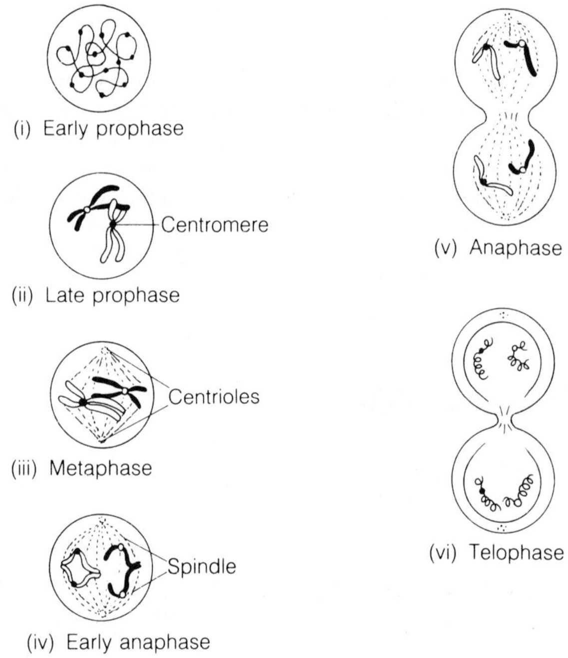

Figure 2.9 *Stages of mitosis (from Hinchliff SM, Montague SE, 1990, with permission).*

Indeed, cells can remain in this phase for days, weeks and even years before resuming proliferation.

In conditions that favour growth, the total protein content of a typical cell increases continuously throughout the cell cycle (Alberts et al 1994, Richards 1991). Similarly, RNA synthesis continues at a steady rate, except during the mitotic phase when the chromosomes are too condensed to permit transcription. Analysis of the pattern of individual protein synthesis suggests that the vast majority of proteins are synthesised throughout the cell cycle. Therefore, cell growth is a steady and continuous process, interrupted briefly by the mitotic phase when the nucleus and then the corresponding cell compartment divide into two.

Meiosis

Meiosis, meaning diminution, is a special kind of nuclear division in which the chromosome complement is precisely halved. Meiosis involves two nuclear divisions rather than one.

With the exception of the sex chromosomes (different in male and female), a **diploid** nucleus contains two similar versions of each of the **autosomes** (alike in both male and female). One set of these chromosomes is paternal and one set maternal in origin. The two sets of chromosomes are known as the **homologues**. In most cells they maintain a separate existence as independent chromosomes.

In contrast, a mature **haploid gamete** produced by the divisions of a diploid cell during meiosis must contain half the

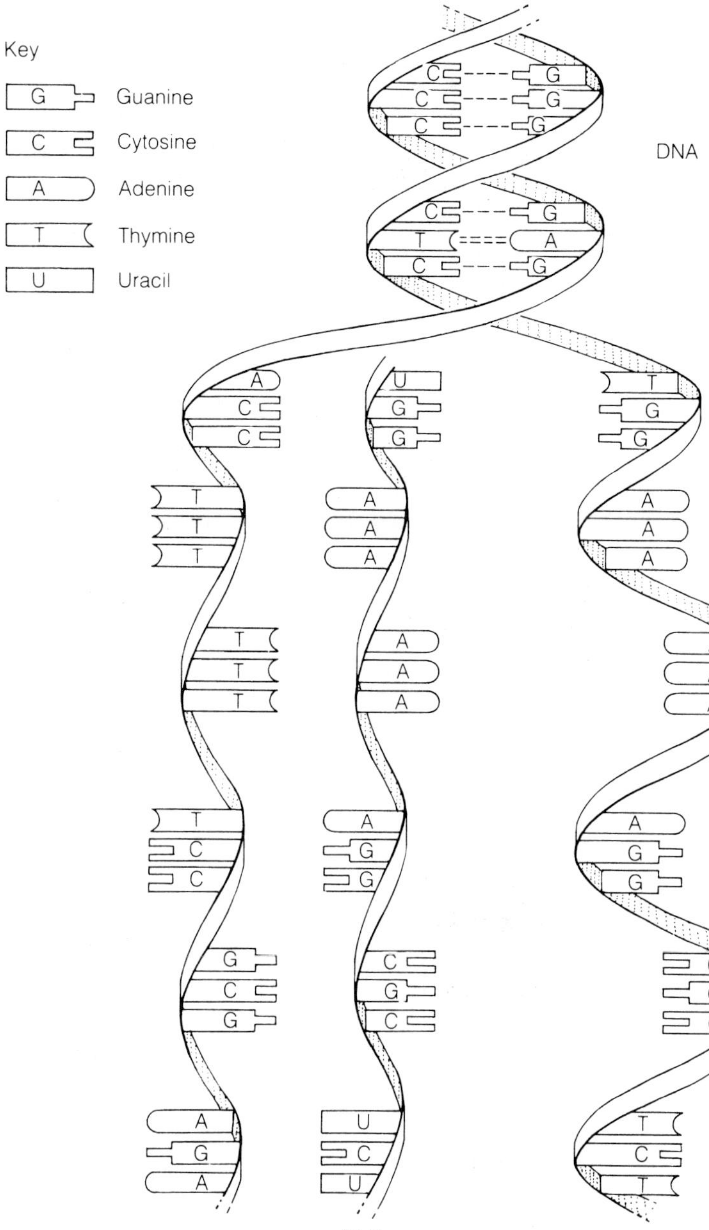

Figure 2.10 *Transcription of a strand of DNA by messenger RNA (mRNA)(from Hinchliff SM, Montague SE, 1990, with permission).*

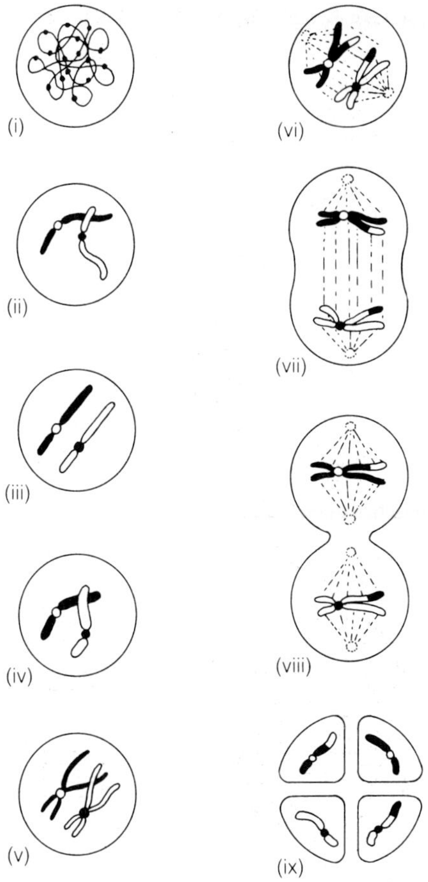

Figure 2.11 *The stages of meiosis. (Only one chromosome pair is shown for clarity).*
(i) Interphase. (ii) Prophase I: leptotene.
(iii) Zygotene. (iv) Pachytene. (v) Diplotene.
(vi) Metaphase I. (vii) Anaphase I.
(viii) Telophase I. (ix) Second meiotic division (from Hinchliff SM, Montague SE, 1990, with permission).

original number of chromosomes. This means that only one chromosome from each homologous pair of chromosomes is present, ensuring that either the maternal or the paternal copy of each gene is present but not both. This specific requirement makes an extra demand on the natural processes governing cell division.

Evidence suggests that a mechanism has evolved to accomplish the additional sorting of the chromosomes which appears to involve the homologues recognising each other and becoming physically paired prior to lining up on the mitotic spindle. This pairing of the maternal and the paternal copy of each chromosome is unique to meiosis. The highly complex mechanisms which facilitate chromosomal recognition in meiosis remain unclear.

Evidence suggests that it is only after the DNA replication has been completed that the special feature of meiosis becomes evident. Rather than separating, the **sister chromatids** behave as a unit, giving the impression that the earlier chromosome duplication has not occurred and duplicated homologous pairs form a structure which contains four chromatids. This allows **genetic recombination** to occur when a fragment of a maternal chromatid is exchanged for a corresponding fragment of a homologous paternal chromatid.

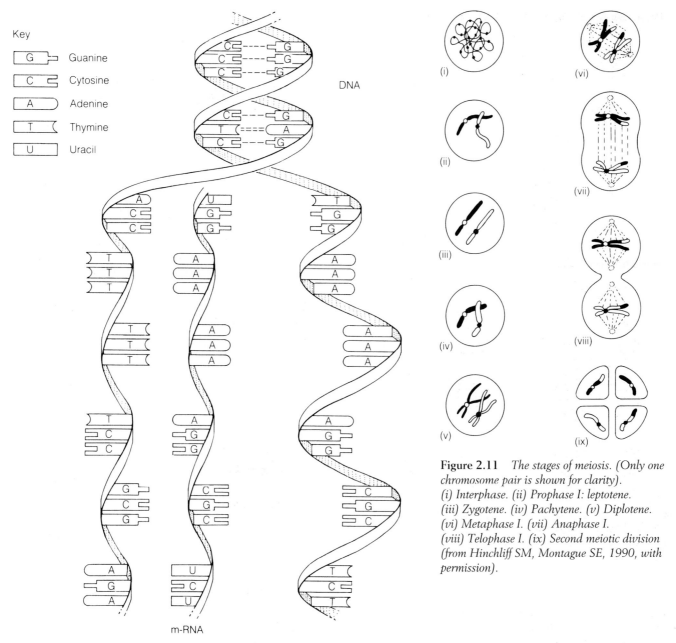

Summary of main points

- The mammalian cell is a fundamental unit of life. Its morphological and functional features are governed by its genetic blueprint contained in its nucleus. Numerous physiological processes such as diffusion of gases, ions and the transport of nutrients depend on the size of the surface area of the individual cell.
- Most cells in the human body have a high but carefully balanced metabolic rate. One of the major physical advantages of a particular cell may be identified in its capacity to permit selective but rapid diffusion of substrates over short distances of up to 50 nm. The benefit of this phenomenon is that it ensures that the metabolic needs of the active cells are easily sustained.
- In larger cells the metabolic and physiological challenges appear to be overcome to some extent by a significant increase in the cell's surface area. This is achieved by either folding the plasma membrane and forming microvilli or other surface protrusions or flattening the entire cell body. In each case the cells generate a larger surface area for selective transport and diffusion.
- Most cells display a characteristic capacity for motility which generally involves the movement of the cytoplasm or specific organelles from one part of the cell to another. However, cell motility is by and large influenced by environmental factors such as tissue injury which stimulates migration of phagocytic white blood cells. A similar example of cell migration is manifested by fibroblasts which migrate during embryonic development to take up an important role in histiogenesis which contributes to the construction of the embryonic neural crest and muscle tissue.
- Fibroblasts also interact with collagen by means of adhesion plaques and so exert traction on the tissue matrix. This process, amongst others, plays a key role in efficient wound healing.
- All three germ layers, the ectoderm, the endoderm and the mesoderm, contribute to the formation and development of some form of epithelium. The major anatomic position of the epithelium is to provide an internal and external covering for body surfaces. Consequently, the epithelia protect the underlying tissue from dehydration, chemical or mechanical injury. However, some forms of epithelia also function as sensory surfaces.
- For functional purposes, the widely diverse epithelia are classified into groups according to their morphological and functional characteristics. Each epithelial cell type may be identified in terms of size, shape, cell volume and density. Consequently, where cells are small the volume of the cytoplasm is relatively low, containing few organelles, and the metabolic activity is invariably low.
- Complex organ structures such as the liver or the placenta, which are largely derived from the epithelia, show an elaborate capacity to absorb, transport and secrete substrates necessary to the normal function of the entire human organism.
- The most common feature of the epithelia, and other cell types, is the plasma membrane. This highly specialised membrane encloses the cellular content and defines its boundaries and so maintains the essential differences between the cytosol and the extracellular environment. In common with all biological membranes, the plasma membrane is constructed of a very thin lipid bilayer containing protein molecules. The plasma membrane is capable of considerable adaptation because of the ability of most of its molecular structures to move about within the membrane.
- The lipid bilayer provides the universal basis for the refined, highly specific construction of the plasma membrane. The lipid molecules consist of a hydrophilic polar head and a hydrophobic non-polar tail. The shape and nature of the lipid molecules contribute to the spontaneous formation of these bilayers in aqueous solutions.
- The lipid bilayer is not exclusively composed of phospholipids; it also contains proteins, cholesterol, glycoproteins and glycolipids. Each of the molecular structures contributes to the structural specificity and corresponding functional scope of the cell-specific plasma membrane.
- Most of the specific functions of the plasma membrane are carried out by the membrane proteins. Many membrane proteins rotate about an axis which is perpendicular to the plane of the lipid bilayer, facilitating the process of rotational diffusion. Some membrane proteins are also capable of lateral movement within the membrane itself, whilst others may be confined to specific domains of the plasma membrane such as the apical, basal or lateral surfaces.
- The selective permeability of the plasma membrane facilitates free passage of gases and water but restricts the movement of larger ions such as sodium, potassium, calcium, chloride and bicarbonate to their specific protein channels which can be opened or closed in order to regulate transmembrane traffic.
- The main stimuli that are known to cause specific ion channels to open and close are a change in the voltage across the membrane (voltage-gated channels), a mechanical stress (mechanically gated channels) or the reversible binding of a ligand (ligand-gated channels).
- The most common form of ion channels present in a plasma membrane are those that are permeable to potassium ions. The function of these channels is to ensure that a critical plasma membrane potential is maintained, thereby enabling the cell to function normally. The critical concentration of potassium ions may be 10–20 times higher in the cytoplasm than the concentrations found in the extracellular fluid whilst the reverse is true of sodium. These significant ionic concentration differences are maintained by sophisticated sodium–potassium pumps found in the plasma membrane of cells.
- The gel-like cytoplasm acts as an effective reservoir for the suspension of small molecular structures, large particles and organelles. Some of the most important organelles are the endoplasmic reticulum, the Golgi apparatus, the mitochondria, the lysosomes and the peroxisomes.
- The endoplasmic reticulum plays a central role in lipid and protein biosynthesis. The Golgi apparatus is found in close proximity to the endoplasmic reticulum and its main function is to process various proteins for eventual intra- and extracellular use.
- Lysosomes are vesicular organelles formed by the Golgi apparatus. They are dispersed throughout the cytoplasm where they form the digestive system of the cell. The lysosomes are surrounded by a membranous lipid bilayer and are filled with a granular protein aggregate which forms the necessary digestive enzymes.
- Peroxisomes are specialised vesicles containing oxidases which are enzymes capable of catalysing many diverse intracellular reactions. Several oxidases are capable of combining intracellular oxygen with hydrogen ions, thus forming hydrogen peroxide which is used in turn to oxidise substances that might otherwise be poisonous to the cell.
- Mitochondria are power centres of the cell capable of generating ATP which is a form of energy currency essential to normal cellular function. Mitochondria vary in their size and shape but their structure is constant, mainly composed of two limiting membranes. Mitochondria are self-replicating and contain their own DNA.
- The cytoskeleton consists of a complex network of protein filaments which appears to facilitate cell movement. The chief constituents of the protein filaments are actin, microtubules and intermediate filaments.
- The nucleus is the largest structure of the cell. Its position and number may vary in each cell type. Nuclei contain large quantities of DNA which holds the cell's genetic blueprint. The nuclear genome determines the characteristics of proteins and enzymes contained in the cytoplasm of a specific cell type. Through these, it controls cytoplasmic activities and cell reproduction.

- Controlled cell division is vital to human reproduction, tissue growth, repair and other processes. To produce a pair of genetically identical daughter cells, the nuclear DNA must be precisely replicated and the replicated chromosomes must be separated into two genetically identical cells.
- Meiosis is a special form of cell replication leading to gamete formation where the chromosome numbers are halved. After exchanging genetic material, one of each pair of homologous chromosomes is represented in the mature gamete.

References

Alberts B, Bray D, Lewis J et al 1994 The Molecular Biology of the Cell. Garland Publishing, New York.

Bannister L, Berry M, Collins P et al 1995 Gray's Anatomy. Churchill Livingstone, Edinburgh.

Bray J, Cragg P, MacKnight A et al 1994 Lecture Notes on Human Physiology. Blackwell Scientific Publications, Oxford.

Cross P, Mercer K 1993 Cell and Tissue Ultrastructure – A Functional Perspective. WH Freeman, New York.

Devlin T 1990 Textbook of Biochemistry with Clinical Correlations. John Wiley, Chichester.

Evans WH, Graham JM 1991 Membrane Structure and Functions. Oxford University Press, Oxford.

Guyton A 1994 Textbook of Medical Physiology. WB Saunders, Philadelphia.

Hinchliff SM, Montague SE 1990 Physiology for Nursing Practice. Baillière Tindall, London.

Hinchliff SM, Montague SE, Watson R 1996 Physiology for Nursing Practice. Baillière Tindall, London.

Laskey RA 1987 Basic molecular and cell biology – the cell nucleus. British Medical Journal, 295, 1121–1123.

McKee T, McKee J 1996 Biochemistry. WC Brown, London.

Mueller R, Young I 1995 Emery's Elements of Medical Genetics. Churchill Livingstone, Edinburgh.

Murray A, Kirschner M 1991 What controls the cell cycle? Scientific American, 3, 34–41.

Preston TM 1990 The Cytoskeleton and Cell Motility. Blackie and Son, Glasgow.

Richards F 1991 The protein folding problem. Scientific American, 1, 34–41.

Schmidt R, Thews G 1987 Human Physiology. Springer-Verlag, Berlin.

Sherwood L 1993 Human Physiology – From Cells to Systems. West Publishing, St Paul, Maine.

Stossel T 1994 The machinery of cell crawling. Scientific American, 9, 40–47.

Warren G 1987 Basic molecular and cell biology – sorting signals and cellular membranes. British Medical Journal, 295, 1259–1261.

Recommended reading

Austin B, Westwood O 1991 Protein Targeting and Secretion. Oxford University Press, Oxford.

Chan L, Seeburg P 1995 RNA editing. Science and Medicine, 2(2), 68–77.

Glover DM, Gonzalez C, Raff JW et al 1993 The centrosome. Scientific American, 6, 32–38.

Hoffman A, Thanh H 1996 Genomic imprinting. Science and Medicine, 3 (1), 52–61.

Linder M 1992 G proteins. Scientific American, 7, 36–43.

Richards F 1991 The protein folding problem. Scientific American, 1, 34–41.

Welch W 1993 How cells respond to stress. Scientific American, 5, 5–64.

Chapter

3 The female reproductive system

In this chapter

INTRODUCTION

The biological function of the reproductive system is to ensure the future of the species by producing the **gametes** – male **spermatozoa** and female **oocytes** or **ova** – essential for transferring combined and reshuffled genes from the parents to the next generation. This reshuffling ensures the genetic variability needed to provide adaptation to changing environments. In the female the role is extended to include provision of optimum conditions for fertilisation and development of the embryo and fetus and providing nourishment and protection until it is able to survive independently. Finally expulsion from its mother's body at the correct gestation must occur and lactation must be initiated. The non-pregnant female reproductive system will be described below and the male reproductive system in Chapter 4.

SEXUAL DIFFERENTIATION

In the early embryo there is no anatomical evidence of sexual difference internally or externally prior to the seventh week of development. This is often referred to as the **indifferent stage** of the reproductive organs (Moore 1989). Two pairs of genital ducts are present in all embryos, the **paramesonephric** or **Mullerian ducts** with the potential to develop into female genitalia and the **mesonephric** or **Wolffian ducts** with the potential to develop into male genitalia. If the genetic make-up of the embryo is XY, a gene influences the development of testes and in the presence of testosterone the male duct develops into male genitalia. If the genetic make-up of the embryo is XX ovaries will form and the female ducts develop into female genitalia. The ducts not required to develop degenerate.

This influence on the indifferent tissues leads to homologous structures, i.e. structures differing in male and female that have developed from the same origin. Examples include testis and ovary, penis and clitoris. Rarely, the tissues develop in such a way as to make instant recognition of the sex of the baby difficult or impossible without genetic testing.

THE FEMALE REPRODUCTIVE TRACT ANATOMY

The soft tissues forming the female internal genitalia are situated in the pelvic cavity. It is sensible to study the organs separately whilst remembering they form a continuous tract (Fig. 3.1). The organs described below are: vulva, vagina, uterus and cervix, uterine tube and ovary. It is customary and logical, as well as acting as an aid to memory, to follow a pattern in writing about the anatomy and physiology of an organ. The following style of presentation will be used in this chapter wherever possible:

- description, to include development, shape, size and situation;
- structure – gross and microscopic;
- relations to other organs;
- supports;
- blood supply, lymphatic drainage and nerve supply;
- functions.

The vulva

The labia majora

These are two folds containing sebaceous and sweat glands embedded in adipose and connective tissue. They are covered with skin and form the lateral boundaries of the vulval cleft. They are homologues of the scrotum. They unite anteriorly to form the **mons veneris**, an adipose pad over the symphysis pubis. Hair covers the mons veneris and terminates cephalically in a horizontal upper border. Posteriorly, the labia majora unite to form the posterior commissure. Hair grows on the outer surface of the labia majora but not on the inner surface.

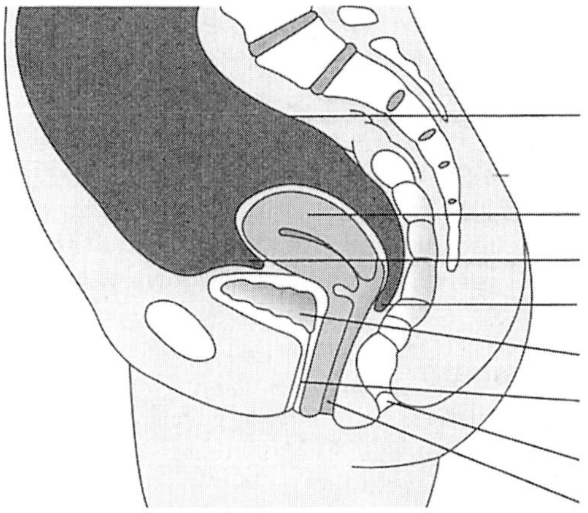

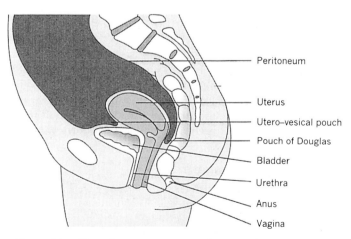

Figure 3.1 *The pelvic organs in sagittal section (from Sweet B, 1997, with permission).*

The labia minora

These are two delicate folds of skin containing connective tissue, some sebaceous glands but no adipose tissue. On the medial aspect keratinised skin epithelium changes to squamous epithelium with many sebaceous glands. Anteriorly the labia minora split into two parts. One passes over the clitoris to form its prepuce and the other beneath the clitoris to form a homologue of the frenulum in the male. Posteriorly the two labia minora unite to form the fourchette. The size of the labia minora varies between women but this is of no significance.

The clitoris

This is the homologue of the male penis. It is composed of erectile tissue and can enlarge and stiffen during sexual excitement. Only the glans and prepuce are normally visible but the corpus can be palpated as a cord-like structure along the lower surface of the symphysis pubis.

The vestibule

This is the cleft between the labia minora onto which open the urethral meatus, the vaginal orifice and Bartholin's glands which are homologues of Cowper's glands in the male. These two pea-sized glands embedded in connective tissue are connected to the

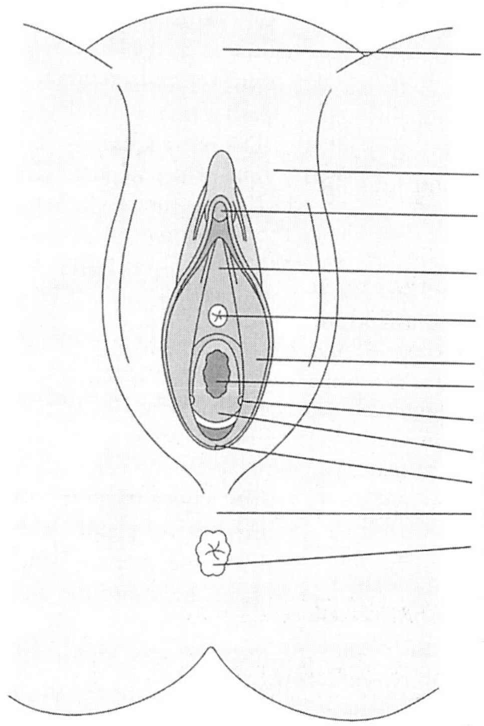

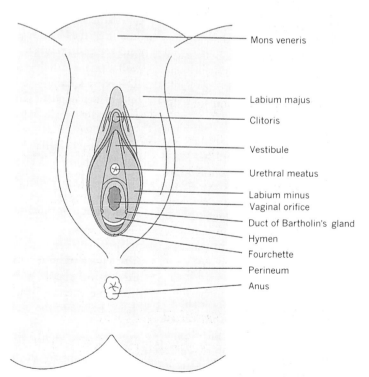

Figure 3.2 *The external genitalia (from Sweet B, 1997, with permission).*

vestibule by ducts that are 2 cm long. The ducts are lined with columnar epithelium which produces a mucoid secretion onto the vestibule for lubrication during coitus.

Blood supply, lymphatic drainage and nerve supply

Blood supply

The vulva is very vascular, receiving its arterial supply from the internal pudendal arteries branching off the internal iliac arteries and the external pudendal arteries branching off the femoral arteries. Venous drainage is usually by corresponding veins which accompany the arteries but from the clitoris a plexus of veins joins the vaginal and vesical plexi.

Lymphatic drainage

Lymphatic vessels form interconnecting meshwork through the labia minora, prepuce, fourchette and vaginal introitus. These drain into the superficial and deep femoral nodes, inguinal nodes and the internal iliac nodes.

Nerve supply

Branches of the pudendal nerve and the perineal nerve supply the vulva.

The vagina

The vagina is a fibromuscular sheath and a potential canal which extends from the vulva to the uterus. The walls are normally in apposition. The widest diameter is anteroposterior in the lower third and transverse in the upper two-thirds of the vagina. This is an important point to remember when inserting vaginal specula. The vagina runs upwards and backwards from the vestibule at 85° to the horizontal when the woman is standing erect. This is parallel to the plane of the pelvic brim.

The vagina is surrounded and supported by the pelvic floor muscles. The cervix projects into the anterior wall of the vagina, making it shorter than the posterior wall. The anterior wall is 7 cm long and the posterior wall, which ends blindly to form the vault of the vagina, is 9 cm long. The projection of the cervix into the anterior vaginal wall divides the vault of the vagina into four fornices: shallow anterior and lateral fornices and a more capacious posterior fornix.

The entrance to the vagina is partially covered by the membranous **hymen** which has one or two uneven perforations to allow flow of the menses. This membrane varies in elasticity and is usually torn at the first coitus and more so at the first birth. Imperforate hymen is a possible cause of failure to menstruate. Once ruptured, remnants are left called **carunculae myrtiformes**. The walls of the vagina fall into transverse folds or rugae to allow for distension. These run in a circumferential manner from two longitudinal columns running sagitally the length of the anterior and posterior walls.

Structure

Layers of the vagina from inner to outer are as follows.

The lining is made of **stratified squamous non-keratinised epithelium** 10–30 cells deep resting on a basement membrane. This is continuous with the epithelium of the infravaginal cervix. The cells are divided into three layers, all derived from the basement membrane and changing as they get nearer to the surface:

1 parabasal cells;
2 intermediate cells;
3 superficial cells.

Superficial cells and some intermediate cells contain glycogen. The entire epithelium shows cyclical changes with the ovarian and menstrual cycles and develops and differentiates further during pregnancy in response to circulating oestrogens, progesterone and androgens. The vaginal epithelial cells do not secrete mucus but secretions seep between the cells to moisten the vagina. Superficial cells are continuously exfoliated and release their glycogen. Doderlein's bacillus metabolises the glycogen and produces lactic acid as a waste product. This results in the normal vaginal acid medium of 4.5. Pathogenic organisms are less likely to invade in this pH. The cells can also absorb drugs, in particular oestrogen.

The **vascular connective tissue** contains elastic tissue, nerves, lymphatics and blood vessels.

The **involuntary muscle coat** has inner muscle fibres which are more oblique than circular while the outer are longitudinal. The vagina varies in size functionally, mainly as a result of muscle tone and contraction in the above muscle layer which is under voluntary control (vaginismus).

Fascia or loose connective tissue surrounds the vagina.

Relations

The lower half of the anterior wall is in contact with the urethra to which it is tightly bound. The upper half is in close contact with the base of the bladder. The lower third of the posterior wall is separated from the anal canal by the perineal body (see Chapter 24), the middle third is in apposition with the rectum and the upper third with the pouch of Douglas. Laterally, the upper third of the vagina is supported by pelvic connective tissue, the middle third by the levatores ani and the lower third by the bulbocavernosus (see Chapter 24).

Blood supply, lymphatic drainage and nerve supply

Blood supply

Arterial supply is from the vaginal and uterine arteries, both branches of the internal iliac artery. Venous drainage is by rich venous plexi in the muscular layer. These communicate with pudendal, vesical and haemorrhoidal plexi and then with the internal iliac vein.

Lymphatic drainage

Vessels from the lower third drain to inferior gluteal nodes and the upper two-thirds to internal iliac, obturator and sacral nodes.

Nerve supply

Via the pudendal nerve to voluntary vaginal muscle.

Functions

- Menstrual flow escapes via the vulva.
- Coitus with entry of the male penis.
- Birth with exit of the fetus, placenta and membranes.

The non-pregnant uterus

The uterus develops from fusion of the two Mullerian ducts in the embryo. It lies in the pelvic cavity in an anteverted and anteflexed position. It is a thickwalled, muscular, hollow, pear-shaped organ flattened in its anteroposterior diameter. Its apex forms the cervix which projects into the vault of the vagina through its anterior wall. Sources give the measurements slightly differently but many books for students of nursing and midwifery (e.g. Bennett & Brown 1996, Hinchliff et al 1996) give the following measurements:

Length	7.5 cm
Breadth	5.0 cm
Depth	2.5 cm
Average thickness of walls	1.5 cm
Weight	60 g

The uterus actually varies in size and is largest during the reproductive years. In women who have had children, all dimensions increase by 1.5 cm.

Structure

The uterus consists of the body (two-thirds of its length), the narrow isthmus (just 0.5 cm long in the non-pregnant uterus) and the cervix (one-third of its length) (Fig. 3.3). The area lying above the uterine tubes is called the **fundus** and where each uterine tube joins the uterus is known as the **cornu** (plural cornua). A constriction at the upper end of the isthmus is called the **anatomical internal os** whilst where the endometrium meets the columnar cervical epithelium is called the **histological internal os**. The cavity has a triangular shape when viewed in coronal section.

Although the cervix is continuous with and part of the uterus, it differs in structure and function from the body of the uterus and therefore some aspects of cervical anatomy and physiology will be described separately. The cervix is barrel-shaped and penetrated by the cervical canal. It is 2.5 cm long and separated from the body of the uterus by the isthmus. It is divided into two equal parts. The supravaginal cervix is that part which lies above the vaginal vault and is surrounded by pelvic fascia – the parametrium – except posteriorly where it is in apposition to the pouch of Douglas. The cone-shaped infravaginal cervix is the part that projects into the vagina and is covered by stratified squamous epithelium continuous with the vaginal epithelium, joining the columnar epithelium of the cervical canal at or near the external os at the squamocolumnar junction.

Lining of the body (corpus)

The mucous lining or **endometrium** builds up from a layer of basal cells. It consists of vascular connective tissue known as **stroma** and contains many mucus-secreting tubular glands which open into the uterine cavity. The stroma is covered by a layer of cuboid cells which dip into the stroma to form the glands. The cells are ciliated on the surface. The thickness varies depending on the phase of the menstrual cycle and is thinnest at the isthmus.

Lining of the cervix

The cervical canal is spindle-shaped and connects the cavity of the uterus at the internal os with the vagina at the external os. The cervix is lined by columnar mucus-secreting epithelium. The mucus membrane is thrown into anterior and posterior folds from which circular folds radiate like branches from the trunk of a tree. This has led to it being known as the **arbor vitae** or tree of life. The epithelium dips into the stroma in a complex

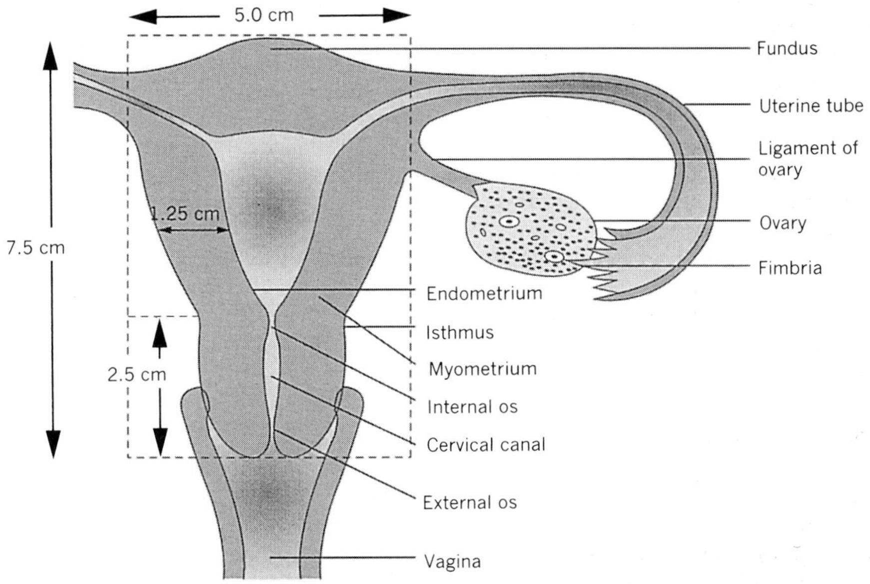

Figure 3.3 *The uterus and the left uterine tube and ovary (from Sweet B, 1997, with permission).*

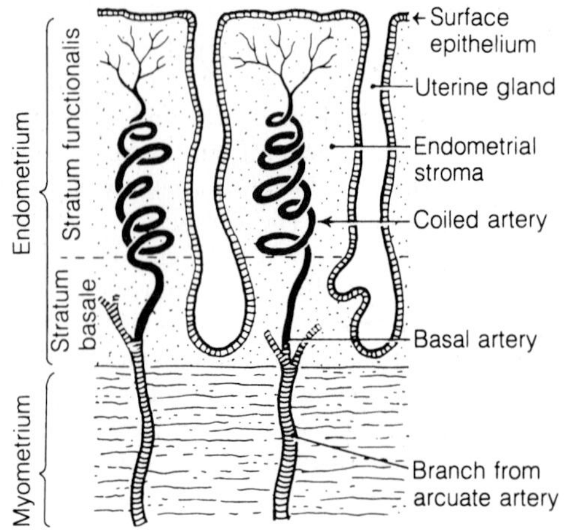

Figure 3.4 *The vascular supply to the endometrium (from Hinchliff SM, Montague SE, 1990, with permission).*

system of crypts and tunnels. These are separated by ridges of stroma covered by epithelium. The stroma consists of 80% collagen, 10% muscle fibre and 10% blood vessels. Compound racemose glands secrete cervical mucus which varies in quality and quantity under the influence of the sex hormones.

Muscle layer

The muscle layer or **myometrium** is made up of bundles of smooth muscle fibres. The outer longitudinal layer and inner circular layer are not well developed in the non-pregnant uterus so that the bulk of the myometrium is made up of fibres that run obliquely and interlace to surround blood vessels and lymphatic vessels. The proportion of muscle begins to diminish in the isthmus, being replaced by connective tissue. The cervix has only 10% muscle content with the fibres running in a circular fashion. It is mainly made of collagen fibres.

Peritoneal layer

The peritoneal layer is a double serosal layer known as the **perimetrium**. It covers the anterior and posterior surfaces but is absent from the narrow lateral surfaces. It is reflected off the uterus onto the superior surface of the bladder at the level of the anatomical internal os, an important point for understanding the technique of lower segment caesarean section.

Relations

- Anterior – uterovesical pouch and bladder
- Posterior – pouch of Douglas and rectum
- Lateral – broad ligaments uterine tubes and ovaries

■ *The squamo-columnar junction and cervical screening*

The squamocolumnar junction is between the columnar epithelium of the cervical canal and the squamous epithelium, continuous with the vaginal epithelium. Sometimes this is an abrupt transformation but the two tissue types may merge in a transformation zone which is the usual site for cervical carcinoma to arise. The position of this junction is determined by the amount of stroma. This in turn is influenced by the level of the hormones oestrogen and progesterone. Oestrogen softens the cervical collagen by binding water to the molecules. This increases the volume of stroma which causes the clefts and tunnels to unfold. The squamocolumnar junction is displaced downwards and out of the cervical canal. This is called **eversion**. Exposure of the columnar epithelium causes the tissues to hypertrophy (**squamous metaplasia**). This leads to the development of the transformation zone. This appearance of the cervix used to be categorised as pathological but now treatment is not considered to be always necessary. However, the squamocolumnar junction is the main site for development of carcinoma of the cervix.

The cervix is readily accessed and tissue samples are easily obtained. Therefore the squamous epithelium has been studied widely. In some women the cervical epithelium seems unstable and cells with abnormal appearance of the nucleus (**nuclear dyskaryosis**) and abnormal cell growth (**cellular dysplasia**) are likely to lead to cervical carcinoma. These abnormalities are due to infection with the human papillomavirus (HPV) types 16, 18 and 6. Evidence from epidemiology has indicated that up to 30% of sexually active women have been affected by HPV by age 30. HPV is sexually transmitted and is a cause of genital warts.

Early recognition of these precancerous changes allows successful surgical treatment to be done so that screening women on a regular basis can be life saving. The technique is called **cervical exfoliative cytology** and is offered to antenatal patients who have not been recently screened. A special spatula called an Ayres spatula is used to obtain cells from both outside (**exocervix**) and inside the cervical canal (**endocervix**).

The cells are examined under the microscope and reported as:

1. unsatisfactory – insufficient cells or incorrect processing of the slide;
2. inflammatory or inconclusive – cells distorted by other infections such as *Monilia*;
3. normal;
4. mild dyskaryosis (CIN 1) (CIN means cervical intraepithelial neoplasia);
5. moderate dyskaryosis (CIN 2);
6. severe dyskaryosis (CIN 3).

Over 90% of smears will be reported as normal. Categories 1, 2 and 4 need a repeat smear after 3–4 months following treatment for infection if necessary. Categories 5 and 6 need direct vision examination by colposcopy followed by a tissue biopsy. The extent of surgical treatment will depend on the results of the biopsy and whether the woman wishes to have more children. It will vary from destruction of the abnormal cells by laser or cryosurgery to cone biopsy to hysterectomy. Invasive carcinoma of the cervix, where the cancer has spread beyond the epithelial tissues, is more serious and likely to lead to death of the woman.

- Superior – intestines
- Inferior – vagina

Supports

Four pairs of ligaments support the uterus. Three pairs support its position in relation to the vagina:

1 the cardinal ligaments: origin, cervix; insertion, side walls of pelvis;
2 the pubocervical ligaments: origin, cervix; insertion, under the bladder to the pubic bones;
3 the uterosacral ligaments: origin, cervix; insertion, sacrum. One pair of ligaments maintains anteversion and anteflexion:
4 the round ligaments: origin, cornu; insertion, via inguinal canal to labia majora.

In addition, the so-called broad ligaments are not actually ligaments but thickened folds of peritoneum running from the uterus to the side walls of the pelvis.

Blood supply, lymphatic drainage and nerve supply

Blood supply

The blood supply to the uterus is complex and rich and contributed to by both ovarian and uterine arteries. The uterine artery, which is a branch of the internal iliac artery, enters at the level of the internal os and sends a small branch downwards to join the vaginal arteries in supplying the cervix and vault of the vagina. The main branch turns upwards and takes a tortuous path anteriorly and posteriorly to anastomose with the ovarian artery which enters along the broad ligament to supply the ovaries and uterine tubes before anterior and posterior divisions travel to anastomose with the opposite side. Branches are then given off at right angles to these vessels to penetrate and supply blood to the myometrium and enter the endometrium as basal arteries.

Venous drainage is by the uterine and ovarian veins after the blood has been collected into **pampiniform plexuses** (tendril-like), some of which communicate with veins from the bladder.

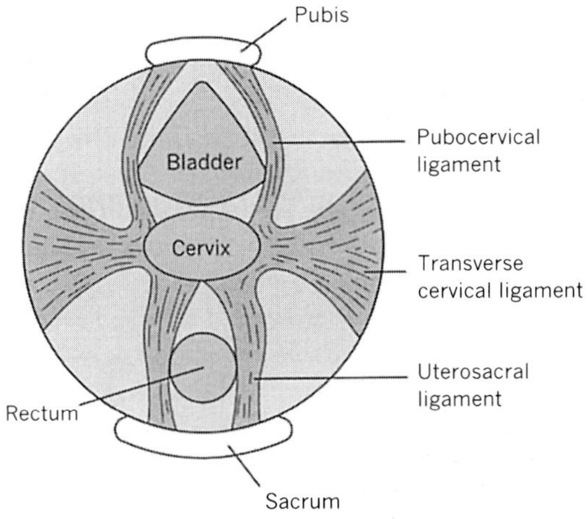

Figure 3.5 *The uterine supports seen from above (from Sweet B, 1997, with permission).*

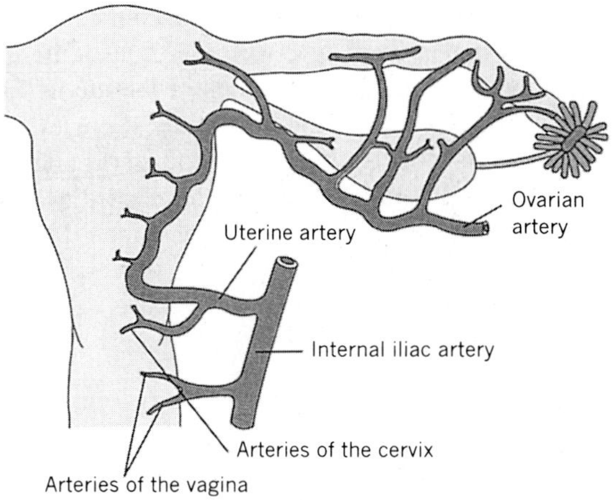

Figure 3.6 *The blood supply to the uterus and its appendages as below (from Sweet B, 1997, with permission).*

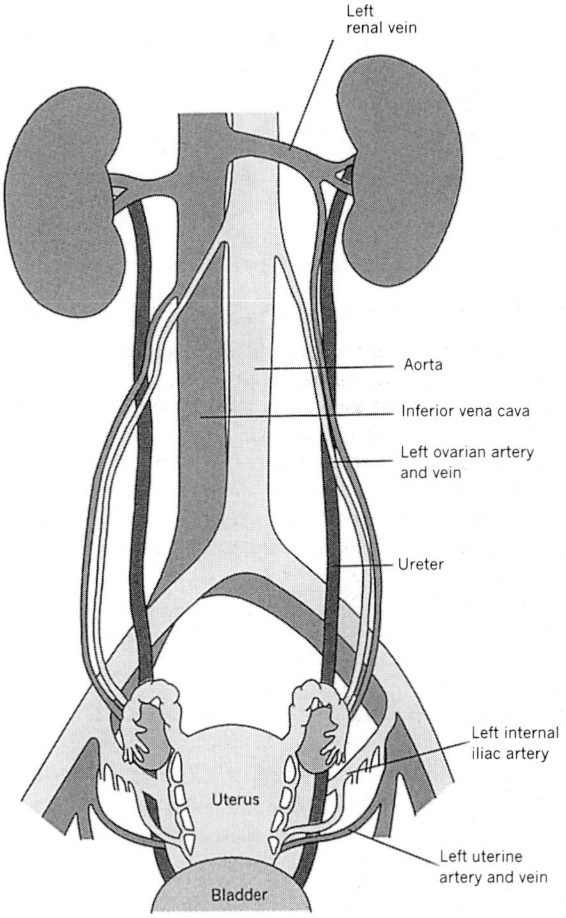

Figure 3.7 *The blood supply to the uterus. Note where the ovarian vein terminates (from Sweet B, 1997, with permission).*

Lymphatic drainage

There is very good lymph drainage of the uterus which acts as a defence against uterine infection, especially following birth. There are three communicating networks of vessels and small

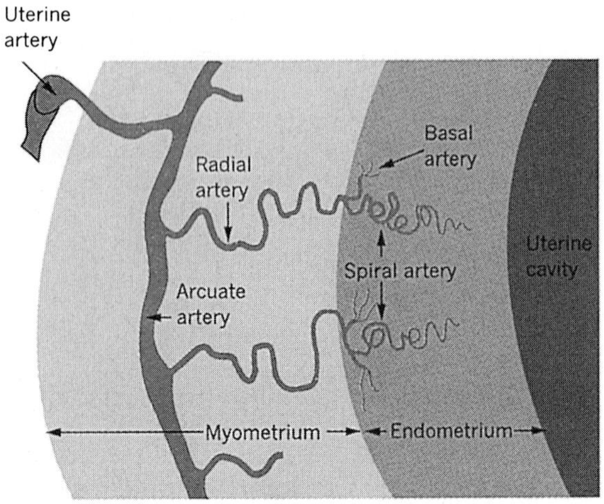

Figure 3.8 *The arterial supply to the uterine endometrium. (Reproduced with permission from Studd 1989.)*

nodes at the level of the endometrium, myometrium and subperitoneal layers of the uterus. The lymph is then collected into major ducts and taken to lumbar and sacral nodes centrally and inguinal, internal and external iliac nodes laterally.

Nerve supply

The body of the uterus is supplied by autonomic nerves originating in thoracic 11 and 12 and lumbar 1 vertebrae. Sensation from the body of the uterus is perceived as pain in response to stretch, infection and contraction. The cervix is innervated by the sacral plexus from sacral 2, 3 and 4 vertebrae nerves which pass through the transcervical or Lee Frankenhauser nerve plexi. Pain sensation from the cervix is in response to rapid dilatation.

Functions

- To receive the fertilised ovum.
- To nurture and protect the developing embryo and fetus.
- To expel the fetus and placenta.

The uterine tubes (fallopian tubes or oviducts)

The uterine tubes develop from the right and left Mullerian ducts in the embryo. They are two small, muscular, hollow tubes 10 cm long. Each tube extends from a cornu of the uterus and travels to the side walls of the pelvis but turns downwards and backwards before reaching them. The tubes lie within the broad ligament and communicate with the uterus at their medial end and the ovaries at their lateral end. Note that there is a direct pathway between the vagina and the peritoneal cavity, risking entry of ascending infection to the peritoneal cavity.

Structure

Sections

Each uterine tube is divided into four sections:

1. The interstitial part is the narrowest part of the tube. Its lumen is only 1 mm in diameter and it runs within the uterine wall.
2. The isthmus is a straight, narrow, thick section extending 2.5 cm laterally from the uterine wall.
3. The ampulla is the longest and widest section. It extends 5 cm from the isthmus to the side walls of the pelvis. Its lumen is tortuous, relatively thin and distensible.
4. The infundibulum or fimbriated portion is trumpet-shaped and ends in the fimbriae or finger-like processes. It is the lateral 2.5 cm of the tube which turns downwards and backwards. Although the fimbriae have little or no contact with the ovary, they become very active during ovulation and sweep the ovarian surface.

Layers

The uterine tubes are constructed of three layers of tissue.

1. An inner epithelial layer of cuboid cells arranged in **plicae** (folds), most pronounced in the ampulla. The complexity of the folds and the diameter of the lumen increase from the interstitial portion to the infundibular portion. Many of the cuboid cells are ciliated but goblet cells, which are secretory, are non-ciliated. About half the cells secrete mucus and the other half are ciliated.
2. Involuntary muscle fibres in two layers, inner circular and outer longitudinal, continuous with the fibres make up the middle wall of the tube in the body of the uterus. These undergo peristaltic contractions during ovulation.
3. There is an outer covering of peritoneum on the superior, anterior and posterior surfaces but absent on the inferior surface.

Relations

- Anterior, posterior and superior – peritoneal cavity and intestines
- Lateral – side walls of the pelvis
- Inferior – broad ligaments and ovaries
- Medial – uterus

Supports

The uterine tubes are held in position by their attachment to the uterus and the broad ligaments.

Blood supply, lymphatic drainage and nerve supply

These are shared with the ovaries and are described below.

Functions

- The mucus, cilia and peristaltic movements of the uterine tubes move the ovum towards the uterus.
- Fertilisation normally takes place in the ampulla.
- The mucus secreted by the uterine tubes may provide nourishment for the ovum.

The ovary

The pair of ovaries develop from the gonadal ridges of the embryo. Undifferentiated primitive germ cells that begin life on the wall of the yolk sac migrate into the gonadal ridges using amoebic movements at about 4 weeks of embryological development. In the female, the ovary is recognisable as such slightly later than the male testis, at about 10 weeks of development

The ovaries are small, almond-shaped glands measuring 3 × 2 × 1 cm and weighing just 6 g. They have a dull pinkish grey, uneven external appearance. They lie in a shallow peritoneal fossa adjacent to the lateral pelvic wall, outside the posterior layer of the broad ligaments and inside the peritoneum. The long axis of each ovary is in the vertical plane but the position is influenced by movements of the uterus and broad ligament. If the uterus is retroverted they may lie in the uterorectal pouch or pouch of Douglas and cause pain during coitus. The uterine tubes arch over the ovaries.

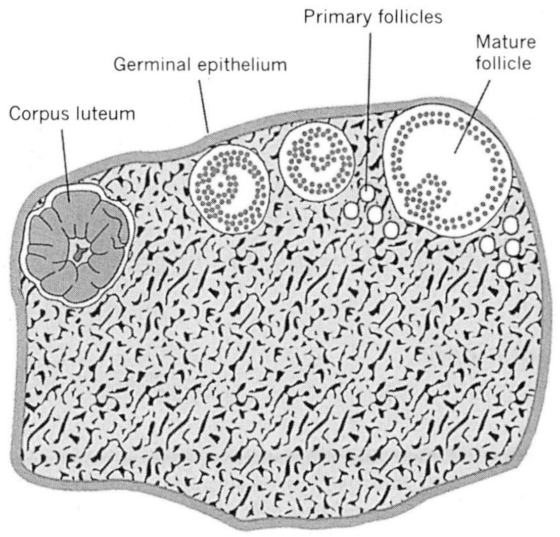

Figure 3.9 *Diagrammatic section of an ovary. (Reproduced with permission from Williams et al 1989)*

Macroscopic structure

- The **medulla** is the inner part of the ovary which is directly attached to the broad ligament by the mesovarium. It consists of fibrous tissue containing blood vessels, lymphatics and nerves carried by the infundibulopelvic ligament.
- The **cortex** is the functional part of the ovary and consists of highly vascular dense connective tissue (stroma) in which the ovarian follicles are embedded (see Microscopic structure below).
- The **tunica albuginea** is a tough fibrous capsule forming the outer part of the cortex.
- The **germinal layer** consists of cuboidal cells and is modified peritoneum continuous with the broad ligament. It forms an outer covering for the ovary.

Microscopic structure – the follicles

Tiny sac-like structures at different stages of maturation called ovarian follicles are embedded in the ovarian cortex. These stages of maturation, shown in Figure 3.9, are brought about by neurohormonal changes (see Physiology section below) and recognisable by the structure of the follicle. The **primordial follicle** contains an immature egg or oocyte encased in a single layer of squamous-like follicle cells. Over 2 million primordial follicles, consisting of the ovum surrounded by a single layer of flattened cells, are present in the fetal ovary prior to birth. However, by the menarche about 200 000 remain. This means that more than 80% have regressed. Only 300–400 will be shed at ovulation.

The primary follicles are surrounded by two or more layers of cuboidal granulosa cells. Secondary follicles develop when tiny fluid-filled spaces that appear between the granulosa cells coalesce to form a central cavity called an **antrum**. An outer layer of cells develops, probably from the interstitial cells of the stroma, known as the **thecal layer**.

The main change from then on is an increase in size as granulosa and theca cells proliferate and differentiate and the oocyte increases in size by a factor of 300. The granulosa cells divide to become several layers thick and gap junctions develop which allow easy transfer of molecules between cells. Secretion of fluid droplets leads to the formation of a single pool, separating the granulosa cells into distinct layers. A dense layer called the **cumulus** surrounds the oocyte whilst a thin outer layer lines the theca. A stalk of granulosa cells to which the mature oocyte is attached connects the two layers. The theca cells differentiate into the **theca interna**, which is a highly vascularised layer, and the **theca externa** which is the dense, fibrous outer capsule of the follicle (McNabb 1997a).

Glycoproteins secreted from the cell surface of the oocyte form a transparent layer called the **zona pellucida**. The mature **vesicular** or **Graafian follicle** has the oocyte placed at the end of a stalk of granulosa cells at one end of the antrum. It then breaks away and floats free in the liquor folliculi. The follicle bulges out from the surface of the ovary with the ovum on the outer wall and the stroma overlying it becomes thin. Each month from the menarche to the menopause, in this dynamic, ever-changing population of oocytes, a cohort of about 12 growing follicles emerges from the primordial follicles. One or occasionally more of the ripe follicles is selected for final maturation, ruptures and the oocyte escapes. After ovulation the ruptured follicle is transformed into a structure called the **corpus luteum** (yellow body) which, in the absence of a pregnancy, will degenerate in about 6 months into a **corpus albicans** (white body).

Relations

- Anterior – broad ligaments
- Posterior – intestines
- Lateral – infundibulopelvic ligaments and the side walls of the pelvis
- Superior – uterine tubes
- Medial – uterus and ovarian ligament

Supports

The ovary is held suspended in position by the following structures:

- attached to the uterus by the ovarian ligament;
- attached to the posterior surface of the broad ligament by the mesovarium, which is modified peritoneum carrying blood vessels and nerves;
- attached to the side walls of the pelvis by the suspensory or infundibulopelvic ligament, another modified peritoneal structure.

Blood supply, lymphatic drainage and nerve supply

Blood supply

The long slender ovarian arteries arise from high up on the aorta, immediately below the renal arteries, demonstrating the joint developmental history of the renal and reproductive systems. The ovarian arteries cross over the pelvic brim laterally and enter the broad ligament where branches supply the uterine tube and the ovary. They then anastomose with the uterine artery to form a rich blood supply to the uterus. Venous drainage is different: the right ovarian vein drains into the inferior vena cava while the left ovarian vein joins the left renal vein which then joins the inferior vena cava.

Lymphatic drainage

Lymph drainage is into the lumbar glands.

Nerve supply

The nerve supply of the ovary is well developed and via the ovarian plexus. Sympathetic fibres and sensory nerves from the ovary run with the arteries to be relayed in the 10th thoracic segment of the spinal cord. The ovaries, like the testes, are extremely sensitive organs if handled or squeezed.

Functions

1 To produce ova.
2 To produce the female hormones oestrogen and progesterone.

PHYSIOLOGY OF THE FEMALE REPRODUCTIVE TRACT – CYCLICAL CONTROL OF REPRODUCTION

The ovarian cycle

In each menstrual cycle stromal cells surrounding the developing follicle take on an endocrine function. Developmental changes are much more complex than those that occur during spermatogenesis and the sequence of events is still being researched. It involves preparation of an ovum for release at ovulation, fertilisation and implantation. At the same time changes occur within the woman's body, both in reproductive and non-reproductive tissues, depending on the cyclical presence of specific hormone receptors on the tissue cells, to prepare it for a possible pregnancy and the subsequent lactation (McNabb 1997b).

Ovulation

Meiosis and the development of an ovum are discussed fully in the first section of Chapter 8 so that the process can be compared with that of spermatogenesis, prior to discussing fertilisation. The mature ovum consists of the haploid cell with its 23 chromosomes. The ovarian capsule stretches until it bursts, the follicle ruptures and the ovum with its surrounding tissues and liquor is flushed into the abdominal cavity. There it is picked up by the fimbriae of the uterine tubes. These waft the ovum into the ampulla of the tube where it awaits fertilisation. Some women feel a pain at this time called *Mittelschmertz*. The follicle now collapses to become the corpus luteum. The lining cells of the follicle, granulosa and theca interna absorb fluid, swell and proliferate until the corpus luteum is 1–2 cm across.

Neurohormonal control of the ovarian cycle

Although the cyclical changes which occur are an integrated process, they can be discussed at various levels to achieve understanding of the whole process. McNabb (1997b) discusses how the interactions between the oocyte and the follicular cells lead to oocyte growth and that early work stressing the formation of receptors on follicle cells in response to alterations in circulating hormone levels has been extended by examination of the importance of local intraovarian regulators.

The following aspects will be considered:

1 the hormonal function of the hypothalamic-pituitary-ovarian axis;
2 growth and development of the oocyte;
3 the menstrual cycle;
4 non-endometrial sites of hormone action.

The hormonal function of the hypothalamic-pituitary-ovarian axis

The average ovarian cycle lasts 28 days with ovulation on day 14. However, the cycle shows considerable variation, both from cycle to cycle in an individual woman and between women. The cycle is known to be responsive to stress, disease, allergies, physical activity and also to nutritional deficiencies (Bradley & Bennett 1995; see Chapter 5 on infertility). It is usually the duration of the follicular phase leading up to ovulation that is variable. These variations must be taken into account when advising women about the rhythm method of contraception.

The hypothalamus

The control of the rhythmicity of the ovarian cycle and thus the menstrual cycle is via the hypothalamus and anterior pituitary gland (Fig. 3.10). Hormonal interactions between the hypothalamus and the pituitary occur by vascular and neuronal pathways (McNabb 1997b). The larger anterior lobe of the pituitary or **adenohypophysis** has no direct neural connections with the hypothalamus whilst the posterior lobe or **neurohypophysis** consists mainly of axons whose cell bodies are situated in the hypothalamus. The hormone oxytocin released by the posterior pituitary gland will be discussed in the chapters on the physiology of labour in Section 3.

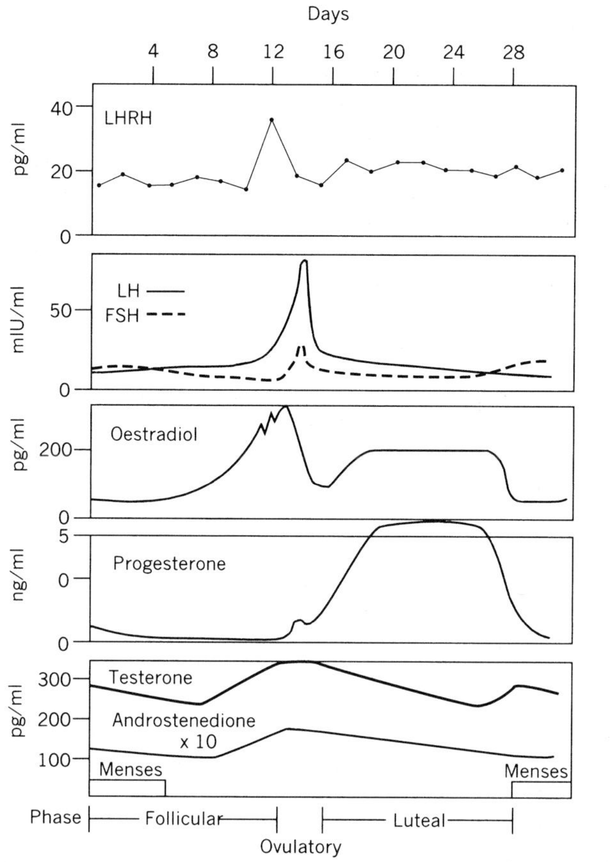

Figure 3.10 *Profile of plasma hormone levels throughout the menstrual cycle. (Reproduced with permission from Berne & Levy 1993.)*

The anterior pituitary gland

At least five groups of hormone-producing cells are found in the anterior lobe of the pituitary. Their function is regulated by neuronal substances from the hypothalamus. Those concerned with reproduction include:

- follicle-stimulating hormone (FSH);
- luteinising hormone (LH);
- adrenocorticotrophic hormone;
- prolactin.

A detailed consideration of the many interactions involved in the process of cyclical changes can be found in Johnson & Everitt (1995). Hypothalamic gonadotrophic-releasing hormone (GnRH) is a neuropeptide (see neurotransmitters, Chapter 25) which is transferred via a portal blood system to the anterior lobe of the pituitary where it interacts with specific cell receptors to bring about the release of the gonadotrophins FSH and LH.

The ovary

In turn, rising plasma levels of the ovarian hormones oestrogen and progesterone, especially oestrogen, can reduce the production of GnRH in a negative feedback mechanism. There are three main oestrogens. The most important is oestradiol with oestrone second and oestriol third in potency. Progesterone and the oestrogens are synthesised in the body from a **precursor**, which is cholesterol. If pregnancy does not occur the corpus luteum begins to degenerate and both FSH and LH begin to rise on day 1 of the cycle and steadily increase towards the late follicular phase.

Ovulation is dependent upon a midcycle surge of LH and FSH, occurring 24 h after the surge. Although plasma levels of

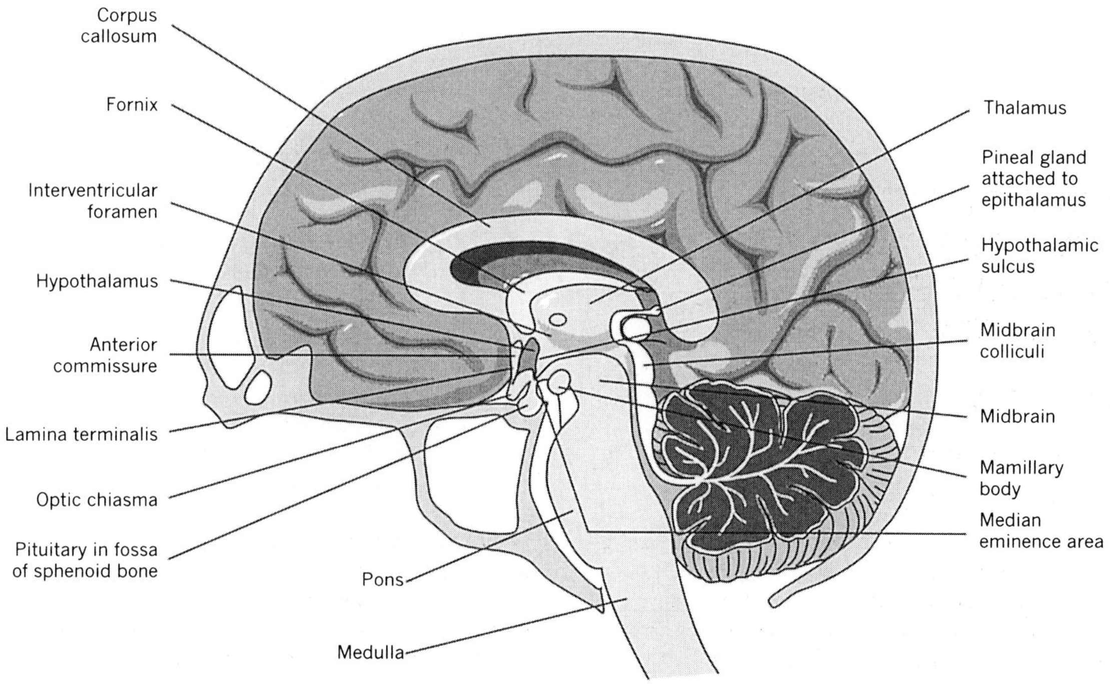

Figure 3.11 *Sagittal section of the human brain with the pituitary gland attached. (Reproduced with permission from Johnson & Everitt 1995.)*

both hormones rise, the level of LH is higher and this hormone appears to be more important in causing ovulation (see Assisted reproduction in Chapter 6). Generally only a single ovum is released in each cycle and the others that have begun developing regress to become **corpora atretica**, possibly following the development of a corpus luteum as rupture of the most advanced follicle causes negative feedback to the anterior pituitary gland and a fall in FSH. If two follicles develop simultaneously with double ovulation, **dizygotic twinning** occurs. The frequency of double or even multiple ovulation increases with age. There is a racial difference in this with black women more likely and Asian women least likely to have multiple ovulation. The incidence of **monozygotic twinning** (from one ovum) is invariable.

After 14 days, in the absence of a pregnancy, the corpus luteum will begin to regress. During this regression production of oestrogen and progesterone declines rapidly. When the plasma levels of these ovarian steroids become low enough, the anterior pituitary begins to produce FSH and LH and the cycle begins again.

Local control of growth and development of the oocyte

Within the follicle, local activities aimed at the growth and development of the dominant follicle are carried out, some by theca cells, some by granulosa cells and some involving cooperation between both types of cells.

Oestrogen and progesterone

During follicular development LH stimulates the theca cells to produce the steroid hormones androstenedione and testosterone which are transported to the granulosa cells which contain the necessary enzymes to convert them to oestrogen. This oestrogen causes proliferation of the granulosa and theca cells and the follicles enlarge further. The follicle(s) that develop more rapidly, i.e. the dominant follicle(s), may be able to produce larger amounts of oestrogen which then inhibits the release of FSH so that further growth of the remaining follicles is prevented. Further growth of the dominant follicle results in the surge of oestradiol that immediately precedes ovulation. Within 12 h progesterone takes over as the dominant steroid hormone produced by the theca and granulosa cells.

Some other hormones involved locally

Research into the causes of infertility and the techniques of in vitro fertilisation has shown that some peptide hormones, as well as the better known steroid hormones, have major influences on follicular development. In particular, two that have been found in follicular fluid are worth mentioning – inhibin and growth hormone.

Inhibin is known to have an effect on sperm production (see below). It has also been found in relatively high quantities in follicular fluid and may be one of the factors that determines the number of follicles released at ovulation (Herbert 1996). The rise in concentration of inhibin in follicular fluid may be a response to the surge in GnRH from the hypothalamus (Mitchell et al 1996; Yding Andersen et al 1993).

Kotarba et al (1997) summarise research into the effect of **growth hormone** in follicular development. Growth hormone may increase the intraovarian production of insulin-like growth factor 1(IGF1), which in turn amplifies the response of the granulosa cells to gonadotrophins (Adashi et al 1985). The GH

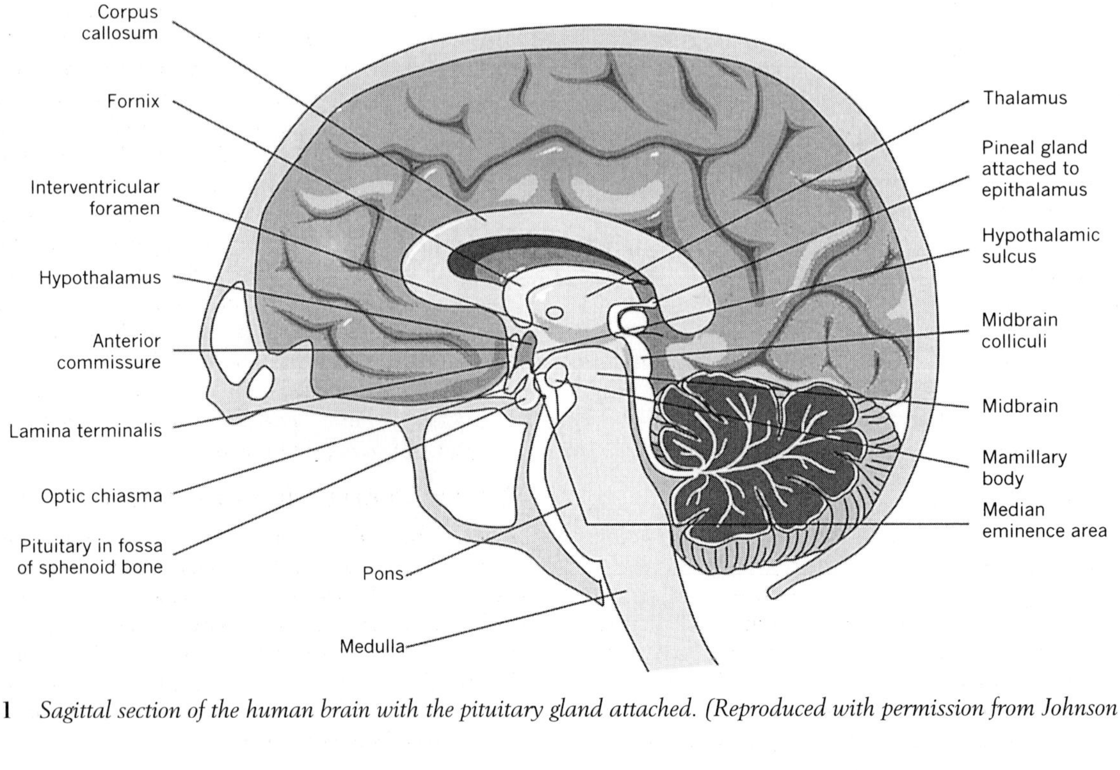

Figure 3.11 *Sagittal section of the human brain with the pituitary gland attached. (Reproduced with permission from Johnson & Everitt 1995.)*

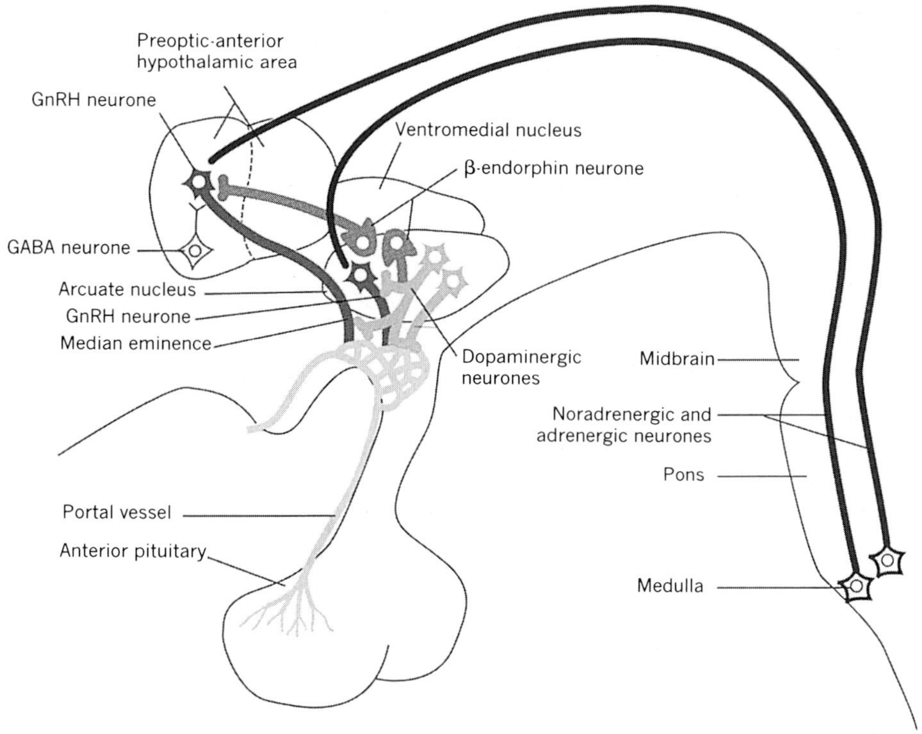

Figure 3.12 *Schematic diagram to show some of the postulated neurochemical reactions which may control GnRH secretion. (Reproduced with permission from Johnson & Everitt 1995.)*

receptor gene and GH binding sites have been found in human granulosa cells (Carlsson et al 1992). However, GH augmentation does not improve the rate of pregnancies in women with a poor follicular development response to gonadotrophin treatment (Tulandi et al 1993).

Triggering of ovulation

Meanwhile, the actions of FSH and oestrogen combine to induce the development of LH receptors on the outer layers of the granulosa cells, which coincides with the FSH and LH surge from the anterior pituitary brought about by GnRH from the hypothalamus. Ovulation then occurs. Ovulation is facilitated by the local release of prostaglandin E_2 (PGE_2) and the vasodilatory substances histamine and bradykinin. PGE_2 initiates breakdown of the collagen of the follicular wall whilst the vasodilatory substances set up a local inflammation. Proteolytic enzyme activity breaks down the wall of the follicle, allowing ovulation to occur.

The menstrual (endometrial) cycle

The changing levels and interactions between oestrogen and progesterone lead to alterations in the tissues of the endometrium and selected tissues elsewhere, depending on the presence of hormone receptors in the tissue cells. The endometrium is itself an endocrine organ and secretes oestrogens, progesterone and prolactin. It is therefore not totally dependent on hormones supplied by the ovary. The menstrual cycle is divided into three phases – menstrual, proliferative and secretory. The menstrual and proliferative phases coincide with the follicular phase of the ovarian cycle and the secretory with the luteal.

Menstrual phase – days 1 to 5

As the corpus luteum degenerates, plasma progesterone, which has a shorter half-life than oestrogen, falls more rapidly, changing the balance of the two hormones in favour of oestrogen. This causes the endometrium to become unstable. Fluid is lost from the tissues which shrink, compress the spiral arteries and cause endometrial anoxia. Tissue **autolysis** begins and the upper endometrium sloughs away from the basal layer with extensive bleeding into the tissues. Oestrogen also increases the excitability of the myometrium which further increases the anoxia and expels the sloughed tissue and blood. Menstrual fluid does not normally clot due to high levels of plasmin which breaks down fibrin as it forms. Blood loss is normally between 10 and 80 ml, with a mean of 35 ml and an average loss of about 0.5 ml of iron. At this point the endometrium is thin and poorly vascularised and only the bases of the endometrial glands remain.

The proliferative phase – days 6 to 14

During this phase rising oestrogen levels cause rapid proliferation of cells of the stroma with some oedema and the endometrium thickens from 1 to 6 mm by ovulation. The outer epithelium remains one cell thick throughout the cycle. At the same time the glands lengthen and eventually become tortuous. The blood vessels regrow and begin to show a spiral formation. The epithelial cells and the cells of the glands begin to synthesise and store glycogen.

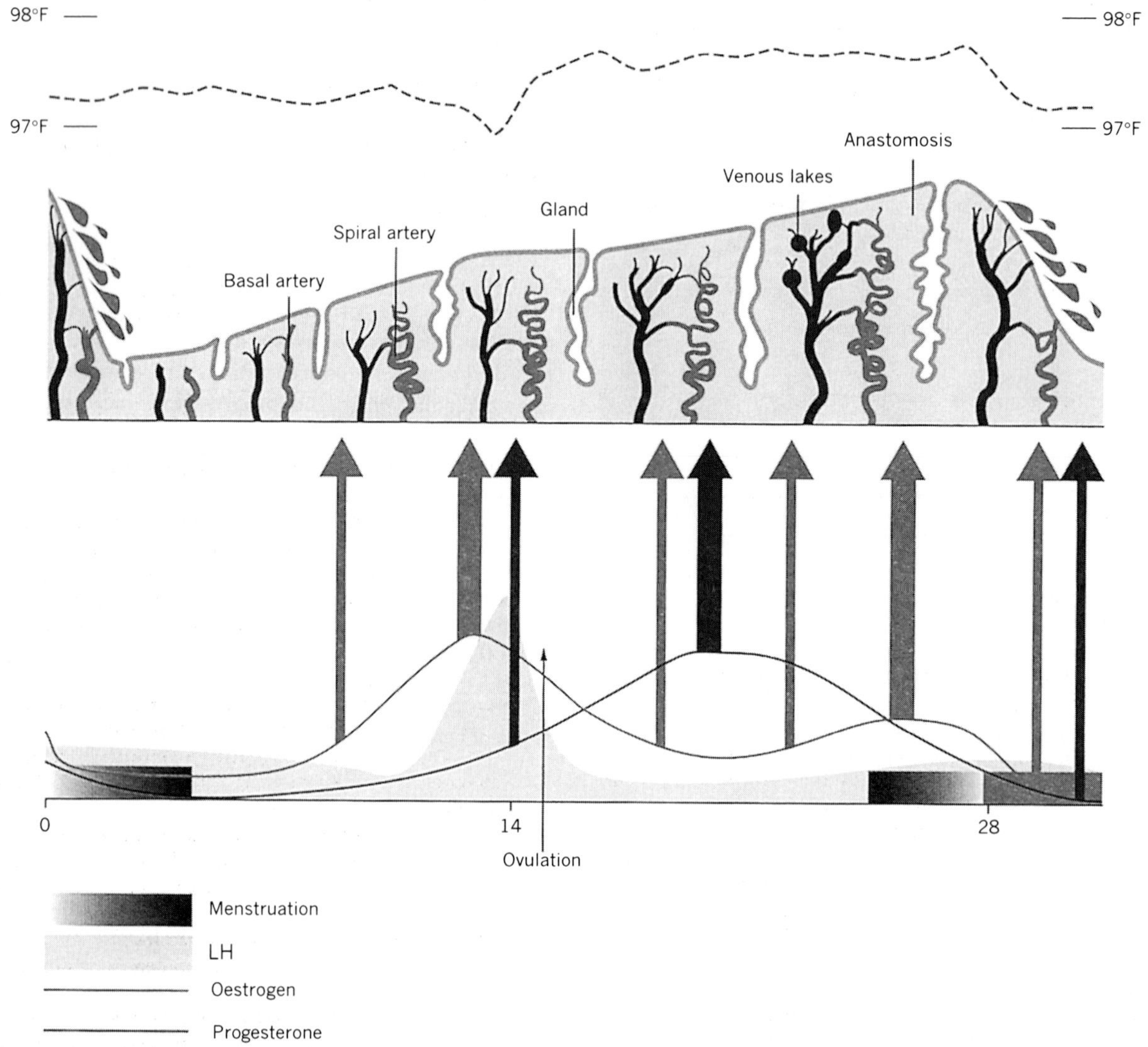

Figure 3.13 *Changes in human endometrium during the menstrual cycle. (Reproduced with permission from Johnson & Everitt 1995.)*

The secretory phase – days 15 to 28

After ovulation the corpus luteum secretes large amounts of progesterone. This acts on the oestrogen-primed endometrium to convert it to a secretory tissue. The endometrium is now highly vascular, the arteries have developed pronounced spiralling and venous lakes are formed. The stroma becomes even more oedematous and the cells themselves become larger and there is a further thickening of the endometrium to 6 mm. The endometrial glands are highly convoluted and begin to secrete glycogen into the lumen. The endometrial surface becomes folded and is prepared for implantation. This would normally occur 7 days after ovulation and be completed 14 days after ovulation, i.e. at the time of the next expected menstrual cycle.

Non-endometrial sites of hormone action

The myometrium

Excitability of myometrium is dependent on the balance between progesterone and oestrogen. Oestrogen increases bring about cyclical changes in the thickness of the myometrium and muscle excitability and stimulate spontaneous contractions, whilst progesterone reduces excitability. High levels of oestrogen also increase myometrial response to **oxytocin**.

The cervix

The mucus secreted by the cervical glands during the follicular phase is watery and turbid whilst that secreted after ovulation is thicker and clearer. Mucus secreted at the time of ovulation will crystallise in a fern-like pattern if left to dry on a glass slide.

The vagina

During the follicular phase the cells of the vaginal epithelium are large and flat with an acidophilic cytoplasm. During the luteal phase they become polygonal and more basophilic. There is an increase in the glycogen content of the vagina, partly due to the secretory activity of the endometrium and partly due to vaginal epithelium cell activity. Lactobacilli present in the vagina metabolise the glycogen to lactic acid, lowering the pH (increasing acidity) of the vagina from 6.5 during the follicular phase to 4.5 in the luteal phase.

The uterine tubes

During the follicular phase there is an increase in the number of ciliated cells and in the frequency and coordination of the peristaltic contractions of the muscle, reaching a maximum at the time of ovulation. Following this, the tubes become more quiescent.

Other actions

Oestrogen governs:

- development of the typical female shape;
- growth of breasts and nipples;
- development of the adult vulva, vagina and uterus;
- control of FSH production by feedback mechanism.

Progesterone governs:

- development of the secretory endometrium;
- development of alveolar breast tissue prior to menstruation;
- increased body temperature of 0.5°C following ovulation.

Summary of main points

- In the early embryo there is no evidence of sexual differentiation prior to the seventh week of development. If the genetic make-up of the embryo is XY the testis-determining factor influences the development of testes and testosterone causes the development of male genitalia. If the genetic make-up of the embryo is XX ovaries will form and female genitalia develop.
- The tissues forming the female internal genitalia are situated in the pelvic cavity. It is important to remember that this continuous tract has a direct opening to the peritoneal cavity from the external environment, necessary to allow fertilisation of the ovum. This increases the risk of pelvic infections.
- The vulva consists of the labia majora, labia minora, the clitoris and the vestibule onto which opens the urethral meatus and the vaginal orifice. The vagina is a fibromuscular sheath and a potential canal which extends from the vulva to the uterus. The projection of the cervix into the anterior vaginal wall divides the vault of the vagina into four fornices. The entrance to the vagina is partially covered by the membranous hymen which is usually torn at the first coitus and more so at the first birth to leave the carunculae myrtiformes. The walls of the vagina fall into transverse folds or rugae to allow for distension.
- The lining of the vagina is stratified, squamous, non-keratinised epithelium. Superficial cells are continuously exfoliated and release their glycogen which Doderlein's bacillus metabolises to produce lactic acid to ensure an acid medium of 4.5 which minimises the risk of invasion by pathogenic organisms. Functions of the vagina are the escape of menstrual fluid, the entry of the penis during coitus and to act as part of the birth canal.
- The uterus develops from fusion of the two Mullerian ducts in the embryo. It lies in the pelvic cavity in an anteverted and anteflexed position. It is a thickwalled, muscular, hollow, pear-shaped organ flattened in its anteroposterior diameter. Its apex forms the cervix which projects into the vault of the vagina through its anterior wall.
- The endometrium of the body of the uterus consists of vascular connective tissue containing mucus-secreting tubular glands which open into the uterine cavity. The stroma is covered by a layer of cuboidal cells which dip into the stroma to form the glands. The cells are ciliated on the surface. The thickness varies depending on the phase of the menstrual cycle.
- The cervix is barrel-shaped and penetrated by the cervical canal. It is divided into two equal parts: the supravaginal cervix and the cone-shaped infravaginal cervix. The cervical canal is spindle-shaped and lined by columnar mucus-secreting epithelium. The mucus membrane is thrown into anterior and posterior folds from which circular folds radiate called the arbor vitae.
- The epithelium dips into the stroma in a complex system of crypts and tunnels. These are separated by ridges of stroma covered by epithelium. Compound racemose glands secrete cervical mucus which varies in quality and quantity under the influence of the sex hormones.
- The squamocolumnar junction is between the columnar epithelium of the cervical canal and the squamous epithelium continuous with the vaginal epithelium. In some women the cervical epithelium seems unstable and cells with certain abnormalities may lead to cervical carcinoma. Early recognition of these precancerous changes allows surgical treatment so that screening women on a regular basis can be life saving.
- The myometrium is made up of bundles of smooth muscle fibres, the bulk of which run obliquely and interlace to surround blood vessels and lymphatic vessels. The proportion of muscle diminishes in the isthmus, being replaced by connective tissue so that the cervix has only 10% muscle content.
- The peritoneal layer or perimetrium covers the anterior and posterior surfaces but is absent from the narrow lateral surfaces. It is reflected off the uterus onto the superior surface of the bladder at the level of the anatomical internal os.
- The functions of the uterus are to receive the fertilised ovum, to nurture and protect the developing fetus and to expel the fetus and placenta.
- The two uterine tubes develop from the right and left Mullerian ducts in the embryo. The tubes communicate with the uterus at their medial end and the ovaries at their lateral end. Each uterine tube consists of three layers of tissue. About half the cells secrete mucus whilst the other half are ciliated. Involuntary muscle fibres – inner circular and outer longitudinal – are incompletely covered by the outer layer of peritoneum.
- Fertilisation takes place in the ampulla and the involvement of the epithelial layer in providing nutrition for the sperm and fertilised ovum is important. The functions of the uterine tubes are to secrete mucus which may provide nourishment for the ovum, move the ovum towards the uterus and provide a site for fertilisation.
- The pair of ovaries develop from the gonadal ridges of the embryo. They are small, almond-shaped glands measuring 3 × 2 × 1 cm and weighing just 6 g. They have a dull, pinkish grey, uneven external appearance and lie in a shallow peritoneal fossa next to the lateral pelvic wall, outside the broad ligaments and inside the peritoneum. The ovaries consist of the medulla, cortex, tunica albuginea and germinal layer. They produce ova and the female hormones oestrogen and progesterone.
- The mature ovum consists of the haploid cell with its 23 chromosomes floating in liquor folliculi surrounded by the zona pellucida and the follicular cells of the corona radiata. The ovarian capsule stretches until it bursts, the follicle ruptures and the ovum with its surrounding tissues and liquor is flushed into the abdominal cavity. There it is picked up by the fimbriae of the uterine tube.

- The average ovarian cycle lasts 28 days with ovulation on day 14. The ovaries produce the oestrogens, progesterone and small quantities of androgens. The control of the rhythmicity of the ovarian cycle and thus the menstrual cycle is via the hypothalamus and anterior pituitary gland.
- The development of the dominant follicle with its oocyte to maturity and the subsequent ovulation are complex processes involving local as well as distant steroid and peptide hormonal changes. Research into infertility management and in vitro fertilisation has added greatly to the understanding of this complexity.
- The changing levels and interactions between oestrogen and progesterone lead to alterations in the tissues of the endometrium. The menstrual and proliferative phases of the menstrual cycle coincide with the follicular phase of the ovarian cycle and the secretory with the luteal. The steroid hormones also affect the myometrium, the cervix, the vagina, the uterine tubes and the development of secondary sexual characteristics.

References

Adashi EY, Resnick CE, D'Ercole AJ, Svoboda ME, Van Wyke J. 1985 Insulin-like growth factors as intra-ovarian regulators of granulosa cell growth and function. Endocrine Review, 6, 400–420.

Bennett VR, Brown LK. 1996 Myles Textbook for Midwives, 12th edn. Churchill Livingstone, Edinburgh.

Berne, Land, Levy. 1993 Principles of Physiology. Mosby Yearbook, St Louis.

Bradley SG, Bennett N. 1995 Preparation for Pregnancy. Argyll Publishing, Argyll, Scotland.

Carlsson G, Bergh C, Bentham J et al. 1992 Expression of functional growth hormone receptors in human granulosa cells. Human Reproduction, 76, 1205–1209.

Herbert RA. 1996 Reproduction. In Hinchliff SM, Montague SE, Watson R (eds) Physiology for Nursing Practice, 2nd edn. Baillière Tindall, London, pp 679–734.

Hinchliff SM, Montague SE. 1990 Physiology for Nursing Practice. Baillière Tindall, London.

Hinchliff SM, Montague SE, Watson R. 1996 Physiology for Nursing Practice, 2nd edn. Baillière Tindall, London.

Johnson MH, Everitt BJ. 1995 Essential Reproduction. Blackwell Scientific, Oxford.

Kotarba D, Kotarba J, Hughes E. 1997 Growth hormone in in vitro fertilisation. In Lilford R, Hughes E, Vandekeckhove P (eds) Subfertility module of The Cochrane Database of Systematic Reviews, updated 3.6.97, Issue 3. Update Software, Oxford.

McNabb M. 1997a Male and female reproduction – early development. In Sweet BR with Tiran D (eds) Mayes Midwifery, 12th edn. Ballière Tindall, London 48–56.

McNabb M. 1997b Neurohormonal regulation of female reproduction. In Sweet BR with Tiran D (eds) Mayes Midwifery, 12th edn. Ballière Tindall, London 57–72.

Mitchell R, Buckler HM, Matson P et al. 1996 Oestradiol and immunoreactive inhibin-like secretory patterns following controlled ovarian hyperstimulation with urinary (Metrodin) or recombinant follicle stimulating hormone (Puregon). Human Reproduction, 11, 962–967.

Moore KL. 1989 Before We are Born, 3rd edn. WB Saunders, Philadelphia.

Studd J. (ed) 1989 Progress in obstetrics and Gynaecology. Churchill Livingstone, Edinburgh, p 28.

Sweet B. 1997 Mayes' Midwifery. Baillière Tindall, London.

Tulandi T, Falcone T, Guyda H et al. 1993 Effects of synthetic growth hormone-releasing factor in women treated with gonadotrophin. Human Reproduction, 8, 525–527.

Williams PL, Warwick K, Dyson M et al (eds) 1989 Gray's anatomy 37th Edn, Churchill Livingstone, Edinburgh.

Yding Andersen C, Westergaard LG, Figenschau Y, Bertheussen K, Forsdahl F. 1993 Endocrine composition of follicular fluid comparing human chorionic gonadotrophin to a gonadotrophin-releasing hormone agonist for ovulation induction. Human Reproduction, 8, 840–843.

Recommended reading

Espey LL, Ben-Halim IA. 1990 Characteristics and control of the normal menstrual cycle. Obstetrical and Gynecological Clinics of North America, 19 (2), 275–298.

Knobil E, Neill JD, Greenwald GS et al. (eds) 1994 The Physiology of Reproduction. Raven Press, New York.

Yen SSC, Jaffe RB. (eds) 1991 Reproductive Endocrinology. WB Saunders, Philadelphia.

Wynn M, Wynn A. 1991 The Case for Preconception Care for Men and Women. A B Academic Publishers, Oxford.

Chapter 4

The male reproductive system

In this chapter

INTRODUCTION

An understanding of the anatomy and physiology of the male reproductive system is essential knowledge for the extended role of the practising midwife. Many aspects of fertility, infertility and preconception care depend on the general and sexual health of both partners. The three abovementioned aspects of reproduction will be discussed in the following chapters. This chapter ends with a brief discussion of the physiology of sexual intercourse in both men and women.

THE MALE REPRODUCTIVE SYSTEM ANATOMY

Because of the necessity for both production and transfer of spermatozoa, the male genitalia are mainly outside the body cavity. The organs to be described below are: scrotum, testis, rete and epididymis, ductus deferens, seminal vesicles, prostate gland, bulbourethral glands and penis with the urethra (Fig. 4.1) (Herbert 1996). Unlike the female urinary system, where the urethral orifice is separate from the vagina, the male genital and urinary systems share a common outlet through the urethra.

The scrotum and testes

In the embryo the testes develop high up on the posterior wall of the abdominal cavity (Moore & Persaud 1993). In the last few months of fetal life they begin to descend through the abdominal cavity and down the inguinal canal into the scrotal sac outside the body cavity. This descent is completed under the influence of the male hormone testosterone and is completed by birth in 98% of baby boys. At maturity each testis measures 4 cm long and 2 cm in diameter and is surrounded by two coats. The outer is the **tunica vaginalis**, derived from peritoneum. The inner is a thick fibrous capsule – the **tunica albuginea**. One testis sits in each pocket of the scrotal sac. The scrotum is a thinwalled sac covered with hairy rugose skin well supplied with sebaceous glands. The scrotal skin is highly vascularised and has a large surface area (Marieb 1992).

The temperature of the testes is maintained 2–3°C below that of the body core to facilitate spermatogenesis. The position of the scrotum in relation to the body can be adjusted by a spinal reflex in order to regulate testicular temperature. In a cold environment, contraction of the scrotal dartos muscle wrinkles the scrotal skin and reduces the size of the sac whilst the skeletal cremaster muscle, arising from the internal oblique muscle, contracts and lifts the testes nearer to the body. Relaxation of these muscles allows the testes to be held away from the body to facilitate cooling.

Structure

Each testis is divided into 200–300 wedge-shaped lobules by

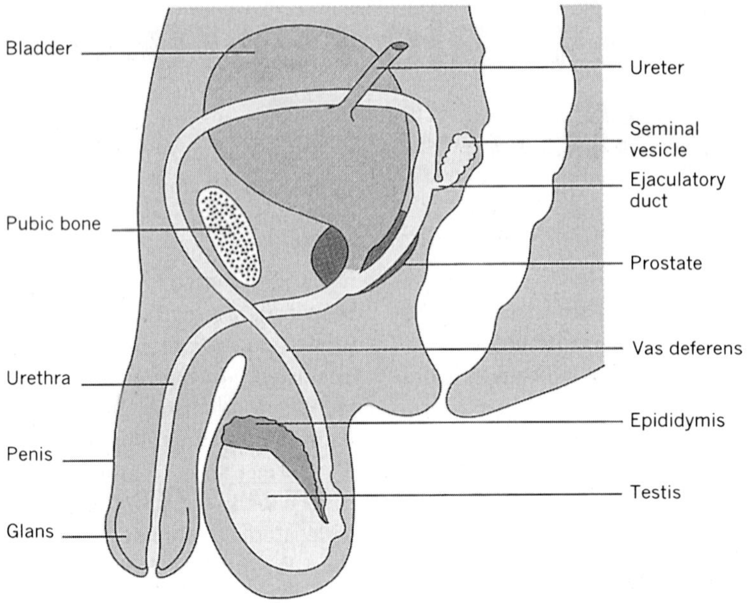

Figure 4.1 *The male reproductive system (from Sweet B, 1997, with permission).*

thin fibrous partitions which are extensions of the tunica albuginea (Fig. 4.2). Each lobule contains up to four seminiferous tubules which are highly coiled loops. About 80% of the testis by weight consists of **seminiferous tubules**, in which develop spermatozoa. The seminiferous tubules of each lobule converge to form a straight tubule or **tubulus rectus** that conveys the sperm into the **rete testis**, a tubular network on the posterior aspect of the testis. From here sperm enter the **epididymis** which is in close apposition to the external surface of the testis. Macrophages that phagocytose dead sperm are found in the lumen of the epididymis. Interstitial tissue is packed around the seminiferous tubules and contains blood vessels and endocrine Leydig cells which secrete testosterone. Seminiferous tubules contain developing spermatozoa and Sertoli cells which provide the sperm with nutrition and support (Fig. 4.3).

Blood supply, lymphatic drainage and nerve supply

Blood supply

The testes are supplied by the testicular arteries that arise from the abdominal aorta. The testicular veins form a network around the testicular artery, called a **pampiniform plexus** (tendril-like). This absorbs heat from the artery before the blood enters the testis.

Lymphatic drainage

Lymph drainage is by the inguinal nodes.

Nerve supply

Innervation is via the autonomic system – both sympathetic and parasympathetic. There is also a rich sensory nerve supply,

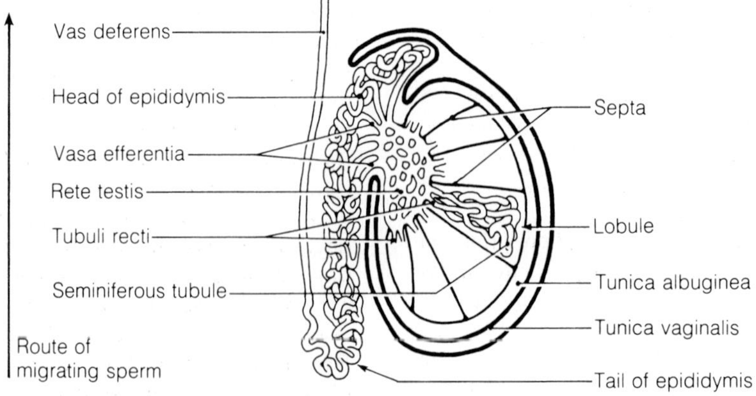

Figure 4.2 *The testis (from Hinchliff SM, Montague SE, 1990, with permission).*

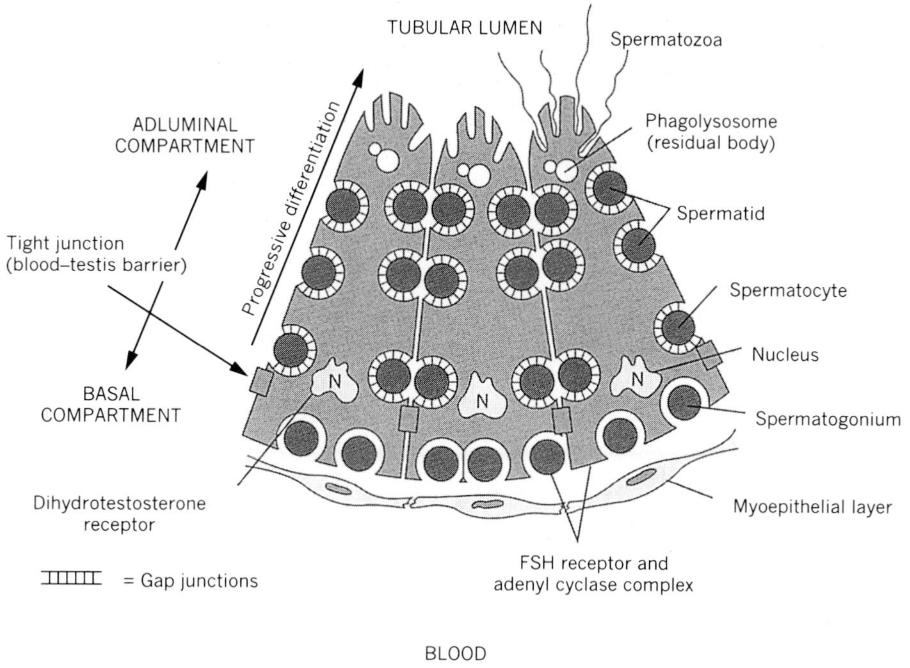

Figure 4.3 *Sertoli cells with developing germ cells. (Reproduced with permission from Tepperman & Tepperman 1987.)*

resulting in much pain and nausea if the testes are struck. The nerve fibres run with the blood vessels and lymphatics in the fibrous connective tissue sheath called the spermatic cord.

Functions

- To produce spermatozoa.
- To produce the hormones testosterone and inhibin.

Spermatogenesis, the process of sperm production, will be discussed fully in Chapter 8 so that it can be compared with **oogenesis** – the production of ova. When the spermatozoa are fully formed they are pushed along the duct system to the epididymis by the cilia in the lining of the tubuli recti and the smooth muscle in the tubal wall. Here they mature and become motile prior to ejaculation. The columnar epithelium of the epdidymis is thought to secrete hormones, enzymes and nutrients to enable the sperm maturation. Sperm can be stored in the epididymis for as long as 42 days which has implications for preconception advice on the environmental effects present for at least 2 months before the ejaculation event which results in fertilisation of an ovum.

Recently scientists have noticed that the number of spermatozoa in a single ejaculate has reduced drastically and this may have caused an increase in the number of men who are infertile. Other problems with the male reproductive tract include an increase in testicular cancer in young men, an increase in prostatic cancer in older men and malformations of the penis in babies. A deeper discussion of these issues can be found in Chapter 7.

The duct system

The epididymis is a comma-shaped tightly coiled tube about 6 metres long. The head of the comma which caps the superior aspect of the testis receives sperm from the efferent ductules of the testis. During ejaculation, the smooth muscle in the wall of the epididymis contracts strongly, expelling sperm from the tail portion into the ductus deferens.

The vas (ductus) deferens

This is a muscular tube which runs upwards from the epididymis, through the inguinal canal into the pelvic cavity. It can be felt easily as it passes over the pubic bone. Its terminus expands to form the ampulla and joins with the duct from the seminal vesicle to form the short ejaculatory duct. The two ejaculatory ducts pass into the prostate gland and empty into the urethra.

The wall of the vas deferens is composed of an outer layer of loose connective tissue and three layers of smooth muscle which can undergo rapid peristaltic contractions during ejaculation to pass the sperm forward. This movement is facilitated by the autonomic nerve supply. The cells of the mucosal layer are pseudostratified epithelium arranged in longitudinal ridges. In the extraabdominal portion, the ductus is accompanied by the testicular artery, the pampiniform plexus of veins, a nerve plexus, lymphatic vessels and the cremaster muscle. The whole complex is called the **spermatic cord**.

If no ejaculation occurs the spermatozoa in the epididymis degenerate and phagocytic cells in the epithelial layer remove them. Male sterilisation involves ligating and cutting the vas deferens, an operation called a **vasectomy**. Fertility may remain for 6–8 weeks because of the presence of viable spermatozoa above the sectioned segment. Although the operation prevents the presence of spermatozoa in the ejaculate, normal ejaculation still occurs because of the presence of fluids from the accessory glands (see below).

The urethra

This is the terminal portion of the duct system and serves both urinary and reproductive systems. It is divided anatomically into three regions:

1 the prostatic urethra which exits from the bladder and is surrounded by the prostate gland;
2 the membranous urethra which passes through the urogenital diaphragm;
3 the spongy (penile) urethra which passes through the penis to exit at the external urethral meatus. The spongy urethra is about 15 cm long and is 75% of the total urethral length.

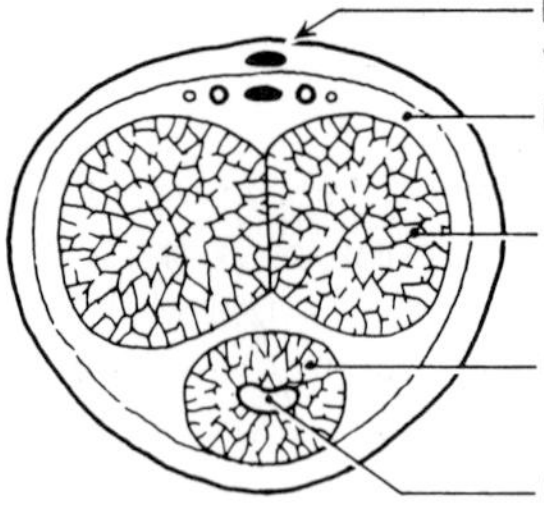

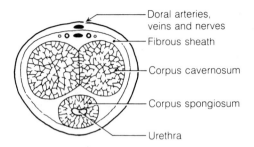

Figure 4.4 *Cross-section of the penis (Hinchliff SM, Montague SE, 1990, with permission).*

Accessory glands

These include the paired seminal vesicles, the bulbourethral glands and the single prostate gland. They provide a transport medium and nutrients and the bulk of the ejaculate.

The seminal vesicles

These lie behind the prostate gland and are finger-shaped and sized. They have a capacity of 3 cubic cm. They secrete an alkaline, sticky yellowish fluid containing fructose, globulin, ascorbic acid and prostaglandins which accounts for 60% of the semen. Sperm and seminal fluid mix in the ejaculatory duct and enter the urethra together during ejaculation.

The bulbourethral (Cowper's) glands

These are tiny pea-sized glands situated inferiorly to the prostate which secrete a thick clear mucus that drains into the spongy urethra. This mucus acts as a lubricant prior to ejaculation.

The prostate gland

This organ is situated around the bladder neck and first part of the urethra. It is about 3 cm in diameter in the normal adult and may involute or hypertrophy after middle age, resulting in urological problems. It produces a thin, acidic, milky fluid containing enzymes, calcium and citrates. This fluid may act to stimulate motility in the sperm.

Semen

This is a milky white, sticky fluid mixture of sperm and accessory gland secretions. The liquid is a transport medium and provides nutrients and chemicals that activate the sperm. The prostaglandins in semen are thought to decrease the viscosity of the cervical mucus and to cause reverse peristalsis in the uterus, facilitating movement of the sperm up the female reproductive tract. It is relatively alkaline with a pH of 7.2–7.6 which helps to neutralise the acid medium of the vagina to protect the sperm and maintain their motility. There is also a bacteriostatic chemical called seminal plasmin present and clotting factors, including fibrinogen, coagulate the semen shortly after it has been ejaculated. Once established in the vault of the vagina, the fibrinolysin also contained in the semen causes it to liquefy so that the sperm can swim free into the female duct system. The average ejaculate is about 3–6 ml and contains 60–200 million sperm, of which at least 60–80% should be normal and 50% motile after 1 h at 37°C.

The penis

The structure of the penis is shown in Figure 4.4. This is the organ of copulation which normally hangs flaccidly from the perineum in front of the scrotum. It has an attached root and a free shaft that ends in an enlarged tip – the **glans penis**. Internally it has three long columns of erectile tissue consisting of two dorsal corpora cavernosa side by side and one corpus spongeosum containing the urethra. The erectile tissue is a spongy network of connective tissue and smooth muscle full of vascular spaces. The root of the penis is broad and firmly fixed to the pubic rami by the proximal ends of the corpora cavernosa, known as the **crura**. Each crus is surrounded by an ischiocavernosus muscle. The terminal glans penis is perforated by the urethral meatus and is very well supplied with sensory nerve endings and is the main erogenous zone in the male. In the resting state the glans penis is covered by a folded cylinder of skin known as the **prepuce** or foreskin.

HORMONAL CONTROL OF MALE REPRODUCTIVE FUNCTION

Control is via the hypothalamus, anterior pituitary lobe and testis. Gonadotrophic-releasing hormone (GnRH) from the hypothalamus influences the anterior pituitary to produce the same two gonadotrophic hormones as in the female – follicle-stimulating hormone (FSH) and luteinising hormone (LH). In the male, plasma levels of LH are usually three times higher than FSH.

Actions of LH

LH acts on the interstitial tissue to cause synthesis and release of testosterone and plasma testosterone levels are directly related to plasma LH levels. **Testosterone** is a steroid molecule synthesised from cholesterol (as are the female hormones oestrogen and progesterone). It binds loosely to plasma proteins to be taken to its target organs. The functions of testosterone are shown in Table 4.1.

Inhibin is a non-steroidal factor which has been isolated in the testis and may inhibit FSH secretion. It is possibly produced by the Sertoli cells and acts by a negative feedback loop.

Table 4.1 *Functions of testosterone*

Action	*Functions*
Before birth	Masculinisation of the reproductive tract and external genitalia Promotion of testicular descent
Sex-specific tissues	Growth and maturation at puberty Maintenance of reproductive tract throughout adult life Essential for spermatogenesis
Other reproductive effects	Increased libido and sex drive Control of gonadotrophic hormone secretion
Secondary sexual characteristics	Development of male distribution of body and facial hair Deepening of the voice due to thickening of the vocal cords and enlargement of the larynx
Other effects	Anabolic effect on protein production Growth of the long bones at puberty and fusion of epiphyses Increased secretion from sebaceous glands Possible role in aggressive behaviour

Actions of FSH

FSH seems to act on the later stages of sperm maturation and cannot initiate spermatogenesis in the absence of LH.

The role of prostaglandins in reproduction

The group of chemical messengers known as the prostaglandins are active in multiple sites in the body and are involved in many physiological processes. Some have been found to act on smooth muscle, for example in both bronchodilation and bronchoconstriction. Prostaglandins also promote pain and inflammation and modulate platelet aggregation. The common drug aspirin is a prostaglandin inhibitor and this is why it also has many pharmaceutical uses. Prostaglandins are fatty acid derivatives and are produced wherever they occur in the body from arachidonic acid. They act locally, after which local enzymes rapidly inactivate them so that they do not gain access to the circulatory system. They were first identified in semen and were thought to be produced by the prostate gland, hence the name.

In the reproductive system prostaglandins have the following effects:

- increase uterine activity during menstruation;
- play a role in ovulation by influencing follicular rupture;
- promote sperm transport by causing smooth muscle contraction in the male and female reproductive tracts;
- mediate the renal vasodilation of pregnancy;
- involved in preparing the cervix for labour by softening it;
- are probably the final mediator in the regulation of uterine contractions.

THE PHYSIOLOGY OF SEXUAL INTERCOURSE

Stated simply, this is the process by which male and female gametes are brought together. In evolutionary terms, in order to ensure that sperm meets ovum the behaviour must be pleasurable so that male and female are willing to take part. There is necessarily in men and women an enormous psychological and social input to sexual behaviour and arousal includes both cognitive and emotional aspects, equally as important as the physiological context (Haeberle 1983). A classic study of human sexual response was undertaken by Masters & Johnson (1966) who described the response in both sexes as having the four phases: excitement, plateau, orgasm and resolution.

The male response

In the male two stages can be described – erection and ejaculation.

Erection

The erection reflex is a spinal reflex triggered by local stimulation of sensitive mechanoreceptors in the tip of the penis (Fig. 4.5). When the man is sexually excited increased parasympathetic and decreased sympathetic activity cause the arterioles in the erectile tissue of the corpora cavernosa and the corpus spongeosum to dilate and engorge. Normally there is no parasympathetic control over blood vessels. It is the variation in sympathetic stimulation that causes vasodilation or vasoconstriction in blood vessels in other sites of the body. This is the major instance in which both branches of the autonomic nervous system control blood vessels and vasodilation is accomplished much more rapidly than usual.

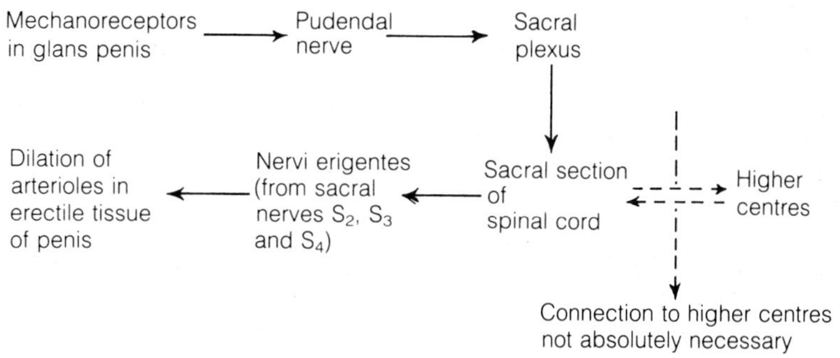

Figure 4.5 *The nervous pathways (simplified) involved in the erection reflex (Hinchliff SM, Montague SE, 1990, with permission).*

Ejaculation

Ejaculation is also controlled by a spinal reflex with a patterned sequence of events following the efferent nerve messages. Sympathetic nerve impulses cause sequential contractions of smooth muscle in the prostate, epididymis, ductus deferens, ejaculatory duct and seminal vesicles. This activity causes emission when the genital ducts and accessory glands empty their contents into the posterior urethra. This is followed by the expulsion phase of ejaculation when the semen is expelled from the penis by a series of rapid muscle contractions. Filling of the urethra with semen triggers nerve impulses that activate skeletal muscle at the base of the penis. These contract at about 0.8 s intervals to expel the semen forcibly.

During ejaculation the sphincter at the base of the bladder is closed so that spermatozoa do not enter the bladder and urine cannot be voided. Orgasm occurs, which is a feeling of intense pleasure accompanied by involuntary rhythmic action of the pelvic muscles and generalised contraction of skeletal muscle throughout the body. This is followed by resolution which is the physical and usually psychological relaxation. Loss of erection follows due to vasoconstriction of the penile arterioles and venous drainage. There is now a latent or refractory period during which further erection cannot occur. This varies, depending on circumstances, from a few minutes to several hours.

The female response

In the female there is erection of the clitoris and the erectile tissue in the labia minora. Nipples also have erectile tissue and respond to sexual excitement. Lubrication from Bartholin's glands facilitates intromission. Orgasm may occur following movement of the penis in and out of the vagina. During the plateau phase vasocongestion of the outer third of the vagina occurs which tightens the introitus around the penis. The uterus is raised upwards, lifting the cervix and enlarging the upper two-thirds of the vagina. This is called ballooning and increases the space for deposition of the ejaculate.

If orgasm takes place, the same pelvic muscle contractions occur as in the male, mostly in the outer engorged section of the vagina. This region is sometimes called the **orgasmic platform**. The uterus may contract, beginning at the fundus (Walton 1994). Unlike males, females do not have a refractory period and may experience more than one orgasm. During resolution, vasocongestion and the cardiac and respiratory changes return to normal. Stimulation of the clitoris can enhance the pleasure and contribute to female orgasm.

Orgasm is similar in both sexes but may not occur with the same regularity in females. Whilst female orgasm is not necessary for fertilisation, contractions of the uterus may aspirate semen and help the sperm on their journey.

Cardiovascular and respiratory changes

In both sexes there are changes in the cardiovascular and respiratory systems. There is a marked increase in heart rate to between 100 and 170 beats per minute, systolic blood pressure may increase by 30–80 mmHg and diastolic by 20–40 mmHg. Respiration may double to 40 per min and flushing of the chest, neck and face occurs.

Summary of main points

- The male genitalia are mainly outside the body cavity. The organs are: scrotum, testis, rete and epididymis, ductus deferens, seminal vesicles, prostate gland, bulbourethral glands and penis with the urethra. Unlike the female urinary system, the male genital and urinary systems share a common outlet through the urethra.
- In the embryo the testes develop high up on the posterior wall of the abdominal cavity. In the last few months of fetal life they begin to descend through the abdominal cavity and down the inguinal canal into the scrotal sac outside the body cavity. One testis sits in each pocket of the scrotal sac. The temperature of the testes is maintained 2–3°C below that of the body core to facilitate spermatogenesis.
- Each testis is divided into 200–300 wedge-shaped lobules by thin fibrous partitions which are extensions of the tunica albuginea. Each lobule contains up to four seminiferous tubules which are highly coiled loops where the spermatozoa develop. The functions of the testes are to produce spermatozoa and to produce the hormones testosterone and inhibin.
- The seminiferous tubules of each lobule converge to form a straight tubule that conveys the sperm into the rete testis. From here sperm enter the epididymis. Interstitial tissue is packed around the seminiferous tubules and contains blood vessels and endocrine Leydig cells which secrete testosterone.
- During ejaculation the smooth muscle in the wall of the epididymis contracts, strongly expelling sperm from the tail portion into the ductus deferens. This joins with the duct from the seminal vesicle to form the ejaculatory duct which then passes into the prostate gland to empty into the urethra.
- The accessory glands of the male reproductive system include the paired seminal vesicles, the bulbourethral glands and the single prostate gland. They provide a transport medium and nutrients and the bulk of the ejaculate.
- Semen is a milky white, sticky fluid mixture of sperm and accessory gland secretions. The liquid is a transport medium and provides nutrients and chemicals that activate the sperm. The average ejaculate is about 3–6 ml and contains 60–200 million sperm. There are currently anxieties about the number of men with reduced sperm counts.
- The penis normally hangs flaccidly from the perineum in front of the scrotum. Internally it has three long columns of erectile tissue consisting of a spongy network of connective tissue and smooth muscle full of vascular spaces – two dorsal corpora cavernosa side by side and one corpus spongeosum containing the urethra. The terminal glans penis is perforated by the urethral meatus and is very well supplied by sensory nerve endings and is the main erogenous zone in the male. In the resting state, the glans penis is covered by a folded cylinder of skin known as the prepuce or foreskin.
- Control of the male reproductive system is via the hypothalamus, anterior pituitary and testis. Gonadotrophic-releasing hormone influences the anterior pituitary to produce the same two gonadotrophic hormones as in the female – FSH and LH.
- LH acts on the interstitial tissue to cause synthesis and release of testosterone and plasma testosterone levels are directly related to plasma LH levels. Inhibin may inhibit FSH secretion. It is possibly produced by the Sertoli cells and acts by a negative feedback loop to

prevent sperm manufacture.

- The group of chemical messengers known as the prostaglandins are active in multiple sites in the body and are involved in many physiological processes. Some have been found to act on smooth muscle, for example in both bronchodilation and bronchoconstriction. Prostaglandins also promote pain and inflammation and modulate platelet aggregation.
- In the reproductive system prostaglandins increase uterine activity during menstruation, influencing follicular rupture and promotion of sperm transport by causing smooth muscle contraction in the male and female reproductive tracts.
- Sexual activity in humans is more than a physiological response. Psychological and social factors are important in developing the relationship between partners. In the male, sexual activity has two stages – erection and ejaculation. Higher brain centres can inhibit or facilitate the process. Research has found that there are similar stages in the male and female physiological sexual response although the psychosocial attitudes differ between the sexes.

References

Haeberle EJ. 1983 The Sex Atlas. Sheridan Press, London.

Herbert RA. 1996 Reproduction. In Hinchliff SM, Montague SE, Watson R (eds) Physiology for Nursing Practice, 2nd edn. Baillière Tindall, London, pp 679–734.

Hinchliff SM, Montague SE. 1990 Physiology for Nursing Practice. Baillière Tindall, London.

Marieb EN. 1992 Human Anatomy and Physiology, 2nd edn. Benjamin/Cummings Publishing

Masters W, Johnson V. 1966 Human Sexual-Response. J and A Churchill, London.

Moore KL, Persaud TVN. 1993 The Developing Human. WB Saunders Philadelphia.

Tepperman and Tepperman. 1987. Metabolic and Endocrine Physiology. Yearbook Medical, Chicago, p 119.

Sweet B. 1997 Mayes' Midwifery. Baillière Tindall, London.

Walton I. 1994 Sexuality and Motherhood.

Recommended reading

Johnson MH, Everitt BJ. 1995 Essential Reproduction. Blackwell Scientific, Oxford.

Knobil E, Neill JD, Greenwald GS et al. (eds) 1994 The Physiology of Reproduction. Raven Press, New York.

Wynn M, Wynn A. 1991 The Case for Preconception Care for Men and Women. AB Academic Publishers, Oxford.

Yen SSC, Jaffe RB (eds). 1991 Reproductive Endocrinology. WB Saunders, Philadelphia.

Chapter

5 Fertility control

In this chapter

WORLD POPULATION

A key question being asked at global level is whether the world can sustain the accelerating growth of human population. Bromwich & Parsons (1990) introduced their book on contraception with an overview of the world situation. It is probable that the agricultural revolution that began about 15 000 years ago led to a trend to larger families and an increase in population. From time to time as travel became easier, world pandemics such as bubonic plague reduced specific populations by up to 50% (McNeill 1976). In Europe from the end of the 16th century, there was a steady increase in population.

Table 5.1 *World population figures adapted from Bromwich and Parsons (1990)*

1650	600 million
1850	One billion (1000 million)
1930	Two billion
1960	Three billion
1974	Four billion
1987	Five billion
2000	Six billion??

Causes of population increase

The changes are not necessarily caused only by a surfeit of births. In some countries improving health is reducing the number of children dying in infancy and early childhood and preventing early adult deaths. Many of the world's population are young and have still to produce children and there is concern that unless something can be done to slow down this increase in humanity, famine, infections and wars may intervene.

Thomas Malthus (1773) believed that the ability of humans to produce enough food to prevent mass starvation would eventually fail but currently the 'green revolution', with the development of high-yielding strains of grain, seems to be effective in delaying this problem. Contraception should be able to curb population growth and the destruction of the environment but people have to be assured that the children they have will survive.

Two further concepts involving the status of women and their ability to make decisions about their fertility are important. The first is the equal right of girls and women to education and the second is the involvement of women in paid employment (Dasgupta 1995). Obviously population problems differ from country to country and some Western countries such as Britain have a problem with an ageing population as the number of children born drops.

Various countries are involved in contraceptive trials to combat overpopulation. China has been conducting research into a 'male pill' and the Indian National Institute of Immunology has been testing a female immunocontraceptive vaccine targeting human chorionic gonadotrophin. The World Health Organization (WHO) is also testing such a vaccine (Alexander 1995). Such methods will have to be cheap, easily accessible to rural as well as urban dwellers and acceptable to both partners and to the culture in which they live. Currently, worldwide, the contraceptive effect of breast/feeding probably has as much impact as all the other forms of contraception put together.

THE EFFECTIVENESS OF CONTRACEPTION

Contraception has probably been an issue for people ever since the link was made between sexual behaviour and pregnancy. It certainly occupied the minds of the first cultures such as the Egyptians, Greeks and Romans. However, in modern times it is only during the latter half of the 20th century that contraception has been openly discussed, used and legal in most countries. There are religious, moral and cultural issues to be considered and therefore it is unlikely that any one method would ever become universal. The ideal contraceptive would be 100% effective. However, it would also need to be painless, easy to use independently of the user's memory, cheap and accessible independently of medical control. It would be completely safe medically and acceptable to the individuality and the culture of its user.

Great strides have been made in the development and refinement of contraceptive methods but there has also been anxiety about the safety of some methods. What is certain is that the death rate from childbearing-related problems has been extremely high in the past and risk must be measured against the physical, social and psychological effects of unwanted or too frequent pregnancies.

Calculating effectiveness

A mathematical concept used to assess the effectiveness of contraceptive methods is the calculation of the failure rate per 100 woman-years (HWY). This is the number of women who would become pregnant if 100 women used the method for 1 year (Bromwich & Parsons 1990). In a perfect world this would be truly representative of the effectiveness of the method but it is complicated by factors such as changes in fertility with age, the motivation of the individual to use the method correctly every time and the fact that about 10% of women are infertile anyway, some of whom will not know it whilst they are using contraception. It is difficult to differentiate between failure of the method and failure of the user to comply with instructions. Also failure often occurs in the early months following commencement of any method. As people become more skilled in using the method so the method becomes more reliable.

Individual needs

Although the above information places contraception in a global context, health professionals in the main are involved in caring for individuals. Books covering the social and cultural meaning and acceptance of the available methods of contraception are easily obtained. The following section explains the physiological significance of the methods and, although it will not always be possible to exclude social factors and it is certainly not intended to belittle these important considerations, in order to keep within the context of the rest of the book these are deliberately kept to a minimum. The information on contraceptive usage will be presented in a way that follows the physiological factors necessary for fertilisation. It is possible by this means to look into future possibilities for prevention of conception.

Table 5.2 *The methods and their failure rates per HWY. The variations in numbers reflect the commitment and skill with which the method is used:*

Method	*Failure rate per HWY*
The combined oestrogen with progestogen pill	0.1 to 7
The progestogen-only pill	0.5 to 7
Injectable progestogen	0 to 1
Female barrier methods	2 to 15
The male condom	2 to 15
The female condom	Not yet known
The intrauterine device	0.3 to 4
Spermicidal preparations (used alone)	14 to 25
The contraceptive sponge	9 to 25
Symptothermal method (temperature + cervical mucus)	1 to 4
Coitus interruptus	25
Male sterilisation	0 to 0.2
Female sterilisation	0 to 0.2

Table 5.3 *The means of prevention of conception*

Prevention of gamete production	Sperm Ovum
Prevention of fertilisation	Altering cervical mucus, female barrier methods Condoms, withdrawal, timing, IUD, male sterilisation, female sterilisation
Prevention of embedding/ development of conceptus	IUD, postcoital pill, abortion
Future advances	Vaccine – immunocontraceptives

PREVENTION OF GAMETE PRODUCTION

Ovum

All the ova available to the woman for reproduction are already present in her ovary at birth. It is therefore not a matter of prevention of ova production but of preventing their maturation and thus preventing ovulation by suppressing luteinising hormone (LH) and follicle-stimulating hormone (FSH). This is the basis for the combined oral contraceptive, so-called because the preparations combine oestrogens and progestogens (a synthetic progesterone). The concept of hormonal control of fertility arose in the late 1940s when it was realised that the roots of the wild Mexican yam contained a chemical from which steroid hormones could be produced. Unfortunately natural hormones are expensive to produce and are digested if taken orally.

In 1954 clinical trials of the pill took place in Puerto Rico, chosen because of its high birth rate and accessibility to the pharmaceutical industry. The pill became available to women in the United States of America in 1960 and in Britain in the early 1960s. These first pills contained quite high amounts of hormone. In 1968 studies were published showing a link between the use of oral contraceptives and thrombosis. This was thought to be due to the high level of oestrogen and the content of the pills was changed. However, it has since been realised that oestrogen is not the only risk factor and that cigarette smoking is probably significant. Obesity, a sedentary way of life and family history of thrombosis are also important factors increasing the risk of thrombosis.

The combined pill

The modern pill is a mixture of the same two hormones as the original. One is a derivative of oestrogen and the other is a progesterone mimic – a progestogen. Two types of oestrogen are used in the pill: ethinyl oestradiol and a derivative called mestranol. The dose of oestrogen is fairly constant amongst all preparations at a maximum of 30–35 μg. There are several different progestogens including norethisterone and norgestrel. The dose of progestogen is more variable and progestogens add to the contraceptive effect by causing thickening of the cervical mucus (Billings et al 1972), making the endometrium unsuitable for implantation, and by reducing the motility of the uterine tubes (Alexander 1996).

Benefits

- Couples with sexual difficulties because of a fear of pregnancy are relieved of that fear and may find themselves able to relax and enjoy a better sex life.
- There is no direct action to be taken during the sexual act as there is in putting on a condom so that the flow of behaviour is not interrupted.
- The pill does not cause spotting between periods nor does it cause a woman to have heavy periods. It can also be used to combat irregular, painful or heavy periods often found in younger women. For some people this may be of value in preventing anaemia.
- Some men find that using a condom is embarrassing and distasteful; they may even lose their erection during the attempt or ejaculate prematurely.
- The combined pill seems to offer protection against ovarian cancer, possibly due to the cessation of ovulation and quiescence of the ovary. A similar protection has been noticed against cancer of the endometrium.
- Bromwich & Parsons (1990) suggest that the pill protects against some forms of pelvic infection by its alteration of cervical mucus and, because it prevents ovulation and tubal infection (salpingitis), it reduces the risk of **ectopic pregnancy**.

Side effects

For some women the pill is contraindicated and may be dangerous. The reasons can be divided into those related to oestrogen and those related to progestogen although it is not always possible to be as simplistic and the two hormones do interact (Bromwich & Parsons 1990). Oestrogen side effects are due to the amount of oestrogen in the pill and are less severe and less frequent in low-dose preparations. Headaches, dizziness, nausea and water retention are reported and there may also be a rise in blood pressure. The most serious side effect is the increased risk of blood clotting.

Progestogens may predispose women to long-term weight gain, tiredness, depression and reduced libido. It may be the progestogen content in the presence of oestrogen that predisposes to arterial thrombosis rather than venous thrombosis. Any side effect reported by women should be considered as soon as possible by a medical practitioner so that the treatment can be reviewed and contraception usage changed.

- **Thrombosis** – Some of the side effects of taking the combined pill occur because of the altered physiology, which mimics that of pregnancy, and it is worth reminding ourselves that all drugs work by altering physiological parameters. The risk of arterial or venous thrombosis has already been mentioned and occurs because of increased clotting factors, platelet aggregation and serum lipids. This will be discussed in relation to pregnancy adaptation in Section 2 of the book. The risk is thought to be low in slim women under 35 who are not hypertensive, do not smoke and have no previous personal or family history of thrombosis. The consequences of thrombosis are serious and include deep vein thrombosis, pulmonary embolism and cerebral ischaemia. However, it is worth considering that the effects of an unwanted pregnancy on the physical health alone are far greater.
- **Cancer** – Evidence for the link between taking the pill and cancer is mixed. Research indicates that women taking the pill have a reduced incidence of ovarian and endometrial cancer but there is mixed evidence, complicated by other factors, on the increased incidence of cervical cancer and breast cancer. Women taking oral contraceptives lose the protection that barrier methods give to the cervix. Whilst there may have been an increase in breast cancer since the 1960s and it may be related to taking oestrogenic compounds, it may also possibly be due to earlier diagnosis, postponement of the first pregnancy and increased fat consumption, all known risk factors for breast cancer.
- **Hypertension** – The risk increases with age and is more likely in those who smoke.
- **Migraine** – Some women find their migraines improve whilst they take the pill and some find a deterioration. However, a serious problem occurs when women experience focal migraine with transient weakness, numbness of part of the body or loss of part of the visual field. These symptoms may be a sign of reduced blood flow to the brain.
- **Jaundice** – The pill has to be metabolised by the liver and has effects on liver function. Most women have a change in composition of bile and this may lead to the formation of gallstones. This may be due to an acceleration of the problem rather than being the sole cause. A few women may develop

jaundice and intense itching of the skin and even fewer women may develop liver tumours.

- **Effect on pregnancy** – Large-scale studies fail to find a link between taking the pill in early pregnancy and congenital abnormality (Alexander 1996, Bromwich & Parsons 1990). However, because of the past link between women who were given diethylstilboestrol (DES) in pregnancy and clear cell carcinoma in their teenage daughters (see Environmental issues in Chapter 7), it is safer to discontinue taking the pill once pregnancy has been confirmed, although no such link has been seen with other oestrogenic compounds. Women who have taken the pill have no increase in absolute infertility but may take longer to become pregnant, with 98% of women resuming normal periods within 3 months of discontinuing the pill.
- **Effect on lactation** – Oestrogen suppresses the hormone prolactin secreted by the anterior pituitary gland. Prolactin acts on the alveoli of the breast to stimulate milk production. The result will be diminished milk production and a shorter duration of lactation (see The progestogen-only pill below).
- **Drug interactions** – Briefly, synthetic oestrogens can be taken orally and are well absorbed by the intestinal tract. Unlike natural oestrogens which are rapidly broken down by the liver, synthetic compounds take longer to be metabolised and degraded (Rang & Dale 1991). The combined pill is probably effective for up to 36 h.

It is important to consider other medication that the woman may be taking as some drugs interfere with the contraceptive action of the combined pill. Broad-spectrum antibiotics such as ampicillin may impair intestinal absorption whilst most anticonvulsant drugs increase liver enzyme production and hasten drug breakdown. A further consideration is the problem of absorption. Vomiting and diarrhoea may prevent absorption and the pill should be considered non-effective for that cycle. Women with malabsorption disorders such as those with an iliostomy should not be prescribed the oral combined pill.

Contraindications

Because of the above side effects, those advising women about contraception or prescribing the pill to women may be guided by the following contraindications although these must be considered in the context of each woman's needs.

Box 5.1 Contraindications against prescribing the combined contraceptive pill

- A history of thromboembolic conditions or abnormal clotting factors
- Hypertension
- Familial hyperlipidaemia
- Valvular heart disease
- Diabetes mellitus with complications
- Oestrogen-dependent malignancy
- Gross obesity
- Smokers over the age of 35
- Current liver disease
- A history of idiopathic jaundice of pregnancy
- Puerperal psychosis
- During lactation

Sperm

Testosterone

Men typically generate 1000 sperm a minute and this is controlled by hormones. The hormones involved are gonadotrophin-releasing hormone from the hypothalamus which controls pituitary production of LH and FSH. LH stimulates the testes to produce testosterone which, together with FSH, induces sperm production. Alexander (1995) mentions that the WHO is currently interested in injectable testosterone which theoretically would act as a negative feedback mechanism to reduce the production of GnRH. However, there are problems with this because of the side effects of high levels of circulating androgens, namely irritability, increased risk of cholesterol production with risk of vascular disease and acne. Adding a synthetic form of progesterone (progestogen) seems to allow a lower dose of testosterone to be given without reducing the contraceptive effect. However, it may be another 10 years before such a drug reaches the market because of the need for safe trials.

Gossypol

Other drugs have been considered for male contraception, the most famous of these being gossypol discovered by researchers in China in the 1980s. People in a certain part of China were cooking their food in cotton seed oil and were infertile. Following this the compound has been studied intensively but there are two major problems (Alexander 1995, Bromwich & Parsons 1990). First, the effects of gossypol in reducing sperm production are not always reversible and second, some men experience a fall in serum potassium which could endanger their lives. Alexander points out that many drugs that are successful in preventing sperm production have proved toxic to the spermatogonia in the testes, leading to irreversible sterility.

PREVENTION OF FERTILISATION

The progestogen-only pill

It has already been noted that progestogens in the combined pill thicken cervical mucus and prevent sperm penetration. The endometrium is also made inhospitable to a possible embryo. Uterine tube contractions become less coordinated so that sperm that have managed to penetrate the cervical mucus now find it impossible to journey up the uterine tubes to the ovum. Ovulation may be suppressed in 50% of women but this is not the main mode of action.

Because of the chance that ovulation will occur, there has been discussion about the relative effectiveness of the progestogen-only pill (often called the mini pill) and the combined pill. Progestogen's effects last about 27 h so that women must take their pills at the same time each day. Missing out one tablet may rapidly result in alteration of cervical mucus so that sperm can penetrate it. Therefore if more than 3 h elapse beyond the 24 h other forms of contraception should be used. This may be the reason for the belief that the progestogen-only pill is less effective than the combined pill. Also there may be a few women for whom the dosage of progestogen is insufficient to produce effective contraception.

Benefits

Cervical mucus thickens after a few hours so that contraceptive protection will be achieved 48 h after starting to take this pill. Besides preventing sperm penetration, there is protection against some of the bacterial pathogens so that the risk of pelvic inflammatory disease is lessened.

Milk production is not diminished and few hormones seem to cross into breast milk. Therefore this pill is useful in women who are breastfeeding.

Children of some of the first women to be given this pill, when hormone content was much higher than at present, are now adult and no health or reproductive problems have been identified in them.

In the combined pill it is the oestrogen that increases the likelihood of blood clotting problems. Women taking progestogens have been shown to have no higher incidence of bloodclotting than those taking no medication. The very small doses of progestogen used in the pill are unlikely to have an effect on blood vessels so that this pill is considered a safe option for some women who could not be prescribed the combined pill.

Cigarette smokers are more likely to develop blood vessel changes, especially of the vessels supplying the heart. Whilst stopping smoking is the best option this pill will not add to the risk. The same applies to those women who have reached the age of 35. Their fertility is already reduced and their motivation to prevent a pregnancy is high. The progestogen-only pill is often prescribed for perimenopausal women. Hypertension may indicate the use of the progestogen-only pill. All oestrogen pills are likely to raise blood pressure and this may lead to heart disease.

Side effects

This form of contraception has been taken by limited numbers of people compared to the combined pill so that far fewer studies have been carried out. Nevertheless, the progestogen-only pill has been prescribed for as long as the combined pill and there have been sufficient studies to indicate that no significant problems occur.

Alteration in menstrual bleeding patterns is the most common side effect. Progestogen alone cannot control periods and its use can lead to breakthrough bleeding and spotting between periods. The endometrium grows irregularly and bits of it may be shed, producing the bleeding. This usually settles down after the first 3 months but some women find the bleeding troublesome and discontinue the medication. Some women find their periods stop altogether and become anxious about a pregnancy occurring. Whilst rapid and accurate pregnancy tests are available over the counter, most women may find the constant worry too stressful. Changing to a different preparation may work for some.

Progestogen-only pills may alter the way that glucose is handled in women who have diabetes although the effect is not as strong as that produced by the combined pill.

Besides the risks of any pregnancy, there is an important extra risk of becoming pregnant whilst taking the progestogen-only pill. The pregnancy is more likely to occur outside the uterus (ectopic) and the commonest site is the uterine tube. Bromwich & Parsons (1990) believe this is a rare but dangerous complication. If the pregnancy continues there is a risk of rupture of the uterine tube with heavy internal bleeding sufficient to threaten life. Treatment requires an emergency operation to remove the uterine tube and the woman's fertility is permanently reduced. Whilst no clear factor is known to account for this link, it must be remembered that ovulation is not always suppressed. The motility of the uterine tubes is reduced so that the embryo cannot reach the uterine cavity before it begins to increase in size. It will not be able to pass through the narrow part of the tube and so implants into the tubal wall.

Long-acting progestogen injections

Because progestogens are rapidly broken down by the liver, leaving a small margin of time safety, ways of keeping them in the body longer have been tried. Two preparations available in Britain are Depo-Provera and Noristerat. The action of these substances is similar to the progestogen-only pill but there is a more profound effect on the ovary. Ovulation and menstrual cycles cease.

Benefits

At present, in some countries, these drugs are only licensed to be used when other forms of contraception are not possible. Progestogens increase the stability of red cells and women with sickle cell disease may benefit. Women who cannot take oral preparations, because absorption is poor or large areas of intestine have been removed, may benefit from an injectable preparation. There has been controversy over the treatment of women who have learning difficulties and are thought not able to cope with pregnancy and childrearing. The concept of informed consent must be a prime consideration. Worldwide, these drugs have been controversial when used in developing countries. However, the risk of repeated pregnancies may outweigh the side effects of the progestogen injection.

Side effects

Irregular bleeding may occur and has been heavy enough in some women to require hospitalisation. Other women have no bleeding at all. Bleeding is the most problematic when the injections are commenced following the birth of a baby. As with the mini pill bleeding settles down after the first 3 months. Some medical practitioners believe the bleeding is easily treated and the benefits of delayed return of fertility outweigh the risks. The drugs need to be repeated every 8 weeks to ensure efficacy.

Other methods of progestogen delivery

Other methods of progestogen delivery are under development

and should be ready within the next 5 years. These include subcutaneous implant (such as Norplant), by release from intrauterine device (see below) and by vaginal ring which can be kept in place for 3 weeks and removed to allow menstruation to occur (Alexander 1995). Alexander also anticipates 3-monthly injectable contraceptives for men which consist of a progestogen with an androgen to stop sperm production.

Barrier methods of contraception

The aim of these methods is to prevent sperm deposited in the vagina from ascending the cervix and reaching the ovum. This type of method has a long history and some of the methods have been found to be reasonably successful. For example, Egyptian women placed pessaries coated in honey into their vaginas and honey is known to kill both spermatozoa and bacteria. Similar acidic preparations have been used.

The female diaphragm

The female diaphragm, a thin rubber dome, is the most commonly used of the female rubber barriers (Fig. 5.1). It must be fitted to the individual and any loss or gain in weight of more than 7 pounds necessitates refitting. Cervical and vault caps which adhere to the cervix by suction are less commonly used. Diaphragms are normally used in conjunction with a spermicidal preparation and should be left in situ long enough for the sperm to be killed.

Benefits of the diaphragm

It is an efficient alternative to hormonal contraception and the woman is able to take responsibility for avoidance of pregnancy. It may also be protective against some sexually transmitted diseases.

Side effects

Despite its simplicity, there are a few problems with the diaphragm. Some women may be allergic to the rubber or to the spermicide and those with a degree of uterine prolapse may find the diaphragm uncomfortable and difficult to maintain in place.

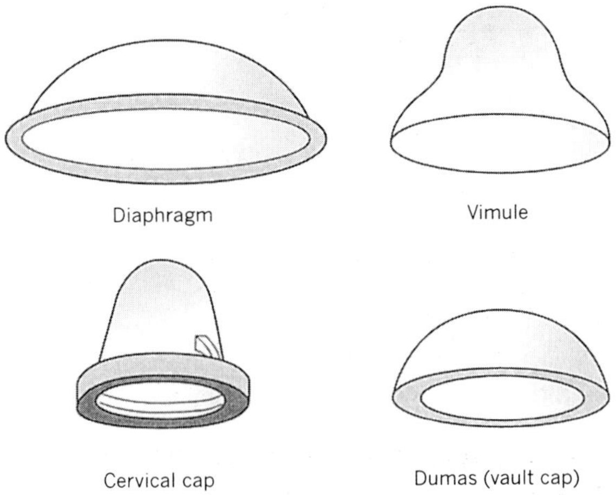

Figure 5.1 *Examples of female barrier methods. (Reproduced with permission from Cowper & Young, 1989.)*

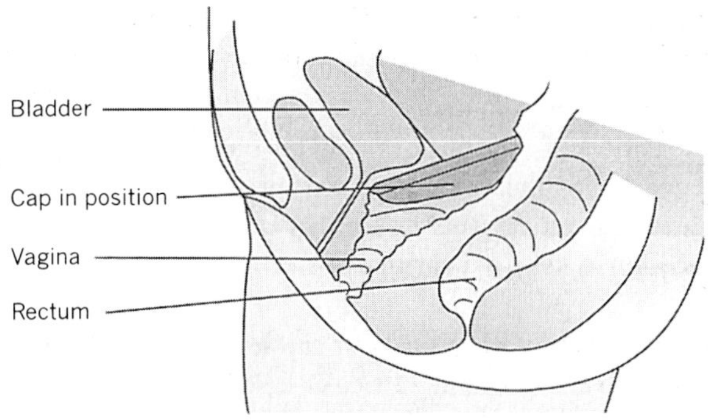

Figure 5.2 *Diaphragm cap in position. (Reproduced with permission from Cowper & Young, 1989.)*

The diaphragm predisposes to vaginal candidiasis (thrush) especially in diabetic women, and some women may develop recurrent cystitis. Using the diaphragm may be distasteful to some women who object to its messiness and the need to handle their bodies or to remember to insert it prior to coitus.

The contraceptive sponge

This consists of a one-size sponge impregnated by spermicide. One side has an indentation and the other side has a ribbon for removal of the sponge. It is moistened with water and inserted high into the vagina with its indented side against the cervix and can be left in situ for 24 h. It must be left in place for at least 6 h after intercourse. It can be purchased without prescription. When it was developed in the early 1980s it was seen as the answer to the modern young woman as it needed no contact with professionals and its failure rate was given by the manufacturer as reasonable – between 9 and 11 HWY. However, research by Bounds & Guillebaud (1984), using well-motivated young women, suggested the true rate was nearer to 25 HWY. It may be that the method is more suitable to women who are spacing their families and would not be too concerned if they became pregnant or to perimenopausal women whose fertility is low. A further problem is that it is less successful when used by women who have had children.

The male condom

These tubular closed-ended devices have also had a long history. They have been made of lambs' intestines (still available), oil-soaked cloth and more recently of rubber. They must be placed on the erect penis prior to sexual contact as there may be sperm in the fluid released from the tip of the penis following arousal. After the event, the penis must be removed from the vagina before the erection is lost and no further genital contact must occur. They have the advantage of being cheap, easily purchased and successful. Most condoms are meant to be used once and then disposed of.

The female condom

These have been introduced under the trade name of Femidom and are made of polyurethane which is both tougher and finer than rubber. The device lines the vagina with an inner rim that fits into the vaginal fornices and an outer rim around the vulva. They are also lubricated to aid insertion of the penis. It is thought that they will provide an efficient barrier to sexually transmitted disease and should be as efficient as the diaphragm or condom.

Spermicidal preparations

These chemical preparations may come in the form of foaming tablets, aerosols, films, creams, pessaries and jellies. Whilst they all contain chemicals efficient at killing sperm it must be remembered that hundreds of millions of sperm may be released per ejaculate. Therefore it is not recommended that they be used alone. Spermicides may reduce the incidence of sexually transmitted organisms, such as the gonococcus and spirochaete of syphilis, and also viruses. This is because they do not differentiate between the single-celled sperm and single-celled microorganisms, killing them all. Also some microorganisms hitch a ride into the female genital tract through the channels in the cervical mucus made by the sperm. The commonest spermicidal agent is called nonoxynol-9. The substance attaches itself to the surface of the spermatozoa and prevents them taking in oxygen. It also destroys the surface tension of the outer membrane so that the sperm bursts.

Natural methods

Preventing ejaculation into the vagina

Various techniques of preventing ejaculation into the vagina are practised. Withdrawing the penis from the vagina, or coitus interruptus, avoiding ejaculation or coitus reservatus and coitus intracrura where the penis is placed between the thighs of the woman are all still used as contraceptive techniques. A more unusual practice is coitus saxonicus where hard pressure to the male perineum just prior to ejaculation results in retrograde ejaculation into the bladder, a difficult technique but effective. Anal intercourse is also used by some couples. These methods are easy to use and do not need medical supervision so that, despite their relatively high failure rate, they will continue to be used.

Timing, temperature and cervical mucus

For some people physiological techniques of contraception are the only acceptable methods (Cowper 1997, Rider 1993). There is a very brief window in each ovulatory cycle when the ovum is available for fertilisation. If this window can be pinpointed and intercourse avoided at that time, it is reasonable to assume that a pregnancy will not occur. In women with a

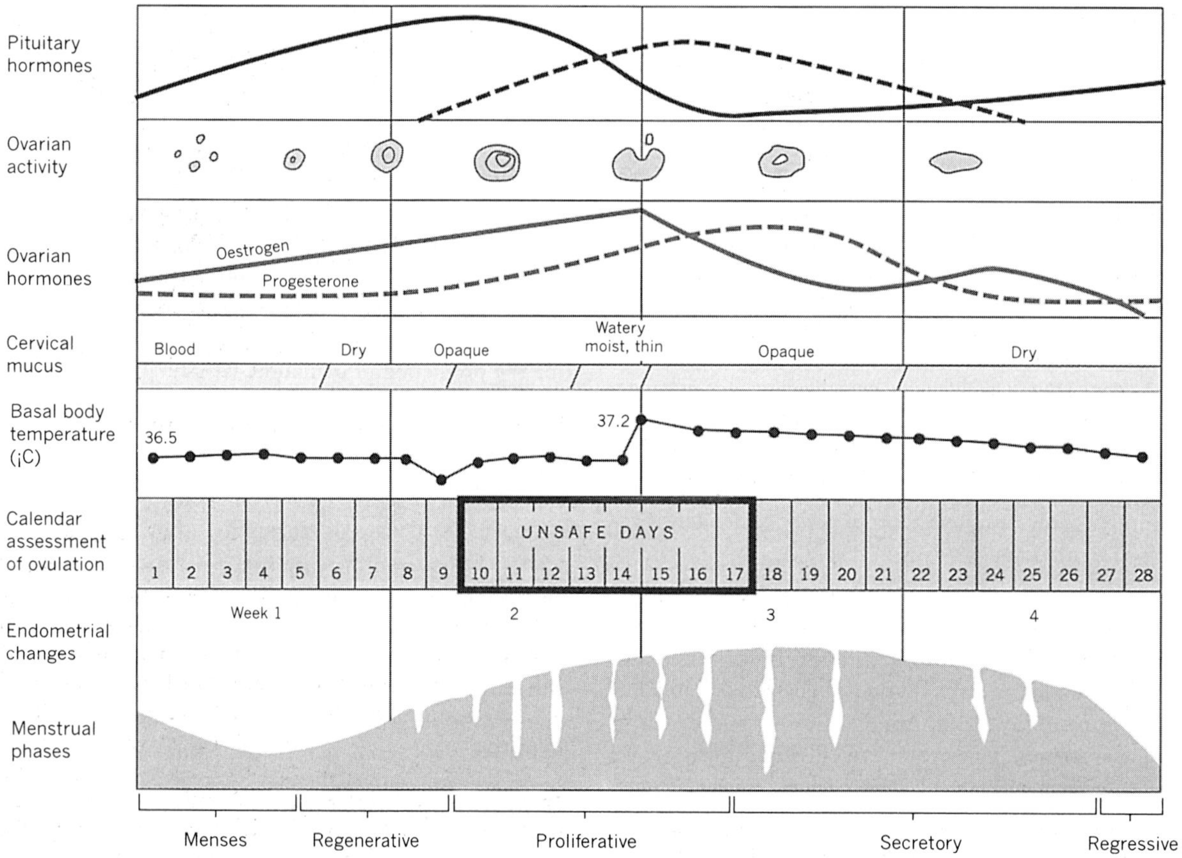

Figure 5.3 *Physiological changes in the menstrual cycle in conjunction with physiological methods of birth control. (Reproduced with permission from Cowper & Young, 1989.)*

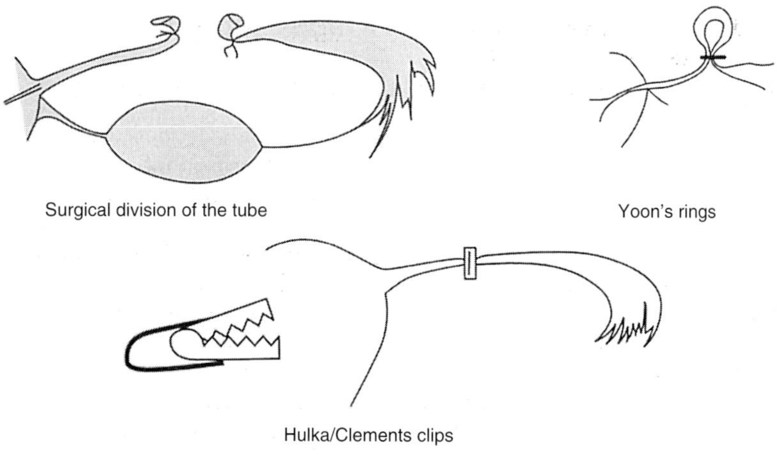

Figure 5.4 *Sterilisation methods. (Reproduced with permission from Cowper & Young, 1989.)*

regular menstrual cycle the calendar or timing method can be used. There is always the possibility of ovulation occurring irregularly so methods of pinpointing ovulation have been discovered. These rely on the changes brought about by the secretion of progesterone (see Chapter 2). The first is the change in cervical mucus and the second is the rise in core temperature. A combination of the two, the symptothermal method, is quite successful for highly motivated women.

Sterilisation

Fertilisation occurs in the ampulla of the uterine tube and the zygote then travels down the tube to the uterus. The aim of female sterilisation is to remove sections of the uterine tubes to prevent the sperm reaching the ovum (Fig. 5.4).

Spermatozoa travel up the vas deferens towards the urethra to be ejaculated into the vagina. The aim of male sterilisation or **vasectomy** is to remove a section of the two vasa to prevent the sperm entering the ejaculatory fluid (Fig. 5.5). The application of clips has been tried to increase the chances of reversal.

These are not difficult operations but the techniques must be considered permanent as reversal may be very difficult, involving microsurgery. Despite this, recanalisation of the ducts can occur in up to two in 1000 men or women, resulting in a pregnancy. Following vasectomy, it may take up to 20 ejaculations to clear sperm from the ducts and specimens of ejaculate should be tested until two clear specimens are obtained. In certain parts of the world where it would be difficult to carry out these tests, 20 condoms are given to the man and he is told that when these have been used he can begin unprotected intercourse. There may be a short-term risk of infection or haematoma, as there is with any surgery, but despite multiple studies no statistical link with long-term health problems has been made.

Intrauterine device (IUD)

Intrauterine devices for the purpose of contraception began in the 1950s with the development of the plastics industry. Many different shapes have been tried but they must be small enough to insert through the cervix but large enough to fill the small uterine cavity (Fig. 5.6). Practically, this has involved a device that can be reduced in diameter during insertion and will recoil to its effective shape once in the uterus. In the past IUDs big enough to prevent pregnancy have caused problems of discomfort, bleeding and rejection so that the so-called 'third generation' devices have been developed. These are smaller and the plastic is there to hold substances that will prevent pregnancy, the most successful of which, are copper and progesterone. Most women now have a copper-containing device inserted. IUDs work by reducing the likelihood of the sperm being able to swim through the uterine cavity. They also alter the contractability of the uterine tubes, reducing the chances that a fertilised ovum will reach the uterine cavity (but increasing the risk of ectopic pregnancy). Finally, they prevent a

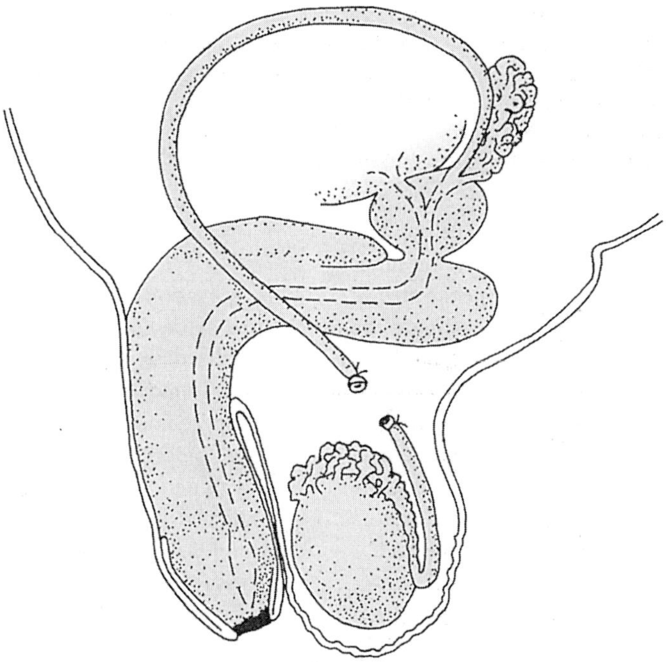

Figure 5.5 *Ligation of the vas deferens (from Sweet B, 1997, with permission).*

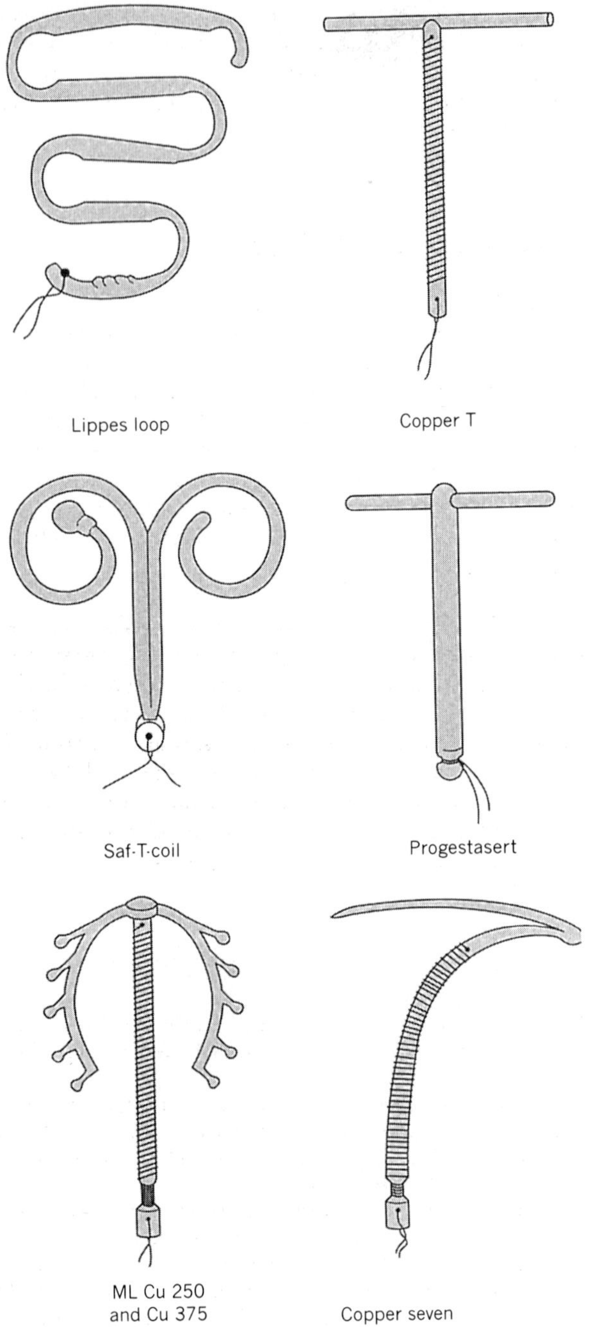

Figure 5.6 *Intrauterine devices. (Reproduced with permission from Cowper & Young, 1989.)*

fertilised ovum from embedding in the uterus. This last fact is unacceptable to some people who see it as a form of early abortion.

Benefits

The advantage of these devices is that once inserted they can be forgotten about, except for periodic checking that they are still in situ.

Side effects

One of the main complaints following insertion of an IUD is the increase in the duration of menstruation and blood loss that results. This is not a straightforward lengthening of the menstrual phase of the cycle but an annoying light loss beginning 2 or 3 days before true bleeding commences and a similar tailing off at the end of the period. The only IUD without this effect is the progesterone-containing type.

An increased tendency to pelvic infection is probably the most important problem that may occur when an IUD is in place. Although the increased risk is only 1% or 2%, pelvic infections are dangerous and lead to heavy, irregular menstrual bleeding, infertility, miscarriage and ectopic pregnancy. Some experts estimate the increase to be five fold that of a woman with no IUD in situ. This is not related to promiscuity as some of the organisms are commonly found in the bowel. Women in the steadiest partnerships are equally at risk. There is no physical, chemical or hormone-induced barrier to bacteria. These organisms accompany the sperm through the cervical mucus and carry on to cause infection. Research has shown that contraceptive practices that prevent sperm from reaching the cervix are associated with a reduced incidence of pelvic infection. Vasectomy is also associated with a reduced incidence of infection, suggesting that the bacteria hitch a ride through the female genital tract on the sperm. Some people advocate the addition of a spermicide to reduce the risk of infection.

Although the IUD is a very efficient type of contraceptive, it can fail. IUDs fail because they have become displaced or expelled from the uterus so that about two people per 100 would become pregnant per year. Although no damage has been seen to a baby conceived with an IUD in situ, there are some pregnancy problems. Miscarriage is more common, occurring in about 50% of the pregnancies, and ectopic pregnancy may be more likely. If the IUD remains in situ and the pregnancy continues, premature onset of labour may occur.

PREVENTION OF EMBEDDING/DEVELOPMENT OF CONCEPTUS

IUD

The probable effect on prevention of embedding of a fertilised ovum has been discussed above.

Postcoital contraception

Amongst professionals, there is a distinct dislike of contraception 'after the event'. However, not all acts of intercourse are premeditated and planned for. Postcoital contraception only became legal in the United Kingdom in 1983 although abortion in certain circumstances had been legal since 1967. Modern methods interrupt implantation or even ovulation, depending on the time in the menstrual cycle. They include:

- insertion of an IUD;
- taking four tablets of the combined pill or an equivalent preparation;
- antiprogesterone pills such as RU486.

Abortion

It is not the intention to discuss this in depth but for some women it may be the only answer to an unwanted or dangerous pregnancy. Not all requests for abortions are due to lack of prevention. As failure occurs in most of the methods discussed above, there is always likely to be a demand. The 1967 Abortion Act requires that two doctors state that they have formed the opinion that one of four circumstances applies to this pregnancy:

1 continuing the pregnancy would involve risk to the life of the pregnant woman greater than if the pregnancy were terminated;
2 continuing the pregnancy would involve risk of injury to the physical or mental health of the pregnant woman greater than if the pregnancy were terminated;
3 continuing the pregnancy would involve risk of injury to the physical or mental health of the existing child(ren) of the family of the pregnant woman greater than if the pregnancy were terminated;
4 there is substantial risk that if the child were born it would suffer from such physical or mental abnormalities as to be seriously handicapped.

Menstrual extraction or suction emptying of the uterus following an endometrial scrape can be performed when the period is 10–14 days late. This is not as popular now as it used to be because of the discomfort to the woman. Dilatation of the cervix and curettage of the endometrium (D & C) can be used followed by vacuum aspiration of the products of conception up to 12 weeks from the last menstrual period (10 weeks from conception). After 12 weeks prostaglandin induction of uterine contractions is used to expel the fetus. These contractions are painful and the placenta may be retained in the uterus, necessitating a trip to theatre and a D & C.

FUTURE ADVANCES

Vaccines that will give contraceptive protection for up to a year may be ready for use in 10–15 years. These could be targeted against selected proteins involved in reproduction. Nancy Alexander (1995) suggests antibody production could be raised against GnRH in men but as this would prevent testosterone production, replacement therapy would be necessary. Female vaccines currently being developed target human chorionic gonadotrophin (HCG), the hormone produced by the conceptus that is necessary for implantation. Antisperm antibodies could also be a possibility.

As yet there is no perfect contraceptive method that could be used globally. Also, there are some countries where for social, cultural or religious reasons, contraception is either forbidden or frowned upon. It is not just an academic problem as the ability of countries to produce food or avoid war is compromised by growing populations. Perhaps the saddest result of uncontrolled population growth is the effect on the health of children. For this reason it is important to maintain the research into ever simpler and more acceptable contraception and to support people in their chosen optimum spacing of their children.

Summary of main points

- The growth of the human population is occurring rapidly. The world population in 1987 was 5 billion and may increase to 6 billion by 2000. The changes are not brought about totally by a surfeit of births. In some countries improving health is reducing the number of children dying and preventing early adult deaths.
- Various countries are involved in contraceptive trials to combat overpopulation. China has been conducting research into a 'male pill' and the Indian National Institute of Immunology has been testing a female immunocontraceptive vaccine targeting human chorionic gonadotrophin. The World Health Organization is also testing such a vaccine.
- Contraception has been an issue for people ever since the link was made between sexual behaviour and pregnancy but there are religious, moral and cultural issues to be considered and therefore it is likely that no one method would ever become universal.
- A mathematical concept used to assess the effectiveness of contraceptive methods is the calculation of the failure rate per 100 woman years (HWY). This is the number of women who would become pregnant if 100 women used the method for 1 year.
- All the ova available to the woman for reproduction are already present in her ovary at birth. It is therefore not a matter of prevention of production of ova but of preventing their maturation and thus preventing ovulation. This is the basis for the combined oral contraceptive.
- The modern pill is a mixture of two hormones: one is a derivative of oestrogen and the other is a progesterone mimic (a progestogen). Risks of taking the contraceptive pill include its oestrogen content, cigarette smoking and obesity; a sedentary way of life and family history of thrombosis are also important factors increasing the risk of thrombosis. This information should be considered before prescribing the pill and women should be fully informed of the risks and benefits.
- The dose of progestogen is more variable and progestogens add to the contraceptive effect by causing thickening of the cervical mucus, making the endometrium unsuitable for implantation and reducing the motility of the uterine tubes.
- It is important to consider other medication that the woman may be taking as some drugs interfere with the contraceptive action of the combined pill. Broad-spectrum antibiotics such as ampicillin may impair intestinal absorption whilst most anticonvulsant drugs increase liver enzyme production and hasten drug breakdown.
- Vomiting and diarrhoea may prevent absorption and the pill should be considered non-effective for that cycle. Women with malabsorption disorders such as those with an iliostomy should not be prescribed the oral combined pill.
- The WHO is currently interested in injectable testosterone which prevent sperm production but the side effects of high levels of circulating androgens include irritability and increased risk of cholesterol production with risk of vascular disease and acne. Adding a synthetic form of progesterone seems to allow a lower dose of testosterone to be given without reducing the contraceptive effect.
- Other drugs that might suppress sperm production have been considered, the most famous of these being gossypol. Many drugs that are successful in preventing sperm production have proved toxic to the spermatogonia in the testes, leading to irreversible sterility.
- Progestogens have the effect of thickening cervical mucus and preventing sperm penetration. The endometrium is also made inhospitable to a possible embryo. Uterine tube contractions become

less coordinated so that sperm find it impossible to journey up the uterine tubes. Ovulation may be suppressed in 50% of women but this is not the main mode of action.

- Milk production is not diminished when breastfeeding women take progestogen only and little hormone seems to cross into breast milk. This form of contraception may cause alteration in menstrual bleeding patterns, changes in the way that glucose is handled in women who have diabetes, and ectopic pregnancy.
- Because progestogens are rapidly broken down by the liver, leaving a small margin of time safety, ways of keeping them in the body longer have been tried. Two preparations available in Britain are Depo-Provera and Noristerat. Methods of progestogen delivery by subcutaneous implant, by release from intrauterine device and by vaginal ring are being developed.
- The aim of barrier methods is to prevent sperm deposited in the vagina from ascending the cervix and reaching the ovum. Methods include the diaphragm, the contraceptive sponge, the male condom, the female condom and spermicidal preparations.
- Other methods include preventing ejaculation into the vagina, timing, temperature and cervical mucus, control of coital frequency, male and female sterilisation and insertion of an IUD.
- Postcoital contraception became legal in the United Kingdom in 1983. Modern methods interrupt implantation or even ovulation, depending on the time in the menstrual cycle. They include insertion of an IUD, taking four tablets of the combined pill or an equivalent preparation and antiprogesterone pills such as RU486.
- Not all requests for terminations of pregnancy are due to lack of prevention. As failure occurs in most of the methods discussed above, there is always likely to be a demand. The 1967 Abortion Act legalises abortion by requiring that two doctors agree that one of four circumstances applies to the pregnancy.
- Menstrual extraction or suction emptying of the uterus following an endometrial scrape can be performed when the period is 10–14 days late. Dilatation of the cervix and curettage of the endometrium can be used, followed by vacuum aspiration of the products of conception up to 12 weeks from the last menstrual period. After 12 weeks prostaglandin induction of uterine contractions is used to expel the fetus.
- As yet there is no perfect contraceptive method that could be used globally. Also there are some countries where for social, cultural or religious reasons contraception is either forbidden or frowned upon. The ability of countries to produce food or avoid war is compromised by growing populations. Possibly the saddest result of uncontrolled population growth is the effect on the health of children.

References

Alexander J. 1996 Family planning. In Bennett VR, Brown LK (eds) Myles Textbook for Midwives. Churchill Livingstone, Edinburgh.

Alexander NJ. 1995 Future contraceptives. Scientific American 273(3) 71–77.

Billings EL, Billings JJ, Brown JB, Burger HG. 1972 Symptoms and hormonal changes accompanying ovulation. Lancet I 282–284.

Bounds W, Guillebaud J. 1984 Randomised comparison of the use-effectiveness and patient acceptability of the Collatex (Today) contraceptive sponge and the diaphragm. British Journal of Family Planning 10, 69–75.

Bromwich P, Parsons T. 1990 Contraception, The Facts. Oxford University Press, Oxford.

Cowper A. 1997 Family planning. In Sweet BR with Tiran D (eds) Mayes Midwifery, 12th edn. Baillière Tindall, London, pp 748–761.

Dasgupta PS. 1995 Population, poverty and the local environment. Scientific American 272(2) 26–31.

Malthus TR. 1973 (reissue) An Essay on the Principle of Population. Dent, London.

McNeil WH. 1976 Plagues and Peoples. Penguin, Harmondsworth.

Rang HP, Dale MM. 1991 Pharmacology, 2nd edn. Churchill Livingstone, Edinburgh.

Rider REJ. 1993 'Natural family planning': effective birth control supported by the Catholic Church. British Medical Journal 307 (6906), 723–726.

Sweet B. 1997 Mayes' Midwifery. Baillière Tindall, London.

Recommended reading

Alexander NJ. 1995 Future contraceptives. Scientific American

Bromwich P, Parsons T. 1990 Contraception, The Facts. Oxford University Press, Oxford.

Cowper A. 1997 Family planning. In Sweet BR with Tiran D (Eds) Mayes Midwifery, 12th edn. Baillière Tindall, London, pp 748–761.

Family Planning Association 1992 Contraceptive Handbook. FPA, London.

Loudon N. (ed) 1991 Handbook of Family Planning, 2nd edn. Churchill Livingstone, Edinburgh.

Chapter

6 Infertility

In this chapter

INTRODUCTION

Despite the numbers of people currently alive, the fertility of human beings is quite low compared with other mammals. Most mammals would achieve a pregnancy following one mating but even at the peak of fertility when both partners are between 20 and 30 years old, human fertility is as low as 25–30%. Bromwich & Parsons (1990) put this simply as 'If a fertile couple have intercourse with no contraception on the most fertile day possible, the woman has a 1 in 4 chance of a baby'. It appears also that fertility in Western couples is declining at present and some of the possible causes will be discussed in Chapter 7.

NATURAL PATTERNS OF FERTILITY

The frequent pregnancies and births found in developing nations are not typical of the normal human pattern. The !Kung people have no taboos about avoiding sexual intercourse following birth as some cultures do, where the woman returns to the home of her parents for a length of time with her new baby. Fertility limitation in the !Kung appears to rely totally on the patterns of breastfeeding (Bromwich & Parsons 1990). !Kung women have their menarche later than the better fed women of the developed world. They also have an earlier menopause.

Babies are fed on demand, extremely frequently, day and night for up to 3 years. This intensive breastfeeding behaviour keeps the level of prolactin in the women's blood high enough to block the development of ovarian follicles. Five children seems to be the norm and 50% of them may die before reproductive age. Thus the population would remain stable. The !Kung woman may only have a dozen or so periods throughout her life and ovulate equally as infrequently. This pattern is also protective against cancer of the ovary and breast.

THE CAUSES OF MALE AND FEMALE INFERTILITY

All practitioners involved in the care of pregnant women will encounter women who have had treatment for infertility. It is therefore necessary to be aware of the investigations and treatments likely to have been used in order to have all the knowledge needed to plan care for the woman and take appropriate decisions.

The World Health Organization (1988) defined subfertility as failure to achieve a pregnancy after 1 year of unprotected intercourse. The implications of the definition are that one in six couples will be rated as infertile. If a further 6 months elapses then the rate drops to one in 10. Llewellyn-Jones (1990) states that of those couples that are persistently infertile, about 55% will achieve a pregnancy following appropriate treatment.

A worthwhile analysis was undertaken by Llewellyn-Jones (1990) who examined the causes in Table 6.1 as a percentage of the total. From this a clear picture begins to emerge and an indication of the areas of investigation can be planned.

Table 6.1 *Causes of infertility*

Male	*Female*
Defective spermatogenesis ■ Endocrine disorders – dysfunction of the hypothalamus, pituitary, adrenal glands or thyroid gland ■ Systemic disease such as diabetes mellitus ■ Testicular disorders – trauma or environmental	*Defective ovulation* ■ Endocrine disorders – dysfunction of the hypothalamus, pituitary, adrenal glands or thyroid gland ■ Systemic disease such as renal disease ■ Ovarian disorders – hormonal or cystic disorders such as Stein–Leventhal syndrome or ovarian endometriosis
Defective sperm transport ■ Obstruction or absence of seminal ducts ■ Impaired secretions from accessory glands	*Defective transport* ■ Ovum because of tubal obstruction or fimbrial adhesions ■ Sperm because of thick cervical mucus or loss of tubal patency
Ineffective sperm delivery ■ Impotence due to psychosexual problems	*Defective implantation* ■ Due to hormone imbalance, congenital anomalies, fibroids or infection
■ Drug–induced problems either prescription or recreational drugs ■ Physical anomalies	

TREATMENT OF INFERTILITY

For both men and women it is important to rule out any past or present systemic disease as a cause of infertility before proceeding to a detailed examination of the reproductive systems. A discussion of frequency and behavioural aspects of coitus is necessary. Unusual though it may seem, this author recollects a couple under investigation for infertility in whom penetrative sex was said to be impossible. Vaginismus (thought to be responsible for about 1% of infertility) had been suspected and it was during a pelvic examination of the woman under general anaesthetic, followed by an X-ray of the pelvis, that the true problem of abnormal bony pelvic structure (absent sacral alae) was ascertained. Whilst the couple were able to psychologically come to terms with their alternative sexuality it was still a problem in that they dearly wished for a family. Artificial insemination using the husband's sperm followed by a caesarean section to deliver the baby resulted in a happy couple.

The list of possible causes of infertility shown in Table 6.1 indicates that investigations should be centred around the following aspects, ensuring that:

1 adequate numbers of sperm are deposited around the cervix;
2 ovulation occurs;
3 the fallopian tubes are patent;
4 the endometrium is in an appropriate state to receive the fertilised ovum;
5 the woman is psychologically prepared for pregnancy.

MALE INFERTILITY

Semen analysis and sperm deposition

Specimens of semen for analysis are deposited into a clean dry glass jar by coitus interruptus or by masturbation following 2 days of abstinence from coitus and examined in the laboratory within 1 h of collection. If a couple objects to this mode of obtaining semen, the woman may agree to a postcoital test (see below) but this will not allow a full semen analysis to be made. Ideally an average of three specimens at 2–3 week intervals allows a semen value to be calculated.

Table 6.2 *The percentage range of infertility factors (from Llewellyn-Jones 1990)*

Male factors	%
Defective spermatozoon production and insemination difficulties	25–40
Female factors	
Gross female pelvic pathology	5–12
Cervical factor	1–5
Uterine factor	< 4
Tubal factor	30–50
Ovarian factor	3–10
Unexplained after investigation	10–20

Postcoital test

A specimen of cervical mucus taken at the fertile part of the woman's cycle and within 6 h of intercourse is examined. This test can be used to ascertain the following points.

- What is the quality of the cervical mucus?
- Have the sperm been able to penetrate the cervical mucus?
- Has effective intercourse taken place?
- Are immunological problems present?

Normal values for semen are (WHO 1988):

- volume 2–6 ml;
- total sperm count more than 40 million per ml;
- motility – more than 60% should be moving steadily;
- morphology – more than 60% should appear normal on examination.

Llewellyn-Jones (1990) suggests a memory aid for these values as 2–2–6–6, substituting the lowest possible sperm count value of 20 million sperm per ml.

Defective spermatogenesis

This is a worrying problem and little seems effective in increasing the number of sperm produced. Absence of sperm (**azoospermia**), which may be due to defective spermatogenesis or damage to the transport ducts, is usually untreatable. Defective spermatogenesis may follow abnormal development of the testes, late or non-descent of the testes, damage to the testicular blood supply or mumps infection. Damage to the duct system is usually due to gonococcal infection of the epididymis. Biopsy of the testes will show whether sperm are being produced at all and chromosome studies will indicate whether the problem is the presence of **Klinefelter's syndrome** (XXY karyotype).

A reduced sperm count (**oligospermia**) may be caused by deficient spermatogenesis or by raised testicular temperature. Wearing tight underpants and trousers or working in a hot atmosphere are two environmental factors that could be altered. If a varicocoele is the cause of raised testicular temperature, surgical correction can be made. Sperm production may be increased by eating a healthy diet and an improvement in general health and by reducing alcohol intake and smoking.

Blood tests for hormone levels sometimes indicate possibilities for treatment. Reduced FSH may respond to clomiphene. Abnormally high levels of prolactin may respond to bromocriptine. Direct treatment with testosterone appears to be of little use in stimulating sperm production.

Some authorities recommend that fructose, zinc and acid phosphatase levels in seminal fluid should also be measured when the sperm count is reduced. Low levels of fructose and zinc or high levels of acid phosphatase suggest a low-grade vesiculoprostatitis. Treatment with antibiotics may improve sperm count and motility. Prostatic infection, if present, can also be treated by antibiotics.

Poor sperm delivery

A sperm penetration test can be carried out by introducing fresh sperm into a sample of cervical mucus on a glass slide to determine whether sperm function or mucus hostility is the problem. At the same time crossed hostility tests can indicate whether the woman is producing antisperm antibodies to her partner's sperm. Other causes of infertility include impotence and retrograde ejaculation into the bladder. Artificial insemination by the husband's semen (AIH) may be of use in these cases. Artificial insemination by donor sperm (AID or DI) is frequently used in azoospermia or severe oligospermia. In vitro fertilisation with sperm injection may be helpful for couples where sperm are actually being produced.

FEMALE INFERTILITY

Following the general health questions mentioned above, a pelvic examination is made to rule out any gross abnormalities of the genital tract such as imperforate hymen, vaginismus, partial or complete absence of the vagina or uterus, as was found in some young women whose mothers had been treated with DES or in those with an XY chromosome genetic karyotype. Any tubal or ovarian swelling could also be detected. If not recently done, cervical cytology for suspicious or malignant cells should be carried out. The uterus may be a cause of infertility because of a malformation, infection or because of poor endocrine control of endometrial development. Llewellyn-Jones (1990) states that a belief that retroverted uterus can cause relative infertility is not borne out by research findings.

Tubal patency

Fertilisation takes place in the outer third of the fallopian tube and the zygote then takes 4 days to reach the uterine cavity. A hysterosalpingectomy can be carried out, preferably just prior to ovulation, where an oily or water-soluble radiopaque contrast medium is injected through the cervix. Its passage through the uterus and fallopian tubes can be monitored. Laparoscopy can also be carried out to examine the pelvic organs and to check on tubal function.

A common cause of loss of tubal patency is infection which generally ascends through the cervix and uterus to affect the fallopian tubes (**salpingitis**), the ovaries and the pelvic peritoneum. This is known as **pelvic inflammatory disease** or PID. Protective mechanisms which reduce the risk of ascending infection include the fact that the vulval cleft is normally closed and the vaginal walls in apposition. Also, the normal acidity of the vagina inhibits bacterial growth and finally, as postulated by Profet (1993), the monthly shedding of the endometrium may reduce the risk of long-standing infection. Infection is usually introduced at coitus and childbirth or following illegal abortions. Infection following coitus is usually due to the gonococcus or *Chlamydia*, whilst streptococci, staphylococci and anaerobes are more likely following childbirth or abortion. Pelvic tuberculosis can also be a cause of PID.

Pelvic inflammatory disease

Chronic PID seems to be occurring with greater frequency and may be so mild as to be symptomless. This may result in pelvic adhesions that distort the fallopian tubes or the endothelial folds lining the tubes may be functionally damaged with reduced or absent ciliated cells or peristaltic movements. The tubal lumen may become blocked. As the number of infections increase, so a woman's fertility reduces and following three attacks, more than 50% of women will be infertile. Tubal microsurgery may be useful following antibiotic treatment but the operation may need to be radical. Restoring or preserving patency is difficult and the results are poor. Also, it is necessary to inform patients of the increased risk of ectopic pregnancy and spontaneous abortion. In vitro fertilisation techniques to bypass the blocked fallopian tubes are more successful.

Endometriosis

Gynaecologists have found that 40% of patients with endometriosis have involuntary infertility and that 10% of women attending infertility clinics have endometriosis (Llewellyn-Jones 1990). However, this does not imply a direct causal factor unless tubal occlusion is present. The relationship needs clarification. There is no evidence that mild or moderate endometriosis affects fertility. The involvement of the immune system is being researched, in particular of macrophages inhibiting fertilisation. A combination of hormone treatment and surgery, depending on individual needs, may be offered if infertility persists.

Ovulation

There are specific tests to establish whether or not ovulation is occurring, some of which can be carried out in the woman's home while others require hospital involvement. These relate to the physiological changes accompanying ovulation. Cervical mucus should become clear, copious and stretchy and show a ferning pattern when dried on a glass slide. Basal body temperature drops slightly before ovulation and then should rise about 0.3°C but this method may be difficult to ascertain. There are ovulation predictor kits available over the counter which work by measuring levels of luteinising hormone. More detailed assays of hormone changes checked throughout a cycle examine the changing relationships of the four hormones oestrogen, progesterone, FSH and LH. Hyperprolactinaemia, which antagonises oestrogen and prevents ovulation, should be excluded. Ultrasound scanning can detect a ripening Graafian follicle and a thickening endometrium.

Stimulation of ovulation

Medical treatments

Depending on the results of investigations and where in the normal cycle the failure of ovulation is thought to originate, various drug treatments may be successful in stimulating ovulation. Clomiphene citrate (Clomid) will stimulate FSH production. Human chorionic gonadotrophin (HCG) is identical to LH and can be used to trigger ovulation, often in conjunction with clomiphene. Human menopausal gonadotrophin (HMG or Pergonal) or FSH (Metrodin) may be used if clomiphene has failed or in cases of polycystic ovary disease. Bromocriptine (Parlodel) can be used to inhibit prolactin release by the pituitary gland.

Surgical treatments

Surgical removal of cysts or tumours may help to trigger ovulation. Correction of endometriosis, if present, can be of value.

THE NEW REPRODUCTIVE TECHNOLOGIES

Artificial insemination by husband – AIH

This is useful where there are cervical problems, problems with sperm delivery or antisperm antibodies and where semen has been stored prior to chemotherapy or radiotherapy.

Artificial insemination by donor – AID/DI

This is of value where there is azoospermia, severe oligospermia, non-motile or abnormal sperm, a risk of transmission of a hereditary disease or rhesus incompatibility and when no male partner is available. Donors are carefully selected for health and family history of disease. Sexually transmitted diseases are excluded and the semen is frozen and stored for at least 3 months to ensure that repeated tests for HIV presence in the donor are negative.

In vitro fertilisation/embryo transfer – IVF/ET

This is the method of choice when there is tubal damage, too few sperm, cervical problems or endometriosis. It is also used where there is no satisfactory explanation for the infertility. Steinberg (1990) discusses four phases to the technique of IVF labelled superovulation, egg recovery, fertilisation and embryo transfer. Superovulation involves using the drugs discussed above to stimulate multiple ovulation. The investigations necessary to ensure that the phase of egg recovery results in mature ova involve frequent blood tests for oestradiol levels and ultrasound scans for follicle tracking. At least six eggs are usually recovered by various methods including laparoscopy. The highest number recorded in any one cycle was 22 ova.

The ova are then placed in a Petri dish in an optimum environment for fertilisation and the donor sperm are added, hoping that most or all will be fertilised. The embryos that begin to develop will be kept in vitro for 24 h while the woman receives more hormones to prepare the endometrial lining for pregnancy. Finally three embryos are placed directly into the uterus of the woman via the cervix. Any spare embryos are frozen in case further attempts are necessary. The success rate is quite poor and may not exceed 25% even in the best clinics. Some couples undergo repeated attempts.

Gamete intrafallopian transfer – GIFT

Where there are cervical barriers to conception but there is a patent fallopian tube, ova and sperm are placed in the distal end of the tube when it is hoped fertilisation will occur. There is an increased risk of ectopic pregnancy.

Zygote intrafallopian transfer – ZIFT

Here the ova are fertilised in vitro and the zygote placed in the fallopian tube.

Intracytoplasmic sperm injection – ICSI

The collection of multiple ova is carried out as for IVF. Sperm are obtained from the man and put into a solution that slows down motility to make them easier to work with. Each egg is sucked up into a holding pipette A microneedle whose diameter is seven times smaller than a human hair is used to inject a sperm directly into the centre of each ovum and then the technique continues exactly as for IVF and ET. This technique has been successful in men who are paralysed because of spinal injury when 85% are unable to ejaculate and the sperm are often of poor quality. The sperm are collected by electroejaculation technology (Stacey 1995).

Ovum donation

This is helpful if a woman is not ovulating but could carry a pregnancy. Most ova are donated by women undergoing IVF treatment. The menstrual cycles of the two women, donor and recipient, must be synchronised by the use of hormones. In Britain the law concerning ovum donation is the same as for sperm donation.

Surrogacy

The baby is carried to term by one woman with the intention of handing the new baby over to a second woman after birth. It is legal in Great Britain as long as no payment is involved. Legislation concerning this practice is clearly laid out in the Human Fertilisation and Embryology Act 1990 mentioned below.

Social implications

These techniques have resulted in much public concern and the report of the Committee of Enquiry into Human Fertilisation and Embryology (1984), commonly known as the Warnock Report, led to the Human Fertilisation and Embryology Act 1990. The Human Fertilisation and Embryology Authority (HFEA) was set up by the act to regulate any research or treatment involving the creation, keeping and use of human embryos and the storage and donation of human eggs and sperm. This is achieved by a licensing system. An informative sociological approach to the new reproductive technologies has been edited by McNeil et al (1990) with essays gathered on different sociological implications of controlling reproduction.

Whilst sperm donation is accepted, ovum donation appears to cause more anxiety in people. Acceptance may vary from legal acknowledgement that there is in principle no difference between ovum and sperm donation, as in New Zealand, to total rejection of ovum donation, as in Sweden. A register of donors must be maintained so that any child born following sperm or ovum donation has access to details about the biological parent-age. It is not clear whether access to the donor will be allowed. Confidentiality is a major consideration for most donors.

Summary of main points

- The frequent pregnancies and births found in developing nations are not typical of the normal human pattern. Fertility limitation in the !Kung appears to rely totally on the patterns of breastfeeding. Babies are fed on demand, extremely frequently, day and night for up to 3 years. This intensive breastfeeding behaviour keeps the level of prolactin in women's blood high enough to block the development of ovarian follicles.
- The World Health Organization defined subfertility as failure to achieve a pregnancy after 1 year of unprotected intercourse. The implications of the definition are that one in six couples will be rated as infertile. If a further 6 months elapses, then the rate drops to one in 10. Of those couples that are persistently infertile, about 55% will achieve a pregnancy following appropriate treatment.
- Male causes of infertility include defective sperm production and insemination difficulties. Up to half of female causes of infertility involve the fallopian tubes and up to 20% remain unexplained after investigation. The remaining causes are uterine, ovarian and pelvic pathology.
- For both men and women, it is important to rule out any past or present systemic disease as a cause of infertility before proceeding to a detailed examination of the reproductive systems. A discussion of frequency and behavioural aspects of coitus is necessary.
- Fresh specimens of semen for analysis are deposited into a clean dry glass following 2 days of abstinence from coitus. A postcoital test may be utilised but this does not allow a full semen analysis to be made. Ideally an average of three specimens at 2–3 week intervals allows a semen value to be calculated.
- The environmental effects on diminishing sperm counts are worrying and little seems effective in increasing the number of sperm produced. Azoospermia, which may be due to defective spermatogenesis or damage to the transport ducts, is usually untreatable. Defective spermatogenesis may follow abnormal development of the testes, late or non-descent of the testes, damage to the testicular blood supply or mumps infection. Damage to the duct system is usually due to gonococcal infection of the epididymis.
- Biopsy of the testes will show whether sperm are being produced at all and chromosome studies will indicate whether the problem is Klinefelter's syndrome. Oligospermia may be caused by deficient spermatogenesis or by raised testicular temperature. If a varicocoele is the cause of raised testicular temperature, surgical correction can be made. Sperm production may be improved by eating a healthy diet and reducing alcohol intake and smoking.
- Blood tests for hormone levels may indicate possibilities for treatment of oligospermia. Reduced FSH may respond to clomiphene. Abnormally high levels of prolactin may respond to bromocriptine. Direct treatment with testosterone appears to be of little use. Low levels of fructose and zinc or high levels of acid phosphatase in semen suggest a low-grade vesiculoprostatitis. Treatment with antibiotics may improve sperm count and motility. Prostatic infection, if present, can be treated by antibiotics.
- A sperm penetration test can be carried out by introducing fresh sperm into a sample of cervical mucus on a glass slide to determine whether sperm function or mucus hostility is the problem. At the same time, crossed hostility tests can indicate whether the woman is producing antisperm antibodies to her partner's sperm.
- A pelvic examination of the woman is made to rule out any gross abnormalities of the genital tract such as imperforate hymen, vaginismus, partial or complete absence of the vagina or uterus.
- The uterus may be a cause of infertility because of a malformation or infection or because of poor endocrine control of endometrial development. A hysterosalpingectomy can be carried out, preferably just prior to ovulation. Laparoscopy can also be carried out to examine the pelvic organs and to check on tubal function.
- A common cause of loss of tubal patency is ascending infection, known as pelvic inflammatory disease. Chronic PID seems to be occurring with greater frequency. This may result in pelvic adhesions that distort the fallopian tubes or the endothelial folds lining the tubes may be functionally damaged with reduced or absent ciliated cells or peristaltic movements. The tubal lumen may become blocked.
- Gynaecologists have found that 40% of patients with endometriosis have involuntary infertility and that 10% of women attending infertility clinics have endometriosis. However, this does not imply a direct causal factor unless tubal occlusion is present.
- The involvement of the immune system is being researched, in particular of macrophages inhibiting fertilisation. A combination of

hormone treatment and surgery, depending on individual needs, may be offered if infertility persists.

- There are specific tests to establish whether or not ovulation is occurring. Cervical mucus should become clear, copious and stretchy and show a ferning pattern when dried on a glass slide. Basal body temperature drops slightly before ovulation and then should rise about 0.3°C.
- More detailed assays of hormone changes checked throughout a cycle examine the changing relationships of the four hormones oestrogen, progesterone, FSH and LH. Hyperprolactinaemia, which antagonises oestrogen and prevents ovulation, should be excluded. Ultrasound scanning can detect a ripening Graafian follicle and a thickening endometrium.
- Depending on the results of investigations and where in the normal cycle the failure of ovulation is thought to originate, drug treatments may be successful in stimulating ovulation. Surgical removal of cysts or tumours may help to trigger ovulation. Correction of endometriosis, if present, can be of value.
- New reproductive techniques have resulted in much public concern and the report of the Committee of Enquiry into Human Fertilisation and Embryology (1984) led to the Human Fertilisation and Embryology Act 1990 and the setting up of the HFEA to regulate any research or treatment involving the creation, keeping and use of human embryos and the storage and donation of human eggs and sperm.
- Whilst sperm donation is accepted, ovum donation appears to cause more anxiety in people. Acceptance may vary from legal acknowledgement that there is in principle no difference between ovum and sperm donation, as in New Zealand, to total rejection of ovum donation, as in Sweden.
- A register of donors must be maintained so that any child born following sperm or ovum donation has access to details about the biological parentage. It is not clear whether access to the donor will be allowed. Confidentiality is a major consideration for most donors.

References

Bromwich P, Parsons T. 1990 Contraception, The Facts. Oxford University Press, Oxford.

Llewellyn-Jones D. 1990 Fundamentals of Obstetrics and Gynaecology, Volume 2 Gynaecology, 5th edn. Faber and Faber, London.

McNeil M, Varcoe I, Yearley S. (eds) 1990 The New Reproductive Technologies, Macmillan, Basingstoke.

Profet W. 1993 On the costs and benefits of menstruation. Quarterly Review of Biology 68, 335–386.

Stacey S. 1995 You never imagine you won't be able to father your own children. Mail on Sunday YOU magazine, 11th June.

Steinberg DL. 1990 The depersonalisation of women through the administration of 'in vitro fertilisation'. In McNeil M, Varcoe I, Yearley S (eds) The New Reproductive Technologies. Macmillan, Basingstoke, pp 74–122.

World Health Organization 1988 Laboratory Recommendations. WHO, Geneva.

Recommended reading

Botting BJ, Price FV, MacFarlane AJ. 1990 Three, Four and More: A Study of Triplet and Higher Order Births. HMSO, London.

Brinsden PR, Rainsbury P. 1992 A Textbook of In Vitro Fertilisation and Assisted Reproduction. Parthenon, Carnforth.

Lilford R. 1992 How general practitioners can help subfertile couples. British Medical Journal 305, 1376.

Winston R. 1994 Infertility, a Sympathetic Approach, Optima, London.

Chapter 7 Preconception matters

In this chapter

INTRODUCTION

Biological science concepts that have traditionally not played much part in human health sciences are becoming increasingly relevant to the survival of humans, especially in reproductive terms. If reproduction fails the species will die out but smaller problems may affect individual couples. This is the background for the development of preconception counselling and of groups such as Foresight.

Abercrombie et al (1992) define ecology as 'derived from the Greek word for house or place to live: the study of relationships of organisms or groups of organisms in their environments both animate and inanimate'. Evolution is defined as 'changes in the phenotype (functional body type) occurring in populations from one generation to the next'. It involves random changes in genes acted on by selective environmental forces; for instance, the random change which led to the altered haemoglobin molecule of sickle cell disease, selected for because it is protective against malaria.

Over the last decade a scientific concept applying Darwinian evolutionary theory to human health and disease has been developed. This is outlined in a well-written and accessible book by Nesse & Williams (1995), several chapters of which are especially valuable to those caring for men and women during their reproductive events. For some health-care professionals the book may indicate new areas for research.

AIMS OF PREPREGNANCY CARE

Chamberlain (1992) gives the aims of prepregnancy care as:

- to bring the woman and her partner to pregnancy in the best possible health;
- to provide the means of ensuring that preventable factors are attended to before pregnancy starts – for example, rubella inoculation;
- to give advice about the effects of preexisting disease and its treatment on the pregnancy and unborn child;
- to consider the likelihood and effects of any recurrence of events from previous pregnancies and deliveries.

He goes on to outline some of the practical management issues that could be introduced before conception. Besides ascertaining any health treatments that may need modifying to safeguard the fetus, dietary habits, cigarette and alcohol consumption could be discussed and changes suggested. Of current interest is the prepregnancy commencement of folate supplements to women who have had a child with a previous neural tube defect such as spina bifida.

This chapter is concerned with the extent to which child-bearing can be affected by the lifestyle of individuals and the environment in which they live. Concepts from the disciplines of ecology and evolution will be utilised to discuss the implications of radiation, toxic waste and drug ingestion. A difficulty inherent in the concept of preconceptual care is that while planned parenthood is acceptable to many people, one-third of babies are still conceived accidentally.

Following conception there is usually a gap of 10 weeks before women seek professional care. By this time organogenesis is mostly complete and advice on healthy living may be too late. For instance, folic acid intake around conception and for the first 4 weeks of pregnancy would probably prevent many neural tube defects. Few couples currently approach health professionals for preconceptual advice and few consider the need to change their lifestyles before conception. Research by Ward (1995) suggests that pregnancy outcome is improved markedly when couples are screened and advised prior to conception.

THE HEALTHY GAMETE

Bradley & Bennett (1995) have a sentence in the introduction to their book which is worth considering in the context of preconceptual health.

> In a biological sense the life process begins about 100 days before conception when the sperm and the ova begin their maturation process. During these processes both ova and sperm are extremely vulnerable to nutritional disturbances, toxins and radiation.

Ward mentions that scientific evidence indicates that genetic, microbial, biochemical, dietary and environmental factors play a major role in affecting fertility and fetal outcome. Although these categories are interwoven each will be explored in terms of the health of spermatozoa and ova. In terms of outcome there is no clear cut-off point between the health of the gametes immediately prior to conception and the developing embryo. In both instances cells are developing rapidly and are vulnerable to disruption. Even when pregnancies are planned it is unlikely that a couple will consider the importance of those 100 days of gamete formation.

The sensitive sperm

The continuously produced sperm are seemingly most at risk of environmental insult. McCloy (1989) reminds us that in the female fetus the primary oocytes have already undergone their first reduction division early in the first trimester and no further ova will be generated after the 5th month of gestation. In this arrested stage of development they are relatively resistant to mutagenic damage. It is just prior to ovulation that sensitivity increases and the mutation rate from radiation may rise sharply.

Following fertilisation, the zygote becomes resistant to genetic injury whilst undergoing cleavage but after 16 days intense organogenesis begins. Sensitivity is high but so few cells are present that either the fetus will be affected and aborted spontaneously or not affected and normal. This may account for the high rate of early pregnancy loss (within the first 6 weeks) reported.

PERSONAL HEALTH

General health check

In an ideal world couples who intend to start a family would present themselves for health screening. The history of both man and woman would be taken and known personal or familial health problems would be discussed. A clinical examination would ensure that there are no hidden health problems. A gynaecological examination of the woman and screening of blood and urine and in some cases hair, stool and semen analysis would also be carried out. Any infections could be treated, dietary problems discussed and possible work and lifestyle hazards considered.

There are some long-term health problems, such as diabetes mellitus, where stabilisation of the condition should occur prior to conception. In other conditions which are treated with known teratogenic drugs, such as epilepsy, a discussion of the risks and possible alteration of treatment may be necessary. The age of the prospective parents, especially the mother, is important as the frequency of all reproductive problems, including the occurrence of chromosome abnormalities, increases with maternal age.

Hair mineral analysis

Hair analysis for mineral content is an interesting concept that is still regarded as fringe research by some practitioners but studies confirm its usefulness. Barnes (1995) presents evidence to show that both excess of toxic minerals and shortage of essential minerals may cause reproductive problems. Hair mineral analysis involves taking a sample of scalp hair and measuring contaminants present at levels of 0.1 parts per million or less.

Some toxins are eliminated from blood and stored in body tissues. Hair grows slowly and will show traces of whatever has passed into the follicle in the previous 6–8 weeks. Hair analysis can therefore be a useful addition to blood and urine tests to screen for minerals (Bradley & Bennett 1995). Foresight include testing for the following minerals and advice would be given depending on the findings. Either supplementation of essential minerals or removal of toxic minerals by such methods as chelation may be offered.

- Essential minerals – calcium, magnesium, potassium, iron, chromium, cobalt, copper, manganese, nickel, selenium, zinc
- Toxic minerals – aluminium, cadmium, mercury and lead. The last two are discussed below.

Inherited disorders

Some couples may be anxious to discuss the possibility of inherited conditions, i.e. those where genetic mutations have led to abnormalities serious enough to be a health or even life threat to the child. Such couples may need referring to genetic counsellors so that an accurate family tree can be obtained and the genetic risk calculated (see Chapter 15).

Nutrition and weight

Dallison & Lobstein (1995) state that 'Over recent years there has been increasing evidence about the importance of nutrition to a satisfactory birth'. In developed countries it is rare to find overt malnutrition except in people with eating disorders such as anorexia nervosa. However, suboptimal dietary deficiencies are common, especially in areas of high unemployment and poverty. Some cultures may inadvertently suffer from dietary deficits because of religious food restrictions. More people are becoming vegetarian but if this is undertaken without the correct knowledge of nutrient content, suboptimal nutrition may occur.

A further complication is the high level of prepared and processed foods making up a large part of the normal British diet. Processing may destroy essential nutrients whilst chemical additives such as preservatives, artificial colourings and flavourings are added to increase the shelf-life of food and its attractiveness for purchasers. The effects of artificial fertilisers and pesticides used to increase crop production will be considered in the section on environmental issues. The increase in food allergy and the possibility of sensitisation of the fetus in utero are growing concerns.

Another problem is excessive weight, mainly due to a combination of ingesting too many calories for the diminished amount of exercise brought about by labour-saving devices in the home and increased car transport. This has introduced the concept of dieting to reduce weight and the value placed upon excessive thinness can lead to underweight and anorexia nervosa, especially in young women.

Vines (1995) states that one in two adult Britons is overweight and one in seven obese. She summarises research to show that the increase in obesity seen in Great Britain must be due to a decrease in physical activity as, despite the increase in types of available food, British people actually eat less than their grandparents did but exercise less. Healthy eating is discussed in Chapter 23.

Prepregnancy weight is known to influence pregnancy outcome. Women who are outside the optimal weight range may develop amenorrhoea and infertility. Being underweight is associated with fetal abnormality and low birth weight whilst being overweight brings the risk of complications of pregnancy, especially hypertension. A helpful guide to ascertaining the optimum weight for a woman is the **Quetelet index** or **body mass index**. This is obtained by using the formula weight in kilograms divided by height in metres squared and the following range is used for a guide:

< 20 = underweight
20–24.9 = desirable weight
25–29.9 = moderate obesity
30 and over = severe obesity

Heredity and obesity

Heredity, diet and energy expenditure are all components of an individual tendency to develop and maintain overweight and obesity (Bouchard 1991, Miller 1991). Bouchard (1991) discusses two factors that influence body fat deposition and states that both have an inherited component: activity and metabolic rate and response to overfeeding. Miller (1991) talks of a disequilibrium in energy balance. People tend to eat more calories than their energy expenditure requires and those with an inherited tendency to obesity will lay down adipose tissue.

Nesse & Williams (1995) discuss this in evolutionary terms and consider the life of 'stone age' man. It would have been adaptive to conserve valuable energy by being as lazy as possible and to take in energy by eating as many high-calorie foods as were available. In times of plenty, adipose tissue would be stored to use in a famine situation. In an era when fats, sugar and salt are freely available this would tip the energy balance towards excess and adipose tissue would be stored with no opportunity to lose it. Therefore, the population is being encouraged to exercise more. A social comment made by Vines (1995b) is that as exercise becomes something to be actively sought in leisure time, poor people are more likely to become obese.

Infection

Commensal organisms, such as the lactobacillus that produces a mild acid that increases the acidity of the vagina, are helpful. However, many organisms are pathogenic and cause infection and damage to the individual; the most virulent pathogens may kill. Systemic infections may cause reproductive problems such as infertility and congenital defects (see Chapter 15). There are methods of combating organisms and offering protection to vulnerable women. Vaccination may be available, such as for rubella, or advice on how to minimise the risk of infection during pregnancy for those where no vaccine is available. Most bacteria are too large to cross the placenta but viruses are very small and the spirochaete of syphilis can penetrate the placental membrane.

Drugs

Drugs are naturally occurring or synthesised chemicals that alter biological systems by affecting the functioning of cells, tissues, organs and systems. Drugs may affect reproductive health at different times in the lifecycle. They may damage sperm or ova and may have an adverse effect on nutrient absorption so that essential nutrients are absent at crucial times during embryonic development. They often have a wider range of effects than is medically optimal and may be teratogenic, interfering in normal growth and development. The placenta is not a complete barrier against all kinds of chemicals. A further anxiety is the amount of drugs and environmental pollutants that reach babies via their mothers' breast milk.

A higher percentage of the population is exposed to drugs used to treat medical conditions. Drugs may be essential treatment and difficult to withdraw or reduce or they may be replaced by less toxic drugs or stopped altogether during pregnancy. Women of childbearing age should not take medicines except under medical supervision and medical practitioners should be alert to the teratogenic side effects of any drugs they prescribe. Many drugs taken for minor problems such as pain relief and indigestion are purchased from a chemist by people without their doctor's knowledge and drugs may be prescribed that exacerbate the effects of the over-the-counter drugs. The general public should be informed about the danger of taking drugs in pregnancy.

Drugs may be taken for recreational reasons because of their mood-altering abilities, in which case it is sometimes difficult to ascertain whether they are being taken and to help people to stop taking them. Such substances include the socially acceptable alcohol, tobacco and caffeine as well as addictive drugs such as cocaine and its derivative crack, marihuana and heroin.

Smoking

Tobacco smoking with the inhalation of smoke for its pharmaceutical and psychoactive effects originated at least 5000 years ago, possibly in religious magical and ceremonial practices

(Tuormaa 1994). Smoking amongst the population of Europe and now Africa and Asia has spread, mainly because of the rapid effects of nicotine on the central nervous system. Thousands of other chemicals, including polycyclic aromatic hydrocarbons, carbon monoxide, cyanide, lead and cadmium, are inhaled in cigarette smoke, many of them known to be harmful to the smoker and to cross the placenta to damage the developing fetus.

Once the baby is born, contact with these chemicals through secondary smoking continues to have harmful effects on the child. Tuormaa (1994) has summarised the effects of tobacco smoking in a literature review. Smoking is probably the most dangerous avoidable risk taken by people and it is essential that men and women thinking about starting a family should stop smoking, both for the child's sake and for their own safety.

Box 7.1 The major effects of tobacco smoking on reproduction

- Male and female infertility
- Reduced length of gestation
- Low birth weight
- Spontaneous abortions
- Increased perinatal mortality (stillbirths + neonatal deaths in the first week)
- Fetal malformations
- Reduced immunocompetence

Infertility

Besides experiencing infertility, women who smoke often undergo an early menopause (Jick et al 1977). In men, smoking reduces testosterone levels, reduces the number and motility of sperm and increases the number of abnormal sperm (Evans et al 1981). A further problem with sperm production is alcohol consumption. Alcohol is a direct testicular toxin, causing atrophy of seminiferous tubules and Leydig cells. A reduction in the synthesis of testosterone occurs and similar effects on sperm are seen as those from tobacco smoking.

Fetal malformations

Tuormaa (1994), summarising findings from multiple studies, states:

> As maternal smoking reduces both the rate of cell replication and protein synthesis, it is therefore speculated that maternal smoking may cause most of its damage during the first weeks of gestation when the rates of embryonic and fetal cell replication are the most active, leading to various congenital malformations.

Conditions associated with smoking include hare lip and cleft palate, nervous system abnormalities and congenital heart defects.

ENVIRONMENTAL ISSUES

Toxins

Toxins can be divided into natural and manufactured. In both cases, they form part of the ecological system in which humans live and reproduce. Natural toxins have evolved alongside humans and a degree of mutual tolerance exists, allowing the interacting species to live together. Manufactured toxins have mainly been developed since the beginning of the industrial revolution and have not been present for sufficient time to allow tolerance to develop. These substances are increasingly causing concern to the public and to scientific researchers, leading to the setting up of international pressure groups such as Greenpeace.

Natural toxins

As poisons and teratogenic substances

Natural toxins are part of the ecological environment in which humans have always lived. It is probable that they were developed by plants as a defence against being eaten and examples include the tannins and alkaloids found in oak acorns. Acorns have often been eaten in desperation during famines and may have caused almost as many deaths as the famines themselves. Some plants make cyanide as part of their defence system. These include apple and apricot seeds and whilst the flesh is nutritious the seeds in quantity are poisonous. Cassava, the staple diet in some cultures, also contains cyanide but these toxins can be neutralised by special preparation and cooking.

Defence systems

Evolution can be seen as a competition for survival and members of the animal kingdom, including humans, have developed defence systems of their own against plant toxins. The first line of defence is avoidance mediated by the senses of sight, smell and taste. On the whole people avoid eating mouldy or rotten food as a defence against the toxins produced by bacteria and fungi. Penny Profet (1992), an American researcher, is very interested in evolutionary aspects of reproduction and has developed a theory to explain why 80% of pregnant women suffer from nausea and morning sickness during the early weeks of pregnancy. In particular, she mentions the aversion to bitter-tasting foods as a protection against possible teratogenic effects of naturally occurring toxins.

Despite sensory detection of toxins, some are hidden and the next line of defence is to expel ingested toxins from the body by vomiting and diarrhoea. People are very reluctant to eat foods that have previously affected them in that way and may develop a lifetime avoidance. In the stomach acids and enzymes play a part in neutralising some toxins. There are two other cellular defence mechanisms. Cells in the epithelial lining of the stomach secrete a thin layer of protective mucus to keep the toxins away. However, should the toxin breach this mucus layer and damage the cells, they are quickly replaced by the high turnover of epithelial tissue.

The role of the liver

The main organ responsible for the detoxification of ingested substances is the liver (see Chapter 22). Toxins that are absorbed by the gastrointestinal tract are taken via the portal vein directly to the liver where a wide range of enzymes can render them harmless. The detoxified substances can then be excreted via the kidneys. Dozens of naturally occurring toxins can be dealt with and many turn out to be useful as therapeutic drugs in the correct dose. This is only so if the amount is carefully controlled which is why herbal recipes may be dangerous. Examples include digitalis from the foxglove, which affects the heart rate and rhythm, opioids from the poppy and caffeine from the coffee bean, which affect the nervous system, and antibiotics produced by fungi which are lethal to bacteria.

Low levels of toxin

Plants tend to produce low levels of toxin, insufficient to have major effects on humans. The potato produces diazepam but in too small an amount to produce relaxation when eaten. There are two very interesting side issues to this. The first is the continuous bombardment of low levels but multiple types of toxin that would occur in a typical varied 'stone age' diet. Whilst many of the toxins are potentially damaging, some actually increase enzyme production in the liver. Johns (1990) believes that reducing the level of exposure to everyday toxins may reduce the preparedness of liver enzyme systems to a sudden toxic overload. Dietary diversification can help limit the risk of such an overload. Think how a diet of nothing but broccoli would affect you, even if you like broccoli in reasonable amounts!

With the development of society from about 10 000 years ago trends have conspired to increase our vulnerability to toxins in foods. Plants have been refined to contain fewer toxins than their wild ancestors and all cultivated brassicas are far less bitter than their wild cousins. At the same time the variety of different plants in the modern diet is much smaller than forest dwellers eat. Social learning plays an enormous part in what cultures find acceptable in their diets and people are often reluctant to eat foods that their parents did not give them.

Food preparation and toxins

Cooking and food preparation can make some toxic substances safe to eat. Nesse & Williams (1995) mention that the Pomo Indians of California detoxify acorns by cooking bread made from acorn meal in a type of red clay that binds sufficient tannin to make the food safe. Low levels of tannin taste good and may act as a mild central nervous system stimulant and in low amounts tannin may aid digestion by promoting the production of the proteolytic enzyme trypsin. However, cooking may produce new dangerous toxins. Meat has been cooked over open fires for many thousands of years and barbecued meat is very popular, but still the body cannot combat the carcinogenic toxins produced which may cause stomach cancer (Cooper 1992).

As contraceptives

Naturally occurring oestrogens are produced by plants and the effect may be to control the numbers of animals grazing on the plants. At least 20 such substances are known in over 300 plants, many of which are staple human foods such as wheat, oats, barley, rice, potatoes and soy beans. The contraceptive effect of this type of plant was recognised by the Greeks who advocated eating pomegranates to reduce fertility.

Manufactured toxins

The development of the chemical industry has resulted in contamination of the environment by vast quantities of synthetic pollutants such as DDT and polychlorinated biphenyls (PCBs) (Colborn et al 1996). We need to examine the effect of environmental toxins on the formation of the gametes. It must be pointed out that much of the data is new and needs more research. However, implications for changes in lifestyle may become apparent and at times worrying.

In the foreward to the book *Our Stolen Future* (Colborn et al 1996), Al Gore referred to the 30th anniversary edition of the book *Silent Spring* (Carson 1962). Carson was amongst the first to raise the issue of pollution and the effect on reproduction and the book led to the withdrawal of a class of pesticides called organochlorides such as DDT. In one of her last speeches she said:

> We are subjecting whole populations to exposure to chemicals which animal experiments have proved to be extremely poisonous and in many cases cumulative in their effects.
> These exposures now begin at or before birth and – unless we change our methods – will continue through the lifetime of those now living. No one knows what the results will be because we have no previous experience to guide us.

Scientists in America, including Theo Colborn, began to suspect that pesticides such as DDT and other chemical pollutants such as PCBs were disrupting sexual development by mimicking the effect of the female hormone oestrogen on tissues. The result was a feminisation of male reproductive organs across species of fish, reptiles, birds and mammals. The effect was seen on younger rather than older animals.

These chemicals were found in high levels in human blood and body fat and Colborn was shocked by the high levels found in human breast milk. She called them 'hand-me-down poisons' and warned that studies on the effects on humans should concentrate on children and younger people. Thirty years on, these chemicals are still pumped into the environment and are found in humans and in food. Many of them are not biodegradable and will linger as pollutants for a very long time. One of the most recent major concerns is the presence of phthalates in artificial baby milk and the possible risk of similar chemicals in breast milk.

Infertility in humans

Meanwhile, similar patterns of reproductive problems in humans began to alert medical and scientific researchers, although many failed to consider that humans share a common ancestry and environment with the rest of the animal kingdom. In 1992 Niels Skakkebaek at the University of Copenhagen found male reproductive problems such as reduced sperm counts with an increase in abnormal sperm and a threefold increase in the rate of testicular cancer in Denmark. A review of the literature, which included 61 studies of 15 000 men in 20 countries worldwide, indicated a 50% fall in sperm count between 1938 and 1990. The findings included the following.

1. The average male sperm count dropped 45% from 113 million per ml in the 1940s to 66 million per ml in 1990.
2. This drop was seen to occur in younger men; the younger the man, the lower the sperm count.
3. The average volume of ejaculate had dropped by 25%.

4 The number of men with an internationally agreed extremely low sperm count of under 20 million per ml had increased from 6% to 18%.

Possible culprits

At first, there was scepticism but recent research has confirmed these findings. Sharpe, at the Medical Research Council's Reproductive Biology Unit in Edinburgh, found similar problems and is of the opinion that prenatal events may be responsible. He believes that oestrogenic compounds affect fetal testes by preventing development of the full complement of Sertoli cells. This reduces sperm counts as the number of sperm produced depends on how many can be nurtured by Sertoli cells.

Vines (1995a) reviewed the effect of six industrially produced oestrogenic compounds:

- polycyclic aromatic hydrocarbons (PAHs);
- polychlorinated biphenyls (PCBs);
- dioxins;
- phthalates used in plastics, paints, inks and adhesives;
- breakdown products of alkylphenol polyethoxylates (APEs) used as surfactants in detergents (such as nonylphenol);
- organochlorine pesticides such as DDT, aldrin and dieldrin.

Oestrogenic mimics

Associated problems of oestrogenic compounds under investigation include:

- in men – increased incidence of prostatic cancer, undescended testicles and penile abnormalities such as hypospadias;
- in women – increased incidence of endometriosis and oestrogen-dependent breast cancer (an increase of 32% between 1980 and 1987 in America).

The final answer may be complex but oestrogenic compounds are probably an important factor. Some research is available to suggest that in children contaminated in utero there may be behavioural effects much more subtle than external sexual appearance. In North Carolina maternal breast milk levels were checked as a yardstick to measure likely exposure and children were found to have weaker reflexes, clumsier motor skills, poorer memories, attention deficit and higher aggression (Colborn et al 1996). Media attention so far has focused on the reduction of sperm volume in first world countries and other problems with male development and fertility which arise. There is less data available on female problems and children's behaviour.

Leaching from plastics

Accidental discoveries seem to be as important as targeted research in the attempt to find the chemical(s) likely to be responsible for the effect on male reproductive health. Soto and Sonnenschein (Soto et al 1991) were investigating growth inhibition in cell cultures and had set up an experiment to examine the role of oestrogen. They had cultures growing in various strengths of oestrogen including an oestrogen-free culture. When they examined the cultures, cell division had occurred in all of them at an unprecedented rate. This happened again when the experiment was repeated and the scientists suspected that the dishes holding the cultures must be acting as an oestrogenic source. Although the plastics manufacturer was reluctant to say which chemicals were used in the manufacture of the dishes, nonylphenol was found to be leaching out of the plastic into the tissue culture. This oestrogen-acting compound was widely used in domestic cleaners but many countries have banned its use. Others will discontinue it in the year 2000. Similarly bisphenol-A has been found to leach from polycarbonates. It is difficult to say how important this is but these substances, unlike naturally occurring oestrogens, are not biodegradable.

River pollution

In Britain anglers became aware that it was difficult to tell the sex of fish that they caught. Most fish appeared to be female or to have some female characteristics. Sumpter of Brunel University found that male fish were producing huge quantities of a substance called vitellogenin necessary for egg production, normally only produced by females in response to ovarian release of oestrogen (Sumpter & Jobling 1995). At first Sumpter postulated that oestrogens in the urine of women taking the contraceptive pill were to blame but no trace of these was found in the water. Having read of the findings of Soto and Sonnenschein, he decided that nonylphenol entering the rivers in detergents was responsible. This is not yet confirmed and now Sumpter thinks a wider range of chemicals acting together may be responsible. Another source of bisphenol-A is found in the plastic lining of food cans.

Unto the third generation

Perhaps the most important message is that environmental factors are equally as important as genes in gametogenesis and fetal development. The more rapidly developing cells will be the most affected. It is important to realise the need to consider the effect over three generations. The ova of today's childbearing woman were developed whilst she was still in her own mother's uterus, as were the numbers of Sertoli cells currently present in the testicles of today's prospective fathers.

Data given by Colborn et al (1996) show the importance of taking these findings seriously and acting quickly. Around the world 100 000 synthetic chemicals are on sale. Some banned in developed countries, such as DDT, are still used in the third world countries. This amount is being increased by 1000 new chemicals a year. Worldwide use of pesticides is increasing annually so that the problem is likely to be with us for years ahead. Colborn et al state:

> Wildlife data, laboratory experiments, the DES experience and a handful of human studies support the possibility of physical and behavioural disruption in humans that could affect fertility, learning ability, aggression and conceivably even parenting and mating behaviour.

Heavy metals

Lead

Lead has been known to be toxic to the fetus for at least 100 years. McCloy (1989) reminds us that the United Kingdom Lead Regulations (HMSO 1985a) legislate for 'a woman of reproductive capacity to be withdrawn from work which exposes her to a specific blood level of lead (40 micrograms per 100 ml)' and for pregnant women to be suspended from any work involving exposure to lead. Day (1996) quotes Jamieson of the National Institute of Environmental Health Sciences (NIEHS) who stated that 'a girl growing up in a lead-polluted environment might years later pass that lead on to her offspring'. Lead is stored in the bones and may reenter the woman's bloodstream and so the fetus, along with calcium mobilised from bone to supply fetal skeletal needs. Exposure to lead in early life is known to affect mental development.

Mercury

Organic mercury was shown to be exceedingly toxic when methyl mercury was discharged into the Minamata Bay area of Japan. The mercury entered the food chain in fish and Nelson (1971) reported that 6% of all births resulted in children with severe neurological abnormalities resembling cerebral palsy. Bradley and Bennett (1995) stated that there is a 'major controversy ... containing mercury-containing amalgams used in dentistry'. Women desiring to become pregnant or who are already pregnant should avoid dental work involving mercury amalgams.

Radiation

Radiation can be divided into ionising radiation, such as is emitted by X-rays, nuclear medicine and atomic weapons testing, and non-ionising radiation, emitted as ultraviolet and infrared rays and by microwaves. Visual display units are now widely used in both home and workplace and release low levels of mixed wavelength radiation.

Ionising radiation

Ionising radiation has the ability to damage DNA by transferring its energy into living cells (Jones 1996). Atoms lose electrons and develop an electric charge. These charged particles can penetrate the body and damage molecules, producing free radicals and oxidising agents which break and destroy the DNA chain. An intense dose can kill cells during their actively dividing state. This function of radiation is useful against the rapidly dividing cells of a cancer.

Diagnostic X-ray

Because of the known dangers of radiation during childbearing years, X-ray examinations of the abdomen, pelvis or hips of women should only be made during the 10 days following a menstrual period to avoid irradiating the early embryo. Modern techniques of shorter wavelength X-rays, as well as shielding the gonads of both men and women whenever possible during diagnostic X-rays, are helpful in preventing possible damage to ovum and sperm. Radiology during pregnancy has been much reduced because of the development of new ultrasound techniques (Proud 1996).

Natural radiation

Humans are exposed to low-level natural background radiation. Edwards (1996) quotes Neilson of Brunel University who believes this low-level radiation, stemming mainly from natural γ-radiation from uranium in the ground, may be more dangerous than originally thought. High doses are statistically associated with deaths from anaemia, respiratory infections, diseases of the nervous system and problems at birth. In England and Wales, high levels are more likely to people in Cornwall, South Yorkshire, Northumberland, Tyne and Wear, West Glamorgan and Derbyshire. However, the National Radiological Protection Board, which advises the British government, has been critical of the statistical relevance of Neilson's findings.

Risks of radiation

Can radiation damage actively maturing sperm and ovum and the rapidly dividing cells of the fetus? Fetuses were found to be very sensitive to radiation when many of the babies of mothers who had survived the atomic bomb were born dead or deformed. Pochin (1988) states that the critical exposure time seems to be between 8 and 15 weeks post conception. Bithell & Stewart (1975) found a link between prenatal irradiation of the fetus and childhood leukaemia. The United Kingdom Ionising Radiations Regulations (HMSO 1985b) legislated dose limits for women 'of reproductive capacity' and for the 'abdomen of a pregnant woman who is at work'.

Whilst the rapidly developing fetus is known to be at risk, the Radiation Effects Research Foundation has checked the children of Japanese bomb survivors and found no evidence to indicate genetic damage to the gametes of those exposed to radiation (Jones 1996). There has been no sign of damaged chromosomes amongst children conceived after the bomb had fallen. No new mutations have been found but leukaemia, lung cancer and particularly thyroid cancer have increased amongst bomb survivors. It had been known since the discovery of X-rays that radiation could cause cancer and Marie Curie, who carried radium around in her pocket, died of cancer.

The atom bomb

Jones (1996) discussed what has been described as the 'most cynical scientific experiment ever' – the dropping of atom bombs on Hiroshima and Nagasaki in Japan on 6 August 1945. The Atomic Bomb Casualty Commission, set up in 1947 and now renamed the Radiation Effects Research Foundation, has studied the long-term effects of ionising radiation on bomb survivors and their children.

Many science fiction stories about life after a nuclear holocaust painted a picture of a severely malformed population where each child conceived was born with horrific appearance. This fear of damaged sperm and ova has been a legitimate concern and Japanese people do not find it easy to accept reassurances that this scenario will not happen. Even with the evidence against such gamete damage, it is still a concern.

Chernobyl

Is there any evidence from other nuclear accidents such as Chernobyl in 1986? Scherbak (1996) calls this 'the worst technogenic environmental disaster in history'. Following the explosion, hot air carried fission products far more reactive than uranium and plutonium into the atmosphere. Amongst the most dangerous were iodine 131, strontium 90 and caesium 137. These travelled thousands of miles to the North and West, affecting The Ukraine, Russia, Poland, Sweden, Germany,

Turkey, Great Britain and the USA. The immediate effects mirrored the Japanese bombings with radiation burns and sickness. Children were immediately evacuated and villages within a 30 kilometre range have been abandoned. Greenpeace Ukraine estimate there have been 32 000 deaths.

A long-term problem has been deficient immunity with reduced numbers of natural killer cells, which tend to attack tumours and virally infected cells. The syndrome has been nicknamed 'Chernobyl AIDS'. Results have been increased rates of leukaemia, cancer, cardiac conditions and common respiratory tract infections. Iodine 131 has a short half-life of only 8 days compared to years for strontium 90 and caesium 137. Exposure to iodine 131 caused children to develop chronic inflammation of the thyroid gland and many are developing thyroid cancer.

Scherbak reports that scientists found that one-third of the workers who attempted to contain the explosion, mainly men in their 30s, have developed sexual or reproductive disorders, including impotence and sperm abnormalities with reduced fertilising capacity of the sperm. There has also been an increase in the number of pregnancies with complications.

To summarise the above findings, radiation has its worst effect on the DNA of rapidly dividing cells. This includes the spermatozoa, the ovum in the early menstrual cycle and the early embryo, as well as tissues that divide rapidly such as skin cells and epithelial linings.

Non-ionising radiation

Non-ionising rays include ultraviolet, infrared, lasers, microwaves, radar and radiofrequency waves. The relation of the incidence of leukaemia to electromagnetic fields produced by high-voltage power lines and transformer stations is currently being researched. Nordstrum (1983) found that men working near high-voltage systems fathered more congenitally malformed children than would be expected. This may indicate an increased level of mutation in the DNA carried by their sperm. The government is at last beginning to take the problem seriously (personal discussion, G. Stables 1997).

Many people are now exposed to visual display units (VDUs) at work and at home. VDUs may release low levels of radiation including X-rays, microwaves, ultraviolet and infrared light. McCloy (1989) summarised the work done in the 1970s and 1980s, finding no consistent evidence for any link between reproductive risk and VDU emissions. However, some studies have revealed clusters of effects including increased miscarriages, stillbirths and congenital defects. Interpretation of these studies is complicated by the possible effects of work stress as some of the women worked uninterrupted for long periods of time.

Microwaves have also been implicated in causing Down's syndrome in the children of men exposed to microwaves. It is necessary to indicate that research into these issues is far from convincing and it is difficult to isolate the effect of non-ionising radiation from other environmental hazards but it should be considered carefully by couples wishing to begin a family. Safeguards such as the distance of the person from the equipment and the length of time spent at the equipment should be discussed. Further research is ongoing and better designed protocols may result in clearer risk identification.

Summary of main points

- Following conception there is a gap of at least 10 weeks before many women present themselves for professional care. By this time organogenesis is mostly complete and advice on healthy living may be too late. Research suggests that pregnancy outcome is improved markedly when couples are screened and advised prior to conception.
- The continuously produced sperm are most at risk of environmental insult. The ova are in a state of arrested development and are relatively resistant to mutagenic damage until just prior to ovulation. Following fertilisation, the zygote becomes resistant to genetic injury whilst undergoing cleavage. After 16 days a period of intense organogenesis begins and sensitivity is high but so few cells are present that if the fetus is affected it will be aborted spontaneously.
- Preconception care should include taking the history of both man and woman, a clinical examination to ensure that there are no hidden health problems, a gynaecological examination of the woman and screening of blood and urine and possibly hair, stool and semen analysis.
- Any infections should be treated, dietary problems discussed and possible work and lifestyle hazards considered. Long-term health problems should be stabilised prior to conception. In other conditions which are treated with known teratogenic drugs, such as epilepsy, a discussion of the risks and possible alteration of treatment may be necessary.
- The age of the prospective parents could be important as the frequency of all reproductive problems, including the incidence of chromosome abnormalities, increases with maternal age. Some couples may be anxious to discuss their risk of inherited conditions and may need referring to genetic counsellors.
- In developed countries malnutrition is rare except in people with eating disorders such as anorexia nervosa. However, suboptimal dietary deficiencies are common. Some cultures may inadvertently suffer from dietary deficits because of associated religious food restrictions. Prepared and processed foods make up a large part of the normal diet in Great Britain.
- Processing may destroy essential nutrients whilst chemical additives such as preservatives, artificial colourings and flavourings are added to increase the shelf-life of the food and to increase its attractiveness for purchasers. A growing concern is the increase in food allergy with possible sensitisation of the fetus in utero.
- Excessive weight is probably due to a combined problem of the ingestion of too many calories and diminished amount of exercise brought about by labour-saving devices in the home and increased car transport. Prepregnancy weight is known to influence pregnancy outcome. Women who are outside the optimal weight range may develop amenorrhoea and infertility.
- Commensal organisms live in and on the human body and are helpful. However, many organisms are pathogenic and cause infection and damage to the individual. Some of the most virulent pathogens may kill. Systemic infections may cause reproductive problems such as infertility and congenital defects. Vaccination should be offered, if available, or advice on how to minimise the risk of infection during pregnancy.
- Drugs may damage sperm or ova. They may have an adverse effect on nutrient absorption so that essential nutrients are absent at crucial times during embryonic development. They may be teratogenic,

adversely affecting the fetus by interfering in normal growth and development.

- Tobacco smoking concerns the inhalation of smoke for its pharmaceutical and psychoactive effects. Smoking amongst the population of Europe and now Africa and Asia has spread, mainly because of the rapid effects of nicotine on the central nervous system. Thousands of other chemicals are inhaled in cigarette smoke and many have been shown to cross the placenta to damage the developing fetus.
- Toxins, natural or manufactured, form part of the ecological system in which humans live and reproduce. Natural toxins have evolved alongside humans and a degree of mutual tolerance exists, including human defence systems against plant toxins. The first line of defence is avoidance mediated by the senses of sight, smell and taste. The next line of defence is to expel toxins by vomiting and diarrhoea. People are reluctant to eat foods that have previously affected them in that way.
- Manufactured toxins have mainly been developed since the beginning of the industrial revolution and there has been insufficient time for tolerance to develop. These substances cause concern to the public and to scientific researchers. The main organ responsible for the detoxification of ingested substances is the liver and detoxified substances are excreted via the kidneys.
- Cooking and food preparation make some toxic substances safe to eat but cooking may produce new dangerous toxins. Carcinogenic toxins may be produced which may cause stomach cancer. Low levels of tannin act as a mild central nervous system stimulant. Tannin in low amounts may aid digestion by promoting the production of the proteolytic enzyme trypsin.
- Naturally occurring oestrogens are produced by plants to control the numbers of animals grazing on the plants. At least 20 such substances are known in over 300 plants, many of which are staple human foods.
- The development of the chemical industry has resulted in release into the environment of vast quantities of synthetic materials. These may be disrupting sexual development by mimicking the effect of the female hormone oestrogen, resulting in a feminisation of both animal and human male reproductive organs.
- Associated problems of oestrogenic compounds include, in men, increased incidence of prostatic cancer, undescended testicles and penile abnormalities such as hypospadias and, in women, increased incidence of endometriosis and oestrogen-dependent breast cancer.
- Scientists suspected that plastic dishes holding cultures they were studying were an oestrogenic source. Nonylphenol was found to be leaching out of the plastic into the tissue culture. In Britain anglers became aware of a problem in telling the sex of fish. Most fish appeared to be female or to have female characteristics. Nonylphenol in detergents poured into rivers may be responsible.
- Environmental factors are important in gametogenesis and fetal development. It is important to look back over three generations. The ova of today's childbearing woman were developed whilst she was still in her own mother's uterus, as were the numbers of Sertoli cells currently present in the testicles of today's prospective fathers.
- The heavy metals lead and mercury are exceedingly toxic to the developing nervous system of the fetus and young child.
- Ionising radiation has the ability to damage DNA, the blueprint for cellular structure and activity, by transferring its energy into living cells. Humans are exposed to low-level natural background radiation from radon gas. Fetuses are very sensitive to radiation. Many babies of mothers who survived the atomic bomb were born dead or deformed. The critical exposure time may be between 8 and 15 weeks of development.
- The Radiation Effects Research Foundation checked the children of Japanese bomb survivors, finding no evidence to indicate genetic damage to the gametes of those exposed to radiation. Leukaemia, lung cancer and particularly thyroid cancer have increased amongst the bomb survivors.
- Following nuclear accidents such as occurred at Chernobyl in 1986, hot air carried highly reactive fission products into the atmosphere. Scientists found that one-third of the men who attempted to contain the explosion have developed sexual or reproductive disorders including impotence, sperm abnormalities and reduced fertilising capacity.
- Non-ionising rays include ultraviolet, infrared, lasers, microwaves, radar and radiofrequency waves. Electromagnetic fields produced by high-voltage power lines are currently being researched in relation to leukaemia. Men working near high-voltage systems were found to father more congenitally malformed children than would be expected, possibly indicating an increased level of mutation in the DNA carried by their sperm.
- VDUs may release low levels of radiation. Some studies have revealed clusters of effects including increased miscarriages, stillbirths and congenital defects. Microwaves have also been implicated in causing Down's syndrome in the children of men exposed to microwaves. Research into these issues is not convincing but should be considered carefully by couples wishing to begin a family.

References

Abercrombie M, Hickman M, Johnson ML, Thain M. 1992 New Penguin Dictionary of Biology, 8th edn. Penguin, Harmondsworth.

Barnes B. 1995 Hair Mineral analysis, supplementation and cleansing. In Bradley SG, Bennett N (Eds) Preparation for pregnancy Argyll Publishing, Argyll.

Bithell JF, Stewart AM. 1975 Prenatal irradiation and childhood malignancy: a review of British data from the Oxford survey. British Journal of Cancer 31, 271–287.

Bouchard C. 1991 Heredity and the path to overweight and obesity. Medicine and Science in Sport and Exercise 23(3), 285–291.

Bradley SG, Bennett N. 1995 Preparation for Pregnancy. Argyll publishing, Argyll.

Carson R. 1962 Silent Spring. Houghton Mifflin, Boston.

Chamberlain G. 1992 ABC of Antenatal Care. BMJ Books, London.

Colborn T, Myers JP, Dumanoski D. 1996 Our Stolen Future. Little, Brown, Boston.

Cooper GM. 1992 Elements of Human Cancer. Jones and Bartlett, Boston.

Dallison J, Lobstein T. 1995 Poor Expectations. Poverty and Undernourishment in Pregnancy. The Maternity Alliance, London.

Day M. 1996 Past lead pollution poisons unborn children. New Scientist, 150(2038) p 4.

Edwards R. 1996 Natural radiation may kill thousands. New Scientist, 150 (2031) pp 4.

Evans HJ, Fletcher J, Torrance M, Hardgreave TB. 1981 Sperm abnormalities and cigarette smoking. Lancet 1, 627–629.

HMSO 1985a Control of Lead at Work Regulations 1980: Approved Code of Practice – Control of Lead at Work. HMSO, London.

HMSO 1985b The Ionising Radiations Regulations (SI 1985 No 1333). HMSO, London

Jick H, Porter J, Morrison AS. 1977 Relation between smoking and age of natural menopause. Lancet 1, 1354–1355.

Johns T. 1990 With Bitter Herbs They Shall Eat It. University of Arizona Press, Tucson.

Jones S. 1996 In the Blood: God, Genes and Destiny. HarperCollins, London.

McCloy EC. 1989 Work, environment and the fetus. Midwifery 5, 53–62.

Miller WC. 1991 Diet composition, energy intake and nutritional status in relation to obesity in men and women. Medicine and Science in Sport and Exercise 23 (3), 280–284.

Nelson N. 1971 Hazards of mercury. Environmental Research 4, 1–69.

Nesse RM, Williams GC. 1995 Evolution and Healing. Weidenfeld and Nicolson, London.

Nordstrum S. 1983 Genetic defects in offspring of power-frequency workers. Bioelectromagnetics 5 p 91.

Pochin EE. 1988 Radiation and mental retardation. British Medical Journal 297, 154–156.

Profet M. 1992 Pregnancy sickness as adaptation: a deterrent to maternal ingestion of teratogens. In Barkow J, Cosmides L, Tooby J (eds) The Adapted Mind: Evolutionary Psychology and the Generation of Culture. Oxford University Press, New York, pp 327–365.

Proud J. 1996 Specialised antenatal investigations. In Bennett VR, Brown LK (eds) Myles Textbook for Midwives Churchill Livingstone Edinburgh: 660–674.

Scherbak YM. 1996 Ten years of the Chernobyl era. Scientific American, 1274(4) 32–37.

Soto A, Justicia H, Wray J, Sonnenschein C. 1991 p-Nonylphenol: an estrogenic xenobiotic released from 'modified polystyrene'. Environmental Health Perspectives 92, 167–173.

Sumpter J, Jobling S. 1995 Vitellogenesis as a biomarker for oestrogen contamination of the aquatic environment. Proceedings of the Estrogens in the Environment Conference.

Tuormaa TE. 1994 The adverse effects of tobacco smoking on reproduction. Foresight. AB Academic Publishers. Tacoma, Washington.

Vines G. 1995a Some of our sperm are missing. New Scientist, 147(1992), 22–25.

Vines G. 1995b Fighting fat with feeling. New Scientist, 147(1987), 14–15.

Ward NI. 1995 Preconceptional care and pregnancy outcome. Journal of Nutritional and Environmental Medicine 5, 205–208.

Recommended reading

Carlsen E, Giwercman A, Keiding N, Skakkebaek N. 1992 Evidence for decreasing quality of semen during past 50 years. British Medical Journal 305, 609–613.

Colborn T, Myers JP, Dumanoski D. 1996 Our Stolen Future. Little, Brown, Boston.

Dallison J, Lobstein T. 1995 Poor Expectations. Poverty and Undernourishment in Pregnancy. The Maternity Alliance, London.

Doughty S. 1996 AIDS is no risk to most, admit gays. Daily Mail, 20.6, p 2.

Jones S. 1996 In the Blood. God, Genes and Destiny. HarperCollins, London.

McCloy EC. 1989 Work, environment and the fetus. Midwifery 5, 53–62.

Nesse RM, Williams GC. 1995 Evolution and Healing. Weidenfeld and Nicolson, London.

Ward NI. 1995 Preconceptional care and pregnancy outcome. Journal of Nutritional and Environmental Medicine 5, 205–208.

Section 2A

PREGNANCY – THE FETUS

Section contents

The care of the childbearing woman now includes complex screening tests for fetal wellbeing. The midwife must have knowledge and experience of these procedures in order to inform clients. This section is concerned with the development and growth of the fetus, placenta and membranes. Chapters 8 to 15 cover the important subject of embryology and feto-placental development. The topic is presented in some detail because developments in infertility treatment and treatment of fetal abnormalities are expanding rapidly. The style is easy to follow and the diagrams clarify three-dimensional developmental concepts. Chapter 8 discusses general points about development, chapters 9 and 10 examine the development of individual systems, chapter 11 looks in detail at the important fetal organ, the placenta and chapter 12 explores the nature of amniotic fluid.

Chapter 13 explores fetal growth and development whilst chapter 14 discusses some common fetal problems. Finally the very important topic of causes and management of some of the more common congenital abnormalities is discussed in chapter 15.

Chapter

8 General embryology

In this chapter

INTRODUCTION

This section of the book is concerned with the developmental processes that take the human from one fertilised cell to a fetus ready to be born and survive. The theories and general principles of embryology, as far as current science can explain them, will be outlined in this chapter. In Chapter 9 the processes involved in the development of the skeletal system will be outlined and Chapter 10 will discuss the development of the internal organs. Chapter 11 examines the structure and function of the placenta whilst Chapter 12 considers the nature of amniotic fluid. Chapters 13 and 14 discuss the nature of fetal growth and fetal problems. The section ends with Chapter 15, a discussion of congenital abnormalities and what happens when the processes go wrong.

Human embryology involves the study of human development. As more is discovered about the disciplines of developmental biology, molecular biology and genetics, it becomes difficult to separate them. There is much overlap and a need for researchers to share information. Discoveries about the nature of development in the human embryo are gained from research into the development of other species. There are similarities and parallels can be drawn but little is known about the development of the human embryo because of the problem of unethical experimentation.

The Human Fertilisation and Embryology Act (HMSO 1990) laid down strict prohibitions in connection with embryos and states that:

> A licence cannot authorise keeping or using an embryo after the appearance of the primitive streak … the primitive streak … is to be taken to have appeared in an embryo not later than the end of the period of 14 days beginning with the day when the gametes are mixed, not counting any time during which the embryo is stored.

Why study embryology?

One good reason for understanding embryology is that light is cast on the possible causes of congenital abnormalities that are present in about 6% of live births, half of which are detectable at birth and most of the others during the first year of life (Fitzgerald & Fitzgerald 1994). Malformations vary from minor to major in their effects on the well-being and health of the individual. At least half of all conceptuses are malformed but in most cases these lead to spontaneous abortions.

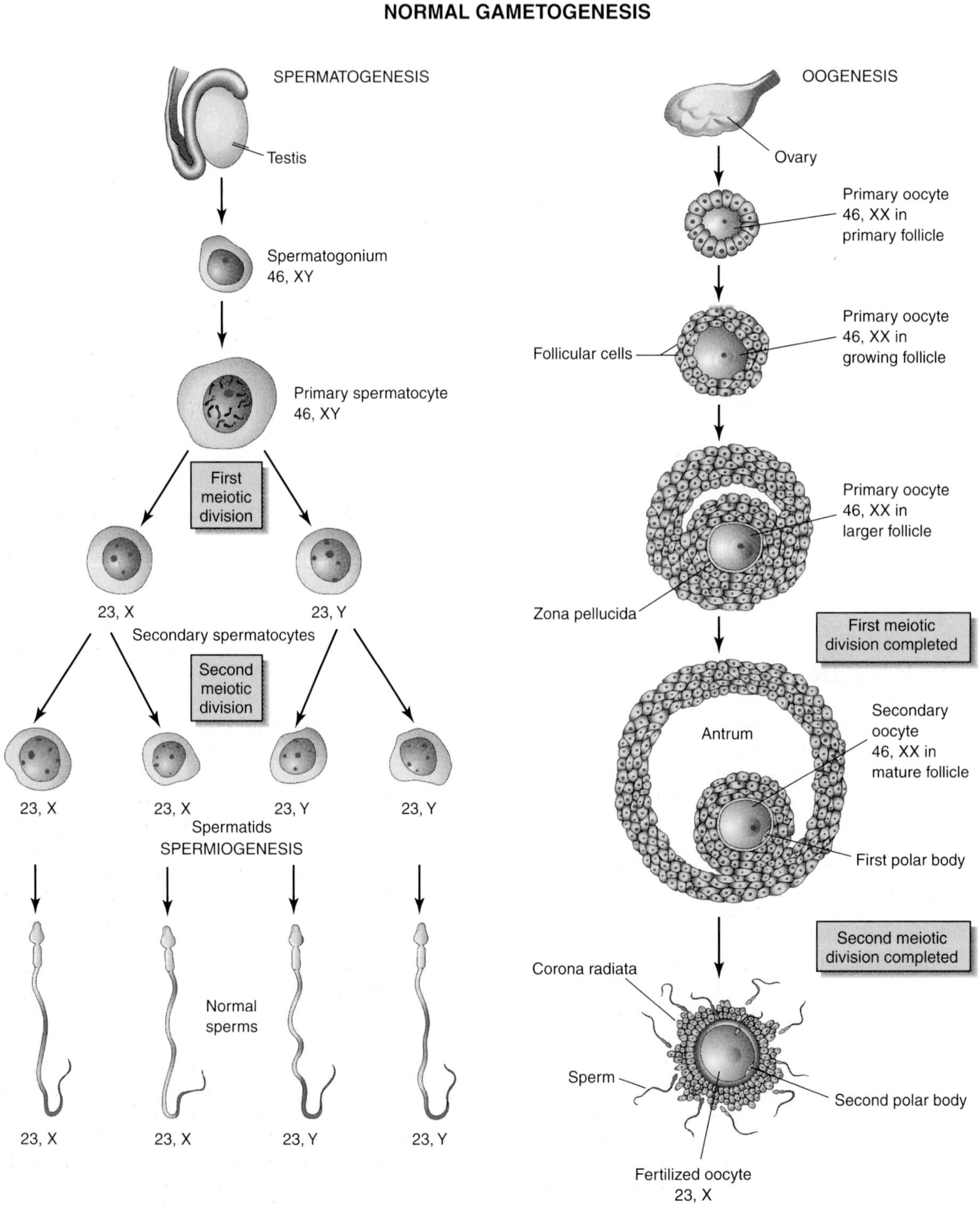

Figure 8.1 *Normal gametogenesis. (Reproduced with permission from Moore 1989.)*

GAMETOGENESIS

Meiosis

In Chapter 2 the concept of mitosis, by which every daughter cell is assured of its full complement of 46 chromosomes during cell division, was discussed. Following fertilisation of an ovum by a sperm, the resulting zygote must have 46 chromosomes and therefore the gametes must undergo a process of halving of the chromosomes before they are mature. This process is called reduction division or meiosis and at the end of it each ovum or sperm will have 23 chromosomes, one from each pair. The immature germ cells, i.e. the primary spermatocyte and the primary oocyte, have the usual complement of 46 chromosomes. This is called the **diploid number**. Meiosis consists of two cell divisions, resulting in the reduction of the diploid number of chromosomes to the **haploid number** of chromosomes (23) found in the mature sperm and ovum (Fig. 8.1).

Meiosis allows the independent assortment of maternal and paternal chromosomes amongst the gametes. It also allows crossing over by relocating segments of the maternal and paternal chromosomes. This 'shuffles' the genes, producing recombination of genetic material. Each gamete is a mixture of its owner's maternal and paternal genes. Therefore at fertilisation a zygote is produced which has a mixture of genes from its mother and father and its grandparents. The production of ova and spermatozoa by meiosis differs in the number of gametes produced, resulting in only one mature ovum but four sperm.

Oogenesis

The ova have been present as primary oocytes in the woman's ovaries since she was a developing embryo in her mother's uterus. Oogenesis is the process of transforming oocytes into ova. It begins before a woman's birth but is not completed until after puberty and is a recurring process in each menstrual cycle. By the time a baby girl is born all her primary oocytes have undergone the prophase of the first meiotic division (meiosis 1).

The ovarian cycle is divided into two parts – a preovulatory phase in which the follicles develop (the **follicular phase**) and, following ovulation, the ovary enters the **luteal phase**. The first 4–6 days of the follicular phase coincide with menstruation. As a follicle begins to mature the follicular epithelium develops into cuboid granulosa cells. This occurs in a few primordial follicles in each ovary during the luteal phase of the preceding cycle. Cell division results in a multilayered follicle and a clear zone, the **zona pellucida**, laid down between the ovum and its surrounding epithelium.

Just before ovulation, with maturation of the ovum (Fig. 8.2), the first meiotic division is completed (Fig. 8.3). This results in a secondary oocyte, which receives most of the cytoplasm, and a non-functional cell called the **first polar body**. The secondary oocyte receives 23 chromosomes, all carrying an X chromosome, and the first polar body receives the other 23 chromosomes but degenerates. At ovulation the secondary oocyte now begins the second meiotic division but becomes arrested in metaphase of secondary meiosis (Fig. 8.4). If penetrated by a sperm this division completes and one mature ovum with a second polar body results. This second polar body also degenerates.

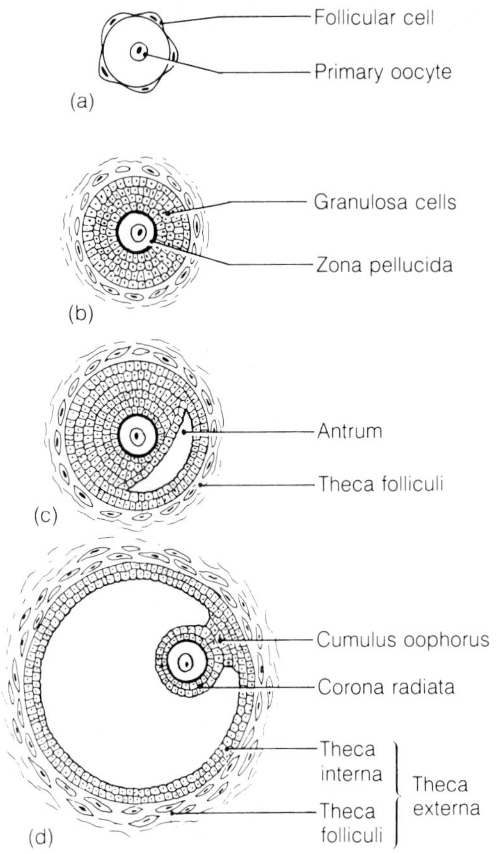

Figure 8.2 *The stages of development in the follicle: (a) primordial follicle, (b) primary follicle, (c) secondary follicle, (d) Graafian follicle (from Hinchliff SM, Montague SE, 1990, with permission).*

Spermatogenesis

The production of spermatozoa occurs in the seminiferous tubules of the testes. Seminiferous tubules contain two types of cell: the germ cells and the Sertoli cells. Primary germ cells are dormant in the testis from the fetal period of life and begin to increase in number at puberty. In a functioning testis germ cells will be present at various stages of development, all originating from spermatogonia. Spermatogonia divide by mitosis continuously to ensure a constant supply of cells maturing towards spermatozoa. After undergoing several mitotic divisions, they mature, become larger and are known as **primary spermatocytes** which contain 46 chromosomes (23 pairs) and are therefore diploid cells.

Primary spermatocytes undergo the first meiotic division to form two secondary spermatocytes which have only 23 chromosomes, one of each pair. Half will receive the X chromosome of the male cell genotype and half will receive the Y chromosome. Secondary meiosis results in four haploid cells called **spermatids**. The spermatids are found in close association with Sertoli cells – polymorphic cells attached to a basement membrane but extending into the lumen of the seminiferous

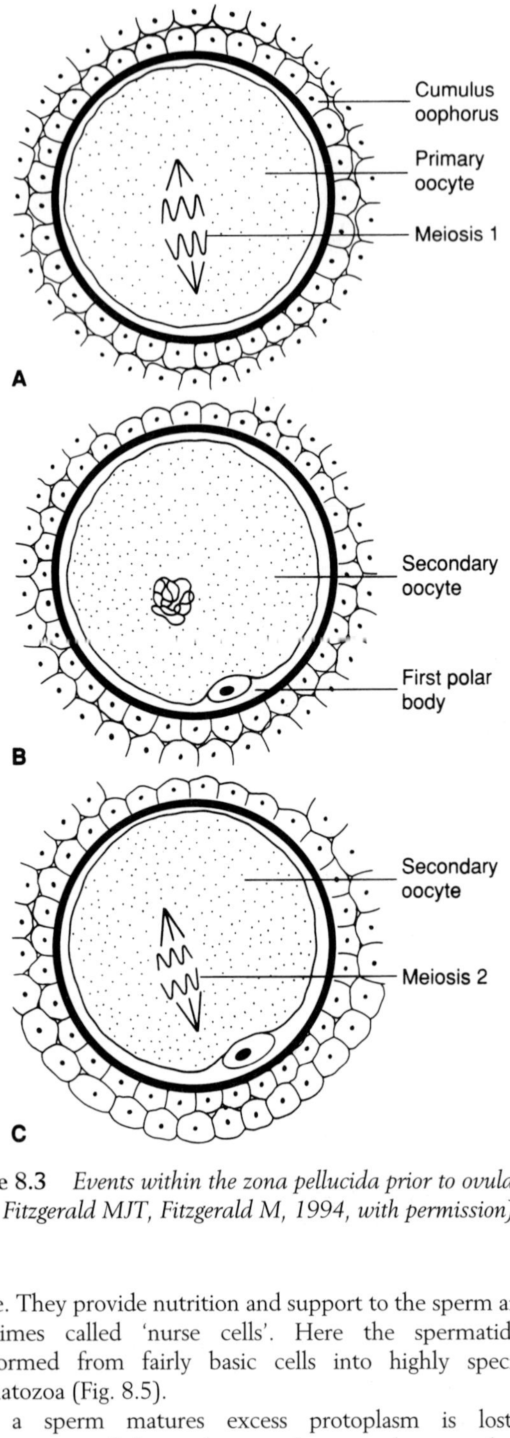

Figure 8.3 *Events within the zona pellucida prior to ovulation (from Fitzgerald MJT, Fitzgerald M, 1994, with permission).*

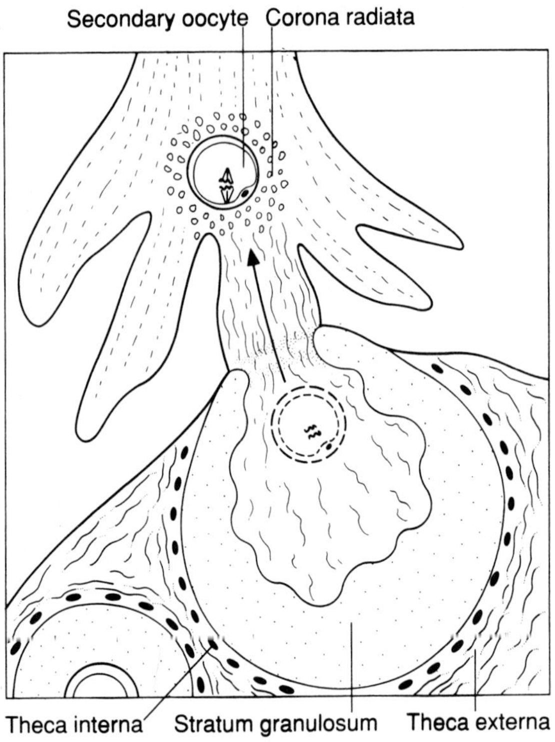

Figure 8.4 *Ovulation (from Fitzgerald MJT, Fitzgerald M, 1994, with permission).*

tubule. They provide nutrition and support to the sperm and are sometimes called 'nurse cells'. Here the spermatids are transformed from fairly basic cells into highly specialised spermatozoa (Fig. 8.5).

As a sperm matures excess protoplasm is lost and the chromatin of the nucleus condenses to become the head of the spermatozoon. One centriole develops into the tail which is composed of a central filament of two microfibrils surrounded by a circle of nine fibrils. Mitochondria aggregate into the neck region and the Golgi apparatus helps to form the acrosome cap which develops over the head of the sperm and contains enzymes called hyaluronidases and proteases (Fig. 8.6). The process takes about 70 days and several hundred million a day are produced continuously from puberty. However, as men become older the seminal tubules do undergo involution and by 70 years extensive atrophy may be present. Germ cells may have been reduced in number but the Sertoli cells remain.

Gamete size

The oocyte is a very large cell and usually only one is released at ovulation. It must contain all the material necessary for the beginning of growth and development of the embryo following fertilisation. In sharp contrast, during their development sperm lose most of their cytoplasm. They are very small and millions of them are released during ejaculation. About 1000 of the ejaculated sperm will reach the ovum (oocyte) and these will all be needed to allow just one to enter. When one male sperm enters a secondary oocyte the first cell of a new human being, with the full complement of 46 chromosomes, is formed. This is called a **zygote** and is a very large cell, just visible to the unaided eye.

FERTILISATION

Capacitation

Freshly ejaculated sperm are unable to fertilise a secondary oocyte and must undergo a process of maturation called capacitation whilst travelling through the female genital tract. This usually occurs in the uterus or uterine tubes. Glycoproteins are removed from the surface of the acrosome. When a capacitated sperm meets the corona radiata of the oocyte the

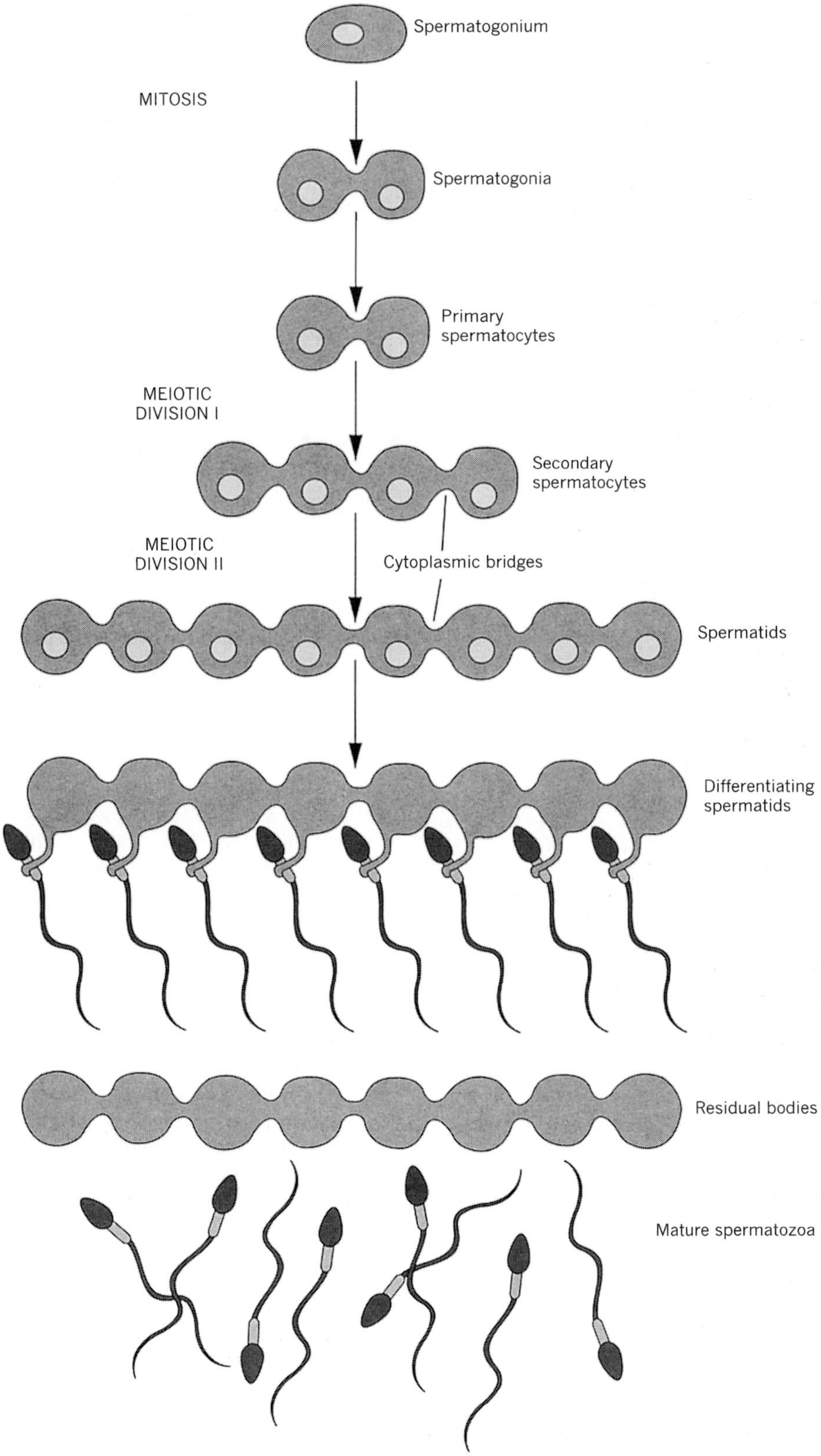

Figure 8.5 *The progeny of a single maturing spermatogonium remain connected to one another by cytoplasmic bridges throughout their differentiation into mature sperm. (Reproduced with permission from Alberts et al 1994.)*

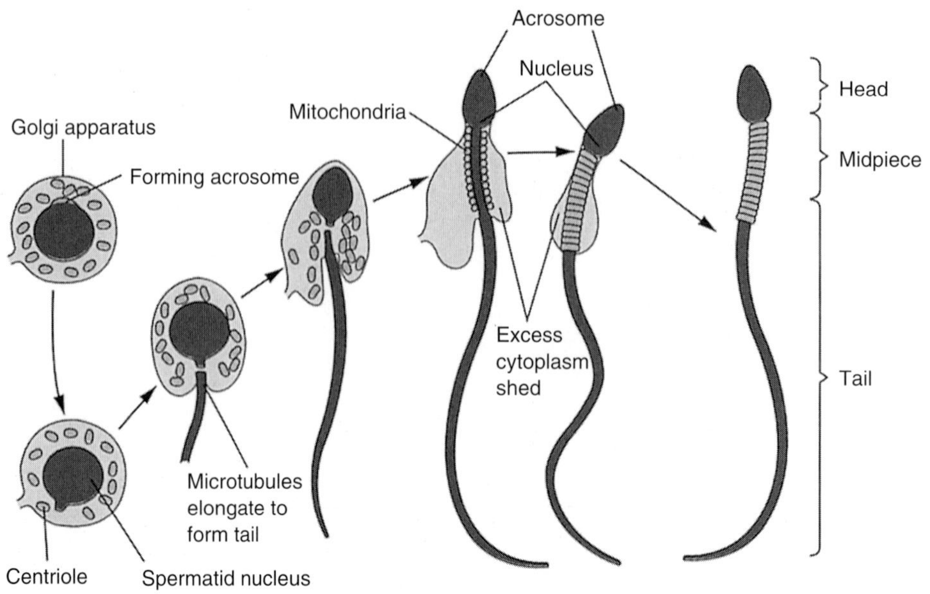

Figure 8.6 *Sperm formation. (Reproduced with permission from Chiras 1991.)*

acrosome develops perforations in it. This is known as the **acrosome reaction**.

The acrosome reaction

Binding of a sperm to the zona pellucida of the oocyte is species specific. Lytic (digestive) enzymes such as hyaluronidase are released around the oocyte and it takes the enzymes from many sperm to create a passageway for one sperm to enter. These enzymes disperse the follicular cells of the corona radiata, allowing the head of the sperm to make contact with the zona pellucida. Other enzymes, one of which is acrosin, are now released and these produce an opening in the zona pellucida. This is followed by fusion of the sperm cell membrane with the oocyte cell membrane and the nucleus of one sperm passes into the oocyte (Fig. 8.7). This occurs in the ampulla of the fallopian tube.

Blocks to polyspermy

The ability of the oocyte to fuse with the sperm must immediately be reversed following entry of the first sperm, to prevent the entry of multiple sperm (**polyspermy**). This ensures that the fertilised oocyte will contain only 46 chromosomes. There are two mechanisms by which entry of more sperm is prevented.

Fast block

The oocyte plasma membrane electrical resting potential is normally negatively charged at –70 millivolts (mV), a potential that sperm can readily fuse with. Immediately after the entry of one sperm this rises to become positively charged at +20 mV. The entry of the sperm opens sodium channels in the cell membrane and extra sodium ions which carry a positive charge are allowed into the oocyte cytoplasm. Sperm are now prevented from entering the oocyte. However, this reaction is brief and resting potential soon returns to the normal –70 mV.

Slow block (cortical reaction)

The brief depolarisation described above has two other effects. First, it allows subcortical granules lying just under the oocyte plasma membrane to rupture and release chemicals which bind water into the cytoplasm. The oocyte swells and detaches any remaining sperm in contact with it. Second, the secondary oocyte is activated to complete the second meiotic division and expel the second polar body and the ovum is now mature. Its nucleus is now called the **female pronucleus**. Once the head of the sperm enters the cytoplasm of the ovum, it enlarges to form the **male pronucleus**. The male and female pronuclei fuse and paternal and maternal chromosomes intermingle.

Mitochondrial deoxyribonucleic acid (MtDNA)

Cells have small organelles situated in the cytoplasm, each performing its own function. Those that produce energy for the cell are called **mitochondria**. The more active the cell is, the more mitochondria it contains so that busy cells like muscle and liver cells have hundreds of them. Each mitochondrion is surrounded by two lipid bilayer membranes. The outer membrane is smooth and the inner membrane has shelf-like inward folds called **cristae** where glucose is broken down to release energy. This process requires oxygen and is called **cellular respiration**. Enzymes are also required.

Our mitochondria are all inherited from our mothers' ovum as the sperm mitochondria used in motility are shed with the tail and do not enter the oocyte. They have their own DNA separate and distinct from nuclear DNA. In humans this MtDNA is a circular shape and is very compact, being one of the smallest known in the animal kingdom. It has 37 genes of which 13 code for proteins acting as enzymes during cellular respiration. These include the cytochromes. The remaining genes code for RNA molecules. Unlike nuclear DNA, nearly all the MtDNA is functional.

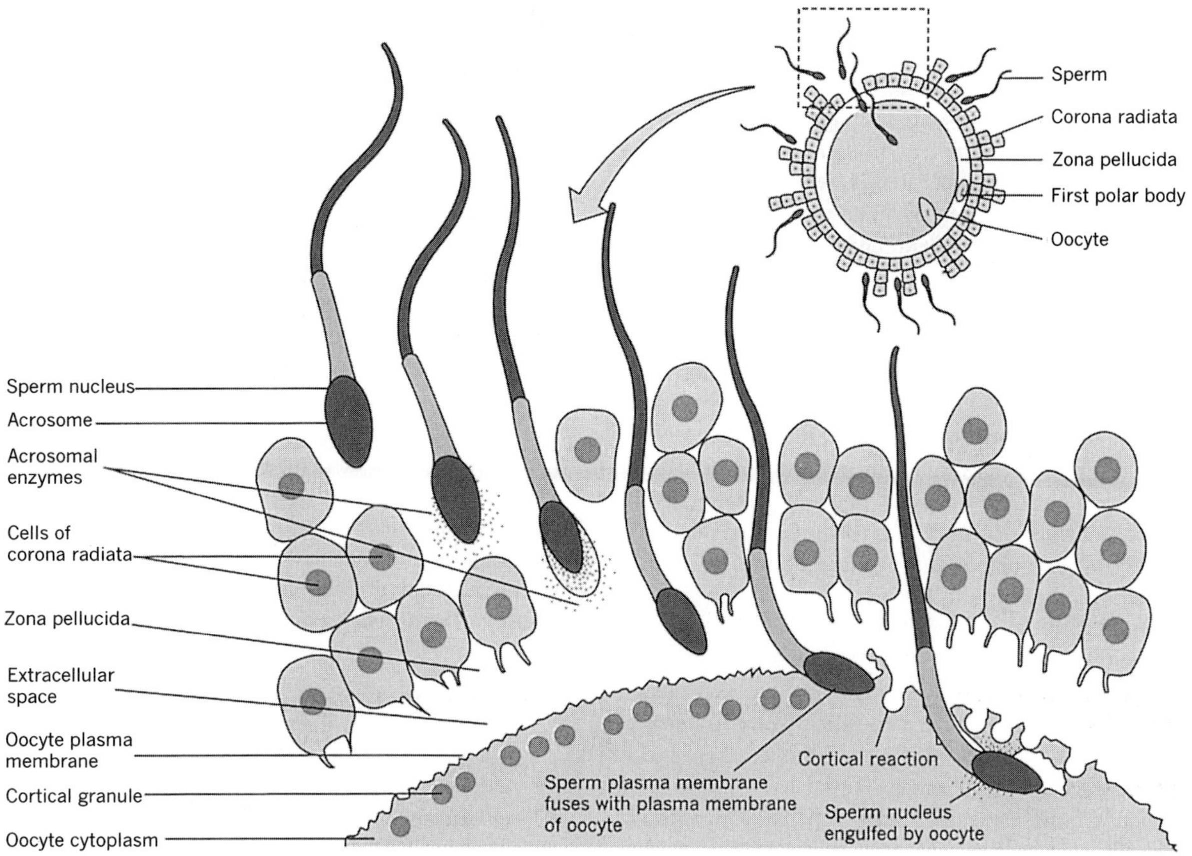

Figure 8.7 *Fertilisation and cortical reaction. (Reproduced with permission from Chiras 1991.)*

Mitochondrial DNA may also contain mutations that lead to congenital disease in humans. One series of diseases involves muscle weakness and is known as the **mitochondrial myopathies**. The muscle weakness is present because of changes to enzymes responsible for energy production. These changes result in insufficient energy being available for muscle function. The pattern of inheritance of such diseases is carriage by the mother and sons and daughters are equally affected.

Results of fertilisation (Fig. 8.8)

- The number of chromosomes is restored to the diploid 23 pairs or 46 chromosomes.
- The new individual inherits a unique set of genes from its parents.
- Sex determination occurs depending on which type of sperm fertilises the ovum.
- Initiation of cleavage stimulates the zygote to begin mitotic cell division.

THE EMBRYO

Terminology

The term **conceptus** refers to the products of fertilisation and comprises the embryo with its supporting tissues or adnexae. The developmental process is divided into discrete sections of time according to the process that is occurring in the pregnancy. The **preimplantation period** between fertilisation and implantation lasts about 6 days. The conceptus is called an **embryo** from the commencement of implantation until the end of the 8th week after fertilisation when it becomes known as a **fetus** until the moment of birth. The size of embryos is expressed as the **crown–rump length** from the crown of the head to the terminal part of the caudal end. Once the embryo has developed into the fetus, the **standing length** from crown to heel is used.

General concepts used in embryology

It is important to develop an understanding of the general concepts of embryology as well as some detail about the development of specific systems. Whilst knowledge of anatomy is necessary to understand embryology, it is also important to understand the processes involved. What decisions do cells have to make? How does one cell develop into millions of cells and hundreds of variations? What kind of information or instructions does the cell use and what processes are available for carrying out the instructions? Three books have been used as major sources of material for this chapter. To save the continual referencing of agreed data, they are Fitzgerald & Fitzgerald (1994), Moore (1989) and Wolpert (1991).

There are three important concepts in understanding embryology.

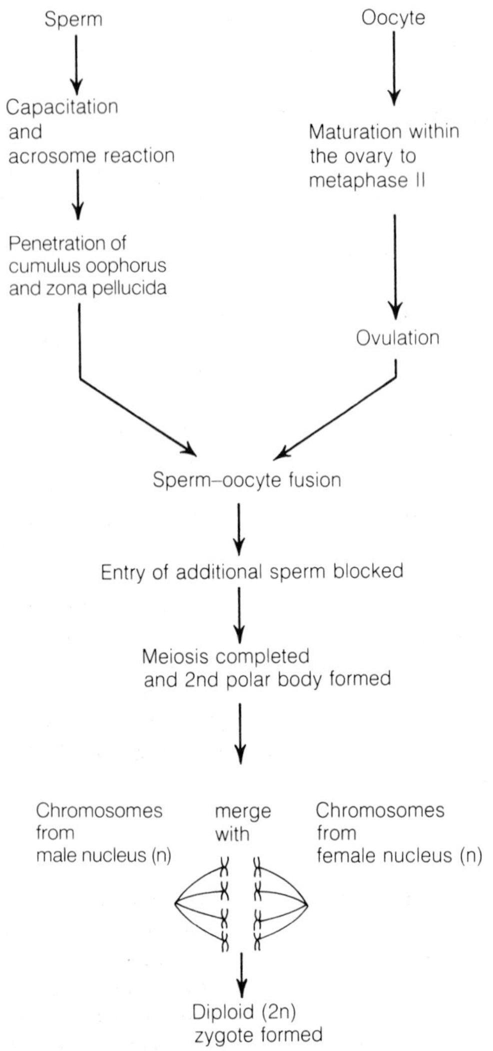

Figure 8.8 *Events in the female reproductive tract leading up to fertilisation (from Hinchliff SM, Montague SM, Watson R, 1996, with permission).*

1 A programme of simple instructions can generate complex forms.
2 Most developmental processes depend upon a coordinated interaction of genetic and environmental factors.
3 Each system in the body has its own developmental pattern (Moore 1989).

Programming the embryo

The information to make an embryo is located in the deoxyribonucleic acid (DNA) of the zygote and is contributed to by the ovum and sperm. The sperm and ovum each contribute 23 chromosomes but the ovum also contributes organelles and the mitochondrial DNA of the new individual. Only the head of the sperm enters the ovum at fertilisation so that only the maternal organelles are present in the zygote. As well as the 23 pairs of chromosomes present in the nucleus of the cell, mitochondria contain genes that synthesise a small amount of their protein for them. As in the nuclear genes, mistakes in the mitochondrial genome can lead to human disease (Lewin 1990).

Cells in the embryo seem to 'know' where and when to change shape and position and this pattern of cell movements is part of the embryo's developmental programme. Wolpert (1991) describes this as a set of instructions, not so much for describing the final form but for creating shapes. A parallel can be made with knitting a garment. The knitting pattern is the code or instruction manual but does not itself resemble the finished article. In order to translate the words into a garment, the knitter must interpret the code and apply energy, intelligence, order, control and a variety of stitches.

Cellular processes include:

- somatic cell division where the daughter cells receive identical genetic information;
- cell differentiation to make up the different tissues of the embryo;
- induction – cell interaction where one type of cell influences another;
- the migration of cells;
- programmed cell death to remove redundant cells

Early cell division

Cleavage

Early in pregnancy growth and development are very similar in any human embryo. It is possible to pinpoint the days when certain embryonic features develop. It is important to understand that when days of development are given these are days from fertilisation, not from the last menstrual period. The first event is the splitting of the very large zygote (fertilised ovum) into smaller cells, each with the full complement of maternal and paternal chromosomes, through the process of mitosis. This is called **cleavage**. The daughter cells are called **blastomeres** (Fig. 8.9).

There is synthesis of new DNA but no increase in the amount of cytoplasm so that the size of the blastomeres diminishes progressively. The fertilised ovum continues its journey down the uterine tube and by the 4th day after fertilisation there are between 16 and 20 cells and the conceptus is known as the **morula** (Fig. 8.10). The cells at this stage are said to be **totipotent** and could contribute to any part of the embryo. If the cells are separated there is the potential for multiple identical individuals. This property of the cells must last quite a while in humans as the formation of identical twins (or more fetuses) occurs when hundreds of cells are present.

Differentiation

In the early embryo there is little difference in the cells except their shape and the cells are not specialised. Wolpert (1991) reminds us that animals are made up of specialised cells and that humans have about 350 different cell types. A simpler animal such as the hydra has only 10–20 cell types. Cells carry out an amazing variety of functions from carrying oxygen to making and secreting hormones and chemicals and transmitting messages.

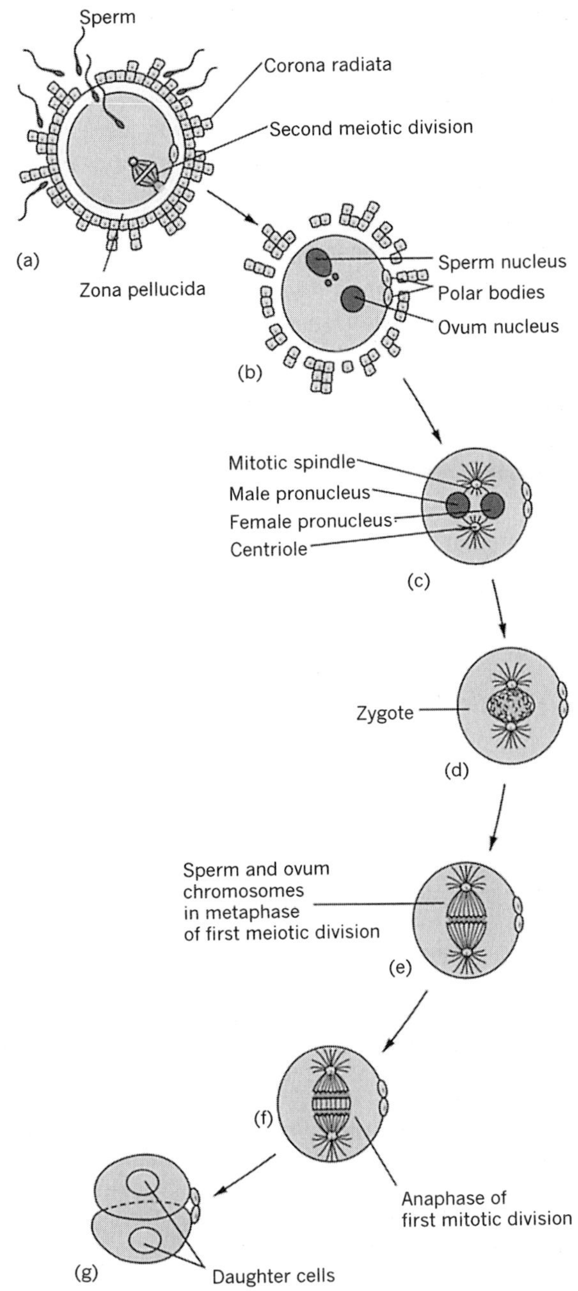

Figure 8.9 *The zygote prepares for division. (Reproduced with permission from Chiras 1991.)*

The epigenetic landscape

The type of cells that develop depends on their position in the embryo. The concept of **epigenesis** means that each embryo develops to the adult shape of its species from undifferentiated cells. Wolpert (1991) reported Waddington's (1940) description of the process of this diversification. Waddington suggested imagining the cells in an undulating landscape with multiple pathways down which they could 'roll'. He called this the epigenetic landscape. What type of cell develops depends on which path in the landscape it 'rolls' down as it migrates. These pathways represent gene activity and the pathway a cell selects depends on extracellular signals wherever a pathway branches.

Regulatory genes

The cells in different parts of the embryo have to change their shape and function so that they can carry out their role in the developing multicelled embryo. Genes in the nuclei of the cells interact with environmental factors, as described in the epigenetic landscape, to bring about this huge variety in cell types that make up tissues, organs and systems. De Robertis et al (1990) introduce their paper on embryology with the following sentence: 'Starting as a fertilised egg with homogeneous appearance an embryo made of skin, muscles, nerves and other tissues gradually arises through the division of cells'. They were able to write that sentence because of a line of research that began when Thomas Hunt Morgan initiated the use of *Drosophila* (fruit flies) for experiments on embryology in the early part of this century. Something in the environment of the embryo turns on developmental genes. It is important to have control so that the cells divide, multiply and move around in the embryo in an organised manner. Research has identified regulatory genes that control patterning in the embryo of the fruit fly. Regulation of the complex development of the embryo appears to be by a cascade of gene products. The most important discovery was of a discrete portion of DNA called the **homeobox**.

The homeobox

Since then the homeobox has been found not only in the chromosomes of fruit flies but in many other species, including humans. The genes control segmentation in the developing embryo so that the correct positioning of organs is brought about. Whilst much of the research has been carried out on *Drosophila*, the presence of the homeobox is likely to indicate similar functions in human embryos.

Wolpert (1991) says that a number of **homeotic** (meaning alike) genes have been found to be active in specific positions controlling patterning in the brain in the developing nervous system. These genes are referred to as **HOM genes** in invertebrates such as the fruit fly and **Hox genes** in vertebrates such as humans (McGinnis & Kuziora 1994) and are responsible for cell patterning locally. De Robertis et al (1990) describe how different homeobox genes produce different protein products which subdivide the embryo into discrete **homeodomains** prior to differentiation into specific types, organs and systems.

Morphogens

Homeobox genes may be switched on to produce their protein products sequentially by chemical gradients. Cytoplasm with special genetic properties is located at the ends of the zygote, setting up gradients called **morphogens** which activate other genes at specific concentrations. Nusslein-Volhard (1996) discusses these gradients in relation to the development of the *Drosophila* embryo, saying that 'Cells in a developing field respond to a special substance – a morphogen – the concentration of which gradually increases in a certain direction, forming a gradient'.

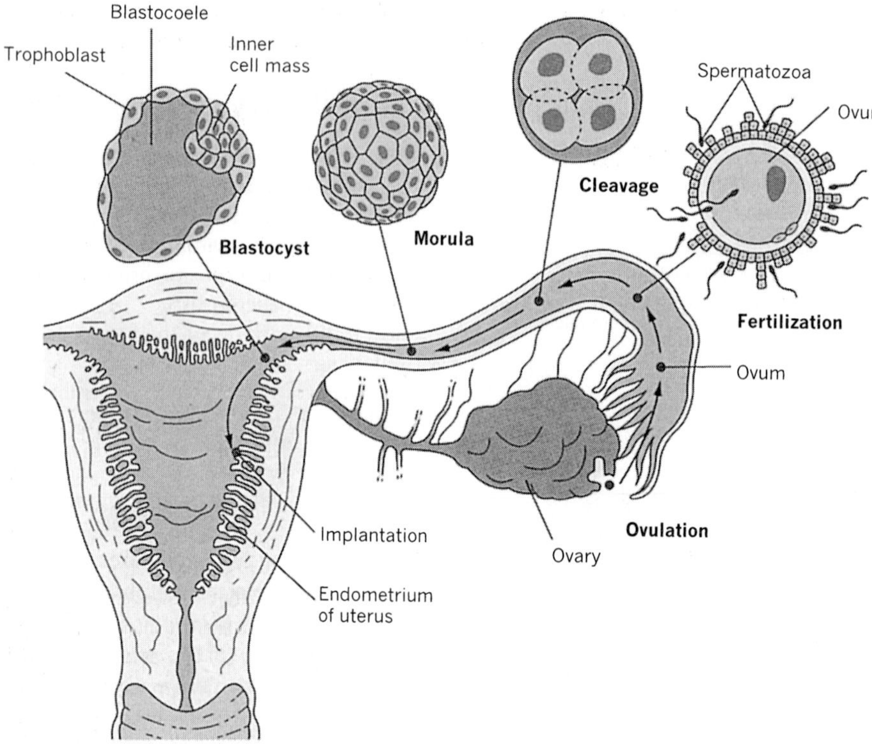

Figure 8.10 *Fertilisation and early embryonic development. (Reproduced with permission from Chiras 1991.)*

Induction

Hans Spemann won the only Nobel Prize so far awarded in embryology for discovering what organises the embryo's development. He found that cells taken from the gastrula of a newt would form a whole new embryo if grafted onto another embryo. He also demonstrated that a nervous system will only develop if future muscle and adjacent cells move from the outside underneath the outer layer. The cells that have migrated produce a signal that causes the overlying sheet of cells to develop into a nervous system.

During a limited time in early development, some embryonic tissues can influence the development of adjacent tissues. In the case of the nervous system, inward movement of the outer cells is said to induce its development. These influencing tissues are called **inductors** or **organisers**. The inductor needs to be near but not necessarily in contact with the tissue to be induced. Primary organisers establish the basic body plan and then a chain of secondary inductions occurs. Whilst the process of induction is not fully understood, it is generally accepted that some signal passes from the inductor to the induced tissue. The cells need to be in a community of sufficient size for induction to occur. This is referred to as the **community effect**. A further example of induction is the development of the lens of the eye from an invaginated sheet of cells exactly at the spot where the eyecup reaches the surface of the embryo (see the development of the eye in Chapter 9).

Cell communication

Cells communicate with each other in different ways. The induction signal varies between tissues and may take the form of a diffusible molecule passing directly from one tissue to another. In other tissues the message is mediated by a non-diffusible extracellular matrix (ECM) secreted by the inductor and with which the reacting tissue comes into contact. An extracellular matrix or ground substance is a network of cells from the mesoderm which provides pathways for cells to crawl along. As described in the section on morphogens, chemicals appear and disappear in the ECM.

Some tissues react when there is direct physical contact between the inducing and reacting tissues (Moore 1989) and cells receive cues from their neighbours about where they should be and how they should behave. Tissue-specific proteins create cell recognition and accumulation. The originators of a group of cells may specify where it travels to in the embryo and the tissue it forms.

Programmed cell death

Programmed cell death plays a major part in the final pattern of cells. Cells in some tissues are overproduced and some must die (Gilbert 1988). Cell death is a normal feature of development of the nervous system, limbs, skeleton and heart. The following three examples help to explain this. Cell death occurs in limb formation, helping to achieve the final shape of the limb, for instance the disappearance of webbing between the fingers. In the developing brain and nervous system over 50% too many axons arrive at target cells. The first to arrive make the best connection and start sending signals back in the form of **nerve growth factor** (NGF) which sustains neurones. There is no room for late arrivals and they cannot obtain nourishment from the muscle cells so they die. Cell death is also important in the development of tubes such as blood vessels. Too many cells are made and the tube is pruned by cell death.

DEVELOPMENT OF THE EMBRYO

The blastocyst

The group of cells carries on cleaving during the next 4 days during which time the conceptus passes through the uterine tubes into the uterine cavity. Whilst the first three cleavages are synchronous, later cleavages are asymmetrical. There is also **polarisation** where the inner cells divide less frequently and remain large and round whilst the outer cells in contact with the zona pellucida become flattened. At this point the cells lose their totipotency and begin to differentiate and their fate is determined. They are destined to become specific parts of the embryo. On the 5th day after fertilisation the zygote 'hatches' as the zona pellucida is digested by uterine secretions. Fluid accumulates in the space between the peripheral and central cells of the morula and the conceptus has now become a

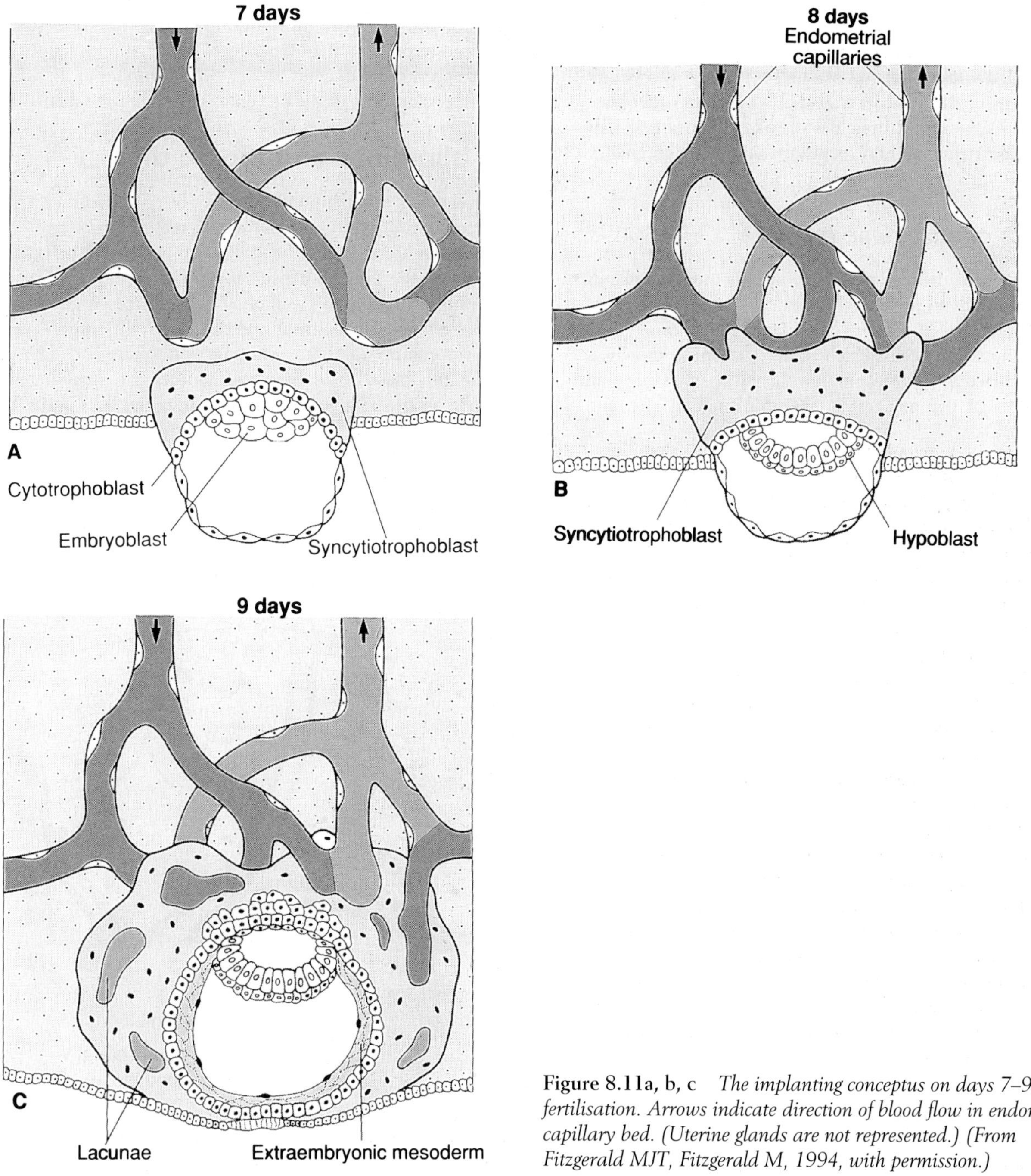

Figure 8.11a, b, c *The implanting conceptus on days 7–9 after fertilisation. Arrows indicate direction of blood flow in endometrial capillary bed. (Uterine glands are not represented.) (From Fitzgerald MJT, Fitzgerald M, 1994, with permission.)*

blastocyst. The inner cell mass of the blastocyst is the **embryoblast** and will become the embryo and the flattened outer layer of cells is called the **trophoblast** which will form the placenta.

Implantation

On the 6th day the blastocyst begins to implant into the endometrium during the secretory phase of the menstrual cycle. The site of implantation is most commonly on the posterior wall of the uterus. The part of the blastocyst where the embryo has begun to develop, the embryoblast, settles onto the endometrium. Where the trophoblastic cells make contact with the endometrium, they undergo rapid DNA synthesis and become cuboid in shape to form the **cytotrophoblast**. The daughter cells shed their plasma membranes to form a mass of protoplasm filled with nuclei and organelles, called a **syncytium**. The mass of tissue is therefore called the **syncytiotrophoblast** (Fig. 8.11). The syncytiotrophoblast produces enzymes that attack the endometrium and hormones that allow the pregnancy to continue.

The effects of enzymatic erosion

As the enzymes erode the endometrium, the uterine glands release their content to nourish the embryo and the blastocyst begins to enlarge as it obtains nutrition. Nutrition is also provided by the stroma cells which undergo changes known as the **decidual reaction** and become swollen with glycogen and lipid. The change commences at the implantation site and spreads within a few days throughout the whole endometrium except the lining of the cervix. The endometrium is now known as the **decidua**.

At the implantation site there is development and dilatation of new blood capillaries fed by branches of the spiral arteries and drained by the endometrial veins (Fig. 8.12). The conceptus is completely embedded in the compact layer of the endometrium by the 12th day after fertilisation and is covered by the overlying uterine epithelium. Erosion of these sinuses results in maternal blood entering the syncytiotrophoblast to collect in a labyrinth of little pockets of blood called **lacunae**. The hormone human chorionic gonadotrophin (HCG) is secreted into the lacunae by the trophoblast, enters the maternal circulation and is taken to the ovary. The HCG maintains the corpus luteum to ensure the continued production of oestrogen and progesterone for maintenance of the pregnancy until the placenta produces sufficient of the two hormones at 12 weeks. Further development of the placenta is discussed in Chapter 11.

The bilaminar embryonic disc

The following descriptions should be studied with the accompanying diagrams. Perhaps the greatest problem is that the diagrams are two-dimensional sections through a flattened disc which is the three-dimensional embryo. By the 2nd week of development the cells are well organised and the inner cell mass forms a flattened disc consisting of two layers. The inner layer or **epiblast** is composed of tall columnar epithelium and the outer layer or **hypoblast** of low cuboidal epithelium. Together they are known as the bilaminar embryonic disc (Figs 8.13 and 8.14).

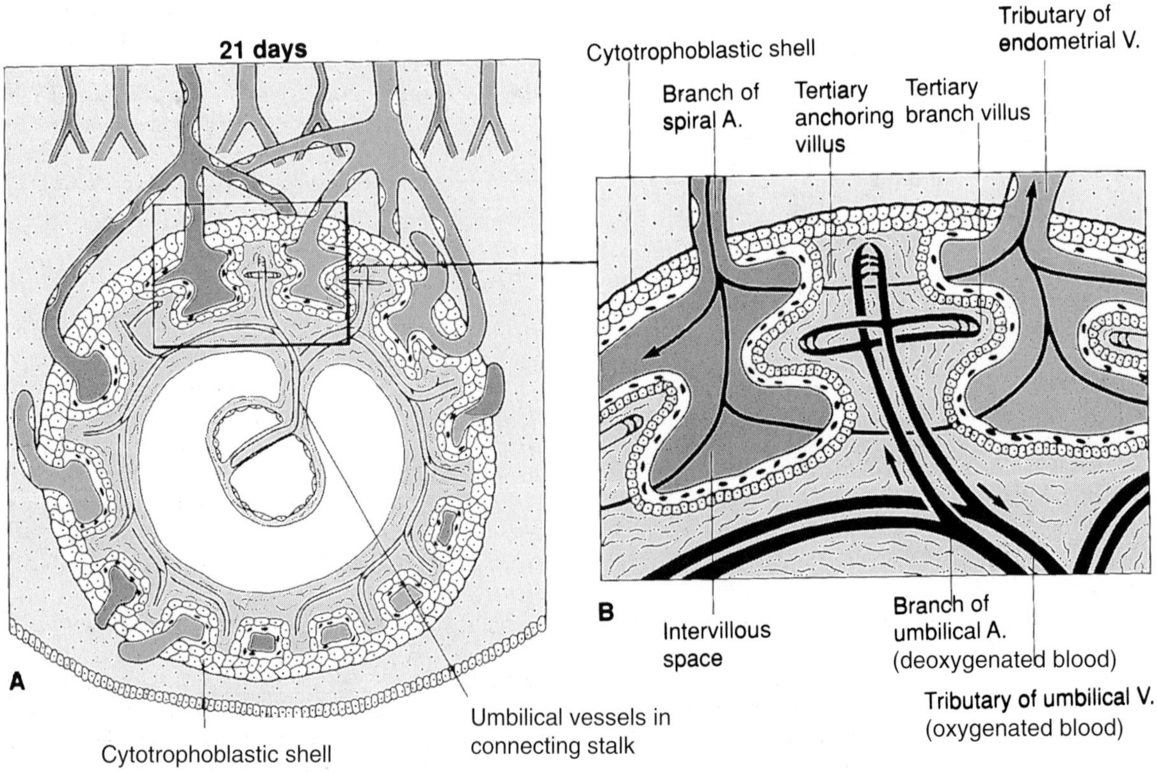

Figure 8.12a & b *Chorionic vesicle at 21 days. (b) Enlargement of upper part of (a) showing the circulation of embryonic and maternal blood (from Fitzgerald MJT, Fitzgerald M, 1994, with permission).*

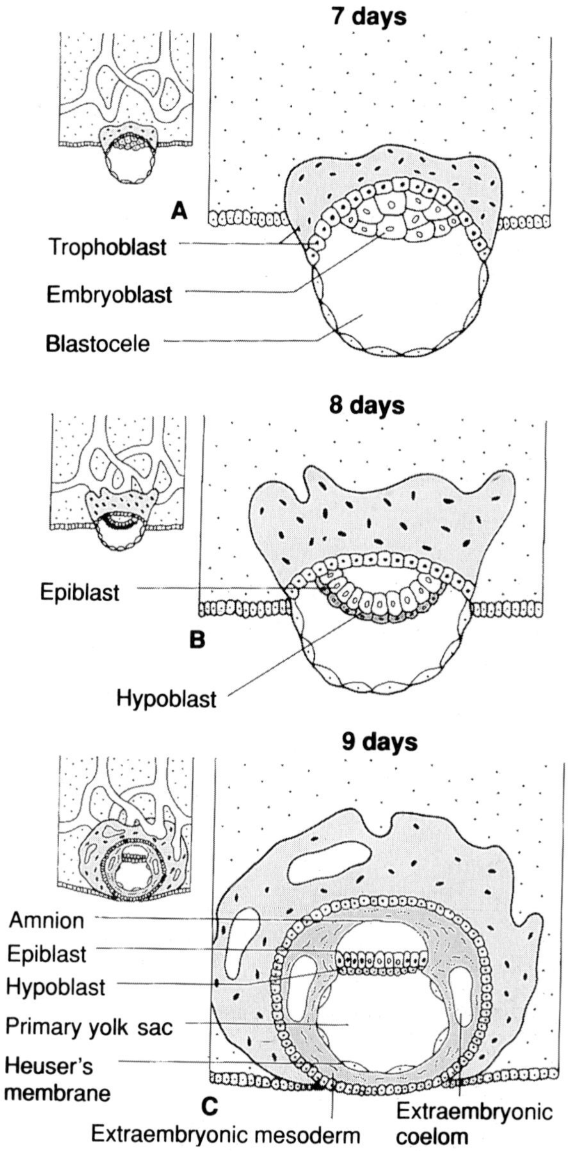

Figure 8.13a, b, c *Early steps in differentiation of the blastocyst (from Fitzgerald MJT, Fitzgerald M, 1994, with permission).*

The margins of the epiblast create a thin epithelial layer, the **amnion**, and the epiblast and amnion form the amniotic sac. This sac grows more rapidly than the embryo to surround the embryo for protection. The cell margins of the hypoblast also divide rapidly to form branched cells that line the cavity of the blastocyst. This lining is called the **extraembryonic mesoderm**. Spaces develop within the mesoderm and coalesce to become the **extraembryonic coelom** (a coelom is a cavity).

This cavity splits the mesoderm into a visceral layer, which is included in the yolk sac, and a parietal layer, which contributes to the **chorion** together with the trophoblast. The visceral innermost cells become flattened and form an epithelium called **Heuser's membrane** which encloses the cavity known as the primary yolk sac. The visceral and parietal extraembryonic mesoderm are linked by a connecting stalk that will develop into the umbilical cord. Towards the end of the 2nd week the

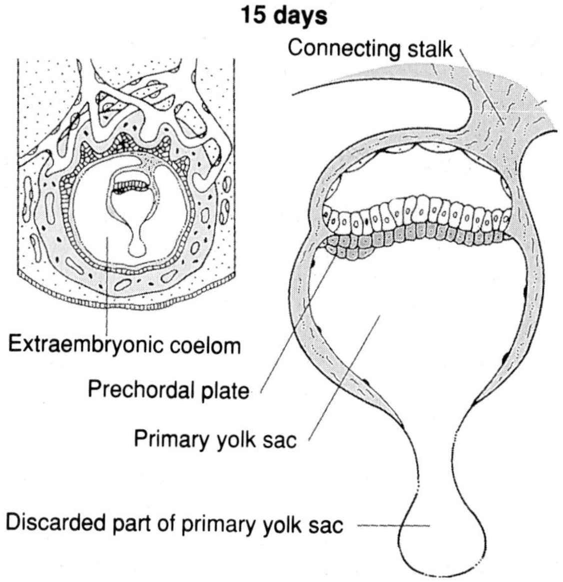

Figure 8.14 *Prechordal plate; connecting stalk; reduction of primary yolk sac (from Fitzgerald MJT, Fitzgerald M, 1994, with permission).*

flattened disc becomes ovoid. The cranial part of the hypoblast thickens to form the **prechordal plate**.

The trilaminar embryo

There is an immense amount of cellular activity that occurs during embryogenesis and organogenesis. Cells migrate and move about the embryo and then differentiate into specific cell types to form organs and systems. The three processes of formation of the primitive streak, gastrulation and formation of the notochord are extremely important in creating the body plan (Figs 8.15 and 8.16). They will be described separately although this is artificial as they occur simultaneously and are interlinked in the embryo.

The primitive streak

At the beginning of the 3rd week a thick linear band of embryonic epiblast appears caudally in the dorsal aspect of the embryonic disc. This is the primitive streak and results from cells of the epiblast heaping up and migrating to the centre of the embryonic disc. It is the site of enormous cell activity when the first wave of migration forms the middle third layer of the embryo and the basic body plan is laid down with a head or **cranial** (rostral) end and a tail or **caudal** end. As the primitive streak elongates by adding cells to its caudal end, the cranial end enlarges to form a **primitive node** (Fig. 8.17).

The primitive streak continues to form mesodermal cells until the end of the 4th week by which time it has retreated to the caudal end of the embryo. Rarely, it may persist and give rise to a tumour called a **sacral teratoma** containing tissue derived from more than one germ layer. Embryonic mesodermal cells migrate in three directions from the primitive streak: laterally to the margins of the embryonic disc, cranially alongside the notochord and caudally around the **cloacal membrane** (see below).

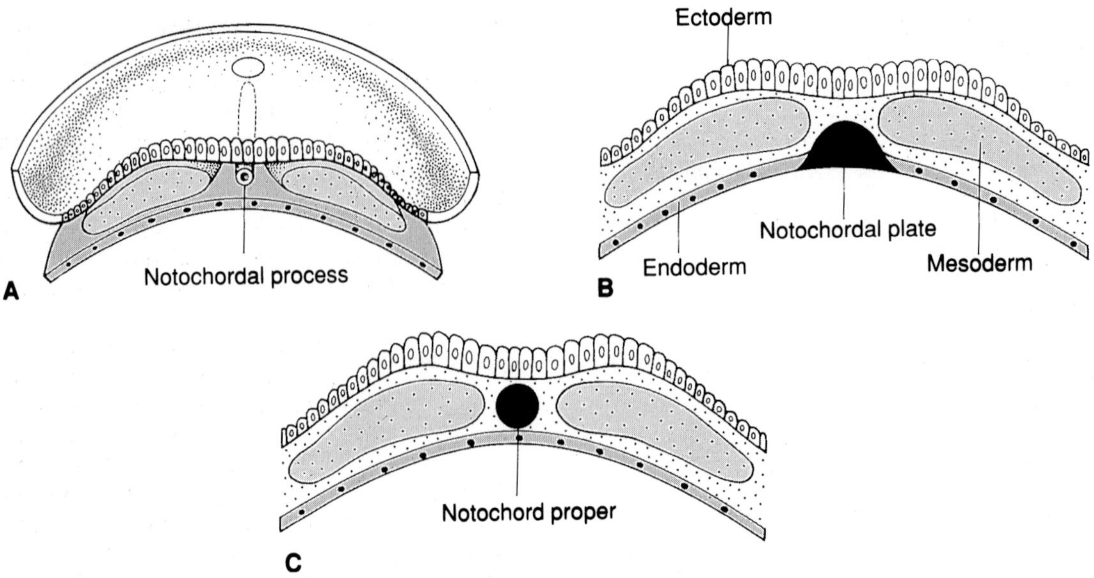

Figure 8.15a, b, c *Transverse sections taken rostral to the primitive node, showing (a) the hollow notochordal process; (b) the notochordal plate fused with the endoderm; (c) the notochord proper (from Fitzgerald MJT, Fitzgerald M, 1994, with permission).*

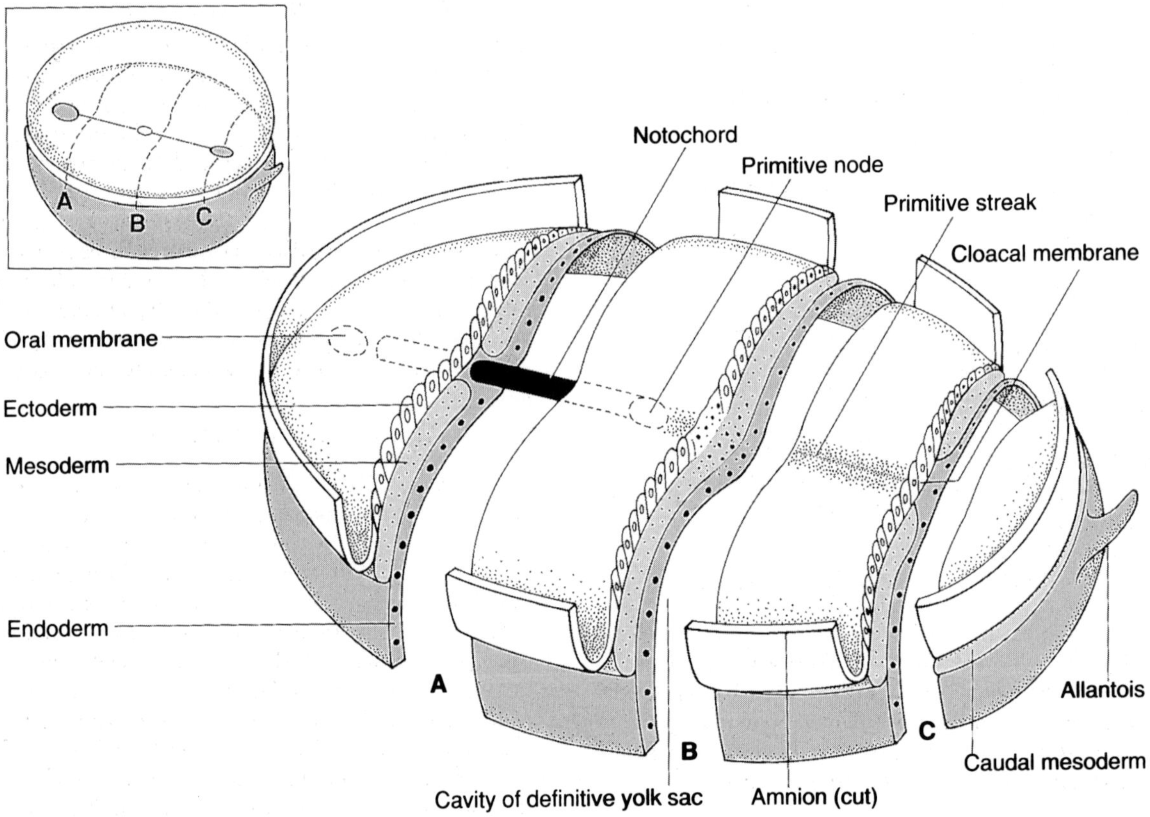

Figure 8.16 *Stereosections of the trilaminar embryonic disc, viewed obliquely from above (from Fitzgerald MJT, Fitzgerald M, 1994, with permission).*

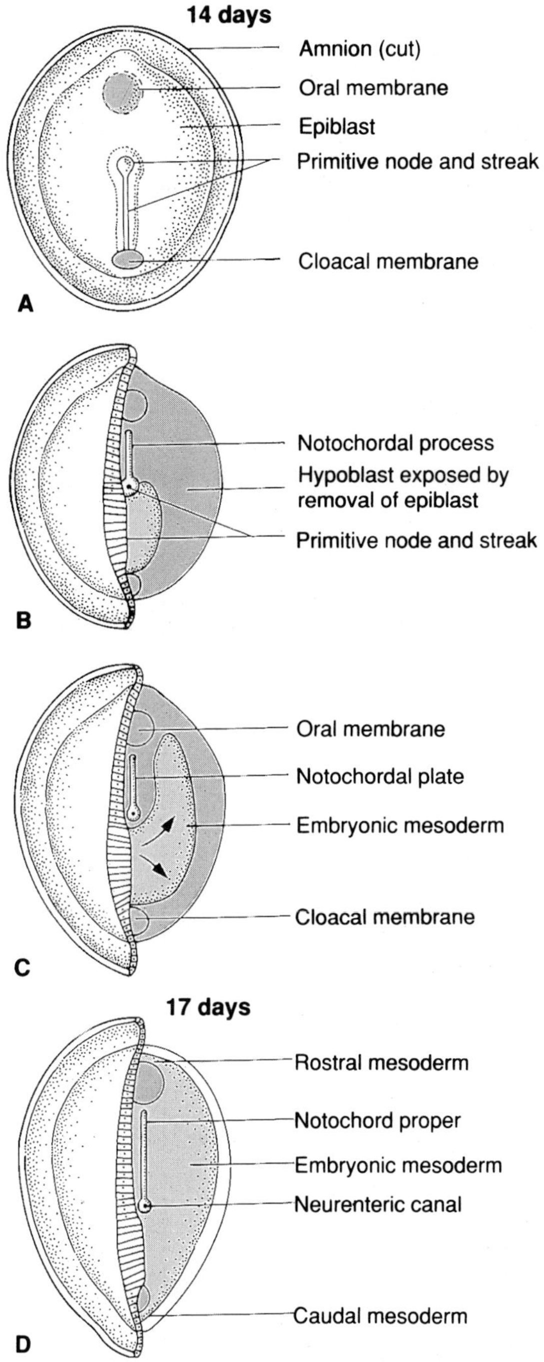

Figure 8.17a, b, c, d *Dorsal views of the embryonic disc. (a) represents the floor of the amniotic sac. In (b–d), the epiblast has been removed from the right side, to show migration of the embryonic mesoderm over the surface of the hypoblast (from Fitzgerald MJT, Fitzgerald M, 1994, with permission).*

Gastrulation

Wolpert (1991) has been quoted as saying 'It is not birth, marriage or death, but gastrulation which is truly the important event in your life'. Gastrulation, which is a process of invagination, occurs in all species of animal and is the process by which the inner cell mass becomes the trilaminar embryo. The process actually begins in the 1st week with the formation of the hypoblast, continues during the 2nd week with the formation of the epiblast and is completed during the 3rd week when the three primary germ layers of **ectoderm, mesoderm** and **endoderm** are in situ and the embryo has become a trilaminar disc. It may help to visualise a simple hollow animal such as a sea urchin. The inner layer or lining is epithelium, surrounding that is a layer of muscle and outside that is a layer of skin. A human being is a complex elaboration of the three layers.

Epiblastic cells dip through the primitive streak and spread laterally beneath it. Wolpert (1991) describes the cell movements in the following words: 'Movements occur simultaneously over many parts of the embryo with sheets of cells streaming past each other, contracting and expanding'. Some of the cells displace the underlying hypoblast to form the embryonic endoderm whilst the remainder form the embryonic mesoderm or **mesenchyme**. Epiblastic cells that do not migrate and remain on the surface form the embryonic ectoderm. The endoderm migrates inside the wall of the primary yolk sac to become the secondary yolk sac, usually just referred to as the yolk sac. A finger-like projection of the yolk sac called the **allantois** becomes pinched off and extends into the connecting stalk.

Development of body cavities

Late in the 2nd week fluid-filled spaces appear in the cranial half of the embryonic mesoderm. The spaces coalesce during the 3rd week to form the U-shaped embryonic coelom. The bend of the U at the cranial end of the embryonic coelom is called the **pericardial coelom** and is divided by the **septum transversum** from the caudal two arms of the U which form the **pericardioperitoneal canals** (pleural canals) leading to two branches of the **peritoneal coelom** which open into the extra-embryonic coelom. Three body cavities will soon become recognisable: a large pericardial cavity around the heart, two smaller pleural canals and a large peritoneal cavity. The septum transversum will be incorporated into the diaphragm.

Formation of the notochord

The **notochordal process** grows out cranially from the primitive knot beneath the ectoderm until it reaches the prechordal plate and can extend no further. Where the prechordal plate is firmly attached to the ectoderm and remains bilaminar, it forms the **oropharyngeal membrane** which is the future site of the mouth. Caudal to the primitive streak is a circular area which also remains bilaminar, called the **cloacal membrane**, which is the future site of the anus and urogenital orifices. The notochord is a rigid cellular rod stretched out along the embryo that develops from the notochordal process. Mesodermal cells gather around it to form the vertebral column. The notochord is almost completely formed by the end of the 3rd week and will degenerate and disappear once it is surrounded by the vertebral bodies.

Organogenesis

From 3 weeks the embryo enters the vulnerable stage of organogenesis (see also Chapter 7). The zygote is now

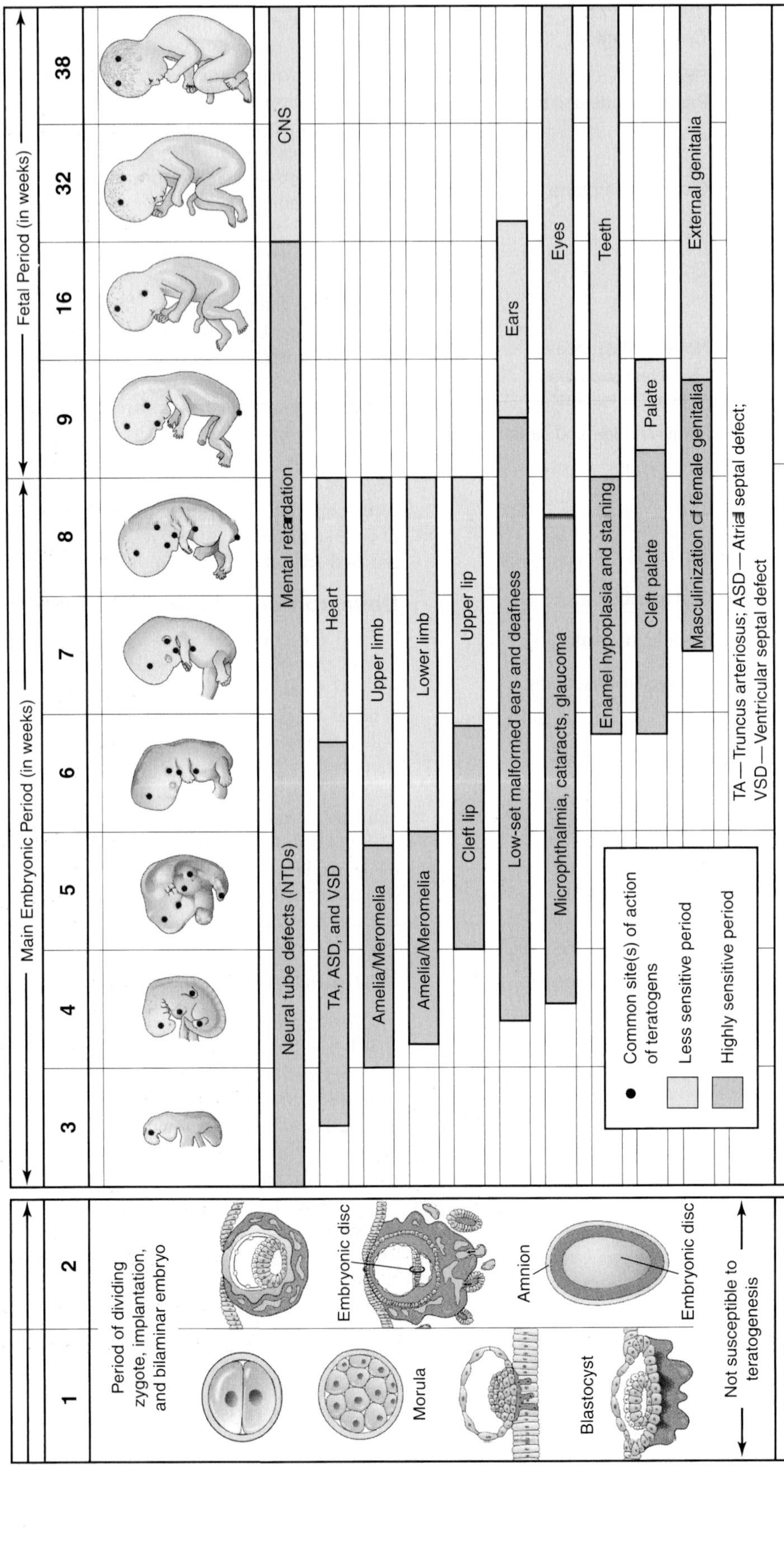

Figure 8.18 *Schematic illustration of critical periods in human prenatal development, showing periods of sensitivity to teratogens. (Reproduced with permission from Moore 1989.)*

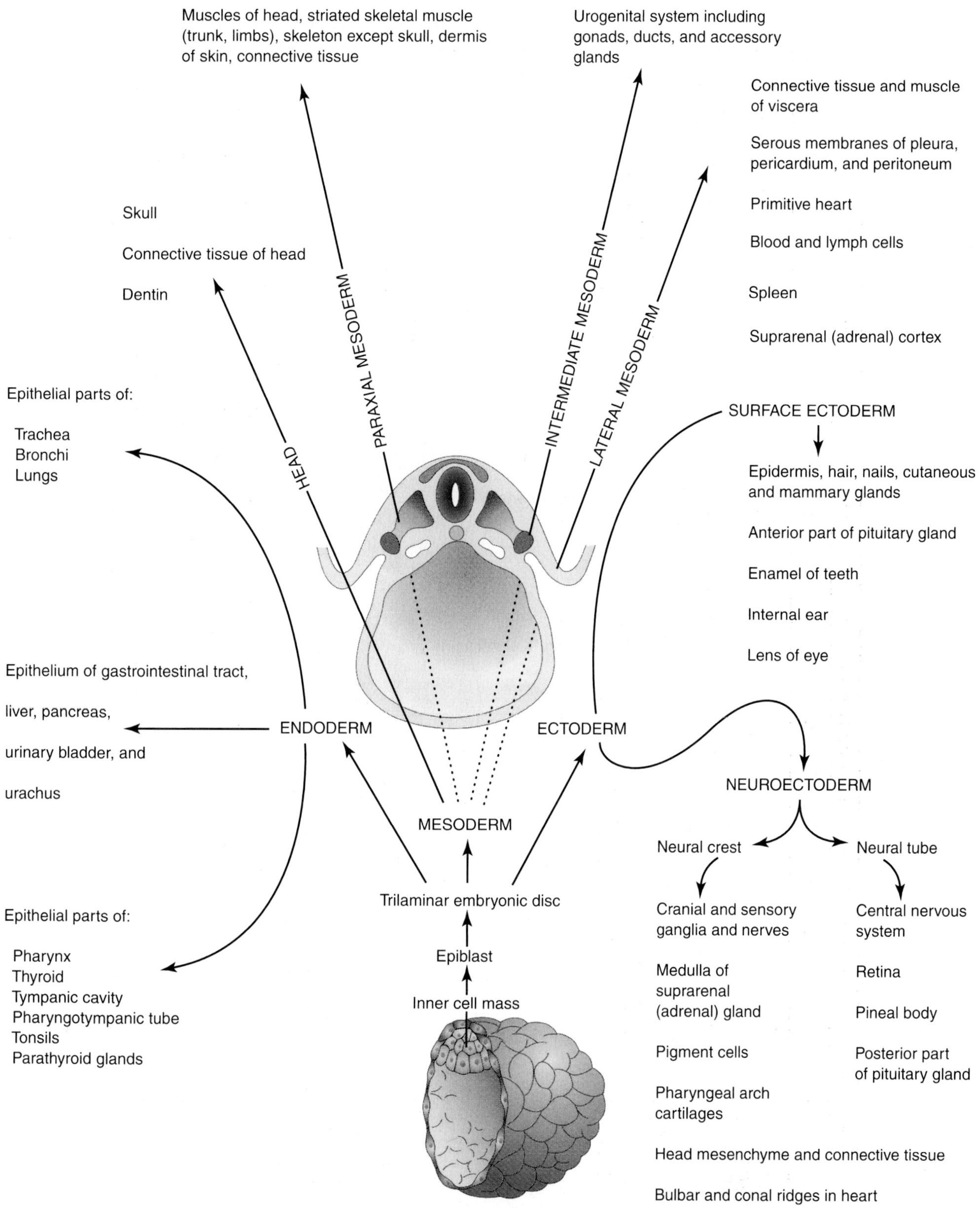
Muscles of head, striated skeletal muscle (trunk, limbs), skeleton except skull, dermis of skin, connective tissue
Urogenital system including gonads, ducts, and accessory glands
Connective tissue and muscle of viscera
Serous membranes of pleura, pericardium, and peritoneum
Primitive heart
Blood and lymph cells
Spleen
Suprarenal (adrenal) cortex
Skull
Connective tissue of head
Dentin
PARAXIAL MESODERM
INTERMEDIATE MESODERM
LATERAL MESODERM
HEAD
Epithelial parts of:
Trachea
Bronchi
Lungs
SURFACE ECTODERM
Epidermis, hair, nails, cutaneous and mammary glands
Anterior part of pituitary gland
Enamel of teeth
Internal ear
Lens of eye
Epithelium of gastrointestinal tract,
liver, pancreas,
urinary bladder, and
urachus
ENDODERM
ECTODERM
NEUROECTODERM
MESODERM
Neural crest
Neural tube
Trilaminar embryonic disc
Epithelial parts of:
Pharynx
Thyroid
Tympanic cavity
Pharyngotympanic tube
Tonsils
Parathyroid glands
Epiblast
Inner cell mass
Cranial and sensory ganglia and nerves
Central nervous system
Medulla of suprarenal (adrenal) gland
Retina
Pineal body
Pigment cells
Posterior part of pituitary gland
Pharyngeal arch cartilages
Head mesenchyme and connective tissue
Bulbar and conal ridges in heart

Figure 8.19 *Schematic drawing illustrating the derivatives of the three germ layers. (Reproduced with permission from Moore 1989.)*

technically known as the embryo until it has completed organogenesis by 8 weeks, when it becomes known as the fetus (Fig. 8.18). Organogenesis involves many processes and much simultaneous cell movement. Organs are made up of cell types that may originate from different sources and obey different instructions. From about day 20 until day 30, the dorsal surface of the embryo develops a segmented aspect with the appearance of **paired somites** which are clumps of embryonic tissue. From the somites develop the vertebral column and the segmentally innervated muscles of the trunk. The somites are still visible at 6 weeks but have differentiated by 8 weeks.

Differentiation of the germ layers

Figure 8.19 summarises the tissues and organs developing from the three layers.

Ectoderm

Tissues derived from **neuroectoderm** include the central and peripheral nervous systems, the retina of the eye and the posterior lobe of the pituitary gland.

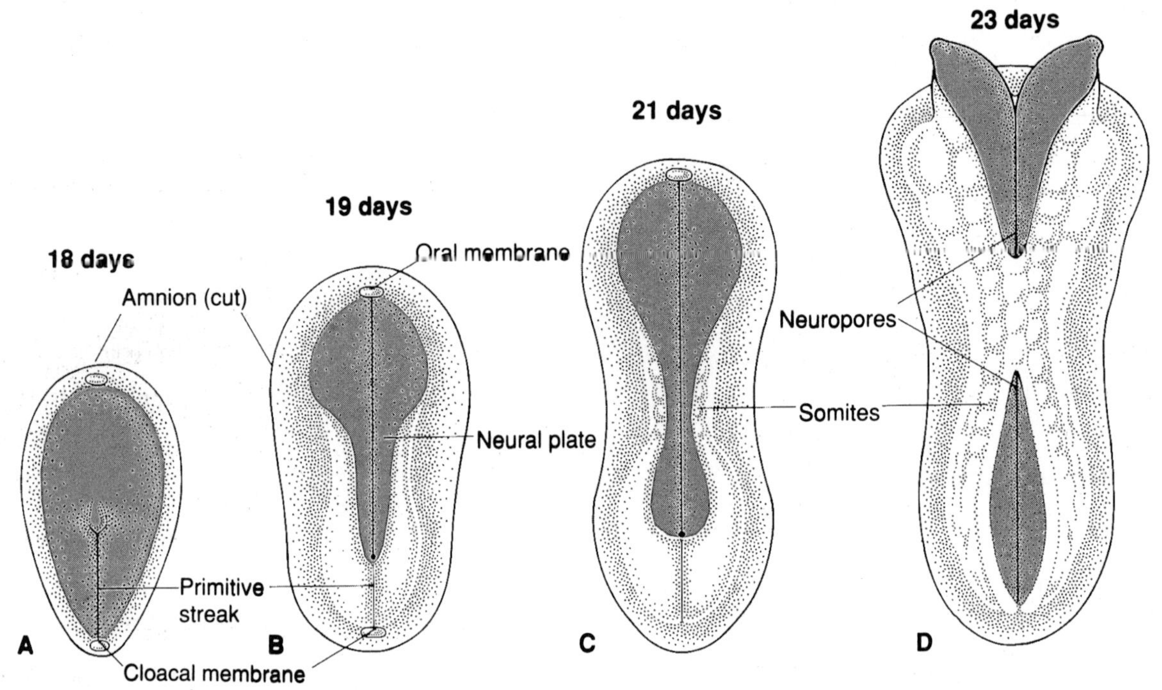

Figure 8.20a, b, c, d *Dorsal views of the floor of the amniotic sac (from Fitzgerald MJT, Fitzgerald M, 1994, with permission).*

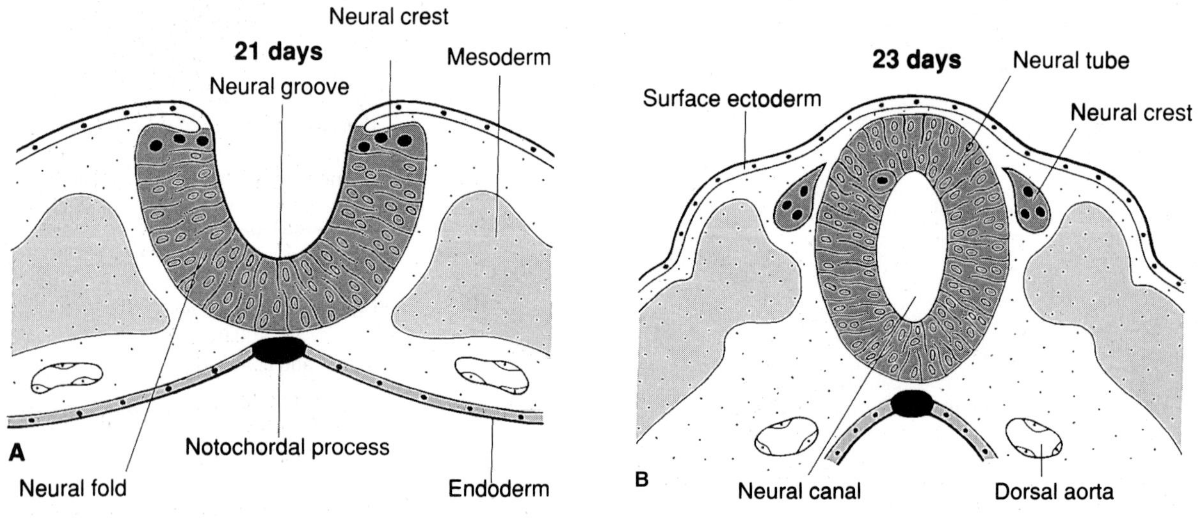

Figure 8.21a & b *Transverse sections of the mid-region of embryos (c) and (d) in Fig. 8.20 (from Fitzgerald MJT, Fitzgerald M, 1994, with permission).*

Tissues derived from **surface ectoderm** include the outer layer of the skin, called the **epidermis**, with its hair follicles and cutaneous glands, the breasts, the lens of the eye, the special sense cells of the inner ear, the anterior lobe of the pituitary gland and the enamel of the teeth.

Neurulation

The process of development of the human brain and nervous system is known as neurulation (Figs 8.20–8.25). The notochord induces its overlying ectoderm to thicken and form a neural plate known as the neuroectoderm which differs from the remaining surface ectoderm. A flat sheet of cells on the upper surface of the embryo folds up into a tube which will develop into the brain and spinal cord. On about day 18 the neural plate develops a midline **neural groove** with lateral **neural folds**. At the beginning of the 4th week the folds come together to form the **neural tube**.

Fusion of the folds begins at the level of the 4th pair of somites and proceeds simultaneously in cranial and caudal directions. Cells near the crests of the neural folds escape from the neural tube during closure and come to lie on either side of the neural tube, forming the **neural crest**. The two ends of the neural tube, termed **neuropores**, are open. The cranial neuropore closes on day 25 or 26 and the caudal neuropore on day 27 or 28. The neural tube becomes the brain and spinal cord and the neural canal within the tube becomes the ventricular system of the brain and the central canal of the spinal cord. This early closure of the neural tube has implications for the causation and prevention of a common congenital abnormality – open neural tube defects.

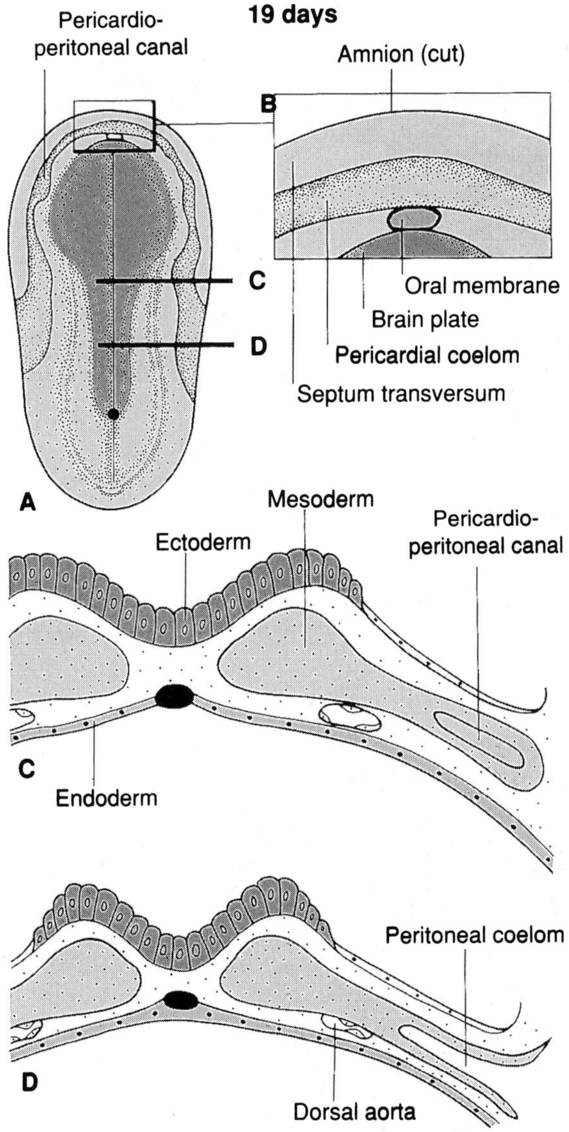

Figure 8.22a, b, c, d *(a) Dorsal view of a 19-day embryonic disc. (b) Enlargement from the rostral part of (a). (c,d) Transverse sections at the levels indicated in (a) (from Fitzgerald MJT, Fitzgerald M, 1994, with permission).*

Mesoderm

The mesoderm nearest the midline axis of the embryo is called paraxial mesoderm and undergoes segmentation to form

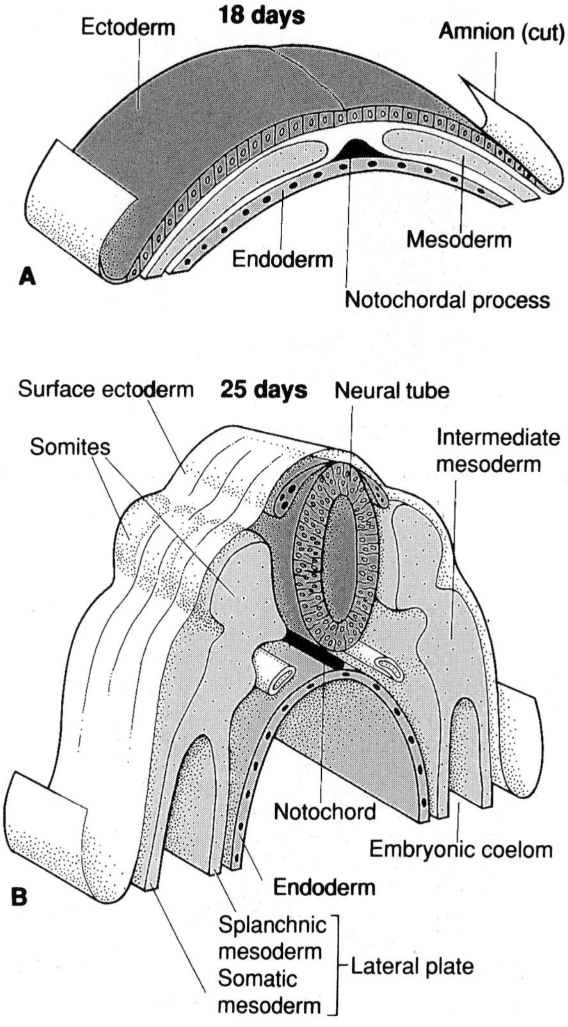

Figure 8.23a & b *Early differentiation of the embryonic mesoderm (from Fitzgerald MJT, Fitzgerald M, 1994, with permission).*

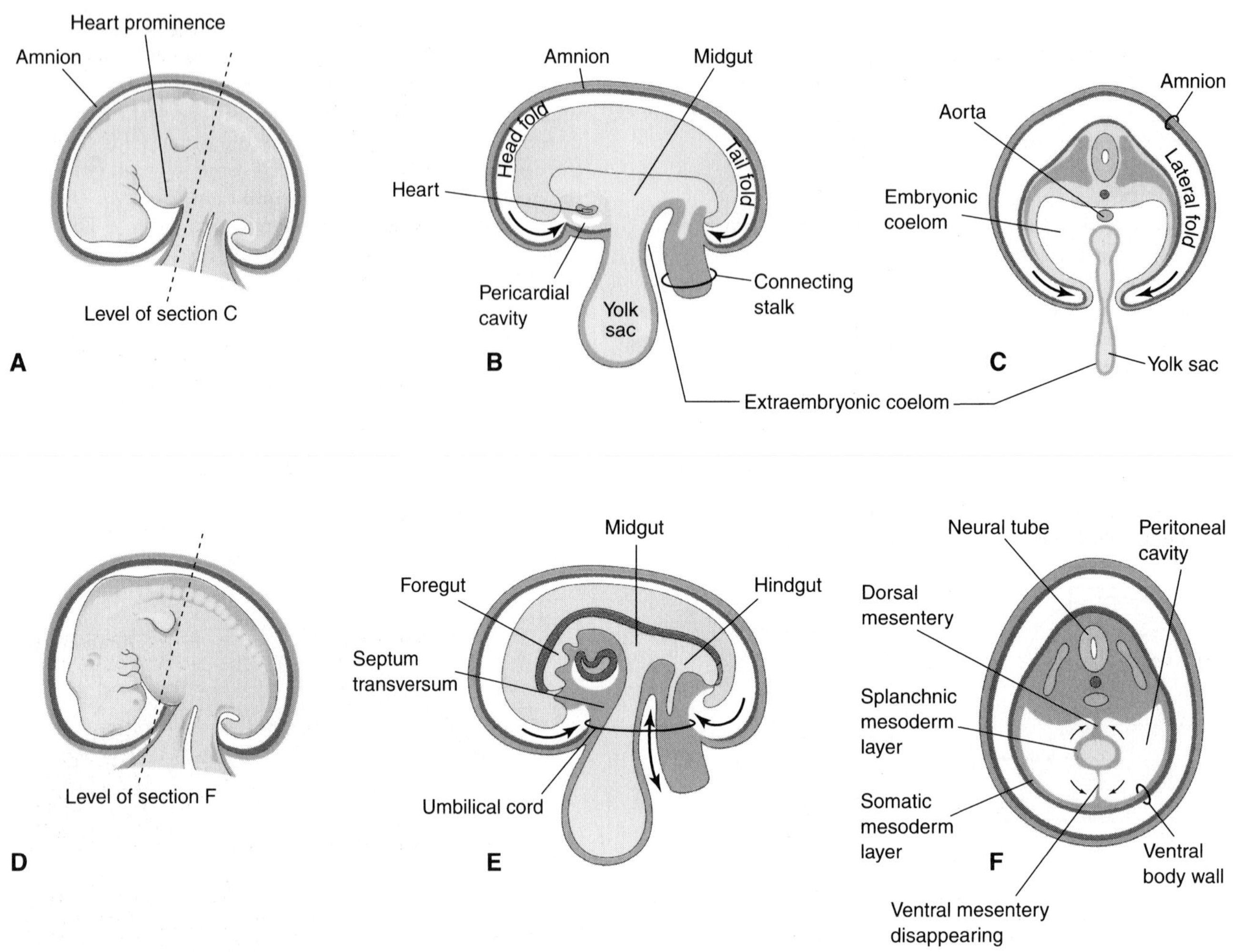

Figure 8.24 *Drawings illustrating embryonic folding and its effects on the intraembryonic coelom and other structures. (Reproduced with permission from Moore 1989.)*

somites. Next to the somites is the intermediate mesoderm, which does not undergo segmentation, and outside that is the **lateral plate**. The lateral plate is divided into somatic mesoderm, that lies just beneath the body wall, and the splanchnic mesoderm lying next to the endoderm of the yolk sac.

- Tissues derived from the paraxial mesoderm cranial to the somites include part of the skull and the muscles of the face and jaws.
- Tissues derived from the somites include the vertebral column and the skeletal musculature of the trunk and the connective tissue or dermis of the skin.
- Tissues derived from the intermediate mesoderm include the kidneys and ureters, the gonads, the ductus deferens and the uterus and fallopian tubes.
- Tissues derived from the somatic mesoderm include the skeleton and muscles of the limbs, the sternum and the anterior part of the ribs.
- Tissues derived from the splanchnic mesoderm include the cardiovascular system and the blood, the spleen and the smooth muscle of the gastrointestinal tract.

Endoderm

Tissues derived from the endoderm include the epithelial linings of the alimentary tract and its glands, the liver and pancreas, the epithelial lining of the lower respiratory tract and of the bladder and urethra.

Folding of the embryo

Folding of cell sheets forms the basis of the early development of organs and folding of the embryo changes its shape and the relationships of the organs (Figs 8.24 and 8.25). Again, there is the problem of describing three-dimensional changes in words and two-dimensional drawings. The process of development of the human brain and nervous system known as **neurulation** is a good example. A flat sheet of cells on the upper surface of the embryo folds up into a tube which will develop into the brain and spinal cord.

Fitzgerald & Fitzgerald (1994) describe events in the longitudinal and transverse planes separately.

Longitudinal folding

Longitudinal folding brings about flexion and development of the head and tail folds (Figs 8.26 and 8.27). A major effect of this folding is to bring about an hourglass constriction on the yolk sac. There is partial extrusion of the yolk sac with the

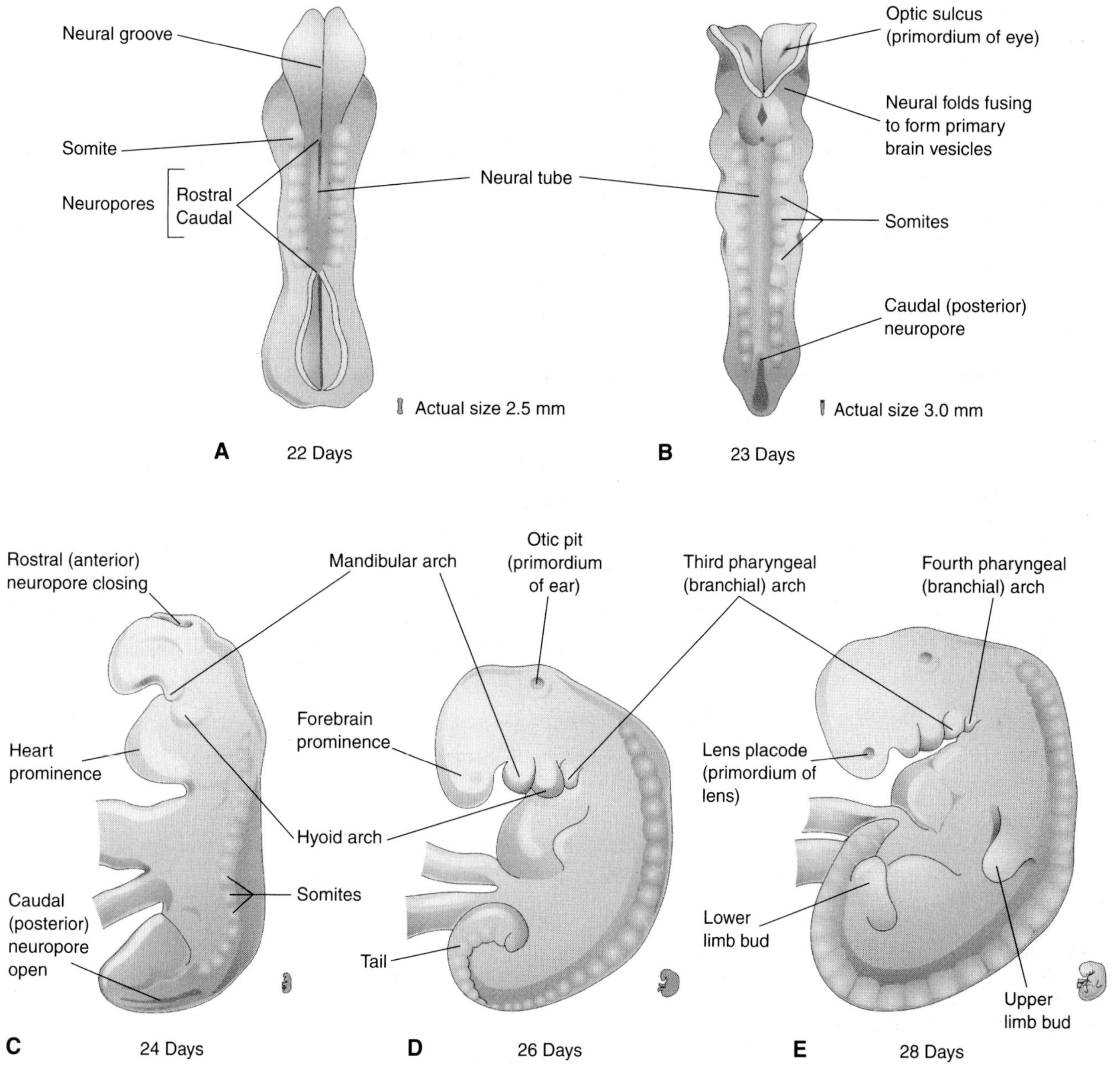

Figure 8.25 *(a,b) Dorsal views of embryos early in the 4th week showing 8 and 12 somites respectively. (c,d,e) Lateral views of older embryos showing 16, 27 and 33 somites respectively. The rostral neuropore is normally closed by 25–26 days and the caudal neuropore by the end of the 4th week. (Reproduced with permission from Moore 1989.)*

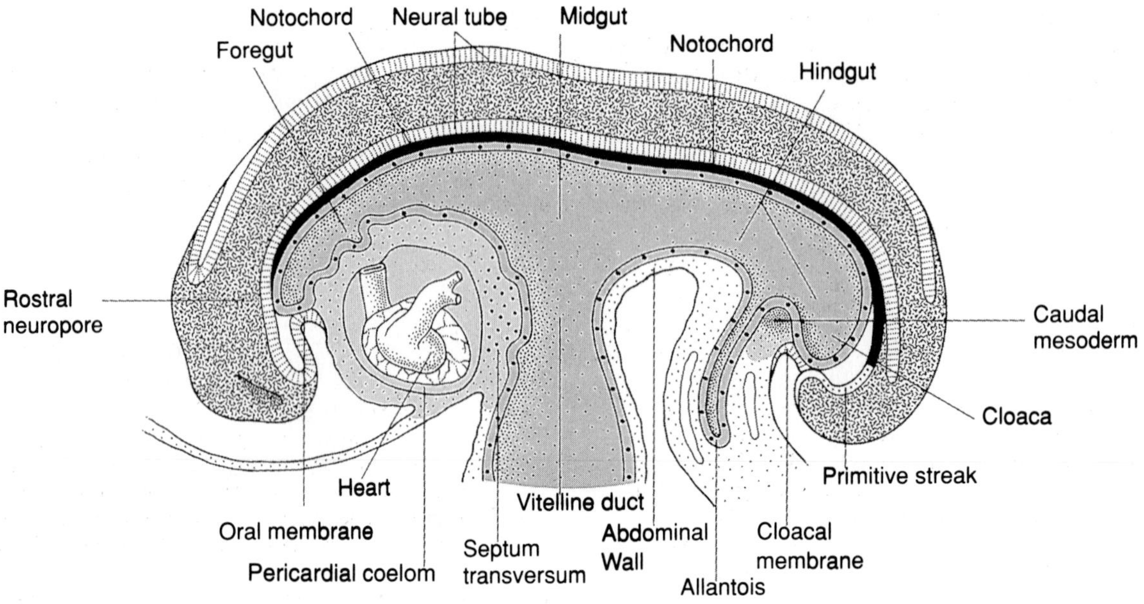

Figure 8.26 *Longitudinal section of a 25-day embryo (from Fitzgerald MJT, Fitzgerald M, 1994, with permission).*

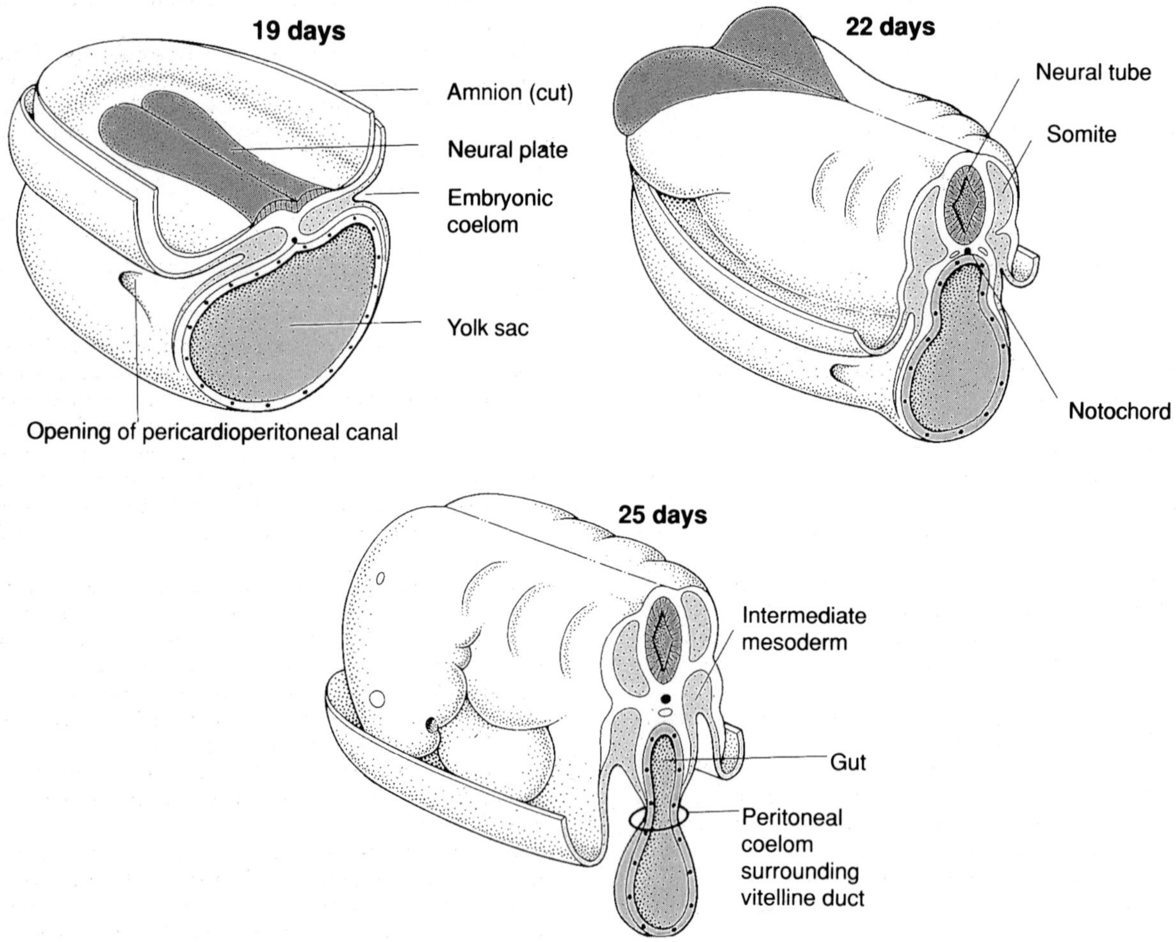

Figure 8.27 *Schematic transverse sections depicting formation of the lateral body folds (from Fitzgerald MJT, Fitzgerald M, 1994, with permission).*

portion retained within the embryo being the gut. The portion of the yolk sac extruded from the embryo is called the **vitelline duct**. It remains attached to the gut at the **vitellointestinal communication**. The vitelline duct disappears later on. At the conclusion of the flexion process the brain overhangs the developing heart and the heart is ventral to the foregut. The midgut faces into the vitelline duct and the hindgut extends from the vitellointestinal communication to the cloacal membrane.

Transverse folding

The lateral margins of the embryonic disc form the lateral body folds which turn the embryo from a flattened disc into a cylinder. The peritoneal coelom on each side initially opened out into the extraembryonic coelom. Transverse folding directs these openings ventrally and with the constriction of the yolk sac the two openings communicate across the midline to form the peritoneal cavity.

Summary of main points

- Gametogenesis is the production of ova and spermatozoa by meiosis. This allows the independent assortment of maternal and paternal chromosomes with their genes amongst the gametes.
- Oogenesis begins before a woman's birth but is not completed until after puberty and is a recurring process in each menstrual cycle. The ovarian cycle is divided into two parts: a preovulatory phase in which the follicles develop (the follicular phase) and the luteal phase following ovulation.
- The production of spermatozoa occurs in the seminiferous tubules of the testes. In a functioning testis germ cells will be present at various stages of development, all originating from spermatogonia. The process takes about 70 days and several hundred million a day are produced continuously from puberty. As men become older the seminal tubules undergo involution. Germ cells are reduced in number but the Sertoli cells remain.
- The oocyte is a very large cell and usually only one is released at ovulation. It must contain all the material necessary for the beginning of growth and development of the embryo following fertilisation. Sperm are very small and millions of them are released during ejaculation. About 1000 of the ejaculated sperm will reach the ovum. When one sperm enters a secondary oocyte the first cell of a new human being, with 46 chromosomes, is formed.
- Freshly ejaculated sperm are unable to fertilise an ovum and must undergo capacitation whilst travelling through the female genital tract. When a capacitated sperm meets the corona radiata of the oocyte the acrosome develops perforations in it. This is known as the acrosome reaction.
- Lytic enzymes are released around the oocyte and it takes the enzymes from many sperm to create a passageway for one sperm to enter. There is dispersal of the follicular cells of the corona radiata, allowing the head of the sperm to make contact with the zona pellucida.
- Other enzymes are released and these produce an opening in the zona pellucida. This is followed by fusion of the sperm cell membrane with the oocyte cell membrane and the nucleus of one sperm passes into the oocyte. The ability of the oocyte to fuse with the sperm must immediately be reversed following entry of the first sperm to prevent the entry of multiple sperm (polyspermy). There is a fast block and a slow block to polyspermy.
- Cells have small organelles that produce energy for the cell, called mitochondria. The more active the cell is, the more mitochondria it contains so that busy cells like muscle and liver cells have hundreds of them. Mitochondria are inherited from our mothers' ovum as the sperm mitochondria used in motility are shed with the tail and do not enter the oocyte. MtDNA may contain mutations that lead to congenital disease in humans.
- The preimplantation period between fertilisation and implantation lasts about 6 days. The conceptus is called an embryo from the commencement of implantation until the end of the 8th week after fertilisation when it becomes known as a fetus.
- There are three important concepts in understanding embryology: there is a programme of simple instructions that can generate complex forms; most developmental processes depend upon a coordinated interaction of genetic and environmental factors; and each system in the body has its own developmental pattern. The information to make an embryo is located in the deoxyribonucleic acid (DNA) of the zygote and is contributed to by the ovum and sperm.
- Cells in the embryo change shape and position and this pattern of cell movements is part of the embryo's developmental programme. Cellular processes include somatic cell division, cell differentiation, induction, cell migration and programmed cell death to remove redundant cells.
- When days of development are given these are days from fertilisation and not from the last menstrual period. The first event is the splitting of the very large zygote into smaller cells through the process of mitosis, a process called cleavage. The daughter cells are called blastomeres.
- By the 4th day after fertilisation, there are between 16 and 20 cells and the conceptus is known as the morula. The cells at this stage are said to be totipotent and could contribute to any part of the embryo. If the cells are separated there is the potential for multiple identical individuals.
- Humans have about 350 different cell types. Cells carry out an amazing variety of functions. Research has identified regulatory genes that control patterning in the embryo of the fruit fly. Regulation of the complex development of the embryo appears to be by a cascade of gene products. The most important discovery was of a discrete portion of DNA called the homeobox. These genes control segmentation in the developing embryo so that the correct positioning of organs is brought about. Homeobox genes may be switched on to produce their protein products sequentially by chemical gradients.
- During a limited time in early development some embryonic tissues can influence the development of adjacent tissues. In the case of the nervous system, inward movement of the outer cells is said to induce its development. These influencing tissues are called inductors or organisers. The induction signal varies and in some tissues may take the form of a diffusible molecule passing from one tissue to another. In other tissues the message is mediated by a non-diffusible extracellular matrix secreted by the inductor with which the reacting tissue comes into contact. Programmed cell death plays a major part in the final pattern of cells.
- The group of cells carries on cleaving during the next 4 days during which time the conceptus passes through the fallopian tubes into the uterine cavity. There is also polarisation where the inner cells divide less frequently and remain large and round whilst the outer cells in contact with the zona pellucida become flattened.
- On the 5th day after fertilisation the zygote 'hatches' as the zona pellucida is digested by uterine secretions. Fluid accumulates in the space between the peripheral and central cells of the morula and the conceptus has now become a blastocyst. The inner cell mass of the

blastocyst is the embryoblast which becomes the embryo and the flattened outer layer of cells is called the trophoblast which forms the placenta.

- On the 6th day the blastocyst begins to implant into the endometrium, most commonly on the posterior wall of the uterus. Where the trophoblastic cells make contact with the endometrium they undergo rapid DNA synthesis and become cuboid in shape to form the cytotrophoblast. Daughter cells shed their plasma membranes to form the syncytium. This mass of tissue, called the syncytiotrophoblast, produces enzymes that attack the endometrium and hormones that allow the pregnancy to continue.
- At the implantation site there is development and dilatation of new blood capillaries fed by branches of the spiral arteries and drained by the endometrial veins. The hormone HCG enters the maternal circulation and maintains the corpus luteum to ensure continued production of oestrogen and progesterone for maintenance of the pregnancy until the placenta produces them at 12 weeks.
- By the 2nd week of development the cells are well organised and the inner cell mass forms a flattened disc consisting of the inner layer or epiblast and the outer layer or hypoblast. Together, they are known as the bilaminar embryonic disc.
- The cell margins of the hypoblast divide rapidly to form branched cells that line the cavity of the blastocyst – the extraembryonic mesoderm. Spaces develop within the mesoderm and coalesce to become the extraembryonic coelom, splitting the mesoderm into a visceral layer which is included in the yolk sac and a parietal layer which contributes to the chorion together with the trophoblast. The visceral and parietal extraembryonic mesoderm are linked by a connecting stalk that will develop into the umbilical cord.
- An immense amount of cellular activity occurs during embryogenesis and organogenesis. Cells migrate and move about the embryo and then differentiate into specific cell types to form organs and systems. The three processes of formation of the primitive streak, gastrulation and formation of the notochord are extremely important in creating the body plan.
- From 3 weeks the embryo enters the vulnerable stage of organogenesis. The zygote is now technically known as the embryo until 8 weeks when it becomes known as the fetus. Organogenesis involves many processes and much simultaneous cell movement.
- From about day 20 until day 30 the dorsal surface of the embryo develops a segmented aspect with the appearance of paired somites which are clumps of embryonic tissue. From the somites develop the vertebral column and the segmentally innervated muscles of the trunk.
- Tissues derived from neuroectoderm include the central and peripheral nervous systems, the retina of the eye and the posterior lobe of the pituitary gland. Tissues derived from surface ectoderm include the outer layer of the skin, called the epidermis, with its hair follicles and cutaneous glands, the breasts, the lens of the eye, the special sense cells of the inner ear, the anterior lobe of the pituitary gland and the enamel of the teeth.
- The process of development of the human brain and nervous system is known as neurulation. The notochord induces its overlying ectoderm to thicken and form a neural plate. A flat sheet of cells on the upper surface of the embryo folds up into a tube which will develop into the brain and spinal cord. The cranial neuropore closes on day 25 or 26 and the caudal neuropore on day 27 or 28. This early closure of the neural tube has implications for the causation and prevention of open neural tube defects.
- Folding of cell sheets forms the basis of the early development of organs and folding of the embryo changes its shape and the relationships of the organs. Longitudinal folding and transverse folding of the sheets of cells both occur in the early embryo.

References

Alberts B, Bray D, Lewis et al. 1994 Molecular Biology of the cell. Garland, New York.

Chiras DD. 1991 Human Biology. West, New York.

De Robertis EM, Oliver G, Wright CVE. 1990 Homeobox genes and the vertebrate body plan. Scientific American, 263 (1) 26–32.

Fitzgerald MJT, Fitzgerald M. 1994 Human Embryology. Baillière Tindall, London.

Gilbert SF. 1988 Developmental Biology, 2nd edn. Sinauer Associates, Massachusetts.

Hinchliff SM, Montague SE. 1990 Physiology for Nursing Practice. Baillière Tindall, London.

Hinchliff SM Montague SE, Watson R. 1996 Physiology for Nursing Practice, Bailliere Tindall, London.

HMSO 1990 Human Fertilisation and Embryology Act 1990. HMSO, London

Lewin R. 1990 A new type of genetic disease. New Scientist, 126 (1720) 41.

McGinnis W, Kuziora M. 1994 The molecular architects of body design. Scientific American, 270 (2) 36–42.

Moore KL. 1989 Before We Are Born, 3rd edn. WB Saunders, Philadelphia.

Nusslein-Volhard C. 1996 Gradients that organise embryo development. Scientific American 275 (2) 38–43.

Sweet B. 1997 Mayes' Midwifery. Baillière Tindall, London.

Waddington C. 1940 quoted in Wolpert L. 1991 The Triumph of the Embryo. Oxford University Press, Oxford.

Wolpert L. 1991 The Triumph of the Embryo. Oxford University Press, Oxford.

Recommended reading

De Robertis EM, Oliver G, Wright CVE. 1990 Homeobox genes and the vertebrate body plan. Scientific American, 263(1) 26–32.

Fitzgerald MJT Fitzgerald M. 1994 Human Embryology. Bailliére Tindall, London.

McGinnis W, Kuziora M. 1994 The molecular architects of body design. Scientific American, 270 (2) 36–42.

Moore KL. 1989 Before We Are born, 3rd edn. WB Saunders, Philadelphia.

Nusslein-Volhard C. 1996 Gradients that organise embryo development. Scientific American, 275 (2) 38–43.

Wolpert L. 1991 The Triumph of the Embryo. Oxford University Press, Oxford.

Chapter 9 Embryological systems 1 – trunk, head and limbs

In this chapter

INTRODUCTION

This chapter and the next are intended to help the student understand when and how normal systems develop and to act as a knowledge base for the understanding of congenital abnormalities. Explanations will be kept as simple as possible as the student is not expected to be an expert in the field. Each system will be discussed separately. In order, these are the trunk, skeletal and soft tissues, the skull, the brain, the spinal cord, structures of the head and neck, the ears and eyes, the limbs, the cardiovascular system, the respiratory system, the alimentary tract and the genitourinary systems. Fitzgerald & Fitzgerald (1994) and Moore (1989) are the major sources for this chapter and are useful for students who wish to deepen their knowledge. The fetal skull is discussed in Chapter 24.

THE TRUNK

Skeletal features

The vertebral column

There are four phases in the development of the vertebral column: mesenchymal, blastemal, cartilaginous and bony.

Mesenchymal

The precursors of the vertebrae are called sclerotomes and are derived from the somites. Mesenchymal cells surround the notochord to form the segmented mesenchymal vertebral column.

Blastemal

The cranial end of each mesenchymal vertebra has a thinned out appearance because of the relative sparseness of cells. The caudal end is denser. The cells at the interface between the two tissues will form an intervertebral disc and the remainder of the condensed element merges with the vertebra caudal to it. This means that the centrum of the blastemal vertebra is formed from two sclerotomes on each side of it. From the condensed upper part of the centrum, a pair of neural arches grows and surrounds the neural tube. The neural arches give rise to paired costal and transverse processes. The meninges are laid down in the blastemal period. Cells from inside the rim of the neural arches form the dura mater and the arachnoid mater and pia mater are formed from cells of the neural crest.

Cartilaginous

Chondrification centres appear in the centrum and the neural arch late in the 5th week. In the 12 thoracic vertebrae the cartilaginous costal processes which will develop into the ribs become detached from their parent neural arches by the formation of synovial joints. Synovial joints also appear between the costal and transverse processes. At other levels in the spine the costal processes become incorporated into the vertebrae.

Bony

During the 8th week ossification centres appear in the central and neural arches and in the ribs.

Ribs and sternum

As the lateral body folds develop in the 4th week, the somatic mesoderm is penetrated by the thoracic costal processes which induce the mesoderm to add to their tips, completing the formation of the blastemal ribs. The sternum begins with the development of two sternal bars in the ventral part of the somatic mesoderm. The bars meet in the midline and unite from above downward to form a mesenchymatous sternum. The xiphisternum often remains bifid. The ventral ends of the cranial seven costal processes fuse with the sternum and cartilage persists at the junction as the costal cartilages.

Soft tissues

The dermomyotomes are what remains of the somites after the sclerotomes depart to surround the notochord. During the lateral folding of the body the dermomyotomes split into **dermatomes** (Gilbert 1988).

Myotomes

Myotomes give rise to the muscles of the head and trunk. This

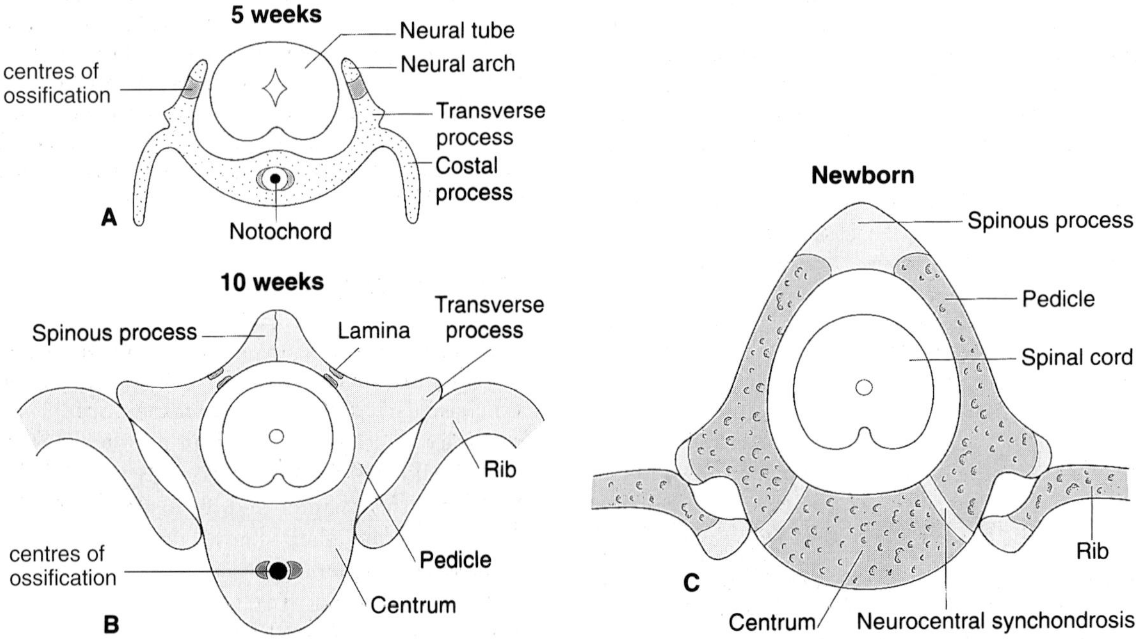

Figure 9.1 *(a) Blastemal vertebra with centres of chondrification (shaded dark). (b) Cartilaginous vertebra with centres of ossification (shaded dark). (c) Bony vertebra (from Fitzgerald MJT, Fitzgerald M, 1994, with permission).*

includes all the muscles that link the vertebrae together and to the skull and the muscles of the abdominal and thoracic walls. The muscles of the limbs, including the muscles that are involved in attachment of the upper limb to the trunk such as the pectoralis, sternomastoid and trapezius muscles, are not formed from the myotomes. Each myotome divides into a dorsal epimere and a ventral hypomere. The corresponding spinal nerves divide into dorsal and ventral rami. Dorsal rami supply the muscles with motor fibres originating in the ventral horn of the spinal cord. The muscles and their overlying dermatomes are supplied via ventral rami with sensory fibres originating in the appropriate dorsal root ganglion.

Dermatomes

The dermatomes merge with each other and migrate to form the connective tissue or dermis layer of the skin. Each dermatome is accompanied by sensory nerve fibres derived from the level in the spinal cord where the dermatome originated. This is why neurologists are interested in dividing the body surface into clinical regions called dermatomes which is the band of skin and its spinal nerve.

The skin and mammary gland

Whereas the dermis develops from the dermatomes, the outer layer of skin or epidermis and its appendages are derived from the surface ectoderm. At first, the surface ectoderm is a single cuboidal layer but it becomes two-layered in the 2nd month. The superficial layer or periderm is now shed, leaving the underlying germinal layer to form the structures of the skin. In the 3rd month the epidermis becomes stratified and its basal layer sends pegs down into the dermis to form the root sheath of the hair follicles. During the 5th month the sebaceous glands bud into the dermis from the root sheath and the sweat glands grow down from the epidermis. **Lanugo**, which is a coat of very fine hair, grows all over the body and the sebaceous glands produce a secretion which, when mixed with peridermal cells and lanugo, becomes the white 'cheesy' **vernix caseosa**. True or **vellus hair** is derived from a second set of hair follicles and replaces the lanugo which is shed shortly before birth.

The mammary gland, whose structure and function will be described in Chapter 54, makes its appearance in the 6th week as paired strips of ectodermal thickening formed longitudinally on the ventral surface of the embryo called the mammary ridge. In humans normally only one pair of breasts forms from the thoracic part of the ridge and the rest of the ridge disappears.

THE SKULL

The adult skull is divided into two parts: the **neurocranium**, which encloses the brain and consists of the vault and base, and the **viscerocranium** making up the bones of the face. The base, called the **chondrocranium**, and viscerocranium develop out of cartilage mainly from ectomesoderm of neural crest origin, whilst the vault bones develop from membrane with a paraxial mesoderm origin.

The vault

The bones making up the vault will be described in detail in Chapter 24. Basic facts will be presented here. Intramembranous ossification begins from the 4th month with separate ossification centres giving rise to the parietal bones, frontal bones, occipital bone and the squamous part of the temporal bone. Fusion of the two frontal bones is not complete until a child is 8 years old.

The viscerocranium

All the facial bones ossify in membrane from neural crest elements. The mandible is the first skeletal part to commence ossification early in the 6th week. A template is laid down in cartilage. The ramus is formed by endochondrial ossification from a **condylar growth centre** that appears in the 14th week. This is responsible for the elongation of the ramus during the first 10 years of life.

The teeth

Tooth buds form from thickened ectoderm called the **dental lamina** – 10 in the upper jaw and 10 in the lower jaw. These are responsible for the deciduous teeth, commonly known as milk teeth. Later the dental lamina forms the buds of the permanent dentition. The permanent molar teeth do not have precursors in the deciduous dentition but develop from a backward extension of the dental lamina.

The crowns of the teeth begin when cells called **odontoblasts** form **predentine**, which later calcifies to become **dentine**. This calcification is a signal for cells called **ameloblasts** to start laying down tooth enamel on the surface of the dentine. The central cells constitute the pulp of the tooth which is richly supplied with blood and sensory nerve endings, as many of us can testify!

Deep to the level of enamel production, the outer and inner enamel epithelia fuse to form the epithelial root sheath. Predentine and dentine are again induced to form the root of the tooth. The mesoderm of the dental sac produces a specialised form of bone called cement and the periodontal ligament which anchors the cement to the wall of the tooth socket. Eruption of the deciduous teeth normally occurs between 6 months and 2 years after birth.

THE BRAIN

The human nervous system begins to form at approximately 19 days after fertilisation and is the earliest system to differentiate. The brain is actually a very complex structure made up of separate sections with very different functions. By 19 days the three expansions of the brain are present (Fig. 9.2). These are known as the primary brain vesicles and the correct terms are (Marieb 1992):

- forebrain – prosencephalon
- midbrain – mesencephalon
- hindbrain – rhombencephalon.

From 4 weeks the major regions of the brain are distinct and neurones begin to differentiate from the epithelium of the

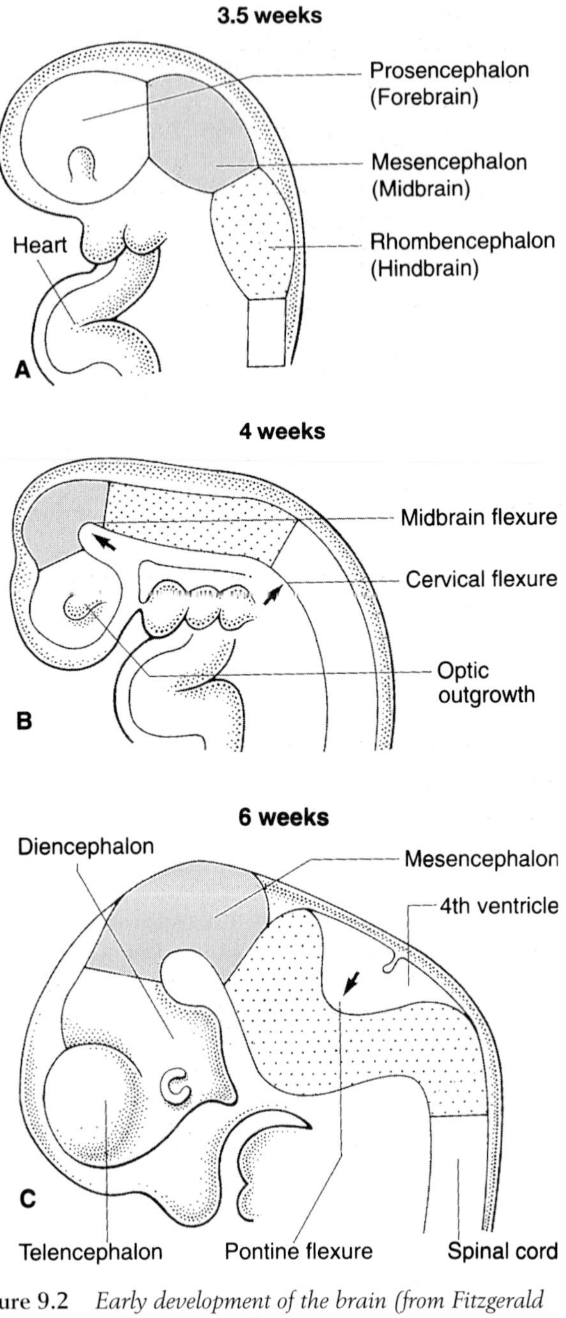

Figure 9.2 *Early development of the brain (from Fitzgerald MJT, Fitzgerald M, 1994, with permission).*

neural tube. The thalamus and hypothalamus are differentiated by the 5th week (Fig. 9.3). By the end of the 8th week the head is equal to half the length of the embryo and controls the first movement of the limbs (McNabb 1997).

The changing shape of the brain

The brainstem buckles and a cervical flexure appears at the junction of the brainstem and spinal cord. A midline flexure moves the mesencephalon to the summit of the brain (Marieb 1992). The rhombencephalon folds on itself, causing the walls of the neural tube to expand into the 4th ventricle. The dorsal region of the prosencephalon expands on either side to form the cerebral hemispheres or **telencephalon**. Within the cerebral hemispheres the neural canal dilates to form the lateral ventricles. The remainder of the prosencephalon which straddles the midline is known as the **diencephalon**. The 3rd ventricle is a cavity within the diencephalon and communicates with the 4th ventricle through the **aqueduct of Sylvius**.

An outgrowth from the diencephalon becomes the two retinas and optic nerves. The cranial end of the rhombencephalon gives rise to the pons and the cerebellum whilst the caudal end becomes the medulla oblongata.

The cerebellum

In the cranial end of the rhombencephalon, paired **rhombic lips** arise. Neuroblasts proliferate to form the cerebellar **primordium**. At first the cerebellum enlarges within the 4th ventricle but later, as the extraventricular portion grows rapidly, the cerebellum seems to evert.

The forebrain

Neurones migrate from the ventricular zone of the telencephalon to the surface where they form the **cerebral cortex**. The frontal, parietal, occipital and temporal lobes are present at 12–14 weeks. Several complex processes give rise to the structures in the cerebral hemispheres such as the hippocampus. Two commissures of nerve fibres link the right and left cerebral hemispheres. These are the **anterior commissure**, which connects the olfactory regions, and the much larger **corpus callosum** linking matched areas of the cerebral cortex.

Other brain structures

The diencephalon gives rise to the **epithalamus** which remains small and forms the pineal gland, the paired and linked **thalami**, which are actually made of about 30 separate nuclei (small discrete sections), and the **hypothalamus**. The basal ganglia develop immediately below the thalamus and are involved in the control of body movement. There are four separate nuclei: the striatum, the pallidum, the subthalamic nucleus and the better known substantia nigra.

Blood supply of the brain

The arterial blood supply develops from cranial segments of the dorsal aortae. These are two internal carotid arteries and two vertebral arteries. The internal carotid arteries run alongside the diencephalon and give off the anterior, middle and posterior cerebral arteries. Each vertebral artery gives off a branch which supplies the cerebellum and medulla oblongata before uniting with its partner to form the basilar artery. The basilar artery gives off two pairs of arteries to the cerebellum and upper brainstem before dividing into two terminal branches that link up with the ends of the internal carotids.

There are differences in the final arrangements of the blood supply, with 25% of the population maintaining three cerebral arteries on both sides of the brain whilst in the majority of people the vertebral arteries take over the posterior cerebral arteries. These intercommunicating arteries at the base of the

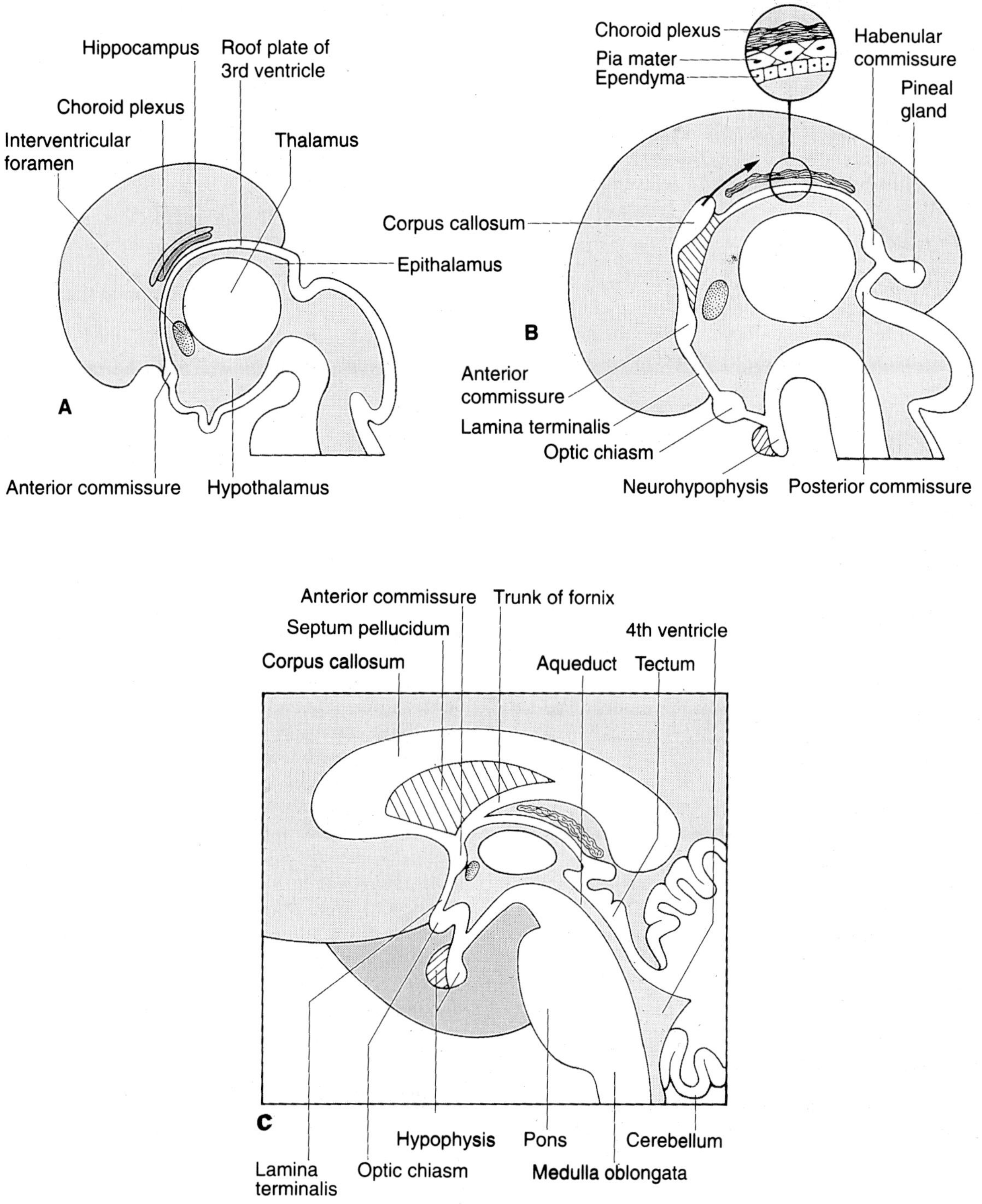

Figure 9.3 *Median sections of the brain. (a) At 8 weeks. (b) At 12 weeks. (c) Postnatal (from Fitzgerald MJT, Fitzgerald M, 1994, with permission).*

brain are known as the **circle of Willis**. The venous drainage will be discussed fully in Chapter 24.

THE SPINAL CORD

Following the closure of the neural tube and the segmentation of the paraxial mesoderm into somites, neural crest cells form clusters corresponding to the somites. When the caudal neuropore closes at about the 28th day the neural tube reaches only as far as the 2nd pair of somites and the rest of the somites differentiate in the following week. Corresponding levels of the neural tube develop from the primitive streak during the process of **secondary neurulation**. At first, the neural tube is solid but it becomes canalised by caudal extension of the neural canal.

Zones of the spinal cord

During the 5th week a shallow sulcus limitans (limiting groove) appears on each side of the neural canal, separating the side walls into the dorsal section called the **dorsolateral (alar) plate** and the **ventrolateral (basal) plate**. It is possible to distinguish three zones in the side walls of the neural tube. These are, from within outwards, the ventricular, intermediate and marginal zones.

The ventricular zone

The inner ventricular zone is where neuroepithelial cells divide. After several cell divisions the daughter cells move out of the ventricular zone. The first cells to move out become neurones and the last to move out become the connective tissue cells called **neuroglia**.

The intermediate zone

The intermediate zone is the forerunner of the grey matter of the spinal cord and is composed of **neuroblasts** that have migrated from the ventricular zone. These differentiate into neurones and grow processes called **neurites**. Once this has happened, the neurones cannot divide. **Glioblasts** enter the intermediate zone and differentiate into **astrocytes**, which provide structural support for the central nervous system (CNS), and **oligodendrocytes** which will form the **myelin sheaths**. **Microglial cells** are phagocytic and develop from the monocytes of the blood and migrate from the capillary bed to enter the CNS during the 3rd month.

The marginal zone

The marginal zone is the forerunner of the white matter. Small neurones invade the marginal zone and emit axons alongside the grey matter to form pathways that link the different levels of the cord.

During the 6th week an accumulation of neuroblasts in the dorsolateral plate gives rise to the dorsal horn of grey matter which has a sensory function. The dorsal horn communicates with neurites of the neural crest cells that have accumulated outside the neural tube to form dorsal root ganglia. Large accumulations of cells in the ventrolateral plate form the ventral horn of grey matter which has a motor function. Axons emerging from the ventral horn form the ventral nerve roots which join with peripheral processes to form the mixed spinal nerves.

The definitive spinal cord

During weeks 7–10 the definitive spinal cord is formed. The neural canal shrinks to become the central canal of the spinal cord. Cells left behind in the ventricular zone develop cilia and become the lining cells of the central canal called **ependymal cells**. The discrete ascending and descending columns in the white matter are finalised. These are the fast-conducting posterior columns which will acquire myelin sheaths and the lateral and ventral columns formed by ascending pathways from neurones in the dorsal grey horns and descending pathways from the brain.

Cells from the neural crest

The neural crest cells are pluripotent, meaning they can give rise to tissues of more than one kind. The following is a list of cell types thought to originate in the neural crest, many of them involved in regulation of body systems.

- Dorsal root ganglia cells
- Autonomic ganglion cells
- Chromaffin cells of the adrenal medulla
- Schwann cells producing myelin sheaths around peripheral neuronal processes
- Pia mater and arachnoid mater around the brain and spinal cord
- Melanocytes of the skin
- Connective tissue in the wall of the heart and great vessels
- Parafollicular cells of the thyroid gland
- Glomus cells of the carotid and aortic bodies
- Much of the craniofacial skeleton
- Odontoblasts of the developing teeth

STRUCTURES OF THE HEAD AND NECK

Branchial arches and placodes

Branchial arches begin to develop early in the 4th week as ridges on the future head and neck region. During the 5th week a side view of the embryo shows the presence of five pairs of branchial (sometimes known as pharyngeal) arches. These are numbered I, II, III, IV and VI in craniocaudal sequence. In vertebrates other than mammals, arch V is important but in mammals the 5th pair of arches is transient. These arches are formed of mesoderm and are the equivalent of the gill arches (branchia) in fishes. However, in mammals there are no gill slits and the arches are linked by mesoderm (Fig. 9.4). On the surface ectoderm there are a number of thickenings called **placodes**. Three of these are the nasal placode, lens placode and otic placode, whilst four others contribute sensory ganglion cells to the underlying cranial nerves. Most malformations of the head and neck happen during transformation of branchial arch structures into their final form.

Sources of the mesoderm

Head and neck mesoderm originates mainly from two sources: the paraxial mesoderm and the neural crest. The paraxial mesoderm is divided into three parts.

- The cranial part does not form somites but forms the bulk of the branchial arch mesoderm.
- The first four occipital somites form sclerotomes that contribute to the occipital bone, myotomes that form the muscles of the tongue and dermatomes that form the dermis in the occipital region.
- The eight pairs of cervical somites form sclerotomes that give rise to the cervical vertebrae, myotomes that form the muscles of the neck and dermatomes that form the dermis of the neck.

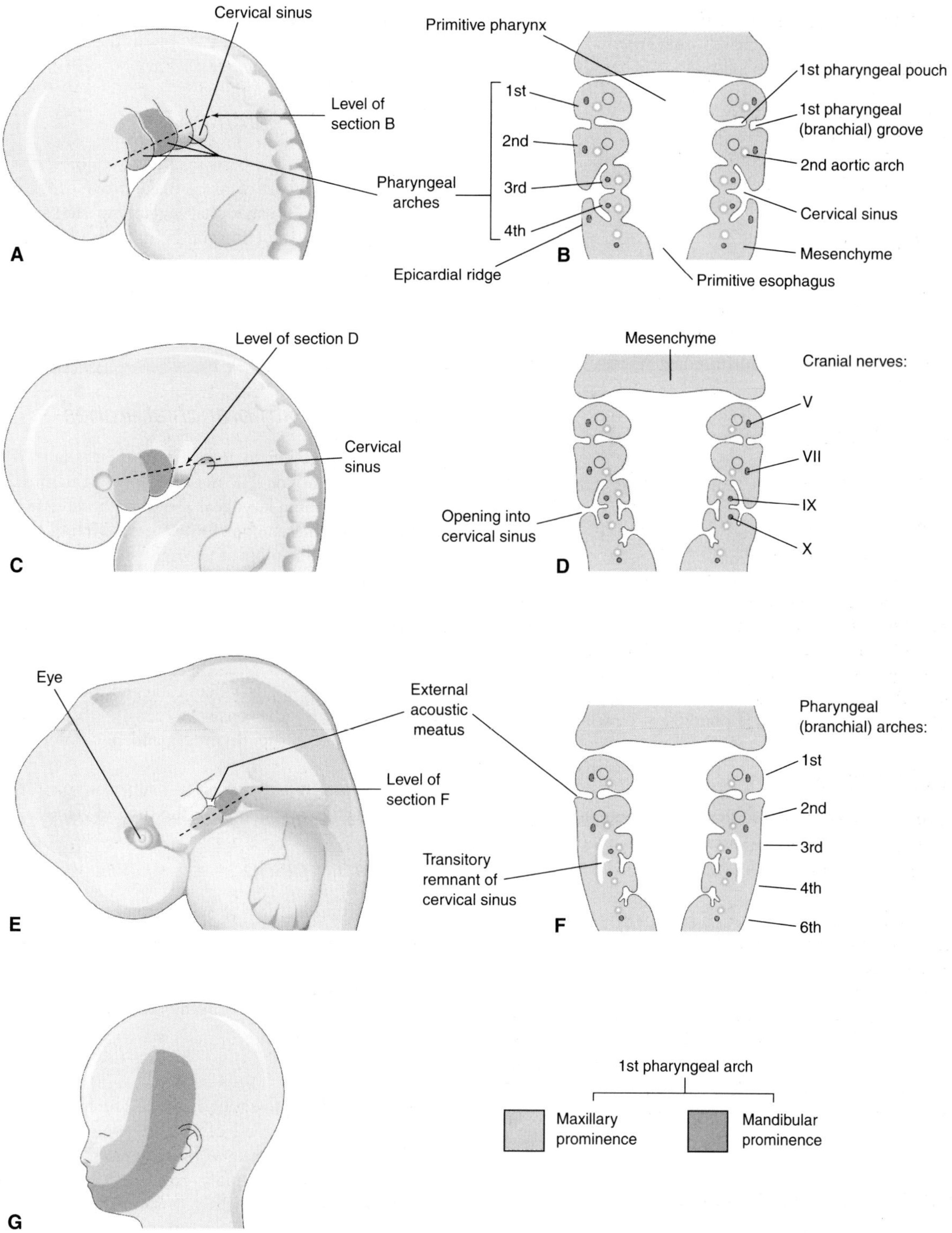

Figure 9.4 *(a) Lateral view of the head, neck and thoracic regions of an embryo (about 32 days), showing the pharyngeal arches and cervical sinus. (b) Diagrammatic section through the embryo at the level shown in (a), illustrating growth of the second arch over the third and fourth arches. (c) An embryo of about 33 days. (d) Section of the embryo at the level shown in (c), illustrating early closure of the cervical sinus. (e) An embryo of about 41 days. (f) Section of the embryo at the level shown in (e), showing the transitory cystic remnant of the cervical sinus. (g) Drawing of a 20-week fetus illustrating the area of the face derived from the first pair of pharyngeal arches. (Reproduced with permission from Moore 1989.)*

The neural crest produces some cells called **ectomesenchyme** which can produce tissues which would normally require mesoderm. These cells migrate as follows.

- From the hindbrain, they enter the branchial arches to become cartilage and bone-forming cells.
- From the midbrain, they contribute to the skeleton and connective tissue of the face and the teeth.
- From the forebrain, they contribute to the vascular and fibrous coats of the eyeball.

Structure of the branchial arches

Every arch contains the following structures.

1 Migrated neural crest cells surrounding a central core of mesenchyme cells.
2 Unsegmented mesoderm which can form muscle and bone.
3 An artery that branches off the dorsal aorta on the same side as the arch.
4 A nerve carrying motor fibres, called **branchial efferents**, to support the striated muscles.
5 An external covering of ectoderm.
6 An internal covering of endoderm.

The cells derived from the neural crest form the skeletal structures that will lead to the bones of the head and neck.

Pharyngeal pouches and branchial grooves

From the endoderm pockets called pharyngeal pouches develop between the branchial arches. There are four well-defined pairs and the 5th pair is rudimentary. The primitive pharynx develops from the foregut and widens cranially. It is lined by the endoderm covering the internal surfaces of the branchial arches. Externally the branchial arches are separated by pockets of ectoderm named branchial grooves.

Derivatives of the branchial arches

First branchial arch

The first pair of arches are the **mandibular arches**, involved in the development of the face. The cartilage of this arch forms **Meckel's cartilage** which serves as a template for the development of the mandible. During the 6th week the mandible develops around the ventral portion of the cartilage by ossification of surrounding membrane and the cartilage mostly disappears. The dorsal end of Meckel's cartilage ossifies and is incorporated into the middle ear to form the malleus and incus. From the dorsal part of each mandibular arch, the mandibular prominence and the maxillary prominence develop.

Second branchial arch

The second arch is called the **hyoid arch** which has a much smaller skeletal component than the first. The hyoid arch undergoes endochondrial ossification at its dorsal end to form the stapes of the middle ear and the styloid process of the temporal bone. Its ventral end forms part of the hyoid bone. Most of its mesoderm migrates to form the muscles of facial expression which are inserted into the skin. The facial nerve carries the branchial efferent supply to the muscles formed from the hyoid arch.

Third branchial arch

The 3rd arch forms the basis for the posterior part of the tongue whilst the ventral part of its cartilage provides the lower half of the hyoid bone. The stylopharyngeus muscle running from the styloid process of the temporal bone to the pharynx is the only muscle formed from this arch. It is innervated by the glossopharyngeal nerve. The sensory nerve fibres for taste at the posterior part of the tongue are also carried by the glossopharyngeal nerve. The artery of this arch persists as part of the internal carotid artery.

Fourth and sixth branchial arches

These come together to form the cartilages and ligaments and muscles of the larynx. The nerve supply to the muscles is via the vagus nerve through laryngeal and pharyngeal branches. The left artery of the 4th arch contributes to the arch of the aorta whilst the right one forms most of the right subclavian artery.

Derivatives of the pharyngeal pouches

Derivatives of the pharyngeal pouches are:

- first pouch – the Eustachian tube and the middle ear cavity;
- second pouch – the tonsils;
- third pouch – the thymus gland and inferior parathyroid gland;
- fourth pouch/5th pouch – superior parathyroid gland, parafollicular and C cells of the thyroid gland.

The thyroid gland

This arises during the 4th week from a thickening of midline endoderm in the floor of the pharynx. It is the first endocrine gland to develop. The median rudiment bifurcates to form two lobes connected by an isthmus. By 7 weeks the thyroid gland reaches its final destination in the neck.

The tongue

This develops from five tongue buds. The first or median tongue bud develops at the end of the 4th week on the floor of the pharynx. Two distal tongue buds develop on each side of the median tongue bud, rapidly grow and overgrow the median tongue bud to merge together to form the anterior or oral two-thirds of the tongue. The posterior part of the tongue develops from mesoderm in the 3rd and 4th branchial arches.

Derivatives of the branchial grooves

The only branchial groove that contributes to final structures is the first, which forms the external canal of the ear. The others come to lie in a depression called the **cervical sinus** formed during the 5th week when the 2nd branchial arch overgrows the 3rd and 4th arches to form a deep ectodermal depression. The

2nd to 4th branchial grooves and the cervical sinus are obliterated during the 6th and 7th weeks as the neck develops, giving the neck a smooth contour. Derivatives of the branchial arches and pharyngeal pouches are described below.

THE FACE

The development of the face is complex and it is not possible to cover every detail in this chapter (Fig. 9.5). The primitive mouth begins as a slight depression of the surface ectoderm called the **stomodeum**. It is separated from the foregut by the **oropharyngeal membrane** which ruptures about day 24 to bring the digestive tract into communication with the amniotic cavity. Early in the 4th week, in the region of the future face, five prominences emerge around the stomodeum. They are the frontonasal prominence and the two pairs of mandibular and

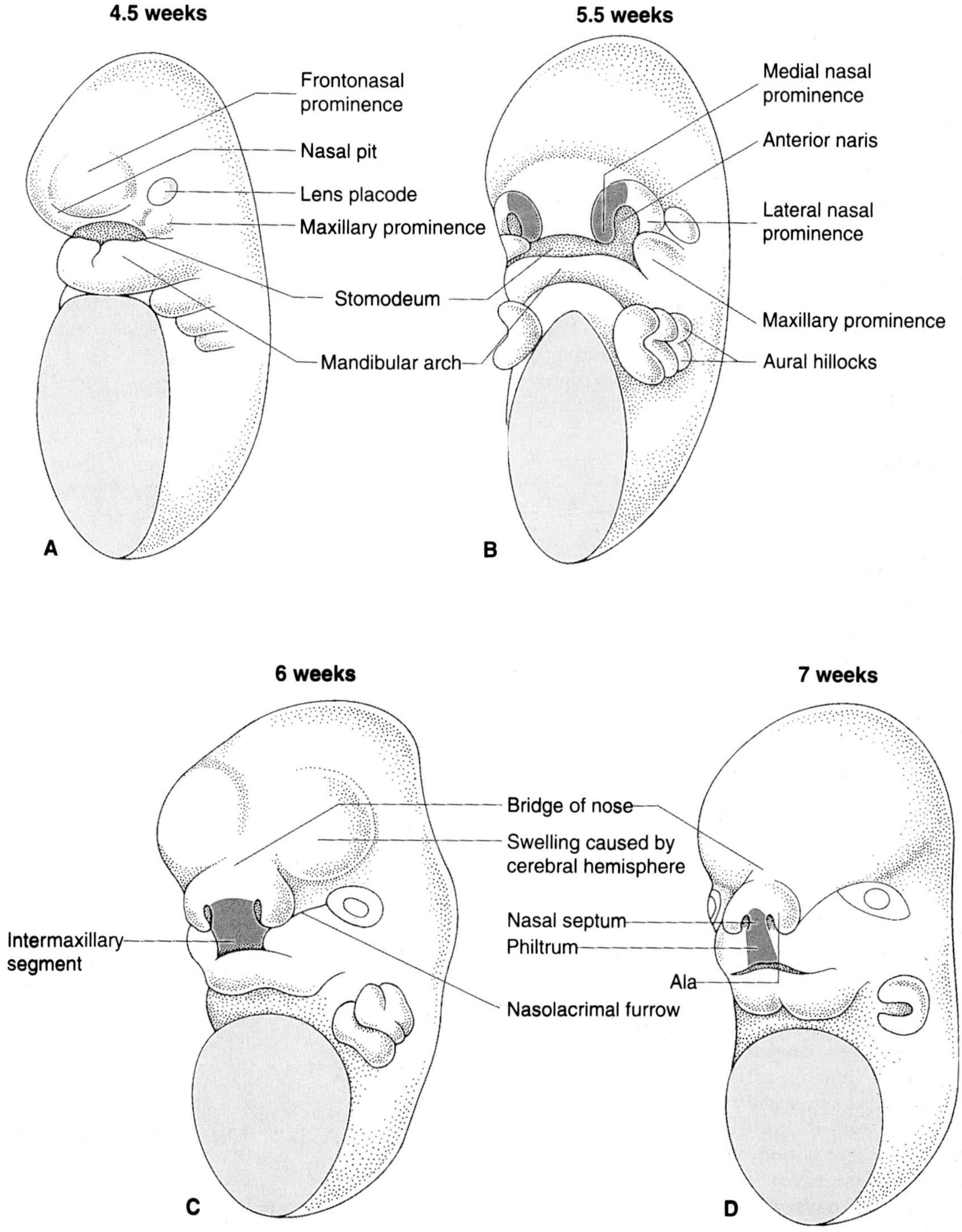

Figure 9.5 a–d *Development of the face. Medial nasal processes and intermaxillary segment are shaded dark (from Fitzgerald MJT, Fitzgerald M, 1994, with permission).*

two pairs of maxillary prominences. These merge with each other and are covered by surface ectoderm. The lens placodes of the future eyes lie over the maxillary prominences.

The mandibular prominence forms the lower jaw or mandible and the maxillary prominence gives rise to the upper jaw or maxilla, the zygomatic bone and the squamous portion of the temporal bone as well as the outer parts of the upper lip. Mandibular arch mesoderm forms the muscles of mastication which are inserted into the mandible. The branchial efferent nerve to the muscles of mastication is the mandibular branch of the trigeminal nerve. The skin of the face and mucous membranes of the mouth are formed from mandibular arch ectoderm. They receive a somatic sensory nerve supply from the three branches of the trigeminal nerve: ophthalmic, maxillary and mandibular.

The formation of the midline portion of the face, including the nose, palate and upper lip, begins early in the 5th week when the two nasal placodes recede into **nasal pits**. A week later the frontonasal prominence extends onto both sides of the nasal pits to form the medial and lateral nasal prominences. The openings to the nasal pits become the nostrils. The two medial nasal prominences merge across the midline to form the intermaxillary segment. During the 7th week this produces three midline structures: the lower border of the nasal septum, the philtrum of the upper lip and the primary palate. Failure of these structures to develop results in cleft lip and palate, among the commoner congenital malformations.

THE EARS

The outer and middle ear

The **pinna** (auricle) of the ear develops from six aural hillocks, three on the first branchial arch and three on the second. It is situated at first in the upper part of the neck and is displaced cranially during development of the mandible. Of the pharyngeal clefts, only the first is of significance. It gives rise to the **external acoustic meatus** (outer ear canal). The middle ear cavity extends outwards from the first pharyngeal pouch during the 5th week. It makes contact with the outer ear canal and where they meet, a thin layer of mesoderm remains to form the tympanic membrane (eardrum). As described above, the ossicles develop from the dorsal ends of the first and second pharyngeal arches.

The inner ear

At the end of the 3rd week, an **otic placode** develops on either side of the head. These sink below the surface to form the **otic vesicles (otocysts)**, which develop a **vestibular sac** and a **cochlear sac**. From the vestibular sac three plate-like expansions become the semicircular canals and the remainder of the sac becomes the utricle. From the cochlear sac the coiled cochlea arises, containing the organ of Corti with its hair cells, and the remainder becomes the saccule. The transformation of the otic vesicles completes the membranous labyrinth. A shell of chondrified mesoderm surrounds the membranous labyrinth and ossifies to become the bony labyrinth. The vestibulocochlear nerve originates when vestibular and cochlear nerve cells differentiate from the walls of the otocyst originating from cells of the neural crest. The inner ear, tympanic cavity and ossicles are almost full size at birth but the outer ear is short and easily damaged by insertion of objects into the canal to clean or inspect it.

THE EYES

In the 4th week two important events happen in the development of the eye (Fig. 9.6).

- The optic vesicle develops as an outgrowth of the diencephalon attached to the diencephalon by the optic stalk.

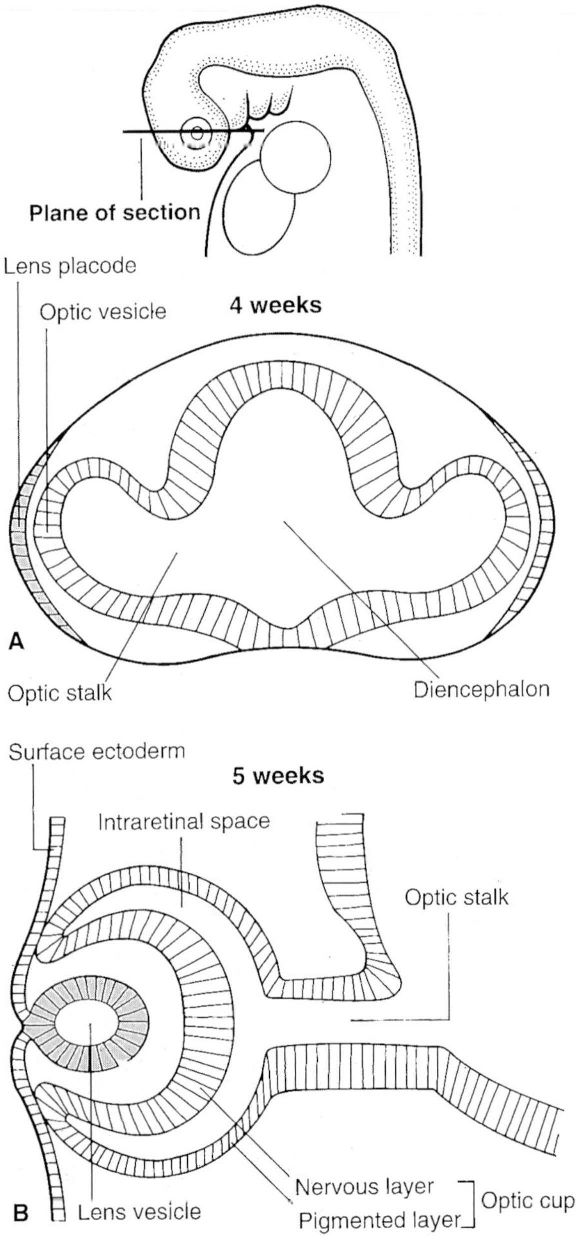

Figure 9.6 *Early development of the eye (from Fitzgerald MJT, Fitzgerald M, 1994, with permission).*

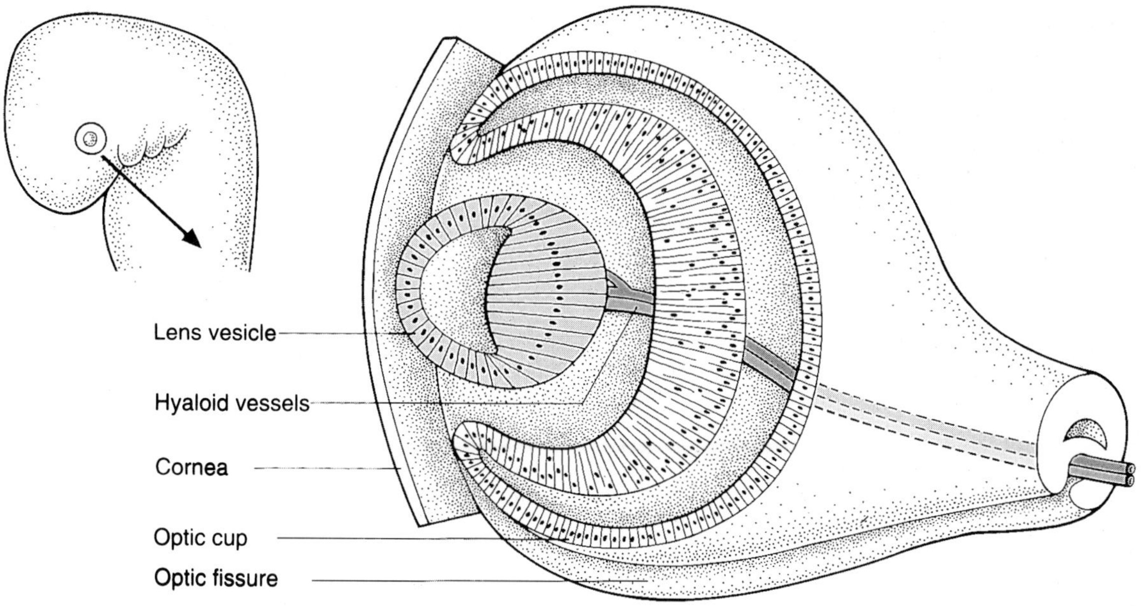

Figure 9.7 *The eye at 6 weeks, showing the optic fissure (from Fitzgerald MJT, Fitzgerald M, 1994, with permission).*

- Under the influence of the optic vesicle, the lens develops as an ingrowth of a thickened patch of surface ectoderm – the lens placode.

As the lens vesicle sinks inwards, the optic vesicle becomes a doublewalled optic cup by invagination. Invagination creates the optic fissure on the undersurface of the optic cup and its stalk. Before the lips of the optic fissure come together during the 6th week, it is infiltrated by mesenchyme (Fig. 9.7). Within the cup the mesenchyme produces a gelatinous secretion that fills the vitreous component of the eye. During the 5th and 6th weeks, a shell of mesenchyme covers the outer surface of the optic cup and differentiates into the vascular choroid coat of the eyeball and the outer fibrous coat, consisting of the sclera and cornea. The extraocular muscles – the four rectus and two oblique muscles – develop from mesoderm. The cells in the posterior wall of the lens vesicle elongate and lay down primary lens fibres. Secondary lens fibres are laid down later by cells migrating into the interior from the margins of the lens.

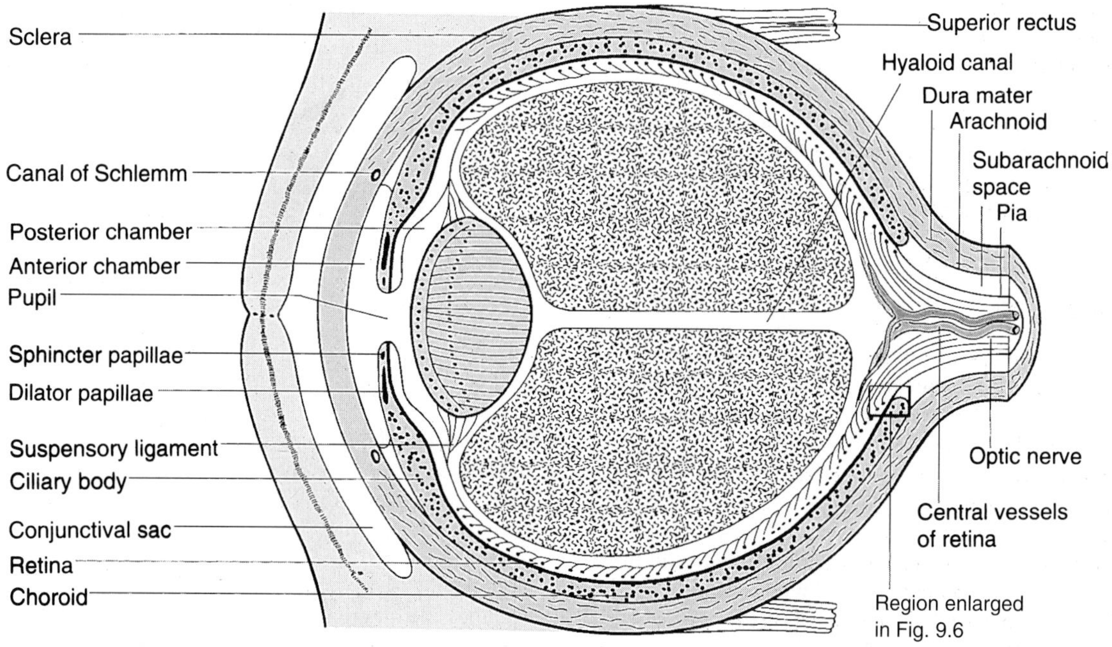

Figure 9.8 *The eye at about 20 weeks (from Fitzgerald MJT, Fitzgerald M, 1994, with permission).*

The optic cup

The outer epithelium of the optic cup accumulates melanin pigment and becomes the pigmented layer of the retina. Around the rim of the cup the outer and inner layers form the ciliary body and the iris. The ciliary muscles develop from ectomesenchymal cells in the ciliary body and the sphincter and dilator muscles of the pupil develop from the posterior epithelium of the iris.

The inner epithelium of the optic cup becomes the nervous layer of the retina, differentiating into the various sensory cells of the eye. The axons of these neurones converge on the optic stalk and escape through the optic fissure to form the optic nerve. About 90% of the fibres terminate in the lateral geniculate nucleus of the thalamus. The optic nerve is not a peripheral nerve but an extension of the white matter of the CNS. It is therefore enclosed in a meningeal sheath. The ciliary processes secrete aqueous humour which accumulates between the cornea and the lens. Between the iris and cornea is the anterior chamber and between the iris and the lens is the posterior chamber. Aqueous humour moves from posterior to anterior chambers through the pupil and then from the anterior chamber into a small vein encircling the eye at the anterior margin of the choroid coat, called the canal of Schlemm.

The eyelids and lacrimal apparatus

The eyelids develop from mesodermal folds lined by surface ectoderm that grow to meet each other in front of the cornea during the 2nd month. From the 3rd to the 6th months the eyelids are fused and this is one of the ways of estimating the gestational age of a very premature baby. The lacrimal glands, which are exocrine, develop from the outer part of the conjunctival sac. It is said that newborns do not produce tears but there is a continuous lacrimal secretion to protect the cornea.

THE LIMBS

When the author was studying for her BA a visiting lecturer asked the class a question. 'How do the limbs know when to stop making one bone and change to two and then to form multiple bones at the wrist and ankle terminating in five digits and how do the two arms end up the same length, as do the two legs?' This is, of course, part of the profound question in developmental biology – what controls the process of development from a single cell to a complete human or any other organism? Some of the answers are becoming clearer and are referred to earlier in this section in Chapter 8. This was the question that fired the author with a lifelong interest in embryology.

Development of the limbs

The limbs form from the somatic mesoderm of the lateral body wall (Figs 9.9–9.13). Minute upper limb buds appear in the middle of the 4th week at the level of the lower cervical somites. The lower limb buds appear 2 days later at the level of the lower lumbar somites. This is one example of the craniocaudal development of the fetus. Proliferation of somatic mesodermal cells is induced in each limb by the **apical ectodermal ridge** (AER) formed by thickening of the surface

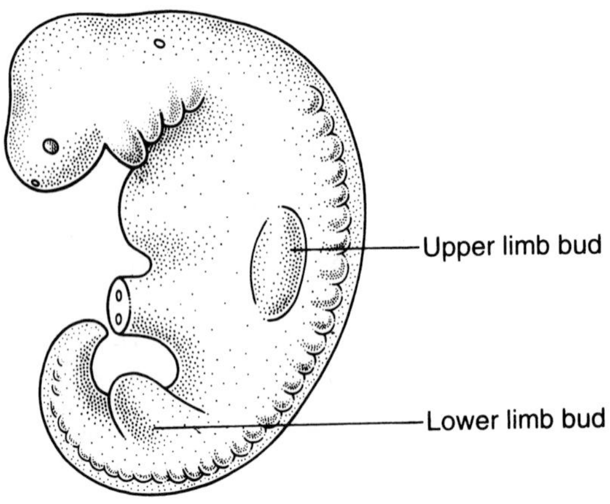

Figure 9.9 *Limb buds at 4 weeks (from Fitzgerald MJT, Fitzgerald M, 1994, with permission).*

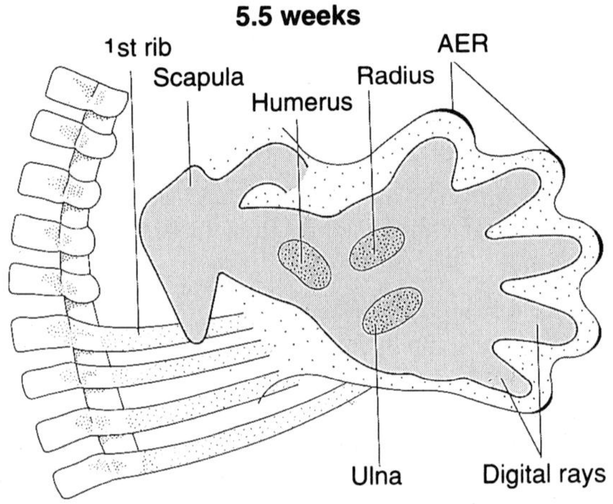

Figure 9.10 *Transilluminated 6-week embryo.*

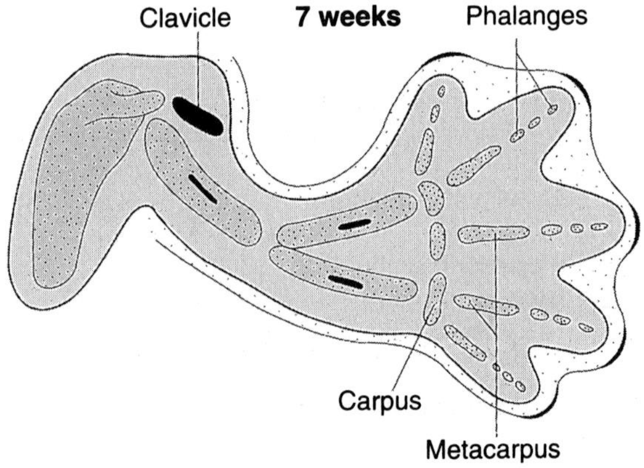

Figure 9.11 *Upper limb skeleton at 7 weeks. Centres of ossification (red) have appeared in the clavicle and in the three major long bones (from Fitzgerald MJT, Fitzgerald M, 1994, with permission).*

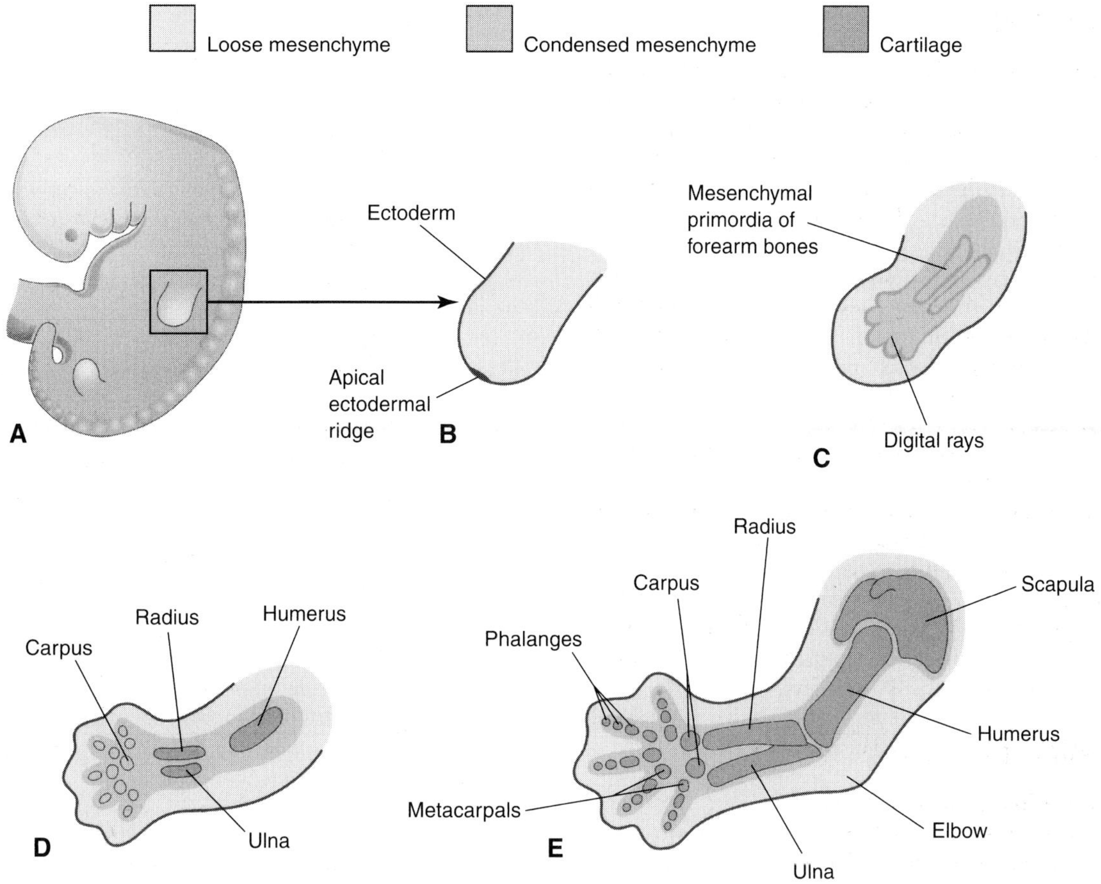

Figure 9.12 *(a) An embryo at about 28 days, showing the early appearance of the limb buds. (b) Schematic drawing of a longitudinal section through an upper limb bud. The apical ectodermal ridge has an inductive influence on the mesenchyme and appears to give it the ability to form specific cartilaginous elements. (c) Similar sketch of an upper limb bud at about 33 days, showing the mesenchymal primordia of the limb bones. The digital rays are mesenchymal condensations that undergo chondrification and ossification to form the bones of the hand. (d) Upper limb at 6 weeks showing the cartilage models of the bones. (e) Later in the 6th week showing the completed cartilaginous models of the bones of the upper limb. (Reproduced with permission from Moore 1989.)*

ectoderm over the limb bud. This covers the whole surface at first but is later confined to the growing tip of the limb. The limb bud is filled with loose mesenchyme. Cell division in the mesenchyme is restricted to a progress zone immediately below the AER. Daughter cells separate out from this zone and add to the limb's length.

Formation of the hands and feet

During the 5th week the primordia of the hands and feet develop in the form of flat limb plates. The AER breaks up into five ridges marking the positions of the future digits. Each of these AERs induces and maintains a progress zone which lays down a rod of mesoderm. The five rods are called **digital rays**. Webs of loose mesenchyme connect the rays but programmed cell death creates interdigital clefts.

Development and rotation of the limbs

As in the vertebral column, the skeleton of the limbs passes through blastemal and cartilaginous stages before undergoing

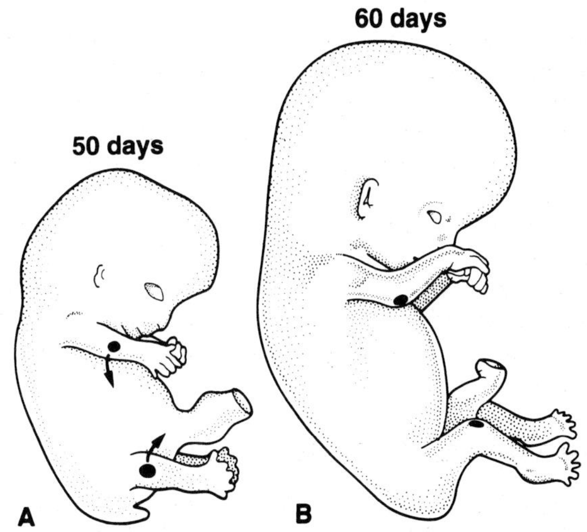

Figure 9.13 *Positions of the extensor aspects (red marks) of elbow and knee. (a) before and (b) after rotation of the limbs (from Fitzgerald MJT, Fitzgerald M, 1994, with permission).*

endochondrial ossification. The exception is the clavicle which develops from membrane. During the 5th week condensations of the limb mesenchyme form a blastemal skeleton giving a rough outline of the bones. By the end of the 7th week this has been converted to cartilage and centres of ossification appear in the three long bones of each limb.

By the end of the 12th week ossification is well advanced in the long bones and has begun in the minor long bones. Ossification of the ankle bones begins late in fetal life but the wrist bones remain cartilaginous until after birth. At first the limbs grow out laterally from the trunk and during the 8th week the limbs rotate to bring them into the expected position. In this same week elbow and knee creases appear.

Muscles and nerves of the limbs

The striated muscle of the arms and legs develops from cells which migrate from the nearest somites whilst tendons develop from somatic mesoderm already present in the limb buds. Spinal nerves called ventral rami invade the limbs in their original positions prior to rotation. The ventral rami are mixed nerves carrying motor fibres from the ventral grey horn of the spinal cord and sensory fibres from dorsal root ganglia. The 31 pairs of spinal nerves exiting from specific sections of the spinal cord are referred to by the first letter of the name in capitals followed by the number of the vertebra from above downwards.

- Cervical = C1–8
- Thoracic = T1–12
- Lumbar = L1–5
- Sacral = S1–5

There is also one coccygeal nerve. There are cervical and lumbar enlargements which accommodate the nerve cells supplying the upper and lower limbs (Fitzgerald 1992). The upper limbs receive nerves from vertebrae C5 to T1 whilst the lower limbs are invaded by nerves from L2 to S2.

Blood supply to the limbs

The limb buds are invaded early in their development by branches of the intersegmental blood vessels. The arterial supply becomes a single axial artery which is later displaced by the developing skeleton and replaced by new blood vessels. In the upper limb these are the axillary, brachial and interosseous arteries with the brachial artery branching into the radial and ulnar arteries to supply the forearm and hand. In the lower limb the popliteal and peroneal arteries replace the axial artery and the femoral artery is a new vessel that develops to join the popliteal artery. The anterior and posterior tibial arteries branch from the popliteal artery to supply the lower leg and foot.

Summary of main points

- There are four phases leading to the development of the bony vertebral column. These are the mesenchymal, blastemal, cartilaginous and bony phases.
- Myotomes give rise to the muscles of the head and trunk. The muscles of the limbs, including those involved in attachment of the upper limb to the trunk such as the pectoralis, sternomastoid and trapezius muscles, are not formed from the myotomes.
- Dermatomes merge with each other and migrate to form the connective tissue or dermis layer of the skin. Each dermatome is accompanied by sensory nerve fibres derived from the level in the spinal cord where the dermatome originated. This is why neurologists divide the body surface into clinical regions called dermatomes which is the band of skin and its spinal nerve.
- Lanugo grows all over the body and the sebaceous glands produce a secretion which, when mixed with peridermal cells and lanugo, becomes the vernix caseosa. True or vellus hair is derived from a second set of hair follicles and replaces lanugo shortly before birth.
- The mammary gland makes its appearance in the 6th week as paired strips of ectodermal thickening formed longitudinally on the ventral surface of the embryo. Normally only one pair of breasts form from the thoracic part of the ridge.
- The adult skull is divided into the neurocranium, which encloses the brain and consists of the vault and base, and the viscerocranium making up the bones of the face. Intramembranous ossification begins from the 4th month with separate ossification centres giving rise to the parietal bones, frontal bones, occipital bone and the squamous part of the temporal bone.
- Tooth buds form from thickened ectoderm called dental lamina. These are responsible for the deciduous teeth. Later the dental lamina forms the buds of the permanent dentition. Eruption of deciduous teeth occurs between 6 months and 2 years after birth.
- The human nervous system begins to form about 18 days after fertilisation and is the earliest system to differentiate. By 19 days the three expansions of the brain are present. These primary brain vesicles are the forebrain or prosencephalon, the midbrain or mesencephalon and the hindbrain or rhombencephalon.
- Neurones migrate from the ventricular zone of the telencephalon to the surface to form the cerebral cortex. The frontal, parietal, occipital and temporal lobes are present at 12–14 weeks. Two commissures of nerve fibres link the right and left cerebral hemispheres: the anterior commissure, which connects the olfactory regions, and the corpus callosum linking matched areas of the cerebral cortex.
- Following the closure of the neural tube and the segmentation of the paraxial mesoderm into somites, neural crest cells form clusters corresponding to the somites. At first the neural tube is solid but it becomes canalised by caudal extension of the neural canal. During the 6th week an accumulation of neuroblasts in the dorsolateral plate gives rise to the sensory dorsal horn of grey matter. Accumulations of cells in the ventrolateral plate form the motor ventral horn.
- During weeks 7–10 the definitive spinal cord is formed. The neural canal shrinks to become the central canal of the spinal cord. Cells left behind in the ventricular zone develop cilia and become the lining cells of the central canal called ependymal cells. The discrete ascending and descending columns in the white matter are finalised.
- Mesodermal branchial arches begin to develop as ridges on the future head and neck region. During the 5th week there are five pairs of branchial arches. These arches are the equivalent of the gill arches in fishes. On the surface ectoderm there are a number of thickenings of ectoderm called placodes. Three of these are the nasal placode, the lens placode and the otic placode.
- The first pair of arches or mandibular arches are involved in the development of the face. The second or hyoid arch forms the stapes of the middle ear and the styloid process of the temporal bone. Its ventral end forms part of the hyoid bone. Most of its mesoderm migrates to form the muscles of facial expression. The 3rd arch forms the basis for the posterior part of the tongue whilst the ventral part of its cartilage provides the lower half of the hyoid bone. The

fourth and sixth arches form the cartilages and ligaments and muscles of the larynx.

- Derivatives of the pharyngeal pouches are first pouch – the Eustachian tube and the middle ear cavity; 2nd pouch – the tonsils; 3rd pouch – the thymus gland and inferior parathyroid gland; and 4th/5th pouch – superior parathyroid gland, parafollicular and C cells of the thyroid gland.
- The development of the face is complex. The primitive mouth begins as a slight depression of the surface ectoderm called the stomodeum. It is separated from the foregut by the oropharyngeal membrane which ruptures about day 24 to bring the digestive tract into communication with the amniotic cavity.
- The pinna of the ear develops from six aural hillocks, three on the first branchial arch and three on the second. The first pharyngeal cleft gives rise to the outer ear canal. The middle ear cavity extends outwards from the first pharyngeal pouch during the 5th week to make contact with the outer ear canal. Where they meet a thin layer of mesoderm remains to form the eardrum. At the end of the 3rd week an otic placode develops on either side of the head. These sink below the surface to form the otic vesicles from which develop the semicircular canals.
- Between the 3rd and 6th weeks development of the eye takes place. The eyelids develop from mesodermal folds lined by surface ectoderm that grow to meet each other in front of the cornea during the 2nd month. From the 3rd to the 6th months the eyelids are fused. The lacrimal glands develop from the outer part of the conjunctival sac.
- The limbs form from the somatic mesoderm of the lateral body wall. Minute upper limb buds appear in the middle of the 4th week at the level of the lower cervical somites. The lower limb buds appear 2 days later at the level of the lower lumbar somites, an example of the craniocaudal development of the fetus.
- During the 5th week the hands and feet develop in the form of flat limb plates. The apical ectodermal ridge breaks up into five ridges marking the positions of the future digits. Each lays down a rod of mesoderm called a digital ray. Webs of loose mesenchyme connect the rays but programmed cell death creates interdigital clefts.
- At first the limbs grow out laterally from the trunk but during the 8th week the limbs rotate to bring them into the expected position. In this same week elbow and knee creases appear.

References

Fitzgerald MJT. 1992 Neuroanatomy: Basic and Clinical, 2nd edn. Baillière Tindall, London.

Fitzgerald MJT, Fitzgerald M. 1994 Human Embryology. Baillière Tindall, London.

Gilbert SF. 1988 Developmental Biology, 2nd edn. Sinauer Associates, Massachusetts.

Marieb EN. 1992 Human Anatomy and Physiology, 2nd edn. Benjamin Cummings, California.

McNabb M. 1997 Embryonic and fetal developments. In Sweet BR with Tiran D (eds) Mayes Midwifery, 12th edn. Baillière Tindall, London, pp 89–105.

Moore KL. 1989 Before We Are Born, 3rd edn. WB Saunders, Philadelphia.

Recommended reading

Bogin B. 1988 Patterns of Human Growth. Cambridge University Press, Cambridge.

Coustan DR. (ed) 1995 Human Reproduction, Growth and Development. Little, Brown, Bostan.

Ferry G. 1989 The nervous system: getting wired up. Inside Science no. 19. New Scientist, 121: 1–4

Larsen WJ. 1993 Human Embryology. Churchill Livingstone, Edinburgh.

Moore KL, Persaud TVN. 1993 The Developing Human. WB Saunders, Philadelphia.

Purves D, Lichtman J. 1985 Principles of Neural Development. Sinauer Associates, Massachusetts.

Tanner JM. 1978 Foetus into Man. Open Books, London.

Wolpert L. 1991 The Triumph of the Embryo. Oxford University Press, Oxford.

Chapter

10 Embryological systems 2 – internal organs

In this chapter

INTRODUCTION

To save repetition of referencing, the two main source books for this chapter are Fitzgerald & Fitzgerald (1994) and Moore (1989). Other works will be referenced as required. The change from fetal to independent circulation will be discussed in Chapter 48.

THE CARDIOVASCULAR SYSTEM

It is important for the cardiovascular system to be in place early in the embryo as it soon becomes too big to receive nourishment by diffusion of nutrients (McNabb 1997). From the end of the 3rd week it must obtain its nutrients directly from the maternal circulation. It is the first embryonic system to function, with a heart pumping blood around vessels early in the 4th week.

The developing heart pumps three circulatory systems:

1 a system that collects red blood cells from their site of manufacture on the wall of the yolk sac;
2 a system that collects oxygen and nutrients from and returns waste products to the placenta;
3 the true embryonic circulation that nourishes the cells.

Blood

Early in the 3rd week blood islands appear in the extra-embryonic mesoderm lining the yolk sac. The central cells of these islands are the **haemacytoblasts** which become primitive nucleated red blood cells. The peripheral cells are called **angioblasts** and form a capillary endothelium around each of the blood islands (Fig. 10.1).

There are three phases of blood cell formation (Fig. 10.2):

1 the yolk sac period from week 3 to week 12;
2 the hepatic period from week 5 until week 36 when clones of blood-forming cells migrate to the spleen;
3 the bone marrow period from week 12 of fetal life and for the rest of the individual's life. During week 12 clones settle in the spleen, liver and bone marrow and produce red blood cells whilst clones settling in the bone marrow, thymus and lymph nodes produce white blood cells.

All red cells contain the red pigment haemoglobin but in cells which originate in the yolk sac and liver, the haemoglobin is fetal or HbF which takes up and releases O_2 and CO_2 more

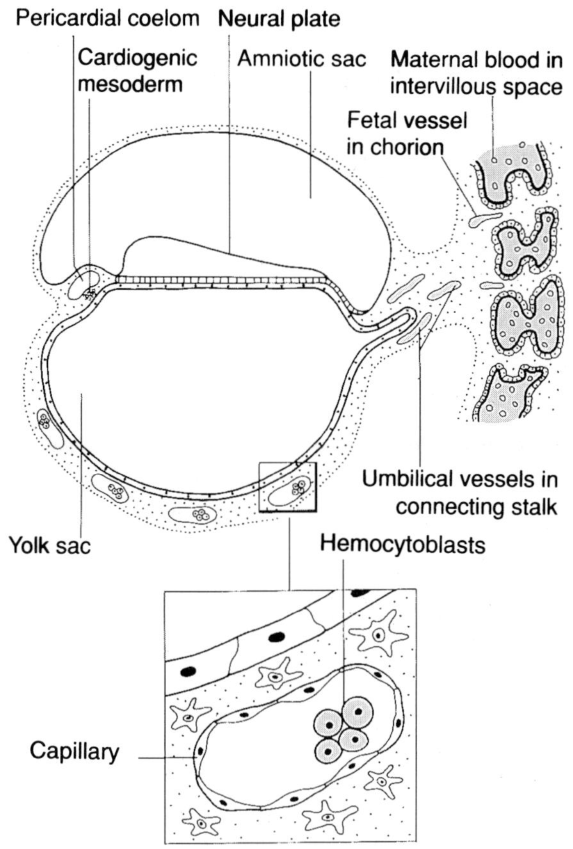

Figure 10.1 *Longitudinal section of 18-day embryo, showing primitive vasculature (from Fitzgerald MJT, Fitzgerald M, 1994, with permission).*

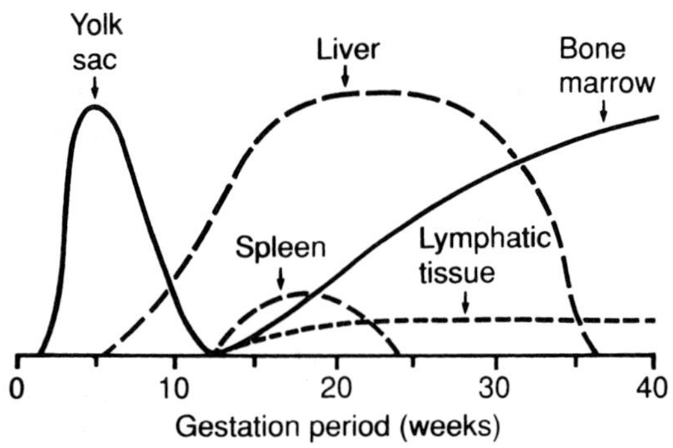

Figure 10.2 *Sites and times of haemopoiesis (from Fitzgerald MJT, Fitzgerald M, 1994, with permission).*

readily than adult haemoglobin. Red cells produced by the bone marrow are mature. They lose their nucleus and contain adult haemoglobin or HbA.

Development of arteries

At the cranial end of the embryo two dorsal aortas form out of paraxial mesoderm (Fig. 10.3). These link by pairs of aortic arches to the **truncus arteriosus** which extends cranially from the heart tube. Six aortic arches can be seen in the embryo at 4 weeks. Naming these 1 to 6 from the cranial end, by the 5th week the first two have disappeared. The third forms the carotid artery system and the 4th left side contributes to the aorta. The 5th aortic arch is also transient and disappears but the 6th is important and gives off branches into the lung buds. The distal portion of the left 6th artery becomes the **ductus arteriosus** which will be described along with the fetal circulation.

The three parts of the embryonic circulatory system develop as follows.

1 A pair of umbilical arteries develop to carry blood to the placenta.
2 Vitelline arteries arise from the dorsal aortas linking up with the capillary bed of the yolk sac, eventually becoming the three mesenteric arteries supplying the gut.
3 Intersegmental arteries supply blood to the somites and neural tube. They link with veins in capillary beds.

Development of veins

Veins form and are linked to the arteries in capillary beds.

1 Two umbilical veins form in the body stalk to link with the arteries in the placental capillary bed.
2 At first numerous vessels carry blood from the yolk sac to the heart tube. The largest pair become the vitelline veins linking with the vitelline arteries in the yolk sac capillary bed.
3 Intersegmental arteries drain the embryo itself, leading to the two main common cardinal veins.

Development of the heart

The heart is derived from mesoderm. Before the head fold develops, **cardiogenic** mesoderm occupies the floor of the **pericardial coelom** and gives rise to a pair of endothelial heart tubes (Marieb 1992). As folding proceeds these unite to form a single heart tube (Fig. 10.4). The pericardial coelom forms a **pericardial sac** around the heart tube.

The heart tube buckles within the sac to form a twisted U shape and four primitive chambers form in the tube. These are not left and right atria and ventricles, as in the fully formed heart, but expansions that cross the full lumen of the tube. The first two dilatations of the heart tube's lumen are the presumptive right and left ventricles (Fig. 10.5). The 3rd expansion is the **common atrium** above and behind the presumptive ventricle and the 4th expansion is the **sinus venosus** at the confluence of the vitelline, umbilical and common cardinal veins. This is shown clearly in Figure 10.5.

The primitive atrium is eventually partitioned into two by the growth and fusion of two septa: the **septum primum** from the dorsocranial wall and the **septum secundum** from the ventrocranial wall. An opening with a flap-like valve remains between the left and right atria to accommodate a left-to-right shunt of blood across the atrial septum. The septum secundum forms the flap of the valve. This opening is the **foramen ovale** and should close at birth.

Division of the primitive ventricle begins at the end of the 4th week with the development of a ridge of tissue called the **interventricular septum**. There is an **interventricular foramen**

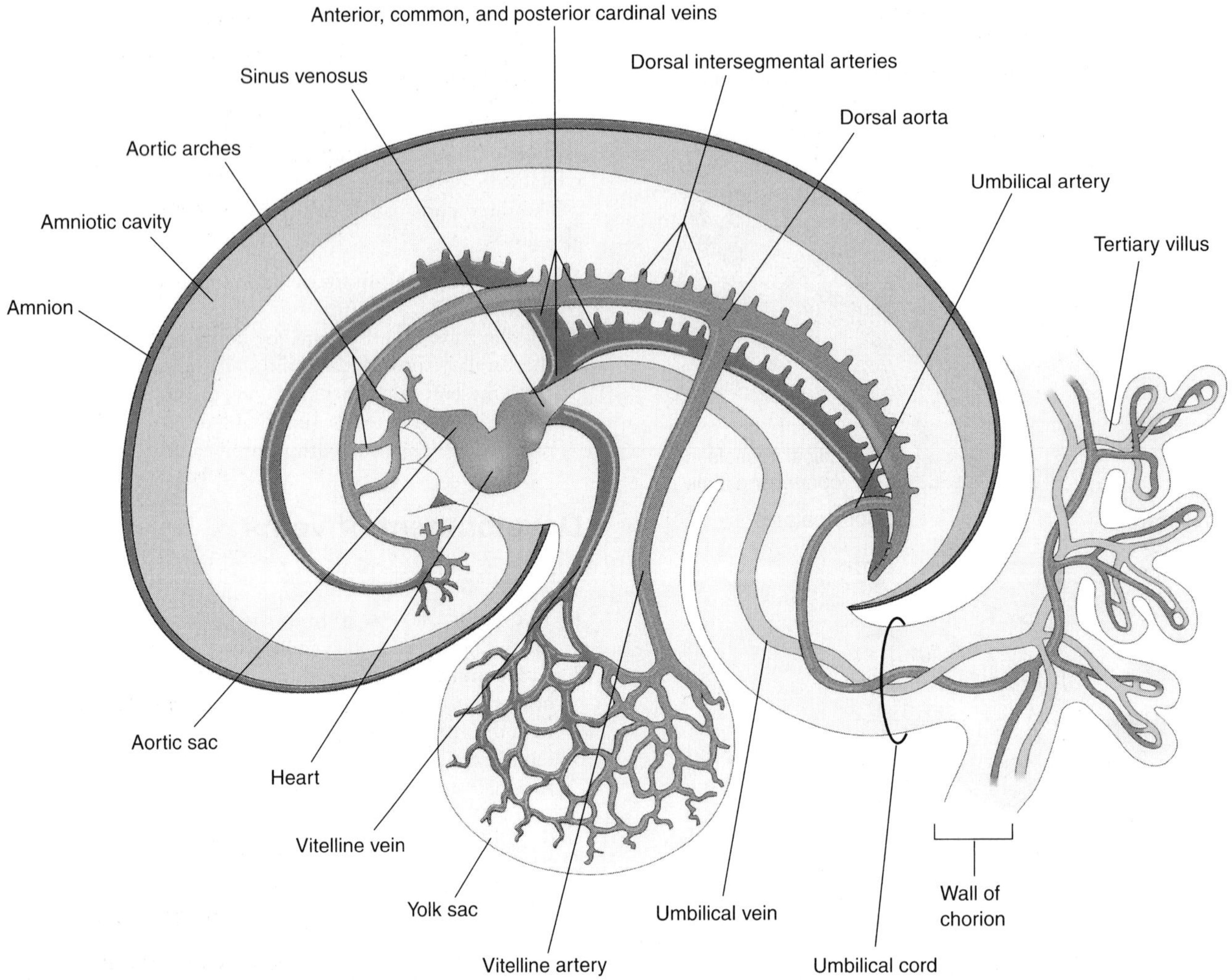

Figure 10.3 *Diagram of the primitive cardiovascular system in an embryo of about 20 days, viewed from the left side. Observe the transitory stage of paired symmetric vessels. Each heart tube continues dorsally into a dorsal aorta that passes caudally. Branches of the aortae are (1) umbilical arteries, establishing connections with vessels in the chorion; (2) vitelline arteries to the yolk sac; and (3) dorsal intersegmental arteries to the body of the embryo. An umbilical vein returns blood from the chorion and divides into right and left umbilical veins within the embryo. Vessels on the yolk sac form a vascular plexus that is connected to the heart tubes by vitelline veins. The anterior cardinal veins return blood from the head region. The umbilical vein carries oxygenated blood and nutrients from the chorion (embryonic part of the placenta) to the embryo. The arteries carry poorly oxygenated blood and waste products to the chorionic villi for transfer to the maternal blood. (Reproduced with permission from Moore 1989.)*

but it usually closes at the end of the 7th week. After closure of the interventricular foramen the pulmonary arterial trunk taking blood to the lungs communicates with the right ventricle and the aorta carrying blood to the body communicates with the left ventricle. Valves and their supporting papillary muscles and chordae tendinae begin developing at about 5 weeks and are in place by the end of organogenesis, as is the tissue forming the conducting system of the heart. Following this second partitioning of the heart into four chambers, two atria and two ventricles, the fetal circulation is established.

Development of the heart and great vessels is a highly complex process leading to the possibility of many different types of malformation with an overall incidence of 0.7% and an incidence in stillborn babies of 2.7% (Moore 1989).

THE LOWER RESPIRATORY TRACT

Development of the laryngeotracheal tube

A median laryngeotracheal groove appears on the floor of the primitive pharynx in the middle of the 4th week. A septum grows into the lumen of the laryngeotracheal groove, converting it into the laryngeotracheal tube with a laryngeal opening into the pharynx. The epithelial lining at the cranial end of this tube, the laryngeal cartilages and the vocal cords develop from the 4th and 6th branchial arches. The epithelium is the primordium of the epithelial lining of the larynx and trachea and the caudal part lines the bronchial tree. Tracheooesophageal folds grow

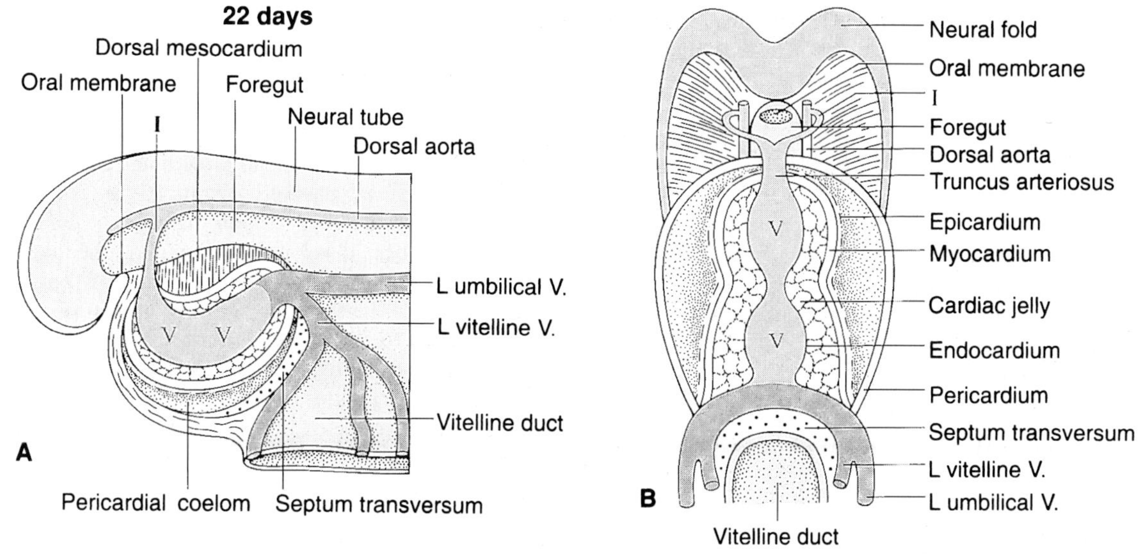

Figure 10.4 *'Straight' heart tube. (a) Viewed from the left. (b) Ventral view. I, first aortic arch; V, V, presumptive ventricles (from Fitzgerald MJT, Fitzgerald M, 1994, with permission).*

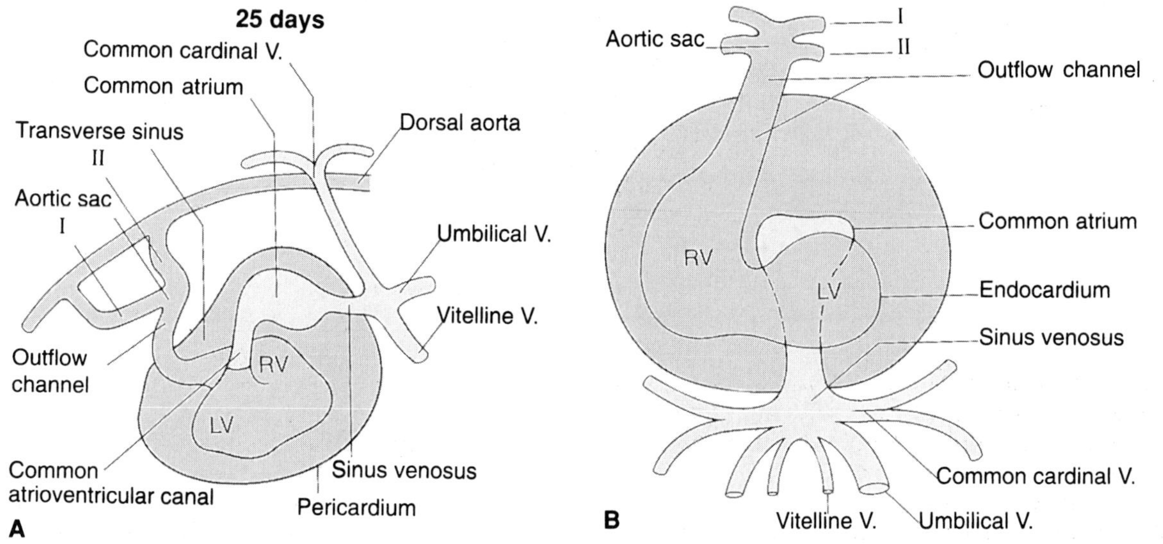

Figure 10.5 *The ventricular loop. (a) Viewed from the left. (b) Ventral view. I, II, first and second aortic arches; LV, RV, presumptive left and right ventricles (from Fitzgerald MJT, Fitzgerald M, 1994, with permission).*

towards each other to form a septum dividing the cranial part of the foregut into the laryngeotracheal tube and the oesophagus (Fig. 10.6).

Development of the lungs

A bulge in the caudal part of the laryngeotracheal tube which is the lung bud splits to form two bronchial buds which give rise to the primary bronchi. The bronchial buds invaginate the pericardioperitoneal canals which then become the pleural cavities. The epithelium covering the outside of the bronchial buds becomes the visceral pleura and the epithelium lining the pericardioperitoneal canals becomes the parietal pleura. The connections between the two pleural cavities and the pericardial cavity containing the heart become closed off. The lungs and heart descend into the thorax with some delay during the 7th week because of the enlargement of the liver and adrenal glands inside the abdomen. The 6th aortic arterial arches give rise to the pulmonary arteries. A venous plexus around the bronchial tree drains into the left atrium of the heart.

Tissues of the lung

The two primary bronchi divide into secondary bronchi. The right pulmonary bronchus divides into three secondary or lobar bronchi to serve the three lobes of the right lung and the left pulmonary bronchus divides into two lobar bronchi to serve the two lobes of the left lung. Each secondary bronchus further splits

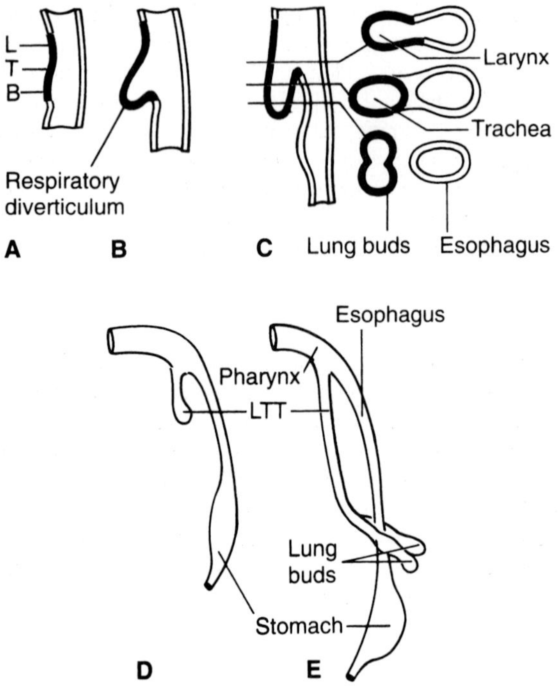

Figure 10.6 *Early development of lower respiratory tract. (a) At 24 days. L, T, B, presumptive epithelial linings of larynx, trachea, bronchial tree. (b) At 25 days. (c) At 26 days. (d) At 4 weeks. (e) At 5 weeks. LTT, laryngotracheal tube (from Fitzgerald MJT, Fitzgerald M, 1994, with permission).*

into tertiary or segmental bronchial subdivisions which have a cuboidal epithelial lining. During the 7th month respiratory bronchioles become more abundant and terminate in alveolar ducts and sacs.

From 5 to 17 weeks the developing lungs are in the **pseudoglandular period** and resemble an exocrine gland. Respiration is not possible. From 16 to 25 weeks is the **canalicular period** when the air passages become patent and blood capillaries develop to surround the future alveoli. Towards the end of this period respiration is possible but the lungs, and the other systems, are very immature and survival is improbable. From 24 weeks until birth is the **terminal sac period** with development of the alveoli. By 28 weeks sufficient terminal sacs are present to permit survival.

At first these are lined by type 1 alveolar cells which will take part in gas exchange. At the end of the 6th month type 2 alveolar cells can be found which secrete **surfactant** to lower the surface tension between the alveolar epithelium and inspired air. At this point the fetus becomes viable. Even then, babies born before 34 weeks may develop respiratory distress syndrome because of insufficient production of surfactant. Budding of fresh bronchioles, alveolar ducts and alveolar sacs continues for the first 8 years of life.

The diaphragm

The diaphragm is quite complex in its origins, with five elements contributing to its formation.

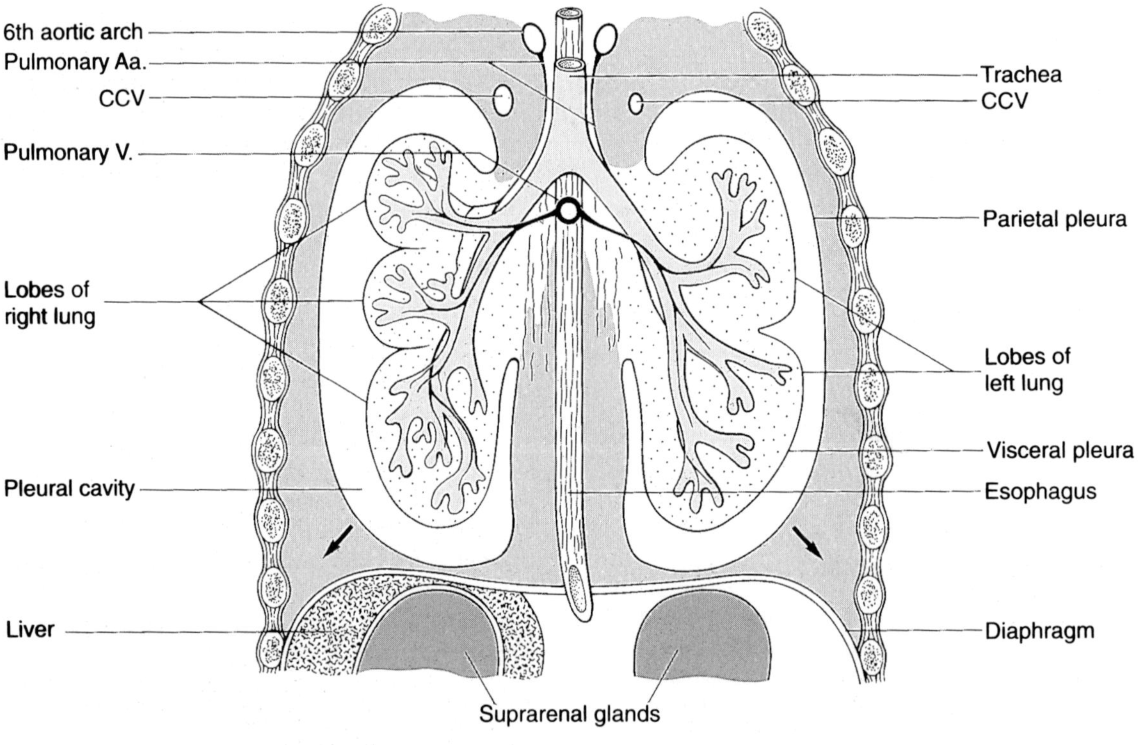

Figure 10.7 *Coronal section of the posterior mediastinum at 7 weeks. CCV, common cardinal vein. Arrows indicate directions of expansion of pleural cavities and lungs. The septum transversum has been incorporated into the diaphragm (from Fitzgerald MJT, Fitzgerald M, 1994, with permission).*

1 Prior to its descent with the heart, the septum transversum lies opposite the 3rd to 5th somites. These somites contribute cells which differentiate to form the muscles of the diaphragm. This is why the nerve supply to the diaphragm is from C3, 4 and 5 in the form of the phrenic nerve.
2 Ventral extension of the pleural sacs creates the fibrous pericardium from a layer of somatic mesoderm. The sacs also peel off a layer of cells to form the connective tissue of the diaphragm.
3 The mesentery of the oesophagus contributes connective tissue to the diaphragm around the oesophagus and inferior vena cava.
4 The septum transversum gives rise to the fibrous tissue of the central tendon.
5 The pleuroperitoneal membranes contribute connective tissue surrounding the central tendon.

THE ALIMENTARY TRACT

The primitive gut begins to form during the 4th week. The dorsal part of the yolk sac becomes incorporated into the embryo during folding. The endoderm of this primitive gut gives rise to most of the epithelial lining and glands of the digestive system. By the middle of the 4th week the alimentary tract consists of foregut, midgut and hindgut. The epithelial linings of the cranial and caudal ends of the gut are derived from ectoderm as the stomodeum (primitive mouth) and anal pit. The muscular and fibrous parts of the digestive tract form from splanchnic mesoderm.

The foregut

The oesophagus

Although the oesophagus is part of the alimentary tract, it is in close proximity to the respiratory tract and its position is as a thoracic structure. The oesophagus extends from the lower limit of the pharynx to the stomach. As the thoracic cavity lengthens and the heart and lungs descend into it, the oesophagus also lengthens. The upper and lower parts of the oesophagus differ in origin. Pharyngeal arch mesoderm contributes striated muscle to its upper part and the vagus nerve gives off recurrent laryngeal branches to supply this part. Splanchnic mesoderm contributes smooth muscle to its lower part and the nerve supply is autonomic from the neural crest.

The stomach

The stomach begins as a spindle-shaped dilatation of the caudal end of the foregut. The stomach is attached to the dorsal wall of the abdominal cavity by the dorsal mesentery or **dorsal mesogastrium**. During the 5th and 6th weeks the dorsal border elongates to form the convex greater curvature of the stomach whilst the ventral border forms the concave lesser curvature. The stomach now rotates clockwise on its axis through 90°, taking the dorsal mesogastrium to the left. This rotation ensures that the liver becomes mainly a right-sided organ and the spleen a left-sided organ.

The duodenum

The duodenum develops from the caudal part of the foregut and the cranial end of the midgut. The junction of the two embryonic parts of the duodenum is just distal to the entrance of the common bile duct.

The liver, gallbladder, pancreas and spleen

On day 24 there is a thickening of the endoderm directly caudal to the septum transversum. This is the **hepatic diverticulum** or **liver bud** which grows out from the duodenum (Fig. 10.9). The liver bud gives off the gallbladder and biliary duct system. The hepatic diverticulum divides into the left and right hepatic buds which will develop into the lobes of the liver. The stalk of the

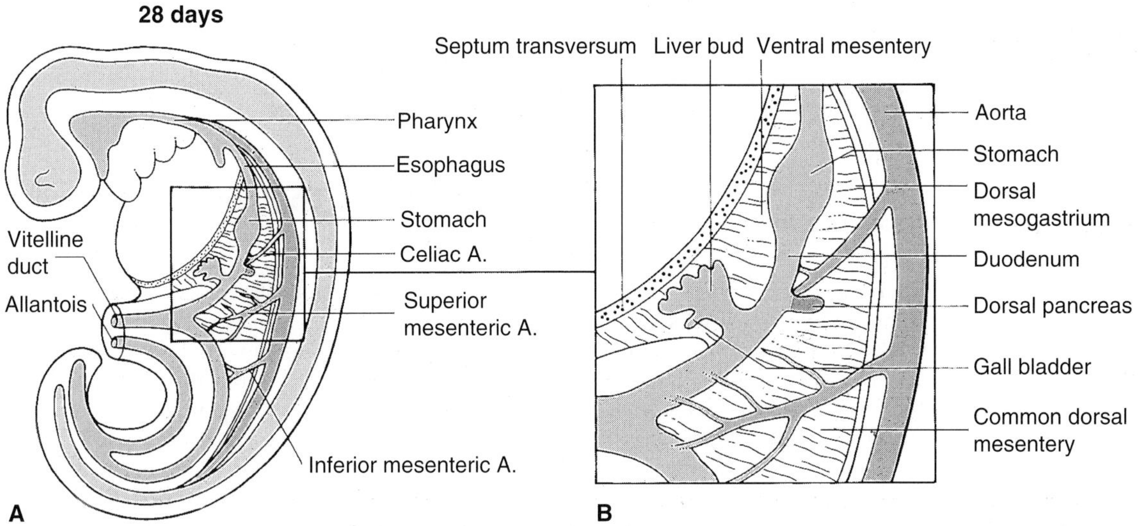

Figure 10.8 *(a) Digestive system at 4 weeks. (b) Enlargement from (a) (from Fitzgerald MJT, Fitzgerald M, 1994, with permission).*

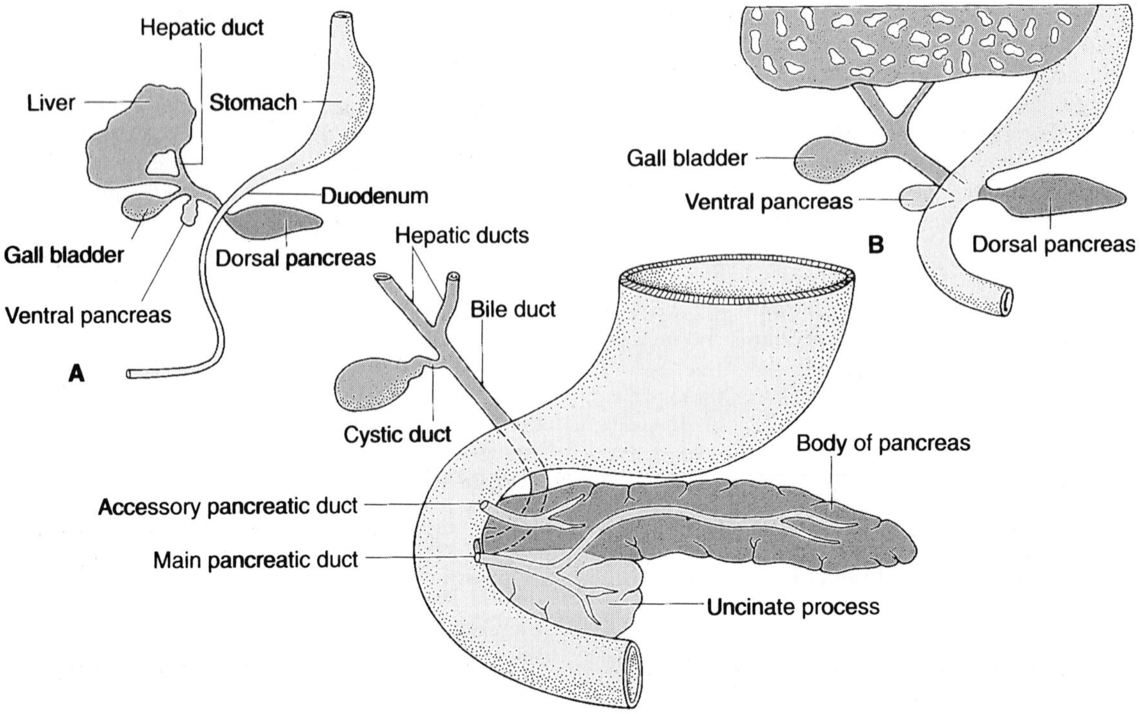

Figure 10.9 *Development of duct systems of liver, gallbladder, and pancreas (from Fitzgerald MJT, Fitzgerald M, 1994, with permission).*

gallbladder becomes the cystic duct and the stalks of the hepatic buds become the hepatic ducts. The bile duct is formed by the union of the conjoined hepatic ducts with the cystic ducts. The hepatic buds produce a network of **hepatocytes** arranged in branching and anastomosing plates.

The **pancreas** actually develops as two separate structures. The smaller ventral pancreas arises from a structure called the **hepatic diverticulum**, which will become the bile duct, to form the **uncinate process** of the pancreas. The larger dorsal pancreas arises from the duodenum to form the head, body and tail. The main pancreatic duct enters the duodenum along with the bile duct.

The **spleen** is a large, vascular lymphatic organ which develops from mesenchymal cells between the layers of the dorsal mesogastrium. It appears about the 5th week and enlarges to take up its position on the left side of the abdomen. The spleen is seeded by haemopoietic cells from the wall of the yolk sac and manufactures both red and white blood cells in the middle trimester of pregnancy.

Development of the veins of the liver

The vitelline veins infiltrate between the hepatocytes to form the **liver sinusoids**. The **portal vein**, which drains the entire gut below the diaphragm, also develops from segments of the two vitelline veins. During the 5th week the right umbilical vein shrinks and disappears whilst the left enlarges to receive the entire return of blood from the placenta. During the 6th to 8th weeks a large vascular shunt diverts oxygenated blood from the left umbilical vein to the right hepatic vein. This is the **ductus venosus** of the fetal circulation which ensures that the highly metabolic fetal liver receives sufficient oxygen and nutrients.

The midgut

The derivatives of the midgut are the small intestine including the main part of the duodenum, jejunum and ileum, the caecum and vermiform appendix, ascending colon and right half or more of the transverse colon. During the 6th week the midgut lengthens to such an extent that it is too big for the abdominal cavity and is found in the umbilical cord (Fig. 10.10). This is called **physiological herniation of the midgut**.

As it enters the umbilical cord, the midgut begins to twist on itself in a counterclockwise direction when viewed from the front. This occurs because of the space taken up by the developing liver and kidneys. By 10 weeks the peritoneal coelom has increased sufficiently to allow the intestines to slide back into the abdomen. The small intestine returns first and fills the central region and the colon follows to frame it. The caecum with its attached appendix enters last and enters on the right side below the liver.

The hindgut: the rectum and anal canal

The hindgut extends from the midgut to the cloacal membrane. It includes the cloaca which is not purely alimentary but will form the bladder and urethra with development of the urorectal septum. Migration of cells from the urogenital tubercle forms the **urorectal septum** which is completed during the 7th week to form the urogenital sinus and the rectum. This divides the cloaca into two parts: the rectum and upper anal canal dorsally and the urogenital sinus ventrally (see Fig. 10.11 and next section). The anal canal lies below the level of the levatores ani muscles. The upper half is lined by columnar epithelium

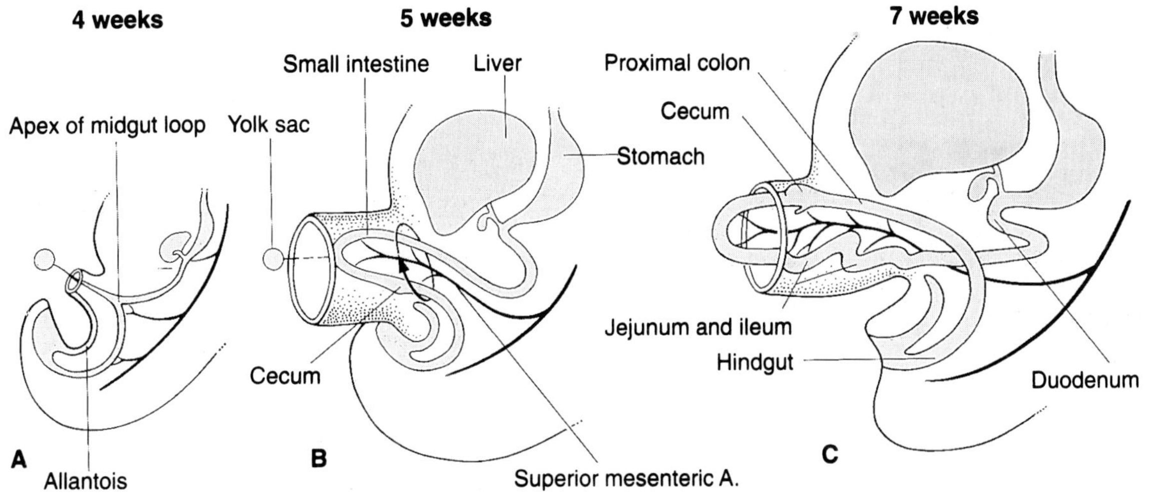

Figure 10.10 *(a) Intestine at 4 weeks. (b) Entry of midgut loop into umbilical cord. Arrow indicates rotation of the midgut loop. (c) Rotation through 180° carries caecum and proximal colon to a cranial position (from Fitzgerald MJT, Fitzgerald M, 1994, with permission).*

continuous with the rectum whilst the lower half develops from the anal pit and is lined by stratified epithelium continuous with the epidermis of the surrounding skin.

The urorectal septum fuses with the cloacal membrane by the end of the 6th week to form the dorsal anal membrane and the larger urogenital membrane. The anal membrane ruptures at the end of the 7th week to form the anal orifice. The mesoderm of the urorectal septum persists as the perineal body. Simple imperforate anus, when the anal membrane fails to rupture, occurs in one in 5000 births. It is easily resolved if noticed early.

THE URINARY TRACT

Both the urinary and genital systems develop from intermediate mesoderm. During embryonic folding the intermediate mesoderm which extended along the full length of the dorsal wall of the embryo is carried ventrally and loses its contact with the somites. There is a longitudinal ridge of mesoderm on either side of the primitive aorta called the **urogenital ridge**. That part of the urogenital ridge that gives rise to the urinary system is known as the **nephrogenic cord or ridge**. The part giving rise to the genital system is called the **gonadal or genital ridge**.

The kidneys and ureter

Three pairs of kidneys appear in succession during embryonic development. These are the **pronephros, mesonephros** and **metanephros**. The pronephros appears early in the 4th week. It is non-functional in mammals and soon degenerates but is functional in some fishes. It is replaced between weeks 4 and 8 by the second type of kidney called the mesonephros which is the kidney form found in adult amphibia (Fig. 10.12). Finally the third type of kidney, the metanephros, appears which is the permanent kidney of mammals.

Development of the collecting system

The metanephros develops from the metanephric diverticulum and a mass of metanephric mesoderm. The metanephric diverticulum is a dorsal bud from the mesonephric (Wolffian) ducts and it grows into the metanephric mesoderm. The stalk of the metanephric diverticulum becomes the ureter. As it advances towards the kidney it acquires a lumen by cell death and its tip hollows out to become the renal pelvis. The ureteric bud keeps dividing into two to form generations of collecting tubules (Fig. 10.13). The first four generations enlarge and coalesce to form the major calyces and the next four become the minor calyces of the kidney. Tubules of generations 9–16 are the actual kidney tubules.

The cells of the intermediate mesoderm surrounding the kidney multiply to form a **metanephric cap** over the renal pelvis. A cluster of metanephric cells forms at the tip of each collecting tubule and these cells form a nephron with its Bowman's capsule and convoluted tubule. Different growth rates within the embryo cause the kidneys to ascend into the abdomen and come into contact with the adrenal glands by the 8th week. The fetal kidney produces small amounts of urine from about 9 weeks and becomes more functional from about 15 weeks. Urine is excreted into the amniotic cavity. Early in their development the kidneys receive their blood supply from the common iliac arteries but by the time they are in their correct position the renal arteries have developed to supply blood.

The bladder and urethra

The urogenital sinus

The urogenital sinus has three parts:

1 a vesical part above the level of entry of the mesonephric ducts which expands to form the bladder and receives the two ureters. Its smooth muscle coat is, as usual, derived from mesoderm;

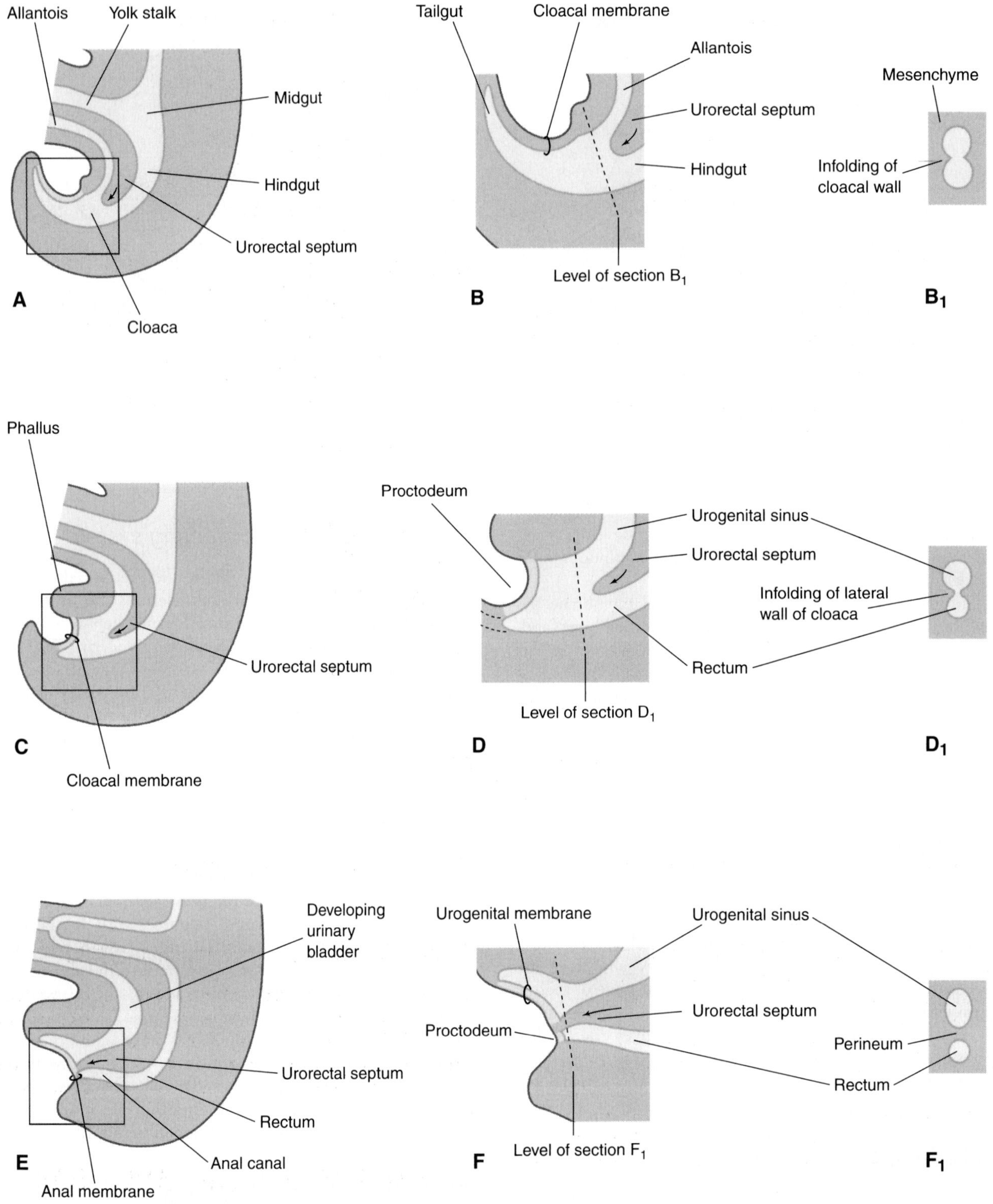

Figure 10.11 *Drawings illustrating successive stages in the partitioning of the cloaca into the rectum and urogenital sinus by the urorectal septum. (a,c,e) Views from the left side at 4, 6, and 7 weeks respectively. (b,d,f) Enlargements of cloacal region. (b_1, d_1, f_1) Transverse sections of the cloaca at the levels shown in (b), (d) and (f), respectively. Note that the tailgut (shown in (b)) degenerates and disappears as the rectum forms from the dorsal part of the cloaca (shown in (c)). (Reproduced with permission from Moore 1989.)*

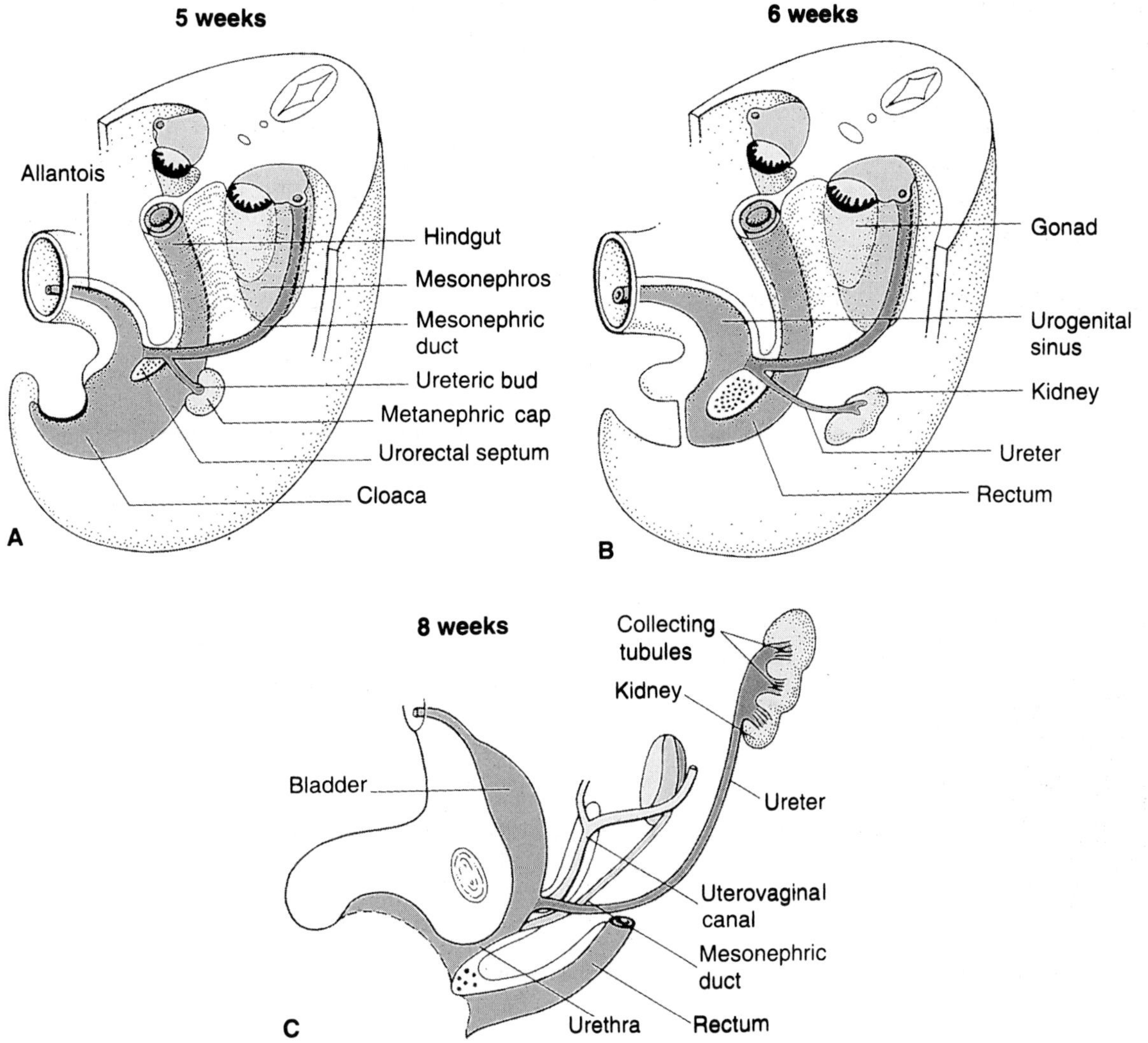

Figure 10.12 *Early development of urinary system (from Fitzgerald MJT, Fitzgerald M, 1994, with permission).*

2 a pelvic part which is narrow and forms the lining epithelium of the prostatic and membranous parts of the urethra. In females the pelvic part forms the lining of the whole of the short urethra;
3 a phallic part extending ventrally beneath the phallus in males. At first, the urethra opens on the underside of the phallus behind the developing glans but during the 4th month an ectodermal invagination grows to form the glandar urethra and the proximal opening closes off so that the urethra opens at the tip of the glans. The prepuce is an outgrowth of skin from the glans.

Between the umbilicus and the cloacal membrane, caudal mesoderm forms a midline swelling called the **genital tubercle**. Migration of cells from this forms the urogenital sinus which gives rise to the bladder and urethra. As the bladder enlarges the caudal parts of the mesonephric ducts are incorporated into its dorsal wall so that the ureters open separately into the urinary bladder.

The adrenal (suprarenal) glands

The **cortex** and the **medulla** of the adrenal glands are formed from separate tissues. The cortex develops from mesoderm and the medulla is derived from cells of the neural crest. The **chromaffin cells** of the medulla are modified sympathetic ganglion cells. The chief secretion of chromaffin cells is **adrenaline** (epinephrine).

THE REPRODUCTIVE SYSTEMS

The gonads can be identified by about the 5th week and develop from three sources: the gonadal ridge is a thickened ridge of tissue including cells from two sources, the **coelomic epithelium** and its underlying **intermediate mesoderm**. The coelomic epithelium releases a chemical that attracts the third source of cells, primordial germ cells, of which about 100 are present on the caudal surface of the yolk sac during the 4th week. These cells migrate into the interior of the gonadal ridge

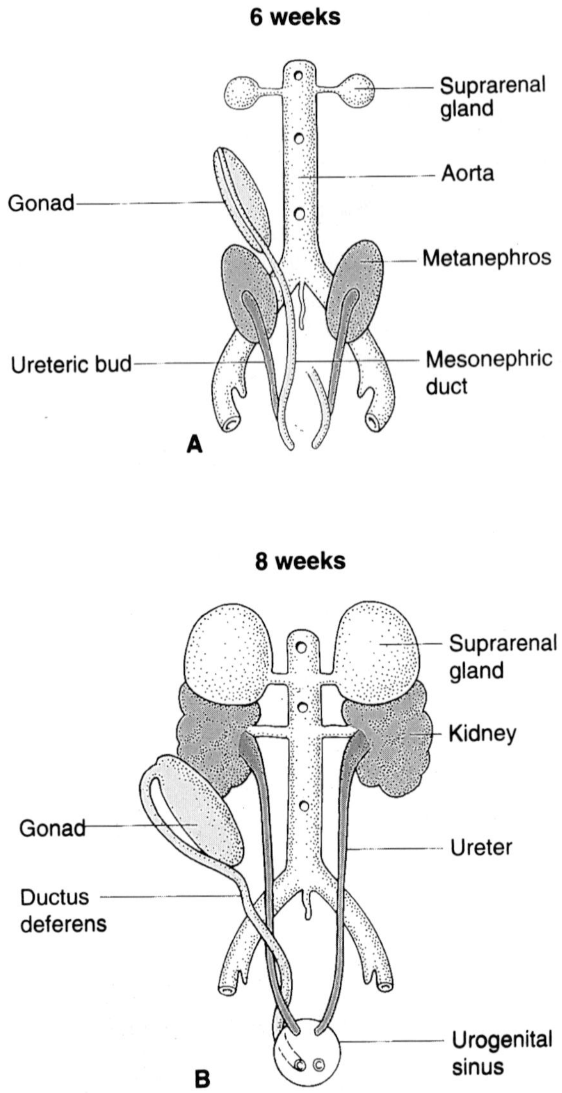

Figure 10.13 *Renal ascent. (a) At 6 weeks. (b) At 8 weeks (from Fitzgerald MJT, Fitzgerald M, 1994, with permission).*

and are enclosed in columns of epithelial cells, called **sex cords**. This is the cell line that will form the next generation by becoming ova or sperm. The gonads are identical in males and females up to the 7th week and are referred to as **indifferent gonads** (Fig. 10.14).

Becoming male or female

Two pairs of genital ducts are present in the embryo. The **mesonephric** (Wolffian) ducts are forerunners of the male genital tract and the **paramesonephric** (Mullerian) ducts are the forerunners of the female genital tract. In the absence of a trigger, all embryos will become female. The short arm of the Y chromosome in male embryos contains a gene which will produce a testis-determining factor (TDF). If this factor is secreted the gonads will become testes. If it is absent, whether in a genetic female or in a male with a non-functioning gene, the gonads will become ovaries (Fig. 10.15).

Testes and the male genital tract

About day 50 the intermediate mesoderm forms a cellular fibrous shell which is the **tunica albuginea**. The sex cords become the testicular cords and the primordial germ cells become prospermatogonia which will produce sperm from puberty. The testicular cords are gathered into lobules separated by testicular septa derived from the tunica albuginea. The inner ends of the cords are linked together in a network called the **rete testis**.

Two sets of endocrine cells form in the lobules.

1 The **Sertoli cells** (sustentacular or nurse cells). These are the most numerous cell type in the early testis. Their earliest function is to produce a **Mullerian duct inhibitory factor** which enters the fetal circulation and causes regression of the paramesonephric ducts during the 9th week. Researchers believe that the current increase in male infertility is caused by insufficient numbers of Sertoli cells being produced in the fetus. This may be caused by an excess of oestrogen mimics in the environment (see Chapter 7).
2 **Leydig cells** (interstitial) arise in the stroma between the lobules and secrete **testosterone** into the fetal circulation. This hormone ensures the survival and growth of the Wolffian ducts and the formation of the epididymis, ductus deferens, seminal vesicle and the ejaculatory duct.

The testes descend gradually from their original site in the lumbar region through the abdomen, into the pelvis and out into the scrotal sac, usually by term. They are accompanied by a pocket of peritoneum called the **processus vaginalis**, which becomes the **tunica vaginalis** on completion of descent, and by the ductus deferens, testicular blood vessels, nerves and lymphatics which constitute the two **spermatic cords**.

In females the Wolffian ducts disappear by programmed cell death without any influence from the ovary. Remnants are normally found in the broad ligament and may form parovarian cysts.

Ovary and the female genital duct

In the absence of a Y chromosome and/or TDF, there is no formation of a tunica albuginea. The sex cords accumulate in the outer region or cortex of the gonadal ridge and this becomes filled with primordial follicles consisting of an oocyte derived from the primordial germ cells, an inner shell of follicular cells derived from cell-cord epithelium and an outer shell, the **theca**, derived from the intermediate mesoderm. The number of primordial follicles reaches a maximum of 6–7 million in the 15th week. Programmed cell death reduces this number drastically so that 2 years after birth only 1 million remain and at puberty only 300 000 are present. The ovary descends from its original site in the lumbar region of the abdomen into the true pelvis after the 12th week.

The upper and middle sections of the Mullerian ducts form the epithelial lining of the fallopian tubes and the lower segments fuse into one during the 9th week to become the uterovaginal canal which eventually forms the epithelial lining of the body and cervix of the uterus. The muscle walls of the fallopian tubes and the myometrium of the uterus are formed from splanchnic mesoderm.

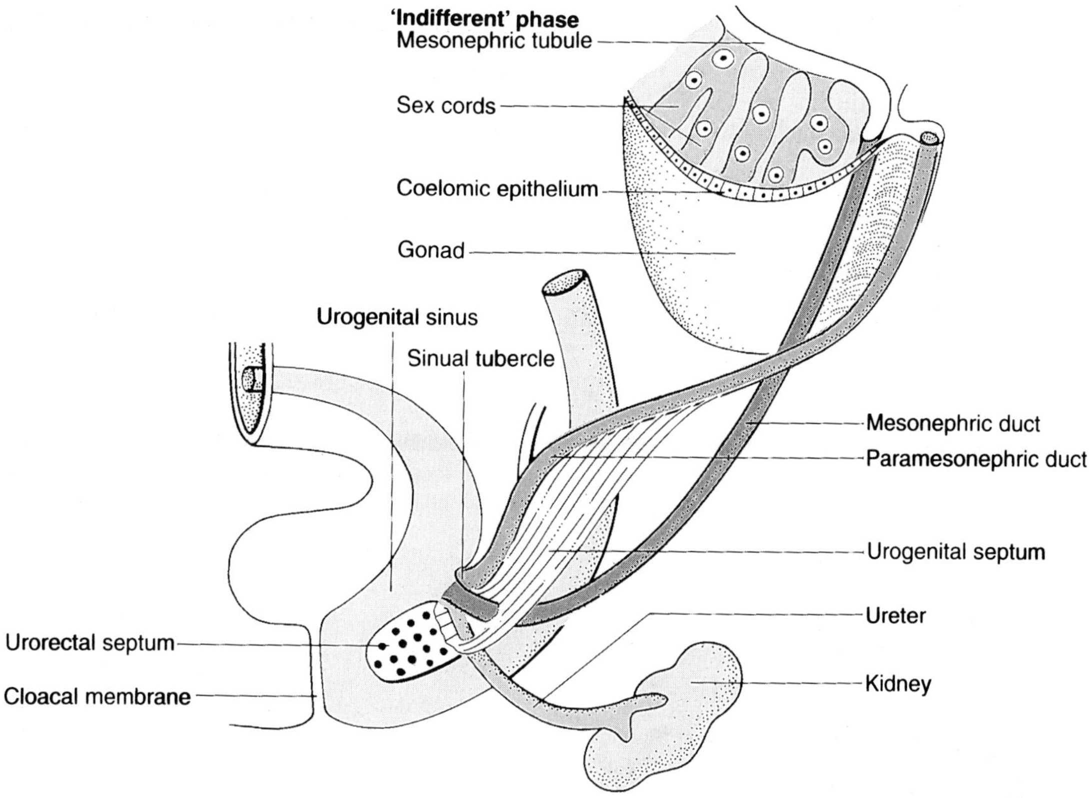

Figure 10.14 *Indifferent gonad and genital ducts at 4 weeks (from Fitzgerald MJT, Fitzgerald M, 1994, with permission).*

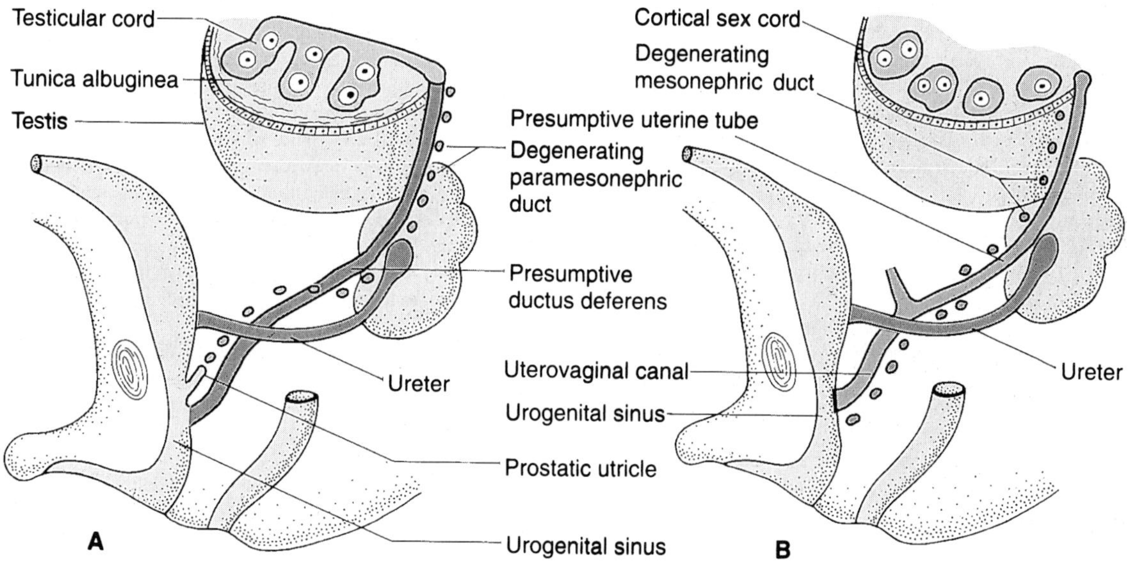

Figure 10.15 *Early sexual differentiation. (a) Male. (b) Female (from Fitzgerald MJT, Fitzgerald M, 1994, with permission).*

The vagina

If the Mullerian system develops, a small tubercle called the **Mullerian eminence** is formed. This gives rise to the vaginal plate which lengthens along the dorsal wall of the urogenital sinus. The lumen of the vagina is formed by canalisation from below upwards. The lumen extends around the cervix to form the fornices. The hymen is left as a partition between the vagina and the vestibule.

The external genitalia

Early in the 3rd month it is not possible to see a sexual difference externally. The phallic urethra is an open urethral groove flanked by paired inner urogenital folds and outer genital swellings derived from mesenchyme.

In males the matching pairs come together under the influence of testosterone. The urogenital folds unite below the urethral groove to complete the spongy urethra and the genital swellings form the two halves of the scrotum. There is a line of union at the junction of the two halves of the scrotum called the **scrotal raphe** and the line of union of the urogenital folds is marked by the **urethral raphe**.

In females they stay apart and there is growth in situ of the urogenital folds and genital swellings. The phallus forms the clitoris with a small glans at its tip. The urethral groove and the phallic part of the urogenital sinus remain open as the vestibule and the urogenital folds become the labia minora whilst the genital swellings become the labia majora.

ESTIMATION OF THE AGE OF THE EMBRYO

By 8 weeks the embryo is recognisably human although the head is more round and very large in proportion to the body. The remaining fetal intrauterine time is concerned mainly with growth although many organs have to mature. Besides the usual calculations of embryonic age made by using the first day of the last menstrual period (LMP), as it is unusual to know the exact day of fertilisation in vivo, there are other ways of estimating the age of an embryo if spontaneously or therapeutically aborted. External features and measurements of the embryo are useful and careful ultrasound scanning can confirm the age of a viable embryo in utero. At 4 weeks after fertilisation (usually 6 weeks from the first day of the LMP), the embryo and its sac measure 5 mm long. A week later discrete embryonic features can be visualised and crown–rump measurements can be made.

Summary of main points

- It is important for the cardiovascular system to be in place early in the embryo as from the end of the 3rd week it must obtain its nutrients directly from the maternal circulation. It is the first embryonic system to function, with a heart pumping blood around vessels early in the 4th week.
- Early in the 3rd week blood islands appear in the extraembryonic mesoderm lining the yolk sac. The central cells of these islands are the haemacytoblasts which become primitive nucleated red blood cells. The peripheral cells are called angioblasts and form a capillary endothelium around each of the blood islands.
- Three parts of the embryonic circulatory system develop: a pair of umbilical arteries develop to carry blood to the placenta, vitelline arteries arise from the dorsal aortas linking up with the capillary bed of the yolk sac, eventually becoming the three mesenteric arteries supplying the gut, and intersegmental arteries supply blood to the somites and neural tube.
- Veins form and are linked to the arteries in capillary beds: two umbilical veins form in the body stalk to link with the arteries in the placental capillary bed, a large pair of yolk sac veins become the vitelline veins linking with the vitelline arteries in the yolk sac capillary bed and intersegmental arteries drain the embryo itself, leading to the two main common cardinal veins.
- The heart is derived from mesoderm by a highly complex process leading to the possibility of many different types of malformation. Valves and their supporting papillary muscles and chordae tendinae begin developing at about 5 weeks and are in place by the end of organogenesis, as is the tissue forming the conducting system of the heart.
- A median laryngeotracheal groove appears on the floor of the primitive pharynx in the middle of the 4th week. A septum grows into the lumen of the laryngeotracheal groove, converting it into the laryngeotracheal tube with a laryngeal opening into the pharynx. Tracheooesophageal folds grow towards each other to form a septum dividing the cranial part of the foregut into the laryngeotracheal tube and the oesophagus.
- The lung bud splits to form two bronchial buds giving rise to the primary bronchi. The bronchial buds invaginate the pericardio-peritoneal canals which then become the pleural cavities. The two primary bronchi divide into secondary bronchi. The right pulmonary bronchus divides into three secondary bronchi to serve the three lobes of the right lung and the left pulmonary bronchus divides into two secondary bronchi to serve the two lobes of the left lung. Each secondary bronchus further subdivides into tertiary or segmental bronchi.
- During the 7th month respiratory bronchioles become more abundant and terminate in alveolar ducts and sacs. At first these are lined by type 1 alveolar cells which will take part in gas exchange. At the end of the 6th month type 2 alveolar cells appear, which secrete surfactant to lower the surface tension between the alveolar epithelium and inspired air.
- The primitive gut begins to form during the 4th week. The dorsal part of the yolk sac becomes incorporated into the embryo during folding. The endoderm of this primitive gut gives rise to most of the epithelial lining and glands of the digestive system. By the middle of the 4th week the alimentary tract consists of foregut, midgut and hindgut. The epithelial linings of the cranial and caudal ends of the gut are derived from ectoderm as the stomodeum and anal pit.
- Although the oesophagus is part of the alimentary tract, it is in close proximity to the respiratory tract and its position is as a thoracic structure as it extends from the lower limit of the pharynx to the stomach.
- The stomach begins as a spindle-shaped dilatation of the caudal end of the foregut and is attached to the dorsal wall of the abdominal cavity by the dorsal mesentery. During the 5th and 6th weeks the dorsal border elongates to form the convex greater curvature of the stomach whilst the ventral border forms the concave lesser curvature. The stomach rotates clockwise on its axis through 90°, ensuring that the liver becomes mainly a right-sided organ and the spleen a left-sided organ.
- On day 24 the hepatic diverticulum or liver bud grows out from the duodenum and gives off the gallbladder and biliary duct system. It divides into the left and right hepatic buds which will develop into the lobes of the liver. The stalk of the gallbladder becomes the cystic duct and the stalks of the hepatic buds become the hepatic ducts. The bile duct is formed by the union of the hepatic ducts with the cystic ducts.
- The pancreas develops as two separate structures. The smaller ventral pancreas arises from the hepatic diverticulum to form the uncinate process of the pancreas. The larger dorsal pancreas arises from the duodenum to form the head, body and tail.

- The spleen appears about the 5th week and develops from mesenchymal cells between the layers of the dorsal mesogastrium. It is seeded by haemopoietic cells from the wall of the yolk sac and manufactures both red and white cells in the middle trimester of pregnancy.
- The derivatives of the midgut are the small intestine, including the main part of the duodenum, jejunum and ileum, the caecum and vermiform appendix, ascending colon and right half or more of the transverse colon. During the 6th week the midgut lengthens and is too big for the abdominal cavity. It is found in the umbilical cord which is called physiological herniation of the midgut. As it enters the umbilical cord, the midgut begins to twist on itself in a counterclockwise direction. The small intestine returns first and fills the central region and the colon follows to frame it.
- The hindgut includes the cloaca which will form the bladder and urethra with development of the urorectal septum. The urorectal septum fuses with the cloacal membrane by the end of the 6th week to form the dorsal anal membrane and the larger urogenital membrane. The anal membrane ruptures at the end of the 7th week to form the anal orifice. The mesoderm of the urorectal septum persists as the perineal body.
- A longitudinal ridge of mesoderm on either side of the primitive aorta called the urogenital ridge gives rise to the urinary system. It is known as the nephrogenic cord or ridge. The part giving rise to the genital system is called the gonadal or genital ridge.
- Three pairs of kidneys appear in succession during embryonic development. These are the pronephros, similar to fish kidneys, the mesonephros, similar to reptilian kidneys, and the metanephros which is the permanent kidney found in all mammals.
- The gonads can be identified by about the 5th week and develop from three sources: the gonadal ridge which is a thickened ridge of tissue including cells from two sources, the coelomic epithelium and underlying intermediate mesoderm.
- The coelomic epithelium releases a chemical that attracts the third source of cells, primordial germ cells, of which about 100 are present on the caudal surface of the yolk sac during the 4th week. These cells migrate into the interior of the gonadal ridge and are enclosed in columns of epithelial cells called sex cords. This cell line will form the next generation by becoming ova or sperm. The gonads are identical in males and females up to the 7th week and are referred to as indifferent gonads.
- Two pairs of genital ducts are present in the embryo. The mesonephric (Wolffian) ducts are forerunners of the male genital tract and the paramesonephric (Mullerian) ducts are the forerunners of the female genital tract.
- In the absence of a trigger all embryos will become female. The short arm of the Y chromosome in male embryos contains a gene which will produce a testis-determining factor (TDF). If this factor is secreted, the gonads will become testes. If it is absent, whether in a genetic female or in a male with a non-functioning gene, the gonads will become ovaries.
- Two sets of endocrine cells form in the lobules in the testes: the Sertoli cells and the Leydig cells. The earliest function of the Sertoli cells is to produce a Mullerian duct inhibitory factor which enters the fetal circulation and causes regression of the paramesonephric ducts during the 9th week. Leydig cells secrete testosterone into the fetal circulation which ensures the survival and growth of the Wolffian ducts and the formation of the epididymis, ductus deferens, seminal vesicle and the ejaculatory duct.
- In females the Wolffian ducts disappear by programmed cell death without any influence from the ovary. Remnants are normally found in the broad ligament and may form parovarian cysts. In the absence of a Y chromosome and/or TDF, the sex cords accumulate in the outer region or cortex of the gonadal ridge and this becomes filled with primordial follicles consisting of an oocyte derived from the primordial germ cells, an inner shell of follicular cells derived from cell-cord epithelium and an outer shell, the theca, derived from the intermediate mesoderm.
- The number of primordial follicles reaches a maximum of 6–7 million in the 15th week. Programmed cell death reduces this number drastically so that 2 years after birth only 1 million remain and at puberty only 300 000 are present.
- The upper and middle sections of the Mullerian ducts form the epithelial lining of the fallopian tubes and the lower segments fuse into one during the 9th week to become the uterovaginal canal which eventually forms the epithelial lining of the body and cervix of the uterus. The muscle walls of the fallopian tubes and the myometrium of the uterus are formed from splanchnic mesoderm.
- The Mullerian eminence gives rise to the vaginal plate which lengthens along the dorsal wall of the urogenital sinus. The lumen of the vagina is formed by canalisation from below upwards. The hymen is left as a partition between the vagina and the vestibule.
- Early in the 3rd month external sexual differentiation is absent. The phallic urethra is an open urethral groove flanked by paired inner urogenital folds and outer genital swellings derived from mesenchyme. In males the matching pairs under the influence of testosterone come together. The urogenital folds unite below the urethral groove to complete the spongy urethra and the genital swellings form the two halves of the scrotum. In females they stay apart and there is growth in situ of the urogenital folds and genital swellings. The phallus forms the clitoris with a small glans at its tip. The urethral groove and the phallic part of the urogenital sinus remain open and the urogenital folds become the labia minora whilst the genital swellings become the labia majora.
- By 8 weeks the embryo is recognisably human although the head is more round and very large in proportion to the body. The remaining fetal intrauterine time is concerned mainly with growth.

References

Fitzgerald MJT, Fitzgerald M. 1994 Human Embryology. Baillière Tindall, London.

Marieb EN. 1992 Human Anatomy and Physiology, 2nd edn. Benjamin/Cummings, California.

McNabb M. 1997 Embryonic and fetal developments. In Sweet BR with Tiran D (eds) Mayes Midwifery, 12th edn. Baillière Tindall, London, pp 89–105.

Moore KL. 1989 Before We Are Born, 3rd edn. WB Saunders, Philadelphia.

Recommended reading

Bogin B. 1988 Patterns of Human Growth. Cambridge University Press, Cambridge.

Coustan DR. (ed) 1995 Human Reproduction: Growth and Development. Little, Brown, Boston.

Larsen WJ. 1993 Human Embryology. Churchill Livingstone, New York.

Moore KL, Persaud TVN. 1993 The Developing Human. WB Saunders, Philadelphia.

Tanner JM. 1978 Foetus into Man. Open Books, London.

Wolpert L. 1991 The Triumph of the Embryo. Oxford University Press, Oxford.

Chapter 11 The placenta

In this chapter

INTRODUCTION

Gilbert (1988) reminds us that most mammals have evolved the strategy of fetal development within the mother's body. The embryo obtains nutrients and oxygen and disposes of waste products via its mother's circulation. It does not use stored yolk as do babies of non-mammalian species. The development that enabled this capacity was the evolution of a fetal organ closely associated with maternal circulation, the placenta (Bennett & Brown 1996). The placenta is a **haemochorial villous organ** derived from embryonic trophoblast cells with the addition of a few mesodermal cells from the inner cell mass. Whilst the embryo proper is developing, the extraembryonic trophoblastic cells are making the uniquely mammalian tissues of the placenta. The chorion, amnion, yolk sac and allantois constitute the fetal membranes.

IMPLANTATION

The initial trophoblastic cells have a normal cellular appearance and are called collectively the **cytotrophoblast**. They soon give rise to a group of cells that have undergone nuclear division without forming daughter cells, the **syncytiotrophoblast** (trophoblast without cells), which invades the uterine lining allowing the embryo to embed. By the 10th day the embryo is completely embedded and a plug of clotted blood and cellular debris closes over its point of entry. The syncytiotrophoblast at the embryonic pole of the zygote forms a thick multinucleated layer.

The uterus grows new blood vessels in the area of embedding. Endometrial capillaries surrounding the embryo swell to form **sinusoids** which are eroded by the invasive syncytiotrophoblast. Small spaces called **lacunae** appear in the syncytiotrophoblast and become filled with a mixture of blood from ruptured maternal capillaries and secretions from the eroded endometrial glands. This fluid is the **embryotroph** and passes to the embryonic disc by diffusion (Moore 1989). The lacunae fuse to form a network which is the beginning of the **intervillous spaces** of the placenta. Maternal blood begins to flow through the network in a primitive uteroplacental circulation. In normal pregnancy decidual and myometrial arteries undergo changes to convert them to uteroplacental arteries. Two types of **migratory cytotrophoblast** (MC) cause this.

1 **Endovascular MC** invades spiral arterioles on the decidua and myometrium and replaces arterial endothelium, destroying muscle and elastic tissues in the tunica media. Tissue is replaced by maternal fibrinoid. The migration takes place in two waves: 6–10 weeks into the decidua and 14–16 weeks into the myometrium.
2 **Interstitial (stromal) MC** destroys the ends of decidual blood vessels, promoting the flow of blood into the lacunae. The maternal arteries are opened up and functionally denervated so that they are completely dilated and unresponsive to circulatory pressor substances or autonomic neural control. Behind this, at uterine radial artery level, local prostacyclin (PG_1) maintains vasodilation.

Soon mesodermal tissue from the developing embryo migrates through the primitive streak and becomes extraembryonic. It joins the trophoblast extensions and forms the narrow connecting stalk. This extraembryonic mesoderm gives rise to the umbilical blood vessels linking the mother to the embryo. The structure will eventually become the **umbilical cord** (Fitzgerald & Fitzgerald 1994).

By the end of the 2nd week the trophoblastic cells have formed finger-like projections all around the embryo. These are the **primary chorionic villi** which will differentiate into the chorionic villi of the placenta. The chorion forms the **chorionic sac** within which the embryo and its yolk sac and early **amniotic sac** are suspended. It consists of a layer of mesoderm nearest the embryo, the cytotrophoblast and the syncytiotrophoblast nearest the endometrium. Moore (1989) describes the structure as 'two balloons pressed together to form the bilaminar embryonic disc, suspended by a cord (the connecting stalk) from inside a larger balloon (the chorionic sac)'. The amniotic sac is nearest to the uterine wall, divided from the chorion by a fluid-filled cavity, the **extraembryonic coelom**.

DEVELOPMENT OF THE CHORIONIC VILLI

Early in the 3rd week a core of loose connective tissue developed from embryonic mesenchyme invades each primary chorionic villus. The villi are now known as **secondary chorionic villi**. Some of the mesenchymal cells in the core differentiate into fetal blood capillaries. By 15–20 days there is a functioning arteriocapillaryvenous network which becomes connected to the embryonic heart vessels. The villi are now fully formed **tertiary chorionic villi**. By the end of the 3rd week fetal blood circulates through the capillaries of the chorionic villi and the exchange of nutrients, wastes and blood gases between maternal and fetal circulations commences (Figs 11.1 and 11.2).

Whilst this development is taking place the cytotrophoblastic cells proliferate and extend through the syncytiotrophoblast to form a cytotrophoblastic shell. This attaches the chorionic sac to the maternal endometrium by specialised chorionic villi called **stem** or **anchoring villi**. Those growing from the sides of the stem villi are called **branch villi**. It is through the branch villi that the main exchange of material between maternal and fetal circulations occurs.

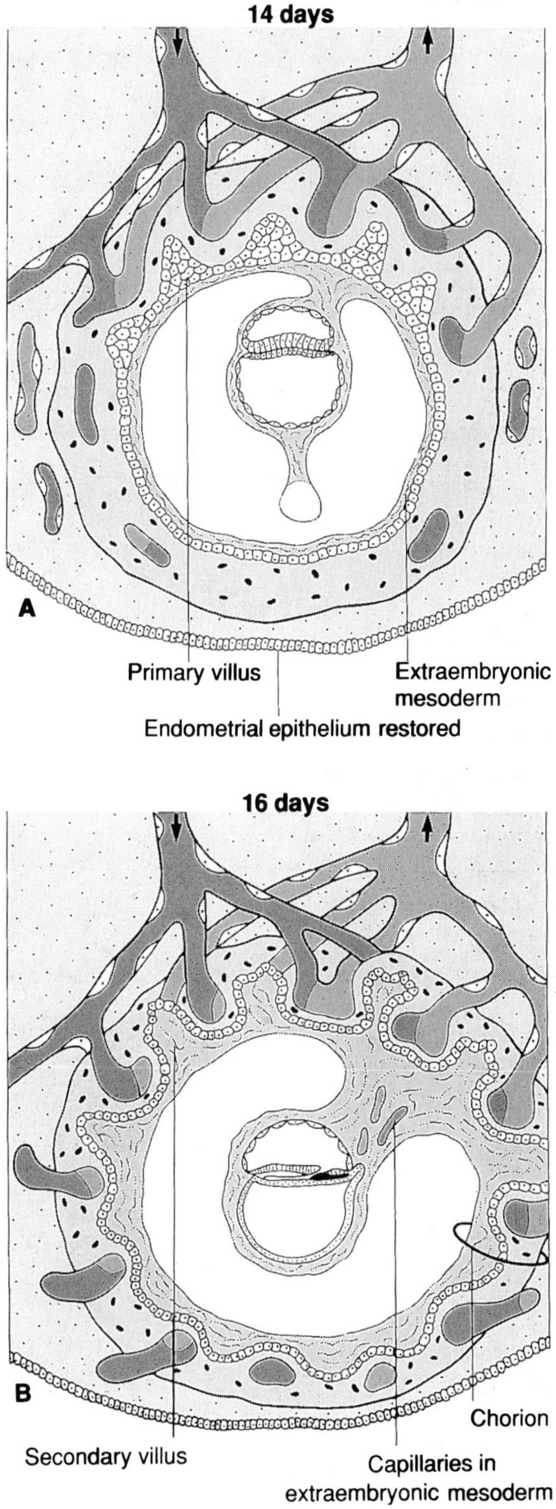

Figure 11.1 *Formation of chorionic vesicle (from Fitzgerald MJT, Fitzgerald M, 1994, with permission).*

Until about 20 weeks the placental membrane (Fig. 11.3) consists of four layers of tissue separating the two circulations, which do not mingle unless there is damage to the villi (Bennett & Brown 1996). These layers are the syncytiotrophoblast, the

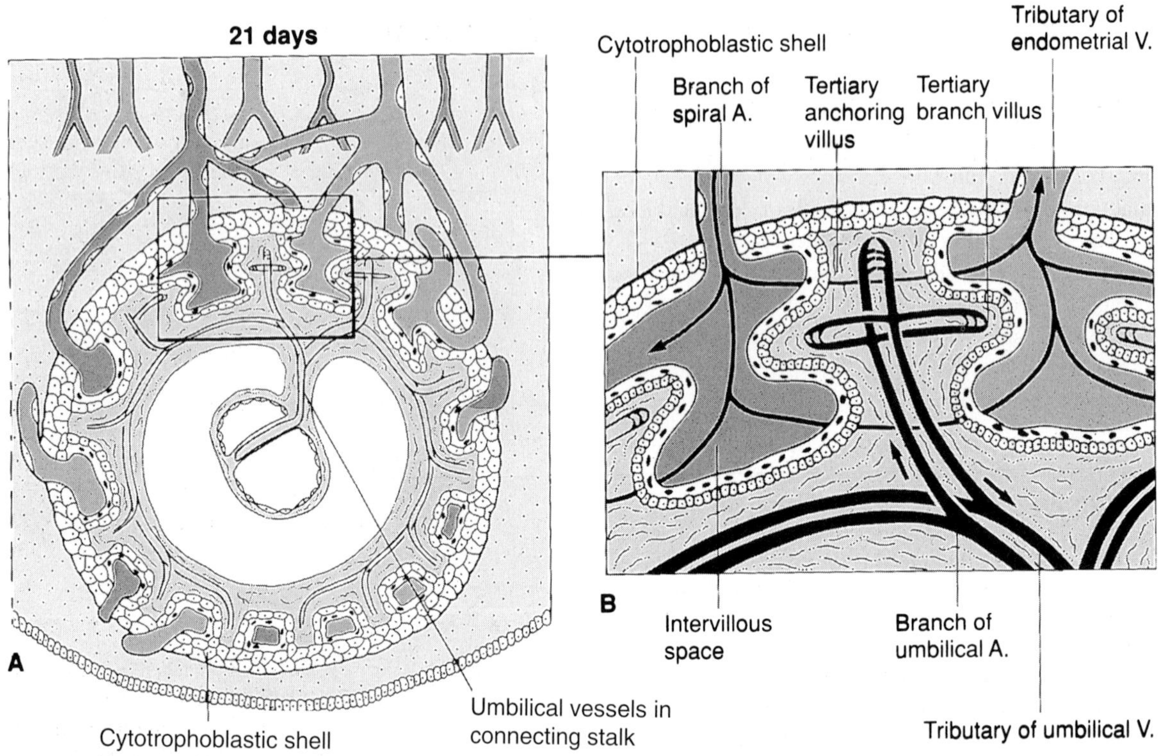

Figure 11.2 *Chorionic vesicle at 21 days. (b) Enlargement of upper part of (a) showing the circulation of embryonic and maternal blood. (From Fitzgerald MJT, Fitzgerald M, 1994, with permission).*

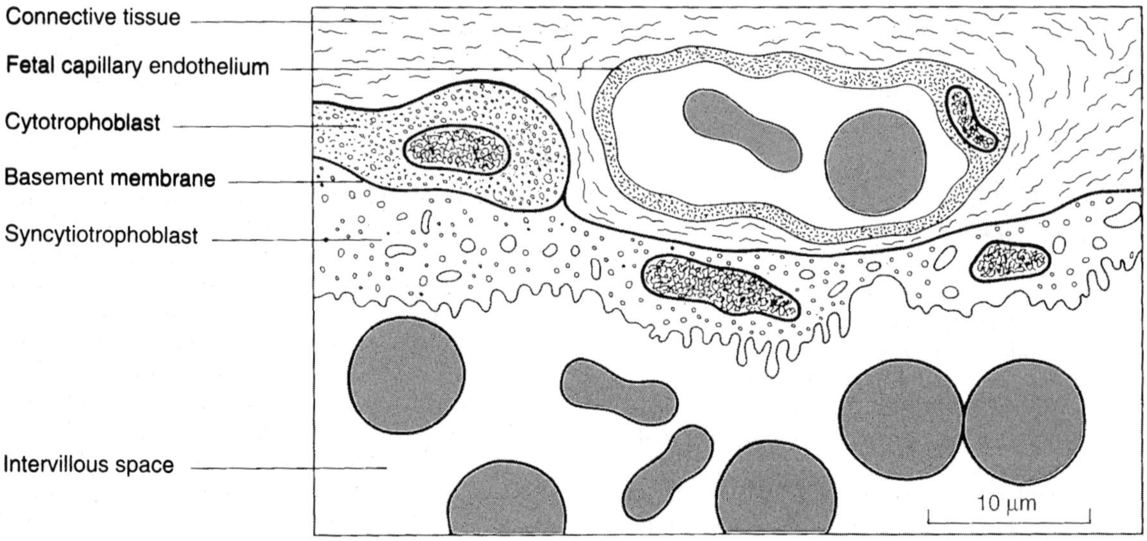

Figure 11.3 *Structure of the placental membrane. All erythrocytes are coloured grey (from Fitzgerald MJT, Fitzgerald M, 1994, with permission).*

cytotrophoblast, the connective tissue of the mesenchymous core and the endothelium of the fetal capillary (Moore 1989). As pregnancy advances this placental membrane becomes thinner and many of the fetal capillaries lie very close to the syncytiotrophoblast.

Later placental development

Once the conceptus has implanted the decidual reaction occurs, spreading outwards from the embedding site. The endometrium is then called the **decidua** because it is shed at the end of pregnancy. Three regions of the decidua are described, based on their relation to the implantation site.

- The **decidua basalis** lies beneath the conceptus, forming the maternal component of the placenta.
- The **decidua capsularis** is the portion overlying the conceptus.
- The **decidua vera** or **parietalis** is the name of the remaining uterine lining.

As the conceptus grows the decidua capsularis bulges into the uterine cavity and eventually fuses with the decidua vera, obliterating the uterine cavity. By 22 weeks the decidua capsularis has degenerated and disappeared (Fig. 11.4)

The entire surface of the chorionic sac is covered by chorionic villi until the 8th week. As the sac grows the chorionic villi associated with the decidua capsularis become compressed. Their blood supply is reduced and they eventually degenerate, leaving a bare area, the **chorion laeve** (smooth), which becomes the chorionic membrane. The chorionic villi of the decidua basalis increase, branch and enlarge rapidly to form the **chorion frondosum**, forming the fetal part of the placenta. By 16 weeks the placenta reaches its full thickness and no new lobes or stem villi develop. Circumferential growth continues with branching of villi. The size and number of maternal capillaries increase, as does the surface area for gas exchange. Cellular proliferation stops at about 35 weeks but cellular hypertrophy continues until term.

THE MATURE PLACENTA

The placenta is a flattened discoid organ about 20 cm in diameter. It is about 2.5 cm thick at the centre and thins out towards its circumference, where it is continuous with the chorion. It is about one-sixth of the baby's weight at term. There are two distinct surfaces: one attached to the maternal decidua and therefore called the maternal surface and one covered with amnion with the umbilical cord inserting into it, called the fetal surface.

The maternal surface

Because of its contained maternal blood, this surface is a dark red colour. Part of the decidua basalis will separate with it during delivery. The surface is formed of about 20 **cotyledons** (lobes) separated by **sulci** (grooves). The decidua dips down into these sulci to form septa. The lobes are made up of lobules each containing a tertiary villus with its branches. Deposits of lime salts may be found on this surface if the placenta is past term.

The fetal surface

Because of the presence of the amnion, this surface has a shiny greyish white appearance. From the insertion of the umbilical cord, branches of the single umbilical vein and two arteries can be seen spreading out from the cord and dipping down into the tissue. The amnion can be peeled off the surface leaving the chorionic plate from which the placenta has developed. This is the portion continuous with the chorion.

The membranes

A double membrane forms the sac containing the fetus in utero, the amnion and chorion. The membranes continue to grow up to about 28 weeks of gestation but then increase their size by stretching. This allows them to resist rupture as the fetus grows, mainly due to the tensile strength of the amnion. Rupture of the membranes in labour is probably brought about by increased intrauterine pressure as contractions reduce the space available for amniotic fluid and fluid cannot be reduced in volume. The forewaters are formed and may resist rupture until additional pressure is provided in the second stage.

The amnion and chorion are not fused and can contain up to 200 ml of amniotic fluid between them. The chorion is relatively fixed in its attachment to the decidua but the amnion moves over it aided by mucus. This may lead to rupture of the amnion with the formation of amniotic bands which may constrict or amputate fetal parts such as limbs (Blackburn & Loper 1992). This author has seen such an amputation of an arm, just below the elbow.

The chorion

The outer membrane is the chorion which is closely adherent to the decidua. This is a thick, opaque, friable membrane that originated as the chorion laeve developing from the trophoblast. It is continuous with the edge of the placenta. At term it varies between about 0.2 and 0.02 mm thick. It consists of four layers of tissue (Fig. 11.6) which atrophy as pregnancy advances but contain no supporting lymphatics or nerves (Anderson 1992). The cells of the chorion laeve are metabolically active, producing enzymes that can reduce the level of locally produced progesterone, a protein that can bind progesterone, and prostaglandins, oxytocin and platelet-activating factor all able to stimulate uterine myometrial activity (McNabb 1997).

The amnion

The inner membrane is the amnion, a tough, smooth, translucent membrane derived from the inner cell mass. It lines the chorion and the surface of the placenta as far as the insertion of the umbilical cord. It is continuous with the outer layer of the umbilical cord. At term it is about 0.02–0.5 mm thick. It consists of five layers (Fig. 11.6) and is lined by non-ciliated cuboid epithelial cells. These cells possibly help in the formation and regulation of the quantity of amniotic fluid, especially the portion of the amnion covering the placenta and umbilical cord (Bennett & Brown 1996 and see Chapter 12). The amnion also produces prostaglandins, in particular PGE_2 (Germain et al 1994). The membranes' role in initiating the onset of labour is discussed in Chapter 35.

The umbilical cord

The umbilical cord or **funis** can be called the 'lifeline' of the fetus. Moore (1989) describes it as 'a vascular cable that connects the embryo or fetus to the placenta'. It is usually attached to the centre of the fetal surface of the placenta but can be located at the edge, when it is called a battledore placenta (after the bat used in a medieval game of bat and ball), or inserted into the membranes (a **velamentous** insertion of cord).

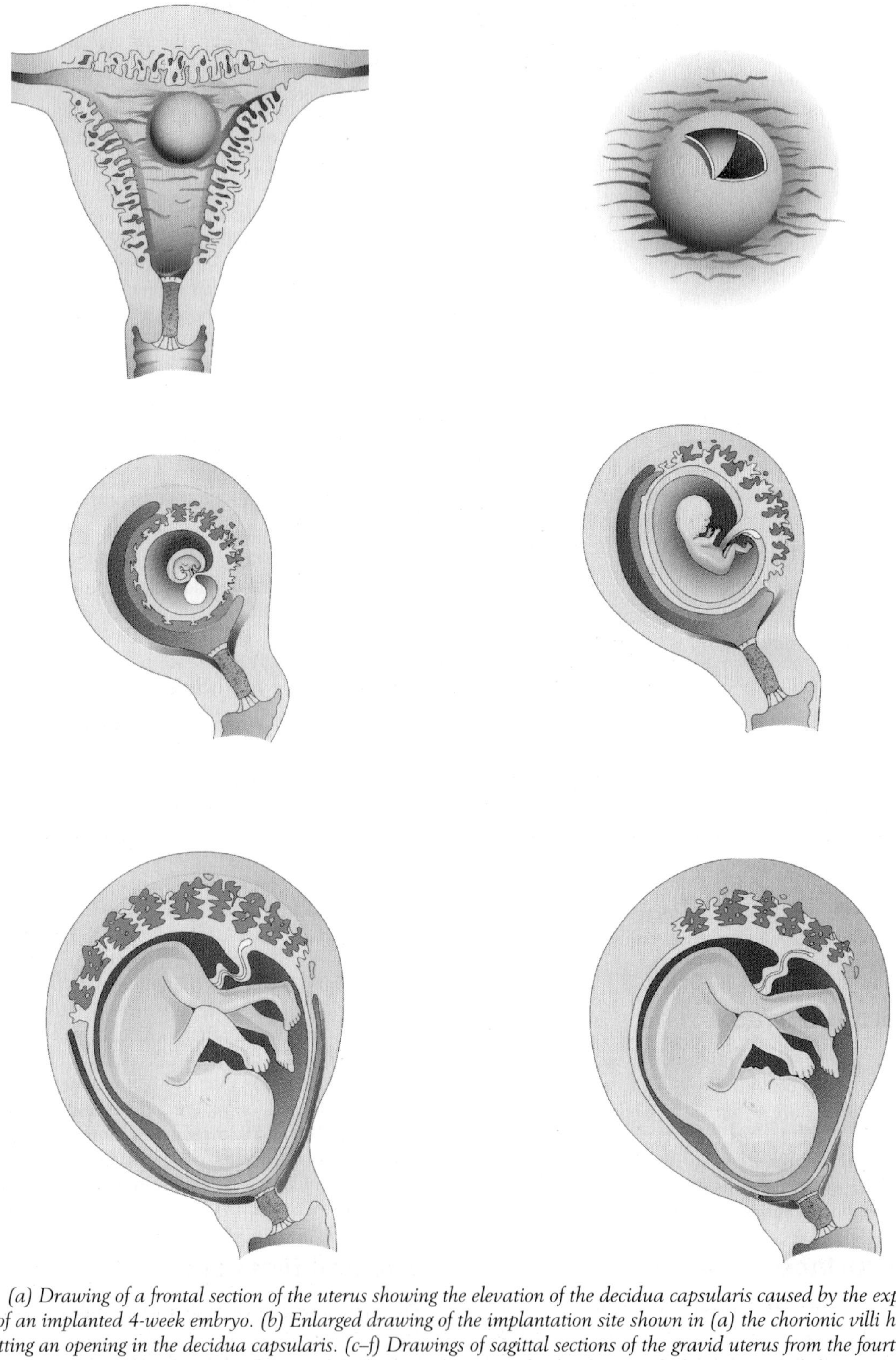

Figure 11.4 *(a) Drawing of a frontal section of the uterus showing the elevation of the decidua capsularis caused by the expanding chorionic sac of an implanted 4-week embryo. (b) Enlarged drawing of the implantation site shown in (a) the chorionic villi have been exposed by cutting an opening in the decidua capsularis. (c–f) Drawings of sagittal sections of the gravid uterus from the fourth to the twenty-second weeks, showing the changing relations of the fetal membranes to the decidua. In (f) the amnion and chorion are fused with each other and the decidua parietalis, thus obliterating the uterine cavity. Note that the chorionic villi persist only where the chorion is associated with the decidua basalis; here they have formed the villous chorion (from Moore K, Persand TVN, 1998, with permission).*

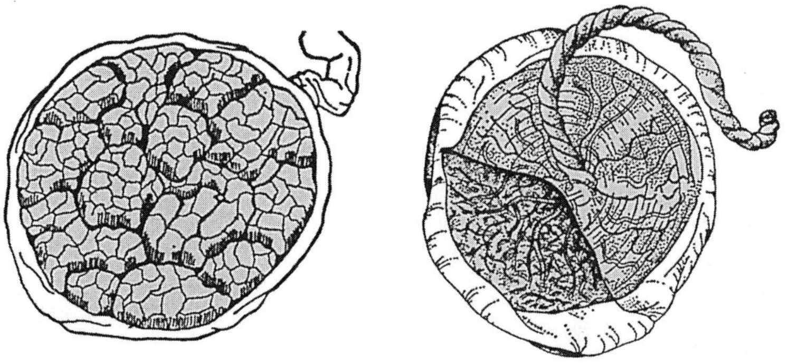

Figure 11.5 *The placenta. (a) The maternal surface, showing cotyledons. (b) The fetal surface (from Sweet B, 1997, with permission).*

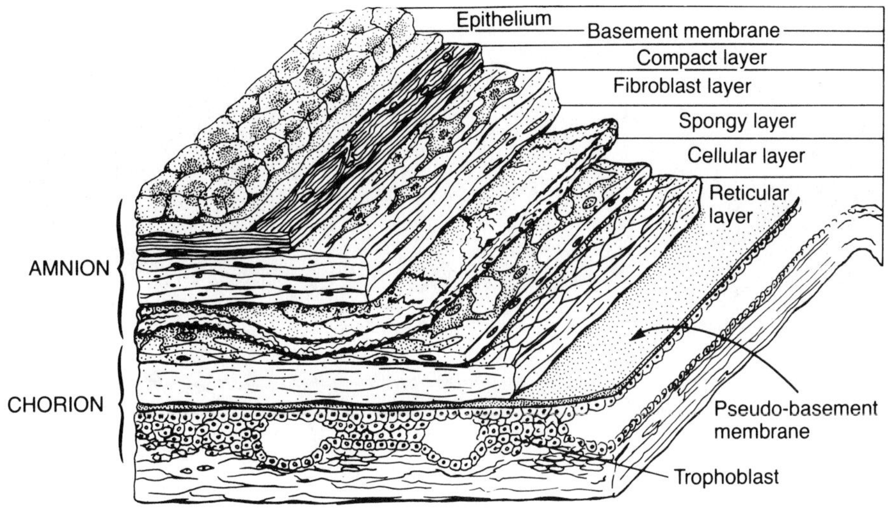

Figure 11.6 *Layers of the human amnion and chorion. (Reproduced with permission from Blackburn & Loper 1992.)*

The umbilical cord is usually 1–2 cm in diameter and varies in length from 30 to 90 cm with an average of 50 cm. It usually contains two arteries and one vein surrounded by a mucoid connective tissue called **Wharton's jelly**. There is an outer covering of amnion. The umbilical vein is longer than the arteries and the vessels are longer than the cord so loops of vessel may be seen inside the Wharton's jelly. These are the non-significant false knots. Lumps of Wharton's jelly are also not significant. Occasionally a true knot may be present and the blood vessels may become occluded, causing fetal distress, especially during the descent of the fetus through the birth canal during labour.

The yolk sac and allantois

By 9 weeks the yolk sac has shrunk to a small pear-shaped remnant about 5 mm in diameter. Once its functions are completed it becomes detached from the gut and remains in the umbilical cord. In about 2% of adults the intraabdominal part of the yolk sac persists as a diverticulum of the ileum known as a Meckel's diverticulum. Once the early functions of the allantois are completed, the extraembryonic part degenerates and the intraembryonic portion runs from the umbilicus to the urinary bladder, forming the **urachus** (the median umbilical ligament).

AMNIOTIC FLUID

Amniotic fluid is fully discussed in Chapter 12. It is thought to be of both fetal and maternal origin. Some is secreted by the part of the amnion which covers the surface of the placenta and cord. Most amniotic fluid is derived from maternal blood. From about the 10th week the fetus also adds to the volume by excreting urine into the amniotic sac.

Amniotic fluid is a clear, pale straw-coloured liquid consisting of 99% water. Most of the remaining 1% is solutes, including food substances and waste. There are also tissues of fetal origin such as skin cells, vernix caseosa and lanugo. Amniotic fluid is normally swallowed by the fetus and absorbed by the gastrointestinal tract. Abnormalities of quantity may occur. Too much amniotic fluid (**polyhydramnios**) may be present if the fetus cannot swallow and too little (**oligohydramnios**) if the fetus cannot pass urine.

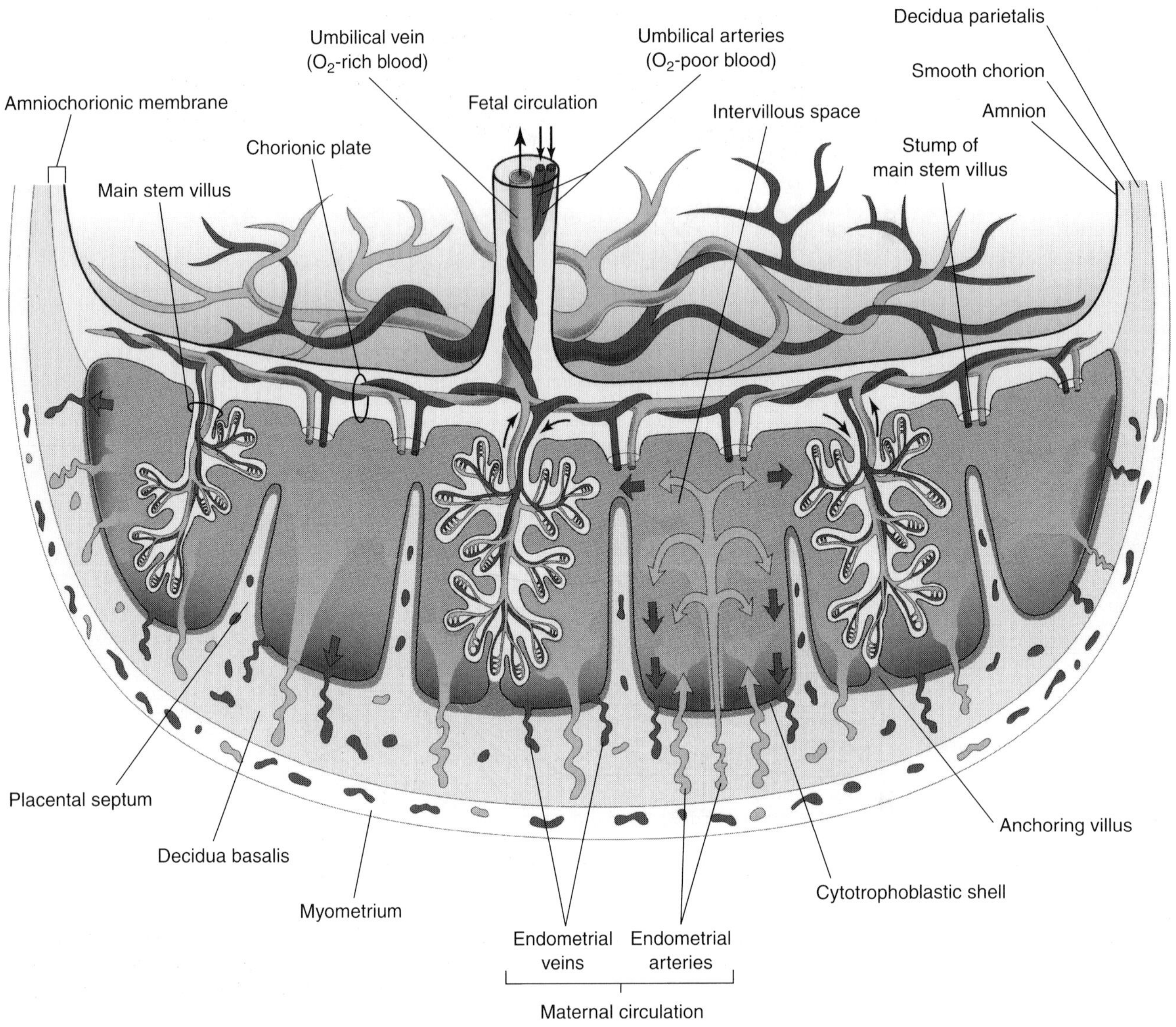

Figure 11.7 *Schematic drawing of a transverse section through a full-term placenta, showing (1) the relation of the villous chorion (fetal part of placenta) to the decidua basalis (maternal part of placenta); (2) the fetal placental circulation; and (3) the maternal placental circulation. Maternal blood flows into the intervillous spaces in funnel-shaped spurts from the spiral arteries, and exchanges occur with the fetal blood as the maternal blood flows around the branch villi. It is through the branch villi that the main exchange of material between the mother and embryo/fetus occurs. The inflowing arterial blood pushes venous blood out of the intervillous space into the endometrial veins, which are scattered over the entire surface of the decidua basalis. Note that the umbilical arteries carry poorly oxygenated fetal blood (shown in dark grey) to the placenta and that the umbilical vein carries oxygenated blood (shown in light grey) to the fetus. Note that the cotyledons are separated from each other by placental septa, projections of the decidua basalis. Each cotyledon consists of two or more main stem villi and their many branches. In this drawing, only one stem villus is shown in each cotyledon, but the stumps of those that have been removed are indicated. (Reproduced with permission from Moore 1989.)*

Functions of amniotic fluid

The embryo floats freely in the amniotic fluid. This:

- allows symmetrical growth and development of the embryo;
- enables free movement to facilitate musculoskeletal development;
- prevents adherence of the amnion to the embryo;
- cushions the embryo against jolts and injury;
- helps to control the embryo's body temperature.

THE PLACENTAL CIRCULATION

The villi of the placenta form an enormous surface area for the exchange of substances between maternal and fetal circulations. The blood is propelled by maternal blood pressure towards the chorionic plate or 'roof' of the placenta. It then flows slowly over the surface of the villi so that an exchange of materials can occur in both directions between the two circulations. The maternal blood eventually reaches the floor of the intervillous space where it drains into the endometrial veins. The placental

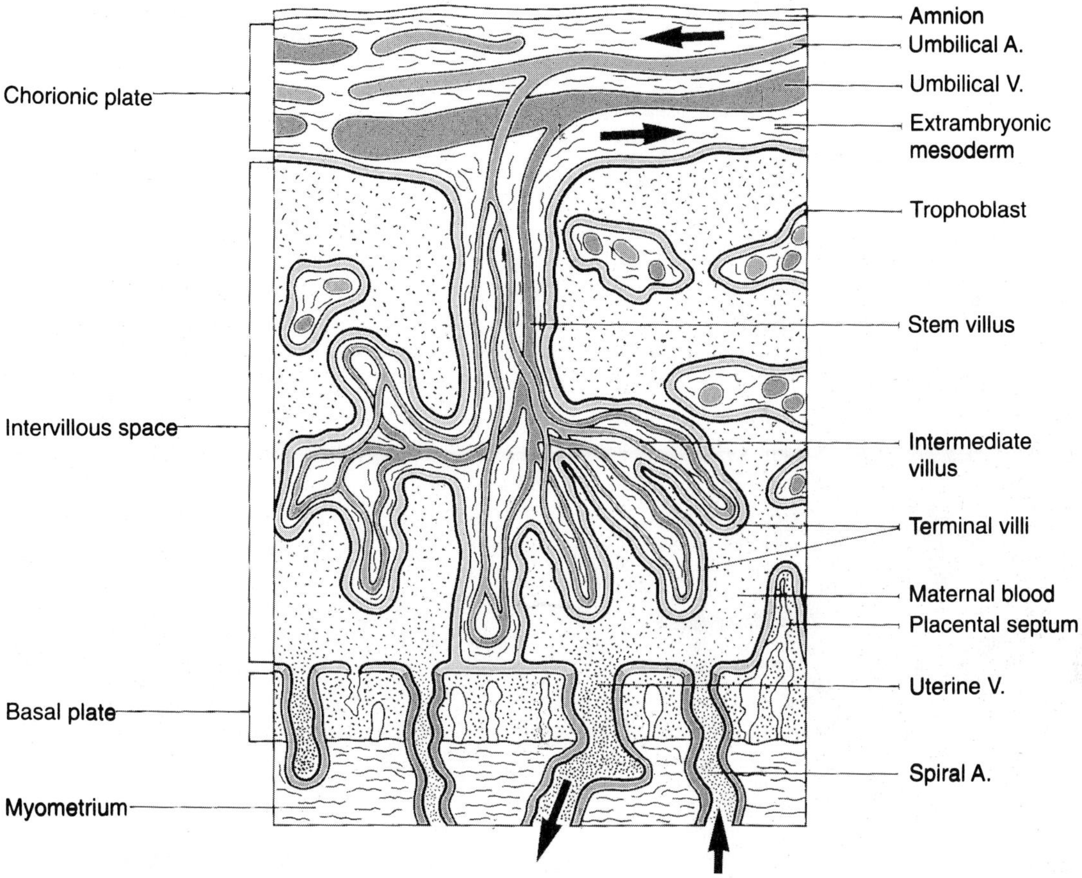

Figure 11.8 *Diagrammatic section through the placenta. The arteries carry deoxygenated blood; the veins carry oxygenated blood. Arrows indicate directions of blood flow (from Fitzgerald MJT, Fitzgerald M, 1994, with permission).*

membrane is called the **placental barrier**. There are few compounds that cannot pass through the membrane, as will be discussed later.

Fetal placental circulation

The fetal circulation is described in full in Chapter 48. Briefly, deoxygenated blood leaves the fetus and passes into the two umbilical arteries which take it to the placenta. Here the blood vessels form the extensive arteriocapillaryvenous system within the chorionic villi. The fetal blood is brought very close to maternal blood. Oxygenated fetal blood then converges in thinwalled veins to enter the umbilical vein which returns it to the fetus.

Maternal placental circulation

Whilst the blood is in the intervillous space it is temporarily outside the maternal circulatory system. It enters the intervillous space in spurts via 80–100 spiral arteries of the endometrium. The system is very like taking a shower. If you imagine yourself to be in a shower, your body will be the tertiary villus, the shower head delivering water is the spiral arteriole delivering blood and the drainage hole in the bottom of the shower is analogous to the endometrial vein. You are covered by a continuous fresh supply of water which drains away down the plug hole. The fetus depends on this maternal blood supply and anything affecting the uteroplacental circulation will result in fetal hypoxia and may interfere with growth or cause death.

ANATOMICAL VARIATIONS OF THE PLACENTA

Placentae may be abnormally shaped and there is a danger that some portion will be left in the uterus at delivery. It is important to examine the placenta for these abnormalities and to record the findings and seek medical aid if it is suspected that the placenta is incomplete.

Succenturiate lobe

Sometimes a small extra lobe, separated from the main placenta by membranes, develops and is linked by blood vessels to the main placenta. There is a danger attached to this otherwise functionally unimportant feature. Failure to deliver the succenturiate lobe may lead to retained placental tissue and infection and haemorrhage may supervene. It is important that the person conducting the delivery examines the placenta to ensure there is no hole in the membranes with blood vessels leading away from it.

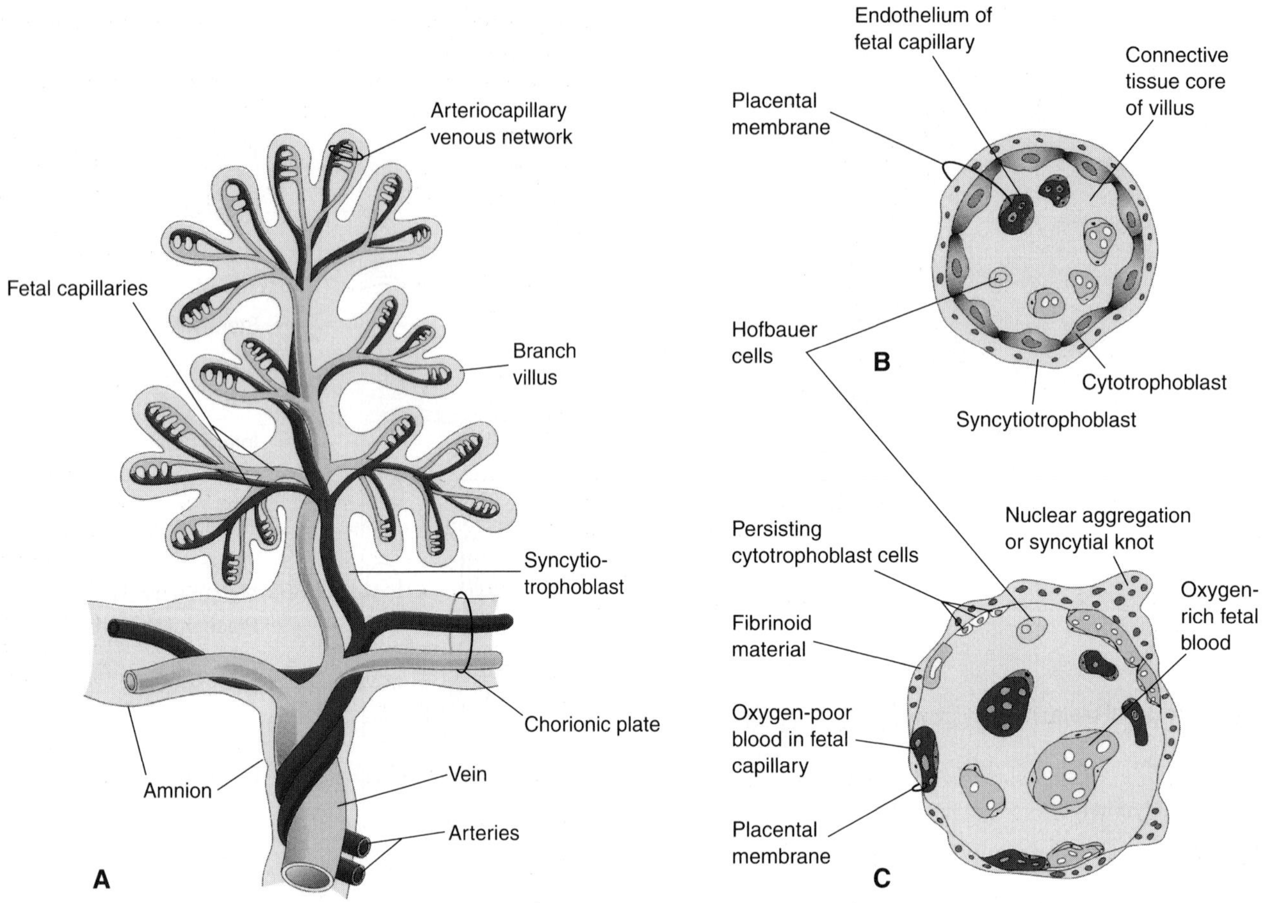

Figure 11.9 *(a) Drawing of a stem chorionic villus showing its arteriocapillary venous system. The arteries carry poorly oxygenated fetal blood and waste products from the fetus, whereas the vein carries oxygenated blood and nutrients to the fetus. (b, c) Drawings of sections through a branch villus at 10 weeks and full term, respectively. The placental membrane, composed of extrafetal tissues, separates the maternal blood in the intervillous space from the fetal blood in the capillaries in the villi. Note that the placental membrane becomes very thin at full term. Hofbauer cells are thought to be phagocytic. (Reproduced with permission from Moore 1989.)*

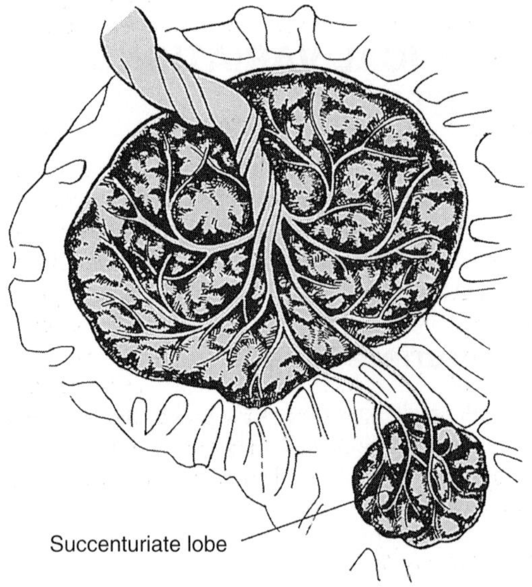

Figure 11.10 *Succenturiate placenta (from Sweet B, 1997, with permission).*

Circumvallate placenta

An opaque thickened ring is seen on the fetal surface of the placenta, caused by doubling back of the membranes. The membranes may leave the placenta nearer to the centre than normal.

Bipartite (tripartite) placenta

A placenta may be divided into two (or three) fairly equal lobes.

Infarcts

Infarcts are red or white patches on the maternal surface of the placenta caused by localised death of placental tissue. This is due to an interruption of blood supply. They are red when newly formed and degenerate into white fibrous patches. Any placenta may contain them but they are more common in women with hypertension of pregnancy.

Calcification

Small greyish white patches may be found on the surface of the

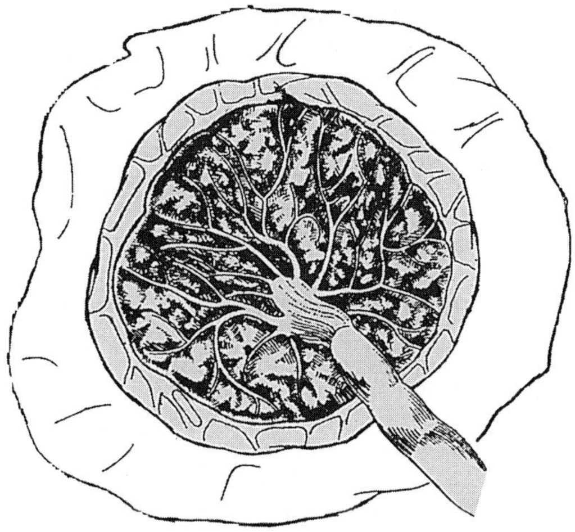

Figure 11.11 *Circumvallate placenta (from Sweet B, 1997, with permission).*

placenta, especially if the pregnancy is post term. These are deposits of lime salts and are of no significance.

FUNCTIONS OF THE PLACENTA

The functions of the placenta are summarised in Box 11.1.

> ### *Box 11.1 Functions of the placenta*
> ### *Endocrine – production of hormones*
> *The protein hormones*
> Human chorionic gonadotrophin (HCG)
> Human placental lactogen (HPL)
> Schwangerschaftsprotein 1 (SP_1)
> Pregnancy-associated protein A (PAPP-A)
> Pregnancy-associated protein B (PAPP-B)
> Placental protein 5 (PP5)
>
> *The steroid hormones*
> Oestrogens
> Progestogen
>
> *Transfer during* **metabolism**
> Respiration
> Nutrition
> Excretion
> Barrier

Endocrine function

Klopper (1991) defines hormones as 'biological signals which modulate metabolic processes'. The fetoplacental unit produces hormones which alter maternal metabolic processes to benefit the fetus. The hormones produced by the placenta can be divided into two groups – steroid hormones and protein hormones. The steroid hormones, such as oestriol, are made in a series of steps by sending molecules backwards and forwards between the fetus and placenta until the final hormone structure is reached. The steroid hormones, such as oestrogens and progesterone, are found in higher concentrations in fetal blood than in maternal blood.

However, the manufacture of protein hormones does not appear to need input from the fetus. They are found only in maternal blood and are implicated in changing maternal physiology. Unlike normal hormone production, there does not seem to be a feedback mechanism controlling their production. Production seems to be linked to the amount of active trophoblastic tissue. The syncytiotrophoblast produces its own luteinising hormone-releasing hormone (LHRH) which controls HCG production in the same cell.

The production of hormones by maternal pregnancy tissue

The maternal part of the placenta and the extraplacental decidua secrete hormones. Prolactin, relaxin and the prostaglandins are secreted by the decidua as well as by other tissues. It is probably the decidual production of these hormones that influences pregnancy. Another hormone produced by the decidua as well as by the placental trophoblast is pregnancy-associated placental protein A (PAPP-A). These decidual hormones are aimed at the fetoplacental unit and bind to the fetal membranes and trophoblast.

The protein hormones

The main protein hormones are:

- human chorionic gonadotrophin (HCG)
- human placental lactogen (HPL)
- Schwangerschaftsprotein 1 (SP_1)
- pregnancy-associated protein A (PAPP-A)
- pregnancy-associated protein B (PAPP-B)
- placental protein 5 (PP5).

The protein hormones of the placenta are analogous to the pituitary hormones. For instance, HCG has a similar structure to luteinising hormone (LH) and HPL is similar to prolactin and growth hormone. In the same way, insulin and relaxin share a similar structure.

Human chorionic gonadotrophin

The hormone HCG is a glycoprotein with a large carbohydrate content. Its molecular weight is about 50 000. It consists of two subunits, α and β, joined by a disulphide bond. The α subunit is the smaller of the two and contains 92 amino acids. The β subunit is larger and contains 147 amino acids. It is probably the β subunit which is biologically active and pregnancy tests are based on its immunological antigenic properties. The test kit contains antibodies which will bind to the β subunit if it is present to show a positive result for pregnancy. If necessary, the β subunit can be detected in maternal blood even before the first menstrual period is missed, as early as the 9th day following ovulation.

Secretion of HCG

The trophoblast secretes HCG and although there is still controversy as to whether it is secreted by the syncytiotrophoblast or cytotrophoblast, Klopper (1991) believes that this is an irrelevant distinction as the syncytiotrophoblast is derived from cytotrophoblastic cells. In early pregnancy there is a rapid increase in HCG production, the urinary excretion rate doubling every 36–48 h (Klopper 1991). The curve then flattens out at about 9 weeks and declines. The lower level is maintained until just before term when there is another rise. The plasma concentration is measured in international units (iu)/ml and rises from 7 to 100 iu/ml.

Function of HCG

Although sensitive measuring tools have demonstrated the production of HCG by many tissues, including cancer cells, secretion by the syncytiotrophoblast far exceeds that of any other cell. Thus HCG can be said to be the primary hormone of pregnancy. However, scientists have found no association between failure to produce sufficient HCG and spontaneous abortion. The fall in HCG levels found in miscarriage occurs after the death of the conceptus. An early pregnancy placental abnormality called **hydatidiform mole** (see below) produces large amounts of HCG.

The ovary contains receptors for HCG and is its prime target. Its role is probably to stimulate extra production of oestrogen and progesterone necessary for the maintenance of pregnancy. It is also probable that HCG controls placental production of progesterone and that the amount of HCG in the trophoblast determines the level of progesterone production.

Human placental lactogen

This hormone was for a short while called human chorionic somatomammotrophin (HCS) and some older books may refer to it by that name. The hormone HPL is a single chain polypeptide with a molecular weight of 22 000 and 190 amino acids. Of these, 163 are the same as those found in human pituitary growth hormone. It is the only placental protein with no carbohydrate in its structure.

Secretion of HPL

The site of production of HPL is the syncytiotrophoblast but it is also secreted by choriocarcinoma (see Placental pathology, p. 140) and by malignant testicular teratoma. Maternal blood HPL level rises from a value of 0.3 μg/ml at 10 weeks to 5.4 μg/ml at 36 weeks. There is then a fall in serum levels until delivery. It is assumed that the fall relates to a corresponding fall in functioning placental tissue and maternal plasma HPL levels have been used to check placental function.

The role of HPL

There is probably a growth-promoting role for HPL in pregnancy, affecting carbohydrate metabolism. It causes the mobilisation of free fatty acids and antagonises the action of insulin. There is thus a greater need for the mother to manuacture insulin in pregnancy. In women in whom the insulin reserve is poor, carbohydrate metabolism may be compromised, particularly in the diabetic woman. This is the reason for labelling HPL as diabetogenic.

Schwangerschaftsprotein 1

SP_1 is another high carbohydrate glycoprotein with a molecular weight of 90 000. It is present in large amounts so that it can be detected in early pregnancy and easily measured in late pregnancy. The shape of the pregnancy maternal plasma curve is similar to that of plasma HPL with a steady rise until 36 weeks followed by a steady decline until delivery. The hormone has been examined as a test of placental function but the large subject-to-subject spread makes it unsuitable. The role of this hormone is unknown but it may be important in the immunosuppressive mechanism, preventing rejection of the placenta as a foreign protein.

Pregnancy-associated plasma proteins A and B

A series of pregnancy-associated plasma proteins (PAPPs) were discovered by Halbert et al in the early 1970s. Of these, PAPP-A and PAPP-B were found to be new proteins produced by the trophoblast. PAPP-A is a large glycoprotein detectable in maternal plasma early in pregnancy with a rising concentration as pregnancy progresses. The values continue to rise until the onset of labour. It probably helps to prevent rejection of the fetoplacental unit by the cellular lymphocyte component of the maternal immune system. PAPP-B is the largest placental glycoprotein with a molecular weight of over 1 000 000. It rises throughout pregnancy with the steepest part of its curve occurring after 30 weeks. It has been used to ascertain the progress of the placenta in such diseases as preeclampsia and diabetes mellitus.

Placental protein 5

This placental hormone has different properties from the others so far discussed. It is found in the stroma of the chorionic villi as well as in the syncytiotrophoblast. It is a small glycoprotein with a molecular weight of 36 000. In studies it has been found to inhibit the proteolytic activity of trypsin so its function may be to inhibit protease activity in the placenta.

The steroid hormones

All the steroid hormones of the ovary, testis and adrenal gland are made by the fetoplacental unit. The main steroid hormones are oestrogens and progesterone.

Oestrogens

Of about 26 different oestrogens three are important, based on the number of attached hydroxyl groups – 1, 2 and 3. These are respectively oestrone, oestradiol and oestriol. In the non-pregnant woman oestriol is built up from oestradiol and oestrone whereas in pregnancy oestriol is synthesised by the fetoplacental unit. The fetal liver and adrenal glands are important in oestriol production and oestriol is a useful direct measure of fetal well-being. The fetus manufactures primitive forms of steroids such as pregnenolone. These are taken to the placenta in the form of sulphates and converted into oestrogens. Pregnenolone sulphate is the precursor of all fetoplacental steroids.

Three enzymes are needed by the placenta for the production of oestrogens – sulphatase, 3β-hydroxysteroid dehydrogenase and aromatase. A typical outline of production steps is:

1 acetate to cholesterol;
2 cholesterol to pregnenolone;
3 pregnenolone to dehydroepiandosterone;

4 16-hydroxylation to 16-hydroxydehydroepiandosterone;
5 16-hydroxydehydroepiandosterone to oestriol.

Oestrogen levels in normal pregnancy

In a normal pregnancy maternal serum levels of all three hormones rises but the curve for plasma oestriol is the most definitive and useful. Plasma oestriol levels show a steep rise from about 34 to 36 weeks but this may not occur if pregnancy pathology affects the fetus. Serial assays of oestriol are therefore useful in monitoring fetal well-being. Instead of rising, the curve may flatten out or even fall away.

Oestriol estimations and fetal well-being

Previously, urinary oestriol assays were used because there was a clear preponderance in urine of oestriol over the other oestrogens. In blood the levels of the different oestrogens are not as clearly defined but test developments have allowed accurate estimations of plasma oestriol levels. As this is a much more convenient method of assessment, maternal blood is now taken. The unit of measurement is nmol/l. It is not quite as simple as could be wished because the overlap between physiological and pathological levels is large. Therefore the best use of the hormone is in serial estimations in a pregnancy known to be at risk rather than as a single screening device to identify at-risk pregnancies.

The role of oestrogens in pregnancy

There is hardly a tissue or organ unaffected by oestrogens in pregnancy. Oestrogens can be considered to be stimulators of growth and the hypertrophy and hyperplasia of uterine muscle is due to the influence of oestrogens. The growth and development of the breasts are similarly caused by oestrogen.

Progesterone

The site of progesterone production is the syncytiotrophoblast. Some of this is sent to the maternal circulation and some to the fetus. The immediate precursor of progesterone is pregnenolone, the common link in all steroid production. The likely pathway of progesterone production in the placenta is from cholesterol through pregnenolone to progesterone. Progesterone is broken down into the inactive substance pregnanediol and excreted via urine.

Progesterone levels in normal and abnormal pregnancy

It used to be thought that progesterone levels were indicative of fetal well-being and that low maternal plasma progesterone was a cause of spontaneous abortion. However, treatment with progesterone was unsuccessful and later research shows that the low level of progesterone follows fetal compromise rather than acting as an underlying cause. Some sources have found a slight drop in maternal progesterone levels at about the 9th week when placental production is possibly taking over from ovarian production. There is a sharp rise in progesterone production from the 10th week onwards.

Plasma concentration is measured in nmol/l but there is no agreement on what constitutes normal levels. Progesterone exists in both the bound and the free state and plasma progesterone levels fluctuate throughout a normal pregnancy. Klopper (1991) gives the average findings of a rise from about 275 nmol/l at 32 weeks to 450 nmol/l at term so that measuring plasma progesterone assay is neither easy nor relevant. Much progesterone is stored in body fat and may act as a buffer against transient low production.

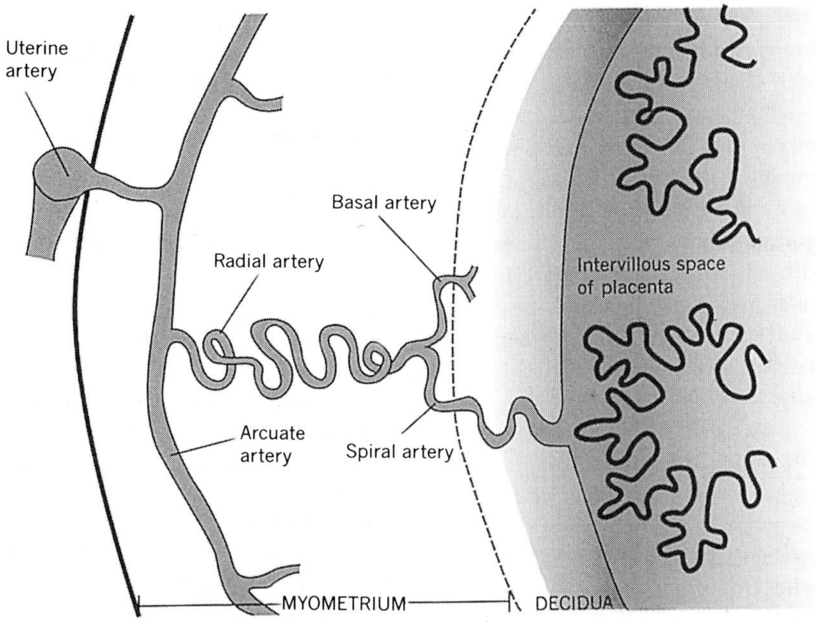

Figure 11.12 *The arterial supply to the placenta in normal pregnancy. (Reproduced with permission from Sheppard B I, Bawwar J 1989. The maternal blood supply to the placenta. Progress in Obstetrics and Gynaecology 7: 27–30.)*

The function of progesterone in pregnancy

Ovarian progesterone plays a part in ovum transport and implantation. It is involved in the development of the endometrium in the second part of the menstrual cycle and in the decidual reaction caused by progesterone secretion for 48 h followed by superimposed oestrogen. Progesterone has a sedative effect on the contractility of uterine muscle, working with **relaxin** to create this effect, possibly by altering membrane potential in the myometrial cells with a reduction in contractile impulses. Progesterone relaxes all smooth muscle during pregnancy and is responsible for many of the minor disorders of pregnancy. It competes with aldosterone for binding sites in the kidney, leading to urinary sodium loss. Aldosterone secretion is increased to counteract this effect.

The role of progesterone in initiating the onset of labour is not as clearcut as used to be thought. If a fall in progesterone influences the onset of labour, it is only part of the complex process of parturition.

Transfer of substances

The fetus is completely dependent on the mother for respiration, nutrition, excretion and protection. The placenta carries out the work of the fetal lungs, alimentary tract, kidneys and endocrine system. There must be sufficient placental transfer to allow the fetus to grow at the necessary fast rate. The placenta continues to grow throughout pregnancy. It weighs about 300 g at 28 weeks gestation and about 900 gm at term. This is slow relative to the growth of the fetus but new villi are still being formed at term. It is worth exploring the nature of the placental membrane that separates maternal and fetal blood. Stacey (1991) describes its unique properties thus:

1 it is the only epithelial membrane to separate two fluids;
2 it is the only syncytium known to exist in the human body.

The surface area of the villi exposed to the maternal circulation is about 11 m^2 at term. By late pregnancy there is thinning of the syncytium in small areas. These areas are called **vasculo-syncytial membranes**. There are fewer microvilli in these areas and the syncytium is closely applied to the capillary basement membrane, possibly enabling the transfer of macromolecules such as immunoglobulins. The structure of the syncytium is complex with a large number of intracellular vesicles which probably allow the active transport of large molecules by **pinocytosis** (see below).

Mechanisms of transfer

Substances such as gases, nutrients, waste materials and drugs are transported across the placental membrane by the usual cellular membrane transport systems. These are summarised in Figure 11.13.

- Simple diffusion of lipid-soluble substances
- Water pores of water-soluble substances
- Facilitated diffusion of substances such as glucose by carrier proteins
- Active transport mechanisms, against a concentration gradient of ions such as calcium and phosphate, of amino acids and some vitamins
- Endocytosis (pinocytosis) of macromolecules.

Transport across the placenta increases during the course of gestation as the placenta increases in size and becomes modified in structure. Increased maternal and fetal blood flow and

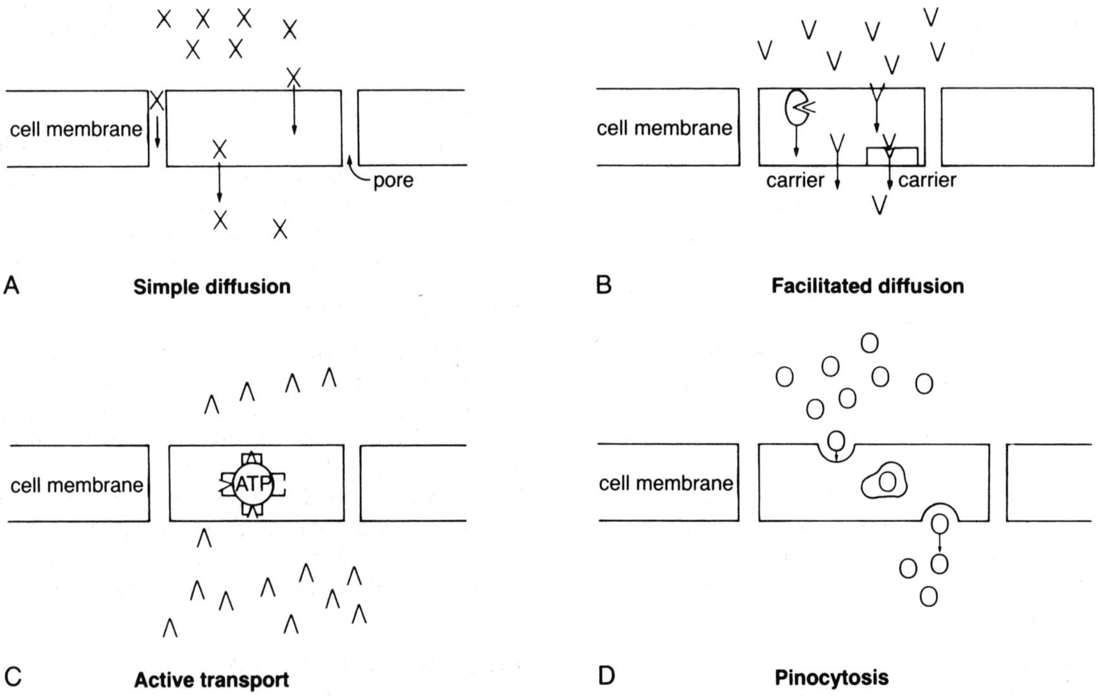

Figure 11.13 *Mechanisms of placenta transfer. (Reproduced with permission from Blackburn & Loper 1992.)*

increased fetal demands also influence the rate of transfer. Transfer across the placental membrane can be modified by maternal nutritional status, exercise and disease. Glucose transfer increases in diabetes mellitus due to maternal hyperglycaemia. Hypertension decreases nutrient transfer because of the reduced placental blood flow and alcoholism impairs placental uptake of glucose and amino acids.

Respiration

The actual transfer of the major respiratory gases such as oxygen and carbon dioxide across the syncytiotrophoblast and fetal capillary epithelium is by simple transfer down a partial pressure concentration gradient. The pattern of transfer is made more complex by the differences in haemoglobin concentration and type. If there is any disorganisation of the blood flows by maternal or fetal disease, respiratory exchange can be compromised.

Oxygen carriage

Most oxygen in the maternal and fetal blood is bound to haemoglobin in the form of oxyhaemoglobin (HbO_2) and there is very little in free solution. A gram of haemoglobin can carry 1.34 ml of oxygen at full saturation. A litre of blood contains about 115 g Hb and can carry about 154 ml of oxygen. One litre of fetal blood contains about 165 g Hb and can carry 221 ml oxygen (Stacey 1991). The interactions between the four subunits of the Hb molecule create a non-linear saturation curve. This is the **oxygen dissociation curve** (see Chapter 16). Because of the different structure, fetal Hb can hold more oxygen per gram than maternal Hb.

Fetal oxygen supply

The membrane separating maternal and fetal blood is permeable to oxygen. Maternal blood arrives in the intervillous spaces of the placenta saturated with oxygen at a high partial pressure. Fetal blood arrives in the placenta on the other side of the membrane with a very low partial pressure and low oxygen content. Oxygen dissociates from the maternal Hb and diffuses readily down the partial pressure gradient from mother to fetus. Maternal blood is not such a good oxygen source as atmospheric air but fetal blood contains more Hb in order to maximise O_2 uptake. The diffusion gradient is enhanced by the increased affinity for oxygen of fetal Hb which combines more readily with oxygen than adult Hb, so that its percentage saturation is greater at the same oxygen tension.

Although the system works in favour of the fetus, oxygen partial pressures in the two circulations never reach equilibrium. One reason for this is that the local consumption of oxygen by the placenta and uterus may utilise 50% of the oxygen extracted from the uterine circulation. Fetal systemic PO_2 is only 25–30 mmHg which is necessary as parts of the vascular tree are extremely sensitive to oxygen. This is a very important mechanism at delivery when a rise in PO_2 due to the onset of respiration leads to closure of the ductus arteriosus and constriction of the umbilical vessels.

Carbon dioxide

Most of the metabolic processes of the fetus are aerobic and depend on a constant oxygen supply. The fetus thus produces carbon dioxide for excretion. The much higher lipid solubility of carbon dioxide over oxygen results in a much more rapid transfer of the gas across cell membranes.

Nutrition

Nutrients pass from maternal to fetal blood through the walls of the villi. The fetus needs amino acids for cell building, glucose for energy, calcium and phosphorus for bones and teeth and iron and other minerals for the formation of blood. Food substances already broken down into simple forms by the mother's digestive system arrive at the placental site via maternal blood. The placenta selects the substances required by the fetus and will even deplete maternal supplies if necessary. Protein is transferred as amino acids, carbohydrate as glucose, fats as fatty acids. Water, electrolytes and water-soluble vitamins cross the placenta (Bennett & Brown 1996).

Carbohydrate transfer

Glucose is a principal substrate for the production of energy which is utilised by the fetoplacental unit for the synthesis of macromolecules not obtained from the mother. The main form of transport for glucose is facilitated diffusion via a carrier protein molecule. Some glucose is stored in the placenta as glycogen and may act as a store for energy for local placental needs. The healthy placenta has a capacity for glucose transfer that far exceeds fetal needs. The transfer is affected by maternal blood glucose levels and by insulin.

Amino acid transfer

Fetal proteins are synthesised from amino acids obtained via the maternal circulation. There is an accumulation of amino acids by the fetus against a concentration gradient and the placenta contains more amino acids than either maternal or fetal circulations (Stacey 1991). There are carrier systems for the transfer of amino acids but the control mechanism is not yet known.

Lipid transfer

The fetus is able to synthesise fatty acids from carbohydrate and short chain organic acids, which helps to compensate for their absence in the diet of strict vegetarians. However, normally it is probable that the fetus obtains and stores fatty acids from the mother by passive transfer. Cholesterol also crosses the placenta.

Vitamin transfer

Although vitamins are often discussed as a group, there is great variation in their molecular structure and therefore in their mechanism of transfer. What unites them is that they cannot be synthesised in the body so that the fetus is dependent on its mother for supply. The lipid-soluble vitamins A, D and E pass from maternal to fetal blood down a concentration gradient to supply the small amounts needed by the fetus. Water-soluble vitamins such as vitamin C appear to be transferred to the fetus against a gradient and cannot be passed back to maternal circulation.

Trace element transfer

Small amounts of these crucial elements are transferred to the fetus. These include iron, zinc and copper.

Water and electrolyte transfer

Water balance is usually achieved by diffusional gradients brought about by hydrostatic pressure and colloid osmotic pressure. Solutes such as sodium, potassium, calcium and phosphate are also freely transferred between maternal and fetal circulations. Research has shown that the fine balance maintained between the maternal and fetal fluid components can be disturbed by the administration to the mother of hypotonic intravenous solutions such as 5% dextrose, especially if it contains the antidiuretic oxytocin. Transfer of water to the fetus will then occur, resulting in fetal hyponatraemia.

Excretion

Besides carbon dioxide discussed above, the placenta must also pass other byproducts of metabolism such as urea, uric acid and bilirubin to the maternal circulation to be excreted.

Protection

The placenta has been considered to be a barrier offering protection against infection. Few bacteria are small enough to penetrate the placental membrane. Two organisms that can cross the barrier to form transplacental infection are those causing syphilis and tuberculosis. Viruses can cross freely. Drugs may also cross to the fetus if they have a small enough molecular structure and some may cause congenital abnormalities, as happened with thalidomide and limb defects. Others may be beneficial, such as the use of antibiotics to treat syphilis. Towards the end of pregnancy there is a transfer by pinocytosis of IgG, conferring passive immunity for the first 3 months of extrauterine life.

PLACENTAL PATHOLOGY

The placenta in pregnancy-induced hypertension (PIH)

PIH is known to be associated with poor invasion of the spiral arteries by the cytotrophoblast. There may be a genetic basis to the problem. There is failure of the second wave of invasion so that the decidual part of the spiral arterioles will be invaded but not the myometrial section. This abnormality leads to:

1 poor perfusion of the intervillous space;
2 the maintenance of sensitivity to pressor agents;
3 hypertension in the uteroplacental arteries;
4 production of thromboxane (TXA) which is a potent vasoconstrictor. It opposes the vasodilatory action of PG_1;
5 a reduction in the production of PG_1;
6 occlusion of villous arterioles;
7 hyperdynamic maternal circulation due to increased cardiac output as early as 11 weeks;
8 severe peripheral vasospasm leading to hypertension;
9 reduced visceral blood flow, including the kidney (Blackburn & Loper 1992).

Other problems

Other pathological conditions affecting the placenta include:

- placental insufficiency;
- abnormal placental separation – abruptio placentae;
- abnormal placental separation in the 3rd stage – retained placenta, morbid adherence of the placenta.
- abnormal location – placenta praevia;

Placental insufficiency is discussed in Chapter 13, abruptio placentae and placenta praevia in Chapter 31 and abnormal placental separation in the 3rd stage of labour in Chapter 40.

Summary of main points

- The placenta is a haemochorial villous organ derived from the embryonic trophoblast cells with the addition of a few mesodermal cells from the inner cell mass. Whilst the embryo proper is developing, the extraembryonic trophoblastic cells are forming the placenta. The initial trophoblastic cells are called collectively the cytotrophoblast. They give rise to a group of cells that have undergone nuclear division without separating into daughter cells, the syncytiotrophoblast, which invades the uterine lining to allow embedding.
- The uterus grows new blood vessels in the area of embedding which swell to form sinusoids. Lacunae appear in the syncytiotrophoblast and become filled with a mixture of blood and secretions from the eroded endometrial glands. The lacunae fuse to form a network which is the beginning of the intervillous spaces. Maternal blood flows through the network in a primitive uteroplacental circulation.
- In pregnancy decidual and myometrial arteries are converted into uteroplacental arteries. They are opened up and functionally denervated so that they are completely dilated and unresponsive to circulatory pressor substances or autonomic neural control. At uterine radial artery level, local prostacyclin maintains vasodilation.
- Mesodermal tissue from the developing embryo joins the trophoblast extensions and forms the narrow connecting stalk. This extraembryonic mesoderm gives rise to the umbilical blood vessels linking the mother to the embryo. The structure will eventually become the umbilical cord.
- By the end of the 2nd week trophoblastic cells have formed the primary chorionic villi which will differentiate into the chorionic villi of the placenta. By the end of the 3rd week fetal blood circulates through the capillaries of the chorionic villi. Cytotrophoblastic cells proliferate and extend through the syncytiotrophoblast to form a cytotrophoblastic shell which attaches the chorionic sac to the endometrium by specialised stem or anchoring villi.

- Until about 20 weeks the placental membrane consists of four layers of tissue which separate the two circulations: syncytiotrophoblast, cytotrophoblast, connective tissue of the mesenchymous core and the endothelium of the fetal capillary. As pregnancy advances this placental membrane becomes thinner.
- The entire surface of the chorionic sac is covered by chorionic villi until the 8th week. The chorionic villi of the decidua capsularis become compressed and degenerate, leaving a bare area called the chorion laeve which becomes the chorionic membrane. The chorionic villi of the decidua basalis branch and enlarge to form the chorion frondosum, the fetal part of the placenta.
- The mature placenta is a flattened discoid organ about 20 cm in diameter. It is about 2.5 cm thick at the centre and thins out towards its circumference where it is continuous with the chorion. There are two distinct surfaces, one attached to the maternal decidua called the maternal surface and one covered with amnion with the umbilical cord inserting into it called the fetal surface.
- A double membrane forms the sac containing the fetus. The outer membrane or chorion is closely adherent to the decidua and is thick, opaque and friable. The inner membrane or amnion is a tough, smooth, translucent membrane derived from the inner cell mass. These membranes are active biologically, producing enzymes and hormones.
- The umbilical cord or funis is usually attached to the centre of the fetal surface of the placenta. It usually contains two arteries and one vein surrounded by a mucoid connective tissue called Wharton's jelly. There is an outer covering of amnion. The umbilical vein is longer than the arteries and the vessels are longer than the cord so loops of vessel (false knots) may be seen inside the Wharton's jelly. Occasionally a true knot may be present and the blood vessels may become occluded, causing fetal distress.
- The placental villi form an enormous surface area for the exchange of materials between maternal and fetal circulations. Maternal blood is propelled towards the chorionic plate. It flows slowly over the surface of the villi to allow materials to be exchanged and eventually reaches the floor of the intervillous space to drain into the endometrial veins.
- Fetal deoxygenated blood leaves the fetus and passes into the two umbilical arteries which take it to the placenta. Here the blood vessels form an extensive arteriocapillary venous system within the chorionic villi where fetal blood is brought very close to maternal blood. Oxygenated fetal blood then converges in thin walled veins to enter the umbilical vein which return it to the fetus.
- The placenta produces protein hormones and steroid hormones. Protein hormones include HCG, HPL, SP_1, PAPP-A and PAPP-B. The steroid hormones are mainly oestrogens and progesterone.
- The fetoplacental unit produces hormones which alter maternal metabolic processes to benefit the fetus. The steroid hormones are made by sending a series of molecules backwards and forwards between the fetus and placenta until the final hormone structure is reached. Oestrogens and progesterone are found in higher concentrations in fetal blood than in maternal blood.
- The protein hormones of the placenta are analogous to the pituitary hormones. For instance, HCG has a similar structure to luteinising hormone (LH) and HPL is similar to prolactin and growth hormone. In the same way, insulin and relaxin share a similar structure.
- In early pregnancy there is a rapid increase in HCG production. The urinary excretion rate doubles every 36–48 h. The curve then flattens out at about 9 weeks and declines. This lower level is maintained until just before term when there is another rise. The ovary contains receptors for HCG and is its prime target. Its role is probably to stimulate extra production of oestrogen and progesterone necessary for the maintenance of pregnancy.
- Human placental lactogen, similar to pituitary growth hormone, is produced by the syncytiotrophoblast. Maternal blood HPL level rises until 36 weeks when there is a fall until delivery and HPL is probably a growth promoter in pregnancy. It causes the mobilisation of free fatty acids and antagonises the action of insulin, resulting in a higher need for the mother to manufacture insulin in pregnancy. This is the reason why HPL is called diabetogenic.
- SP_1 is present in large amounts and can be detected in early pregnancy and easily measured in late pregnancy. There is a steady rise until 36 weeks followed by a steady decline until delivery. This hormone may be important in the immunosuppressive mechanism preventing rejection of the placenta and fetus.
- PAPP-A is detectable in maternal plasma early in pregnancy and its concentration rises as pregnancy progresses. There is no dip at 36 weeks and the values continue to rise up to the onset of labour. It probably helps to prevent rejection of the fetoplacental unit by the cellular lymphocyte component of the maternal immune system. PAPP-B rises throughout pregnancy with the steepest part of its curve occurring after 30 weeks. It has been used to ascertain the progress of the placenta in such diseases as preeclampsia and diabetes mellitus.
- The three important oestrogens are oestrone, oestradiol and oestriol. The fetal liver and adrenal glands are important to the production of oestriol. Plasma oestriol levels rise steeply from about 34 to 36 weeks but this may not occur if pregnancy pathology affects the fetus.
- Progesterone is produced by the syncytiotrophoblast. Some is sent to the maternal circulation and some to the fetus. Progesterone is broken down into the inactive substance pregnanediol and excreted via urine. There is a sharp rise in progesterone production from the 10th week onwards. Much progesterone is stored in body fat and may act as a buffer against transient low production. Therefore measuring plasma progesterone assay is neither easy nor relevant.
- Ovarian progesterone is involved in the development of the endometrium in the second part of the menstrual cycle and in the decidual reaction. Progesterone relaxes all smooth muscle during pregnancy and is responsible for many of the minor disorders of pregnancy.
- The role of progesterone in initiating the onset of labour is not clearcut. If a fall in progesterone influences the onset of labour, it can only be a part of the complex physiological process of parturition.
- The fetus is dependent on sufficient placental transfer of nutrients and oxygen to allow it to grow at the necessary fast rate. Transport across the placenta increases during the course of gestation as the placenta increases in size and becomes modified in structure. Transfer across the placental membrane can be modified by maternal nutritional status, exercise and disease.
- The transfer of the major respiratory gases such as oxygen and carbon dioxide across the syncytiotrophoblast and fetal capillary epithelium is by simple transfer down a partial pressure concentration gradient. The much higher lipid solubility of carbon dioxide over oxygen results in a much more rapid transfer of the gas across cell membranes.
- Nutrients pass from maternal to fetal blood through the walls of the villi. This process is not only by simple diffusion. The fetus needs amino acids for cell building, glucose for energy. Trace elements and vitamins are also transferred to the fetus.
- Water balance is usually achieved by diffusional gradients brought about by hydrostatic pressure and colloid osmotic pressure. Solutes such as sodium, potassium, calcium and phosphate are also freely transferred between maternal and fetal circulations.
- Besides carbon dioxide, the placenta must also pass other byproducts of metabolism such as urea, uric acid and bilirubin to the maternal circulation to be excreted.
- Few bacteria are small enough to penetrate the placental membrane but those causing syphilis and tuberculosis are able to and cause intrauterine transplacental infection. Viruses such as rubella cross freely. Drugs may cross to the fetus if their molecular structure is small. Some may cause congenital abnormalities. Others such as antibiotics may be beneficial.

- PIH is known to be associated with poor invasion of the spiral arteries by the cytotrophoblast. There may be a genetic basis to the problem. There is failure of the second wave of invasion so that the decidual part of the spiral arterioles will be invaded but not the myometrial decidual section.
- Other pathological conditions affecting the placenta include placental insufficiency, abnormal placental separation and abnormal location, such as placenta praevia.

References

Anderson M. 1992 The Anatomy and Physiology of Obstetrics. Wolfe Publishing, London.

Bennett VR, Brown LK. 1996 The placenta. In Bennett VR, Brown LK (eds) Myles Textbook for Midwives. Churchill Livingstone, Edinburgh, pp 43–50.

Blackburn ST, Loper DL. 1992 Maternal, Fetal and Neonatal Physiology – A Clinical Perspective. WB Saunders, Philadelphia.

Fitzgerald MJT, Fitzgerald M. 1994 Human Embryology. Baillière Tindall, London.

Germain AM, Smith J, Casey ML et al. 1994 Human fetal membrane contribution to the prevention of parturition: uterotonin degradation. Journal of Clinical Endocrinology and Metabolism 78(2), 463–470.

Gilbert SF. 1988 Developmental Biology 2nd edn. Sinauer Associates, Massachusetts.

Klopper A. 1991 Placental metabolism. In Hytten F, Chamberlain G (eds) Clinical Physiology in Obstetrics. Blackwell Scientific, Oxford.

McNabb M. 1997 Implantation and development of the placenta. In Sweet BR with Tiran D (eds) Mayes Midwifery, 12th edn. Baillière Tindall, London, pp 81–88.

Moore KL. 1989 Before We Are Born, 3rd edn. WB Saunders, Philadelphia

Stacey TE. 1991 Placental transfer. In Hytten F, Chamberlain G (eds) Clinical Physiology in Obstetrics, 2nd edn. Blackwell Scientific, Oxford. pp 415–437.

Sweet B 1994 Mayes' Midwifery. Baillière Tindall, London.

Recommended reading

Barnea ER, Hustin J, Jauniaux E. (eds) 1992 The First 12 Weeks of Gestation. Springer-Verlag, Berlin.

Redman CWG, Sargent IL, Starkey PM. 1993 The Human Placenta. Blackwell Scientific, Oxford.

Wiley LM, Heyner S. 1990 Early Embryo Development and Paracrine Relationships. Alan R Liss, New York.

Chapter 12

Amniotic fluid

In this chapter

PRODUCTION OF AMNIOTIC FLUID

Amniotic fluid is an alkaline clear, pale, straw-coloured fluid consisting of about 98% water with organic and inorganic substances in solution (Anderson 1992). The exact source of amniotic fluid is not yet known but it appears as droplets early in pregnancy at about 3 weeks postfertilisation. Between 4 and 8 weeks of gestation the production of amniotic fluid increases until there is about 20 ml. This pushes out the amnion until it reaches and lines the chorion (McNabb 1997). Much greater increases in amniotic fluid now occur with the volume being about 400 ml at 20 weeks, reaching a maximum of 800 ml at 36 weeks and declining slightly until term.

The amniotic membrane is composed of a single layer of cuboid epithelial cells on a loose connective tissue membrane. It is not fused to the chorion and up to 200 ml of amniotic fluid can be stored in the intermembrane space (Blackburn & Loper 1992). The cells of the amniotic membrane are separated by intracellular channels that lead directly to the amniotic cavity. Water and solutes can be transferred across the amnion and chorion by hydraulic, osmotic and electrochemical forces (Blackburn & Loper 1992). However, although some of the water in amniotic fluid, along with solutes, is due to a transmembrane pathway from maternal blood to placenta and membranes and into the amniotic cavity, the pathway does not account for a significant amount of the fluid. Fitzgerald & Fitzgerald (1994) include diffusion from the surrounding decidua as a source.

Amniotic fluid is in a constant state of circulation and renewal. The fetal gastrointestinal tract is a major pathway for its removal. It is swallowed by the fetus and absorbed into the fetal bloodstream. Some diffuses across the placental membrane into the intervillous space and some is excreted by the fetus into the amniotic sac. In the second half of pregnancy the fetal kidneys and fetal lungs are chief sources of amniotic fluid, contributing 700 and 350 ml/day respectively.

CONTENT OF AMNIOTIC FLUID

During the first half of pregnancy the fetal skin does not act as a barrier to fluid and the skin is a site for transfer of water and solutes. Hytten (1991) refers to a paper by Lind et al (1972) suggesting that amniotic fluid in early pregnancy can be seen as an extension to the fetal extracellular fluid. The composition of amniotic fluid in early pregnancy is similar to maternal and fetal plasma with little particulate matter and its volume is closely related to fetal weight.

As the fetal skin keratinises after 17 weeks of pregnancy, the continuity between the fetal amniotic fluid and extracellular fluid is lost and the pattern of content and flow changes. Diffusible solutes such as sodium and urea can no longer be equilibrated with fetal or maternal plasma (Hytten 1991). In the latter half of pregnancy osmolality decreases to about 90% of maternal plasma and the composition then resembles that of dilute urine (Blackburn & Loper 1992, Fitzgerald & Fitzgerald 1994).

Mature amniotic fluid contains electrolytes, proteins and protein derivatives such as urea and creatinine, carbohydrates, lipids, hormones, enzymes, desquamated fetal cells, vernix and lanugo. Sodium and chloride content decreases and urea, uric acid and creatinine increases as fetal kidney function matures. Increasing amounts of phospholipids from the lungs appear as the fetal lung matures.

Moore (1989) relates abnormalities of the fetus to abnormalities of amniotic fluid quantity. In fetal conditions where there is obstruction to the flow of urine, such as renal agenesis or urethral obstruction, the volume of amniotic fluid is very low (**oligohydramnios**). If the fetus cannot swallow in conditions such as oesophageal atresia or anencephaly, there is an excess of amniotic fluid (**polyhydramnios**). The clinical implications of these two conditions will be discussed later in this chapter.

REGULATION OF QUANTITY OF AMNIOTIC FLUID

McNabb quotes evidence suggesting that decidual prolactin (Handwerger et al 1992, Kletsky 1992) and prostaglandins (PGE_2) from the amnion and umbilical cord (Demir et al 1991, Gilbert 1991, Kelly 1994) may be active in the regulation of amniotic fluid volume. Concentrations of prolactin in amniotic fluid are up to ten times those of maternal circulation, increasing sharply in the 2nd trimester and declining to a lower plateau by 34 weeks. Prolactin may regulate the volume of amniotic fluid by controlling electrolyte exchange across the chorioamniotic membrane. PGE_2 may regulate amniotic fluid by removing it into the maternal circulation to counterbalance the large volume of fetal urine output in the second half of pregnancy.

FUNCTIONS OF AMNIOTIC FLUID

Amniotic fluid provides the following (Bennett & Brown 1996):

- space for fetal growth and movement;
- an equal pressure on the fetus to protect it from injury;
- a constant temperature for the fetus;
- small amounts of nutrients;
- prevention of placental and cord compression during labour;
- an aid to cervical effacement and dilatation.

POLYHYDRAMNIOS

Arias (1993) comments that one of the commonest anomalies found on ultrasound examination is polyhydramnios, affecting up to 1.5% of all pregnancies. Queenan (1996) defines polyhydramnios as 'a pathological accumulation of amniotic fluid volumes greater than 2000 ml … clinically detectable in the third trimester of pregnancy (which) may or may not be associated with other problems'. Polyhydramnios may be divided into chronic and acute causes (Rankin 1996). Chronic polyhydramnios is more common and is gradual in onset from about the 30th week of pregnancy. Acute polyhydramnios is rare, occurs at about 20 weeks and comes on rapidly over about 4 days. It is most often associated with monovular twins and occasionally with severe fetal abnormality. The pregnancy is usually lost.

Diagnosis

The condition is often diagnosed by ultrasound and should always be confirmed by ultrasound but can be suspected clinically if:

- the uterus is larger than expected for gestational age;
- there is easy ballottement of the fetus;
- fetal parts are difficult to find;
- the fetal heart is muffled;
- maternal symptoms include breathlessness, vulval varicosities, oedema and gastric problems.

Causes

The amount of amniotic fluid present depends on fetal and maternal factors. A disturbance in fetomaternal equilibrium may produce an increase in amniotic fluid volume (Arias 1993). In 65% of cases of polyhydramnios the cause is unknown (idiopathic). Fetal causes are associated with 18%, maternal causes with 15% and placental causes with less than 1% of polyhydramnios cases. These are shown in Box 12.1.

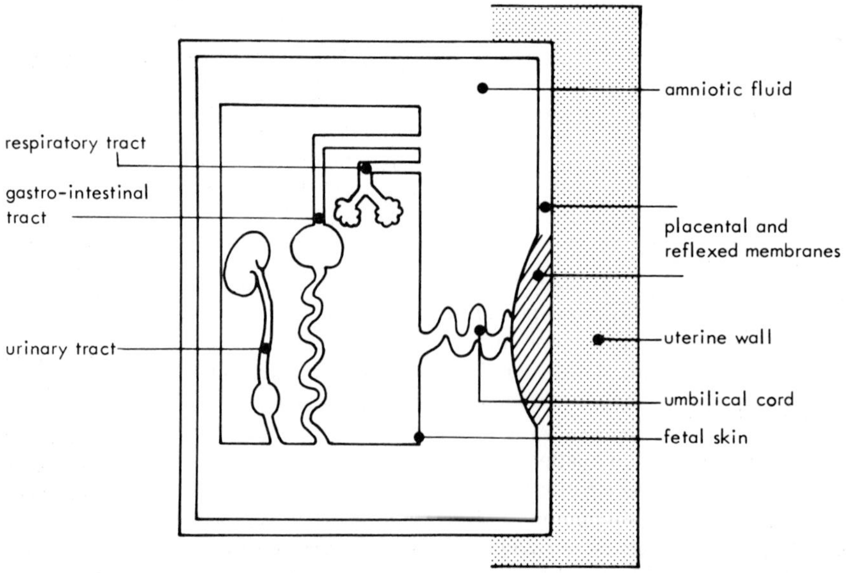

Figure 12.1 *Pathways of amniotic fluid production and exchange. (Reproduced with permission from Wallenburg 1977.)*

Box 12.1 The causes of polyhydramnios

Fetal causes – number of fetuses	Multiple pregnancy
Fetal causes – anomalies	Central nervous system anomalies – anencephaly, hydrocephaly, spina bifida Gastrointestinal anomalies – oesophageal atresia, small bowel atresias, diaphragmatic hernia Cardiac anomalies Haematological abnormalities – α-thalassaemia, fetomaternal haemorrhage Fetal tumours Skeletal malformations – achondroplasia, osteogenesis imperfecta Chromosomal/genetic abnormalities Intrauterine infections – rubella, syphilis, toxoplasmosis
Maternal causes	Diabetes mellitus Rhesus isoimmunisation
Placental causes	Placental chorioangioma Circumvallate placenta syndrome
Idiopathic causes	

Complications

An increase in maternal and fetal mortality is associated with polyhydramnios. Maternal complications include pregnancy-induced hypertension and respiratory discomfort. Fetal mortality is associated with conditions incompatible with life and morbidity with minor abnormalities and preterm birth. Obstetric complications include unstable lie and malpresentation, cord presentation and prolapse, preterm labour, premature rupture of membranes (PROM), placental abruption and postpartum haemorrhage.

Management

Diagnostic tests include:

- ultrasound examination to detect fetal and placental abnormalities and to confirm gestational age;
- studies of fetal karyotype to rule out chromosomal or genetic abnormalities (Barnhard et al 1995);
- fetal swallowing studies;
- TORCH screening for intrauterine infection;
- maternal antibody screening and diabetic screening.

Maternal comfort will be improved if the mother rests in bed in an upright position to relieve dyspnoea. She may require antacids to relieve heartburn and nausea. Amniotic fluid decompression (no more than 500 ml at a time) is carried out as often as necessary to conserve the pregnancy. This will relieve maternal discomfort and reduce intrauterine pressure and the incidence of preterm labour. Risks include infection and provoked onset of labour.

The drug indomethacin has been successful in reducing the amount of amniotic fluid and in preventing preterm labour. Indomethacin is an inhibitor of prostaglandin production and its success demonstrates the involvement of PGE_2 in the regulation of amniotic fluid volume. It may act by reducing fetal urine production or increasing fluid uptake by the lungs (Arias 1993).

Maternal and fetal complications have been noted and more research is necessary (Carmona et al 1993). Maternal complications are nausea, vomiting, diarrhoea, dizziness and headaches. Fetal complications are premature closure of the ductus arteriosus, right-sided heart failure and fetal death. Major et al (1994) suggest that fetal exposure to indomethacin may result in necrotising enterocolitis in low birth weight babies. Arias (1993) suggests the following guidelines for its use:

- a daily dose of 2.2 mg/kg/day administered in divided doses orally every 6 h;
- suspension of treatment at 32 weeks of gestation to avoid fetal haemodynamic complications;
- periodic fetal ultrasound surveillance to avoid constriction of the ductus arteriosus.

Kramer et al (1994) agreed that treatment with indomethacin is associated with serious fetal side effects and a strict therapeutic regime should be adhered to.

OLIGOHYDRAMNIOS

Oligohydramnios is an abnormally small amount of amniotic fluid. This may be less than 500 ml at term but in some cases much less than this is present (Rankin 1996). Oligohydramnios may affect 4% of pregnancies.

Diagnosis

The condition may be suspected on abdominal examination if the following findings are present.

Box 12.2 The causes of oligohydramnios

Postterm pregnancy	
Intrauterine growth retardation	
Premature rupture of membranes	
Fetal renal anomalies	Renal agenesis (Potter's syndrome) Urethral obstruction Prune belly syndrome Multicystic, dysplastic kidneys
Non-renal fetal anomalies	Triploidy Thanatophoric dwarfism Thyroid gland agenesis Skeletal dysplasia Congenital heart block
Chronic abruptio placentae	
Following medical procedures	Amniocentesis Chorionic villus sampling

- The uterus appears smaller than expected for gestational age.
- The mother may have noticed a reduction in fetal movements.
- The uterus feels compact and fetal parts are easily felt.

Ultrasound examination will confirm the absence of amniotic fluid pockets of normal size. Decreased amniotic fluid is one of the serious signs of severe fetal growth retardation, usually associated with maternal disease such as hypertension or chronic renal disease (Arias 1993).

Complications

Prognosis is poor because of the complications of PROM and fetal congenital anomalies. PROM is associated with cervical incompetence and genital tract infection, especially group B haemolytic streptococcus.

Pulmonary hypoplasia affects 60% of fetuses deprived of amniotic fluid for several weeks. It is generally lethal with small anatomically immature lungs, poor surfactant levels and pulmonary hypertension.

Oligohydramnios is often associated with amnion nodosum. Yellow-grey nodules consisting of desquamated fetal epidermal cells, hair and vernix are found in and on the amnion and on the fetal surface of the placenta. The debris is probably pressed into the amnion because of its close application to the fetus.

Management

Management will depend on the length of gestation, the maturity of the fetus, fetal and maternal health and the relative risks to the fetus of conservative management or delivery. Expectant management may be an option depending on the well-being of the fetus (Arias 1993). The means of delivery will, as always, depend on achieving maximum safety for mother and fetus. Amnioinfusion has been used in labour as a means of preventing fetal distress and reducing the incidence of caesarean section.

The role of amnioinfusion

Amnioinfusion is an invasive procedure where saline solution is infused into the amniotic cavity transabdominally or by a transcervical catheter. It can be performed either antenatally or during labour. It can be carried out to:

- improve ultrasound imaging in oligohydramnios with suspected fetal abnormality;
- facilitate rapid fetal karyotyping;
- replace fluid in conservative management of PROM;
- attempt to prevent the development of fetal lung hypoplasia in pregnancies where there is oligohydramnios;
- decrease cord compression and reduce fetal distress during labour;
- reduce recurrent variable decelerations;
- dilute meconium (Telfer 1997).

Hofmeyr (1997) reviewed the use of amnioinfusion 'to assess the effects on perinatal outcome of prophylactic amnioinfusion for oligohydramnios versus therapeutic amnioinfusion only if heart rate decelerations or heavy meconium staining of the liquor became superimposed'. There was no difference in outcomes between the two groups of women, one who received prophylactic amnioinfusion and one where treatment was related to the onset of signs. He concluded that there was no advantage to be gained by prophylactic amnioinfusion over therapeutic amnioinfusion when signs were present.

DIAGNOSTIC USES OF AMNIOTIC FLUID

Biophysical profile

Biophysical profile is a non-invasive test of fetal well-being using ultrasound imaging. It was first described in 1980. Five variables are measured:

1. fetal heart rate
2. fetal tone
3. somatic movements
4. breathing movements
5. amniotic fluid volume (Telfer 1997).

The variables are scored individually and added together to give a total score. It can be an accurate predictor of fetal danger and imminent death but in a metaanalysis of 2839 pregnancies, Hofmeyr (1997) concluded that in comparison with conventional monitoring, usually cardiotocography, there were no effects, beneficial or deleterious, on pregnancy outcome in high-risk pregnancies.

Amniocentesis

Cellular and biochemical components of amniotic fluid change with gestational age and provide useful indicators of fetal well-being and maturity (Blackburn & Loper 1992). Amniotic fluid can be obtained by amniocentesis to obtain knowledge about the fetus as follows.

- Cells can be used for chromosomal and genetic studies.
- α-fetoprotein can be used to assess the likelihood of neural tube defects or as part of the triple test for Down's syndrome.
- Creatinine levels increase as the fetus matures.
- Bilirubin estimates can monitor fetal red cell haemolysis in rhesus incompatibility.
- The ratio of the phospholipids lecithin and sphingomyelin can indicate fetal lung maturity.
- Enzyme studies of cultured cells can help diagnose more than half of the inborn errors of metabolism.

Although the procedure is considered safe when warranted by fetal risk, there are possible complications:

- spontaneous abortion
- infection
- haematoma
- haemorrhage
- leakage of amniotic fluid
- preterm labour.

Summary of main points

- Amniotic fluid is an alkaline clear, pale, straw-coloured fluid consisting of about 98% water with organic and inorganic substances in solution. Both maternal and fetal tissues are involved in its production. Between 4 and 8 weeks of gestation the production of amniotic fluid increases until there is about 20 ml. The volume is about 400 ml at 20 weeks, reaching a maximum of 800 ml at 36 weeks and declining slightly until term.
- The amniotic membrane is composed of a single layer of cuboid epithelial cells on a loose connective tissue membrane. The cells of the amniotic membrane are separated by intracellular channels that lead directly to the amniotic cavity. Water and solutes can be transferred across the amnion and chorion by hydraulic, osmotic and electrochemical forces.
- Amniotic fluid is in a constant state of circulation and renewal. The fetal gastrointestinal tract is a major pathway for its removal as it is swallowed by the fetus and absorbed into the fetal bloodstream. Some diffuses across the placental membrane into the intervillous space and some is excreted by the fetus into the amniotic sac. In the second half of pregnancy the fetal kidneys and lungs are chief sources of amniotic fluid.
- During the first half of pregnancy the fetal skin does not act as a barrier to fluid and the skin is a site for transfer of water and solutes so that amniotic fluid can be seen as an extension to fetal extracellular fluid. The composition of amniotic fluid in early pregnancy is similar to maternal and fetal plasma. As the fetal skin keratinises after 17 weeks of pregnancy, the continuity between the fetal amniotic fluid and extracellular fluid is lost. Diffusible solutes such as sodium can no longer be equilibrated with fetal or maternal plasma. The composition then resembles that of dilute urine.
- Mature amniotic fluid contains electrolytes, proteins, urea and creatinine, carbohydrates, lipids, hormones, enzymes, desquamated fetal cells, vernix and lanugo. Sodium and chloride content decreases and urea, uric acid and creatinine increase as fetal kidney function matures. Increasing amounts of phospholipids from the lungs appear as the fetal lung matures.
- Decidual prolactin and prostaglandins (PGE_2) from the amnion and umbilical cord may be active in the regulation of amniotic fluid volume. PGE_2 may regulate amniotic fluid by removing it into the maternal circulation to counterbalance the large volume of fetal urine output.
- Functions of amniotic fluid include providing space for fetal growth and movement and an equal pressure on the fetus to protect it from injury. A constant temperature for the fetus is provided, as are small amounts of nutrients. In labour, intact membranes prevent placental and cord compression during labour and act as an aid to cervical effacement and dilatation.
- Polyhydramnios affects up to 1.5% of all pregnancies. It is a pathological accumulation of amniotic fluid volumes greater than 2000 ml and may be divided into chronic and acute causes. Chronic polyhydramnios is more common and is gradual in onset from about the 30th week of pregnancy. Acute polyhydramnios is rare, occurs at about 20 weeks and comes on rapidly over about 4 days. It is most often associated with monovular twins and severe fetal abnormality.
- Causes include multiple pregnancy, fetal anomalies, diabetes mellitus and placental abnormalities but in 65% of cases the cause is unknown. An increase in maternal and fetal mortality is associated with polyhydramnios. Obstetric complications include unstable lie and malpresentation, cord presentation and prolapse, preterm labour, premature rupture of membranes, placental abruption and postpartum haemorrhage.
- Useful diagnostic tests are ultrasound examination to detect fetal and placental abnormalities and confirm gestational age, fetal karyotype to rule out chromosomal or genetic abnormalities, fetal swallowing studies, TORCH screening for intrauterine infection and maternal antibody and diabetic screening.
- Maternal comfort will be improved if the mother rests in bed in an upright position to relieve dyspnoea. She may require antacids to help heartburn and nausea. Amniotic fluid decompression (no more than 500 ml at a time) is carried out as often as necessary to conserve the pregnancy.
- Indomethacin may reduce the amount of amniotic fluid and prevent preterm labour but maternal and fetal complications have been noted and more research is necessary. Suspension of treatment at 32 weeks of gestation is necessary to avoid fetal haemodynamic complications and periodic fetal ultrasound surveillance to avoid constriction of the ductus arteriosus.
- Oligohydramnios is an abnormally small amount of amniotic fluid. This may be less than 500 ml at term but in some cases much less than this is present. The condition may be suspected on abdominal examination if the uterus appears smaller than expected for gestational age, the mother has noticed a reduction in fetal movements, the uterus feels compact and fetal parts are easily felt. Ultrasound examination will confirm the absence of amniotic fluid pockets of normal size.
- Decreased amniotic fluid is a serious sign of severe fetal growth retardation, usually associated with maternal disease such as hypertension or chronic renal disease. Causes of oligohydramnios include postterm pregnancy, intrauterine growth retardation, fetal renal and other anomalies, chronic abruptio placentae and amniocentesis ands chorionic villus sampling.
- Fetal complications include pulmonary hyperplasia which is generally lethal with small anatomically immature lungs, poor surfactant levels and pulmonary hypertension. Oligohydramnios is often associated with amnion nodosum; yellow-grey nodules consisting of desquamated fetal epidermal cells, hair and vernix are found in and on the amnion and on the fetal surface of the placenta.
- Management will depend on the length of gestation, the maturity of the fetus, fetal and maternal health and the relative risks to the fetus of conservative management or delivery. Expectant management may be an option depending on the well-being of the fetus.
- Amnioinfusion has been used in labour as a means of preventing fetal distress and reducing the incidence of caesarean section. Hofmeyr (1997) reviewed the use of amnioinfusion and concluded that there was no advantage to be gained by prophylactic amnioinfusion over therapeutic amnioinfusion when signs were present.
- Biophysical profile is a non-invasive test of fetal well-being using ultrasound imaging. It can be an accurate predictor of fetal danger and imminent death but Hofmeyr (1997) concluded that in comparison with conventional monitoring, usually cardiotocography, there were no effects on pregnancy outcome.
- Cellular and biochemical components of amniotic fluid change with gestational age and provide useful indicators of fetal well-being and maturity. Amniotic fluid can be obtained by amniocentesis to obtain knowledge about the fetus. Although the procedure is considered safe when warranted by fetal risk, there are complications of spontaneous abortion, infection, haematoma, haemorrhage, leakage of amniotic fluid and preterm labour.

References

Anderson M. 1992 The Anatomy and Physiology of Obstetrics. Wolfe Publishing, London.

Arias F. 1993 Practical Guide to High Risk Pregnancy and Delivery, 2nd edn. Mosby Year Book, Chicago.

Barnhard Y, Bar-Hava I, Divon MY. 1995 Is polyhydramnios in an ultrasonographically normal fetus an indication for genetic evaluation? American Journal of Obstetrics and Gynecology 173(5), 1523–1527.

Bennett VR, Brown LK. 1996 The placenta. In Bennett VR, Brown LK (eds) Myles Textbook for Midwives, 12th edn. Churchill Livingstone, Edinburgh, pp 43–50.

Blackburn ST, Loper DL. 1992 Maternal, Fetal and Neonatal Physiology, A Clinical Perspective. WB Saunders, Philadelphia.

Carmona F, Martinez-Roman S, Mortera C et al. 1993 Efficacy and safety of indomethacin therapy for polyhydramnios. European Journal of Obstetrics and Gynaecology and Reproductive Biology 52(3), 175–180.

Demir N, Celiloglu M, Thomassen PAB. 1991 Prolactin and amniotic fluid electrolytes. Acta Obstetrica et Gynaecologica Scandinavica 71, 197–200.

Fitzgerald MJT, Fitzgerald M. 1994 Human Embryology. Baillière Tindall, London.

Gilbert SF. 1991 Developmental Biology. Sinauer, Massachusetts.

Handwerger S, Richards RG, Markoff E. 1992 the physiology of decidual prolactin and other decidual protein hormones. Trends in Endocrinology and Metabolism 3(3), 91–95.

Hofmeyr GJ. 1997 Prophylactic versus therapeutic amnioinfusion for intrapartum oligohydramnios. In Neilson LJP, Crowther CA, Hodnett ED, Hofmeyr GJ, Keirse MJNC (eds) Pregnancy and Childbirth module of the Cochrane Database of Systematic Reviews, The Cochrane Library. Update Software, Oxford.

Hytten F. 1991 Weight gain in pregnancy. In Hytten F, Chamberlain G (eds) Clinical Physiology in Obstetrics. Blackwell Scientific, Oxford.

Kelly RW. 1994 Pregnancy maintenance and parturition: the role of prostaglandin in manipulating the immune and inflammatory response. Endocrine Review 15(5), 684–706.

Kletsky OA. 1992 Maternal and fetal prolactin. Seminars in Reproductive Endocrinology 10(3), 282–286.

Kramer WB, Van den Veyver IB, Kirshon B. 1994 Treatment of polyhydramnios with indomethacin. Clinics in Perinatology 21(3), 615–630.

Lind T, Kendall A, Hytten FE. 1972 The role of the fetus in the formation of amniotic fluid. Journal of Obstetrics and Gynaecology of the British Commonwealth 79, 289.

Major C, Lewis D, Harding J, Porto M, Garite T. 1994 Tocolysis with indomethacin increases the incidence of necrotising enterocolitis in the low birth weight neonate. American Journal of Obstetrics and Gynecology 170(1) 102–106.

McNabb M. 1997 Embryonic and fetal developments. In Sweet BR with Tiran D (eds) Mayes Midwifery, 12th edn. Baillière Tindall, London.

Moore KL. 1989 Before We Are Born, 3rd edn. WB Saunders, Philadelphia.

Queenan JT. 1996 Polyhydramnios. Contemporary Obstetrics and Gynaecology 41(5), 11–16.

Rankin S. 1996 Disorders of the pregnancy. In Bennett VR, Brown LK (eds) Myles Textbook for Midwives. Churchill Livingstone, Edinburgh, pp 320–334.

Telfer FM. 1997 Antenatal investigations of maternal and fetal wellbeing. In Sweet BR with Tiran D (eds) Mayes Midwifery, 12th edn. Baillière Tindall, London, pp 246–267.

Wallenburg H. 1977 The amniotic fluid. I water and electrolyte homeostasis. Journal of Perinatal Medicine 5, 193.

Recommended reading

Barnhard Y, Bar-Hava I, Divon MY. 1995 Is polyhydramnios in an ultrasonographically normal fetus an indication for genetic evaluation? American Journal of Obstetrics and Gynecology 173(5), 1523–1527.

Hofmeyr GJ. 1997 Prophylactic versus therapeutic amnioinfusion for intrapartum oligohydramnios. In Neilson LJP, Crowther CA, Hodnett ED, Hofmeyr GJ, Keirse MJNC (eds) Pregnancy and Childbirth module of the Cochrane Database of Systematic Reviews, The Cochrane Library. Update Software, Oxford.

Hytten F. 1991 Weight gain in pregnancy. In Hytten F, Chamberlain G (eds) Clinical Physiology in Obstetrics. Blackwell Scientific, Oxford.

Kramer WB, Van den Veyver IB, Kirshon B. 1994 Treatment of polyhydramnios with indomethacin. Clinics in Perinatology 21(3), 615–630.

Queenan JT. 1996 Polyhydramnios. Contemporary Obstetrics and Gynaecology 41(5), 11–16.

Chapter

13 Fetal growth and development

In this chapter

INTRODUCTION

The general organising principles of embryology were presented in Chapter 8, the development of systems has been discussed in Chapters 9 and 10 and the structure and function of the placenta in Chapter 11. During the development of the zygote into a recognisable human form, the baby is referred to as an embryo. From the beginning of the 9th week of intrauterine life most of the organs are in place even though they may be non-functional. The fetal period is primarily concerned with an increase in size and maturation of the systems begins at week 9 and continues until term. This chapter will outline events in the fetal period and multiple pregnancy will be discussed.

THE FETAL PERIOD

Care must be taken to avoid the confusion caused by the alternative methods of calculating fetal age. Fetal age has traditionally been calculated from the first day of the last menstrual period (LMP) as given by the woman. Increasingly, following the use of ultrasound scanning, it has become more common to calculate the age of the fetus using the estimated day of fertilisation of the ovum. The date of birth is about 266 days or 38 weeks after fertilisation and about 280 days or 40 weeks from the first day of the LMP. Tanner (1978) stated that it is usual to use postfertilisation age when describing organ differentiation and development and this method will be used throughout this chapter.

Moore (1989) reminds us that from the 9th week following ovulation to the 38th week of intrauterine life, 'Development is concerned with the growth and differentiation of tissues and organs that appeared in the embryonic period'. Growth in the first 8 weeks, whilst the organs are forming, is quite slow. There is a remarkable rate of growth of the body, especially during weeks 9–16, but the maximum growth rate occurs between 16 and 24 weeks. Growth then slows a little and remains constant until just before term when it slows again. The increase in size and maturation of the systems is directly linked to the ability of the fetus to survive outside the uterus, a concept known as **viability**.

MATERNAL CONTROL OF FETAL SIZE

Tanner (1978) stated that 'There is considerable evidence that, beginning at 34 to 36 weeks, the growth of the fetus slows down owing to the influence of the uterus, whose available space is by then becoming fully occupied'. He also made the following points. Firstly, twins begin to slow in growth earlier when their combined weight is that of a 36-week fetus. Secondly, this slowing down mechanism allows safe delivery of a genetically large child growing in the uterus of a small mother.

A genetic explanation

Haig (1993) suggests a genetic mechanism for control of fetal size. He hypothesises that how big a baby grows is determined by a conflict between maternal and paternal genes. There is a gene present on chromosome 11 called insulin-like growth factor 2 (IGF2) which is responsible for the regulation of fetal size. The gene on the father's chromosome 11 makes a growth factor which helps the fetus to grow whilst the mother's gene is programmed to be non-functional and to inhibit the effect of the father's gene.

Evidence for this is seen in the genetic condition Beckwith-Wiedemann syndrome where babies are born very large and with enlargement of various tissues in the body. The gene for this syndrome has been found on C11 and, in affected tissues, two paternal genes were found to be present instead of one from each parent. This would cause production of double the amount of the protein product enhancing fetal growth. Evidence for this type of control is seen in the size of foals from horse crosses and calves in cattle crosses. There is also a gene for IGF2 found on C7 of mice where two paternal copies increase the size of the mice pups at birth.

Other explanations

Other possible causes of the slowing of growth in the last few weeks of gestation include compression of uterine blood vessels by the growing fetus, resulting in a reduced maternal blood supply. Differential growth between the placenta and fetus has been suggested by Tanner (1978). From about 30 weeks the growth rate of the placenta falls behind that of the fetus so that the placenta: fetus ratio falls. The placenta may not be able to increase its capacity to sustain the earlier growth rate.

KEY EVENTS IN THE FETAL STAGE OF DEVELOPMENT

The following details of developmental stages are adapted from Moore (1989). Note that there is no absolute time when a fetus can be said to be viable. Dimensional variations increase with age making the judgement of gestational age less accurate (Figs 13.1 and 13.2). It is still unlikely that a fetus of less than 22 weeks or weighing less than 500 g could survive.

Nine to twelve weeks

- At the beginning of the 9th week the fetal head measures half the crown–rump length.
- Body growth now accelerates and by 12 weeks the fetal length has more than doubled.
- Also at the beginning of the 9th week, the lower limbs are short.
- By 12 weeks the upper limbs have attained their relative length in comparison to the body of the fetus but the lower limbs are still short.
- The mature form of the external genitalia appear in the 12th week.
- Intestinal coils are still visible in the proximal end of the umbilical cord until the 10th week.
- There is a decrease of red blood cell formation by the liver and onset in the spleen by 12 weeks.
- The formation and excretion of urine begins by the 12th week.
- The beginnings of fetal muscle movements occur.
- The eyelids fuse.

Thirteen to sixteen weeks

- This is a period of very rapid growth.
- By the end of the period the head is smaller in comparison to the trunk and the lower limbs have lengthened to reach their correct proportions.
- By 16 weeks the skeleton can be seen clearly on X-ray films. By 16 weeks the face has become more human with the eyes facing anteriorly rather than laterally.
- The external ears have moved to their positions on the sides of the head.

Seventeen to twenty weeks

- Growth slows down during this period.
- Fetal movements have become strong enough to be felt by the mother.
- The skin becomes covered with vernix caseosa, a mixture of fatty secretion from the fetal sebaceous glands and dead skin cells. Vernix caseosa protects the skin from the effects of the amniotic fluid.

- Fine downy hair called lanugo has developed over the whole body by the 20th week. It may help to hold the vernix on the skin.
- Head and eyebrow hair become visible.
- Some authorities believe that the highly metabolic brown fat is also formed during this period.

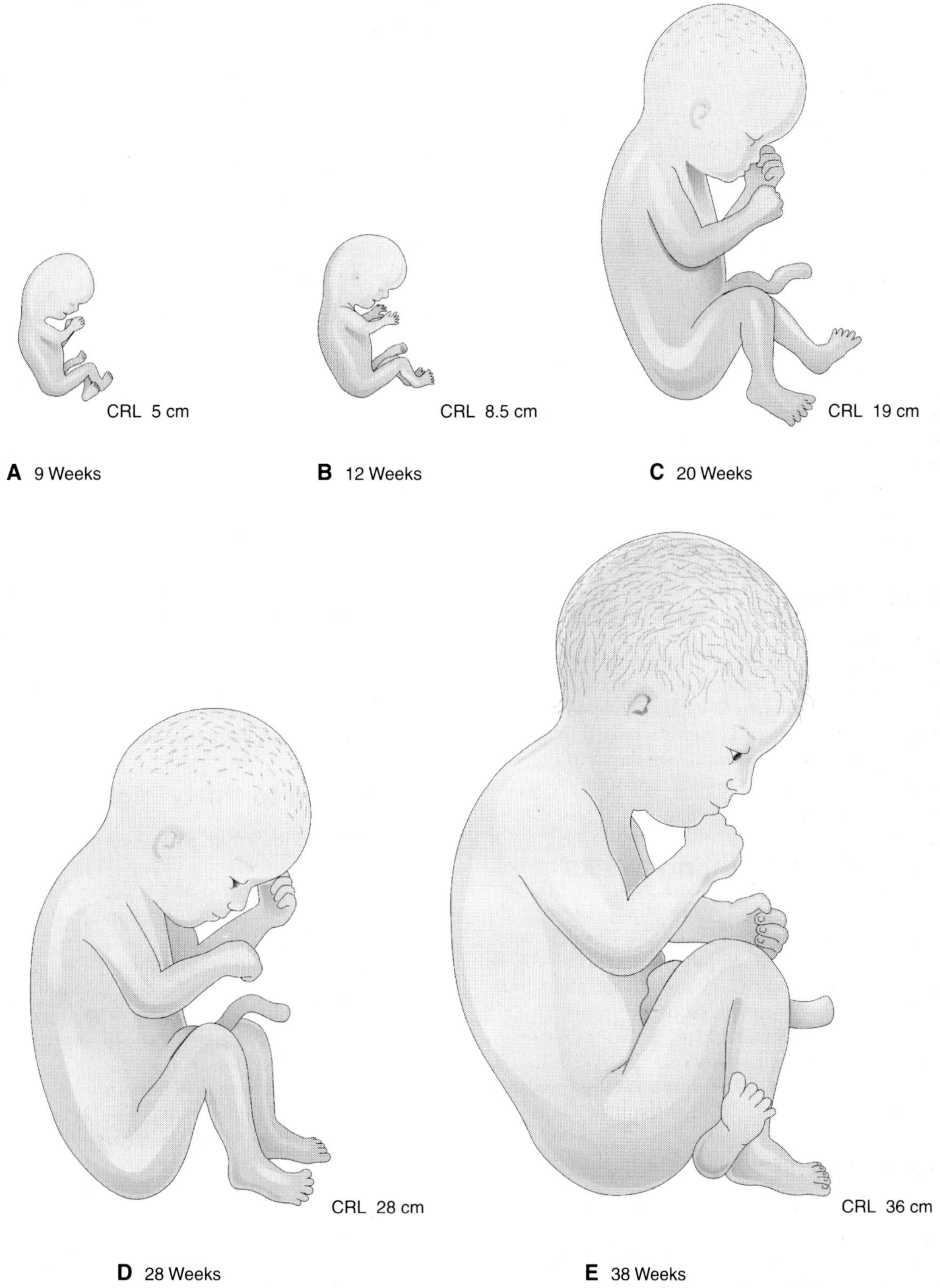

Figure 13.1 *Drawings of fetuses at various stages of development. CRL, crown–rump length. (Reproduced with permission from Moore 1989.)*

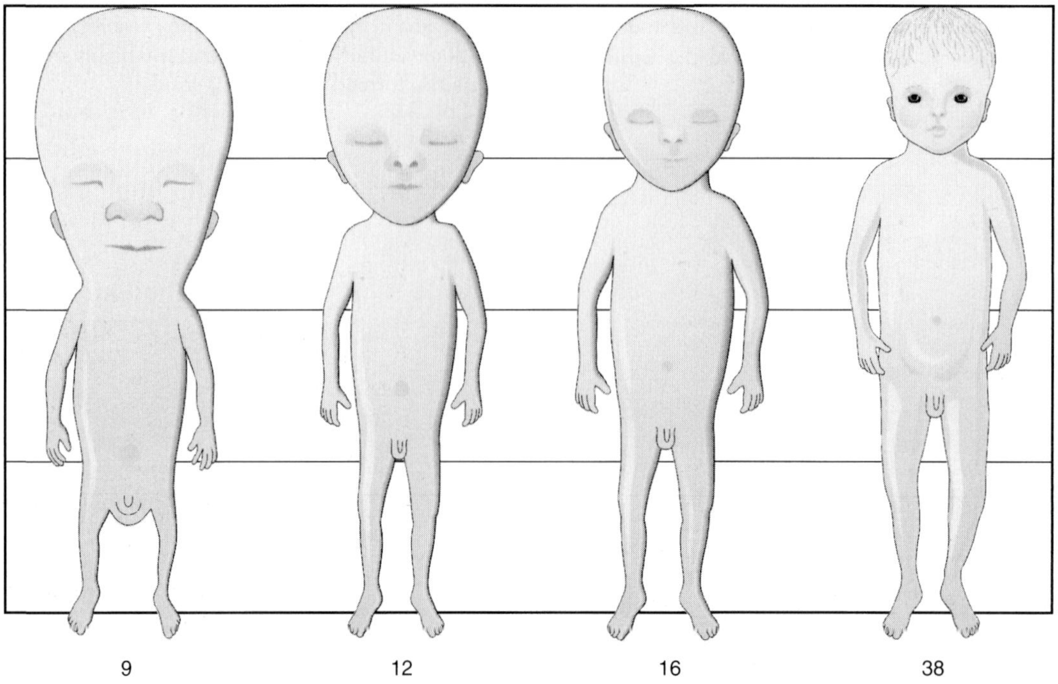

Figure 13.2 *The changing proportions of the body during the fetal period. At 9 weeks the head is about half the crown–rump length of the fetus. By 36 weeks, the circumferences of the head and the abdomen are approximately equal. After this, the circumference of the abdomen may be greater. All stages are drawn to the same total height. (Reproduced with permission from Moore 1989.)*

Twenty-one to twenty-five weeks

- Surfactant production by the alveolar cells in the lungs begins.
- Towards the end of this time there is a chance of survival if the baby is born prematurely.
- The skin lacks subcutaneous fat and is wrinkled. It appears red because of blood capillaries just under the surface.
- The fetus now has periods of sleep and activity and responds to sound.

Twenty-six to twenty-nine weeks

- The lungs are now capable of breathing air and the pulmonary vasculature is sufficient to allow gas exchange. The nervous system has developed to be able to control rhythmic breathing movements and body temperature. Intra-uterine respiratory movements are made.
- The eyes reopen during this time.
- Head and lanugo hair is well developed.
- Until the 26th week most of the increase in fetal weight is due to the accumulation of protein as the main organs and systems of the body are developing. After that period white subcutaneous fat is laid down under the skin (Tanner 1978). The wrinkles are smoothed out.
- At 28 weeks erythropoiesis ends in the spleen and begins in the bone marrow.

Thirty to thirty-four weeks

- The pupillary light reflex is present.
- The quantity of body fat increases to 8% of total body weight and the body begins to appear chubby. The skin is now paler and smooth.
- From 32 weeks most fetuses will survive.
- Lanugo disappears from the face.
- The fetus begins to store iron.

Thirty-five to thirty-eight weeks

- A fetus of 35 weeks will have a firm grasp.
- Most fetuses now become plump.
- At 36 weeks the head and abdominal circumferences are equal but after that the circumference of the abdomen becomes greater.
- Growth slows as term approaches.
- By 38 weeks the body fat content has increased from 30 g at 30 weeks to 430 g. This is about 16% of total weight.
- The skin has become the normal colour depending on the racial background of the parents.
- Breast tissue is present in both sexes.
- The testes are in the scrotum in male infants.
- The nails reach the tips of the fingers.
- Lanugo disappears from the body.

FETAL SIZE

Before birth it is usual to measure the fetus in the form of sitting height or crown–rump length. Table 13.1 is based on postfertilisation age and is derived from Moore (1989).

Table 13.1 *The average size of the fetus related to weeks of gestation*

Age in weeks	*Crown–rump length in mm*	*Weight in grams*
10	61	14
12	87	45
14	120	110
16	140	250
18	160	320
20	190	460
22	210	630
24	230	820
26	250	1000
28	270	1300
30	280	1700
32	300	2100
36	340	2900
38	360	3400

ESTIMATION OF FETAL AGE AND ASSESSMENT OF FETAL GROWTH

Growth curves

A series of measurements can be plotted on a graph and used to calculate growth. Growth can be viewed as a motion through time (Bogin 1988) and if measurements are taken and plotted at regular intervals of time a steady curve called a **distance curve** (Fig. 13.3) is achieved. It is more usual to plot a distance curve when monitoring fetal growth. In order to show how the rate of growth alters over time the speed or velocity of growth is measured and plotted. This will generate a **velocity curve** showing how the rate of growth alters (Fig. 13.4).

Clinical diagnosis

The **medical and obstetric history** of a woman may help to identify a fetus at risk of having poor intrauterine growth. Mothers with certain medical problems, for example, renal disease or hypertension, who are expecting twins or who have a history of a previous small baby should be monitored closely.

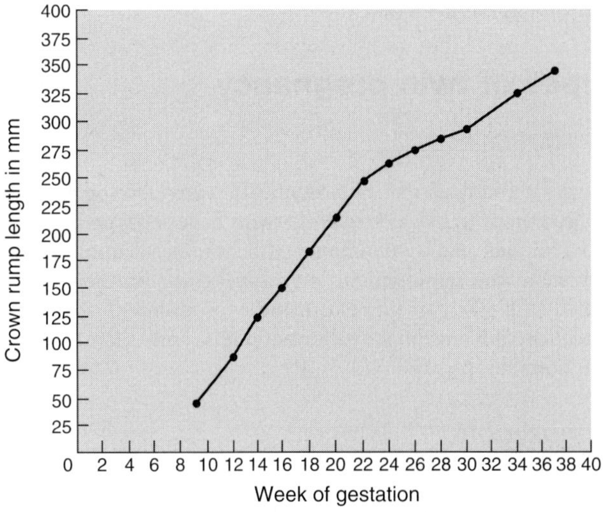

Figure 13.3 *An example of a distance curve using data from fetal crown–rump measurements.*

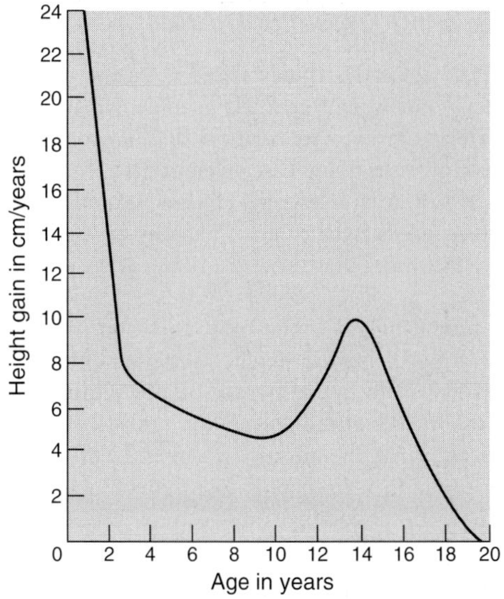

Figure 13.4 *An example of a velocity curve demonstrating the growth of boys from birth to age 18.*

Maternal weight gain has traditionally been used to assess fetal well-being in pregnancy and continued weight gain is thought to be a favourable sign of maternal adaptation and fetal growth and well-being (Thomson 1996). However, weight gain varies widely from a loss to a gain of 23 kg and more (Hytten 1991). Many factors are known to affect maternal weight gain including the presence of oedema, maternal metabolic rate, dietary intake, gastrointestinal problems, smoking and the size of the fetus. Attempts to control maternal weight gain in order to reduce the size of the fetus and make delivery easier have been made but were unsuccessful and had little effect on fetal size. The only components of weight gain available for manipulation are maternal fat and extracellular fluid (Hytten 1990) and Hytten does not believe that either obesity or oedema can be influenced by regular weighing.

An average weight gain appears to be about 12 kg and should be 2 kg in the first 20 weeks and thereafter 0.5 kg until term (Thomson 1996). This can be broken down into its components as shown in Table 13.2.

Table 13.2 *Distribution of maternal weight gain in pregnancy*

Component of weight gain	*Gain in grams*
The fetus	3400
The placenta	600
The amniotic fluid	600
The uterus	900
The breasts	500
Fat stores	3500
Blood volume	1500
Extracellular fluid	1000
Total	12 000

Maternal weight gain and fetal growth

Hytten (1990) reviewed the available literature on weight gain in pregnancy. Poor weight gain has been shown to be associated with intrauterine growth retardation (IUGR) but is not a very sensitive indicator. In many cases weight gain was normal but a baby with IUGR was delivered. Hytten reminds us that daily fluctuations in the weight of a woman can be up to 1% of the total body weight and that there are better ways of assessing the fetus.

Uterine fundal height is the most common method used to assess fetal growth. Fundal height measurements are made in centimetres from the upper border of the symphysis pubis to the top of the fundus of the uterus. Care must be taken to allow for any deviation of the uterus to one side of the abdomen. Error may occur if a woman is too thin or obese or has too much or too little abdominal muscle tone. Breech presentation and trans-verse lie will also result in error. Fundal height can be plotted against a standard curve. Some studies report a 75% correct diagnosis rate using fundal height measurements alone (Belizan et al 1978, Campbell & Dewhurst 1971).

Ultrasound

The gestational age is calculated from the mother's LMP or taken from an early first or second trimester scan. Plotting of later measurements must be charted accurately to avoid wrong diagnosis. The success rate of ultrasound in detecting IUGR may be as high as 95%. Measurements can be taken by ultrasound scan and plotted against a normal curve. Linear and non-linear measurements can be used (Proud 1996).

Linear measurements

Crown–rump length is used to estimate gestational age in the first trimester. The measurement between the two parietal eminences, which is called the **biparietal diameter** (BPD), is a useful estimate of gestation in the second trimester but becomes less accurate later in pregnancy. **Femur length** is also useful in assessing gestational age.

Non-linear measurements

Measurement of the **head circumference** (HC) is preferred in the third trimester when moulding of the head may alter the BPD. **Abdominal circumference** (AC) is measured at the level of the bifurcation of the hepatic vein in the centre of the fetal liver. A reduction in AC suggests a reduction in liver size due to depletion of stores.

Ratios

HC to AC ratio compares the status of the brain to the liver. A raised ratio due to reduced AC suggests IUGR. Femur to AC ratio compares the length of the femur, which is minimally affected by asymmetric IUGR, to the AC. A raised ratio suggests IUGR.

Doppler wave form analysis

Measuring the velocity of blood in the umbilical cord using

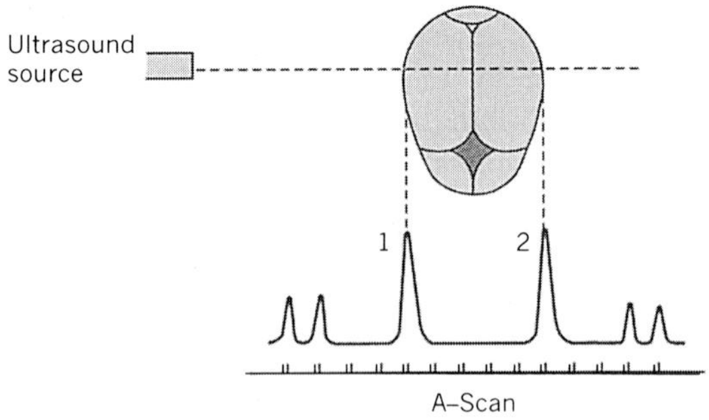

Figure 13.5 *An A-scan sonogram; 1 and 2 indicate the parietal eminences (from Sweet B, 1997, with permission).*

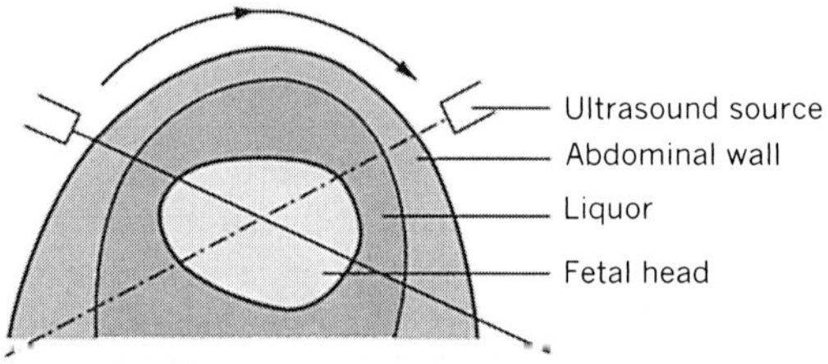

Figure 13.6 *A diagram showing the abdominal wall and the fetal head (from Sweet B, 1997, with permission).*

Doppler ultrasound has been suggested as an additional means of assessing fetal well-being (Almstrom et al 1992). Although ultrasound estimation of fetal weight has been shown to be a better indicator, blood flow measurement may be useful in distinguishing small healthy fetuses from those suffering with IUGR.

MULTIPLE PREGNANCY

Multiple pregnancy (multifetal gestation) is the term used to describe the development of more than one fetus in utero at the same time. Arias (1993) says that there is so much interest and literature on twinning that a new branch of science called **gemellology** has been described.

Types of twin pregnancy

Dizygotic

Dizygotic (binovular or non-identical) twins develop from the fertilisation of two ova. Dizygotic twins have separate placentae, two chorions and two amnions (dichorionic-diamniotic) and only share the same genetic make-up as any brother or sister (Fig. 13.7). They may be the same or different sexes. The incidence of congenital malformation is only slightly greater than normal.

Monozygotic

A rarer form of twinning occurs when a single fertilised ovum divides into two separate fetuses. These are called monozygotic (uniovular or identical) twins. Monovular twins usually share one placenta and chorion and each have their own fetal-derived

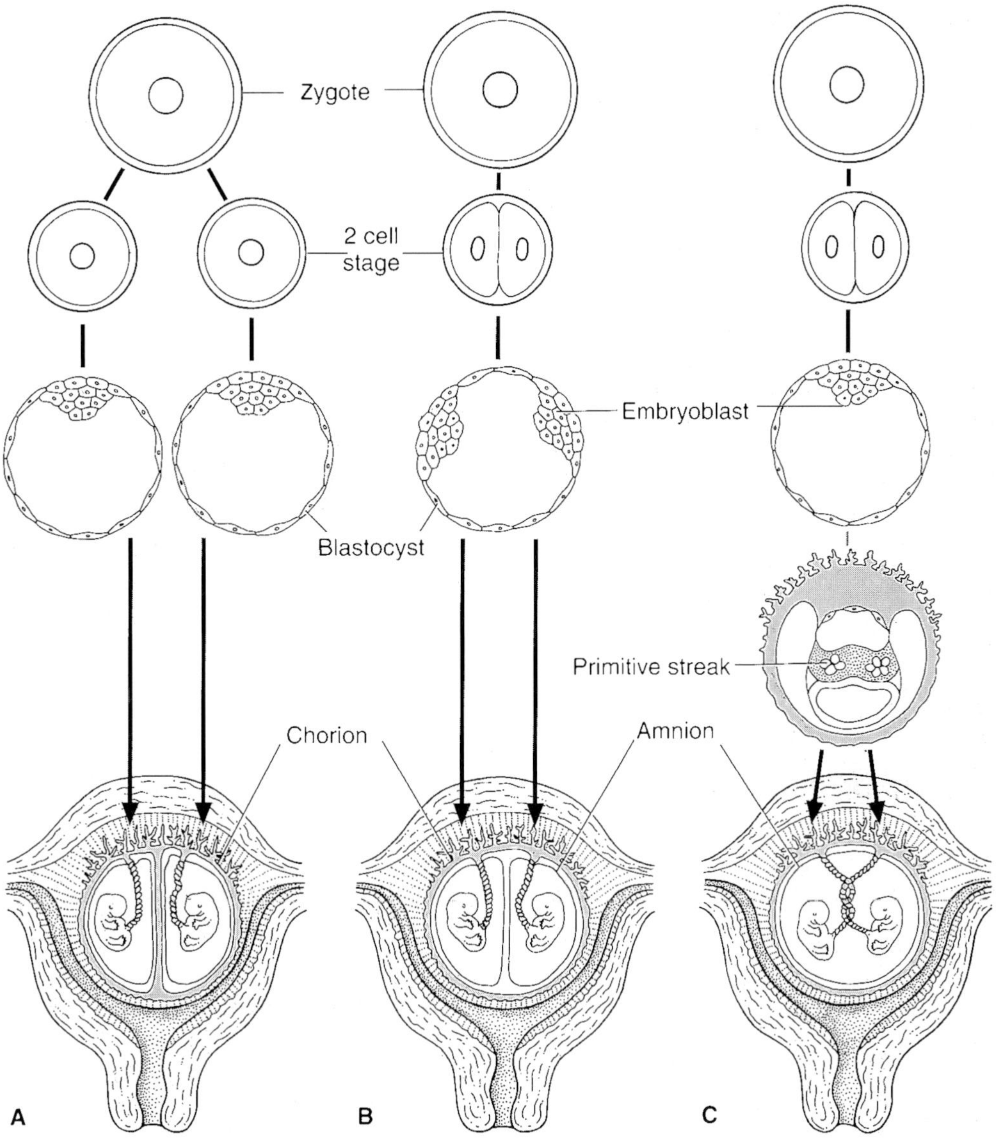

Figure 13.7 *Three kinds of twins. (a) Dichorionic-diamniotic; (b) monochorionic-diamniotic; and (c) monochorionic-monoamniotic (from Fitzgerald MJT, Fitzgerald M, 1994, with permission).*

amnion (monochorionic-diamniotic). Very rarely, the twins will share one amnion (monochorionic-monoamniotic). They are identical in their genetic make-up, having developed from the one fertilised ovum. There is a connection between the two fetal circulations via the placenta and the twins are always of the same sex except in very rare abnormalities of the sex chromosomes (Fig. 13.7). There is a high incidence in errors of development and congenital malformations, which may be linked to the abnormality that caused the twinning. This includes conjoined or Siamese twins.

The incidence of multiple pregnancy

The incidence of multiple pregnancy varies naturally around the world (Arias 1993). In the United Kingdom the incidence of twins is about one in 100 pregnancies. It is higher in black people and lower in Asian people. To support that statement, Arias gives the twinning rate as 57.2 per 1000 in Nigeria, 12.3 per 1000 in Scotland and only three per 1000 in China. Triplets occur in about one in 8000 pregnancies and quadruplets in one in 700 000 pregnancies. The differences in the rates of twinning are the result of variations in dizygotic twinning and the incidence of monozygotic twins is constant at 3.5 per 1000 across all nationalities.

Factors influencing the frequency of dizygotic twinning are:

- maternal age – the incidence increases up to 35 years of age;
- maternal parity;
- conception soon after discontinuing oral contraceptives – if oral contraceptives have been used for more than 6 months and conception occurs within a month of discontinuation, the chance of twins doubles.

The development of ultrasound scanning techniques has shown that the incidence of twin pregnancy in humans may be double the number of eventual twin births. Half may never be recognised as twin pregnancy because of the death of one embryo early in the pregnancy. The embryo may be reabsorbed (vanishing twin) or, rarely, may remain in between the membranes of the second twin as a **fetus papyraceous** (paper fetus).

Grant (1996) reminds us that naturally occurring quintuplets are rare. The introduction of drugs such as clomiphene which stimulate ovulation and are used in the treatment of some infertile couples has led to an increase in pregnancies where 5–8 fetuses are conceived. The outcome of such pregnancies is poor, even with selective termination of most of the fetuses. At the time of writing this chapter, a woman had been in all the popular press and on television because she had conceived eight babies. Furthermore, she had refused selective termination of most of the babies to allow two or three to survive. In the end she lost all eight babies at about 20 weeks into her pregnancy. Arias (1993) gives the incidence of multiple pregnancies following clomiphene as between 6.8% and 17%. If gonadotrophins have been used to stimulate ovulation the rate increases to between 18% and 53%. In the UK assisted pregnancy has led to an increase in the number of multiple births: triplet births have more than doubled since 1989. The implications for maternity and neonatal care where pregnancies carry high risks for mother and babies are a cause for concern (Spillman 1997).

Diagnosis of twin pregnancy

It is apparent that the earlier the diagnosis of twins is made, the more successful the outcome is likely to be. Perinatal losses may be much larger when the diagnosis is made after 28 weeks. Since the development of routine ultrasound scanning, the incidence of undiagnosed twins at delivery has decreased. A family history of twinning or of infertility treatment with ovulation-stimulating drugs should alert the professional carer to the possibility. However, vigilance should be equal in all pregnancies.

Abdominal examination

Inspection

This method is unlikely to diagnose twins before 20 weeks of pregnancy but the uterus may appear larger than expected for the gestational age. It may look large and broad and fetal movements may be very obvious over the whole uterus.

Palpation

The fundal height may be greater than expected for the period of gestation. The presence of two fetal poles in the fundus may help to identify a twin pregnancy. Location of three poles suggests the presence of at least a twin pregnancy. Multiple fetal limbs may also be present. A later clue is the apparent smallness of the fetal head in relation to the size of the uterus. Lateral palpation may find two fetal backs or the presence of fetal limbs on both sides of the uterus.

Auscultation

It is said by some that hearing two fetal hearts simultaneously with a difference of 10 beats per minute is diagnostic of twins. Practically, this is difficult to achieve as the fetal heart of a singleton fetus can be heard over a wide area.

Ultrasound

Ultrasound diagnosis of multiple pregnancy can be made as early as 6 weeks following the last menstrual period with the use of a vaginal probe (Arias 1993). However, it may not be possible to confirm a twin pregnancy until 15 weeks when a clear outline of two heads can be detected (Grant 1996). Placentography should be part of the ultrasound diagnosis to ascertain the number of placentae present. Later in pregnancy, if only one placenta appears to be present, it is possible to identify the number of membranes present. This can be done about 16 weeks into the pregnancy. The sex of the babies can also be identified. Rarely, monoamniotic identical twins will be found.

Complications of pregnancy

Fetal problems

Abortion

Abortion is more commonly associated with multiple pregnancy. This may be due to fetal abnormality in early pregnancy or to overdistension of the uterus in later pregnancy.

Single fetal demise

Single fetal demise may occur. Before 14 weeks this will probably cause no problems for the survivor. A modern dilemma associated with this is the selective termination of several fetuses to ensure two or three survive (see above). Later there may be transfer of thromboplastin released from the tissues of the dead twin which may cause arterial occlusion, brain damage or renal cortical necrosis. A serious problem for the mother may be the onset of disseminated intravascular coagulation (DIC) about 3 weeks after the fetal death. These complications pose a difficulty in management and the surviving twin should be delivered as soon as it is viable.

Fetal abnormality

Congenital malformation is more likely to occur in twin pregnancies. This has been reported to be as high as 17% whilst the incidence is only 2% in singleton pregnancies (Naeye et al 1978). Although the incidence was about the same in monozygotic and dizygotic twins, abnormalities in dizygotic twins tended to be minor whilst those in monozygotic twins were multiple and lethal. The most common abnormalities are cleft lip and palate, central nervous system and cardiac defects (Arias 1993). In monozygotic twins abnormalities also include conjoined twins and fetal acardia.

Monoamniotic twins

It is rare for both babies to share a single amnion. However, when it is present, the perinatal mortality is as high as 50%, mainly because of entanglement of the umbilical cords. Other causes of fetal loss are twin-to-twin transfusion syndrome, congenital abnormalities and preterm birth (Arias 1993). It is possible to diagnose the presence of only one amnion by ultrasound and the babies should be monitored by ultrasound scan every 2 weeks. It is best to deliver the babies by caesarean section to avoid increasing cord entanglement during vaginal birth.

Conjoined twins

The joining of twins by a bridge of tissue affects about one in 200 monozygotic twin pregnancies (Fig. 13.8). This means that one in 900 twin pregnancies and one in 50 000 births are affected. Three out of four pairs of conjoined twins will be female and the cause is unknown. There are two possibilities. First, and considered to be more likely, is incomplete separation of the embryonic cell mass. The second is partial fusion of two separate centres of embryonic growth. It probably happens before the 2nd week following fertilisation.

A diagnosis can be made by ultrasound and suspicion should be raised in the following cases.

- Monoamniotic twins.
- Twins that face each other.
- The heads are at the same level and in the same plane.
- The thoracic cages are in close proximity.
- Both fetal heads are hyperextended.
- There is no change in the fetal positions on a later scan.

Once the diagnosis is confirmed, delivery by caesarean section should be planned. The outcome for conjoined twins is poor:

Table 13.3 *Classification of conjoined twi*

Name	*Percentage of occurrence*	*Desc*
Thoracopagus	40%	Joined at the
Omphalopagus	35%	Joined at the ant abdominal wall
Pygopagus	18%	Joined at the buttocks
Ischiopagus	6%	Joined at the ischium
Craniopagus	2%	Joined at the head

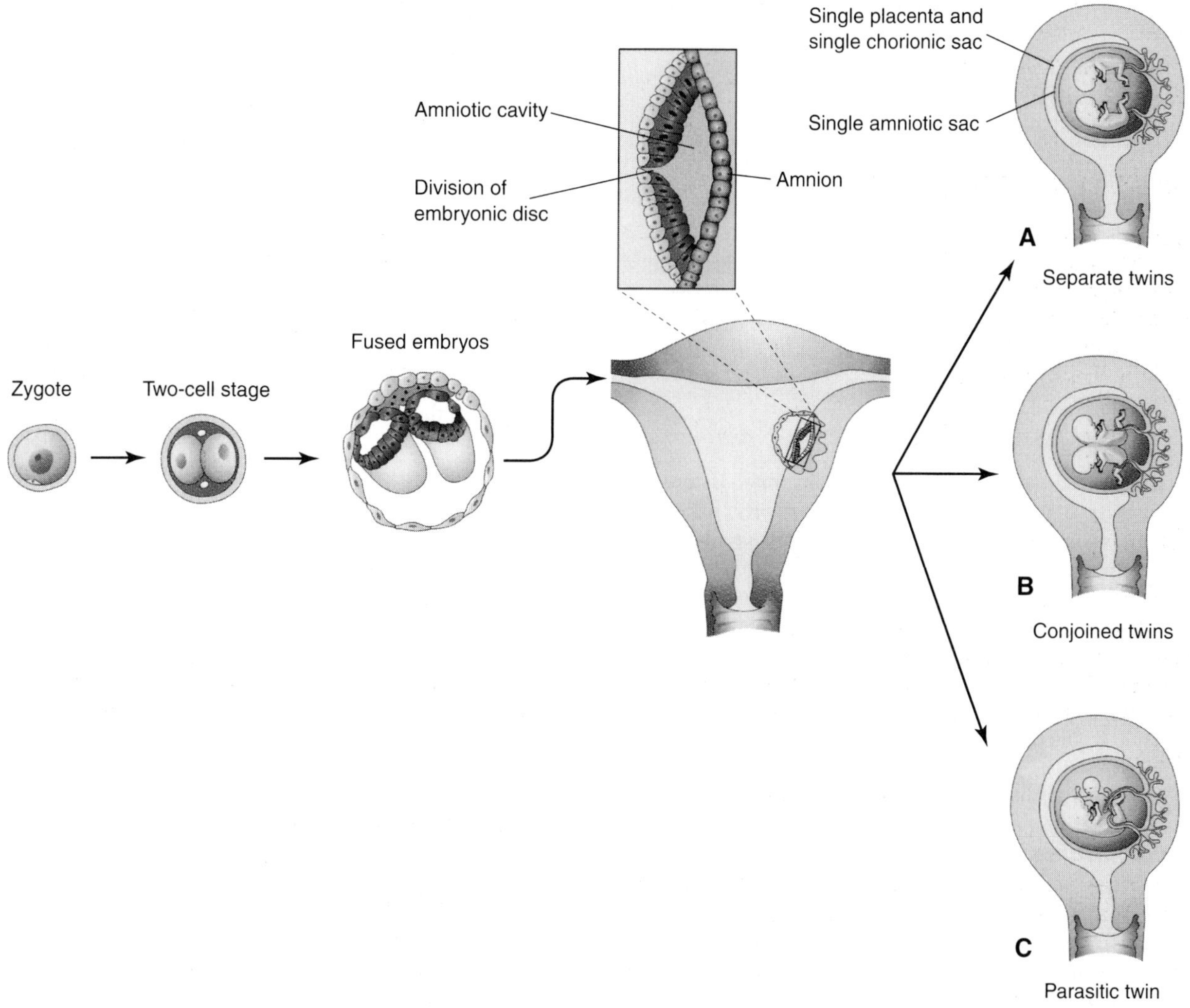

Figure 13.8 *Diagrams showing how some monozygotic (MZ) twins develop. This method of development is very uncommon. Division of the embryonic disc results in two embryos within one amniotic sac. (a) Complete division of the embryonic disc gives rise to twins. Such twins rarely survive because their umbilical cords are often so entangled that interruption of the blood supply to the fetuses occurs. (b, c) Incomplete division of the disc results in various types of conjoined twins. (Reproduced with permission from Moore 1989.)*

vithin 24 h of delivery.
conjoined twins was in
:h independent lives can
d organs may make it

one twin has no heart
oth is maintained by the
overload may lead to heart
ortality rate for the normal

Twin-to-twin transfusion syndrome

This affects between 5% and 17% of monozygotic twins. Vascular communications in the placenta occur between the fetuses with artery-to-vein anastomosis, which causes a circulatory imbalance. This results in anaemia in one twin and polycythaemia in the other.

The criteria for the diagnosis of twin-to-twin transfusion syndrome are:

- a difference in haematocrit of more than 20%;
- a difference in birth weight of more than 20%.

Prenatal diagnosis can be made and the following conditions will be present.

- A single placenta.
- Same-sex twins.
- A thin membrane between the twins showing diamniotic-monochorionic membranes.
- A 20% difference in estimated fetal weight of the twins.
- A discrepancy in the amniotic fluid surrounding the fetuses.
- Fetal hydrops in one or both twins.
- The umbilical cords differ in size.
- Gestational age is less than 28 weeks.

This is a complication with a high mortality rate. Before 26 weeks mortality is 100% while the overall mortality, regardless of gestational age, may be as high as 70%. Attempts to deal with the problem antenatally may reduce the mortality rate to 40%. These include bed rest and preterm delivery, serial amniocentesis or occlusion of the vascular anastomoses by laser coagulation. The recipient of the extra blood may die in utero of cardiomegaly and congestive cardiac failure. This twin also develops hyperbilirubinaemia. The donor twin has retarded growth and, if the anaemia is severe, may develop hydrops fetalis and heart failure. The recipient twin may develop polyhydramnios and the donor twin oligohydramnios.

Polyhydramnios

Polyhydramnios is associated in particular with monozygotic twins and with fetal abnormality. Acute polyhydramnios occurs in midpregnancy and usually leads to abortion. The author remembers one unusual evening when she was recently qualified as a midwife. Two women, both with monozygotic twins, both with acute polyhydramnios, were being cared for in the same room. Both women began to have strong contractions and both delivered identical twin boys within half an hour of each other. All four boys were under 300 g and all died.

Intrauterine growth retardation

Most twins show discordant growth, with one twin being larger than the other. The smaller twin is more at risk of perinatal complications. Discordant growth occurs because one twin obtains less nourishment from the maternal circulation. This is a feature of placental mass and occurs more commonly in dizygotic twins. Genetic conditions and twin-to-twin transfusion syndrome may also result in discordant growth. If preterm delivery of the twins is anticipated to safeguard the smaller twin, weekly injections of betamethasone may be given to the mother to hasten fetal lung maturity.

Maternal problems

Detailed accounts of the diagnosis and management of the following maternal problems are given in other chapters. The aim in this chapter is to provide a reference to alert practitioners caring for women with multiple pregnancy to the possible problems.

Exacerbation of minor disorders

The presence of more than one fetus in utero means a higher level of pregnancy hormones and more pressure from the growing uterus. This will tend to cause an exacerbation of all minor disorders of pregnancy. In particular, morning sickness, nausea and heartburn may be more troublesome than in a singleton pregnancy.

Anaemia

The rate of anaemia in multiple pregnancy is about double that of singleton pregnancies. Iron deficiency and folic acid deficiency occur commonly in multiple pregnancy. Early in pregnancy iron is utilised in the growth of tissues, in particular the expansion of the plasma volume with formation of extra red blood cells. After the 28th week fetal demands deplete the remaining iron stores. If there is a poor response to iron therapy, folic acid deficiency may be present.

Pregnancy-induced hypertension

Hypertension is more common in women with multiple pregnancy. Arias (1993) suggests that both hypertension and oedema develop because of the extra increase in blood volume. Proteinuria is not necessarily a problem with this type of pregnancy-induced hypertension (PIH). With rest, PIH usually improves and pregnancy can be allowed to continue for the sake of the fetuses. A more worrying occurrence is the onset of preeclampsia with proteinuria, vasoconstriction and reduced blood volume.

Antepartum haemorrhage

There is a significant increase in antepartum haemorrhage in multiple pregnancy (MacGillivray & Campbell 1988). Placenta praevia is likely to be present because of the increased size of the placental site and abruptio placentae because of the increased polyhydramnios, with a risk of sudden decrease in uterine size if the membranes rupture early.

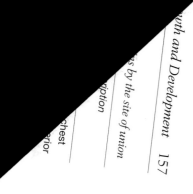

Complications of labour

Fetal malpresentations

Arias (1993) quotes Farooqui et al (1973) who found the percentages of different fetal presentations at the commencement of labour to be as follows.

Vertex-vertex	39.6%
Vertex-breech	27.7%
Vertex-transverse	7.2%
Breech-breech	9.0%
Breech-vertex	6.9%
Breech-transverse	3.6%
Other combinations	6.9%

After delivery of the first twin the lie, presentation and position of the second twin may change and must be checked and the fetal heart listened to before proceeding with the delivery.

Locked twins

Locked twins occur in one in 1000 twin labours. Typically the babies will have presented in a breech-vertex pattern with the head of the first or breech twin obstructed by the head of the second or vertex twin. There are other types of locked twins but they are rarer. If diagnosed before the onset of labour (and this is a situation that should be checked in every breech-vertex combination), an elective caesarean section should be carried out. Undiagnosed locked twins are rare today because of ultrasound scanning.

If, as the author has seen earlier in her career, the body of the first baby has already been born, an attempt to manipulate the babies to free the head should be made quickly. It may be successful as the babies are usually small. Otherwise an emergency caesarean section should be carried out. With one of the sets of twins the author saw, vaginal manipulation was successful and both babies survived with good Apgar scores. Unfortunately, in the second set of twins, vaginal manipulation was unsuccessful and both babies died during the caesarean section. It is pleasant to report that this mother, at the time 40 years old, went on to have a beautiful little girl born by caesarean section, within a year.

Umbilical cord problems

Problems affecting the umbilical cord are more common in multiple pregnancies. These include:

- the presence of a single umbilical artery;
- cord prolapse;
- velamentous insertion of the cord;
- vasa praevia;
- umbilical cord entanglement in monoamniotic twins.

Preterm onset of labour

Labour may begin spontaneously before term or may be induced for maternal or fetal complications. It is unusual for a twin pregnancy to go beyond term. If this happens it is usual to induce labour. Bed rest has been used in an attempt to prevent the preterm onset of labour. If labour threatens a tocolytic drug such as ritodrine or salbutamol may be given to attempt to stop the uterine activity. The rationale is that it prevents pressure on the cervix and also increases uteroplacental circulation. It has been a controversial area but Arias (1993) writes that various studies have shown that bed rest decreases perinatal mortality and morbidity in twins. As the worst mortality is before 30 weeks, Arias concludes that bed rest should be undertaken from 24 to 34 weeks.

Mode of delivery

Many obstetricians believe that indications for an elective caesarean section should include breech presentation or transverse lie of the first twin. However, in 75% of twin pregnancies the first twin presents by the vertex and there is no contraindication to vaginal delivery. The second twin should deliver easily as long as the lie is longitudinal. If the lie of the second twin is oblique or transverse most can be easily converted to longitudinal by external cephalic version. Labour may be prolonged by poor uterine action because of overdistension of the uterine muscle. This can be remedied by oxytocin infusion. Epidural analgesia is the first choice as it does not affect the fetuses and allows any unforeseen manipulative manoeuvres, such as external cephalic version or breech extraction, to be made.

Postpartum haemorrhage

Poor uterine tone because of overdistension and the presence of a large placental site predisposes women giving birth to more than one fetus to postpartum haemorrhage. This condition is more life threatening if the woman's blood has a low haemoglobin level. Prevention of haemorrhage should be a priority. An intravenous infusion of oxytocin should be in situ and intramuscular syntometrine 1 ampoule or intravenous ergometrine 500 μg should be administered.

Undiagnosed twins

If the head of the baby appears small in contrast to the known size of the uterus before delivery, if the uterus still looks large after the delivery of the baby or the baby itself appears small, a second twin should be suspected and the uterus quickly palpated. If an oxytocic drug has already been given delivery of the second twin needs to take place quickly as its life may be in danger. The second baby is likely to be asphyxiated and will need active resuscitation. The author has prevented the administration of an oxytocic drug with the birth of the anterior shoulder in a woman whose uterus was large. A large baby was expected so that on delivery of a tiny head a second twin was suspected and, indeed, was present. Both babies weighed about 1800 g at term but were healthy.

Postnatal care of mother and babies

Care of the babies

Following the birth, once the babies are breathing well, care will depend on the size and maturity of the babies. If the babies are premature or light for dates, appropriate care will be needed.

Some twins may not need any special attention other than helping the mother to care for them. The babies may be breastfed if the mother wishes.

Care of the mother

Involution of the uterus may be painful because of the increased muscle bulk (Grant 1996). Analgesia should be offered. If the mother decides to breastfeed both babies a high-protein, high-calorie diet will be needed. Anaemia should be treated and postnatal exercises to improve muscle tone of the abdominal wall and pelvic floor encouraged. For a deeper discussion of care, the reader is referred to books such as Botting et al (1990), Bryan (1992) and Clay (1989) (see Recommended reading).

Management of pregnancy with a high fetal number

The more fetuses in the uterus, the earlier labour is likely to commence. The mean gestational age at delivery for triplets is 32–33 weeks and for quadruplets, 30–32 weeks (Arias 1993). All complications mentioned above are more likely to occur. Fetal morbidity and mortality are high and are worst for the last babies to be delivered. Caesarean section is the commonest mode of delivery and if the babies are delivered in a centre of excellence, survival is quite good. Alongside this treatment has grown the concept of selective reduction when four or more fetuses are present. This is carried out between 9 and 12 weeks when an intracardiac injection of potassium chloride is given under ultrasound guidance. This ensures the survival of the two or three remaining fetuses but is ethically on shaky ground. The procedure itself may lead to the loss of all the fetuses and Arias (1993) writes that 'when the figures about fetal survival in triplet, quadruplet and quintuplet pregnancies are contrasted with the risk associated with selective feticide it becomes difficult to support a decision to reduce the number of fetuses with fewer than 5 fetuses'.

It never ceases to amaze the author that the Dionne quintuplets, five identical baby girls, were born vaginally in their parents' home in Canada and all survived. Of course, their conception was natural, unlike most of the higher order births of today which occur because of drug treatment for infertility. Sextuplets have survived and grown into healthy children in Britain.

Summary of main points

- Increasingly, following the use of ultrasound scanning, it has become more common to calculate the age of the fetus from the estimated day of fertilisation. The date of birth is about 266 days or 38 weeks after fertilisation and about 280 days or 40 weeks from the first day of the LMP.
- From the 9th week following ovulation there is a remarkable rate of growth of the body. The increase in size and maturation of the systems is directly linked to the ability of the fetus to survive outside the uterus. Maximum growth rate occurs between 16 and 24 weeks. At the cellular level growth occurs through hyperplasia and hypertrophy. Few if any new nerve cells or muscle cells appear after 30 weeks.
- Twins begin to slow in growth earlier when their combined weight is that of a 36-week fetus. This slowing down mechanism allows safe delivery of a genetically large child growing in the uterus of a small mother.
- How big a baby grows may be determined by a conflict between maternal and paternal genes. There is a gene present on chromosome 11 responsible for the regulation of fetal size. The gene from the father makes a growth factor which helps the fetus to grow whilst the mother's gene is programmed to be non-functional and to inhibit the effect of the father's gene.
- Other possible causes of the slowing of growth in the last few weeks of gestation include compression of uterine blood vessels by the growing fetus, resulting in a reduced maternal blood supply. There may be differential growth between the placenta and fetus and the placenta may not be able to increase its capacity to sustain the earlier growth rate.
- There is a pattern of developmental stages clearly seen from the 9th week until delivery. Although there is no clear demarcation between the non-viable and viable fetus, the lungs must be sufficiently developed to utilise oxygen.
- A series of fetal measurements can be plotted on a graph and used to calculate growth. Growth viewed as a motion through time leads to a distance curve. It is usual to plot a distance curve to monitor fetal growth. A velocity curve shows how the rate of growth alters.
- The medical and obstetric history of a woman may help to identify a fetus at risk of having poor intrauterine growth. Maternal weight gain has been used to assess fetal well-being in pregnancy. Continued weight gain is thought to be a favourable sign but many factors are known to affect maternal weight gain. Poor weight gain has been shown to be associated with intrauterine growth retardation but is not a very sensitive indicator.
- Fundal height is the most common method used to assess fetal growth. Fundal height can be plotted against a standard curve. Some studies report a 75% correct diagnosis rate using fundal height measurements alone. The gestational age is calculated from the mother's LMP or taken from an early ultrasound scan. Plotting of later measurements must be charted accurately to avoid wrong diagnosis. The success rate of ultrasound in detecting IUGR may be as high as 95%.
- Dizygotic (binovular or non-identical) twins develop from the fertilisation of two ova. A rarer form of twinning occurs when a single fertilised ovum divides into two separate fetuses. These are called monozygotic (uniovular or identical) twins. There is a high incidence in errors of development and congenital malformations.
- The incidence of multiple pregnancy varies naturally around the world. In the United Kingdom the incidence of twins is about one in 100 pregnancies. It is higher in black people and lower in Asian people. The differences in the rates of twinning are the result of variations in dizygotic twinning and the incidence of monozygotic twins is constant at 3.5 per 1000 births.
- Factors influencing the frequency of dizygotic twinning are maternal age, maternal parity and conception soon after discontinuing oral contraceptives. The development of ultrasound scanning techniques has shown that the incidence of twin pregnancy in humans may be double the number of eventual twin births. Half may never be recognised as twin pregnancy because of the death of one embryo early in the pregnancy. Since the development of routine ultrasound scanning, the incidence of undiagnosed twins at delivery has decreased.
- The introduction of drugs such as clomiphene which stimulate ovulation and are used in the treatment of some infertile couples has led to an increase in pregnancies where 5–8 fetuses are conceived.

The outcome of such pregnancies is poor, even with selective termination of fetuses.

- Twins can be diagnosed by abdominal examination but this is difficult before 20 weeks. Ultrasound diagnosis of multiple pregnancy can be made as early as 6 weeks following the last menstrual period. However, it may not be possible to confirm a twin pregnancy until 15 weeks when a clear outline of two heads can be detected.
- Abortion is associated with multiple pregnancy, possibly due to fetal abnormality in early pregnancy or to overdistension of the uterus later. Single fetal demise may occur. Before 14 weeks this will probably cause no problems for the survivor. Even rarer problems include acardiac twinning and twin-to-twin transfusion syndrome. Acute polyhydramnios is associated in particular with monozygotic twins and with fetal abnormality.
- Most twins show discordant growth, with one twin being larger than the other. The smaller twin is more at risk of perinatal complications. Discordant growth occurs because one twin obtains less nourishment from the maternal circulation.
- The presence of more than one fetus in utero means a higher level of pregnancy hormones and more pressure from the growing uterus. This will tend to cause an exacerbation of all minor disorders of pregnancy, in particular morning sickness, nausea and heartburn. The rate of anaemia in multiple pregnancy is about double that of singleton pregnancies. Iron and folic acid deficiency occur commonly in multiple pregnancy. Hypertension is more common.
- At the commencement of labour most leading twins present by the vertex. After delivery of the first twin the lie, presentation and position of the second twin may change and must be checked and the fetal heart listened to before proceeding with the delivery.
- Locked twins occur in one in 1000 twin labours. Typically the babies present in a breech-vertex pattern with the head of the first, breech twin obstructed by the head of the second or vertex twin. Undiagnosed locked twins are rare today because of ultrasound scanning, allowing planned caesarean section to take place if necessary.
- Problems affecting the umbilical cord are more common in multiple pregnancies. These include the presence of a single umbilical artery, cord prolapse, velamentous insertion of the cord, vasa praevia and umbilical cord entanglement in monoamniotic twins.
- Labour may begin spontaneously before term or may be induced for maternal or fetal complications. It is unusual for a twin pregnancy to go beyond term. Many obstetricians believe that an elective caesarean section should be performed for breech presentation or transverse lie of the first twin.
- Poor uterine tone because of overdistension and the presence of a large placental site predisposes women giving birth to more than one fetus to postpartum haemorrhage. This condition is more life threatening if the woman's blood has a low haemoglobin level.
- If the head of the baby appears small in contrast to the known size of the uterus before delivery, if the uterus still looks large after the delivery of the baby or the baby itself appears small, a second twin should be suspected.
- Following the birth, once the babies are breathing well, care will depend on the size and maturity of the babies. If the babies are premature or light for dates, appropriate care will be needed. The babies may be breastfed if the mother wishes.
- Involution of the uterus may be painful because of the increased muscle. Analgesia should be offered. If the mother decides to breastfeed both babies, a high-protein, high-calorie diet will be needed. Anaemia should be treated and postnatal exercises to improve muscle tone of the abdominal wall and pelvic floor encouraged.
- The more fetuses in the uterus, the earlier labour is likely to commence. Fetal morbidity and mortality are high and are worst for the last babies to be delivered. Caesarean section is the choice for delivery and if the babies are delivered in a centre of excellence, survival is quite good.

References

Almstrom H, Axelsson O, Cnattingius S et al. 1992 Comparison of umbilical-artery velocimetry and cardiotocography for surveillance of small-for-gestational age fetuses. Lancet 340, 936–940.

Arias F. 1993 Practical Guide to High Risk Pregnancy and Delivery, 2nd edn. Mosby Yearbook, Chicago.

Belizan JM, Villar J, Nardin JC. 1978 Diagnosis of intrauterine growth retardation by a simple clinical method: measurement of uterine height. American Journal of Obstetrics and Gynecology 131, 643.

Blackburn ST, Loper DL. 1992 Maternal, Fetal and Neonatal Physiology, A Clinical Perspective. WB Saunders, Philadelphia.

Bogin B (1988) Patterns of Human Growth. Cambridge University Press, Cambridge.

Campbell S, Dewhurst CJ. 1971 Diagnosis of the small-for-dates fetus by serial ultrasound cephalometry. Lancet 2, 1002.

Farooqui MO, Grossman JH, Shannon RA. 1973 A review of twin pregnancy and perinatal mortality. Obstetric and Gynaecological Survey 28, 144–153.

Fitzgerald MJT, Fitzgerald M. 1994 Human Embryology. Baillière Tindall, London.

Grant B. 1996 Multiple pregnancy. In Bennett VR, Brown LK (eds) Myles Textbook for Midwives. Churchill Livingstone, Edinburgh, pp 336–376.

Haig D. 1993 Genetic conflicts in human pregnancy. Quarterly Review of Biology 68(4), 495–519.

Hytten F. 1990 Is it important or even useful to measure weight gain in pregnancy? Midwifery 6, 28–32.

Hytten F. 1991 Weight gain in pregnancy. In Hytten F, Chamberlain G (eds) Clinical Physiology in Obstetrics, 2nd edn. Blackwell Scientific, Oxford, pp 173–203.

MacGillivray I, Campbell DM. 1988 Management of twin pregnancies. In MacGillivray I, Campbell DM, Thompson B (eds) The Stress of Multiple Births. Multiple Births Foundation, London.

Moore KL. 1989 Before We Are Born, 3rd edn. WB Saunders, Philadelphia.

Naeye RL, Tafari N, Judge D et al. 1978 Twins: causes of death in 12 United States cities and one African city. American Journal of Obstetrics and Gynecology 131, 267–272.

Proud J. 1996 Specialised antenatal investigations. In Bennett VR, Brown LK (eds) Myles Textbook for Midwives. Churchill Livingstone, Edinburgh, pp 660–674.

Spillman J. 1997 Multiple pregnancy. In Sweet BR with Tiran D (eds) Mayes Midwifery, 12th edn. Baillière Tindall, London, pp 584–596.

Sweet B. 1997 Mayes' Midwifery. Baillière Tindall, London.

Tanner JM. 1978 Foetus into Man. Open Books, London.

Thomson V. 1996 Psychological and physiological changes of pregnancy. In Bennett VR, Brown LK (eds) Myles Textbook for Midwives. Churchill Livingstone, Edinburgh.

Recommended reading

Barker DJP, Bull AR, Osmond C, Simmons SJ. 1990 Fetal and placental size and risk of hypertension in adult life. British Medical Journal 301, 259–262.

Botting B, MacFarlane AJ, Prince FV. 1990 Three, Four and More: A Study of Triplet and Higher Order Birth. HMSO, London.

Brock DJH, Rodeck CH, Ferguson-Smith MA (eds). 1992 Prenatal Diagnosis and Screening. Churchill Livingstone, Edinburgh.

Bryan E. 1992 Twins and Higher Multiple Births: A Guide to their Nature and Nurture. Edward Arnold, London.

Burton BK, Schultz MS, Burd LI. 1992 Limb anomalies associated with chorionic villus sampling. Obstetrics and Gynaecology 79(5), 730–736.

Chudleigh P, Pierse ML. 1992 Obstetric Ultrasound, How, Why and When. Churchill Livingstone, Edinburgh.

Clay MM. 1989 Quadruplets and Higher Multiple Births. MacKeith, Oxford.

Creasy RK, Resnik R (eds). 1994 Maternal, Fetal Medicine. WB Saunders, Philadelphia.

DOH 1991 While You are Pregnant: Safe Eating and Safe Contact with Pets. HMSO, London.
Enkin M, Keirse MJNC, Renfew M, Neilson J. 1996 A Guide to Effective Care in Pregnancy and Childbirth, 2nd edn. Oxford University Press, Oxford.
Gegor CL. 1993 Third trimester ultrasound for nurse midwives. Journal of Nurse-Midwifery 38(2), S49–S61.
Green J, Statham H. 1993 Testing for fetal abnormality in routine antenatal care. Midwifery 9, 124–135.
James D. 1993 Monitoring the biophysical profile. British Journal of Hospital Medicine 49(8), 561–563.
Richards M. 1989 Social and ethical problems of fetal diagnosis and screening. Journal of Reproductive and Infant Psychology 7(3), 171–185.
Steer P. 1995 Maternal haemoglobin and birth weight. What is the relationship? Maternity Action 69, 3.

Chapter 14 Common fetal problems

In this chapter

INTRAUTERINE GROWTH RETARDATION

Arias (1993) remarks that optimal birth weight depends on an interaction between fetal growth potential and the intrauterine environment. This growth potential varies between races and individuals. As an example, the average birth weight of the Cheyenne Indians is 3700 g whilst that of a tribe in New Guinea is only 2400 g. This creates a problem of diagnosis of IUGR as growth curves developed for one group of babies may not be suitable to screen other groups. The classification of IUGR does not allow for fetuses that are small and healthy. This may lead to inappropriate interference in the course of pregnancy.

Before discussing intrauterine growth retardation (IUGR), it is useful to understand some definitions.

- A **low birth weight baby** (LBW) weighs 2500 g or less at birth.
- A **very low birth weight baby** (VLBW) weighs 1500 g or less at birth.
- A **light-for-dates** or **small-for-gestational-age (SGA) baby** is one whose birth weight is below the 10th centile for its gestational age.
- A **large-for-gestational-age (LGA) baby** is one whose birth weight is above the 90th centile for gestational age.
- A **preterm infant** is a baby born before 37 completed weeks of pregnancy irrespective of the birth weight. A preterm infant may also be SGA or LGA.

Classification

Small fetuses are classified based on the ratio of symmetry between their anatomical parts.

- **Type I IUGR** is the fetus that is symmetrically small but has normal head-to-abdomen and femur-to-abdomen ratios.
- **Type II IUGR** is the fetus whose abdominal circumference is smaller than the head circumference and femur length.
- **Type III IUGR** is a form intermediate between the other two types where fetuses are symmetric initially but become asymmetric later in the pregnancy (Arias 1993).

There is another method of classification:

- **intrinsic IUGR**, where the fetus is small because of fetal conditions such as chromosomal abnormality or intrauterine infection;
- **extrinsic IUGR**, where the growth failure is caused by a factor outside the fetus such as maternal disease or placental pathology;

- **combined IUGR**, where both intrinsic and extrinsic factors are present;
- **idiopathic IUGR**, where the cause of the growth failure is unknown.

Complications

In the antepartum and intrapartum periods there is an increase in the number of stillbirths and cases of, oligohydramnios and fetal distress. Complications in the neonatal period include meconium aspiration syndrome, persistent fetal circulation, hypoglycaemia, hypocalcaemia, hyperviscosity syndrome and poor temperature control. These will be discussed in section 4 of the book.

Factors adversely affecting fetal growth

Fetal growth depends on interacting factors such as genetic determinants, general maternal health and nutrition, availability of growth substrates, the presence of fetal growth hormones and sufficient maternal blood supply to the placenta (Blackburn & Loper 1992). Arias (1993) describes the most essential substrates as oxygen, glucose and amino acids. Any decrease in the availability of substrates caused by pathological conditions affecting the mother, placenta or fetus will result in poor growth.

Maternal factors most frequently associated with poor fetal growth are:

- chronic hypertension;
- pregnancy induced hypertension;
- chronic renal disease;
- diabetes mellitus with vascular lesions;
- sickle cell anaemia;
- severe cardiac disease;
- severe malnutrition;
- smoking;
- alcohol ingestion.

The most common placental problems are:

- abnormal placentation characterised by small placental size and inadequate changes in the spiral arteries;
- placental infarcts;
- placenta praevia.

Fetal problems causing poor growth include:

- chromosomal abnormalities;
- infections;
- multiple pregnancy.

Hypertension, diabetes mellitus, sickle cell anaemia and cardiac disorders are discussed fully in other chapters. Brief discussions of maternal malnutrition, smoking and alcohol consumption are included below.

Maternal malnutrition

Maternal influences associated with a reduction in birth weight but preservation of body length include malnutrition and low weight gain in pregnancy. Barker (1992) mentions that the babies born in the Dutch famine of 1944–45 had a reduced birth weight in proportion to their length. Arias (1993) remarks that severe protein calorie malnutrition, especially during the second half of pregnancy, leads to decreased fetal weight. During the siege of Leningrad in World War II fetal weight reduction was on average 530 g. A more modern cause of IUGR due to malnutrition has been seen in the USA when women have had gastric bypass operations for gross obesity (Arias 1993).

Further analysis of the Dutch famine has shown that women whose mothers were malnourished during pregnancy have themselves given birth to low birth weight babies (Barker 1992). Tanner (1978) mentions that in countries where severe maternal malnutrition occurs some low birth weight babies will result. However, he states that the malnutrition has to be fairly severe.

Smoking

Research into the effects of smoking on fetal growth were carried out in the 1960s and 1970s and smoking has been the subject of health education efforts ever since. Tobacco smoking induces fetal hypoxia by vasoconstrition due to nicotine's effect on adrenergic neurones. This decreases placental blood flow and leads to placental underperfusion. This reduction in blood flow has a direct effect on reducing fetal nutrition, leading to fetal growth retardation (Arias 1993, Kelly et al 1984).

A more prolonged effect on fetal growth results from an increase in carboxyhaemoglobin which causes a sustained reduction of oxygen to the fetus (Longo 1977). This combined effect has also been shown to be associated with reduced length of pregnancy which adds to the problem of low birth weight. The average reported birth weight reduction is quoted as being between 120 and 430 g depending on the number of cigarettes consumed.

Alcohol consumption

A prime example of the effects of a recreational drug on fetal growth is that of alcohol. However, it is only recently that the condition of fetal alcohol syndrome (FAS) has been recognised, first in the USA and latterly in Britain. Alcohol is a low molecular weight substance and as such can cross the placental barrier (see Chapter 11). Alcohol is a known teratogen and alcohol-induced damage to the fetus has been associated with all forms of drinking pattern from heavy to light social drinking. Therefore it is not possible to state how much alcohol will give rise to the abnormalities associated with FAS. It is wise to abstain totally from drinking alcohol during pregnancy. FAS covers a whole spectrum of effects from minor to major and the classic picture may not be present in total. In a few women the secondary factor of alcohol-induced malnutrition will add to the problem for the fetus.

The characteristic features of FAS

- Deficient overall growth, weight, length and head circumference.
- Craniofacial abnormalities including small eyes with inner epicanthic folds, poorly formed nasal bridge, giving the nose

a retroussé appearance, poor or absent vertical groove in a narrow top lip, ears that are large and simple in formation, and cleft palate.
- Musculoskeletal abnormalities including congenital hip lesions and thoracic cage abnormalities.
- Undescended testes, male urethral abnormalities, hypoplastic labia in females and kidney abnormalities.
- Cardiac abnormalities found in up to 50% of children, mainly atrial or ventricular septal defects.
- Cerebellar damage with poor coordination of movement and learning difficulties.
- Alcohol withdrawal symptoms.

Placental insufficiency

The placenta is usually below the 10th centile and there is a reduction in the number of stem and villous capillaries. The muscle layer of the spiral arteries is intact because of incomplete penetration by the trophoblastic cells. These placental changes may occur as an isolated pathology or may be found in the maternal conditions listed above. The extent of the placental changes is related to the severity of the maternal disease. These pathological changes in the placenta have also been found in women with idiopathic (no definable cause) onset of preterm labour.

Multiple pregnancy

Multiple pregnancy is the term used to describe the development of more than one fetus in utero at the same time. Arias (1993) states that IUGR occurs in about 21% of twins, mainly due to abnormal placentation.

Genetic factors and chromosomal aberrations

The prevalence of genetic and chromosomal disorders amongst babies with IUGR is at least 10%. IUGR is particularly common in babies with trisomies such as Down's syndrome (trisomy 21). The majority of affected babies have symmetric growth retardation.

Management of IUGR

Arias (1993) states that the first step in managing IUGR is to identify those women at risk. The second step is to differentiate the small healthy babies from those with genuine IUGR. The third step is to monitor the at-risk fetuses.

Diagnosis of IUGR

Using a combination of the clinical and ultrasound methods outlined in Chapter 13, a diagnosis should be possible in 95% of cases. Measurement of the amount of liquor amnii will demonstrate the presence of oligohydramnios, a late sign of fetal malnutrition. Arias (1993) believes serial estimations of the amount of amniotic fluid are essential and can indicate the need to expedite delivery if used with Doppler assessment and non-stress cardiotocography. Other tests that have been used for monitoring the fetus diagnosed as having asymmetric IUGR have been evaluated by Enkin et al (1996). These are discussed below.

Hormonal tests of placental function

Neither serial oestriol estimation nor human placental lactogen (HPL) assays have been shown to be of value in assessing placental function and fetal well-being. Whilst fundal height measurements alone may not detect all cases of IUGR, it is a method that allows the referral of women to a consultant unit for ultrasonic screening. Monitoring daily fetal movements has also not been shown to be of value as a screening technique.

Contraction stress testing

Continuous cardiotocography recording fetal heart rate and uterine activity is monitored in response to an oxytocin challenge. It has no benefits and some problems. It is time consuming and potentially dangerous for the fetus and its use is contraindicated in at-risk pregnancies such as antepartum haemorrhage, placenta praevia and preterm labour. A similar test using nipple stimulation to induce contractions has proved to be so dangerous that its use is discontinued (Enkin et al 1996).

Non-stress cardiotocography

Antepartum cardiotocography has been used to try and detect the at-risk fetus employing such variables as baseline heart rate, beat-to-beat variability and accelerations of the fetal heart. Readings can be divided into reactive, with a good baseline variability, and non-reactive if there is an inadequate baseline with loss of variability or accelerations in response to fetal movement. There is difficulty in interpreting the printouts and intervention has been carried out too early and inappropriately, causing increased morbidity and mortality (Enkin et al 1996).

Fetal biophysical profile

The method is derived from research into serial ultrasound examinations and antenatal cardiotocography (non-stress test). Five physiological variables are combined in a predictive test to try and reduce the incidence of false-positive diagnoses. These are:

1 fetal movement;
2 fetal tone;
3 fetal reactivity;
4 fetal breathing movements;
5 amniotic fluid volume.

In the small number of studies reported, biophysical profile was a better predictive test than the non-stress test in identifying babies with a low 5-minute Apgar score. However, its use did not result in any improvements in the outcome for the baby. In a metaanalysis, Hofmeyr (1997) found no effect, beneficial or otherwise, on the outcome of pregnancy.

Delivery of the baby

Once fetal lung maturity is achieved and preferably after 34 weeks postfertilisation, the baby should be delivered. Excluding congenital malformations, intrapartum asphyxia is a major cause of morbidity and mortality. A major source of anxiety is the increased incidence of low 5-minute Apgar scores and later neurological deficits.

Every method to avoid asphyxia should be used.

- Direct fetal monitoring by scalp electrode should be utilised to monitor fetal condition.
- Care should be taken with analgesia and an epidural anaesthetic may be best.
- The second stage of labour should be short and a low forceps delivery used if necessary.
- A paediatrician should be present at the delivery.

Long-term prognosis

Most of these babies now survive the neonatal period. However, a universal finding is that IUGR babies remain smaller than their age cohorts for several years after their birth. A major concern is that chronic intrauterine malnutrition may lead to a permanent decrease in brain cell number. Some studies have reported an increased incidence of minimal brain dysfunction and speech defects associated with IUGR whilst others have found no difference in outcome (Arias 1993).

RHESUS ISOIMMUNISATION AND ABO INCOMPATIBILITY

Rhesus isoimmunisation

The reader is advised to read the section on the inheritance of blood groups in Chapter 16 before proceeding. The fetus inherits a gene for the rhesus factor from each parent and as rhesus D is a dominant gene, if either or both genes for rhesus are inherited the baby will be rhesus positive. Only if the baby inherits two d genes will the blood group be rhesus negative (Fig. 14.1).

If there is incompatibility between the mother and fetus in that the mother is Rh– and the fetus Rh+, haemolysis of fetal red cells may occur (Fig. 14.2). However, this would rarely affect the first baby as there are no spontaneous anti-D antibodies present in a woman prior to her first pregnancy unless she has had the misfortune to receive Rh+ blood in a mismatched blood transfusion. During pregnancy and labour there is normally no mixing of maternal and fetal circulation. When the placenta separates the chorionic villi tear and there is a risk of a fetomaternal transfusion; usually between 0.5 ml and 5 ml of fetal blood enters the maternal circulation. If the fetus is Rh+ the small transfusion of blood will stimulate the production of antibodies and memory cells, which can mount a secondary response should the mother become pregnant with a second Rh+ baby. This process is called **isoimmunisation**.

There are other events in pregnancy before delivery which may lead to antibody formation because of a fetomaternal transfusion. These include spontaneous or therapeutic abortion, amniocentesis, antepartum haemorrhage or conversion of a breech presentation to cephalic by a procedure known as external cephalic version. The problem arises in any subsequent pregnancies because anti-D IgG, which is a small molecule, will cross the placenta and begin to haemolyse the fetal red cells. A protective event can occur if the mother and fetus are also ABO incompatible as the naturally occurring anti-A or anti-B will destroy the fetal red cells before the maternal immune system

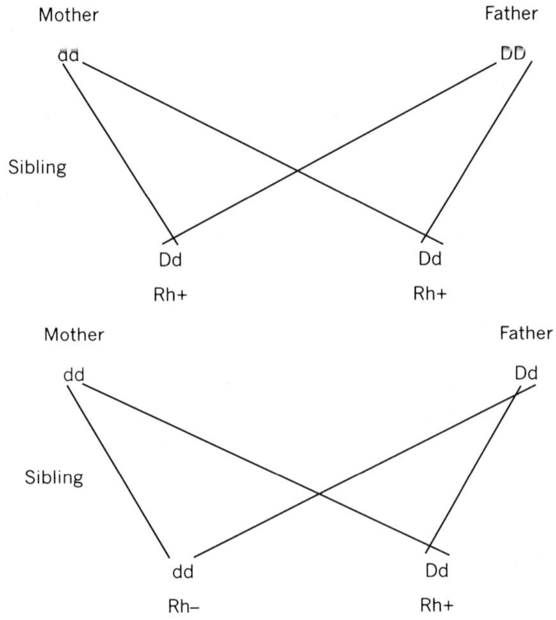

Figure 14.1 *Inheritance of the rhesus factor (from Sweet B, 1997, with permission).*

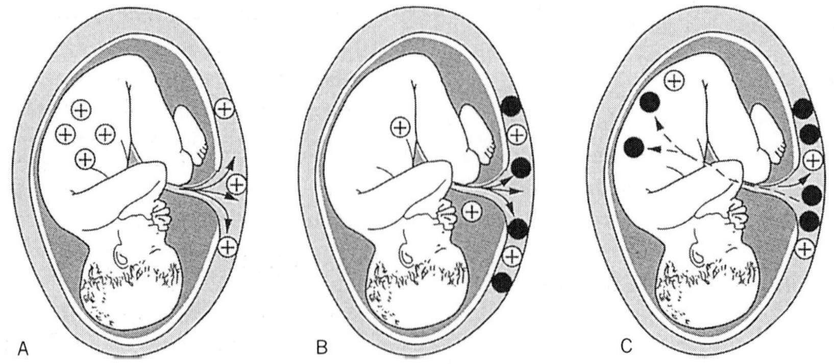

Figure 14.2 *Antibody formation (a) Transfer of rhesus antigen (+) to the maternal circulation. (b) Antibody formation (•) in the rhesus-negative mother (c) Transfer of rhesus antibody to the fetus (from Sweet B, 1997, with permission).*

has time to mount an immune response against the rhesus factor.

Prevention of maternal isoimmunisation

In the past haemolytic disease of the newborn led to fetal or neonatal death but this is now largely preventable if three conditions are met.

1 Rhesus-positive blood should never be used in a transfusion if a woman's blood group is unknown.
2 Unnecessary fetomaternal transfusions by such procedures as placental location prior to amniocentesis should be avoided. Abdominal palpation in women with an antepartum haemorrhage should be kept to a minimum.
3 If an event likely to have caused a fetomaternal transfusion occurs anti-D immunoglobulin (rhesus D antibodies) must be administered to the mother. The immunoglobulin needs to be given within 72 h and will last about 3 months. The antibodies will coat and destroy any fetal red cells in the maternal circulation. The dose of anti-D immunoglobulin is normally 250 IU (international units) before 20 weeks of pregnancy and 500 IU after 20 weeks. Occasionally the fetomaternal haemorrhage is so large that one dose of anti-D immunoglobulin is insufficient to prevent isoimmunisation. For this reason the number of fetal red cells in the maternal blood is estimated by means of a Kleihauer test carried out on maternal blood after delivery. If a second dose is needed the laboratory will inform the doctor.

Antenatal management

Every pregnant woman has her blood tested for ABO and rhesus types early in pregnancy. Any woman who proves to be rhesus negative will be screened for rhesus antibodies. If the test is negative her blood will be retested later, usually at 28 and 34 weeks of pregnancy.

Care at delivery

The cord is clamped at once to minimise the amount of blood with possible maternal antibodies entering the baby's circulation and cord blood is taken for testing. This is best done by using a syringe and needle into a placental vein to avoid the risk of contamination by maternal blood and Wharton's jelly which would lead to difficulty in interpreting the test results. The needle is removed prior to transferring the blood to a bottle to avoid haemolysis. Cord blood is tested from all babies of rhesus-negative women for ABO and rhesus type, direct Coombes test looking for maternal antibodies on fetal red cells and a haemoglobin estimation to check for haemolysis. If the mother is known to have rhesus antibodies the cord blood is also tested for serum bilirubin level.

Management if rhesus antibodies are present during pregnancy

If antibodies are detected, the titre (amount) of antibodies will be checked. Although the level of antibodies present does not relate directly to the fetal condition it at least indicates a more direct test on the amniotic fluid. The amount of bilirubin excreted from the breakdown of red cells can be measured against a **Liley chart** which relates the level to the week of gestation and allows judgement to be made about the future management of the pregnancy. However, the value of this measure should be carefully weighed against the risk of provoking another fetomaternal bleed by performing an amniocentesis. It is usual to delay this examination until after 26 weeks when the fetus is viable (Bennett & Brown 1996). The possible outcomes are as follows.

- The pregnancy is allowed to continue and bilirubin level is estimated at intervals. If the titre is rising it may be necessary to deliver the fetus.
- If the fetus is considered mature enough to survive and if it is considered to be too dangerous to continue the pregnancy, the baby is delivered in a consultant unit at a time when all necessary facilities are available such as the pathology laboratory and paediatrician.
- The fetus may be given an intrauterine transfusion of group O rhesus-negative packed cells to prolong life if it is considered too immature to survive.

Rhesus haemolytic disease

All babies whose mothers have rhesus antibodies should be transferred to a neonatal intensive care unit until the results of cord blood tests are known and care planned. Depending on the percentage of red blood cells destroyed, this disease has varying degrees of severity.

1 Congenital haemolytic anaemia occurs if haemolysis is minimal. There will be slow-onset anaemia and enlargement of the liver and spleen but jaundice will not be severe. If the baby's haemoglobin level is low a small blood transfusion of packed cells can be given.
2 In icterus gravis neonatorum (severe jaundice of the newborn) haemolysis has been present in the fetus and the baby is born with a low haemoglobin level. As the placenta has transferred the bilirubin to the mother for her to excrete, the baby is not jaundiced at birth. After delivery when the baby's liver must cope with the excessive production of bilirubin, he rapidly becomes jaundiced. Treatment is centred on three aspects: restoring the haemoglobin level, reducing the bilirubin level and removing maternal antibodies.
3 Hydrops fetalis is a condition where severe intrauterine anaemia results in congestive cardiac failure. At birth, the baby is pale and oedematous as is the placenta, and may be stillborn. If the baby is born alive an immediate transfusion of packed cells will allow oxygenation of the tissues and an exchange transfusion (Figs 14.3 and 14.4) to remove bilirubin and maternal antibodies will follow when his condition is stable.

ABO incompatibility

In this condition the mother is blood group O and the baby A or B. Note that the baby cannot be group AB as it must have inherited an O gene from its mother. The mother has unprovoked anti-A and anti-B antibodies even in the first pregnancy so the first child may be affected. If the antibodies are

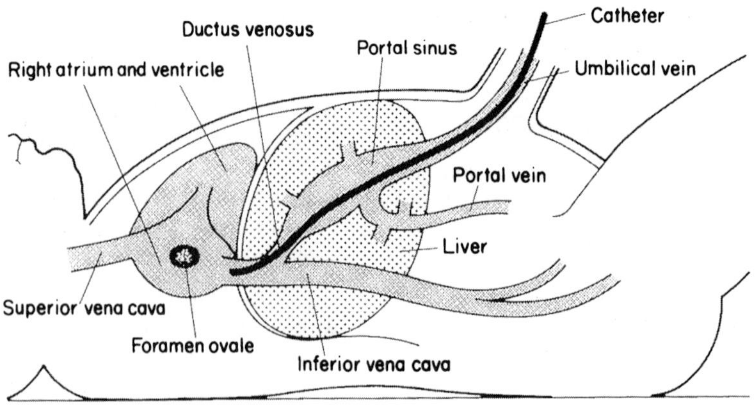

Figure 14.3 *The umbilical vein and its connections in the neonate. The position of the umbilical venous catheter is shown. Note how easy it would be to push it accidentally into the right atrium. (Reproduced with permission from Wallis & Harvey 1979.)*

of the IgM type they are too large to cross the placenta. However, if IgG antibodies are produced they may cross the placenta and haemolyse fetal red cells. Although jaundice appears in the first 24 h it is usually mild. Treatment will depend on the level of bilirubin in the blood and its rate of rise. Other causes of jaundice and their management will be discussed in Chapter 52.

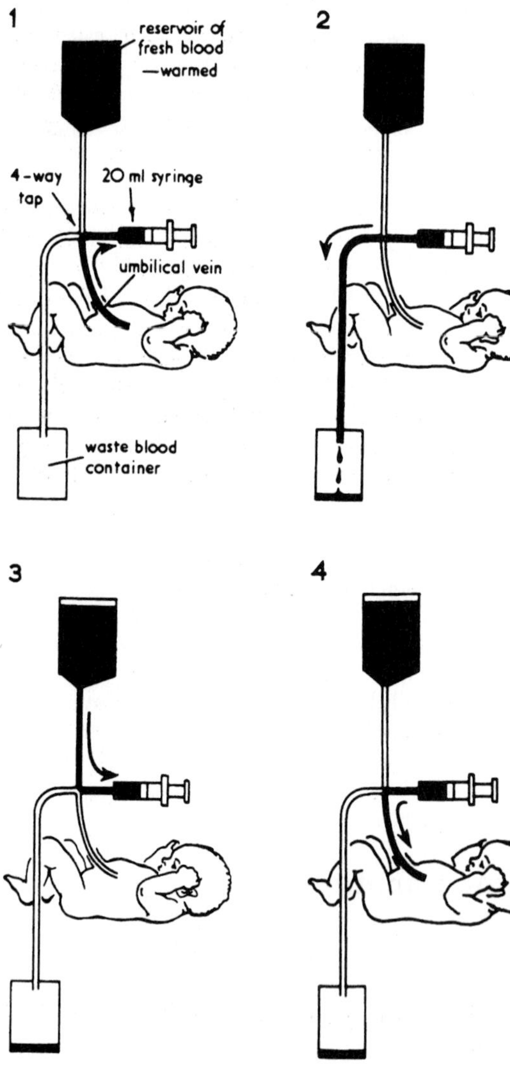

MATERNAL INFECTION IN PREGNANCY

Microbes are small organisms that often live in and on the human body and some of these commensal organisms are helpful, like the lactobacillus that inhabits the vagina and produces a mild acid that increases the acidity of the vagina. However, many can cause infection if the organisms start to multiply and these are called **pathogens**. Over time, the immune system can develop defence systems against pathogens. Microbes can be divided into five major classes: bacteria, viruses, algae, fungi and protozoa. Some of the most virulent pathogens may kill.

Systemic infections may cause reproductive problems such as infertility and congenital defects if the woman is pregnant and some infections are specific to the genitourinary tract. In the vagina other organisms may be present in non-invasive numbers. These would include yeasts, streptococci and sometimes *E. coli*. Some organisms that specifically cause disease in the genital tract will be outlined first, followed by some systemic disorders that may damage the fetus.

Suppression of cell-mediated immunity

Despite the alterations in the maternal immune system in pregnancy most women are not immunocompromised. However, the suppression of cell-mediated immunity means

Figure 14.4 *Exchange transfusion. 1. Blood is drawn out into a syringe via an umbilical vein catheter. 2. This blood is discarded into a waste container. 3. Blood warmed to body temperature is drawn into this syringe. The blood is crossmatched for compatibility with blood from the baby's mother. 4. This blood is injected slowly. The process is repeated until the twice the baby's blood volume has been exchanged. (Reproduced with permission from Wallis & Harvey 1979.)*

that some infections may be more severe in pregnancy, especially viruses and the opportunistic pathogens associated with HIV such as *Pneumocystis carinii* and *Toxoplasma gondii*. The viruses may cause poliomyelitis, influenza and pneumococcal pneumonia. Pregnancy also leads to reactivation of latent cytomegalovirus (CMV) and herpes.

Sexually transmitted diseases

Sexually transmitted diseases (STDs) are a major problem for society and their control constitutes a difficult public health concern. Brock & Madigan (1991) state several reasons for this. First, about a third of cases in developed countries affect teenagers because sexual activity in this age group is increasing and the young person is likely to have more than one sexual partner. Second, many STDs have no symptoms or vague non-specific symptoms. A third reason concerns the social stigma attached to these diseases so that people are less inclined to seek treatment. Untreated, these diseases can have serious long-term health consequences such as pelvic inflammatory disease (PID) with its sequels of infertility, cervical cancer, heart and nerve damage, to mention a few.

Pregnant women infected with a STD may pass the infection on to the fetus resulting in birth defects or even stillbirth. Another problem is that there is often a second disease complicating the treatment. For example, an asymptomatic chlamydial infection may remain after successful treatment for gonorrhoea. This trend is worrying as most of the STDs, with the exception of HIV infection, are treatable. Whilst it is not possible to give a detailed consideration of this major preconception and pregnancy problem, an overview of the more common diseases will be presented.

Gonorrhoea

This infectious disease is still one of the most widespread of human diseases and symptoms are different in males and females. In women the initial symptom is a mild vaginitis which may even go unnoticed whilst in men the organism causes a painful infection of the urethral canal. The organism can also cause a severe eye infection in neonates.

The causative organism is *Neisseria gonorrhoeae* (Fig. 14.5) which is very easily killed outside the body so that the disease can only be transmitted by intimate bodily contact. Severe complications of this disease include PID and damage to heart valves and joint tissues. Most cases will still respond to penicillin but penicillin-resistant strains of the organism are evolving.

Despite the ease with which gonorrhoea can be treated, there are three major reasons for the high level of infection.

1 There are at least 16 types of the organism, causing difficulty in development of immunity and increasing the likelihood of reinfection.
2 Oral contraceptives mimic the pregnant state in women, with reduced glycogen production and reduction in Doderlein's bacillus in the vagina, allowing the gonococcus easier access to the female reproductive tract.
3 Symptoms may go unrecognised in women who may act as a reservoir for infection of men.

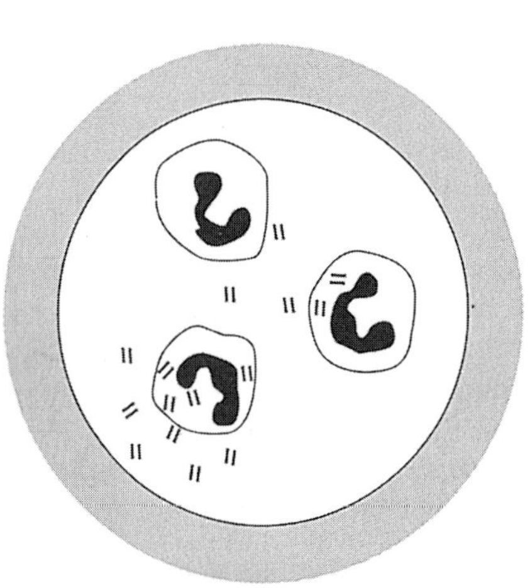

Figure 14.5 *Neisseria gonorrhoeae in pus cells (from Sweet B, 1997, with permission).*

Syphilis

This disease is more serious than gonorrhoea but better controlled as penicillin is very effective against the causative organism, which is the spirochaete (spiral organism) *Treponoma pallidum* (Fig. 14.6). The disease cannot enter the body unless there is a break in the skin or mucous membranes. In men infection is usually on the penis whilst in women it is likely to be hidden in the vagina or on the cervix. In about 10% of cases the infection is extragenital, usually in the oral region. The disease can be transmitted across the placenta to the fetus during pregnancy to cause congenital syphilis.

The organism multiplies within 2–6 weeks at the site of entry to form a primary lesion called a **chancre**. This heals and the organism spreads to other tissues and a generalised skin rash usually develops. This is the secondary stage of the infection. About 25% of people then undergo a spontaneous cure, 25% will remain symptomless although the organism stays in their bodies and about 50% will develop the tertiary stage with possible fatal involvement of the cardiovascular or central nervous systems. Because the symptoms are noticeable in both sexes, sufferers are likely to seek treatment. In Britain it is usual

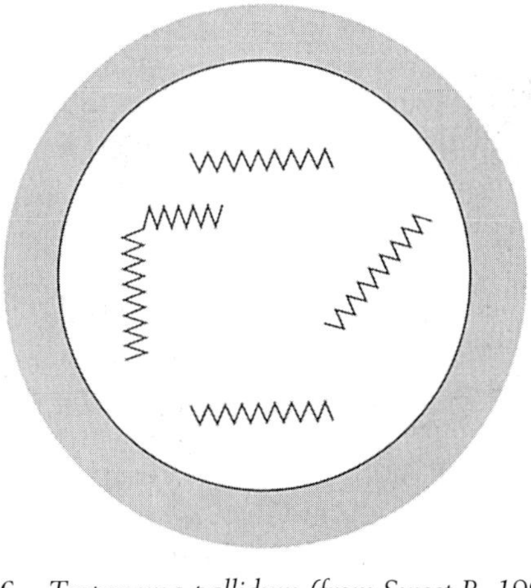

Figure 14.6 *Treponema pallidum (from Sweet B, 1997, with permission).*

to screen pregnant women for the presence of syphilis and offer treatment as this will prevent or treat infection in the fetus in utero.

Chlamydia

The incidence of infection with *Chlamydia trachomatis*, which lives inside cells, probably greatly outnumbers infections with the other two organisms already discussed. One strain can cause severe eye infections but separate strains of the organism cause venereal disease. Contamination of the eyes of the neonate during birth may cause severe conjunctivitis and respiratory distress. Chlamydia can cause non-gonococcal urethritis (NGU) in males and cervicitis and PID in females.

Asymptomatic infection is common in sexually active men and women and in both sexes chlamydial infection can result in infertility. In men, testicular swelling and prostate inflammation can occur whilst in women, fallopian tubes may be damaged or blocked as the cells of the epithelial lining are destroyed, leading to adhesions. Chlamydial infection is difficult to diagnose but is responsive to tetracycline or erythromycin. Chlamydia is often present in people infected with the gonococcus and treatment to eradicate both organisms is best.

Brock & Madigan (1991) discuss the ecology of STDs in Chapter 15 of their book. Their interest lies in the factors common to all diseases transmitted by the physical contact of sexual intercourse. This also includes organisms such as *Trichomonas vaginalis*, a protozoon, the yeast *Monilia albicans*, the herpes viruses and the most dangerous of all STDs – HIV. Features that these organisms have in common are as follows.

- The pathogens are not shed in enormous numbers except during sexual activity.
- Many of the organisms are sensitive to drying and need a moist environment.
- The organisms have lost their ability to survive outside the body.

Group B streptococcus (GBS)

One in three women in Britain may have vaginal carriage of this organism at some time during their pregnancy (Roth 1996). The infection is asymptomatic but it is the organism most often responsible for overwhelming sepsis in neonates. The prevalence is between 0.6 and 3.7 per 1000 live births and Roth quotes Brunham et al (1990) who state that the mortality rate of babies with neonatal GBS is 50%. Screening and treatment of these women are difficult because of the recurrence of the infection but Wang & Smaill (1989) suggest screening women with preterm rupture of the membranes and treatment with intravenous ampicillin or erythromycin if the woman is allergic to penicillin.

Acquired immune deficiency syndrome (AIDS)

There are two reasons why this is designated the most dangerous disease: it is almost always fatal and there is as yet no cure or even treatment. The transmission of the virus is associated with sexual activity where skin or mucous membrane integrity is broken. Promiscuity is a key factor in the spread of the disease, as is blood contamination of needles shared by drug addicts or (in the past in certain countries) in mass vaccinations. Medical instances of HIV transmission include contaminated blood products such as blood transfusion or in factor 8 used to treat haemophilia.

The organism responsible for the eventual development of AIDS is the human immunodeficiency virus (HIV). HIV is a retrovirus carrying its genetic information as ribonucleic acid or RNA, unlike most organisms which contain deoxyribonucleic acid (DNA). Cells of the immune system containing CD4 molecules, which include T lymphocytes, monocytes and macrophages, are the targets of this virus. On entering the target cell the genetic message is converted from RNA to DNA and inserted into the host DNA.

T cells help to stimulate production of antibodies by B lymphocytes so that as the T cell population is reduced over a few years B lymphocyte production of antibodies falls, the immune system becomes crippled and the person becomes ill with opportunistic infections that would have normally been fought successfully. A major problem with HIV is that the mutation rate has resulted in so many different variants that no vaccine against the whole virus can be developed. Trials of vaccines against subunits are under way.

Recent controversy

Much political controversy surfaced in June 1996 about the true nature of pathways of infection in Britain. Concern has been expressed about the publicity surrounding the risks to the heterosexual population. It is now thought that there are as few as 161 heterosexual people not exposed to any known AIDS risk out of a total of 12 565 diagnosed cases of AIDS since 1982.

The sub-Saharan picture

Caldwell & Caldwell (1996) have studied the epidemiological, social and behavioural aspects of the African AIDS epidemic since 1989. They find that the evidence for a heterosexual AIDS epidemic in sub-Saharan Africa is convincing and one factor supporting their belief is that anal intercourse, a high-risk behaviour, is believed to be related to witchcraft and almost completely suppressed in this part of the world. They suggest that two-thirds of the 16 million people worldwide who are infected with HIV live in sub-Saharan Africa.

Half the world's cases are found in the AIDS belt countries in Eastern and Southern Africa where 2% of the world population lives, including the Central African Republic, Southern Sudan, Uganda, Kenya, Rwanda, Burundi, Tanzania, Malawi, Zimbabwe and Botswana. Caldwell & Caldwell base their figures on the urban populations of these countries where nearly 25% of people are infected with HIV whereas other African regions have a rate of infection as low as 1%. The spread of HIV in this part of the world is by heterosexual intercourse, as opposed to the developed world where transmission is still mainly by homosexual intercourse or the sharing of needles by intravenous drug users.

Reducing the risk of transmission

Finally, Caldwell & Caldwell state that a number of unusual conditions may combine to sustain a heterosexual epidemic and it is unlikely that AIDS in developed countries will spread significantly beyond these two high-risk groups. However, the world is becoming a 'global village' and travel is becoming ever easier and it is probably not wise to exclude any mode of transmission from any country. Those caring for a multicultural society, particularly in the inner areas of major cities, need to be aware of the risk factors of virus transmission through contamination with blood and body fluids.

The following recommendations are valid.

1 Avoid mouth contact with penis, vagina and rectum.
2 Avoid sexual activities that may result in tears in the linings of the rectum, vagina and penis.
3 Avoid sexual activity with individuals from high-risk groups. These include male and female prostitutes, homosexual or bisexual individuals and intravenous drug users.
4 If a person has unprotected sexual intercourse with a member of a high-risk group, a blood test should be taken to ascertain whether infection has occurred. If the test is positive future sexual partners should be protected by the use of a condom.

The effect on mothers and babies

Women who are HIV positive may pass the virus across the placenta to affect their unborn child or the baby may be infected by contact with maternal blood during birth. A third way of transmission is through breastfeeding. Transfer from mother to child in this way is referred to as **vertical transmission**. However, this is not inevitable and the risk is usually quoted as one in three (Grimes & Grimes 1994). Brown (1992) quotes the risk to African women as four in 10 whilst in European women it appears to be less, at one in six. Higher rates of perinatal transfer are associated with low CD4 counts, suggesting the risk increases as the disease in the mother progresses.

Pregnancy has not been found to have adverse effects on disease progression although the effect of repeated pregnancies has not been determined. However, the European Collaborative Study (1991) found that there may be protection against vertical transmission if the baby is delivered by caesarean section. Studies suggest that there is a risk of transmission during breastfeeding but this should only be considered when women have access to formula feeds (American College of Obstetricians and Gynecologists 1987).

TORCH organisms and the risk in pregnancy

TORCH is a word derived from the first letters of a series of infections that can cross the placenta to affect the fetus. These are Toxoplasmosis, Others, Rubella, Cytomegalovirus and Herpes. Most of these infections will cause congenital abnormality if acquired in the first trimester and neonatal infection, often affecting the lung, liver, spleen and brain, if acquired late in pregnancy.

Rubella

In 1941 in Australia, Gregg described an association between maternal rubella and congenital cataracts. It is now well established that rubella infection during the first few weeks of pregnancy will inhibit cell division in the embryonic eyes, ears, heart and brain. After the 3rd month the most common defect is congenital deafness. If an infant is born with congenital rubella he will be highly infectious and must be isolated (Bennett & Brown 1996). The virus may remain in his body for up to a year. Rubella vaccination of girls has been carried out in this country and pregnant women are screened so that those who are not immune can be offered vaccination in the postnatal period. Those working with women and their babies should also be screened and offered vaccination if needed.

Varicella

Varicella is chickenpox which is a highly infectious childhood illness transmitted by the respiratory droplet route. If it occurs in pregnancy adult respiratory distress syndrome (ARDS) may develop in the woman with a mortality rate of up to 35% (Arias 1993). Preterm labour and delivery or herpes zoster (shingles) are more common.

Varicella syndrome with developmental abnormalities may be present in the fetus if maternal infection occurred in the first trimester. This includes low birth weight, eye lesions, undeveloped limbs, skin scars and psychomotor retardation. Infection in the 3rd trimester may result in neonatal infection with pneumonitis, hepatitis and disseminated intravascular coagulation (clotting defect). Hyperimmune varicella zoster immune globulin (VZIG) can be offered to susceptible pregnant women who have been in contact with chickenpox or shingles. Lloyd & Lewis (1996) refer to the recommendation by Best & Banatvala (1990) for ultrasound monitoring of the fetus for limb and other external abnormalities. Prophylactic acyclovir can be given to susceptible neonates.

Cytomegalovirus (CMV)

This is one of the herpes group of viruses. Infection is commoner in lower socioeconomic groups and is usually asymptomatic. If the primary infection occurs during pregnancy, CMV may cause abortion, preterm labour, intrauterine growth retardation or fetal death. The greatest risk to the fetus is within the first 20 weeks of pregnancy. The virus may damage the fetal liver and nervous system and microcephaly may be present.

Toxoplasmosis

The causative organism is a protozoon, *Toxoplasma gondii*, found in dog and cat faeces and in uncooked meat. Infection is usually asymptomatic and will occur in one in 500 pregnant women. About 36% of their babies will be affected. Microcephaly, hydrocephalus and hepatosplenomegaly (enlarged liver and spleen) may occur. Screening in pregnancy with treatment by spiramycin could be offered. Blood may be taken from the umbilical cord and tested to see if the fetus is infected. Some women may consider termination of pregnancy.

Herpes simplex

The causative organism is type II *Herpesvirus hominis* or genital herpes. The baby is at risk if the woman has active lesions at the time of delivery and a caesarean section is usually performed. An infected baby may be seriously ill with generalised herpes infection, including septicaemia, and signs include a papular vesicular rash. The antiviral drug acyclovir can be used to treat an affected baby.

Listeriosis

Listeria monocytogenes is a bacterium found throughout the environment. It is a foodborne pathogen which may cause abortion, fetal disease or death. Cook-chill produce, in particular, has been implicated in the transmission of infection. Diagnosis in women or neonates is by culturing the organism from blood and/or cerebrospinal fluid and as it is susceptible to penicillin and erythromycin, large doses can be used to treat anyone with the disease. Health education on safe preparation of food would help to reduce the incidence of infection.

Hepatitis B (serum hepatitis)

The hepatitis B virus (HBV) is highly infectious and can be transmitted by blood, sexual intercourse and vertical transmission to the fetus. Virus particles are found in the blood and body fluids of those infected. Long-term infection can lead to chronic hepatitis, cirrhosis of the liver and liver cancer. It is more commonly carried in people from Asia, sub-Saharan Africa, the Caribbean, Central and South America and Alaska and immigrants from these regions have a one in 10 risk of carrying the virus against a background UK rate of 0.1%. The risk factors for HIV infection are shared by HBV.

Antenatal screening of all pregnant women is recommended so that the baby can be treated and anyone involved in the delivery can take sensible precautions. As with many viruses, the structure includes a central core carrying the genetic material, an outer envelope and an outer surface. This gives rise to three antigenic sites that can stimulate antibody production. The surface antigen (agglutinin) is referred to as **HBs Ag** (this used to be known as the Australia antigen), the envelope antigen as **Hbe Ag** and the core antigen as **HBc Ag**. The presence of Hbe Ag indicates that the disease is highly infectious and these women have a 25% probability of transmitting the virus to their babies (Arias 1993). If women are Hbe Ag positive or have had a late pregnancy infection their babies are given hepatitis B vaccine, the first dose within 24 h of birth and repeated at 1 and 6 months of age. This will protect the babies against the long-term dangers.

Summary of main points

- Optimal birth weight depends on an interaction between fetal growth potential and the intrauterine environment. This growth potential varies between races and individuals, creating a problem of diagnosis of intrauterine growth retardation. The classification of IUGR does not allow for fetuses that are small and healthy and may lead to inappropriate interference in pregnancy.
- In the antepartum and intrapartum periods of pregnancies complicated by IUGR, there is an increase in the number of stillbirths and cases of oligohydramnios and fetal distress. Complications in the neonatal period include meconium aspiration syndrome, persistent fetal circulation, hypoglycaemia, hypocalcaemia, hyperviscosity syndrome and poor temperature control.
- Fetal growth depends on interacting factors such as genetic determinants, general maternal health and nutrition, availability of growth substrates, the presence of fetal growth hormones and sufficient maternal blood supply to the placenta.
- Any decrease in the availability of substrates caused by pathological conditions affecting the mother, placenta or fetus will result in poor growth. Maternal conditions associated with poor fetal growth are pregnancy-induced hypertension, chronic renal disease, diabetes mellitus, sickle cell anaemia, severe cardiac disease, smoking and alcohol ingestion. Placental problems include small placental size, inadequate changes in the spiral arteries, placental infarcts and placenta praevia. Fetal causes of poor growth include chromosomal abnormalities, infections and multiple pregnancy.
- Maternal influences associated with a reduction in birth weight but preservation of body length include malnutrition and low weight gain in pregnancy but the malnutrition has to be fairly severe. Tobacco smoking decreases placental blood flow and leads to placental underperfusion. This reduction in blood flow reduces fetal nutrition, leading to fetal growth retardation. A more prolonged effect on fetal growth is the increase in carboxyhaemoglobin which causes a sustained reduction of oxygen to the fetus.
- Recently fetal alcohol syndrome (FAS) has been recognised, first in the USA and latterly in Britain. Alcohol is a low molecular weight substance and as such can cross the placental barrier and is a known teratogen.
- Placental changes, such as incomplete penetration by the trophoblastic cells of the spiral arteries, may be related to the presence and severity of maternal disease. The prevalence of genetic and chromosomal disorders amongst babies with IUGR is common, particularly in those with trisomies such as Down's syndrome. The majority of these have symmetric growth retardation.
- The first step in managing IUGR is to identify those women at risk. The second step is to differentiate the small healthy babies from those with genuine IUGR. The third step is to monitor the at-risk fetuses. Using a combination of clinical and ultrasound methods, a diagnosis should be possible in 95% of cases.
- Measurement of the amount of liquor amnii will demonstrate the presence of oligohydramnios, a late sign of fetal malnutrition, and can indicate the need to expedite delivery if used with Doppler assessment and non-stress cardiotocography.
- Neither serial oestriol estimation nor human placental assays have been shown to be of value in assessing placental function and fetal well-being. Fundal height measurements may not detect all cases of IUGR but do allow the referral of women to a consultant unit for ultrasonic screening. Monitoring daily fetal movements has also not been shown to be of value as a screening technique.
- Continuous cardiotocography in response to an oxytocin challenge (stress CTG) has no benefits and some problems. A similar test using nipple stimulation to induce contractions has proved to be so dangerous that its use is discontinued. Non-stress cardiotocography is used to detect the at-risk fetus. Intervention carried out inappropriately causes increased morbidity and mortality.
- Biophysical profiling combines five physiological variables – fetal movement, tone, reactivity, breathing movements and amniotic fluid volume. In the small number of studies reported, biophysical profile was a better predictive test than the non-stress test.
- Once fetal lung maturity is achieved and preferably after 34 weeks postfertilisation, the baby can be delivered. Every method should be used to avoid asphyxia. IUGR babies remain smaller than their age cohorts for several years. Some studies have reported an increased incidence of minimal brain dysfunction and speech defects whilst others have found no difference in outcome.

- If a mother is Rh– and the fetus Rh+, haemolysis of fetal red cells may occur. This rarely affects the first baby as there are no spontaneous anti-D antibodies present in a woman prior to her first pregnancy. Fetomaternal transfusion of blood at delivery will stimulate the production of maternal antibodies and memory cells which can mount a secondary response should the mother become pregnant with a second Rh+ baby.
- Other events in pregnancy before delivery which may lead to antibody formation because of a fetomaternal transfusion include abortion, amniocentesis, antepartum haemorrhage or conversion of a breech presentation to cephalic by a procedure known as external cephalic version.
- Haemolytic disease of the newborn is now largely preventable. Rhesus-positive blood should never be used in a transfusion if a woman's blood group is unknown. If an event likely to have caused a fetomaternal transfusion occurs, anti-D immunoglobulin (rhesus D antibodies) must be administered to the mother within 72 h.
- Every pregnant woman has her blood tested for ABO and rhesus types early in pregnancy. Any woman who proves to be rhesus negative will be screened for rhesus antibodies. If the test is negative her blood will be retested later, usually at 28 and 34 weeks of pregnancy.
- If antibodies are detected antenatally the titre will be checked. The level of antibodies indicates a more direct test on the amniotic fluid. The amount of bilirubin can be measured against a Liley chart which relates the level to the week of gestation and allows judgement to be made about the future management of the pregnancy.
- At delivery cord blood is taken for testing from all babies of rhesus-negative women for ABO and rhesus type, direct Coombes test and a haemoglobin estimation. If the mother is known to have rhesus antibodies the cord blood is also tested for serum bilirubin level. All babies whose mothers have rhesus antibodies should be transferred to a neonatal intensive care unit until the results of the tests on the cord blood are known and care planned.
- In ABO incompatibility the mother has unprovoked anti-A and anti-B antibodies even in the first pregnancy so the first child may be affected. IgG antibodies are produced that may cross the placenta and haemolyse fetal red cells. Although the jaundice appears in the first 24 h it is usually mild.
- Systemic infections may cause reproductive problems such as infertility and congenital defects if the woman is pregnant and some infections are specific to the genitourinary tract. In the vagina other organisms such as yeasts, streptococci and *E. coli* may be present in non-invasive numbers.
- Despite the alterations in the maternal immune system in pregnancy, most women are not immunocompromised. However, the suppression of cell-mediated immunity means that some infections may be more severe in pregnancy, especially viruses causing poliomyelitis, influenza and pneumococcal pneumonia. Pregnancy also leads to reactivation of latent cytomegalovirus (CMV) and herpes.
- Sexually transmitted diseases (STDs) are a major problem for society and their control constitutes a difficult public health concern. Untreated, these diseases can have serious long-term health consequences and pregnant women infected with a STD may pass the infection on to the fetus, resulting in birth defects or even stillbirth.
- The causative organism of gonorrhoea is easily killed outside the body so that the disease can only be transmitted by intimate bodily contact. Severe complications of this infection include pelvic inflammatory disease and damage to heart valves and joint tissues. The organism can cause severe ophthalmia in neonates. Most cases will still respond to penicillin but penicillin-resistant strains of the organism are evolving.
- Syphilis is more serious than gonorrhoea but better controlled as penicillin is very effective against the causative organism. The organism cannot enter the body unless there is a break in the skin or mucous membranes. The disease can be transmitted across the placenta to the fetus to cause congenital syphilis.
- The incidence of infection with *Chlamydia trachomatis*, which lives inside cells, greatly outnumbers infections with the other two organisms above. Contamination of the eyes of the neonate during birth may cause severe conjunctivitis and respiratory distress. Chlamydial infection is difficult to diagnose but is responsive to tetracycline or erythromycin.
- Infection with group B streptococcus is asymptomatic in women and the organism is most often responsible for overwhelming sepsis with a high mortality rate in neonates. Screening and treatment of women are difficult because of the recurrence of the infection but screening and giving antibodies to women with preterm rupture of the membranes may be useful.
- The transmission of the HIV virus is associated with sexual activity where skin or mucous membrane integrity is broken. Promiscuity is a key factor in the spread of the disease, as is blood contamination by needles shared by drug addicts or (in the past in certain countries) in mass vaccinations.
- Much political controversy surfaced in June 1996 about the true nature of pathways of infection in Britain. Concern has been expressed about the publicity surrounding the risks to the heterosexual population. It is now thought that there are as few as 161 heterosexual people not exposed to any known AIDS risk out of a total of 12 565 diagnosed cases of AIDS since 1982.
- A very different picture is reported for Africa. Evidence for a heterosexual AIDS epidemic in sub-Saharan Africa is convincing and one factor supporting this belief is that anal intercourse, a high-risk behaviour, is believed to be related to witchcraft and is almost completely suppressed in this part of the world.
- Women who are HIV positive may pass the virus across the placenta to affect their unborn child or the baby may be infected by contact with maternal blood during birth. A third way of transmission is through breastfeeding. There may be protection against vertical transmission if the baby is delivered by caesarean section.
- TORCH is derived from the first letters of a series of infections that can cross the placenta to affect the fetus. These are Toxoplasmosis, Others, Rubella, Cytomegalovirus and Herpes. Most of these infections will cause congenital abnormality if acquired in the first trimester and neonatal infection, often affecting the lung, liver, spleen and brain, if acquired late in pregnancy.
- *Listeria monocytogenes* is a foodborne pathogen which may cause abortion, fetal disease or death. Cook-chill produce in particular has been implicated in the transmission of infection.
- The hepatitis B virus is highly infectious and transmitted by blood, sexual intercourse and vertical transmission to the fetus. Long-term infection can lead to chronic hepatitis, cirrhosis of the liver and liver cancer. It is more commonly carried in people from Asia, sub-Saharan Africa, the Caribbean, Central and South America and Alaska. Antenatal screening of all pregnant women ensures that the baby can be treated and anyone involved in the delivery can take precautions.

References

American College of Obstetricians and Gynecologists. 1987 Prevention of HIV Infection and AIDS. ACOG, Washington.

Arias F. 1993 Practical Guide to High Risk Pregnancy and Delivery. Mosby Year book, Chicago.

Barker DJP. (ed) 1992 Fetal and Infant Origins of Adult Disease. BMJ Books, London.

Bennett VR, Brown LK. (eds) 1996 Myles Textbook for midwives. Churchill Livingstone, Edinburgh.

Best R, Banatuala JT. 1990 Congenital virus infections British Medical Journal, 300: 1151–1152.

Blackburn ST, Loper DL. 1992 Maternal, Fetal and Neonatal Physiology – A Clinical Perspective. WB Saunders, Philadelphia.

Brock TD, Madigan MT. 1991 Biology of Microorganisms, 6th edn. Prentice-Hall, New Jersey.

Brown P. 1992 How does HIV infect babies in the womb? New Scientist 133(1816) 20.

Brunham RC, Holmes KK, Embree JE. 1990 Sexually transmitted diseases in pregnancy. In Holmes KK, Mardh PA, Sparling PF et al (eds) Sexually Transmitted Diseases, 2nd edn. McGraw-Hill, New York.

Caldwell JC, Caldwell P. 1996 The African AIDS epidemic. Scientific American 274(3) 40–49.

Enkin M, Keirse MJNC, Renfrew M, Neilson J. 1996 A Guide to Effective Care in Pregnancy and Childbirth, 2nd edn. Oxford University Press, Oxford.

European Collaborative Study. 1991 Children born to women with HIV-1 infection: natural history and risk of transmission. Lancet 337, 3253–3258.

Grimes DE, Grimes RM. 1994 AIDS and HIV Infection. Mosby Chicago.

Hofmeyr GJ. 1997 Prophylactic versus therapeutic amnioinfusion for intrapartum oligohydramnios. In Neilson LJP, Crowther CA, Hodnett ED, Hofmeyr GJ, Keirse MJNC (eds) Pregnancy and Childbirth module of the Cochrane Database of Systematic Reviews, The Cochrane Library. Update Software, Oxford.

Kelly J, Mathews KA, O'Conor M. 1984 Smoking during pregnancy: effects on mother and the fetus. British Journal of Obstetrics and Gynaecology 95, 111–117.

Lloyd C, Lewis V. 1996 Diseases associated with pregnancy. In Bennett VR, Brown LK. 1996 Myles Textbook for Midwives. Churchill Livingstone, Edinburgh.

Longo LD. 1977 The biological effects of carbon monoxide on the pregnant woman. fetus and newborn infant. American Journal of Obstetrics and Gynecology 129, 69–103.

Roth C. 1996 Genital and sexually transmitted infections in pregnancy. In Bennett VR, Brown, LK. 1996 Myles Textbook for Midwives. Churchill Livingstone, Edinburgh, pp 284–305.

Sweet B. 1997 Mayes' Midwifery Baillière Tindall, London.

Tanner JM. 1978 Foetus into Man. Open Books, London.

Wallis S, Harvey D. 1979 Intensive care of the newborn 3; Disorders in the Newborn 1, Nursing Times, 75(31): 1319–1327.

Wang E, Smaill F. 1989 Infection in pregnancy. In Chalmers I, Enkin M, Keirse MJNC (eds) A Guide to Effective Care in Pregnancy and Childbirth. Oxford University Press, Oxford.

Recommended reading

Blaney CL. 1994 Pregnancy and HIV. Network 14(3), 24–26.

Christie IL, Wolfe CDA, Kennedy J et al. 1995 Voluntary named testing for HIV in a community based antenatal clinic: a pilot study. British Medical Journal 311, 928–931.

Greenhough A, Osborne J, Sutherland S. (eds) 1992 Congenital, Perinatal and Neonatal Infections. Churchill Livingstone, Edinburgh.

McDonald M. 1992 Rhesus incompatibility. Nursing Times 88(19), 42–44.

Meadows J, Catalon J, Gazzard B. 1993 HIV antibody testing in the antenatal clinic: the views of consumers. Midwifery 9(2), 63–69.

Nicoll A, Moisley C. 1994 Antenatal screening for syphilis. British Medical Journal 308, 1253–1254.

Squires K. 1994 HIV infection in women. Journal of Women's Health 3 (5), 383–386.

WHO. 1995 HIV and AIDS in pregnancy. Safe Motherhood 16, 4–8.

Chapter 15 Congenital defects

In this chapter

INTRODUCTION

'Embryology illuminates anatomy and explains how defects develop' (Moore 1989). This chapter is about the causes of congenital defects which are present at birth. They may be visible to the naked eye and involve obvious changes in organs or may be hidden, such as changes in the protein molecules, enzymes, cell receptors or haemoglobin. O'Shea (1995) outlines the terminology used to describe congenital defects as follows.

- A **defect** is a primary aberration in the zygote and is programmed to lead to abnormal development regardless of environmental influences.
- **Disruption** refers to destruction of normally developing tissue by some outside influence such as drug-related defects.
- **Deformation** is the term used for alterations in the development of normal tissues and organs by physical forces, such as occurs in oligohydramnios.
- **Dysplasia** describes abnormal differentiation or organisation of tissues.

Congenital defects now account for most severe illness during infancy and childhood and 25% of childhood deaths. A defect is present in about 2% of liveborn infants but some of them are minor and of no functional significance. Other major problems are incompatible with life and result in early abortion. Recent genetic research shows that some of the diseases that afflict people as they grow older, such as heart disease, hypertension or diabetes, may occur because of structural or functional changes in the embryo and fetus (Barker 1992). General causes of abnormality will be outlined and the more commonly seen defects discussed system by system. Many disorders may be diagnosed by screening techniques and the role of screening technology will be examined.

GENERAL CAUSES OF CONGENITAL DEFECTS

The causes of congenital defects fall into four main groups (O'Shea 1995).

1 Genetic/chromosomal abnormalities.
2 Environmental influences which may be intrauterine or extrauterine.
3 Multifactorial disorders caused by the interaction of environmental effects with genetic inheritance, including neural tube defects and congenital heart disease.
4 Idiopathic defects with no known cause, the largest group.

Teratogens

From the 3rd to the 8th weeks, during organogenesis, the embryo is vulnerable to disruption of development by environmental factors such as radiation, viruses and drugs. These teratogens interfere with different levels of embryogenesis and may affect proliferation, migration or differentiation of cells (Fitzgerald & Fitzgerald 1994):

1 If they occur during the first 17 days, in the pre-differentiation period when cells are proliferating and the three germ layers are being formed, they are usually fatal.
2 During the rest of the embryonic period survival with major defects is likely.
3 During the fetal period following the completion of organogenesis, the effect of teratogens is greatly reduced except in the brain where differentiation is still continuing.
4 Environmental factors usually act together with genetic factors. The genetic mistake predisposes towards defects but the environmental factor is needed to cause the fault.
5 Some teratogens interfere with cell division by affecting nucleic acid synthesis. Others interfere with cell migration or with the synthesis of cell products.

GENETIC DISORDERS

Before considering the nature of genetic disorders, it is worth revising concepts discussed in Chapter 2. The nucleus of every cell contains **deoxyribonucleic acid** (DNA) arranged on 23 pairs of chromosomes. One of each pair originates with the maternal ovum and the other with the paternal sperm. In 22 of the pairs, the chromosomes are identical and these pairs are called **autosomes**. The 23rd pair are the **sex chromosomes**. In the majority of cases (there are exceptions), two X chromosomes are present in females whilst in males an X and a Y chromosome are present.

Each individual has unique DNA unless they happen to have an identical twin and the full complement of DNA is called the **genome**. DNA is arranged in discrete segments called **genes**. Each gene is present at a specific place, called a **locus**, on a pair of chromosomes. Genes can still carry out their function if there are minor differences in the **nucleotides** adenine, cytosine, guanine and thymine (A, C, G and T). These variants of a gene are called **alleles** and there are two alleles present at each locus. Sometimes both parents contribute an identical allele for a locus and the new individual is said to be **homozygous** for that gene. If the two alleles are slightly different the person is **heterozygous**.

Protein code

The role of a gene is to provide the code for a specific body **protein** and there are many tens of thousands of genes. Proteins

First base of codon	Second base of codon: U		C		A		G		Third base of codon
U	UUU	Phenylalanine	UCU	Serine	UAU	Tyrosine	UGU	Cysteine	U
	UUC		UCC		UAC		UGC		C
	UUA	Leucine	UCA		UAA	Terminate	UGA	Terminate	A
	UUG		UCG		UAG		UGG	Tryptophan	G
C	CUU	Leucine	CCU	Proline	CAU	Histidine	CGU	Arginine	U
	CUC		CCC		CAC		CGC		C
	CUA		CCA		CAA	Glutamine	CGA		A
	CUG		CCG		CAG		CGG		G
A	AUU	Isoleucine	ACU	Threonine	AAU	Asparagine	AGU	Serine	U
	AUC		ACC		AAC		AGC		C
	AUA		ACA		AAA	Lysine	AGA	Arginine	A
	AUG	Methionine + initiate	ACG		AAG		AGG		G
G	GUU	Valine + initiate	GCU	Alanine	GAU	Aspartic acid	GGU	Glycine	U
	GUC		GCC		GAC		GGC		C
	GUA		GCA		GAA	Glutamic acid	GGA		A
	GUG		GCG		GAG		GGG		G

Figure 15.1 *Messenger RNA (m-RNA) code words (from Hinchliff SM, Montague SE, 1990, with permission).*

are made up of **amino acids** put together in a specific order determined by the sequence of nucleotides on the gene (Fig. 15.1). A group of three nucleotides called a **codon** spells out each amino acid and the sequence of amino acids makes the particular shape of the protein (Fig. 15.2). Slight differences in a protein brought about by a genetic **mutation** may cause few problems but some changes may lead to devastating diseases such as sickle cell disease or cystic fibrosis by their biochemical influences on cells and tissues. DNA may be involved at the level of the chromosome or at the level of the gene, with mutations leading to abnormal development. Genetic factors are responsible for most of the congenital abnormalities seen. About 50% of spontaneous abortions result from chromosomal defects, such as non-dysjunction during oogenesis.

Mutations

A mutation is an 'alteration in the arrangement or amount of genetic material in a cell' (Abercrombie et al 1992). Mutations can be classified as **point mutations** involving minor changes in DNA such as a simple substitution of one base or **macromutations** involving deletions of large amounts of a chromosome. Mutations occasionally lead to an improvement in development on an evolutionary scale but in the short term they are more likely to result in defects which are harmful and lethal. Point mutations cause amino acid substitutions in protein products, leading to specific functional defects. Macromutations acting at chromosomal level lead to syndromes with multiple effects, often including mental retardation.

Point mutations may occur when a single base is substituted but other events may disrupt the sequences of base pairs on a gene, leading to faulty protein synthesis and disrupted gene function. **Nonsense mutations** involve the creation of a stop codon in an abnormal situation so that the broken gene does not code for a protein product. Additions or deletions of a nucleotide are called **frameshift mutations** and will alter the reading frame of the DNA to the left or right of normal.

Patterns of inheritance

About 8% of congenital defects result from genetic defects brought about by mutations. Genes coding for defects of

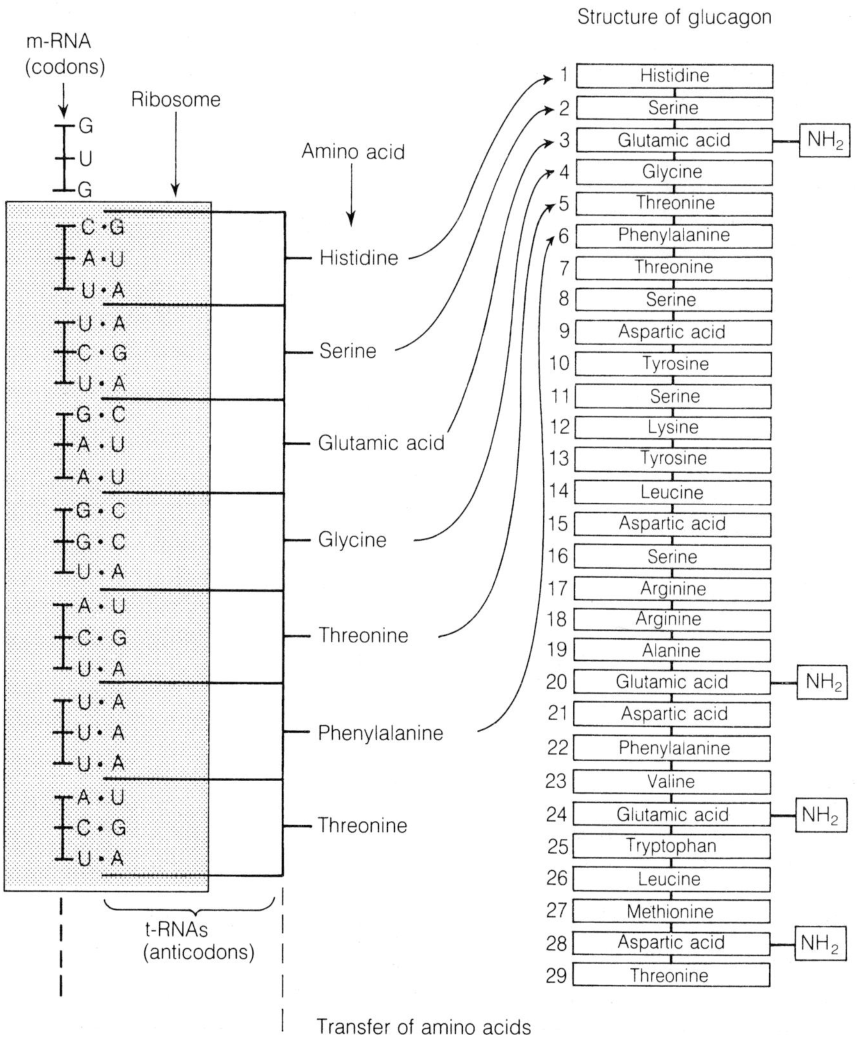

Figure 15.2 *An example of protein synthesis: glucagon (from Hinchliff SM, Montague SE, 1990, with permission).*

structure or function may be present on autosomes or sex chromosomes. They may be inherited as recessive, dominant or sex-linked genes (Figs 15.3–15.5). The terms dominant and recessive were coined by Mendel. A dominant allele manifests its effects in heterozygotes; where there are two different variations of the allele, only one copy is needed to affect the phenotype. Therefore, except in cases of new mutation, every affected child has one affected parent and there is a one in two chance of siblings inheriting the disorder.

A recessive allele only affects the **phenotype** (body appearance) when the individual is homozygous for that allele as two identical copies are necessary to produce the effect. However, there may be no family history if new mutations have occurred in the gametes of one or other parent. People with one copy of the abnormal allele show no symptoms and are said to be **carriers**. The children of two carriers will have a one in four chance of having an affected child and a one in two chance of a child carrying the disorder.

As in all genes, mutant genes are inherited according to Mendel's two laws of inheritance.

1 Genes segregate so that members of the same pair of genes, i.e. the alleles, are never present in the same gamete.
2 Genes assort independently, members of different pairs of genes moving to gametes independently of each other.

Weatherall (1991) puts this succinctly as 'Alleles segregate; non-alleles assort'. The simplicity of these laws means that the likelihood of a child inheriting a disorder can be predicted in many cases. However, genes are often inherited together. If two genes are on the same chromosome situated closely together they may be inherited together. Such genes are said to be **linked**. Parental chromosomes become closely apposed during

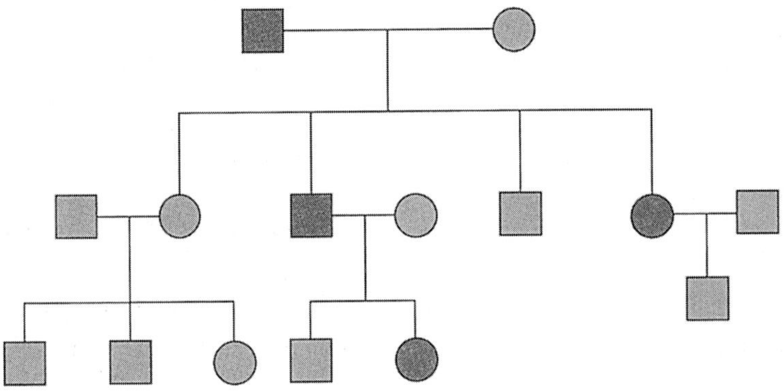

Figure 15.3 *An autosomal dominant pedigree (from Sweet B, 1997, with permission).*

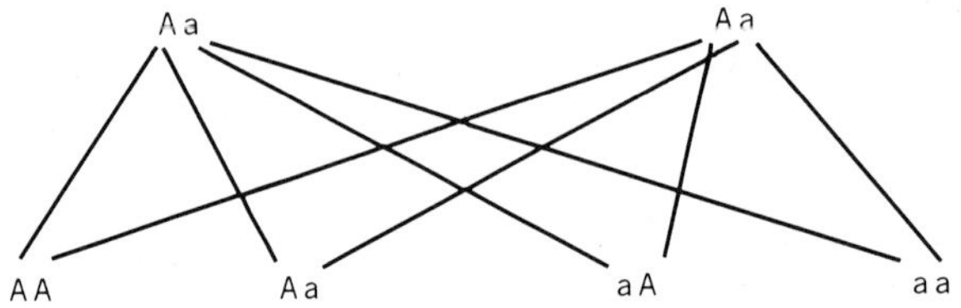

Figure 15.4 *In an autosomal recessive disorder, the disease is only manifest if both members of a pair of chromosomes are abnormal. If both parents are carriers of the abnormal gene (a), then there is a one in four chance that a child will have the disease (from Sweet B, 1997, with permission).*

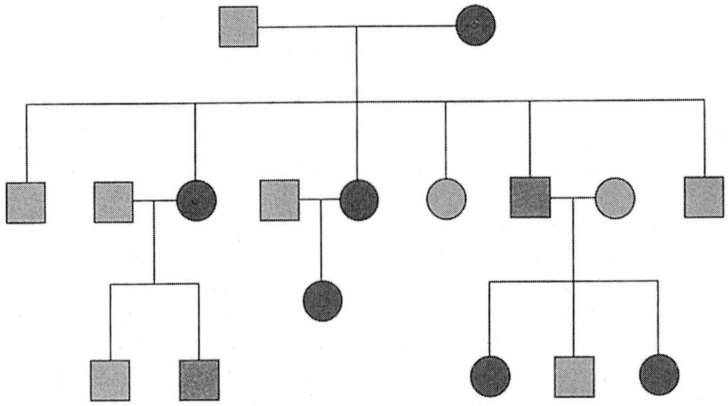

Figure 15.5 *An X-linked pedigree (from Sweet B, 1997, with permission).*

Table 15.1 *Disorders of systems caused by dominant genes*

System	Disorder
Nervous	Huntington's disease
	Neurofibromatosis
Bowel	Polyposis coli
Kidney	Polycystic disease
Eyes	Blindness
Ears	Deafness
Blood	Hypercholesterolaemia
Skeleton	Osteogenesis imperfecta
	Marfan's syndrome
	Achondroplasia
Metabolism	Acute intermittent porphyria

Table 15.2 *Some recessively inherited conditions*

System	Disorder
Metabolism	Cystic fibrosis
	Phenylketonuria
	Tay-Sachs disease
	Galactosaemia
Nervous	Neurogenic muscular atrophies
	Friedreich's ataxia
Blood	Sickle cell anaemia
	β-thalassaemia
Endocrine	Adrenal hyperplasia
Ears	Congenital deafness
Eyes	Recessive blindness

meiosis and crossing over of maternal and paternal genes may occur so that children inherit genes from both their grandparents.

Some inherited conditions

Inherited abnormal genes may affect all systems, as can be seen below. Some genes are **pleiotropic** and have a 'knock-on' effect, that is, an abnormality in the gene product may act as the basis for multiple system effects. For instance, an abnormal gene leads to phenylketonuria, where there is absence of an enzyme that metabolises the amino acid phenylalanine to tyrosine. This causes a build-up of the amino acid in fatty tissue which affects the brain cells. It also causes low tyrosine levels with lack of pigment in hair, skin and eyes because of reduced production of the pigment melanin.

The X chromosome carries a large number of genes involved in many aspects of development and function (Weatherall 1991). Males only have one X chromosome and are therefore **hemizygous** for X chromosome genes. If there is an abnormal X chromosome gene boys will be affected by an X-linked disorder (Table 15.3). Females are usually heterozygous for the X chromosome and will not be affected because of their normal allele. They will be asymptomatic carriers. However, in the rare case of homozygosity, females will be affected. This occurs in a girl born to an affected man and a carrier woman.

An important factor in the inheritance of X chromosomes is the random inactivation of one or other X chromosomes in cells, which occurs early in embryonic life. The descendants of the early cells retain the same activated X chromosome so that half the cells of a female will contain one activated X chromosome and half the other. If there is an abnormal gene carried on either the maternal or paternal X chromosome, the female will be heterozygous for the abnormality; she is a **mosaic** of half abnormal and half normal cells. This effect is called **lyonisation** after its discoverer, Mary Lyon.

Table 15.3 *Some X-linked disorders*

System	Disorder
Locomotor	Duchenne muscular dystrophy
Blood	Haemophilia
Skin	Ichthyosis
Brain	Fragile X syndrome
Eye	Childhood blindness

Most inherited disorders are due to genes on the chromosomes in the cell nucleus. There are also genes in the form of mitochondrial DNA which is inherited only from the mother. Some genetic disorders have been found due to mutations in the mitochondrial DNA. A few disorders, which will not be discussed, are due to abnormal genes on the Y chromosome.

Chromosomal defects

Chromosomal defects may be present in 6% of all zygotes, many of which never implant. Those that do implant will be lost in the first 3 weeks following fertilisation. Chromosomes are subject to two kinds of changes, numerical and structural. The changes may affect the autosomes or sex chromosomes. People with chromosomal defects usually have easily recognisable and characteristic phenotypes. Down's syndrome is an example where the typical features are stronger than family characteristics so that affected children are more similar to each other than to family members.

Numerical chromosomal defects

Human chromosomes are in 23 pairs; 22 of these are alike and are called autosomes and the other pair are the sex chromosomes, XX for a normal female and XY for a normal male. Many of these defects in number arise during failure of **dysjunction**, which is an error in cell division where sister chromatids fail to separate at anaphase. This may occur during meiosis 1, meiosis 2 or during mitosis. The resulting number of chromosomes may be too many or too few.

Polyploidy means the presence of multiples of the normal haploid number of 23 chromosomes. **Triploidy**, the presence of 69 chromosomes, may occur because the chromosomes of the second polar body are not ejected from the ovum or because of the entry of two sperms into the ovum. Triploidy occurs in about 2% of fertilisations, most of them lost early in development.

Monosomy is when one of the chromosomes of a pair is missing so that the chromosomes number 45. This is only compatible with survival if the missing chromosome is a sex chromosome. Survivors have one X chromosome and the syndrome is called Turner's syndrome.

Trisomy is the presence of an extra chromosome. The usual cause is non-dysjunction (see below) so that either the ovum or sperm carries 24 chromosomes instead of 23. At fertilisation the zygote has 47 chromosomes in its cells. The most common condition seen is Down's syndrome where there are three copies of chromosome 21 (see below). Non-dysjunction occurs with increasing frequency as maternal age increases.

Trisomy of the sex chromosomes is quite common and XXX females (triple X) or XXY males (Klinefelter's syndrome) occur. There are also XYY males. There may be **tetrasomy** (four copies) of the X chromosome or even **pentasomy** (five copies). Commonly, mental retardation is associated with increases in sex chromosomes and the greater the number of X chromosomes present, the more severe is the mental retardation.

Mosaicism results when the zygote develops into an individual with two genotypes or cell lines. The condition arises due to non-dysjunction during early mitosis. The defects seen in full monosomic or trisomic disorders are less serious in mosaicism.

Structural chromosomal defects

Environmental factors may induce breaks in chromosomes (see below). Structural rearrangements may also be called macromutations and two of these, inversion and translocation, are likely to be transmitted from parent to child.

Translocation is the transfer of a piece of one chromosome to another non-homologous chromosome. This may be a reciprocal translocation with the two non-homologous chromosomes exchanging pieces. If the translocation is balanced so that the individual receives the normal complement of chromosomal material, there will be no abnormality. However, if the translocation results in extra chromosomal material the abnormality will occur. It is estimated that about 4% of people with Down's syndrome receive their 3rd chromosome 21 attached to another chromosome in a translocation, often chromosome 14 or 15.

Deletion is the loss of part of a chromosome which sometimes follows a break. Loss of the termination of a chromosome number 5 causes a syndrome called cri du chat where affected infants have a weak, cat-like cry, microcephaly, heart defects and mental retardation. A **ring chromosome** is a special type of deletion where both ends have been lost and the broken ends have rejoined to form the ring shape.

Duplication is where a section of a chromosome is repeated, either within a chromosome, attached to another chromosome or as a separate fragment. These are less harmful as there is no loss of chromosome material.

If a segment of a chromosome breaks free and becomes reattached in the reverse position, **inversion** defects may occur. Paracentric inversion involves just one arm of the chromosome whilst pericentric inversion involves both arms and includes the centromere.

In the case of **isochromosome**, the centromere may divide horizontally instead of longitudinally and this appears to occur most often in the X chromosome. Loss of the short arm of the X chromosome, which may follow this type of break, is associated with features of Turner's syndrome.

Molecular genetics

The science of molecular genetics is a fairly recent development. Although the structure of the gene was identified by Watson & Crick (1953), most of the research has taken place since the late 1970s. The history of the development of molecular genetics is told by Bishop & Waldholz (1990). The human genome project has led to identification of many genetic func-tions. Recent developments in gene technology have promised a new type of medicine but have also brought moral and ethical dilemmas. Anxieties about eugenics (Horgan 1993), a concept often misused since Darwin's days when the term was invented by Darwin's cousin Francis Galton, are again prominent. These anxieties raise important questions about the application of genetic engineering to diagnosis and treatment of genetic diseases.

Detection of abnormality

Cell samples can be encouraged to divide in synchrony. The process is then stopped during mitosis and a photograph is taken. The chromosome images are cut out, laid in order and then photographed again to produce a **karyotype** (Fig. 15.6). Chromosomes are identified by their size, banding patterns and the position of the centromere. Gross defects in the chromosomes can be seen (Fig. 15.7). Single gene defects where the identity of the gene is known can be found by using **gene probes**, commercially available synthetic sections of DNA which are attracted to the appropriate gene and can even identify single base changes if present.

Genetic engineering

Genetic engineering techniques allow the removal of a gene from one cell and its insertion into another (Moore 1993). When the gene enters the new cell it may change the way the cell works or the chemicals that the cell secretes. Applications include medical cures, increased food production, crime detection, lessening of pollution and better energy production. The medical applications include preimplantation genetic screening for disease and the sex of the embryo, fetal screening, screening of adults and targeted gene replacement as therapy. Over 5000 human disorders have been attributable to gene defects (Capecchi 1994). Non-therapeutic uses such as selecting attributes for a child or, as has recently been in the news, cloning of a person may present ethical problems as the techniques become more widespread.

ENVIRONMENTAL AND GENETIC INTERACTION

The rate of new mutations can be increased by environmental factors such as genetic, microbial, biochemical, dietary factors, and radiation and many chemicals (Ward 1995). These may interfere with embryonic development at very precise times during organogenesis. Some factors such as the effect of the Rubella virus are easily associated but other, more vague issues such as atmospheric pollutants may be more difficult to ascertain. This interaction is discussed in depth in Chapter 7 but the following section will remind the reader of the main concepts.

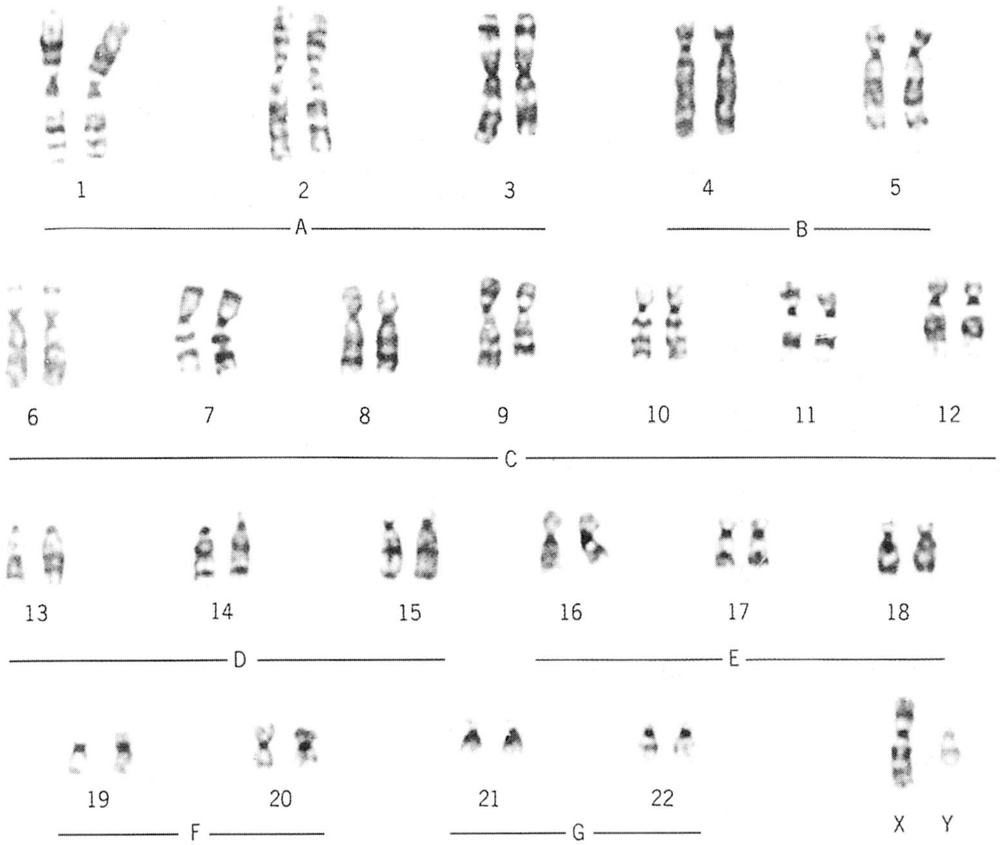

Figure 15.6 *A normal karyotype (from Sweet B, 1997, with permission).*

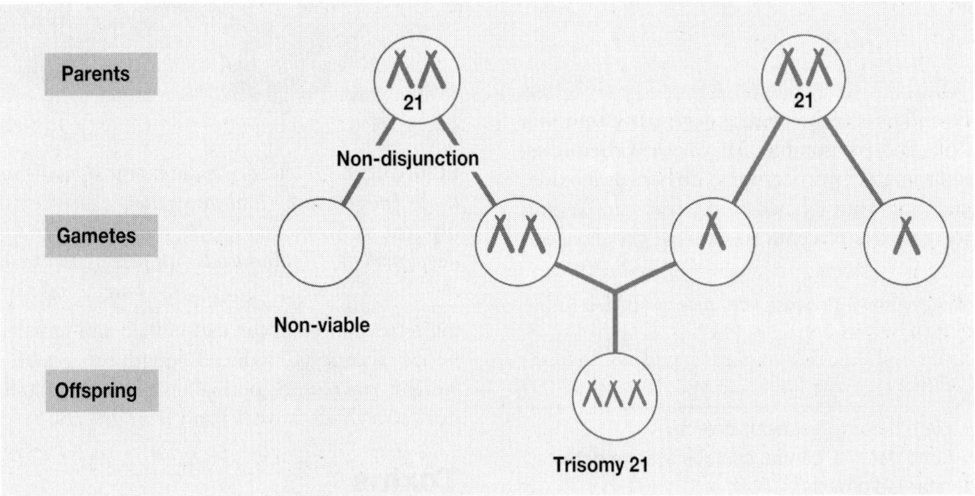

Figure 15.7 *Non-dysjunction of chromosome 21 leading to Down's syndrome (from Hinchliff SM, Montague SE, Watson R, 1996, with permission).*

Infection

Infections causing congenital defects are nearly always viral.

- **Rubella** is a childhood infection and usually insignificant in the adult. The virus crosses the placenta to inhibit cell division, particularly in eyes, ears, heart and brain.
- ***Listeria monocytogenes*** is a bacillus that may cause meningitis and serious respiratory disease in newborn infants.
- **Cytomegalovirus** (CMV) belongs to the herpes virus group. In pregnancy infection with CMV may cause spontaneous abortion, preterm labour, intrauterine growth retardation or fetal death. In the neonate hepatic and neurological damage including microcephaly may occur and respiratory difficulty may be present.

- **Toxoplasmosis** infection is caused by the protozoon *Toxoplasma gondii* which may be found in dog or cat faeces. Maternal infection is usually asymptomatic and one in 500 pregnant women may acquire toxoplasmosis with about one in 1500 babies affected. Typical effects on the baby are microcephaly, hydrocephalus and hepatosplenomegaly.
- Other infections that may be transmitted from mother to neonate during the birth include **herpes simplex, hepatitis B** (which can lead to permanent carriage and later, as an adult, to development of liver cancer), ***Candida albicans*** and the **β haemolytic streptococcus group B**.

Drugs

Medical drugs may be dispensed by practitioners or over the counter from chemist shops. Many drugs taken for minor problems such as pain relief and indigestion are purchased by people without their doctor's knowledge. Drugs may damage gametes or they may have an adverse effect on nutrient absorption so that essential nutrients are absent at crucial times.

The most famous example was thalidomide, a drug taken for morning sickness in the early 1960s which caused major limb reduction deformities as well as other problems. The effects of taking thalidomide in early pregnancy (Fig. 15.8) are still seen in South America where the drug is prescribed for leprosy. Although the drug is not prescribed for pregnant women there is an ongoing problem of lay people offering friends and relatives their drugs. Inevitably some who take drugs in this way will be pregnant. The effect of a drug may be delayed and not show itself for a generation. A further worry is the amount of drugs and environmental pollutants that reach new babies via their mothers' breast milk.

Smoking

Nicotine is addictive and affects the central nervous system in a way that many people find pleasurable. Many other chemicals, including polycyclic aromatic hydrocarbons, carbon monoxide, cyanide, lead and cadmium, are inhaled in cigarette smoke and have been shown to cross the placenta to damage the developing fetus. Smoking can cause male and female infertility, spontaneous abortions, reduced length of gestation and low birth weight, increased perinatal mortality (stillbirths + neonatal deaths in the first week) and fetal defects.

Table 15.4 *Some drugs known to cause fetal defects (BMA/RPS 1990)*

Drug	*Effect*
Thalidomide	Limb deformities, heart defects
Warfarin	Limb defects, central nervous system defects, retarded growth
Corticosteroids	Cleft palate and congenital cataract
Anticonvulsants such as phenytoin	Lip and palate deformities, mental retardation
Androgens	Masculinisation in female fetus
Oestrogens	Testicular atrophy in male
Stilboestrol	Vaginal and cervical cancer at puberty
Cytotoxic drugs (especially folic acid antagonists)	Neural tube defects, cleft palate
Tetracycline	Staining of bones and teeth, thin tooth enamel, impaired bone growth

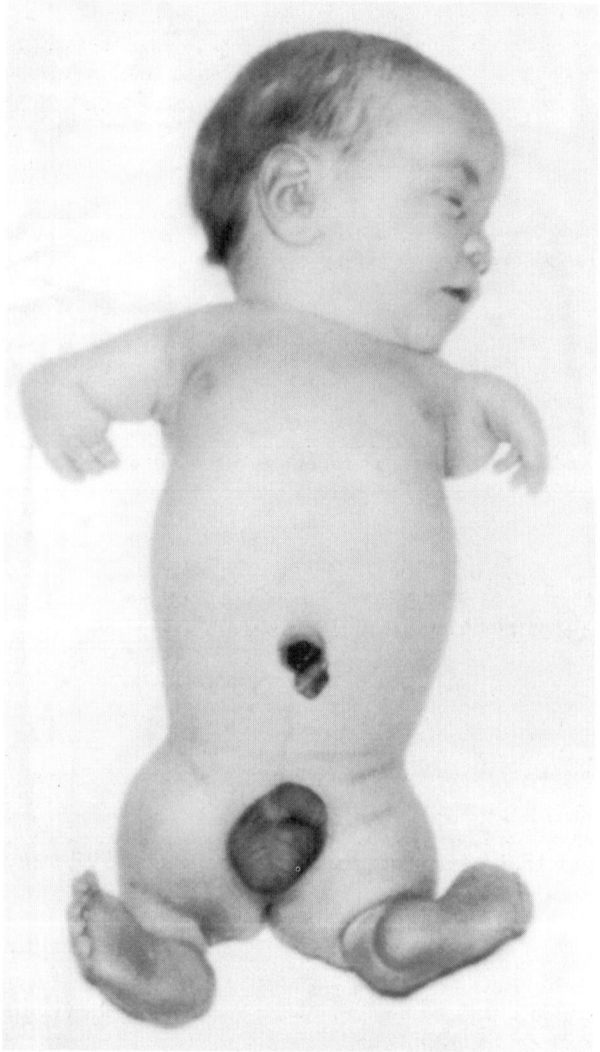

Figure 15.8 *Newborn male infant showing typical malformed limbs (meromelia – limb reduction) caused by thalidomide ingested by his mother during the critical period of limb development. (Reproduced with permission from Moore 1963.)*

Toxins

Toxins can be divided into natural and manufactured substances and form part of the ecological system in which humans live and reproduce. Natural toxins have been developed by plants as a defence against being eaten and examples include the tannins and alkaloids found in oak acorns. Some plants make cyanide as part of their defence system, including apple and apricot seeds, and whilst the sweet flesh is nutritious the seeds in quantity would be poisonous. The development of the chemical industry has resulted in the release into the environment of vast quantities of synthetic pollutants. DDT and polychlorinated biphenyls (PCBs) are just two of many.

Humans have developed defence systems against plant toxins by avoidance mediated by the senses of sight, smell and taste and ejection of toxin by diarrhoea and vomiting. The liver produces a wide range of enzymes which can render toxins harmless so that they can be excreted via the kidney. Cooking and food preparation can make some toxic substances safe to eat.

Radiation

Ionising radiation has the ability to damage DNA, the blueprint for cellular structure and activity, by transferring its energy into living cells (Jones 1996). Atoms lose electrons and develop an electric charge. These charged particles, known as **ions**, can penetrate the body and damage molecules to produce free radicals and oxidising agents. These substances break the DNA chain and destroy the genetic material.

PRENATAL SCREENING FOR CONGENITAL DEFECTS

In an ideal world prevention of congenital defects would be the aim. However, most women are seen for the first time when their pregnancy has already begun. Education and the offer of a preconception service will help to reduce the number of abnormal embryos conceived. Chamberlain (1991) believes that an antenatal service should 'aim at diagnosing congenital defects as early as possible'. The couple may then be offered the choice to terminate the pregnancy.

Any reader wishing to consider the 'human' side of prenatal screening should read Abramsky & Chapple (1994). In this book Turner writes about late pregnancy diagnosis of fetal abnormality and is concerned that medical technology has raced ahead with insufficient consideration given to the ethical, legal and emotional dilemmas raised by an increased ability to detect fetal defects. Couples may not want to terminate the pregnancy and early diagnosis offers them a chance to plan for any possible treatment of the baby after birth.

Screening for congenital defects developed from the detection of central nervous system defects and screening for chromosomal defects such as Down's syndrome. Many other defects can now be detected in specific populations. Techniques include ultrasonography, chorionic villus sampling, amniocentesis and maternal serum screening.

Ultrasound

Most women are offered an ultrasound scan (USS) in pregnancy. Chamberlain (1991) writes that the embryonic sac can be seen as early as 6 weeks following conception and that the embryo can be seen distinctly by 8 weeks. He states that ultrasound screening is probably best carried out at 18–20 weeks gestation so that an accurate fetal age can be confirmed, multiple pregnancy detected and congenital defects diagnosed. Proud (1996) comments that the indications for USS are controversial but that many obstetricians feel the advantages of routine scanning far outweigh the disadvantages. Proud lists the advantages and disadvantages and the author adds a few more.

Advantages

- It is a non-invasive technique.
- The mother requires minimal preparation.
- It provides instant information.
- Movements of the fetus can be seen.
- Parents feel pleased to have seen their baby's image.
- It can support clinical findings.

Disadvantages

- There may be long-term dangers to the fetus.
- Clinical expertise may decline and there may be overreliance on the ultrasound findings.
- Some practitioners have an impersonal approach compared to the midwife's examination.
- It is an expensive form of investigation with little proof of effectiveness.

Neilson (1997) reviewed the use of ultrasound in early pregnancy, finding 'no evidence that it improves substantive clinical outcomes. Where detection of fetal abnormality was a specific aim of the investigation, the number of terminations of pregnancy for fetal anomalies increased'. However, the fetal anomaly data were obtained from centres of excellence and not through routine screening which may be less effective at diagnosis depending on the skill of the scanner. Neilson concluded that pregnant women and their carers must decide whether the results of routine ultrasound screening justify the expense, adding that there is no clear evidence that ultrasound examination in pregnancy is harmful to the fetus.

How ultrasound works

Ultrasound imaging depends on the differences in structure between organs. Sound at a very high pitch is produced by a transducer. Because of its frequency, it travels in a narrow beam. When the transducer is placed on the body sound waves pass into the body until they reach a tissue, when they bounce back. The sound echoes are detected electronically and transmitted onto the screen as dots. The more dense the tissue, the stronger the echo and the whiter the visual display. Weaker echoes produce various shades of grey. Fluid-filled structures reflect no echoes, resulting in a black area.

Common defects diagnosed by ultrasound include:

- anencephaly, microcephaly and hydrocephaly;
- neural tube defects;
- gastrointestinal defects such as atresias and omphalocoele;
- renal tract anomalies such as renal agenesis and polycystic kidneys;
- body defects associated with chromosomal defects.

Obtaining fetal tissue for genetic testing

All invasive techniques carry a risk of infection, haemorrhage and fetal loss. The risks must be weighed against the likelihood of abnormality being present in the fetus. The cells obtained can be used for karyotyping for chromosomal errors such as Down's syndrome, genetic analysis using gene probes as in cystic fibrosis (Weatherall 1991) and sexing the embryo if there is a family history of X-linked disorders such as Duchenne muscular dystrophy. Enzyme assay for detection of an inborn error of metabolism is available in over 50% of disorders.

Amniocentesis

A sample of amniotic fluid is withdrawn from the amniotic cavity through a transabdominal needle. Ultrasound is used to locate and avoid the placenta. Until recently this procedure was not possible until 16 weeks because of insufficient liquor amnii. However, because of improvements in scanning, it can now be carried out between 9 and 13 weeks of pregnancy (Hanson et al 1992). A further problem lies in the culturing of desquamated cells. These may have to be cultured for up to 3 weeks before the chromosomes can be counted. There is a one in 200 chance that amniocentesis may cause a miscarriage and the long waiting period before results are available is distressing to the parents.

Chorionic villus sampling

Chorionic villus sampling (CVS) involves obtaining cells from the chorion frondosum by using a cannula or biopsy forceps under ultrasound guidance. CVS can be performed either transabdominally or transvaginally. This procedure can be carried out as early as 6 weeks but limb reduction defects have increased in such early CVS so it is usually carried out at 10 weeks. The cells are healthy and actively dividing so that results of karyotyping can be obtained quickly. The spontaneous abortion rate following chorionic villus sampling is higher than that following amniocentesis.

Cordocentesis

A needle is guided to the base of the umbilical cord using ultrasound visualisation and a sample of fetal blood withdrawn. This can be used to screen for blood disorders such as haemophilia and haemoglobinopathies, karyotyping for chromosome analysis, DNA analysis, testing for inborn errors of metabolism and assessment of anaemia in rhesus isoimmunisation.

Fetoscopy

An endoscope can be inserted transabdominally and the fetus visualised directly. The procedure is rarely performed and has been superseded by other techniques (Proud 1996). Fetal skin and liver biopsy have been carried out in this way but there is a fetal loss of up to 5% and preterm labour of up to 10%.

Maternal serum screening

This is carried out to search for the small amounts of maternal serum α-fetoprotein (MSAFP) present. Normal values of MSAFP have been assessed and are found to be highest in early pregnancy, decreasing as pregnancy advances. Multiple pregnancy, fetal death, open fetal defects such as spina bifida or exomphalos and Turner's syndrome associated with a cystic hygroma are associated with raised levels of MSAFP. Low MSAFP levels are associated with Down's syndrome if found witha low level of unconjugated oestriol and a high level of HCG. Following the finding of an abnormal level of MSAFP, the fetus can be examined by ultrasound and/or amniocentesis is carried out to check the AFP level.

Comparison of amniocentesis and CVS

Alfirevic et al (1997a) compared CVS with amniocentesis for prenatal diagnosis. They found that there were multiple problems with CVS, probably because it is technically more demanding for both obstetricians and cytogeneticists. The problems included:

- more sampling failures;
- multiple instrument insertions;
- repeated procedures;
- laboratory failures;
- maternal contamination;
- abnormal karyotypes;
- false-positive and false-negative results;
- higher pregnancy loss because of spontaneous abortion;
- increased stillbirths and neonatal deaths.

They concluded that 'Second trimester amniocentesis is safer than CVS and the benefits of earlier diagnosis by CVS must be set against its greater risks'. In a separate review Alfirevic et al (1997b) compared a technique of early amniocentesis (before 14 weeks) with CVS. They found that technical difficulties occurred more often with CVS but laboratory failure was more common in early amniocentesis. Pregnancy loss was also more common in the women allocated to the early amniocentesis group, with an increase in preterm deliveries. They stated that the numbers involved in the trials were too small to be reliable.

Bonner (1996) reported that fetal blood cells leak through the placenta into the maternal circulation. It may be possible in the future to use such cells 'to provide safe and reliable tests for genetic defects such as Down's syndrome'. However, it may be 10 years before the isolating of fetal cells from maternal blood becomes routine enough to provide a screening test.

EXAMPLES OF SOME DISORDERS

The following more common disorders have been selected to represent the major factors in the causation of congenital defects. Some of the implications for society brought about by modern technology will be introduced. A reader wishing to consider the social implications is advised to read Horgan (1993), who warned of the problems that arise when genetic testing followed by termination of affected pregnancies is taken to the extremes of eugenics. Rennie (1994) similarly writes about the effects of population screening for genetic diseases. They include:

- chromosomal disorder – Down's syndrome;
- dominant genetic disorder – Huntington's disease;
- recessive genetic disorder – cystic fibrosis and haemoglobinopathies are discussed in Chapter 28;
- X-linked genetic disorder – haemophilia;
- genetic predisposition with environmental trigger – neural tube defects;
- environmental disorder – rubella (German measles).

Down's syndrome

The natural incidence of Down's syndrome or trisomy 21 is about one in 800 births. Many more are conceived and even without action, three-quarters may be aborted spontaneously. The incidence increases with maternal age and can be as high as one in 40 (Simpson 1997). The main cause, about 95%, is non-dysjunction but translocation 14/21 may occur at any maternal age and is likely to be inherited.

The features of Down's syndrome are easily recognised and include:

- a small head with flattened occiput and a broad flat nose;
- a small mouth cavity with thick gum margins and protruding tongue;
- epicanthic folds;
- Brushfield's spots, which are white flecks seen in the iris;
- short hands with incurving little fingers;
- a single palmar crease;
- a wide deviation of the great toe with a plantar crease between the first and second toes;
- dry skin;
- hypotonic muscles.

Other features include heart defects, increased incidence of duodenal atresia, reduced intelligence, inadequate immune system and a tendency to develop leukaemia. By the age of 40 many Down's syndrome people develop Alzheimer's disease.

Detection of trisomy 21

The risk of a mother carrying a Down's syndrome baby can be estimated using the **Bart's triple test**, developed at St Bartholomew's Hospital. Low MSAFP levels are found with a low level of unconjugated oestriol and a high level of HCG. If the triple test reveals a high risk, karyotyping of the fetal chromosomes is carried out.

Other screening protocols being investigated include the measurement of an enzyme, urea-resistant neutrophil alkaline phosphatase (UR-NAP). This test may prove to be the single best marker for Down's syndrome but is not yet routinely available (Telfer 1997).

A number of ultrasound signs (markers) are significant in the confirmation of Down's syndrome. These are duodenal atresia, cardiac septal defects and thickened nuchal fold (neck). Increased nuchal translucency thickness is associated with chromosomal defects but is not a clear indicator of Down's syndrome.

Huntington's disease

Huntington's disease (HD), caused by a mutant dominant gene, occurs in about one in 2000 births. The gene called G8 was found in 1983, on the terminal band of the short arm of chromosome 4. It affects the basal ganglia and cerebral cortex, resulting in involuntary movements called chorea, which begin in the arms and face and eventually affect the whole body, and dementia with impaired memory and judgement. It affects all races and there is an average age of onset at 45 years. Onset is earlier if the gene is inherited on the paternal chromosome rather than the maternal but the mode is not understood. There is no treatment for halting or even delaying symptoms. Death occurs from cerebral degeneration after 15–20 years.

The onset of HD is delayed until an affected person has already had their own children and might even have grand-

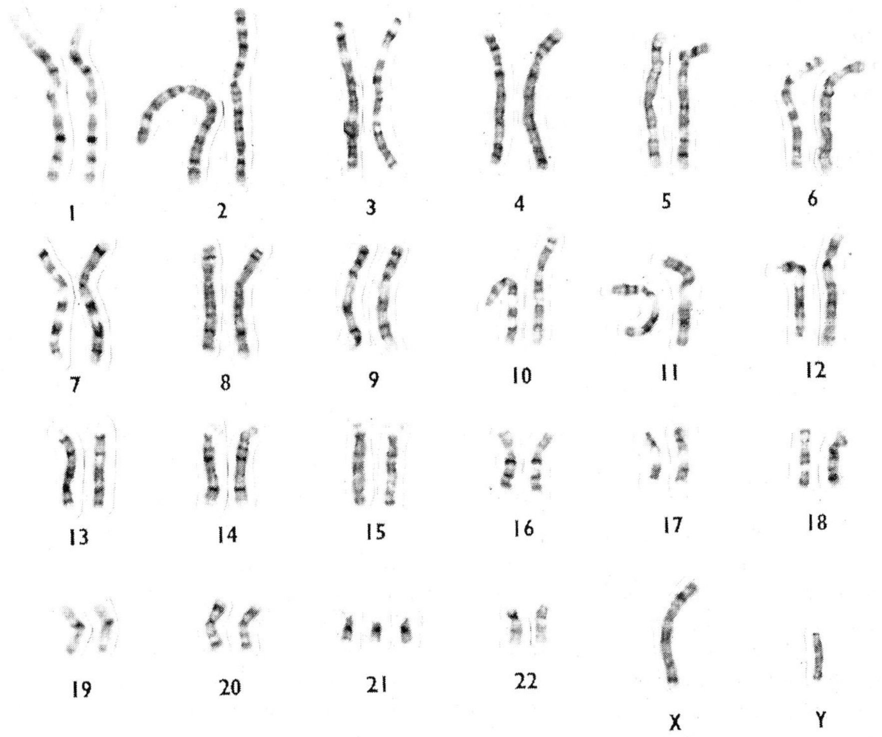

Figure 15.9 *A branded karyotype of Down's syndrome (trisomy 21) (from Kelnar C, Harvey D, Simpson C, 1995, with permission).*

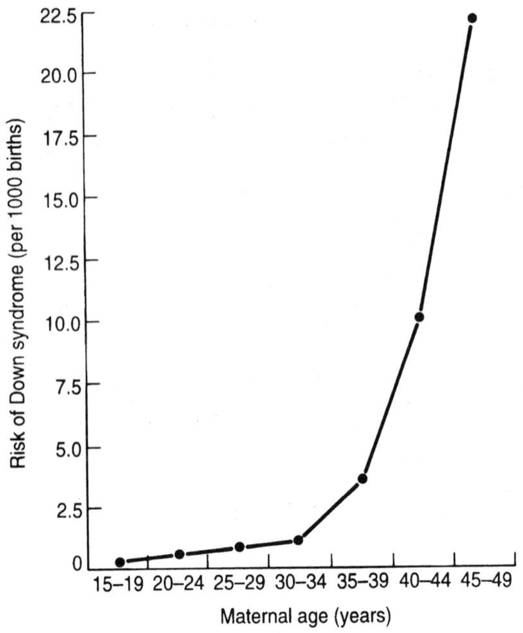

Figure 15.10 *The risk of Down's syndrome at different maternal ages (from Kelnar C, Harvey D, Simpson C, 1995, with permission).*

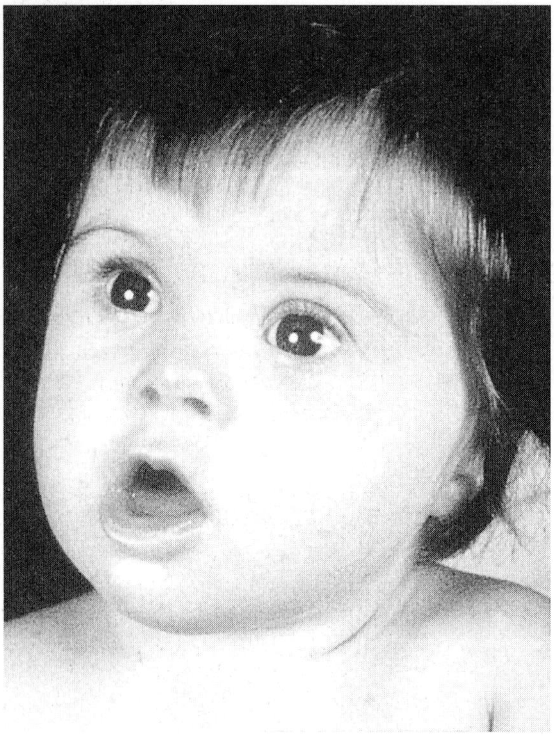

Figure 15.11 *Down's syndrome (from Sweet B, 1997, with permission).*

children. Genetic presymptomatic testing and testing of children are just two of the ethical issues that follow the identification of any gene. There is a detailed consideration of the implications of genetic counselling related to HD in Clarke (1994).

Cystic fibrosis

Cystic fibrosis (CF) is a recessive inherited disease of the exocrine glands with production of thick mucus that obstructs the gastrointestinal tract and the lungs. Although the disease mainly affects white populations slightly different mutations of the gene occur in black and other populations. The gene is located in the middle of the long arm of chromosome 7 and codes for a transmembrane regulator protein. Its full name is the cystic fibrosis transmembrane regulator (CFTR). The CFTR protein is involved in the control of sodium and chloride ions entering the cell. The cells and their secretions lack water. The resulting thick mucus obstructs and dilates the ducts of the pancreas and the lungs, destroying the structure and function of the organs. In the lung secondary bacterial infection is common and there is progressive involvement of the bronchial tree, beginning in the alveolar ducts and resulting in large cystic dilatations involving all bronchi.

Genetic markers allow the prenatal diagnosis of CF and carriers can be detected in over 70% of families with a history of CF. With early diagnosis and active treatment, life expectancy has increased from death in childhood to 30 years. The financial cost of treatment for a person with CF is great and there is the likely need for a heart-lung transplant.

Treatment of CF with a genetically engineered product may be possible. The gene for the CFTR protein could be isolated and attached to a retrovirus for administration to the lungs by a nebuliser. However, the research is still very much at the experimental stage.

Duchenne muscular dystrophy

Duchenne muscular dystrophy (DMD) is the most common of the muscular dystrophies. It occurs only in boys and is an X-linked disorder. The abnormal gene is carried on the short arm of the X chromosome and may be a deletion. This is a severe disorder and sufferers die before they have children of their own. The normal allele at the site codes for a muscle protein called **dystrophin** which is absent in boys with DMD.

Muscle bulk diminishes and connective tissue and fat replace the muscle fibres. DMD presents at about the age of 3 and parents report slow motor development with progressive weakness and muscle wasting. Muscle weakness begins in the pelvic girdle and the boys develop a waddling gait. There is hypertrophy of the calf muscles in 80% of cases (McCance & Huether 1994). Muscular weakness affects pulmonary function and cardiac involvement occurs in over 90% of children. Boys are usually confined to a wheelchair by 12 years and death due to respiratory or cardiac failure occurs before the age of 20. Fetal diagnosis is possible but not as routine screening. Women with an affected son are offered screening in subsequent pregnancies.

Neural tube defects (NTDs)

Most major defects of the brain are the result of defective closure of the anterior neuropore neural canal during the 4th week from conception. The result may be **anencephaly**, with absence of the forebrain and covering skull. Most of the embryonic brain is exposed and extruding from the skull. Life following birth is not possible. Failure of closure of the caudal

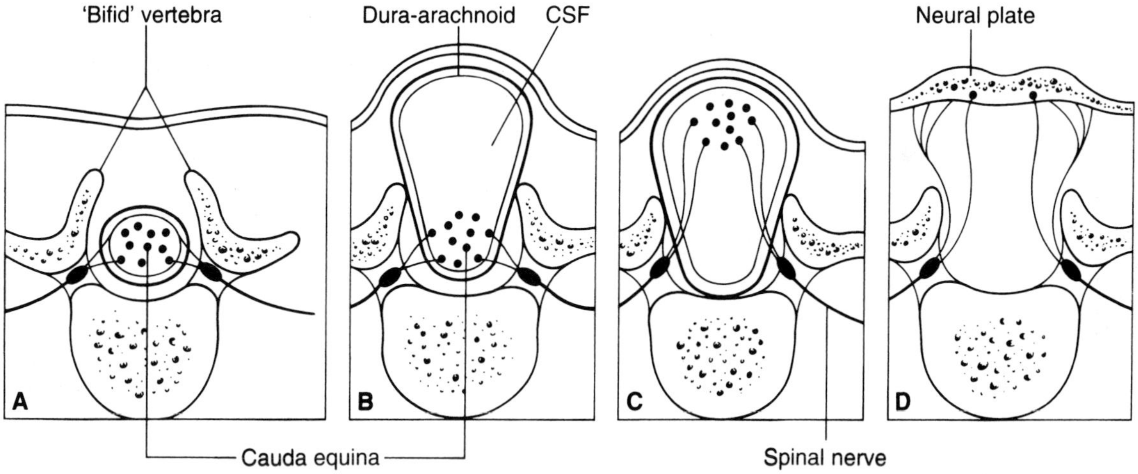

Figure 15.12 *Variants of spina bifida. (a) Spina bifida occulta. (b) Meningocoele. (c) Meningomyelocoele. (d) Myelocoele (from Hinchliff SM, Montague SE, 1990, with permission).*

neuropore at the end of the 4th week results in congenital defects of the spinal cord such as spina bifida.

Severe NTDs involve the tissues lying over the spinal cord – the meninges, vertebral arch, muscles and skin (Moore 1989). Spina bifida occulta may have no external signs and no clinical symptoms. The defect usually involves the vertebrae L5 or S1. The severe types of spina bifida involve protrusion of the spinal cord and meninges through defects in several vertebral arches. This happens only 2 weeks after the woman misses her menstrual period and long before most women present for antenatal care. Once the woman is receiving care, detection of NTD and counselling concerning the termination of pregnancy are offered.

Terminology

If the protruding sac contains only meninges and cerebrospinal fluid, it is called **spina bifida cystica**.

If the spinal cord and nerve roots are included in the sac, as occurs with 75% of fetuses, it is called **spina bifida with meningomyelocoele** (Fig. 15.13). Meningomyelocoeles may be covered with skin or with a thin, easily ruptured membrane and may be associated with talipes (Fig. 15.14).

When all that is present of the spinal cord is a flattened mass of nervous tissue, the condition is called **myeloschisis**.

A meningocoele may be found at the cervical part of the spine (Fig. 15.15).

There has been suspicion that folic acid deficiency (Hibbard & Smithells 1965) was somehow implicated in the causation of NTDs. Two intervention studies (Laurence et al 1981, Smithells et al 1980), where folate was given to women whose previous babies had had an NTD, suggested that supplementation might prevent recurrence. This led to a randomised double-blind trial conducted at 33 centres in seven countries. The results were so clear that the research group recommended that folic acid supplementation should be given to all women who were likely to bear children.

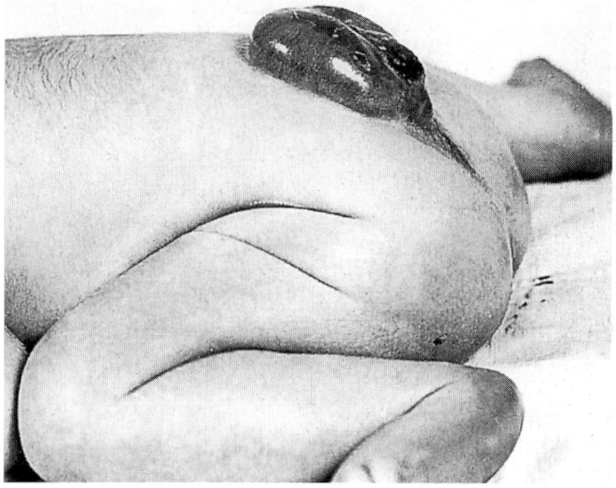

Figure 15.13 *Meningomyelocoele. The 'frog leg' posture is characteristic of combined femoral and sciatic nerve paralysis, with preservation of hip flexion by the ilio psoas muscle (from Hinchliff SM, Montague SE, 1990, with permission).*

Rubella

Rubella in childhood is a mild viral disease. It is now well established that rubella infection during the first few weeks of pregnancy will inhibit cell division in the embryonic eyes, ears, heart and brain. After the 3rd months the most common defect is congenital deafness. If an infant is born with congenital rubella, he will be highly infectious and must be isolated. The virus may remain in his body for up to a year. The diagnosis of maternal rubella is confirmed by tests for a rising antibody titre. Termination of pregnancy should be considered following a positive result.

Rubella vaccination of girls has been carried out in this country and now all children are offered protection in the triple vaccine against measles, mumps and rubella. Pregnant women are screened so that those who are not immune can be offered vaccination in the postnatal period. Women should be advised to avoid becoming pregnant for at least 3 months following immunisation. Those working with women and their babies should also be screened and offered vaccination if needed.

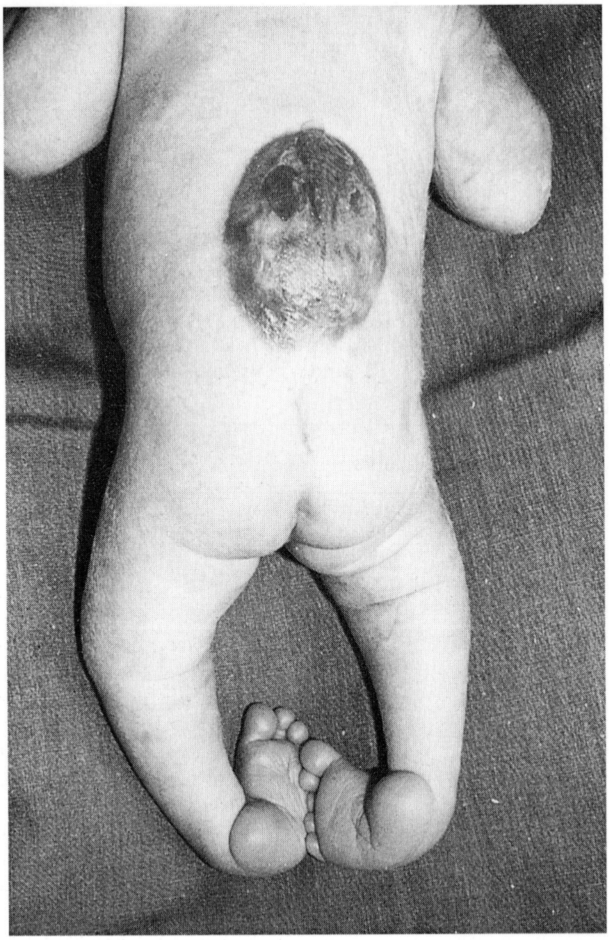

Figure 15.14 *Myelomeningocoele with bilateral severe talipes (from Kelnar C, Harvey D, Simpson C, 1995, with permission).*

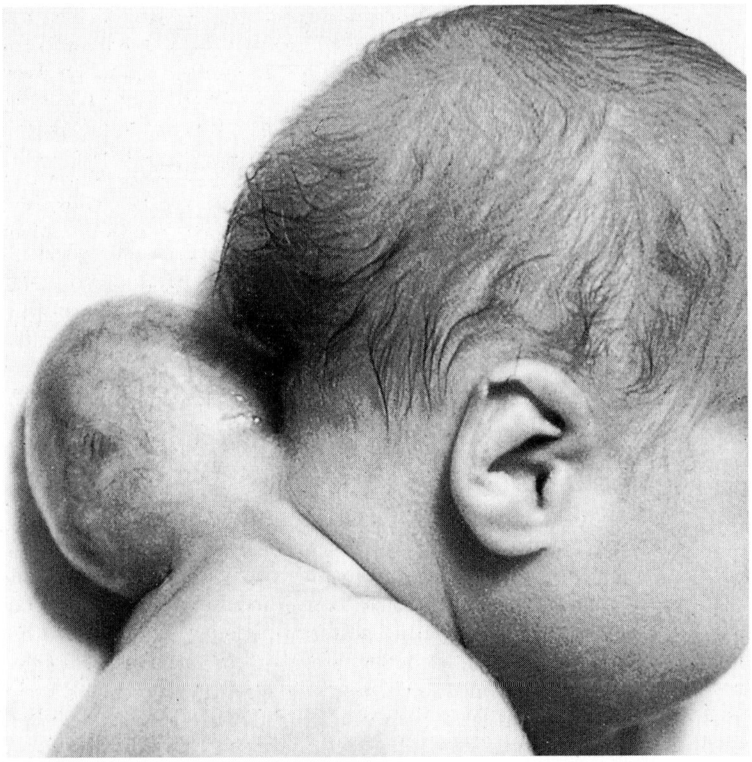

Figure 15.15 *Cervical meningocoele (from Kelnar C, Harvey D, Simpson C, 1995, with permission).*

Summary of main points

- Congenital defects are present at birth. They may be visible to the naked eye or may be hidden, such as changes in protein molecules. Congenital defects account for most severe illness during infancy and childhood and 25% of childhood deaths.
- Chromosomal defects and gene mutations may lead to abnormal development and about 50% of spontaneous abortions result from chromosomal defects. Genetic mutations are responsible for most of the congenital defects seen. Research indicates that some diseases that afflict people as they grow older, such as heart disease, may occur because of structural or functional changes in the embryo and fetus.
- From the 3rd to the 8th weeks, when organogenesis is taking place, the embryo is vulnerable to disruption of development by environmental processes. Such environmental substances are called teratogens and lead to mutations in the genetic material in a cell.
- A dominant allele manifests its effects in heterozygotes where there are two different variations of the allele. Only one copy is needed to affect the phenotype. A recessive allele only affects the phenotype when the individual is homozygous for that allele, i.e. two identical copies are necessary to produce the effect. If two genes are on the same chromosome situated closely together they may be inherited together. Such genes are said to be linked.
- The X chromosome carries a large number of genes involved in many aspects of development and function. Males only have one X chromosome and are hemizygous with respect to X chromosome genes. If there is an abnormal X chromosome gene boys will be affected by the X-linked disorder. Females will be asymptomatic carriers.
- There are also genes in the form of mitochondrial DNA which is inherited only from the mother. Some genetic disorders are due to mutations in the mitochondrial DNA. A few disorders are due to abnormal genes on the Y chromosome.
- Chromosomal defects may be present in 6% of all zygotes, many of which never implant. Chromosomes are subject to two kinds of changes: numerical (too many or too few) or structural. The changes may affect the autosomes, sex chromosomes or both. People with chromosomal defects usually have easily recognisable and characteristic phenotypes.
- Environmental factors may induce breaks in chromosomes. Structural rearrangements may also be called macromutations and two of these, inversion and translocation, are likely to be transmitted from parent to child. Translocation, deletion, duplication and inversion are chromosomal structural rearrangements.
- Recent developments in gene technology have promised a new type of medicine but have brought moral and ethical dilemmas. Anxieties about eugenics have once more become prominent, raising important questions about the application of genetic engineering to the diagnosis and treatment of so-called genetic diseases.
- Cell samples can be encouraged to divide in synchrony. The process is then stopped during mitosis and a photograph is taken. The chromosome images are cut out, laid in order and then photographed again to produce a karyotype. Single gene defects where the identity of the gene is known can be found by using gene probes.
- Applications of genetic engineering include hopes of medical cures, increased food production and crime detection. Medical applications include preimplantation genetic screening for disease and the sex of the embryo, fetal screening, screening of adults and insertion of genes as therapy.
- Drugs may damage sperm or ova or they may have an adverse effect on embryonic nutrient absorption so that essential nutrients are absent at crucial times. They may be teratogenic, adversely affecting the fetus by interfering in normal growth and development. Drugs and environmental pollutants have been found in breast milk.
- Nicotine affects the central nervous system in a way that many people find pleasurable. Many other chemicals are inhaled in cigarette smoke and may cross the placenta to damage the developing fetus. Smoking can cause infertility, spontaneous abortions, reduced length of gestation and low birth weight, increased perinatal mortality and fetal defects.
- Humans have developed defence systems against plant toxins mediated by the senses of sight, smell and taste. Ingested toxins may be expelled by diarrhoea and vomiting. The liver produces enzymes which render ingested toxins harmless so that they can be excreted via the kidney.
- Pesticides such as DDT and other chemical pollutants such as PCBs disrupt sexual development by mimicking the effect of oestrogen, resulting in feminisation of male reproductive organs, reduced sperm count, an increase in abnormal sperm and in the rate of testicular cancer. Oestrogenic compounds may prevent development of the full complement of Sertoli cells in the fetal testis, reducing sperm numbers.
- Ionising radiation damages DNA by transferring its energy into living cells. Atoms lose electrons and develop an electric charge. These charged particles, known as ions, can penetrate the body and damage molecules to produce free radicals and oxidising agents which break the DNA chain and destroy genetic material.
- Most women are seen for the first time when their pregnancy has already begun. Education and the offer of a preconception service will help to reduce the number of abnormal embryos conceived. Couples may not want to terminate the pregnancy and early diagnosis offers them a chance to plan for treatment of the baby.
- Screening for many congenital defects in specific populations is possible. The techniques include ultrasonography, chorionic villus sampling, amniocentesis and maternal serum screening. Fetal tissue obtained by amniocentesis, chorionic villus sampling or cordocentesis can be used for karyotyping for gross chromosomal errors, sexing the embryo if there is a family history of X-linked disorders and enzyme assay for detection of an inborn error of metabolism.
- Maternal serum screening is carried out to search for the small amounts of maternal serum α-fetoprotein (MSAFP) present. Normal values of MSAFP are found to be highest in early pregnancy, decreasing as pregnancy advances. Low levels have been associated with Down's syndrome and high levels with open fetal defects.
- The incidence of Down's syndrome or trisomy 21 is about one in 800 births and increases with maternal age when it can be as high as one in 40. The risk of a mother carrying a Down's syndrome baby can be estimated using the Bart's triple test. Low MSAFP levels are found with a low level of unconjugated oestriol and a high level of HCG.
- Huntington's disease, caused by a dominant gene, occurs in about one in 2000 births. The gene affects the basal ganglia and cerebral cortex, resulting in involuntary movement and dementia from middle life. The onset is earlier if the gene is inherited on the paternal chromosome rather than the maternal but the mechanism of linkage of such diseases is not understood. As the onset of HD is delayed until an affected person has already had children or even grandchildren, genetic presymptomatic testing and testing of children are just two associated ethical issues.
- Cystic fibrosis is a recessive inherited disease of the exocrine glands with production of thick mucus that obstructs the gastrointestinal tract and the lungs. Although the disease mainly affects white populations, slightly different mutations of the gene occur in black and other populations. The gene codes for the cystic fibrosis transmembrane regulator or CFTR which controls the entry of sodium and chloride ions into the cell. The gene for the CFTR protein could be attached to a retrovirus for administration to the lungs by a nebuliser but research is still experimental.

- Duchenne muscular dystrophy is an X-linked, severe disorder and sufferers die before they have children of their own. The normal allele codes for a muscle protein called dystrophin which is absent in boys with DMD. Fetal diagnosis is possible and women who have borne an affected son can be offered screening for subsequent pregnancies.
- Defective closure of the anterior neuropore neural canal results in anencephaly, with absence of the forebrain and covering skull. Failure of closure of the caudal neuropore at the end of the 4th week results in spina bifida. This happens only 2 weeks after the woman misses her menstrual period and long before most women present for antenatal care. Diet, in particular folic acid deficiency, may be implicated in their cause.

References

Abercrombie M, Hickman M, Johnson ML, Thain M. 1992 The New Penguin Dictionary of Biology, 8th edn. Penguin, Harmondsworth.

Abramsky L, Chapple J. (eds) 1994 Prenatal Diagnosis: The Human Side. Chapman and Hall, London.

Alfirevic Z, Gosden C, Neilson JP. 1997a Chorionic villus sampling compared with amniocentesis for prenatal diagnosis. In Neilson JP, Crowther CA, Hodnett ED, Hofmeyr GJ, Keirse MJNC (eds) Pregnancy and Childbirth module of The Cochrane Database of Systematic Reviews, The Cochrane Library. Update Software, Oxford.

Alfirevic Z, Gosden C, Neilson JP. 1997b Early amniocentesis versus chorionic villus sampling. In Neilson JP, Crowther CA, Hodnett ED, Hofmeyr GJ, Keirse MJNC (eds) Pregnancy and Childbirth module of The Cochrane Database of Systematic Reviews, The Cochrane Library. Update Software, Oxford.

Barker DJP. (ed) 1992, Fetal and Infant Origins of Adult Disease. BMJ Books, London.

Bishop JE, Waldholz M. 1990 Genome. Simon and Schuster, New York.

Bonner J. 1996 Simple blood test may replace amniocentesis. New Scientist 149(2053) 24.

British Medical Association and Royal Pharmaceutical Society of Great Britain 1990 British National Formulary, Number 19 (March), Prescribing in Pregnancy. BMA/RPS, London, pp 28–33.

Capecchi MR. 1994 Targeted gene replacement. Scientific American 270(3) 34–41.

Chamberlain G. 1991 Medical problems in pregnancy – 1. British Medical Journal 302, 1262–1264.

Clarke A. (ed) 1994 Genetic Counselling Practice and Principles. Routledge, London.

Fitzgerald MJT, Fitzgerald M. 1994 Human Embryology. Baillière Tindall, London.

Hanson FW, Tennant F, Stacey Hune MS, Brookhyser K. 1992 Early amniocentesis: outcome, risks and technical problems at < 12.8 weeks. American Journal of Obstetrics and Gynecology 166(6,1), 1707–1711.

Hibbard ED, Smithells RW. 1965 Folic acid metabolism and human embryopathy. Lancet in 1254.

Hinchliff SM, Montague SE. 1990 Physiology for Nursing Practice. Baillière Tindall, London.

Hinchliff SM, Montague SE, Watson R 1996 Physiology for Nursing Practice, Ballière Tindall, London.

Horgan J. 1993 Eugenics revisited. Scientific American 268(6) 90–100.

Jones S. 1996 In the Blood: God, Genes and Destiny. Harper Collins, London.

Kelnar C, Harvey D, Simpson C. 1995 The Sick Newborn Baby. Baillière Tindall, London.

Laurenece KM, James N, Miller MH, Tennant GB, Campbell H. 1981 Double-blind randomised controlled trial of folate treatment before conception to prevent recurrence of neural-tube defects. British Medical Journal 282, 1509–1511.

McCance KL, Huether SE. 1994 Pathophysiology. The Biologic Basis for Disease in Adults and Children, 2nd edn. Mosby Yearbook, Chicago.

Moore KL. 1963 The vulnerable embryo. Causes of malformation in man. Manitoba Medical Review 43, 306.

Moore KL. 1989 Before We Are Born, 3rd edn. WB Saunders, Philadelphia.

Moore P. 1993 Genetic manipulation. New Scientist 140(1901) 1–4.

Neilson JP. 1997 Routine ultrasound in early pregnancy. In Neilson JP, Crowther CA, Hodnett ED, Hofmeyr GJ, Keirse MJNC (eds) Pregnancy and Childbirth module of the Cochrane Database of Systematic Reviews, The Cochrane Library. Update Software, Oxford.

O'Shea PA. 1995 Congenital defects and their causes. In Coustan DR, Haning RV, Singer DB (eds) Human Reproduction. Little, Brown, Boston.

Proud J. 1996 Specialised antenatal investigations. In Bennett VR, Brown LK (eds) Myles Textbook for Midwives. Churchill Livingstone, Edinburgh, pp 660–674.

Rennie J. 1994 Grading the gene tests. Scientific American 270(6) 66–74.

Simpson C. 1997 Congenital defects and conditions. In Sweet BR with Tiran D (eds) Mayes Midwifery, 12th edn. Baillière Tindall, London, pp 912–920.

Smithells RW, Shephard S, Schorah CJ et al. 1980 Possible prevention of neural-tube defects by periconceptional vitamin supplementation. Lancet 1; 339–340.

Sweet B. 1997 Mayes' Midwifery. Baillière Tindall, London.

Telfer FM. 1997 Antenatal investigations of maternal and fetal wellbeing. In Sweet BR with Tiran D (eds) Mayes Midwifery, 12th edn. Baillière Tindall, London, pp 246–267.

Weatherall DJ. 1991 The New Genetics and Clinical Practice, 3rd edn. Oxford University Press, Oxford.

Recommended reading

Abramsky L, Chapple J. (eds) Prenatal Diagnosis: The Human Side. Chapman and Hall, London.

Alfirevic Z, Gosden C, Neilson JP. 1997 Chorionic villus sampling compared with amniocentesis for prenatal diagnosis. In Neilson JP, Crowther CA, Hodnett ED, Hofmeyr GJ, Keirse MJNC (eds) Pregnancy and Childbirth module of The Cochrane Database of Systematic Reviews, The Cochrane Library. Update Software, Oxford.

Alfirevic Z, Gosden C, Neilson JP. 1997 Early amniocentesis versus chorionic villus sampling. In Neilson JP, Crowther CA, Hodnett ED, Hofmeyr GJ, Keirse MJNC (eds) Pregnancy and Childbirth module of The Cochrane Database of Systematic Reviews, The Cochrane Library. Update Software, Oxford.

Capecchi MR. 1994 Targeted gene replacement. Scientific American 270(3) 34–41.

Gray J. 1994 Maternal nutrition, fetal environment and adult disease. Modern Midwife 4(8), 13–16.

Medical Research Council Vitamin Study Research Group 1991 Prevention of neural tube defects: results of the Medical Research Council Vitamin Study. Lancet 338 (8760), 131–137.

Neilson JP. 1997 Routine ultrasound in early pregnancy. In Neilson JP, Crowther CA, Hodnett ED, Hofmeyr GJ, Keirse MJNC (eds) Pregnancy and Childbirth module of the Cochrane Database of Systematic Reviews, The Cochrane Library. Update Software, Oxford.

Telfer FM. 1997 Antenatal investigations of maternal and fetal wellbeing. In Sweet BR with Tiran D (eds) Mayes Midwifery, 12th edn. Baillière Tindall, London, pp 246–267.

Turner L. 1994 Problems surrounding late prenatal diagnosis. In Abramsky L, Chapple J (eds) Prenatal Diagnosis: The Human Side. Chapman and Hall, London, pp 134–148.

Ward NI. 1995 Preconceptional care and pregnancy outcome. Journal of Nutritional and Environmental Medicine 5, 2205–2208.

Weatherall DJ. 1991 The New Genetics and Clinical Practice, 3rd edn. Oxford University Press, Oxford.

Section 2B

PREGNANCY – THE MOTHER

Section contents

Women who are pregnant develop an altered normal physiology to compensate for the needs of the developing baby. Section 2B comprises chapters 16 to 29 and is about the physiological adaptation of the woman's body to pregnancy. In anticipation of the needs of those who enter midwifery by the direct route, each system is first described in the non-pregnant state, then the alterations brought about by pregnancy are presented and finally their significance to health are discussed. Related systems have been grouped as far as possible. The chapters also provide revision for those qualified nurses who take up midwifery. Integral to the support of the growing fetus are the haematological system (chapter 16) and the cardiovascular system (chapter 17). Three other systems involved in gas exchange, acid-base (pH) control and fluid balance are next discussed. These are the respiratory system (chapter 18), the renal system (chapter 19) and fluid balance (chapter 20). Chapters 21 to 23 examine the organs of the gastrointestinal tract and nutrition whilst chapters 24 and 25 explore the musculo-skeletal system. The relationship between the nervous, endocrine and immune systems provide much knowledge about human health. The relatively new topic of psychoneuroimmunology is gaining ground. However, for the needs of the midwife each of the systems is given its own space in chapters 26 to 29.

Chapter 16

The haematological system – physiology of the blood

In this chapter

BLOOD AS A TISSUE

During the evolution of multicellular organisms a limitation of size and number of cells was imposed by the inability of cells to maintain direct contact with the external environment. For any further increase in size to occur, a specialised internal transport system, such as the cardiovascular system and circulation of blood, was necessary. Blood carries oxygen and nutrients to the cells and carbon dioxide and metabolic waste from the cells. In an adult human, blood comprises 6–8% of body weight (lower if the person is obese). This is 5–6 litres in a man and 4–5 litres in a woman.

If a sample of blood is placed in a test tube and prevented from clotting, the heavier cellular elements settle out and the plasma rises to the top. As most of the cells are erythrocytes, the resulting separation is equal to the **haematocrit** or red cell content of the blood which averages 45%. White cells and platelets form only 1% and can be seen between the two main layers as a thin cream-coloured layer called the **buffy coat**.

FUNCTIONS OF BLOOD

Montague (1996) outlines the functions of blood as follows.

- Internal transport of substances for respiration, nutrition, excretion, maintenance of water, electrolyte and acid/base balance and metabolic regulation.
- Defence against infection by foreign organisms.
- Protection from injury and haemorrhage.
- Maintenance of body temperature.

Table 16.1 *Specific properties of blood*

Property	*Value*
Specific gravity (relative to water)	1.026
Viscosity (relative to water)	1.5 to 1.75 (cells contribute equally to viscosity)
Ph	7.35 to 7.45
H+ concentration	35 to 45 nmol/l

Table 16.2 *Outline of blood constituents and function*

Constituent	*Function*
Water	Transport medium of nutrients, wastes, gases. Heat distributor
Plasma protein – albumin	Transports many substances. Large contribution to colloid oncotic pressure
Plasma protein globulins – α and β	Transports substances, involved in clotting
Plasma protein globulins – γ	Antibodies
Plasma protein – fibrinogen	Inactive precursor for fibrin
Electrolytes	Osmotic distribution of fluid between compartments

CONSTITUENTS OF BLOOD

Blood is a fluid tissue with living cells in a non-living matrix. It is a sticky, viscous, dark red, opaque fluid consisting of 55% plasma and 45% cells. More than 99% of the cellular component consists of **erythrocytes** (red blood cells). White cells and platelets are present in small quantities. Blood also contains many chemicals in suspension. If blood is exposed to the air it solidifies into a clot and exudes a clear fluid called **serum**.

PLASMA

This is a pale yellow opalescent fluid which acts as a medium for the transport of substances. It contains water (90%), protein (8%), inorganic ions (0.9%) and organic substances (1.1%).

If clotting factors are removed the remaining fluid is called serum. Plasma usually forms about 20% of the body's extracellular fluid. It differs from interstitial fluid in the protein content – plasma has 8%, interstitial fluid only 2%. This is because protein molecules are too large to pass out into the interstitial fluid at the capillary beds. Most protein that does pass into the interstitial fluid is taken up by the lymphatic system and returned to the blood. The main plasma proteins are presented in Table 16.3.

The functions of plasma proteins are to:

- prevent fluid loss from blood to tissues by exerting colloid osmotic (**oncotic**) pressure. This is mainly due to the presence of albumin. Oedema of the tissues will develop if oncotic pressure is lost, as may occur in liver disease, kidney disease, burns, inflammation and allergic disorders;
- transport substances around the body by binding so that they are prevented from being metabolised until they reach their target tissue; for instance, albumin binds bilirubin. Some substances can displace others and compete for binding sites. An example of this is the displacement of bilirubin from albumin by aspirin or sulphonamides;
- aid in clotting and fibrinolytic activities;
- assist in prevention of infection – γ-globulins, also known as immunoglobulins, function as specific antibodies for specific protein antigens such as microbial agents and pollen;
- help regulate acid/base balance by acting in buffering systems;
- act as a protein reserve forming part of the amino acid pool;
- contribute about 50% to the total viscosity of blood.

Table 16.3 *Plasma proteins*

Name	*Origin*	*% of total*
Albumin	Synthesised in the liver	60
Fibrinogen	Synthesised in the liver	4
Globulins (α) and (β)	Synthesised in the liver	36
Globulin (γ)	Synthesised in the immune system	Trace

Other proteins found in the blood in small quantities are hormones, enzymes and most of the clotting factors. There is also a series of plasma proteins called **complement** that assist in the inflammatory and immune mechanisms. Albumin is the smallest of the plasma proteins with a molecular mass of 69 000 and is just too large to pass through the capillary walls in normal circumstances. If the glomerular capillaries in the kidney are damaged albumin can be lost from the blood in large quantities.

THE CELLULAR COMPONENTS OF BLOOD

Three major types of cells are present in blood, each having a very different function: red cells (**erythrocytes**), white cells (**leucocytes**) and platelets (**thrombocytes**).

Normally the proportions of these cells remain constant within narrow limits but can be adjusted to maintain health. Measuring the cellular content of blood is a simple automated basic test carried out on most people at some point in their life, either as part of health screening or for diagnosis of disease. **Haemopoiesis** is the term for blood cell formation.

A pluripotent stem cell, sometimes called a **haemocytoblast**, in the red bone marrow is thought to give rise to progenitor cells for the three main types of cell produced in the marrow. These include the red cells and **megakaryocytes** (leading to platelets). The pluripotent stem cell branches to form myeloid stem cells, leading to the production of granulocytes and monocytes in the bone marrow, and lymphoid stem cells which leave the bone marrow to reside in the lymphoid tissues and produce lymphocytes. Each person has about 1500 g of red bone marrow in the body. Two-thirds of cells are white and one-third are red (Fig. 16.1).

Red blood cells

Erythrocytes or red blood cells (RBCs) are small cells biconcave in shape, i.e. flattened discs with depressed centres. They are about 7.5 micrometres in diameter. Their shape and size

Table 16.4 *Outline of the cellular constituents of blood*

Constituent	*Function*
Erythrocytes (red cells)	Oxygen and carbon dioxide transport
Leucocytes (white cells)	Defence against micro-organisms
Platelets	Haemostasis

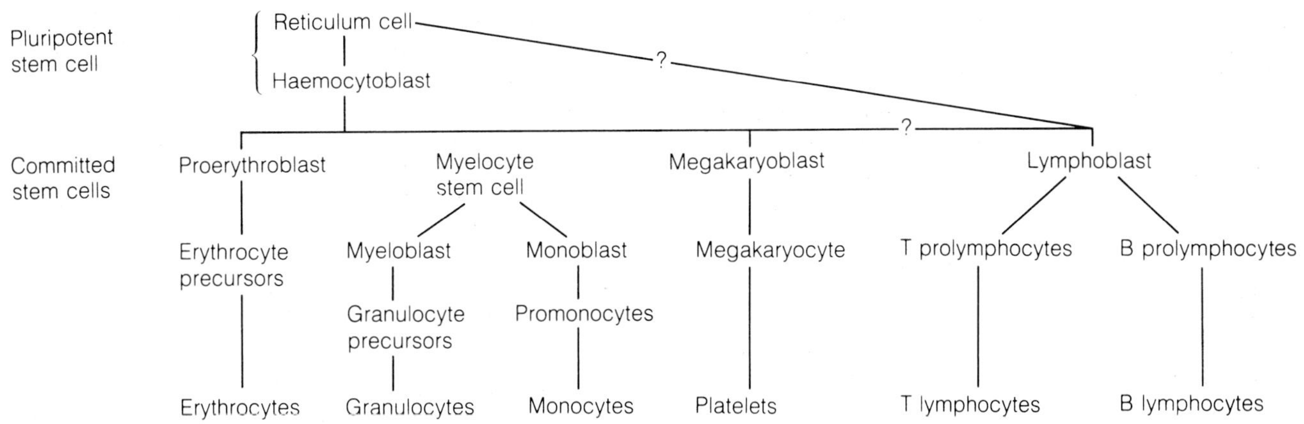

Figure 16.1 *Summary of the major stages of haemopoiesis (from Hinchliff SM, Montague SE, 1990, with permission).*

provide a large surface area relative to their volume. They are filled with haemoglobin and no part of their cytoplasm is far from the cell surface which is ideal for their main function of gas exchange. They are also very flexible and can pass through capillaries whose diameter is smaller than the RBC.

Erythrocytes are normally measured per cubic mm and average 5 million. This value may also be given as 5.0 ×[el] 10^{12}/1. Women have a lower range with 4.3–5.2 per cubic mm and men have a range of 5.1–5.8 per cubic mm (Table 16.5). As RBCs are the main cellular contributor to blood viscosity, any increase above this will increase blood viscosity which may happen when people go to live at high altitude and blood flows more slowly. A decrease, such as is seen in normal pregnancy, will lower viscosity and blood will flow more rapidly.

The main function of erythrocytes is the carriage of oxygen picked up in the lungs to all the cells of the body. Haemoglobin in the blood is measured in grams per decilitre (100 ml) and the normal range of values is 14–20 g/dl in infants, 13–18 g/dl in adult males and 12–16 g/dl in adult females. It also picks up about 20% of carbon dioxide returning from the tissues to form carbaminohaemoglobin but most CO_2 is in solution in blood.

Haemoglobin

Haemoglobin is a red-coloured pigment found in red cells. Each red cell contains 30 pg (picograms) of haemoglobin which equates to 640 million haemoglobin molecules in one cell. This is reported as the mean cell haemoglobin or MCH. Another measure reported is the mean cell concentration of haemoglobin (MCHC) which is 32 g/dl. Each molecule is made up of four protein chains – two α and two β – each of which contains a haem group with an iron atom (Fig. 16.2). The ferrous iron atom has one bond which can enter into loose and reversible association with oxygen to form the bright red oxyhaemoglobin (HbO_2). Once the oxygen has been released in the tissues, it becomes darker red and is known as deoxyhaemoglobin.

Table 16.5 *Red cell laboratory values*

Parameter	*Value*
Red cell count	4.5–6.5 × 10^{12}/l
Haemoglobin	13 g/dl
Mean cell haemoglobin concentration (MCHC)	32 g/dl
Mean cell volume (MCV)	85 femtolitres (fl) – 1000 million millionth/litre

Each haemoglobin molecule can carry four molecules of oxygen. These are picked up one at a time and each binding changes the configuration of globin and increases the affinity of the haemoglobin molecule for oxygen. The affinity for the fourth molecule of oxygen is 20 times that of the first affinity. This aspect of oxygen uptake will be examined in greater detail when respiration is considered.

The pigment haem is made up of ring-shaped organic molecules called **pyrrole rings**. Four of these join together to form a larger ring and a ferrous iron atom is held centrally by

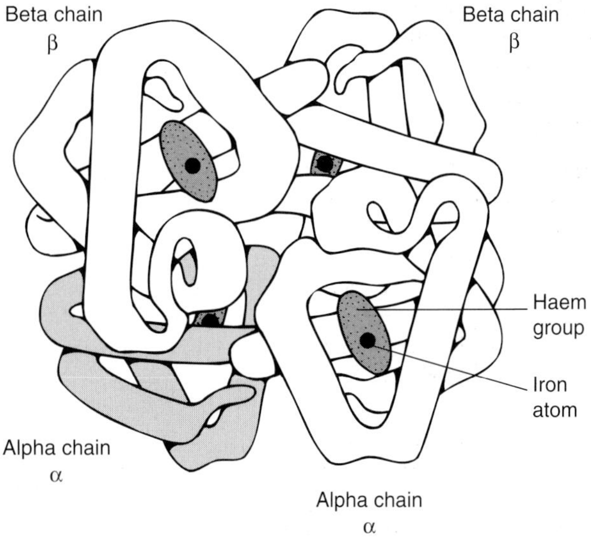

Figure 16.2 *The structure of haemoglobin. Haemoglobin is a protein with four subunits (2 α polypeptides and 2 β polypeptides). Each subunit contains a haem group with an iron atom. (From Jones et al, with permission.)*

the nitrogen atom of each pyrrole ring. The globin proteins consist of long chains of amino acids. There are four types of globin chain, each with slight differences in amino acids: α, β, δ and γ. These four can be varied in pairs to form different types of haemoglobin. Three of these are found normally. At birth HbF makes up two-thirds of the haemoglobin content and HbA one-third. From the age of 5 the adult ratio of HbA > 95%, HbA_2 < 3.5% and HbF < 1.5% is established.

HbA – the major adult haemoglobin	2α	2β
HbA_2 – the minor adult haemoglobin	2α	2δ
HbF – fetal haemoglobin	2α	2γ

Other fetal haemoglobins have substitutions for the β chains which can persist and may be life saving in thalassaemia. Abnormal β chains are made in sickle cell disorders.

Formation of erythrocytes

Mature red blood cells develop from haemocytoblasts in the erythroid tissue in the bone marrow. After 3–5 days they pass into the circulation as cells called **reticulocytes** because they still contain rough endoplasmic reticulum and clumped ribosomes. This disappears when the cell is mature, which normally takes 4 days. There are three or four mitotic cell divisions involved so that each haemocytoblast gives rise to eight or 16 red cells. There is a gradual build-up of haemoglobin made at the ribosomes which appear in the cell. Other organelles and the nucleus are extruded from the cell. There is a reduction in cell size and a change in cell shape. Reticulocytes normally comprise less than 2% of the red cells in the blood of an adult.

The lifespan of red cells

About 1% of erythrocytes are replaced each day. Stimulation of production is by the hormone erythropoietin which originates in the kidney. This is a glycoprotein produced when the kidney cells are hypoxic, for example during haemorrhage, haemolytic crises, at altitude and following exercise. Erythropoietin can only stimulate committed cells and there will be an increase in reticulocytes in the blood if the need is drastic. Red blood cells live about 120 days and are finally ingested and destroyed by macrophages, mainly in the spleen. As the cells circulate, their plasma membrane becomes progressively more damaged until it ruptures. Having no nucleus, they have no mechanism of self-repair. They are fragmented to produce protein and haem, which enter the body stores to be reused, and bilirubin which is excreted in bile (Fig. 16.3).

Very defective cells such as those found in sickle cell-disease may be haemolysed in the circulation and the haemoglobin, which has a molecular mass of 68 000 and is small enough to be excreted in the urine, is released into the plasma. Special plasma proteins called **haptoglobins** bind to free haemoglobin to form larger molecules and prevent it from being excreted. If this mechanism becomes saturated, haemoglobin will appear in the urine (**haemoglobinuria**).

Table 16.6 *Dietary substances needed for erythropoiesis*

Substance	*Utilisation*
Protein	Synthesis of the globin part of haemoglobin and for cellular proteins
Iron	Contained in the haem portion of haemoglobin
Vitamin B_{12} (hydroxycobalamin)	Needed for DNA synthesis
Folic acid	Needed for DNA synthesis
Vitamin C (ascorbic acid)	Facilitates absorption of iron

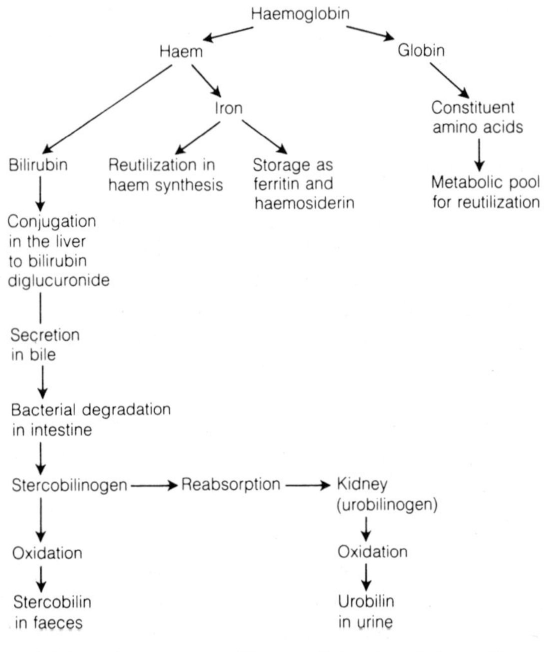

Figure 16.3 *A summary of haemoglobin breakdown (from Hinchcliff SM, Montague SE, 1990, with permission).*

IRON METABOLISM

Absorption

A typical British mixed diet usually contains about 14 mg of iron daily but normally only 1–2 mg is absorbed. The composition of the diet controls how much iron is absorbed and there are two distinct pathways for absorption: iron attached to haem and inorganic iron. Iron attached to haem is found in the haemoglobin and myoglobin protein found in animal products. It is absorbed much more efficiently than non-haem iron and is not influenced by factors affecting the absorption of non-haem iron. In most foods, iron is present in its ferric form and has to be converted to ferrous iron in order to be absorbed.

Absorption is enhanced if reducing agents that can aid this conversion are taken. Hydrochloric acid found in the gastric juice performs this function, as can ascorbic acid (vitamin C). In grain foods iron forms a complex with phytates and only small amounts of soluble iron are available. The iron in eggs is bound to phosphates in the yolk and is poorly absorbed. The amount of iron absorbed depends on the rate of red cell production, the extent of iron stores, the content of the diet and whether or not iron supplements are given. Intestinal absorption of iron is facilitated when there is erythroid hyperplasia, rapid turnover of iron and a high concentration of unsaturated transferrin, as occurs in pregnancy.

Serum iron, transferrin and total iron-binding capacity

Non-pregnant women have a serum iron content of 13–27 μmol/l but this is dynamic and fluctuates widely during 24 h. A low count usually indicates iron deficiency anaemia. The total iron-binding capacity (TIBC) is 45–72 μmol/l. A reduced count is associated with iron deficiency anaemia. **Transferrin** is the protein that specifically binds iron and is usually between 1.2 and 2 g/l. TIBC is usually one-third saturated with iron. Transferrin rises to 4.7 g/l by the 2nd trimester and TIBC increases to 90 μmol/l. This is also seen in women taking oestrogen-containing oral contraceptives so it is probably oestrogen that causes the change. TIBC returns to normal within 3 weeks of delivery.

Serum ferritin

Ferritin is a glycoprotein with a high molecular mass found in cells, where it holds two-thirds of the iron store. It is also found in small amounts in the plasma in a wide range of 15–300 μg/l. It is stable, not affected by iron ingestion and is a good indicator of iron stores (Montague 1996), especially in the lower range as in iron deficiency anaemia in pregnancy.

Marrow iron

Occasionally it is useful to examine bone marrow to assess iron stores. Marrow is taken by aspiration from the iliac crest. A stainable iron/protein complex called **haemosiderin**, which is similar to ferritin, may be seen. No stainable iron will be seen if the serum ferritin has fallen below 40 μg/l. In the absence of iron supplementation, no stainable iron is seen in 80% of women at term. The developing erythrocytes can also be examined for iron deficiency signs. The presence of infection, especially urinary tract infection, can block the incorporation of iron into haemoglobin as the microbes may utilise iron in their own metabolic processes.

FOLATE METABOLISM

Folate is a vitamin found widely in nature, in leafy green vegetables such as spinach and in mushrooms and oranges. Liver is a good source. Folic acid is destroyed by prolonged boiling or by the addition of bicarbonate of soda to the cooking water. Some drugs act as folic acid antagonists and prevent its absorption. A typical Western diet contains 500–800 μg daily and normal daily needs are 100–200 μg (Montague 1996). This excess intake partly compensates for the loss in cooking.

Folates are absorbed in the duodenum and jejunum and stored in the liver. Deficiency is more likely to be seen in the winter months when the foods containing folic acid may be difficult to obtain. It is more common in certain socially and economically deprived groups. It was identified and synthesised in the 1940s. The metabolism of folic acid is the basis for cellular use of folate and it is essential for cell growth (Letsky 1991). Tissue that is active in reproduction and growth is dependent on folate coenzymes and folate metabolism is increased in pregnancy.

BLOOD GROUPS

Red blood cells, like all cells, have **glycoproteins** in their plasma membranes which are genetically coded for and therefore inherited. These can act as **antigens** (see Chapter 29), provoking an immune reaction if an incompatible blood enters the circulation. The red cells are agglutinated and destroyed. There are over 400 different antigens found on the surface of red cells. Some of these cause a more vigorous reaction than others and the two most commonly problematic are those of the ABO system and the rhesus (Rh) system.

The ABO system

The ABO blood groups are based on the presence of two red cell antigens called type A and type B. The O blood group arises if neither antigen (known as **agglutinogens**) is inherited and as the two types are codominant (neither gene masks the presence of the other gene so that both proteins are expressed), a person inheriting both will have the blood group AB. Therefore there are four possible blood groups – A, B, AB and O – depending on which surface antigens are present on the red cells.

A unique factor associated with the ABO system is the presence of preformed antibodies (known as **agglutinins**) in the plasma within 2 months of birth with no previous sensitisation event. A baby cannot have antibodies against any antigen carried on its own red cells or the cells would be destroyed. Therefore a baby who has neither the A or B antigen on its red cells will have both anti-A and anti-B antibodies in the serum whilst a baby with the blood group AB will have neither antibody present in the serum. Those with blood group A will have anti-B antibodies and those with blood group B will have anti-A antibodies.

The Rhesus system

There are eight types of Rh antigens but only three are common. These are called the C, D and E agglutinogens. Each is coded for by a gene and there are two alleles to each gene, giving CDE/cde as the full range of alleles. Rhesus D is by far the most clinically important antigen. The word rhesus is used because agglutinogen D was originally identified in rhesus monkeys.

About 85% of people in the Western world are rhesus positive (Rh+), which means they have the Rh agglutinogen on their red cells, and 15% are rhesus negative (Rh–) and do not have the agglutinogen on their red cells. In Japan 99.7% of people are Rh+ and only 0.3% Rh–. Unlike the ABO system, there are no spontaneously occurring anti-Rh antibodies and these are only formed if there is a sensitisation event with the presence of Rh+ red blood cells in the circulation of an Rh– person. There is a problem associated with the rhesus factor in pregnancy, discussed in Chapter 14.

WHITE CELLS

These cells are the leucocytes and can be referred to as WBCs. Taking all the types together, the average number of WBCs in the circulation is 4000–11 000 per cubic mm which can also be reported as $4–11 \times 10^9$ per litre. They account for only 1% of the blood's cellular content and an increase is called **leucocytosis** and a decrease **leucopenia**. Those white cells present in the blood represent only a small part of the body's total white cell content as the majority are in the tissues.

The reason for the wide variation in the normal count is that cells enter and leave the circulation from hour to hour in response to physiological factors such as exercise. The white cell count of a newborn baby is approximately double that of the adult and reaches adult levels by about 5–10 years of age. These cells are part of the immune defence system and are protective against bacteria, viruses, parasites, toxins and tumour cells. Some undergo **diapedesis** – they can slip out of capillaries with an amoebic action in response to positive **chemotaxis** (chemical call).

Box 16.1 Barr bodies

In normal females whose cells have two X chromosomes, a dense drum-stick projection can be seen on about 5% of polymorphonuclear leucocytes which does not appear on male cells. This was first observed by the Canadian geneticist Barr, hence the name. Mary Lyon, a British geneticist, suggested in 1961 that the drumstick may represent one of the female cell's two X chromosomes lying dormant. She suggested that inactivation of one X chromosome may occur early in embryonic development of the female. This hypothesis has since been confirmed.

The inactivation process is random and half the cells will contain the paternal X chromosome and half the maternal X chromosome. This type of situation with two distinct cell lines is called **mosaicism**. Male cells have only one chromosome which is always functional whilst female cells effectively also have only one functional X chromosome. Thus the number of X chromosomes in a cell is the number of Barr bodies seen plus the active chromosome. This is useful in diagnosing chromosome abnormalities such as Klinefelter's syndrome, essentially males with XXY chromosome constitution.

Types of white cell

Granulocytes (polymorphonuclear leucocytes) contain granules which have substances that can fight infection in their cytoplasm and a lobed nucleus. They are 10–14 micrometres in diameter. They can be further divided into three groups by the size of their granules and the way they take up Wright's stain. All these cells are phagocytic.

Neutrophils contain granules of varying sizes that stain violet because they take up both acidic red dyes and basic blue dyes. They are the most common, accounting for more than 50% of all white cells, and have the most lobular nucleus. Neutrophils are chemically attracted to sites of inflammation and will ingest and destroy bacteria and some fungi.

Eosinophils have large granules which are stained red by acidic dyes. The nucleus usually has two lobes. They make up about 1–4% of the white cell population. Their most important role is to attack parasitic worms such as tapeworms and roundworms. When a worm enters the body the eosinophils surround it and release enzymes from their granules onto the parasite's surface to digest it from the outside. Eosinophils are also involved in dealing with allergy attacks by destroying antigen/antibody complexes.

Basophils have large granules that take up a basic dye and stain blue-black. The nucleus usually has two or three lobes. These are the rarest of the white cells, accounting for only 0.5% of the population. Their large granules contain histamine which is an inflammatory substance that acts as a vasodilator and draws other white blood cells to the site of inflammation. Cells similar to basophils present in connective tissue are called **mast cells**. Both types of cell release histamine when they bind to one of the immunoglobulins (E).

The production of granulocytes

Granulocytes arise from myeloid precursor cells in the red bone marrow and the process takes about 14 days. If cells are urgently needed, such as in an infection, this time can be reduced considerably. Also, there is a pool of cells in the bone marrow and for every granulocyte in the circulation there may be more than 50 in the marrow. During **granulopoiesis**, there is progressive condensation and lobulation of the nucleus. There is loss of organelles such as mitochondria and the development of the granules in the cell cytoplasm.

Within 7 h of reaching the circulation, half the granulocytes will have left to meet tissue needs and will not return to the blood. The normal survival of these cells in the tissues is about 4–5 days. Dead cells are eliminated from the body in faeces and respiratory secretions. Dead neutrophils form the pus at infection sites.

Agranulocytes

These include lymphocytes and monocytes and do not contain visible cytoplasmic granules.

Lymphocytes

Lymphocytes are produced in the bone marrow and immature cells migrate to the thymus and other lymphoid tissue to divide again and mature. The second most common leucocyte, they are round cells with large round nuclei. Large numbers exist in the body but only a small number are found in the circulation as they are more often present in lymphoid tissue. They can be subdivided into small and large lymphocytes and are involved in immune reactions. During the first 2 years of life lymphocytes are the most numerous of the white cells but fall to normal adult levels of 20–40% by the age of 5–10. Functionally, there are two types of lymphocytes – T and B lymphocytes. T cells mature in the thymus gland and are involved in cell-mediated immune responses. B cells are involved in humoral immunity and produce antibodies (immunoglobulins) when needed. Lymphocytes recirculate between the blood and the lymph, returning to the blood via the thoracic duct.

Monocytes

Monocytes are large cells that are produced in the bone marrow. Mature cells spend about 30 h in the blood and then migrate to the tissues where they develop into macrophages. Macrophages are phagocytic although they respond more slowly than the neutrophils. They are also involved in regulating the immune response by activating B and T lymphocytes (see Chapter 29).

PLATELETS

These are small non-nuclear cellular elements produced in the bone marrow. They are colourless discoid bodies and have a diameter of only 2–4 micrometres. There are about 150–400 × 10^9/l.

Production of platelets (**thrombopoiesis**) occurs in the bone marrow. They are formed inside the cytoplasm of large cells called megakaryocytes and bud off from the cell surface. Each megakaryocyte takes about 10 days to mature and produces about 4000 platelets (Fig. 16.4). At any time two-thirds of the body's platelets are in the circulation and one-third in the spleen. The lifespan of a platelet is 7–10 days and they are destroyed by macrophages, mainly in the spleen but also in the liver.

Platelets are complex and have many functions other than being involved in the clotting process by forming a platelet plug. They are able to phagocytose small particles such as viruses and immune complexes. They store and transport histamine and serotonin which are released when platelets are damaged to affect smooth muscle tone in blood vessel walls. They probably supply the endothelial cells of the blood vessels with nutrition and these cells atrophy in platelet deficiency. They secrete platelet-derived growth factor (PDGF) which stimulates proliferation of smooth muscle walls to help healing after injury.

HAEMOSTASIS

If the endothelium of blood vessels is smooth and uninterrupted, blood flow is maintained. However, if a blood vessel is damaged a series of reactions occurs in order to main-

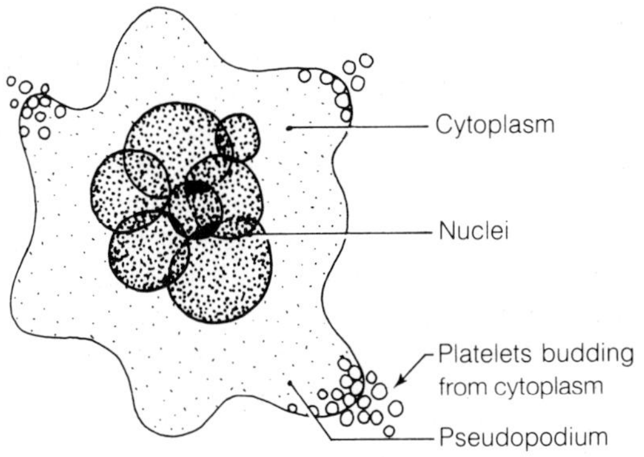

Figure 16.4 *Diagram of megakaryocyte showing platelet budding (from Hinchliff SM, Montague SE, 1990, with permission).*

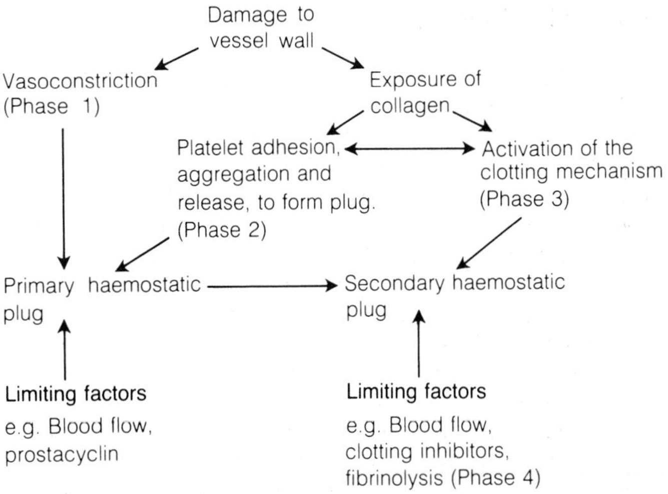

Figure 16.5 *An outline of the events of haemostasis (from Hinchliff SM, Montague SE, 1990, with permission).*

tain haemostasis and minimise blood loss. The mechanism is fast, localised and carefully controlled. Many blood coagulation factors normally present in plasma are involved. Some substances are released by platelets and injured tissues. Haemostasis involves three phases: vascular spasm, platelet plug formation and coagulation of blood (Fig. 16.5).

Vascular spasm

Vasoconstriction after injury is brought about by direct injury to vascular smooth muscle, compression of the vessel by extravasated blood, chemicals released by endothelial cells and platelets and reflexes triggered by pain receptors. A strongly constricted artery can significantly reduce blood loss for up to 30 min. This allows time for platelet plug formation and blood clotting to occur. A blunt injury crushes tissue and is more efficient at causing vascular spasm than a sharp cut.

Formation of a platelet plug

Normally platelets do not stick to each other or to the endothelial lining of blood vessels. Damage or disruption of the endothelium exposes underlying collagen fibres which causes platelets to swell and form spiky processes and stick to the exposed area. Once the platelets have adhered to the endothelium, lipids in the platelet plasma membrane release a shortlived prostaglandin derivative called thromboxane A_2. Degranulation of the platelets occurs and other chemicals are released. These are serotonin, which enhances vascular spasm, and adenosine diphosphate, which attracts more platelets. Within one minute a platelet plug forms (Fig. 16.6). Prostacyclin (PG_{12}) limits the process by confining platelet aggregation to the immediate area of damage.

Coagulation

There are three critical events in coagulation of blood.

1 Prothrombin activator is formed.
2 This converts the plasma protein prothrombin to thrombin.

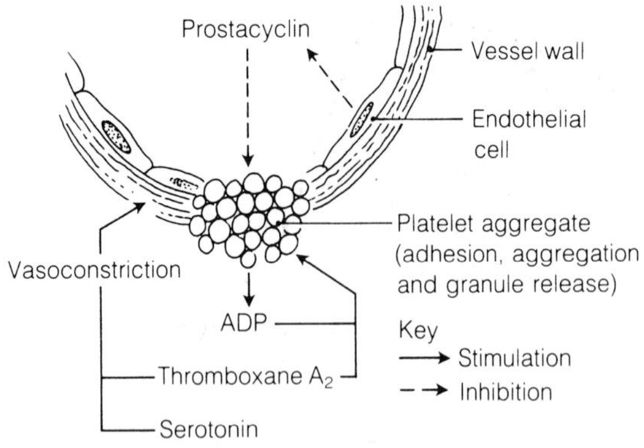

Figure 16.6 *Summary of events in the formation of a platelet plug (from Hinchliff SM, Montague SE, 1990, with permission).*

3 Thrombin causes fibrinogen molecules to form a fibrin mesh. This traps blood cells and seals the hole in the blood vessel.

Over 30 different substances affect the process. There are factors that enhance clot formation, called **procoagulants** (Table 16.7), and those that inhibit clot formation, called **anticoagulants**. Most of the procoagulants are plasma proteins synthesised in the liver – all but for factors III and IV. Many need the presence of vitamin K – factors II, VII, IX and X. The factors are released into the blood where they remain inert until the clotting cascade is triggered.

Clotting may be initiated by either of two pathways. These are the intrinsic and extrinsic pathways. Clotting outside the body is triggered by the intrinsic pathway whilst extravasated blood is clotted by the extrinsic pathway. Clot formation is normally complete within 3–6 min. The extrinsic pathway involves fewer steps and is more rapid than the intrinsic pathway. In severe trauma the extrinsic mechanism can clot blood within 15 s.

Table 16.7 *Procoagulant factors*

Number	*Name*	*Function*
I	Fibrinogen	Converted to fibrin mesh
II	Prothrombin	Converted to thrombin which converts fibrinogen to fibrin
III	Thromboplastin	Catalyses thrombin formation
IV	Calcium ions	Needed at all stages
V	Platelet accelerator	Affects both intrinsic and extrinsic methods
VI	No substance	
VII	Serum prothrombin conversion accelerator (SPCA)	Extrinsic pathway conversion
VIII	Antihaemophilic factor	Intrinsic mechanism. Absence = haemophilia A
IX	Plasma thromboplastin component (PTC, Christmas factor)	Intrinsic mechanism. Absence = haemophilia B
X	Stuart-Prower factor	Both extrinsic and intrinsic pathways
XI	Plasma thromboplastin antecedent (PTA)	Intrinsic mechanism. Absence = haemophilia C
XII	Hageman factor	Intrinsic mechanism
XIII	Fibrin stabilising factor (FSF)	Cross links fibrin to make it insoluble

Clot retraction and fibrinolysis

After 30–60 min a platelet-induced process called **clot retraction** occurs. A contractile protein, **actomyosin**, works as it does in muscle cells. Serum is squeezed out, the clot is compacted and the torn edges of the blood vessel are drawn together. This is the beginning of healing. PDGF released by degranulation of the platelets stimulates smooth muscle and fibroblasts to divide and rebuild the muscle wall.

Unnecessary clots are removed by fibrinolysis. If this did not occur the blood vessels would become occluded. Yet another of the plasma proteins, **plasminogen**, is activated to produce plasmin which is a protein-digesting enzyme. Large amounts of plasminogen may be incorporated into a big clot but remain inactive, producing plasmin only as necessary. Plasminogen activators are released from endothelial cells when clot is present. Factor VII and thrombin are also potent plasminogen activators.

Factors limiting clot growth or formation

- Rapid removal of coagulation factors.
- Inhibitors of activated clotting factors.

Any tendency to clot in rapidly moving blood is usually unsuccessful because any activated clotting factors are diluted and washed away. **Heparin** is a natural anticoagulant normally contained in the granules of the leuckocytes – mast cells and basophils. It is also produced by the endothelial cells. Small amounts released into the plasma normally prevent inappropriate blood coagulation.

MATERNAL ADAPTATIONS TO PREGNANCY

Blood volume and composition

Letsky (1991) writes that 'Plasma volume and total red cell mass are under separate control and bear no fixed relation to one another'. Total blood volume is a combination of plasma volume and red cell volume. The increase in blood volume relates to an increase in cardiac output. The average increase is between 30% and 50% with above 50% in multiple pregnancies. It can be noticed as early as the 6th week of pregnancy, which suggests a hormonal mechanism. Red cell mass increases by 18% whilst plasma volume increases about 50%. This difference results in hypervolaemia, haemodilution and a fall in Hb level often referred to as **physiological anaemia** (Figs 16.7 and 16.8).

Plasma volume

The increase in plasma volume is directly related to the birth weight of the baby. Women with multiple pregnancy have an

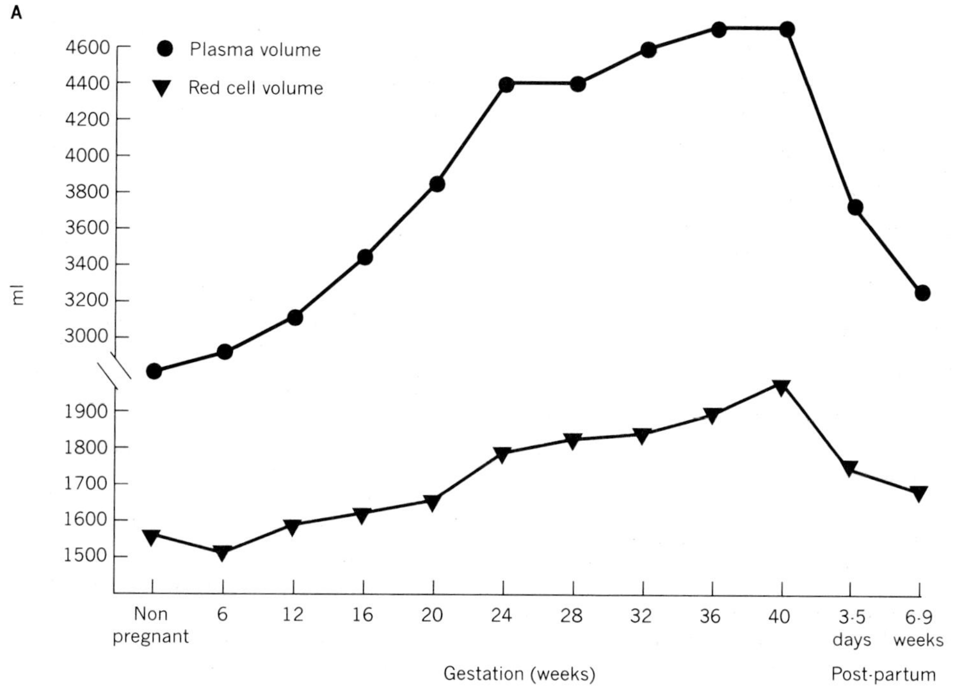

Figure 16.7 *(a) Mean total plasma and red cell volume during normal pregnancy. (Reproduced with permission from Lund & Donovan 1967.)*

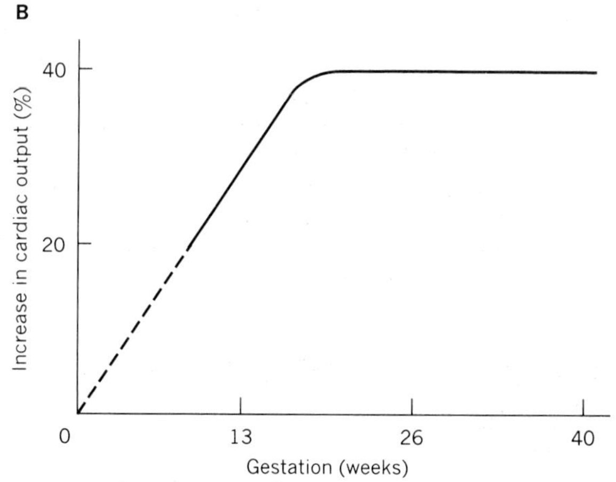

Figure 16.7 *(b) Changes in cardiac output throughout pregnancy. (Reproduced with permission from Hytten & Chamberlain 1991.)*

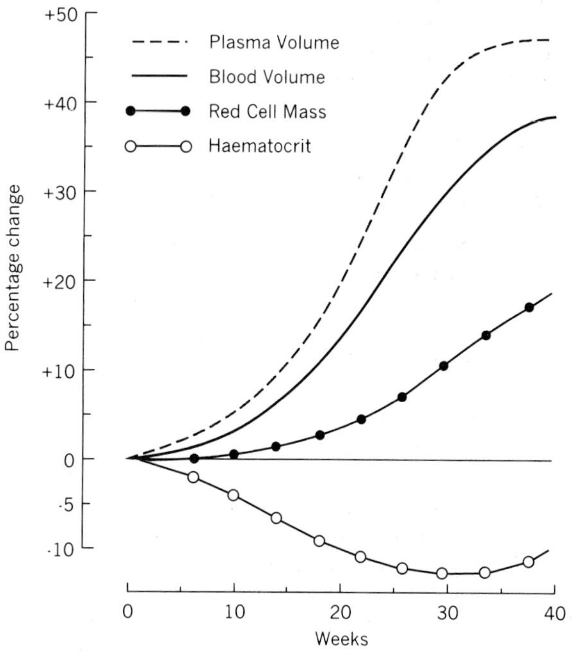

Figure 16.8 *Changes in plasma volume, blood volume, red cell mass and haematocrit during normal pregnancy levels. (Reproduced with permission from Rosso 1990.)*

increase greater than those with a singleton pregnancy and the amount increases with the number of babies in the uterus. There is a further increase in multigravid women which is mirrored by the greater weight of their babies.

The hypervolaemia fulfils the extra demands on the circulation in pregnancy. For instance, the basal metabolic rate increases by 20% in pregnancy with the production of more heat. Blood flow to the skin is increased and this allows heat to be lost. The increased blood volume also helps to maintain blood pressure when blood may be sequestered in the lower part of the body in the last trimester and helps to safeguard the woman against haemorrhage at delivery. The decrease in viscosity with increase in cardiac force leads to a decreased resistance to blood flow. This is essential for placental perfusion.

Red cells

In past research, the increase in red cell content of the blood in a normal pregnancy has been difficult to ascertain because many of the women had been given iron supplements. Letsky (1991) estimates that the increase is about 18% in women not supplemented with iron and 30% for those given iron medication. The red cell mass should expand as oxygen needs increase and as oxygen needs are thought to rise by about 15% in pregnancy, an increase in red cell mass of 18% is adequate. The nature of the increase in red cell production is not fully understood but there is a threefold increase in erythropoietin in the plasma in the 2nd trimester, possibly mediated by human placental lactogen. There is also a slight rise in the production of HbF, reaching a peak at 20 weeks and returning to normal 8 weeks after delivery (Letsky 1991).

Changes in red cell values in pregnancy

- Because the red cell count increase is less than the plasma increase, there is a reduction in red cell count from the normal $4.5 \times 10^{12}/1$ in early pregnancy to $3.6–3.8 \times 10^{12}/1$ by term.
- The haemoglobin level falls about 2 g/dl from a norm of 13 g/dl to about 11 g/dl. The haematocrit falls in parallel with the fall in red cell count.
- Mean cell haemoglobin concentration (MCHC). The average concentration of haemoglobin in each red cell changes little in a normal pregnancy. There is a slight progressive fall in women who are not given iron therapy.
- Mean cell volume (MCV). This is a more sensitive haematological measure of iron status in pregnancy. In normal pregnancy with sufficient iron present, there is an increase in red cell size but in pregnancy complicated by iron deficiency, an early sign is a reduction of cell size.

Iron requirements during pregnancy

In order to meet the expansion in red cell mass and the needs of the fetus and placenta, extra iron is needed in pregnancy. The total requirements throughout pregnancy have been calculated as 700–1400 mg. Overall the requirement is for 4 mg per day but this rises from 2.8 mg/day in early pregnancy to 6.6 mg/day in the last few weeks. The needs can be met from the mobilisation of stored iron as well as from iron intake.

Set against this need is the iron saved during pregnancy and breastfeeding because of amenorrhoea, which is 250–480 mg in total.

Folate metabolism

Requirements for folic acid are increased during pregnancy to meet the needs of the growing fetus and placenta, as well as the increased maternal tissues of the growing uterus and red cell mass. Folate will be transported by the placenta to the fetus even if maternal folate status is deficient.

Table 16.8 *The distribution of the extra iron in pregnancy*

Tissue usage	*Needs in mgms*
Expansion of the red cell mass	570
Fetus	270–370
Placenta	35–100
Blood loss at delivery	100–250
Breast feeding (6 months)	100–180
Loss from skin, faeces, urine	270

Box 16.2 Iron supplementation in pregnancy

There is no agreement on whether women can adapt their iron absorption in pregnancy without iron supplements (Roodenburg 1995). Some recommend iron supplementation of all women during the second half of pregnancy whilst others prefer supplementation only if there is an established iron deficit. Oral iron preparations may cause gastrointestinal upsets such as nausea, constipation and diarrhoea and women may not comply with therapy.

Letsky (1991) makes the point that many authors do not accept that the needs for iron in pregnancy are much higher than the dietary intake even of women who are considered to have a good diet. There is no doubt that women in developing countries often enter pregnancy with their iron stores already depleted, partly due to dietary deficiency but also to chronic infection such as malaria. In these situations iron supplementation can be life saving.

Oral iron supplements may reduce the bioavailability of zinc, important in pregnancy, and fetal intrauterine growth retardation may result. There is still controversy about the interaction between iron intake and zinc absorption. Sheldon et al (1985) found that the decrease of zinc and magnesium is a normal adjustment to pregnancy and therefore is not influenced by oral iron supplementation whereas Barrett et al (1994) believe that prophylactic iron supplements may not only be of no benefit but may be harmful in normal pregnancy by inhibiting zinc absorption.

Letsky reminds us that whilst in evolutionary terms women are adapted to the needs for iron in pregnancy, humans have changed their diet since the beginning of the agricultural revolution about 10 000 years ago. Previous to this people ate a high-protein diet based on fishing and hunting but changed to a mixed diet with grains and a much lower intake of fish and meat. Haem iron found in meats and fish is much easier to absorb than non-haem iron which may also be blocked from absorption by the phytates in grain. It is known that women who eat a vegetarian diet may not have sufficient reserves of iron to cope with a pregnancy. On the other hand, Western women are having many fewer pregnancies than in past centuries and are spacing them over time. This should prevent the continuous depletion of iron stores made by repeated pregnancies.

Letsky concludes that the immediate demands of pregnancy cannot be met by an increased absorption of iron from the diet. Whilst it is possible to screen for iron deficiency anaemia by using serum ferritin as a base and to then supplement only women thought to be at risk, Letsky considers that because of the risks of ill health and the cost of treatment it is safer to give all women iron supplements from 16 weeks of pregnancy.

Box 16.2 (cont'd) Iron supplementation in pregnancy

However, Barrett et al (1994) researched the absorption of iron in pregnancy. They assumed that if there was no change in iron stores during pregnancy then the daily absorption of iron would need to increase, especially to meet the needs of the 3rd trimester. Whilst this was a small study with only 12 women participating, they found that absorption in excess of the demands of pregnancy occurred as a physiological consequence of pregnancy. They suggested that as long as dietary intake was sufficient there was no need to give iron supplements routinely in pregnancy. Montgomery (1990) reminds us that iron supplementation in pregnancy will be augmented in women who take iron supplements and the resultant high haemoglobin levels may interfere with physiological haemodilution and placental perfusion, leading to reduced fetal growth.

Roodenburg (1995) suggests that dietary advice will be essential, preferably before or at the beginning of pregnancy. The advice would have to include not only the foods containing iron but the role of vitamin C in enhancing iron absorption and of the tannins in coffee and tea in inhibiting its absorption. Supplementation with iron will be necessary in diagnosed iron deficiency anaemia.

White cells

The total white cell count rises in pregnancy, mainly due to an increase in neutrophils. The neutrophil count rises in the menstrual cycle at the time of the oestrogen peak and continues to rise if fertilisation of the ovum occurs. A peak is reached at 30 weeks and then a plateau is maintained until delivery. There is a further rise in labour and the count returns to normal by the 6th postnatal day. Circulating oestrogen is probably the cause of the extra neutrophil production.

There is a slight rise in eosinophils in relation to the increased white cell count. There is a sharp fall in circulating eosinophils during labour and they are absent at delivery, returning to normal by the 3rd postnatal day. The basophil and monocyte counts appear to remain unchanged.

Although the lymphocyte count remains unchanged in pregnancy with no change in circulating T cells and B cells, there is profound depression of cell-mediated immunity. This picture is also seen in women taking oral contraceptives containing oestrogen. Oestrogen may increase the number of glycoproteins on the cell surface, leading to impaired response to stimuli. Human chorionic gonadotrophin from the placenta and prolactin from the anterior pituitary are known to suppress lymphocyte function. There seems to be no impairment to the production of immunoglobulins or to humoral mediated immunity. The depression of cell-mediated immunity is essential to the survival of the fetus but may increase susceptibility to viral infections such as rubella, influenza, poliomyelitis and influenza. Worldwide, the increased susceptibility in immune women to malaria leads to an infected placenta with increased fetal mortality.

Haemostasis

Letsky (1991) writes that major changes occur in the haemostatic components of blood during pregnancy, leading to a hypercoagulable state. Adequate haemostasis depends on the interaction between blood vessel wall, platelets, the coagulation system and the fibrinolytic system. Haemostasis in health has three main functions: to keep the circulating blood inside the vascular tree, to maintain the fluidity of blood and to arrest bleeding following injury to vessels.

The following changes are seen in pregnancy.

- Platelet counts decrease slightly in relation to the haemodilution. No change in function has been reported.
- There are increased levels of coagulation factors VII, VIII and X and a marked increase in plasma fibrinogen from as early as the 3rd month of gestation. Plasma fibrinogen levels may double in late pregnancy and labour due to increased synthesis. Factor VII may increase 10-fold (also seen in women taking oral contraceptives containing oestrogen) and the activity of factor VIII doubles (Letsky 1991).
- These changes are consistent with a continuous low-grade coagulation activity with fibrin deposition in the intervillous space of the placenta and in the walls of the spiral arteries. The deposition of a fibrin matrix is the mechanism by which the lumen of the arteries is distended to allow increasing blood flow to the placenta. This hypercoagulability is advantageous following placental separation to help in control of blood loss and to prevent haemorrhage. Following delivery the placental site is very rapidly covered by a fibrin mesh. The fibrinogen utilised represents up to 10% of the total circulating fibrinogen.
- Fibrinolytic activity is decreased during pregnancy, remains low in labour and delivery and returns to normal within 1 h of delivery. Whilst these changes help to combat the hazards of haemorrhage at delivery, the fact that they start early in pregnancy and are accompanied by venous stasis predisposes women to thromboembolic episodes.

The intrapartum and immediate postpartum periods

Blood volume lost at delivery is possibly 500 ml for a singleton pregnancy and up to 1000 ml for a multiple pregnancy or following a caesarean section (Letsky 1991). The normal response to blood loss is vasoconstriction as the blood volume falls. This is followed by an expansion over the next few days back to normal values accompanied by a fall in haematocrit. The hypervolaemia of pregnancy modifies this response. After this loss at delivery blood volume does not increase and stays stable. There is a gradual fall in plasma volume due to a diuresis. The red cell mass gradually reduces to a normal value as red cells are removed from the blood at the end of their lifespan.

Summary of main points

- Blood is a fluid tissue with living cells in a non-living matrix. It is circulated through the body, propelled by the pumping action of the heart, into the capillary beds of the tissues. It carries oxygen and nutrients to the cells and carbon dioxide and metabolic waste from the cells. Blood volume forms 6–8% of body weight which is about 5–6 litres in a man and 4–5 litres in a woman.
- The functions of blood are internal transport of substances for respiration, nutrition and excretion, maintenance of water, electrolyte and acid/base balance and metabolic regulation, defence against infection, protection from haemorrhage and maintenance of body temperature.
- Plasma consists of water, plasma proteins and electrolytes. If clotting factors are removed the remaining fluid is called serum. Plasma proteins prevent fluid loss, transport substances around the body, are involved in clotting and fibrinolytic activities, assist in prevention of infection, help regulate acid/base balance by acting in buffering systems, act as a protein reserve and contribute half of total blood viscosity.
- Red cells, white cells and platelets are present in blood, each having a very different function from the others. Haemopoiesis is the term for blood cell formation. A pluripotent stem cell in the red bone marrow is thought to give rise to progenitor cells for the three main types of cell.
- Red blood cells live about 120 days and are finally fragmented and destroyed by macrophages in the spleen. Protein and haem are produced, which enter the body stores, and bilirubin which is excreted in bile.
- The amount of iron absorbed depends on the rate of red cell production, the extent of iron stores, the content of the diet and whether or not iron supplements are given. Folates are absorbed in the duodenum and jejunum and stored in the liver. Deficiency is more likely to be seen in the winter months when the foods containing folic acid may be difficult to obtain.
- Red blood cells have about 400 inherited glycoproteins in their plasma membranes which act as antigens, provoking an immune reaction if incompatible blood enters the circulation. The ABO blood groups are based on the presence of two red cell antigens, type A and type B. The O blood group arises if neither antigen is inherited. The two types are codominant and if both are inherited, group AB results.
- Only three rhesus antigens are common: the C, D and E agglutinogens. Rhesus D is by far the most clinically important. About 85% of people in the Western world are Rh+ and 15% are Rh–. There are no spontaneously occurring anti-Rh antibodies but these are formed if there is a sensitisation event of Rh+ red cells in the circulation of an Rh– person.
- White cells or leucocytes account for 1% of the blood's cellular content. Those present in blood represent only a small part of the body's total white cell content as the majority are in the tissues.
- In normal females a Barr body can be seen on about 5% of polymorphonuclear leucocytes but not on male cells. This represents a dormant X chromosome and inactivation of one X chromosome in all cells occurs early in embryonic development of the female. The inactivation process is random and half the cells will contain the paternal and half the maternal X chromosome.
- Platelets are produced in the bone marrow inside the cytoplasm of megakaryocytes. They help in the clotting process by forming a platelet plug. They phagocytose small particles such as viruses and immune complexes, store and transport histamine and serotonin, supply the endothelial cells of the blood vessels with nutrition and secrete PDGF which stimulates proliferation of smooth muscle cells to help healing.
- Blood flow depends on a smooth endothelial surface lining blood vessels. If a blood vessel is damaged a series of reactions occurs in order to maintain haemostasis and minimise blood loss. Haemostasis involves vascular spasm, platelet plug formation and blood coagulation.
- Total blood volume is a combination of plasma volume and red cell volume. The increase in blood volume in pregnancy relates to an increase in cardiac output. In pregnancy red cell mass or total volume of red cells increases by 18% whilst plasma volume increases by about 50%. This difference results in hypervolaemia, haemodilution and a fall in Hb level, often referred to as physiological anaemia.
- The increase in plasma volume is related to the birth weight of the baby. Women with multiple pregnancy have an increase greater than those with a singleton pregnancy. The decrease in viscosity with increase in cardiac force leads to a decreased resistance to blood flow which is essential for placental perfusion.
- To meet the expansion in red cell mass and the needs of the fetus and placenta, extra iron is needed in pregnancy but there is no agreement on whether women need iron supplements if well fed. Women in developing countries may enter pregnancy with their iron stores already depleted and iron supplementation can be life saving.
- Requirements for folic acid are increased during pregnancy to meet the needs of the growing fetus and placenta, as well as the increased maternal tissues of the growing uterus and red cell mass. Folate will be transported by the placenta to the fetus even if maternal folate status is deficient.
- The total white cell count rises in pregnancy, mainly due to an increase in neutrophils. The lymphocyte count remains unchanged with no change in circulating T cells and B cells but there is depression of cell-mediated immunity which may be essential to the survival of the fetus but may increase susceptibility to viral infections.
- Major changes occur in the haemostatic components of blood during pregnancy, leading to a hypercoagulable state. Fibrinolytic activity is decreased during pregnancy, remains low in labour and delivery and returns to normal within 1 h of delivery. These changes help to combat haemorrhage at delivery but they are accompanied by venous stasis and predispose women to thromboembolic episodes.
- Blood volume lost at delivery is possibly 500 ml for a singleton pregnancy and up to 1000 ml for a multiple pregnancy or following a caesarean section. After normal loss at delivery, blood volume does not increase as usual in haemorrhage. There is a gradual fall in plasma volume due to a diuresis. The red cell mass gradually reduces to a normal value.

References

Barrett JFR, Whittaker PG, Williams JG, Lind T. 1994 Absorption of haem iron from food during normal pregnancy. British Medical Journal 309, 79–82.

Hinchliff SM, Montague SE. 1990 Physiology for Nursing Practice. Baillière Tindall, London.

Jones S, Martin R, Pilbeam D. The Cambridge Encyclopaedia of Human Evolution, Cambridge University Press, Cambridge.

Letsky E. 1991 The haematological system. In Hytten F, Chamberlain G (eds). Clinical Physiology in Obstetrics, 2nd edn. Blackwell Scientific, Oxford.

Montague SE. 1996 The blood. In Hinchliff SM, Montague SE, Watson R (eds) Physiology in Nursing Practice. Baillière Tindall, London.

Montgomery E. 1990 Iron levels in pregnancy, physiology or pathology? Assessing the need for supplements. Midwifery 6, 205–214.

Roodenburg AJC. 1995 Iron supplementation during pregnancy. European Journal of Obstetrics and Gynaecology and Reproductive Biology 61, 65–71.

Sheldon WL, Aspillaga MO, Smith PA, Lind T. 1985 The effects of oral iron supplementation on zinc and magnesium levels during pregnancy. British Journal of Obstetrics and Gynaecology 92, 892–898.

Recommended reading

Letsky E. 1991 The haematological system. In Hytten F, Chamberlain G (eds). Clinical Physiology in Obstetrics, 2nd edn. Blackwell Scientific, Oxford.

Montague SE. 1996 The blood. In Hinchliff SM, Montague SE, Watson R (eds) Physiology in Nursing Practice. Baillière Tindall, London.

Roodenburg AJC. 1995 Iron supplementation during pregnancy. European Journal of Obstetrics and Gynaecology and Reproductive Biology 61, 65–71.

Chapter 17 The cardiovascular system

In this chapter

INTRODUCTION

Herbert & Alison (1996) state that 'The functioning of the body as a whole depends on the individual and collective functioning of cells'. The cardiovascular system, consisting of the heart and blood vessels, is able to meet those crucial homeostatic needs by maintaining an adequate blood supply to the cells and tissues during varying physiological circumstances. For instance, blood can be preferentially directed to individual systems as required. Flow increases to the muscles during exercise and to the gastrointestinal system following food intake. The system as a whole is controlled by centres in the brain although local events and reflexes may modify the

brain although local events and reflexes may modify the end result. There are three main roles for the cardiovascular system:

1 delivery of nutrients and oxygen;

2 removal of metabolic waste and carbon dioxide;

3 dissipation of heat from active tissues and redistribution of heat around the body.

CIRCULATORY PATHWAYS

Blood flows through the body in two distinct circuits. The **pulmonary circulation** takes deoxygenated blood from the right side of the heart to the lungs and returns oxygenated blood from the lungs to the left side of the heart. The **systemic circulation** takes oxygenated blood from the left side of the heart to all the tissues and returns deoxygenated blood to the right side of the heart. Exchange of nutrients and metabolic waste products takes place in the systemic circulation. In a normal adult at rest, the amount of blood circulated through the heart is 5 litres per minute which is the same as the amount of blood in the circulation.

The force required to move blood around the body comes from the heart which is essentially two separate pumps: the left side supplies the systemic circulation and the right side the pulmonary circulation. As a general principle, veins carry blood to the heart, oxygenated in the pulmonary circulatory system and deoxygenated in the systemic circulation (Fig. 17.1). Arteries carry blood away from the heart, deoxygenated in the pulmonary circulatory system and oxygenated in the systemic circulation.

ANATOMY OF THE HEART

The heart lies in the mediastinum of the thoracic cavity between the two lungs enclosed in their pleural sacs. It is positioned with two-thirds of its mass to the left of the body's midline. It is shaped like a blunt cone with its apex pointing downwards (Fig. 17.2). The heart extends about 12–14 cm from the 2nd to the 5th intercostal space and its base, which points upwards towards the right shoulder, is about 9 cm wide. The heart of an adult normally weighs about 300 g.

Layers

The **myocardium** or contractile wall of the heart consists mainly of cardiac muscle. Connective tissue forms a dense fibrous network which reinforces the myocardium and anchors the muscle fibres. The fibrous network also limits the spread of electrical action potentials to specific pathways.

The inner lining or **endocardium** consists of squamous epithelium resting on connective tissue. This also covers the valves and the tendons that hold them in place. It is continuous with the endothelial lining of the blood vessels entering the heart.

The heart is enclosed in a fibroserous sac or **pericardium** which protects it and anchors it to the large blood vessels, diaphragm and sternal wall. It has two layers – an outer fibrous and an inner serous pericardium. The serous pericardium is also composed of two layers – the outer parietal and the inner visceral layer or **epicardium** next to the myocardium. Between the visceral and parietal layers of the serous pericardium is the **pericardial cavity** which is filled with pericardial fluid. This provides a friction-free area within which the heart can pump.

Chambers and valves

There are four chambers in the heart: two superior atria and two inferior ventricles. The right ventricle forms most of the anterior surface of the heart whilst the left ventricle forms the inferior posterior aspect and the apex. These chambers are separated by septa – the interatrial septum – and the interventricular septum – and the valves.

The valves are attached to papillary muscles by the **chordae tendineae** which anchor them in the closed position. The valves direct and control the flow of blood through the heart by opening as the associated chamber contracts and closing as the chamber relaxes. The valves ensure a one-way flow of blood through the heart.

The atrioventricular valves

The **tricuspid** valve separates the right atrium from the right ventricle.
The **mitral** or bicuspid valve separates the left atrium from the left ventricle.

The semilunar valves

The **pulmonary** valve lies between the right ventricle and the pulmonary artery.
The **aortic** valve lies between the left ventricle and the aorta.

The coronary circulation

Oxygen is carried to the cardiac muscle by the right and left coronary arteries originating from the aorta just beyond the aortic valve. The right coronary artery supplies the right atrium and right ventricle and portions of the left ventricle. The left coronary artery divides near its origin into the left anterior descending branch, supplying the anterior part of the left ventricle and a small part of the right ventricle, and the circumflex branch, which supplies blood to the left atrium and upper left ventricle. Blood returns from the left side of the heart to the right atrium via the coronary sinus and from the right side via small anterior cardiac veins.

PHYSIOLOGY OF THE HEART

Cardiac muscle combines properties of both skeletal and smooth muscle (see Chapter 25). It is striated like skeletal muscle but individual muscle cell membranes have very low

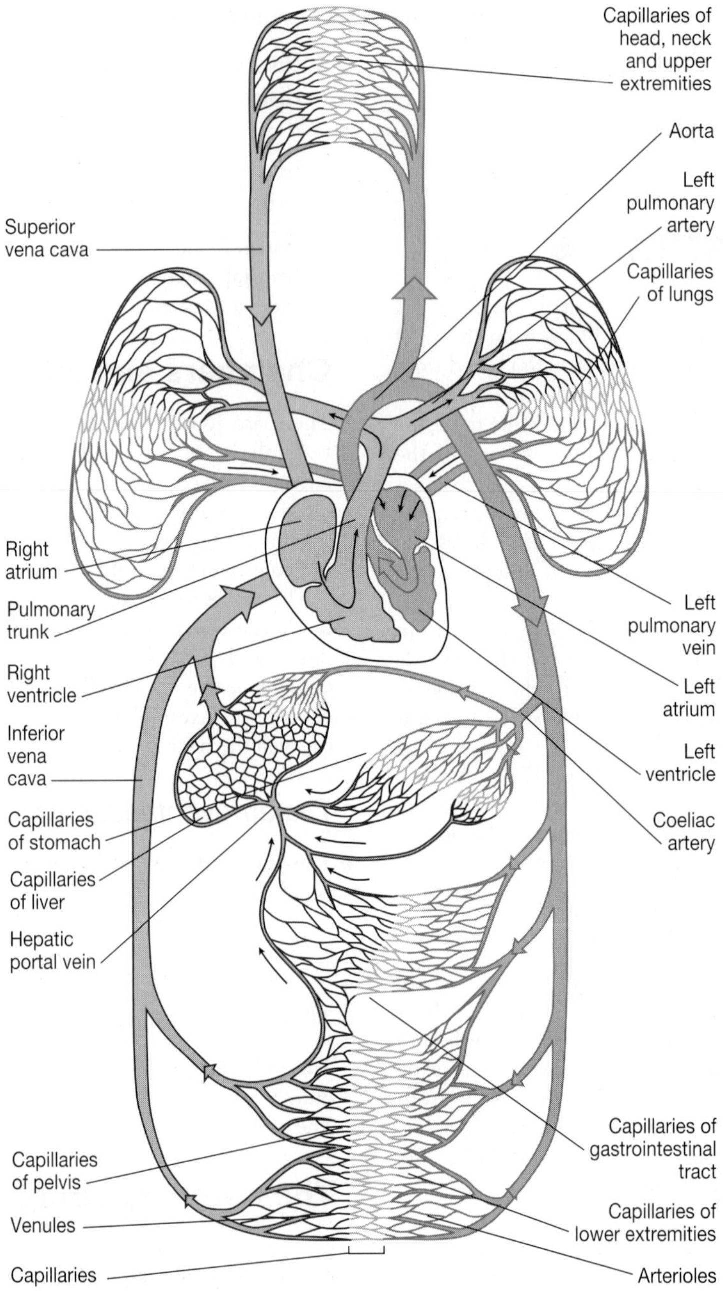

Figure 17.1 *A general plan of the circulatory system (from Hinchliff SM, Montague SE, Watson R, 1996, with permission).*

electrical resistance. Structures called **intercalated discs** (Fig. 17.3) allow action potentials to pass easily from one cardiac muscle cell to another so that the muscle mass functions as a whole. Intercalated discs contain anchoring units called **desmosomes** to hold the fibres together. Gap junctions between the muscle cells allow easy movement of ions to facilitate the spread of action potentials. The action potential is prolonged, allowing the impulse time to travel over the whole atrial or ventricular mass so that the cardiac muscle contracts as a unit. There is then a prolonged refractory period during which the relaxation phase occurs and no further contraction can begin.

The electrical conducting system (nodal system)

The component parts of the electrical conducting system of the heart are:

- the sinoatrial node (SA);
- the atrioventricular node (AV);
- the atrioventricular bundle of His;
- the left and right branch bundles;
- the Purkinje fibres.

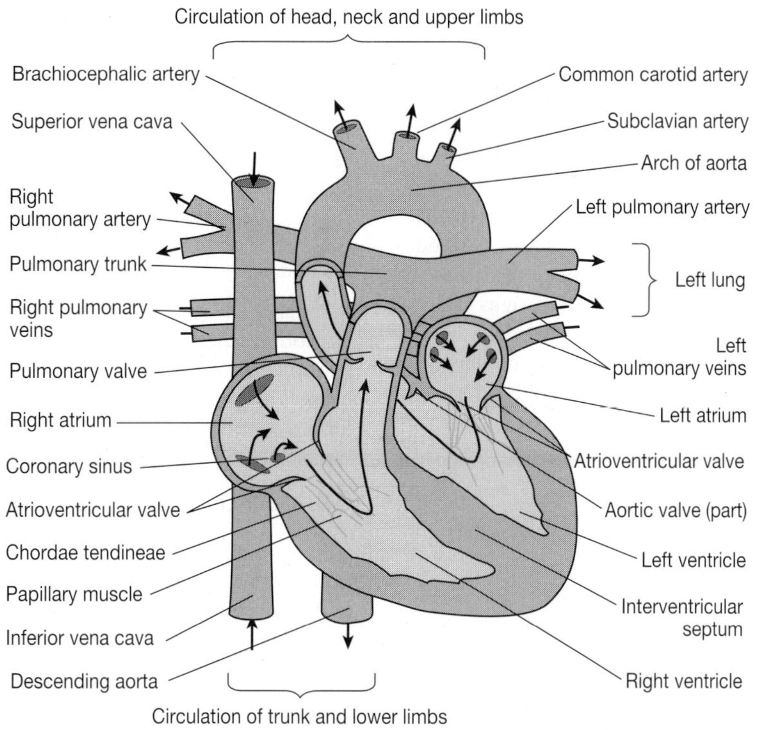

Figure 17.2 *The direction of blood flow within the heart (from Hinchliff SM, Montague SE, Watson R, 1996, with permission).*

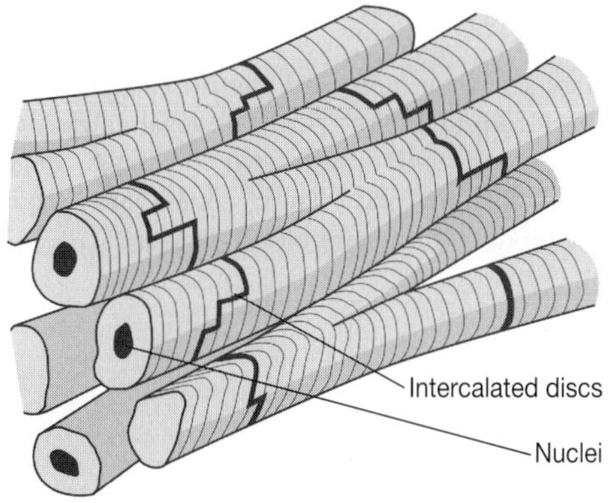

Figure 17.3 *The structure of cardiac muscle showing the intercalated discs (from Hinchliff SM, Montague SE, Watson R, 1996, with permission).*

The action potential which causes contraction is initiated by the SA node, located in the right atrium. It then spreads through both atria and enters the AV node at the base of the right atrium. This plus the bundle of His provides the only conduction link to the ventricles. There is a 0.1 s delay in conduction, allowing the atria to finish contracting and emptying their blood into the ventricles. The wave now spreads via the left and right branch bundles, which lie on either side of the interventricular septum, to the Purkinje fibres and the ventricular muscle. The spread is simultaneous and there is coordinated contraction.

The cardiac cycle

The cardiac cycle is taken from the end of one contraction to the end of the next. It produces two distinct sounds in a single beat, 'lub-dup'. The first heart sound is produced by the closure of the atrioventricular valves at the beginning of ventricular contraction or **systole**. The second sound is produced by the closure of the semilunar valves at the beginning of ventricular relaxation or **diastole**. Each cycle lasts 0.8 s, of which systole is 0.3 s and diastole 0.5 s. The heart rate (HR) is the number of cycles or beats per minute (bpm). The length of one cycle multiplied by the number of seconds in a minute gives the HR of 72 bpm.

CONTROL OF THE HEART RATE

Intrinsic control

The intrinsic conduction system of the heart allows the heart muscle to beat on its own with no external control. The heart's electrical conduction system has **autorhythmicity**. The SA node acts as a pacemaker at about 100 bpm if there are no other influences on heart rate. Other parts of the conducting system also have autorhythmicity. The unopposed AV node can initiate a rate of 40–60 bpm and the rest of the system will initiate a rate of 15–40 bpm.

Extrinsic control

The heart rate is influenced by the autonomic nervous system, hormones such as adrenaline, stretching of the atria, temperature and drugs.

Nervous control

In the medulla oblongata the **cardiovascular centre** (CVC) receives input from baroreceptors, chemoreceptors and higher centres in the brain such as the cortex and hypothalamus (Fig. 17.4). The CVC can be subdivided into the **cardiac centre**, affecting heart function, and the **vasomotor centre**, affecting blood vessels, but these probably function interactively. Sympathetic fibres from the cardiac centre innervate the SA and AV nodes and the myocardium and their stimulation increases the heart rate. Parasympathetic branches from the **vagus nerve** originating in the **nucleus ambiguus** in the medulla also innervate the SA and AV nodes and their action is to decrease the heart rate (Fig. 17.5). This influence, dominant at rest, is sometimes known as the **vagal brake**.

Hormonal control

Adrenaline stimulates β-1 receptors in cardiac muscle and causes the heart rate to increase in response to stress. The hormones noradrenaline and thyroid hormone also enhance the effect of the sympathetic nervous system to increase heart rate.

Stretch

Stretching of the atrial walls by increased venous return or increased blood volume can raise the heart rate by 10–15%. This is the **Bainbridge reflex** which occurs because the stretch receptors in the atrial walls send impulses to stimulate sympathetic output.

Stroke volume

Excess blood also stretches the ventricles (**ventricular end-diastolic volume** (VEDV)). The more the ventricles are stretched before contraction, the greater the force of contraction and the amount of blood leaving the heart. This is **Starling's law of the heart**. The amount of blood leaving each ventricle during one contraction is called the **stroke volume** and is normally 70 ml. When a ventricle contracts, it does not empty completely. The blood left in the ventricle at the end of systole is the **ventricular end-systolic volume** (VESV) and:

$$SV = VEDV - VESV$$

In health the extra VEDV of the next cycle brought about by adding the atrial contents to the remaining blood in the ventricle increases the contraction force, causing the ventricle to empty more completely, thus maintaining SV at a constant level.

Cardiac output

Cardiac output (CO) is usually defined as the volume of blood pumped by the left ventricle into the aorta per minute (Herbert & Alison 1996). It is about 70 ml at rest. An important formula is:

$$CO = SV \times HR.$$

The heart rate is normally 72 bpm so this is 70 × 72 and CO = 5040 ml/min. This can increase to 30 l under extreme conditions. The difference between the cardiac output at rest and what the heart is capable of pumping is called the **cardiac reserve**.

In response to being stretched, the atria secrete a hormone called **atrial natriuretic** factor (ANF) or **atrial natriuretic peptide** (ANP). This is a potent diuretic which causes the kidney to excrete excess sodium and water. This plays a part in the regulation of blood volume and blood pressure.

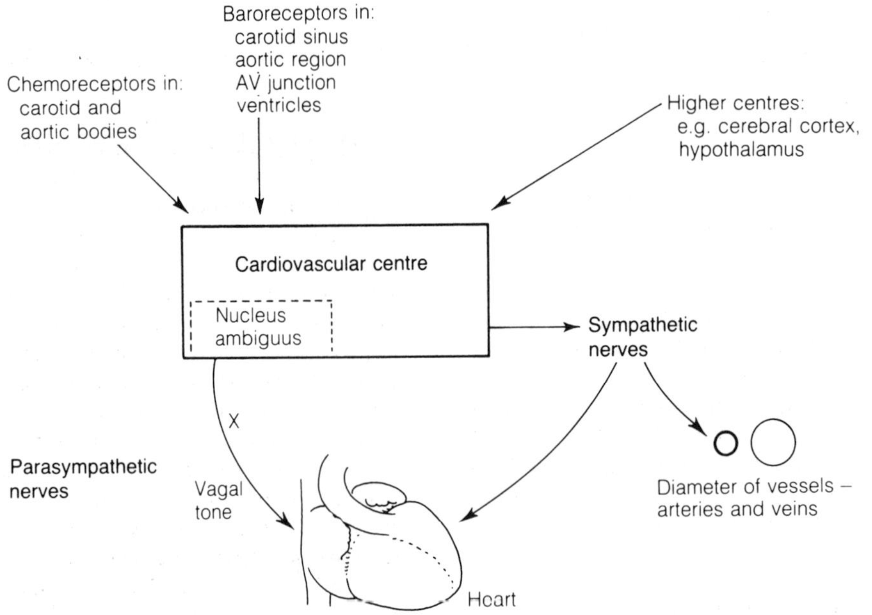

Figure 17.4 *Diagrammatic representation of afferent and efferent pathways associated with the cardiovascular control centre (from Hinchliff SM, Montague SE, 1990, with permission).*

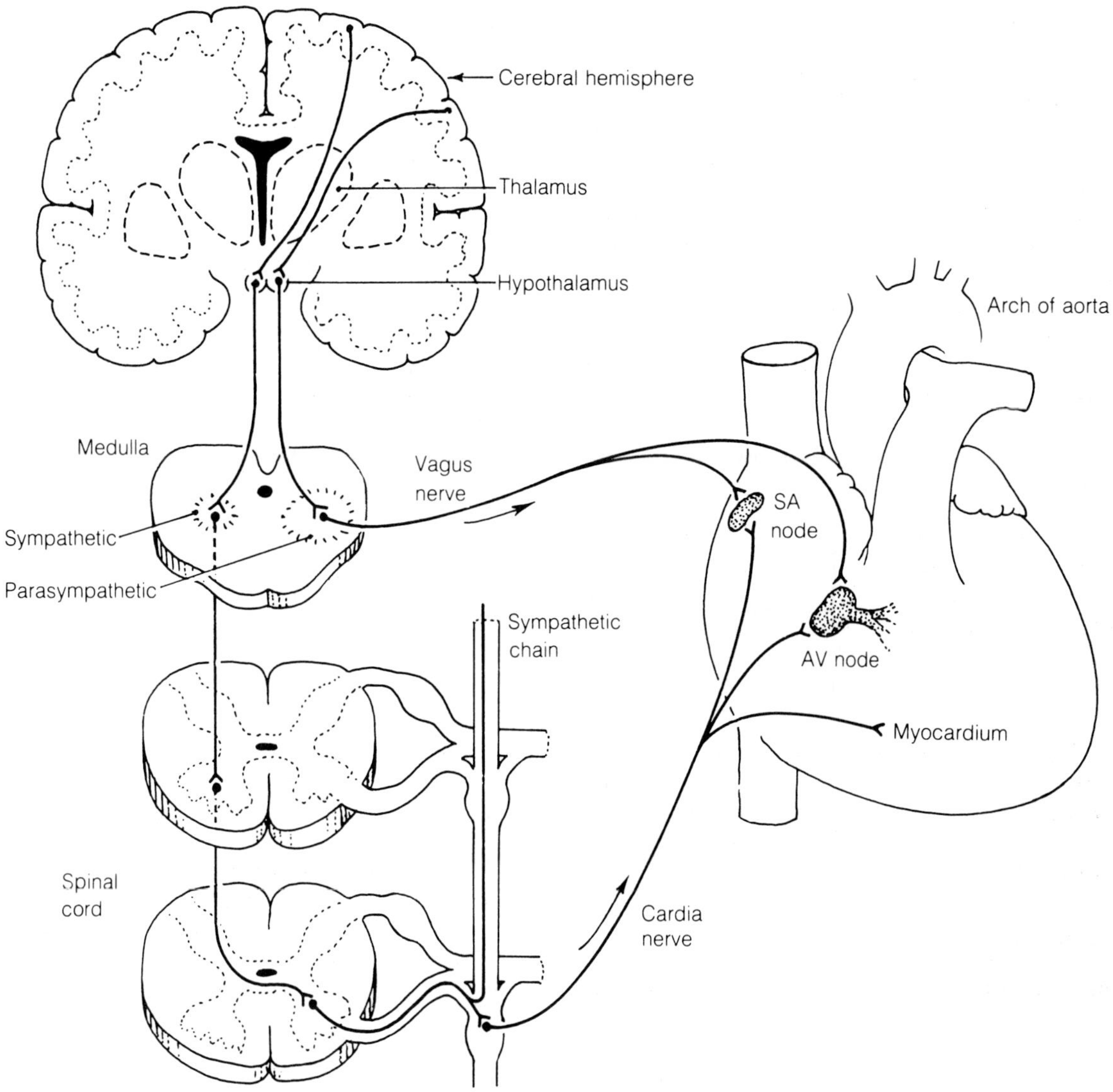

Figure 17.5 *Sympathetic and parasympathetic innervation of the heart (based on Tortora & Anagnostakos 1981).*

Other influences

If core body temperature rises there will be an increase in heart rate whilst a lowering of core body temperature will decrease the heart rate. This latter is seen in people with hypothermia. The changes in body temperature alter the rate of electrical discharge.

Drugs such as isoprenaline or adrenaline can increase the heart rate. Drugs acting as β-adrenergic blockers, such as propranolol, will decrease the heart rate.

A raised arterial blood pressure may decrease SV as the ventricles must exert force against a greater load. A normal heart will adjust to counter this by increasing the force of ventricular contraction. If the blood pressure is chronically raised the left ventricle will hypertrophy and fail.

THE VASCULAR SYSTEM

The vascular system delivers blood to all tissues as needed and returns blood to the heart (Figs 17.7 and 17.8). To achieve this the system must be adaptive to local needs and must change a pulsatile arterial blood flow to a steady capillary flow so that exchange of nutrients and waste can occur effectively.

In the systemic circulation blood leaves the left side of the heart via the aorta which subdivides into smaller arteries. The smallest are **arterioles** which branch into **capillaries** where the exchange of gases, nutrients and metabolic wastes occurs. Capillaries unite to form **venules** which combine to form larger veins. Finally the two largest veins, the **inferior vena cava** returning blood from the lower part of the body and the **superior vena cava** returning blood from the upper part of the body, enter the right atrium of the heart.

In the pulmonary circulation a single pulmonary artery leaves the right ventricle and divides into two branches which deliver deoxygenated blood returning from the tissues to each lung for oxygenation. The division into smaller arteries, arterioles, capillaries, venules and veins is the same as in the systemic circulation. Four pulmonary veins deliver oxygenated blood back to the left atrium.

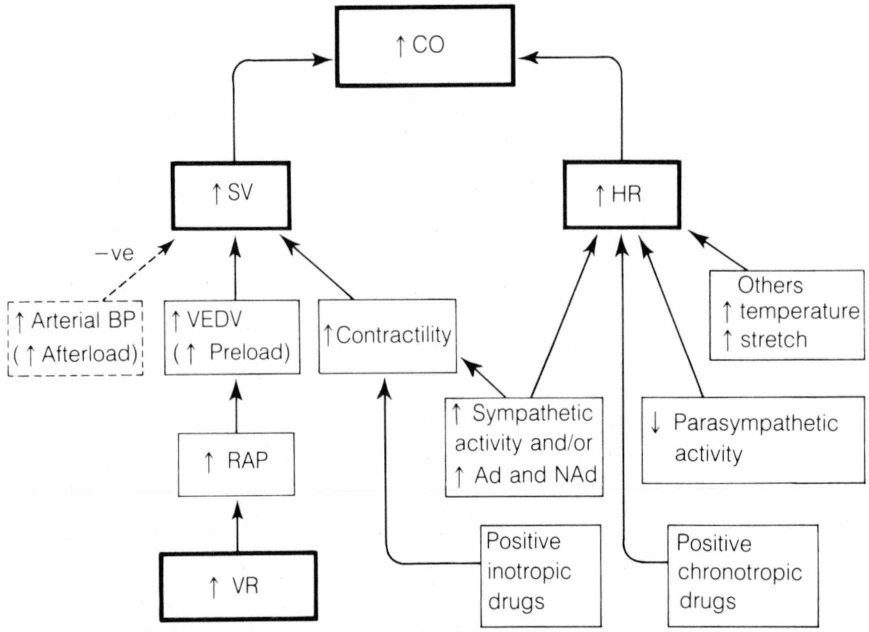

Figure 17.6 *Main factors that can alter cardiac output. An increased arterial blood pressure (i.e. an increased afterload) causes a decrease in stroke volume and consequently a decrease in cardiac output. CO, cardiac output; SV, stroke volume; HR, heart rate; VEDV, ventricular end-diastolic volume; RAP, right atrial pressure; VR, venous return; Ad, adrenaline; NAd, noradrenaline (from Hinchliff SM, Montague SE, 1990, with permission).*

Structure of blood vessels

The structure of the blood vessels varies depending on their specific functions but the walls of the blood vessels, with the exception of the capillaries, contain the same three layers of tissue (Fig. 17.9).

- The **tunica intima** is the innermost layer, called the endothelium, which is a single layer of extremely flattened epithelial cells. This is supported by a basement membrane and some connective and elastic tissue. This is the only layer found in the capillaries.
- The **tunica media** is the middle layer and consists mainly of smooth muscle and elastic tissue. This is the layer that gives rise to the variation throughout the vascular system.
- The **tunica adventitia** is the outer layer and is composed of fibrous connective tissue, collagen and fibroblasts.

The arterial system

Elastic arteries (conducting arteries)

Large arteries contain more elastic tissue and can passively expand and recoil to accommodate changes in blood volume. This allows blood to be kept under continuous pressure rather than starting and stopping with the pulsatile heart beat. When the heart contracts blood is forced into the aorta and distends these vessels. When the heart rests the large arteries return to their normal diameters. They have large diameters, that of the aorta being about 2.5 cm.

Muscular arteries (distributing arteries)

These medium-sized arteries distribute blood to all tissues. They have an average diameter of about 0.4 cm and are still distensible so that resistance to flow is low. As they branch further and become smaller, the amount of elastic tissue decreases and the smooth muscle component increases.

Arterioles

Arterioles are the smallest arteries, less than 0.3 cm in diameter, with a thicker wall mainly made up of muscular tissue in concentric layers. The total resistance to blood flow is mainly determined by the diameter of the arterioles which also determine the distribution of blood flow to different tissues. The **precapillary sphincters** are specialised regions near the junction between the terminal arterioles and the capillaries. These consist of smooth muscle fibres arranged in a circular manner around the vessel which control the amount of blood flowing into a capillary bed. This action may also play a part in the formation of tissue fluid (see below).

Capillaries

Capillaries form a dense network of very narrow short vessels. Red blood cells pass through them in single file and may have to fold to negotiate their lumen. They are the exchange vessels where gases, nutrients and metabolic waste products pass between individual cells and the vascular system. There are up to 50 million capillaries in the body but only 25% of these may be patent at rest. Some modified, wider capillaries are known as **sinusoids**. They are found mainly in the liver, bone marrow, lymphoid tissues and endocrine organs and are lined by phagocytic white cells. Blood flows slowly through sinusoids to allow modification of its content; for instance, in the liver nutrients are extracted.

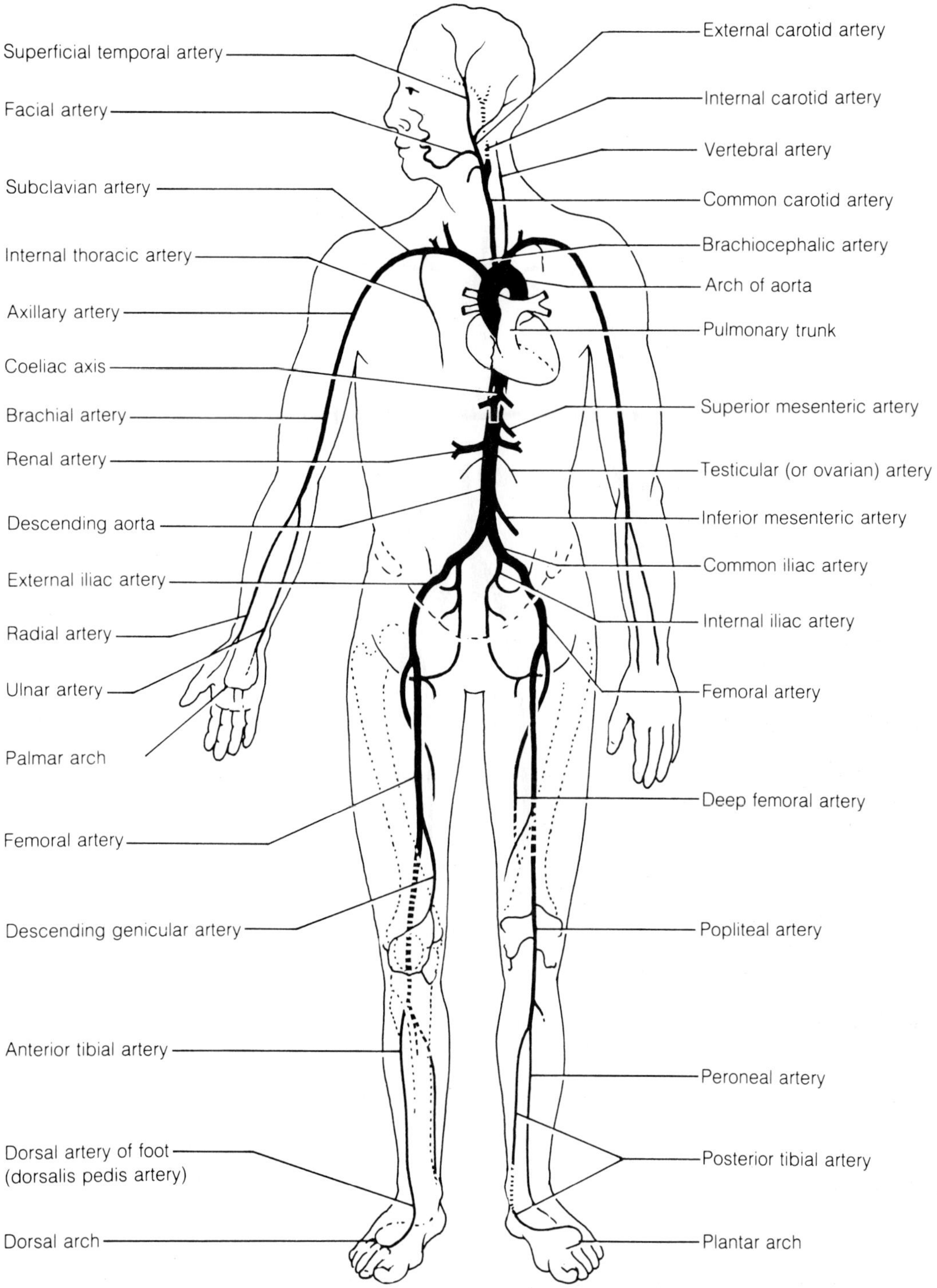

Figure 17.7 *Major arteries of the human body (anterior view) (from Hinchliff SM, Montague SE, 1990, with permission).*

The microcirculation

Each cell must have access to a capillary supply if it is to remain healthy. Substances need to travel a very short distance to enable adequate **diffusion**. Different tissues have varying amounts of capillaries depending on their metabolic needs. There may also be **arteriovenous shunts**, connections between the arteries and veins that bypass the capillaries. Blood can flow rapidly through the shunts but this mechanism does not allow exchange of nutrients and gases. They facilitate dissipation of heat from the body via the skin if needed.

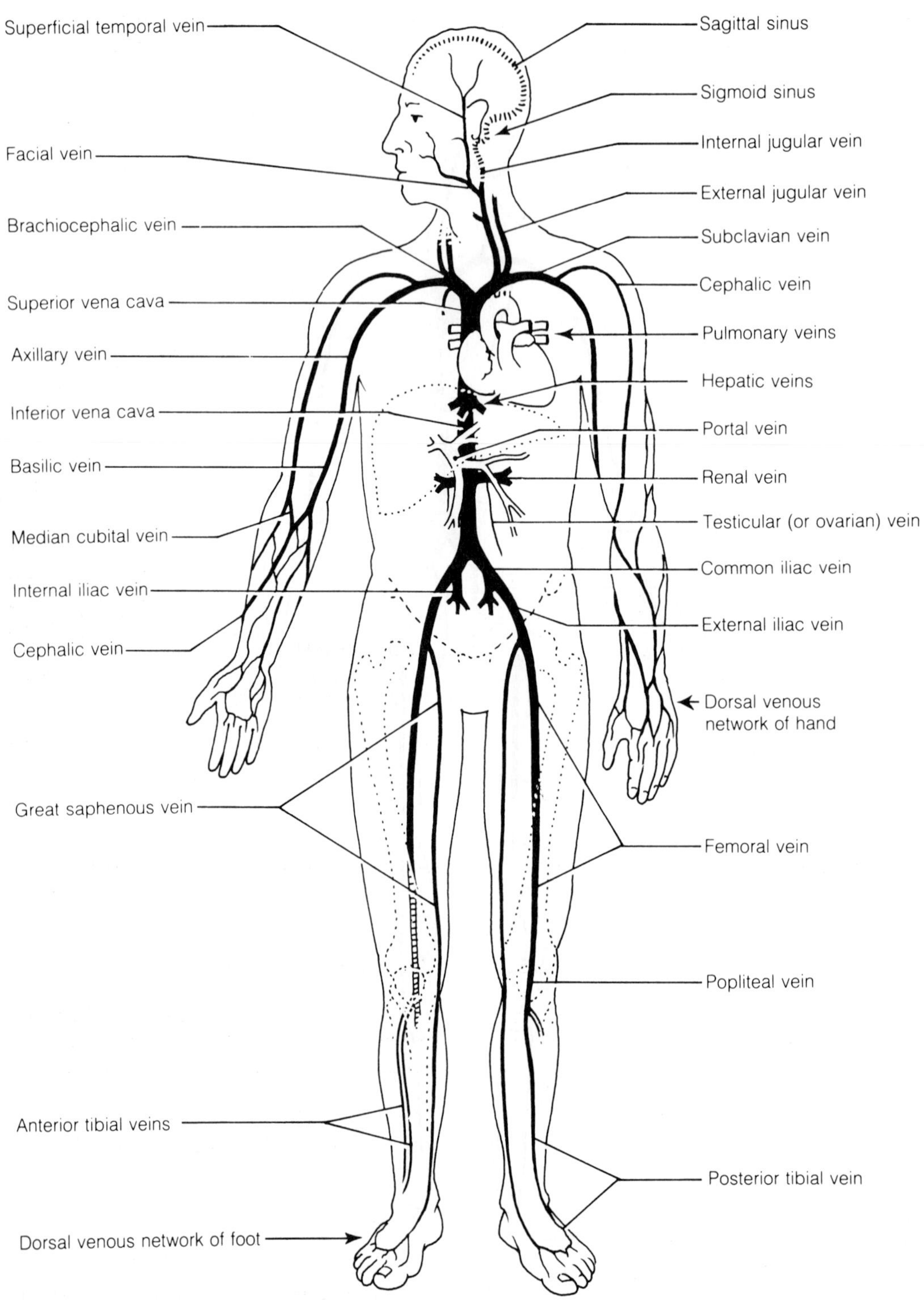

Figure 17.8 *Major veins of the human body (anterior view) (from Hinchliff SM, Montague SE, 1990, with permission).*

The venous system

Veins return blood from the capillary beds to the heart passively along a pressure gradient. As the veins become fewer and larger, resistance to flow decreases. Vein walls have the same three layers as arteries but they are thinner and more distensible than arteries. Some veins, such as those in the legs, have folds in the endothelium which act as valves to ensure that blood flows in one direction towards the heart. These valves may be damaged if overstretched by high pressures, for instance in pregnancy, and this may lead to oedema and varicose veins. The larger part of the circulating blood, about 60%, is contained in the venous

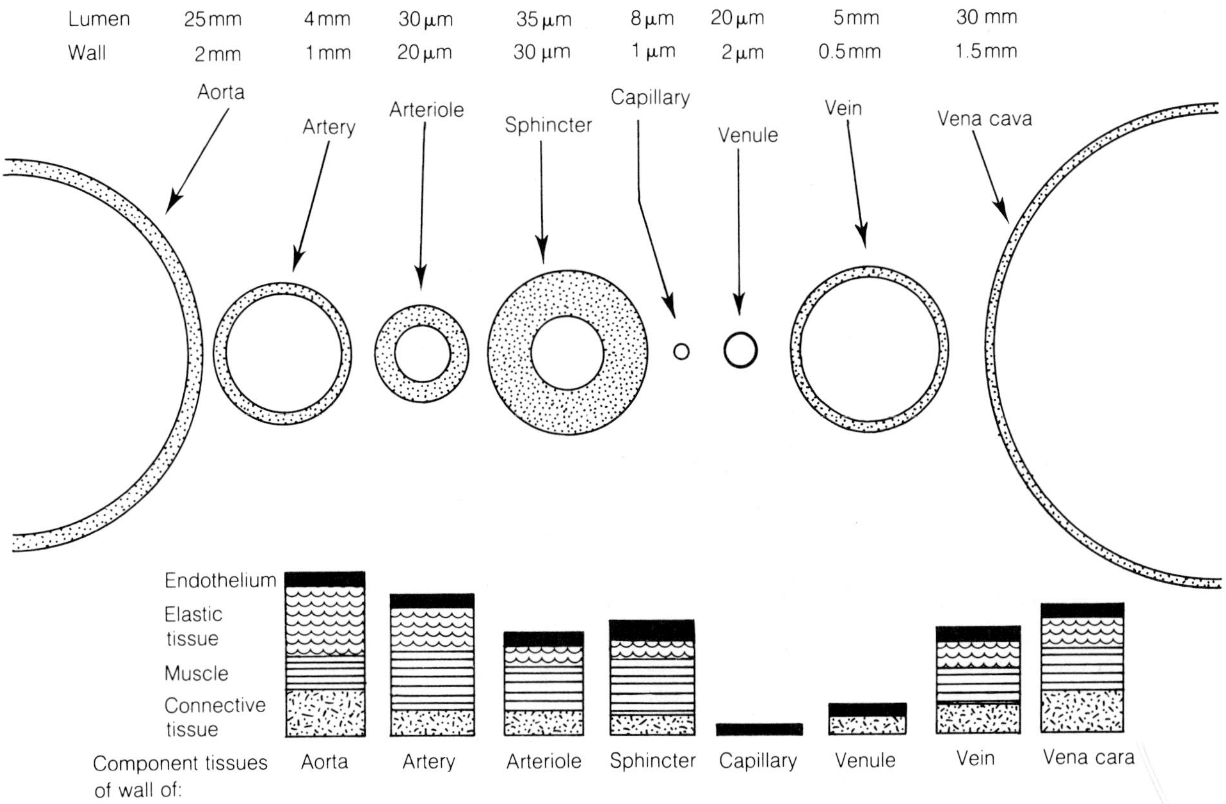

Figure 17.9 *The variations in size and components of the walls of the various blood vessels in the circulatory system (from Hinchliff SM, Montague SE, 1990, with permission).*

system. Veins are sometimes known as capacity vessels and can change their capacity by altering the diameters of the vessels.

THE PHYSIOLOGY OF CIRCULATION

Blood vessel diameter

Altering blood vessel diameter is important for controlling tissue blood flow and helps to regulate blood pressure. Blood vessel diameter is changed by altering the degree of smooth muscle contraction in the tunica media. Increasing contraction of the circular muscle fibres reduces blood vessel diameter (**vasoconstriction**). When the muscle relaxes the diameter increases (**vasodilation**). The smooth muscle of the blood vessel walls is normally in a state of contraction known as **vasomotor tone**. Control of the smooth muscle involves nervous and chemical factors.

Nervous control

The smooth muscle in the tunica media is innervated by sympathetic nerve fibres from the vasomotor centre. These nerve endings are more densely distributed in the arterioles, precapillary sphincters and venules. Sympathetic nerve discharge increases muscle contraction, causing vasoconstriction. A decrease in the frequency of nerve impulses brings about vasodilation. Vasoconstriction from heightened sympathetic activity increases total vascular resistance and venomotor tone and reduces venous capacity and venous return.

Chemical control

Vascular smooth muscle is influenced by hormones and locally produced metabolites. Adrenaline and noradrenaline cause vasoconstriction. Angiotensin II, formed by the action of kidney renin on angiotensinogen, is also a potent vasoconstrictor. Histamine and plasma kinins released from inflamed local tissues cause vasodilation of small vessels. Local prostaglandins may also be involved in vasodilation.

Endothelial-mediated regulation

The endothelium produces **endothelial-derived relaxing factor** (EDRF) that causes relaxation of vascular smooth muscle and vasodilation. One form of EDRF is **nitric oxide** which is a free radical and a chemical messenger carrying signals from cell to cell. Nitric oxide is released from the endothelial cells and diffuses into the blood vessel muscle wall. This local chemical control is extremely important when there is localised increase in metabolism. Control of circulation to the brain and the heart is largely mediated by local chemicals with a major factor being response to oxygen. The blood flow to the skin is mainly under sympathetic nervous control.

BLOOD PRESSURE

Fluid pressure

Hydrostatic pressure is the force a liquid exerts against the walls of its container. In the vascular system, this is the pressure the blood exerts on the blood vessel walls or blood pressure (BP). Pressure will also vary with the height of the liquid column. This is related to gravity. Venous pressure in the feet of a standing human is higher than that in the head. A third factor influencing hydrostatic pressure is the distensibility of the container; pressure is less in a distensible container than in a rigid one. The heart generates a head of pressure which is highest in the aorta and falls throughout the vascular system along the path to the tissues.

Fluid flow

The flow of a fluid through a vessel is determined by the pressure difference between the two ends of the vessel and the resistance to flow. **Resistance to flow** is a measure of the ease with which a fluid flows through a tube. In the vascular system, this is described as vascular resistance but for practical purposes most resistance is generated in the small peripheral vessels, referred to as peripheral resistance (PR). PR is affected by:

- **viscosity**, which is the internal friction within a fluid. In blood it is affected by the ratio of red cells and plasma proteins to plasma fluid. Reduction in plasma fluid, such as in dehydration, or an increase in cell content will increase viscosity whilst an increase in plasma fluid will decrease viscosity. The greater the viscosity, the more force is required to move the fluid along the vessel;
- **blood vessel length** – the longer the blood vessel, the greater the resistance to flow;
- **arteriolar diameter** – small changes in diameter can lead to large changes in PR. The smaller the diameter, the greater the resistance to flow as particles in the fluid are more likely to collide with the vessel walls;
- **the lining** also affects flow. A smooth lining in a blood vessel will create a smooth laminar flow whilst a rough lining will cause a turbulent flow.

Blood pressure is the force exerted on the wall of a blood vessel by its contained blood. It is measured in millimetres of mercury (mmHg). Typical values vary in different parts of the vascular tree, for arterial blood pressure, capillary blood pressure, venous blood pressure and so on. These gradients facilitate blood flow around the systems. The pressure in the systemic circulation falls in blood's journey from the aorta to the right atrium. Pressures in the pulmonary circulation are lower than in the systemic circulation but there is still a falling gradient from right ventricle to left atrium.

Venous return

Following the distribution of blood through the capillary beds, pressure is very low. Mechanisms are needed to ensure blood returns to the right atrium. Blood pressure in the venules is greater than that in the right atrium but gravity retards venous return when a person is upright and blood may pool in the feet and legs. In contrast, blood returning from the head is aided by gravity when in the upright position and dizziness may occur due to a temporary reduction in brain blood supply if a person stands up too quickly. If venous return to the heart is impeded or fails, cardiac output will fall.

There are several mechanisms to ensure adequate blood flow.

- Increasing **venomotor tone** will reduce the capacity of the venous system.
- The **skeletal muscle pump** – contractions of the skeletal muscles, especially in the limbs, squeeze the veins and push the blood towards the heart. Backflow is prevented by the venous valves, most effectively when a person is walking. Standing still means the muscle pump cannot act and venous return is not as good. People may faint if they stand still for long periods.
- The **respiratory pump** – as a person breathes in, pressure in the thorax and the right atrium is lowered. This increases the pressure gradient and assists venous return.

The arterial blood pressure is of most value clinically as it ensures an adequate blood supply to the tissues. The main parameter affecting blood pressure is the relationship between cardiac output (CO) and peripheral resistance (PR), shown by the simple formula

$$BP = CO \times PR$$

Arterial blood pressure

Arterial blood pressure changes through the cardiac cycle. Contraction of the ventricles during systole ejects blood into the aorta and raises the arterial pressure. This is the **systolic pressure** which is determined by the stroke volume and the force of the contraction. Systolic pressure will be raised if the arterial walls are stiffer as the vessels cannot distend to accommodate the extra blood. As the heart relaxes during diastole, blood leaves the main arteries and the blood pressure falls. This is the **diastolic pressure** which is affected by peripheral resistance. Diastolic pressure therefore depends on the level of systolic pressure, the elasticity of the arteries and the viscosity of blood. If the heart rate is slow diastolic pressure will fall as there is more time for extra blood to flow out of the artery. An increase in heart rate will raise the diastolic pressure.

Pulse pressure and mean arterial pressure

Each ventricular contraction initiates a pulse of pressure through the arteries. The difference between the systolic and diastolic pressure is called the **pulse pressure**. A typical blood pressure would be 120/70 mmHg, giving a pulse pressure of 120 –70 = 50 mmHg. The main factors influencing pulse pressure are stroke volume and the rigidity of the arteries.

An average or mean value for arterial pressure is useful as it represents the pressure driving the blood through the arteries. **Mean arterial pressure** (MAP) is more useful as a guide to tissue perfusion than the usual systolic/diastolic BP reading. It is estimated by the following formula:

$$\text{Diastolic pressure} + 1/3\text{rd of the pulse pressure}$$

For a blood pressure of 120/70 mmHg, MAP = (1/3 of 50) + 70 = 87 mmHg.

The regulation of blood pressure

Neural, chemical and renal controls act to modify blood pressure by influencing cardiac output, peripheral resistance and/or blood volume.

Neural system

This system can either alter blood distribution to achieve specific functions or maintain adequate systemic blood pressure. The system operates by spinal reflex. The vasomotor centre sends sympathetic nerve impulses via vasomotor efferent fibres to the muscular walls of the arterial system and acts mainly on the arterioles. The more impulses from these neurones, the more constricted are the arterioles. The vasomotor centre activity is modified by baroreceptors and chemoreceptors.

Baroreceptors are situated in the tunica adventitia of the internal carotid artery (especially in the carotid sinus), the transverse section of the aortic arch and most large vessels in the neck and thorax. These provide a short-term feedback mechanism responding to changes in posture and activity levels. Nerve fibres run from the baroreceptors via the glossopharyngeal cranial nerve (IX) and the vagal nerve (X). The nerve endings respond to stretching of the arterial wall. The normal action of these nerves on the CVC is inhibitory, slowing the heart rate and decreasing the force of ventricular contraction as well as causing arterial vasodilation.

Chemoreceptors are situated in the aortic arch and carotid bodies and respond to a fall in blood oxygen or an increase in blood acidity. The main effect is on the respiratory system but in severe hypoxia they will produce powerful sympathetic effects to increase heart rate and blood pressure. Brain centres such as the cortex and the hypothalamus also affect blood pressure.

Chemical control

Hormones from the adrenal medulla, namely adrenaline and noradrenaline, act to increase sympathetic activity (the flight or fight response). From the posterior pituitary, the antidiuretic hormone, which is released into the circulation during pain, low blood pressure and in response to some drugs such as morphine, alcohol and nicotine, will increase the blood volume by preventing renal excretion of fluid.

The renal system

The kidney responds to altered blood volume by altering the amount of urine excreted via the **renin – angiotensin mechanism** (Chapters 19 and 20). A reduction in blood pressure and kidney blood flow results in the excretion of renin into the circulation by the kidney juxtaglomerular apparatus. Renin acts on angiotensinogen to release angiotension I. Enzymes convert this to angiotensin II which is a powerful vasoconstrictor and also triggers the release of aldosterone from the adrenal cortex to cause retention of sodium and increased excretion of potassium. Water is retained passively by the increased amount of sodium. Blood volume has a direct effect on blood pressure; the higher the volume, the higher the blood pressure.

Table 17.1 *Blood pressure values (from Durkin 1979)*

Age in years	*BP systolic*	*BP diastolic*
Newborn	80	46
10	103	70
20	120	80
40	126	84
60	135	89

Blood pressure values

Blood pressure is highly variable both between individuals and within an individual. It is difficult to quote a normal blood pressure for a population but it is possible to find a typical value for an individual. Both physiological and genetic factors and a range of external influences can affect blood pressure. It is therefore of more value to consider a normal range.

Normal adult blood pressure is considered to be between 100/60 mmHg and 150/90 mmHg. Maturation and growth as well as age, sex and race can influence blood pressure. Durkin (1979) obtained blood pressure readings from 250 000 healthy people and Table 17.1 illustrates the range.

THE FORMATION OF TISSUE FLUID

In the tissues blood contained in the capillaries is separated from the interstitial fluid between the cells and the intracellular fluid. Capillary walls consist of a single layer of endothelial cells resting on a basement membrane. Slit-like spaces appear to be present between the cells. These are known as **pores** and represent only a small proportion of the total surface area of the capillary wall. Water and solutes diffuse to and from the blood and interstitial fluid. Although there is a high rate of substance diffusion between the two compartments, the fluid content of the plasma and the interstitial fluid normally changes very little. The volume of fluid moving out of the capillaries is equal to the amount returned. The hydrostatic pressure on each side of the capillary wall and the osmotic pressure of protein in the plasma and tissue fluid (Fig. 17.10) help to ensure this equilibrium.

Hydrostatic pressure

Hydrostatic pressure is the mechanical force of water pushing against cell membranes. In the vascular system, it is generated by the blood pressure. In the capillaries a hydrostatic pressure of 25 mmHg is sufficient to push water across the capillary membrane into the extracellular space. It is partly balanced by **osmotic pressure**. The excess water moves into the lymph system.

Blood pressure falls from the arteriolar end of the capillary to the venous end. Fluid with its dissolved solutes will also cross the capillary wall, being forced out at the arteriolar end and returning in the blood at the venous end. Capillary hydrostatic pressure (HPc) is higher at the arteriolar end (about

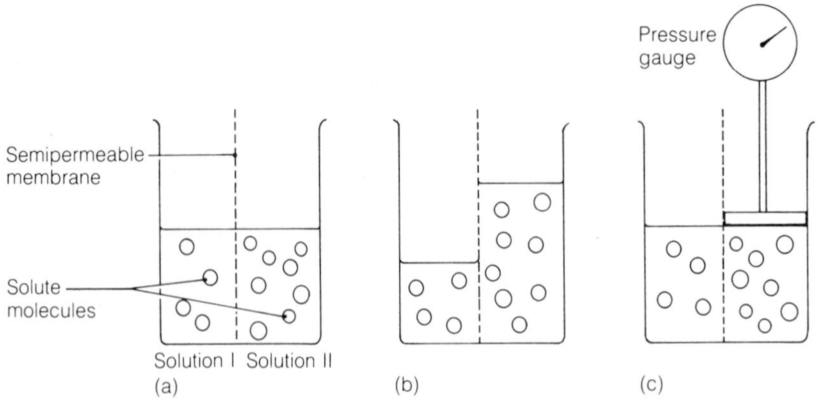

Figure 17.10 *In (a) two solutions of equal volume but differing concentrations are separated by a semipermeable membrane. Solution I is less concentrated than solution II. Soluble molecules are too large to pass through the pores in the semipermeable membrane, but solvent molecules can pass through freely. In (b) solvent has moved across the semipermeable membrane from solution I to solution II, until the concentration of the two solutions is equal. This movement of solvent is called osmosis. Osmotic pressure is the pressure required to stop the movement of solvent by osmosis (c). The greater the difference in concentration between the solutions on either side of the semipermeable membrane, the greater is the pressure required to halt the osmotic movement of solvent across the membrane (from Hinchliff SM, Montague SE, 1990, with permission).*

25–35 mmHg) than at the venous end (10–15 mmHg). Hydrostatic pressure in the interstitial space (HPif) has usually been rated as 0 mmHg because there is very little fluid present as most of it is drawn into the lymphatic system. Current research sited in Marieb (1992) suggests this pressure may have a negative value (about –6 mmHg). The net hydrostatic pressure is HPc – HPif.

Osmotic pressure

Osmosis is the movement of water down a concentration gradient across a semipermeable membrane from a high water content to a lower one. Osmosis is directly related to hydrostatic pressure and solute concentration but not to particle size. Osmotic pressure is created by the presence of large non-diffusible substances in a fluid. In blood, this is provided by plasma proteins (mainly albumin molecules) which apply osmotic pressure if the water concentration near them is less than the water content on the opposite side of the capillary membrane (Fig. 17.11). Capillary osmotic pressure (OPc) is about 25 mmHg whilst interstitial fluid, which contains few proteins, has a much lower pressure at OPif 0.1–5 mmHg. The net osmotic pressure is OPc – OPif.

Fluid will leave the capillary where the net hydrostatic pressure is greater than the net osmotic pressure. Hydrostatic forces dominate at the arteriolar end at about 35 mmHg whilst net osmotic pressure is about 25 mmHg (+10 mmHg). Osmotic pressure dominates at the venous end of the capillary with a net hydrostatic pressure of 13 mmHg and net osmotic pressure of 23 mmHg (–10 mmHg). Therefore fluid is forced out of the circulation at the arteriolar end of the capillary beds and back in at the venous end.

About 1.5 ml/min is lost from the circulation, picked up from interstitial fluid by the lymphatic system. This fluid, with any lost protein, is returned to the vascular system. The opening of precapillary sphincters will increase capillary pressure and force fluid into the tissues and their closure will decrease capillary pressure, ensuring that osmotic force draws fluid back into the capillary. In the pulmonary circulation the same mechanism applies but the pressures are much lower.

Diffusion

Movement of substances always occurs along a concentration gradient, from high to low concentration. Oxygen and nutrients will pass from blood to the interstitial fluid and then to cells. Carbon dioxide and waste products of metabolism will flow from the cells into the capillary blood.

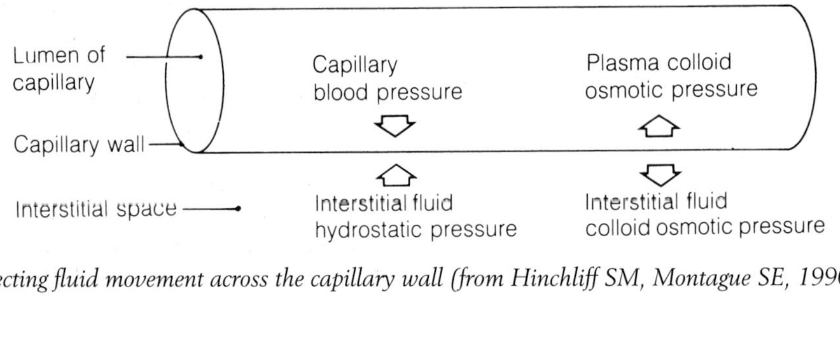

Figure 17.11 *Forces affecting fluid movement across the capillary wall (from Hinchliff SM, Montague SE, 1990, with permission).*

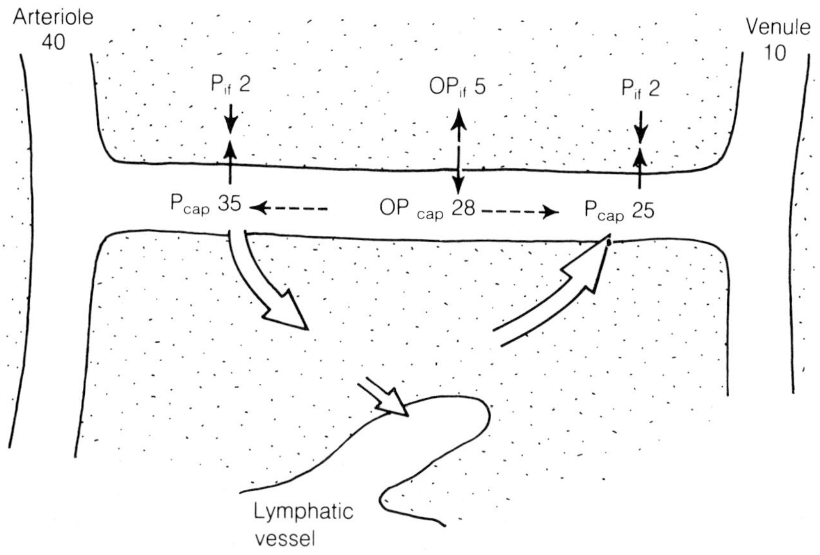

Figure 17.12 *Diagram summarising the forces contributing to the formation and reabsorption of tissue fluid in the systemic circulation (all figures refer to pressures in mmHg). NB: P_{cap} is the only pressure for which magnitude alters. P_{cap}, capillary blood pressure; P_{if}, interstitial fluid pressure; OP_{cap}, plasma colloid osmotic pressure; OP_{if}, interstitial fluid colloid osmotic pressure (from Hinchliff SM, Montague SE, 1990, with permission).*

MATERNAL ADAPTATIONS TO PREGNANCY

In pregnancy the maternal cardiovascular system undergoes enormous changes to meet the demands of the fetus (Blackburn & Loper 1992, de Swiet 1991, Duvekot & Peeters 1994). Exchange of gases, nutrients and waste products between mother and fetus occurs via the uteroplacental circulation. These fetal requirements place an enhanced load on the cardiovascular system added to by the expanded circulating blood mass, placental circulatory system and gradual increase in body weight. Normally these changes are tolerated well but if cardiovascular disease exists they could be dangerous for the mother and fetus. On the other hand, no change could compromise fetal health as research has indicated a link between low blood volume and poor fetal growth (Chapter 13).

Haemodynamic changes

There is a hyperdynamic circulation with high cardiac output. Changes occur in position and size of the heart, cardiac output, heart rate, blood volume, systemic blood pressure, vascular resistance and distribution of blood flow. Clark et al (1989) studied 10 healthy primiparous women between 36 and 38 weeks of gestation and between 11 and 13 weeks postpartum using pulmonary artery catheterisation. They found that the main changes in the pregnant woman were:

- decreased peripheral vascular resistance;
- decreased pulmonary vascular resistance;
- decreased colloid oncotic pressure;
- increased cardiac output;
- increased pulse rate.

Size and position of the heart

As pregnancy progresses, the heart is pushed upwards by the elevation of the diaphragm and the apex is opposite the 4th rather than the 5th intercostal space. The heart volume increases from 70 to 80 ml (about 12%) between early and late pregnancy. There is little change in wall thickness so that increased venous filling rather than muscle hypertrophy causes the expansion in heart size.

The increase in atrial size causes more ANP production which has a diuretic effect, helping to cope with the increased blood volume of pregnancy. Systolic or diastolic murmurs can be detected from as early as 12 weeks and may mimic pathology. Systolic murmurs are common because of the increased cardiovascular load. In the non-pregnant population a diastolic murmur would indicate disease but in pregnant women it may not be significant because of increased blood flow through the tricuspid or mitral valves. Myometrial contractility increases due to greater stretching of the heart muscle.

Cardiac output

Cardiac output (CO) is one of the most significant changes and increases in the first trimester of pregnancy. This is not solely to supply the uterus, as is indicated by the early increase before the uterus has enlarged significantly. An initial rise in heart rate of 15 bpm occurs as early as 4 weeks from conception, resulting in an increased myocardial oxygen requirement which could be significant in women with heart or lung disease. This is followed by a small increase in stroke volume occurring progressively during the first and 2nd trimesters to about 30% over the non-pregnant rate. It is the prime instigator of cardiac output after 20 weeks (Blackburn & Loper 1992).

The maximum increase in CO occurs by the end of the 2nd trimester, when it reaches a plateau; there is some controversy about whether there is a late decline or not. Duvekot & Peeters (1994) say that recent research using modern techniques suggests there is a fall in CO after the 35th week of pregnancy because of reduced stroke volume but the increased heart rate remains constant. From 32 weeks, if the woman lies supine hypotensive syndrome may make her CO seem to fall because venous return is impeded (de Swiet 1991). In a multiple pregnancy CO increases even more.

Total blood volume

The increase in total blood volume, due to a rise in plasma volume and red cell volume occurring simultaneously, probably explains the increase in CO. Uterine blood flow rises from 100 ml/min at the end of the first trimester to 500 ml/min at term. But again, this does not parallel the early changes in CO. Red cell mass or total volume of red cells increases by 18% whilst plasma volume increases about 50%. This difference results in haemodilution of pregnancy and a fall in Hb level, often referred to as physiological anaemia.

Arterial blood pressure

The slight decrease in systolic blood pressure accompanied by the greater increase in diastolic blood pressure leads to an increase in pulse pressure. This is probably due to hormonal vasodilation. It is important to measure BP accurately with the right size of cuff and standardised technique, e.g. the cuff must be level with the left atrium. Taking the BP with a woman lying supine has been shown to have a considerable influence with a profound fall sometimes occurring (**supine hypotension**).

Excluding women with hypertension of pregnancy, the following data have been noticed. There is relatively little change in the systolic reading but a marked fall in the diastolic reading for the first two trimesters which is lowest at midpregnancy, with a rise in the 3rd trimester to non-pregnant levels by term. At the beginning of labour blood pressure rises slightly and uterine contractions are associated with a rise in mean BP of 10 mmHg which mirrors the rise in CO.

Age and parity can affect blood pressure. As parity increases, regardless of age, both the systolic and diastolic blood pressures decrease with the greatest difference being between the first and 2nd pregnancies. As age increases (after 35 years) systolic blood pressure remains unchanged but diastolic BP increases.

Systemic vascular resistance

This is the MAP divided by cardiac output and decreases during pregnancy. Because cardiac output is raised in pregnancy and arterial BP changes with a slight decrease in MAP, systemic vascular resistance is decreased. It rises towards a point midway between the lowest and normal as blood pressure increases in the last trimester. The change is due both to the establishment of new vascular beds, such as the low resistance uteroplacental circulation, and to a general relaxation of peripheral vascular tone.

Venous pressure

Venous pressure increases markedly in the femoral veins in pregnancy and as there is no similar rise in right atrial pressure, this indicates venous obstruction between the two points. In pregnancy this is brought about by:

- mechanical pressure from the weight of the uterus on the iliac veins and on the inferior vena cava;
- the pressure of the fetal head on the iliac veins;
- hydrodynamic obstruction due to the outflow of blood at relatively high pressure from the uterus (de Swiet 1991).

The rate of blood flow in the leg veins is much reduced. This contributes to a risk of varicosities developing in the leg veins and vulva as well as haemorrhoids in susceptible women. Another side effect is the development of gravitational oedema.

Regional distribution of increased blood flow

The uterus

The increased circulation of pregnancy mainly targets the uterus although this is difficult to measure. Estimating the blood flow to the placental site has been tried. It is generally believed that the uterine vascular bed is widely dilated so that oxygen consumption is dealt with by increases in extraction rather than by increases in blood flow. This is a feature of the changes in the uterine blood vessels. Both steroid hormones and the renin-angiotensin system may contribute to the uterine blood flow of pregnancy.

The kidneys

Renal blood flow rises in early pregnancy to about 400 ml/min above non-pregnant levels. This may fall towards the end of pregnancy (see Chapter 18).

The skin

Blood flow to the skin, particularly that of the hands and feet, is greatly increased in pregnancy. Women feel warm and often complain about the heat. Finger and toe temperature are increased.

Peripheral vasodilation

Increased blood supply causes nails to grow faster and more hairs to be in the growth phase rather than the resting phase. After delivery there are more hairs at the end of their lives and there is increased hair fallout. This has led to the old wives tail of 'hair coming out in handfuls' in the puerperium (de Swiet 1991). Increased blood supply to the nasal mucous membrane increases nasal congestion. Nose bleeds may occur, as does increased snoring.

The liver

The research into increased blood flow through the liver is not clear but it is likely because of the increased metabolic rate during pregnancy (see Chapter 23).

The breasts

Mammary blood flow is probably increased (see Chapter 54).

Control of cardiovascular changes

Control of cardiovascular changes is partly hormonal, with increased circulating levels of oestrogen, progesterone and prostaglandins, and partly mechanical, with changes of growth and development of organs necessitating increased blood supply. Vasodilation of peripheral blood vessels is the primary haemodynamic alteration followed by increases in circulating blood volume and cardiac output. Duvekot & Peeters (1994) examined the literature, finding that generalised vasodilation of pregnancy is unlikely to be induced by prostaglandins. Neither do they believe that the pregnancy hormones oestrogen, progesterone, prolactin, human chorionic gonadotrophin or human placental lactogen are the primary stimulus for vasodilation. They postulate that an endothelial-derived relaxing factor such as nitric oxide may be the cause of the vasodilation.

EXERCISE AND THE CARDIOVASCULAR SYSTEM

There are social and cultural determinants of activity levels during pregnancy Artal & Wiswell 1986, Carbon 1988). Women in developing countries may work in the fields until delivery while in Western society they are expected to take more rest as pregnancy progresses. Over the last decade an increasing interest in physical fitness has led more women to exercise throughout pregnancy. However, research into the safety aspects is still not extensive. It is important to ascertain the type of exercise being undertaken as serious training on a regular basis differs from the gentle exercises performed by most pregnant women.

All exercise places increased demands on cardiorespiratory function. Blackburn & Loper (1992) remind us that there is a need for more research into the effect of the following issues concerning exercise in pregnancy:

- the redistribution of weight;
- the hormone changes of pregnancy;
- hyperthermia and fetal normality;
- hypoxia and the fetus;
- increased cardiac workload;
- differences between women who train and those who do not;
- the difference between hard physical work and exercise.

The increased amount and distribution of weight gained make effort and balance more difficult. Most of the weight gain is anterior to the centre of gravity which increases lumbar lordosis and the pelvis tilts to allow the woman to retain an upright position. Evidence suggests that when body weight does not have to be lifted, as in seated exercise, pregnancy does not make much difference to exertion. Where body weight influences the cost of exercise, for instance in oxygen consumption, 'The increased cost in pregnancy is proportional to the increase in body weight' (de Swiet 1991). Sufficient calories should be ingested to supply the needs of the pregnancy as well as the exercise.

Joint instability due to softening of the ligaments means that jumping movements or deep flexion or extension of joints may lead to injury. However, there is good evidence to show that at least for the first half of pregnancy, women in good physical condition should be unaffected by pregnancy. In support of this, de Swiet (1991) wrote that 10 female Soviet athletes out of the 26 who competed in the 1956 Olympic Games were pregnant at the time. Generally no contraindication has been found for healthy women to undertake physical exercise and training and Carbon (1988) summarises studies which show that pregnancy is no longer a barrier to exercise. This may be true for serious athletes such as Liz McColgan, the long-distance runner who trained throughout her pregnancy.

Cardiac reserve lessens as the extra needs of pregnancy develop. It appears that most women spontaneously decrease their physical activity during pregnancy. Reasons for this include fatigue, musculoskeletal strains, lower abdominal discomfort and concern about the pregnancy. Nausea, urinary frequency and embarrassment are also mentioned by Carbon as reasons for discontinuation of exercise.

Uterine blood flow is reduced by exercise, especially in hypertensive women. The usual fetal response to maternal exercise is to increase the heart rate by 10–30 bpm with a return to normal within 15 min. However, if exercise is prolonged or strenuous, fetal bradycardia may occur. There appears to be no adverse fetal outcome associated with this phenomenon (Artal et al 1984). Studies on aerobically healthy mothers have not shown any adverse effect on mother or baby.

Increased oxygen extraction may counter the effect of reduced uterine circulation in fit women. Cardiotocography studies have shown no adverse fetal outcome although mild fetal tachycardia after 30 min of aerobic exercise has been reported (Collings & Curet 1983).

Exercise may be beneficial as it could reduce constipation and varicose veins, improve circulation, reduce backache because of better posture and weight gain because of the increased calorific expenditure and improved attitude to nutrition. Carbon (1988) cautions that the exercise should be undertaken under guidance from a trained person.

Clapp (1991) found no adverse effect of exercise on early pregnancy outcome. Moderate exercise 3–4 times a week is of value to health but pregnant women should be discouraged from taking part in competitive sports. If a pregnant woman wishes to continue her sport, there is good evidence to show that she should but the following guidelines from Carbon (1988) should be followed.

- Consult your doctor first and often.
- Exercise at levels appropriate to previous fitness and taper off in the last 3 months.
- Always warm up and cool down.
- Avoid dehydration and overheating.
- Maintain an adequate weight gain.
- Do not set long-term goals and be prepared for change.

Summary of main points

- The cardiovascular system has three main roles: delivery of nutrients and oxygen, removal of metabolic waste and carbon dioxide and distribution of heat around the body. Blood flows through the body in two distinct circuits: the pulmonary circulation and the systemic circulation. The systemic circulation is much larger than the pulmonary circulation and the force generated by the left side of the heart is much greater than that of the right side.
- The myocardium is mainly composed of cardiac muscle. There is an inner lining called the endocardium and the heart is enclosed in a fibroserous sac called the pericardium. There are four chambers in the heart, two superior atria and two inferior ventricles, separated by septa and valves. Valves direct and control the flow of blood through the heart by opening as the associated chamber contracts and closing as the chamber relaxes.
- Oxygen is carried to the cardiac muscle by the right and left coronary arteries which originate from the aorta just beyond the aortic valve. Blood returns from the left side of the heart to the right atrium via the coronary sinus and from the right side of the heart via small anterior cardiac veins.
- Cardiac muscle combines properties of both skeletal and smooth muscle; it is striated like skeletal muscle but individual muscle cell membranes have very low electrical resistance. Action potentials pass from one muscle cell to another to allow the muscle mass to function as a whole.
- The cardiac cycle is taken from the end of one contraction to the end of the next. It produces two distinct sounds in a single beat. Each cycle lasts 0.8 s, of which systole is 0.3 s and diastole 0.5 s. The intrinsic conduction system of the heart allows it to beat on its own with no external control. The heart rate is influenced by the autonomic nervous system, hormones such as adrenaline, stretching of the atria, temperature and drugs. In the medulla oblongata the cardiovascular centre receives input from baroreceptors, chemoreceptors and higher centres in the brain such as the cortex and hypothalamus.
- Cardiac output, the volume of blood pumped by each ventricle per minute, is about 5 l/min. This can increase to 30 l under extreme conditions. The difference between the cardiac output at rest and what the heart is capable of pumping is called the cardiac reserve.
- In response to being stretched, the atria secrete a hormone called atrial natriuretic factor (ANF) or atrial natriuretic peptide (ANP). This is a potent diuretic which causes the kidney to excrete excess sodium and water and plays a part in the regulation of blood volume and blood pressure.
- The structure of the blood vessels varies depending on their specific functions. The diameter of blood vessels is changed by altering the degree of smooth muscle contraction in the tunica media. Muscle contraction will bring about vasoconstriction and muscle relaxation causes vasodilation. The smooth muscle of the blood vessel walls is normally in a state of contraction and this is known as vasomotor tone.
- The smooth muscle in the tunica media is controlled mainly by sympathetic nerve fibres from the vasomotor centre but it is also influenced by hormones and locally produced metabolites. Adrenaline and noradrenaline will cause vasoconstriction, as will angiotensin II. Histamine and plasma kinins released from local tissues during inflammation will cause vasodilation of small vessels. Locally prostaglandins may be involved in vasodilation.
- The endothelium secretes endothelial-derived relaxing factor (EDRF) that can cause relaxation of vascular smooth muscle, so producing vasodilation. There is now strong evidence that one form of EDRF is nitric oxide.
- The flow of a fluid through a vessel is determined by the pressure difference between the two ends of the vessel and the resistance to flow. Peripheral resistance is affected by viscosity, blood vessel length, arteriolar diameter and the nature of the lining in a blood vessel.
- Blood pressure is the force exerted on the wall of a blood vessel by its contained blood. It is measured in millimetres of mercury. The main parameter affecting BP is the relationship between cardiac output and peripheral resistance; hence the formula: BP = CO × PR.
- Contraction of the ventricles during systole ejects blood into the aorta and pulmonary artery and raises the arterial pressure. This is known as the systolic pressure. As the heart relaxes during diastole blood leaves the main arteries and the blood pressure falls to give the diastolic pressure. The mean arterial pressure or MAP is a useful guide to tissue perfusion.
- Neural, chemical and renal controls modify blood pressure by influencing cardiac output, peripheral resistance and/or blood volume. Blood pressure is highly variable both between individuals and within an individual. Both physiological and genetic factors as well as a wide range of external influences can affect a blood pressure.
- In the tissues blood is contained in the capillaries and is separated from the fluid between the cells and within the cells but pores appear to be present between the cells of the capillary wall. Movement of substances occurs along a concentration gradient from high to low concentration. Oxygen and nutrients will pass from blood to the interstitial fluid and then to cells. Carbon dioxide and waste products of metabolism will flow from the cells into the capillary blood.
- In pregnancy the maternal cardiovascular system changes to meet the demands of the fetus. Exchange of gases, nutrients and waste products between mother and fetus occurs via the uteroplacental circulation. A hyperdynamic circulation with high cardiac output is present. Changes occur in position and size of the heart, cardiac output, heart rate, blood volume, systemic blood pressure, vascular resistance and distribution of blood flow.
- The heart volume increases from 70 to 80 ml between early and late pregnancy. There is little change in wall thickness and it is greater venous filling rather than muscle hypertrophy that causes the increase. The increase in atrial size causes more ANP production which has a diuretic effect, helping to cope with the increased blood volume of pregnancy.
- Myometrial contractility increases because of greater stretching of the heart muscle. Cardiac output rises in the first trimester of pregnancy. The maximum increase in CO occurs by the end of the 2nd trimester, reaches a plateau and there may be a late decline. An initial rise in heart rate of 15 bpm occurs as early as 4 weeks from conception, followed by a small increase in stroke volume.
- There is haemodilution of pregnancy and a fall in Hb level referred to as physiological anaemia. There is little change in the BP systolic reading but a marked fall in the diastolic reading for the first two trimesters, which is lowest at midpregnancy with arise in the 3rd trimester to non-pregnant levels.
- Venous pressure increases markedly in the femoral veins in pregnancy with no similar rise in right atrial pressure. This indicates venous obstruction between the two points. The rate of blood flow in the leg veins is much reduced, sometimes leading to varicosities in the leg veins and vulva as well as haemorrhoids in susceptible women. Gravitational oedema may occur.
- The increased circulation of pregnancy mainly targets the uterus. Renal blood flow rises in early pregnancy but this may fall towards the end of pregnancy. Blood flow to the skin, particularly that of the hands and feet, is increased. Mammary blood flow is probably increased.
- Control of the cardiovascular changes is partly hormonal and partly mechanical as changes of growth and development of organs

necessitate increased blood supply. Vasodilation of peripheral blood vessels is the primary haemodynamic alteration followed by increases in circulating blood volume and in cardiac output.

- There are social and cultural determinants of activity levels during pregnancy. Women in developing countries may work in the fields until delivery while in Western society it is expected that women take progressively more rest as pregnancy progresses. There appears to be no adverse effect of exercise on pregnancy outcome in fit women. Over the last decade an increasing interest in physical fitness has led more women to keep exercising throughout pregnancy.

References

Artal R, Wiswell R. 1986 Exercise in Pregnancy. Williams and Wilkins, Baltimore.

Artal R, Romem Y, Paul RH, Wiswell R. 1984 Fetal bradycardia induced by maternal exercise. Lancet 2 (8397), 258–260.

Blackburn ST, Loper DL. 1992 Maternal, Fetal and Neonatal Physiology. A Clinical Perspective. WB Saunders, Philadelphia.

Carbon R. 1988 Exercise and pregnancy. EXCEL 5, 6–10.

Clapp JF. 1991 Maternal exercise performance and early pregnancy outcome. In Mittelmark RA, Wiswell RA, Drinkwater BL (eds) Exercise in Pregnancy, 2nd edn. Williams and Wilkins, Baltimore.

Clark SL, Cotton DB, Lee W. 1989 Central haemodynamic assessment of normal term pregnancy. American Journal of Obstetrics and Gynecology 161, 1439–1442.

Collings CMS, Curet LB. 1983 Foetal heart rate response to maternal exercise. American Journal of Obstetrics and Gynecology 155, 498–450.

de Swiet M. 1991 The cardiovascular system. In Hytten F, Chamberlain G (eds) Clinical Physiology in Obstetrics, 2nd edn. Blackwell Scientific, Oxford pp 3–38.

Durkin N. 1979 An Introduction to Medical Science. MTP Press, Lancaster.

Duvekot JJ, Peeters LL. 1994 Maternal cardiovascular haemodynamic adaptation to pregnancy. Obstetrical and Gynaecological Survey 49(12, 2), S1–S14

Herbert RA, Alison JA. 1996 Cardiovascular function. In Hinchliff SM, Montague SE, Watson R (eds) Physiology for Nursing Practice, 2nd edn. Baillière Tindall, London.

Hinchliff SM, Montague SE. 1990 Physiology for Nursing Practice. Baillière Tindall, London.

Hinchliff SM, Montague SE. Watson R. 1996 Physiology for Nursing Practice. Baillliѐre Tindall, London.

Marieb EN. 1992 Human Anatomy and Physiology, 2nd edn. Benjamin/Cummings Publishing, California.

Tortora GJ, Anagnustakos NP 1981 Principles of Anatomy and Physiology. Harper & Row, New York.

Recommended reading

Clark SL, Cotton DB, Lee W. 1989 Central haemodynamic assessment of normal term pregnancy. American Journal of Obstetrics and Gynecology 161, 1439–1442.

de Swiet M. 1991 The cardiovascular system. In Hytten F, Chamberlain G (eds) Clinical Physiology in Obstetrics, 2nd edn. Blackwell Scientific, Oxford, pp 3–38.

Duvekot JJ, Peeters LL. 1994 Maternal cardiovascular haemodynamic adaptation to pregnancy. Obstetrical and Gynaecological Survey 49(12, 2), S1–S14.

Herbert RA, Alison JA. 1996 Cardiovascular function. In Hinchliff SM, Montague SE, Watson R (eds) Physiology for Nursing Practice, 2nd edn. Baillière Tindall, London.

Chapter 18 Respiration

In this chapter

INTRODUCTION

Respiration is the process by which the body exchanges gases with the atmosphere in order to provide for the changing needs of cell metabolism. Oxygen (O_2) is taken from the atmosphere and transported in the blood to the tissues. Carbon dioxide (CO_2), produced as metabolic waste by the cells, is returned to the lungs and excreted into the air. Efficient respiration depends on the interactions of respiratory, cardiovascular and central nervous system functions which alter the rate and depth of respiration as needed. An adult utilises about 250 ml of oxygen per minute and this can increase by a factor of 30 in severe exercise.

ANATOMY OF THE RESPIRATORY SYSTEM

The respiratory system consists of the airways from the nasal passages to the pharynx and larynx as well as the bronchi, bronchioles and alveoli of the lungs (Fig. 18.1). The chest structures necessary for moving air in and out of the lungs are part of the system. It is usual to divide the respiratory system into the upper and lower airways at the level of the cricoid cartilage.

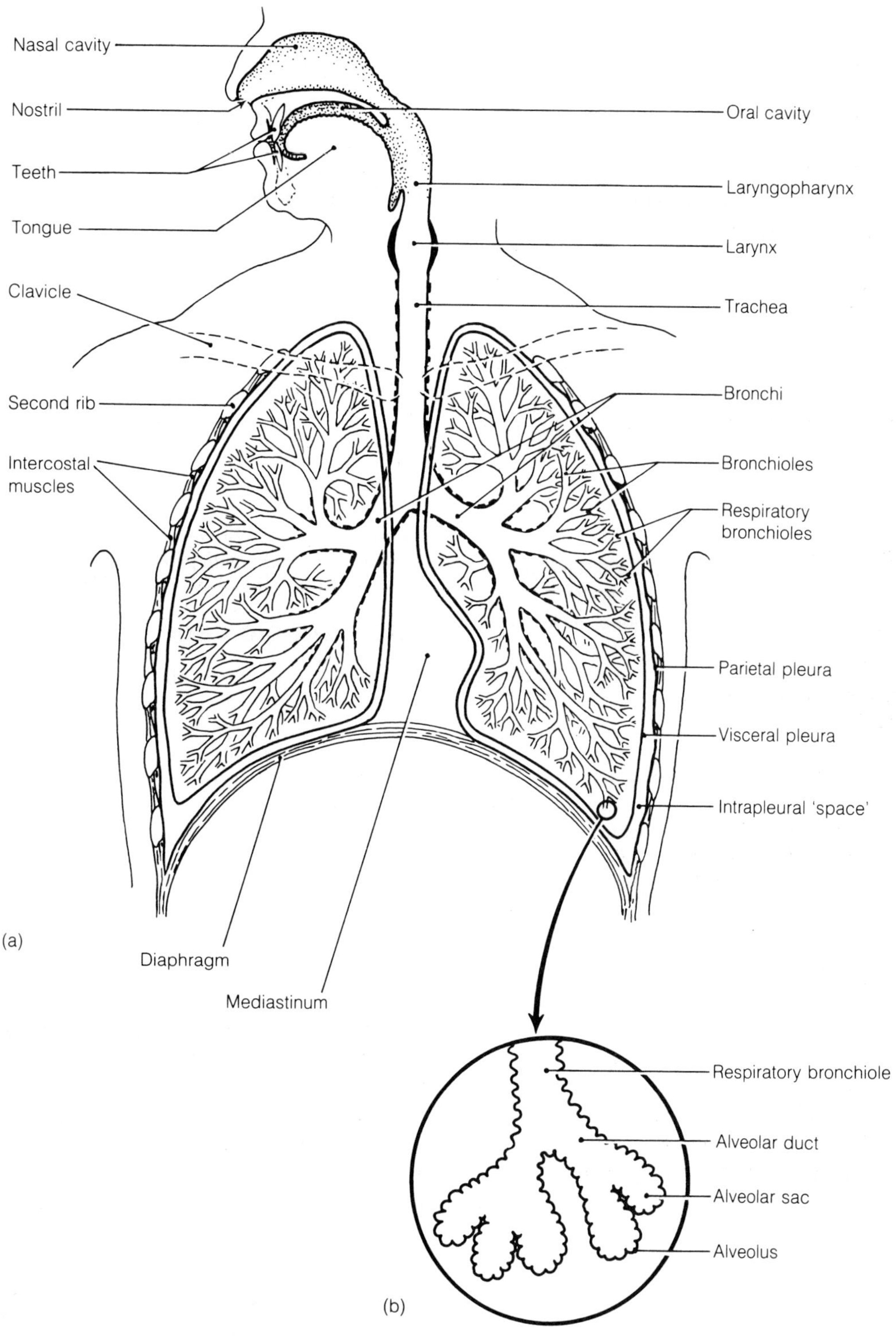

Figure 18.1 *Organisation of the respiratory system (from Hinchliff SM, Montague SE, 1990, with permission).*

The upper airways

The **nasal cavity** is a large, irregularly shaped cavity divided into two by a septum. Bony structures called the **turbinates** increase the surface area of the cavity and it is lined with ciliated epithelium which warms, filters and moistens the incoming air. The air enters the upper pharynx through two internal nares.

The **pharynx** is a common passageway for water and food as well as air. It is a funnel-shaped tube which extends from the internal nares to the level of the cricoid cartilage. The auditory or **Eustachian tubes** open into the upper pharynx and the mouth opens into the central portion or oropharynx. The tonsils and adenoids, which are organs of the lymphatic system, are found in the larynx. The oropharynx divides into the **oesophagus**, which transports food and water into the stomach, and the **trachea**, which transports air into the lungs.

The **larynx**, commonly called the voice box, is composed of pieces of cartilage connected by ligaments and moved by muscles. It is lined with mucous membrane continuous with the pharynx and trachea. In the larynx are the **vocal cords** responsible for the production of sound and between the vocal cords is the **glottis** through which air passes. The **epiglottis** is a leaf-shaped piece of cartilage anchored to the thyroid cartilage. It moves up and down during swallowing to cover the glottis and prevent food and water being inhaled into the larynx and lungs.

The lower respiratory tract

The lower part of the airway is also called the **bronchial tree** because of its resemblance to a trunk and branches (Fig. 18.2). The trachea is a cylindrical tube 10–12 cm long made up of 16–20 C-shaped cartilaginous rings joined together by fibrous and muscular tissue. This gives the trachea a firm structure to prevent the collapsing of the airway during inspiration. The posterior aspect of the cartilaginous rings is absent, which facilitates the passage of food down the oesophagus which lies immediately behind the trachea. The trachea extends from the larynx to the level of the 5th vertebra where it divides into the two **primary bronchi**. The right primary bronchus is wider and shorter and more vertical than the left so that inhaled objects tend to enter the right lung rather than the left. The primary bronchi enter the lungs at the **hilum** where the right bronchus divides into three, the right upper, middle and lower bronchi, to serve the three lobes of the right lung. The left primary bronchus divides into two, the left upper and lower bronchi, to serve the two lobes of the left lung.

The lower branches of the airway are known as bronchi whilst they still have cartilage in their structure. After this they are known as **bronchioles** which have smooth muscle in their walls. The smooth muscle is able to respond to stimuli by causing dilatation or constriction of the lumen of the bronchioles. This function is mainly under the control of the autonomic nervous system with sympathetic impulses causing bronchodilation and parasympathetic impulses causing bronchoconstriction. There are about 8–13 divisions from the trachea to the smallest bronchi and another 3–4 before the terminal bronchioles are reached. Each terminal bronchiole divides into about 50 respiratory bronchioles. About 200 sac-like **alveoli** are supplied with air by each respiratory bronchiole.

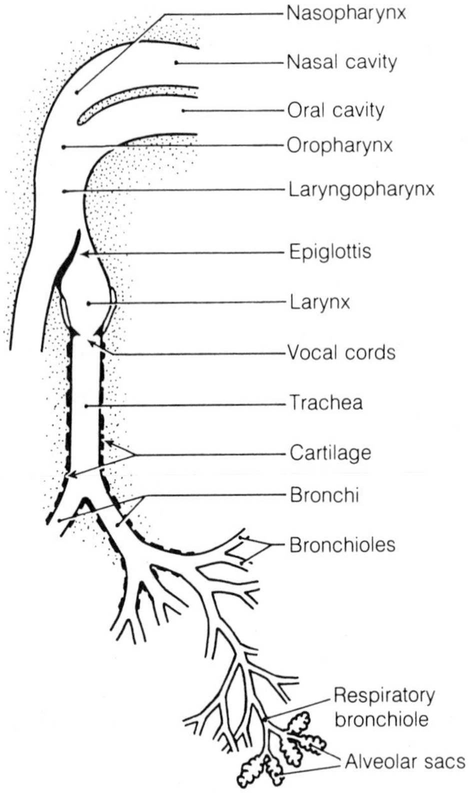

Figure 18.2 *Organisation of the airways (from Hinchliff SM, Montague SE, 1990, with permission).*

The thoracic cage

The thoracic cage forms the cavity which contains the two conical lungs and the heart. The organs are separated from each other by the mediastinum and its contents. Each lung is surrounded by a double-layered fluid-filled sac called the **pleura** which also attaches it to the inner surface of the thorax. The inner or visceral pleura covers the outer surface of the lung and is reflected back to become the outer or parietal pleura which is attached to the inner surface of the thoracic cavity.

PHYSIOLOGY OF THE RESPIRATORY TRACT

The epithelial lining

The upper airway protects the alveolar tissues by warming, filtering and moistening the air. The structure of the epithelial lining is particularly good as a filter. It contains glands that secrete thick sticky mucus to trap particles and is ciliated to waft excess mucus and foreign particles towards the pharynx where they can be swallowed. The cilia beat about 600–1000 times a minute. Large numbers of phagocytic cells will engulf and destroy debris and bacteria trapped by the mucus.

Reflex mechanisms

Coughing is a forceful expiration reflex under the control of the respiratory centre in the medulla which will expel irritant particles from the larynx. Air rushes out at a speed of 500 miles per hour! It is instigated by messages from a sensitive part of the airway at the bifurcation of the trachea, called the **carina**. **Sneezing** is a similar reflex instigated by irritation of the nasal mucosa. The **swallowing reflex** is extremely important for respiration. Absence of this reflex, as is seen in unconscious or anaesthetised patients, may result in inhalation of food or water particles into the larynx or lung. The airway may be obstructed or infection and pneumonia may occur.

Structure and function of the alveoli

The terminal bronchioles feed into respiratory bronchioles which branch into the alveolar ducts. These lead into alveolar sacs and the alveoli where most of the gas exchange occurs (Fig. 18.3). The alveoli are expansions off the alveolar sacs making the latter resemble bunches of grapes. Alveoli open into a common chamber called the **atrium** at the terminus of the alveolar duct (Marieb 1992). There are about 300 million alveoli in the lungs which provides an enormous area for gas exchange.

The alveolar wall (Fig. 18.4) consists of a single layer of flattened squamous epithelial cells called type I cells. The external surfaces of the alveolus have a few elastic fibres around their openings. There is a dense network of pulmonary capillaries surrounding each alveolus providing a continuous encircling sheet of blood. Each capillary wall is also only one cell thick so that the interstitial space between the alveolus and its capillary network, forming the air–blood interface, is very thin. This interface is called the **respiratory membrane** and has blood flowing on one side and gas on the other. Gas exchanges occur by simple diffusion across the respiratory membrane and depend on the existence of pressure gradients between the lungs and the atmosphere. The total surface area for gas exchange is about 75 square metres (Sherwood 1988).

Surfactant

In addition to the type I cells forming the alveolar wall, the alveolar epithelium contains cuboidal type II alveolar cells which secrete pulmonary surfactant. This is a phospholipid that helps to keep the membrane moist and also maintains the patency of the alveolus. Macrophages called dust cells, which are part of the defence system of the body, are also present in the lumen of the alveoli, mopping up bacteria, dust and other inhaled particles. The alveolar surface is usually sterile. There are minute pores of Kohn present in the alveolar walls which allow air flow between adjacent alveoli (**collateral ventilation**), useful if the terminal airways are blocked by disease.

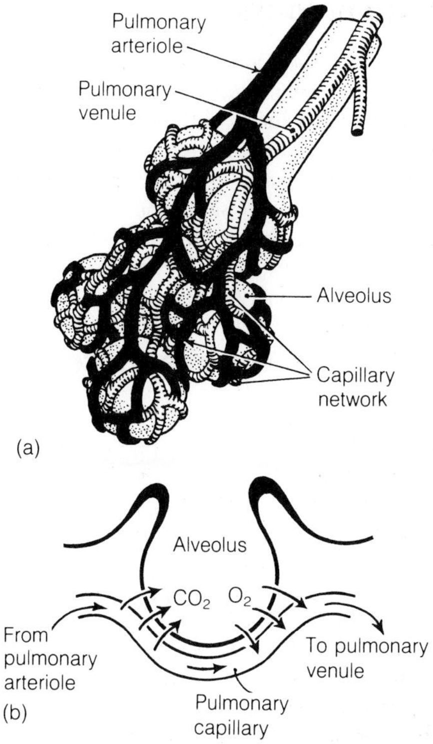

Figure 18.3 *Relationship between alveoli and blood vessels. Gas exchange can occur across the vast surface area provided by the dense network of capillaries (from Hinchliff SM, Montague SE, 1990, with permission).*

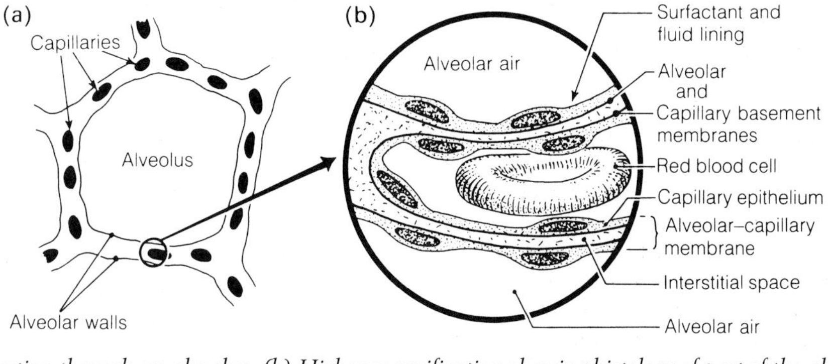

Figure 18.4 *(a) Cross-section through an alveolus. (b) Higher magnification showing histology of part of the alveolar-capillary membrane. The dense network of capillaries forms an almost continuous sheet of blood in the alveolar walls, providing a very efficient arrangement for gas exchange (from Hinchliff SM, Montague SE, 1990, with permission).*

Blood supply to the lungs

The lungs oxygenate the blood but they also need their own blood supply to maintain healthy tissue. The blood to be oxygenated reaches the lungs by branches of the pulmonary arteries, is reoxygenated in the pulmonary capillary network surrounding the alveoli and returns to the heart via the pulmonary veins. The blood supplying the lung tissue with oxygen is provided by the two left and one right bronchial arteries arising from the aorta. Venous return is by both bronchial veins and pulmonary veins.

Nerve supply to the respiratory muscles

The respiratory muscles are innervated by the phrenic nerve to the diaphragm, which originates in cervical nerves 3, 4 and 5, and the intercostal nerves to the intercostal muscles, which originate in the thoracic nerves 1–12. This is why severance of the spine above C3 results in total respiratory paralysis but below that, diaphragmatic breathing can occur although the intercostal muscles will be paralysed.

PHYSIOLOGY OF PULMONARY VENTILATION (BREATHING)

There are two phases to breathing: **inspiration** or breathing in and **expiration** or breathing out. Mechanical factors and neural factors are involved in the control of respiratory rate. Atmospheric air contains about 21% oxygen and 79% nitrogen with traces of inert gases, carbon dioxide and water vapour. Alveolar air exchanges oxygen for carbon dioxide and water vapour. By the time alveolar air reaches the point of expiration it will have been mixed with the atmospheric air in the dead space so that the content of expired air will be between the two extremes of atmospheric and alveolar air.

Mechanical factors

Under normal conditions and pressure gradients, oxygen passes from the alveolus into the blood and carbon dioxide from the blood into the alveolus. The movement of gases flowing from a high to a lower pressure down a gradient is said to occur by bulk flow. Air flows in and out of the lungs during breathing by bulk flow. Expansion of the thoracic cage by contraction of the respiratory muscles during inspiration increases lung volume and causes a temporary drop in the pressure in the alveoli so that atmospheric air flows in until pressure inside the lung is equal to the atmospheric pressure. Relaxation of the respiratory muscles causes expiration by reducing the volume of the thoracic cage, creating a temporary rise in pressure within the lung to above atmospheric pressure.

Inspiration

The diaphragm, the most important muscle of inspiration, is a strong dome-shaped sheet of muscle separating the thoracic and abdominal cavities from each other. When the diaphragm contracts, it flattens. This presses down the abdominal contents and lifts the rib cage, enlarging the thoracic cavity both from top to bottom and from front to back. Normally the external intercostal muscles, which are accessory muscles of respiration lying between the ribs, play little part in this expansion of the rib cage but help to stabilise it. However, during any need for extra oxygen, such as in exercise and in upper airway obstruction, the upper intercostal muscles as well as other accessory muscles of respiration help to enlarge the rib cage and so enhance lung expansion.

Expiration

Under resting conditions, expiration is a passive process brought about by the relaxation and elastic recoil of the diaphragm and accessory muscles if in use. The elastic lung returns to its original volume (the **functional residual capacity**) as air is pushed out of the lung as the reduction in volume makes the alveolar pressure temporarily exceed atmospheric pressure. Active expiration may occur when the need for gas exchange increases, as in exercise or constriction of the airways.

Pulmonary ventilation

Respiratory parameters

Respiratory volumes and capacities can be described and measured using a **spirograph**. The measurements given below are taken from Marieb (1992) and are given for the standardised healthy young male weighing 70 kg.

Respiratory volumes

- **Tidal volume** (TV) is the volume of air that passes in and out of the lungs during each breath under resting conditions and is 500 ml.
- **Inspiratory reserve volume** (IRV) is the maximum amount of air which can be inspired beyond the normal tidal inspiration and is about 3100 ml.
- **Expiratory reserve volume** (ERV) is the maximum amount of air that can be forcibly expired after a normal tidal volume exhalation and is 1200 ml.
- **Residual volume** (RV) is the volume of gas remaining in the lungs at the end of maximal expiration and is 1200 ml.

Respiratory capacities

- **Total lung capacity** (TLC) is the amount of air in the lungs at the end of a maximum inspiration. It includes TV + IRV + ERV + RV and is 6000 ml.
- **Vital capacity** (VC) is total capacity minus RV and is 4800 ml or about 80% of TLC.
- **Inspiratory capacity** (IC) is the maximum volume of gas which can be inspired after a normal expiration and is 3600 ml.
- **Functional residual capacity** (FRC) is the amount of gas remaining in the lungs after a normal expiration and is about 2400 ml.

Minute volume

The total volume of air exchanged with the atmosphere in one minute is called the minute volume or **pulmonary ventilation**. This depends on tidal volume and respiratory rate and varies considerably in different states of health and according to age. An average tidal volume in a resting adult is about 500 ml with a respiratory rate of 12 breaths per minute. Therefore pulmonary ventilation would be 6000 ml/min. Of this, about 150 ml of each breath is trapped in the dead space above the respiratory tissue and is breathed out with its composition unchanged.

Alveolar ventilation

The volume of fresh air entering the alveoli each minute is called the alveolar ventilation. The calculation from the parameters mentioned above is as follows:

Respiratory rate × (tidal volume – dead space) = alveolar ventilation:
12 × 500 – 150 = 4200 ml/min.

Shallow, rapid breathing is not as efficient as slower, deeper respiration because of the greater proportion of each breath wasted in the dead space.

TRANSPORT OF GASES AROUND THE BODY

Gas exchange in tissues

Gas exchange in the tissues occurs at capillary level and the constant usage of oxygen and production of carbon dioxide by the cells creates the necessary pressure gradients, as discussed in Chapter 17. Oxygen is not very soluble in water and must therefore be carried around the blood in association with haemoglobin. Carbon dioxide is about 20 times more soluble than oxygen and dissolves in water to form carbonic acid. However, if all the carbon dioxide was carried in solution the blood would be too acid to sustain life so a more complex mechanism is needed.

Transport of oxygen

About 99% of oxygen in the blood is bound to haemoglobin. There is a small quantity of oxygen dissolved in the blood which helps determine the partial pressure of oxygen in the blood (PO_2) and maintains the pressure gradients as the bound oxygen is not free to exert pressure. The oxygen content of the blood is determined partly by the haemoglobin level but the hydrogen ion content of the blood also plays its part. As more oxygen is available, the PO_2 rises and haemoglobin will take it up. At a certain PO_2 when oxygen content is equal to oxygen capacity, the haemoglobin will be unable to take up any more oxygen and is said to be **fully** or **100% saturated**.

Partial pressure gradients and gas diffusion

The partial pressure gradient needed for the diffusion of oxygen is steep. For instance, the PO_2 of pulmonary blood is only 40 mmHg (5.3 kPa) whilst the PO_2 in the alveoli is 100 mmHg (13.3 kPa). Oxygen diffuses from the alveoli into the pulmonary capillary blood until there is equilibrium, with a PO_2 of 100 mmHg (13.3 kPa) on both sides of the respiratory membrane. Carbon dioxide moves in the opposite direction down a much gentler gradient from about 45 mmHg (6.1 kPa) to 40 mmHg (5.3 kPa) with equilibrium at 40 mmHg (5.3 kPa). Although the gradients are so different, both gases are exchanged equally well because carbon dioxide has a solubility in plasma and alveolar fluid 20 times that of oxygen.

The oxygen dissociation curve

When measured and placed on a graph, the relationship between haemoglobin saturation and PO_2 does not make a straight line (linear) but is S-shaped or sigmoid (Fig. 18.5). Although each of the four haem groups in a haemoglobin molecule can take up a molecule of oxygen, they vary in their affinity. The first haem group in the molecule to take up oxygen does so with difficulty but also holds on to its oxygen tightly. This association changes the shape of the haemoglobin molecule so that the 2nd and 3rd haem molecules take up oxygen readily for a relatively small increase in PO_2 as oxygen saturation goes from 25% to 75%. This is shown on the graph as the steep part of the sigmoid curve. The fourth haem group takes up oxygen more slowly and only at high PO_2. The unloading of oxygen at the tissues is also efficient with the unloading of one molecule facilitating the unloading of the next.

Effects of the sigmoid curve on oxygen uptake

Physiological effects of the oxygen dissociation curve include the following aspects. First, oxygen diffuses into the blood at the alveoli and, by increasing the plasma PO_2, creates a pressure gradient so that oxygen can enter the red cell. Within the erythrocyte, the PO_2 rises more slowly as the dissolved oxygen is rapidly bound to the haemoglobin molecules so the pressure gradient is maintained. Loading to 90% saturation occurs rapidly at a PO_2 of 60 mmHg (8 kPa). However, loading from 90% saturation to full saturation is slower and needs a higher erythrocyte PO_2 of 100 mmHg (13.3 kPa). Second, this flattened upper portion of the curve provides a safety factor in illness or at altitude as the blood leaving the lungs will still reach 90% saturation even when PO_2 remains moderate at 60 mmHg (8 kPa).

Effects of the sigmoid curve on oxygen release

Blood enters the capillary circulation with a PO_2 of 100 mmHg (13.3 kPa) and is exposed to a tissue PO_2 of only 40 mmHg (5.3 kPa). This tissue pressure lies on the steep part of the oxygen dissociation curve so that up to 80% of the bound oxygen is readily released into the blood so that it can diffuse to the tissues. Below 10 mmHg (1.3 kPa), the affinity of haemoglobin for oxygen is increased so that the last molecule of oxygen associated with haemoglobin is lost with difficulty.

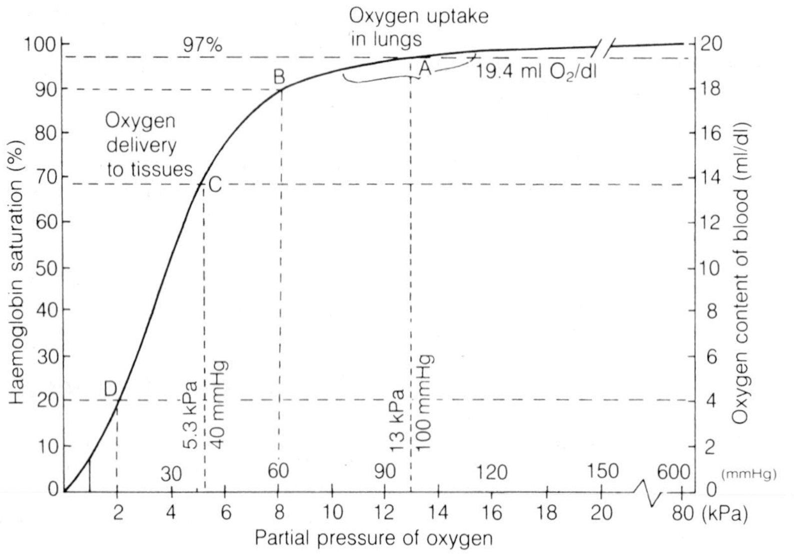

Figure 18.5 *The oxygen-haemoglobin dissociation curve. This applies when pH is 7.4, PCO_2 is 40 mmHg (5.3 kPa) and blood is at 37°C. The total blood oxygen content is shown, assuming a haemoglobin concentration of 15 g/dl blood (i.e. O_2 capacity of 20 ml/dl) (from Hinchliff SM, Montague SE, 1990, with permission).*

However, this low level is very rarely reached. In working muscles, PO_2 of this low level may occur but **myoglobin**, a special oxygen-carrying molecule, can extract all the oxygen.

Factors influencing the oxygen-haemoglobin dissociation curve

Several factors can influence the affinity of haemoglobin for oxygen at any given PO_2. These include factors that move the oxygen dissociation curve to the right, enhancing oxygen unloading, and those that move it to the left, inhibiting unloading.

Increase in carbon dioxide

An increase in carbon dioxide will reduce the ability of haemoglobin to bind oxygen, called the **Bohr effect**. Blood entering the tissues with a PCO_2 of 46 mmHg (6.1 kPa) will release more of its oxygen than blood with a PCO_2 of 40 mm Hg (5.3 kPa). This will shift the oxygen dissociation curve to the right.

Increase in hydrogen ions

As acidity increases in the blood, e.g. addition of lactic acid to the extra carbon dioxide during anaerobic cell metabolism in exercise, oxygen release to the tissues is facilitated by the presence of extra hydrogen ions.

Increase in 2,3-diphosphoglycerate

This substance is a product of red cell metabolism and binds reversibly to haemoglobin, reducing its affinity for oxygen. As the red cells reach the tissues, 2,3-DPG is produced in more quantity and oxygen release is facilitated.

Increase in temperature

Local elevation of temperature due to muscle cell metabolism in exercise or other actively metabolising cells will enhance the release of oxygen from the red cells.

The effects are reversed in the lung where the extra CO_2 is blown off and the local temperature is cooler. Haemoglobin therefore has a higher affinity for oxygen in the pulmonary capillaries, an appropriate effect!

Carbon monoxide

Carbon monoxide (CO) and oxygen compete for the same binding site on haemoglobin but the affinity of haemoglobin for CO is 240 times that of oxygen (Sherwood 1988). The product of haemoglobin combined with CO is carboxyhaemoglobin (HbCO). Even small amounts of CO will block the uptake of oxygen and shift the oxygen dissociation curve to the left. The amount of oxygen in the blood is reduced and the cells die from oxygen deprivation. CO is odourless, colourless and tasteless and is produced during the incomplete combustion of carbon products. If introduced into a small space, it is lethal as the victim has no sense of breathlessness.

Transport of carbon dioxide

There are three ways in which carbon dioxide is carried around the blood.

1. About 5% is carried in simple solution.
2. About 5% is carried in combination with the globin rather than the haem part of haemoglobin as carbamino-haemoglobin.
3. About 90% is transported as hydrogen carbonate (bicarbonate) ions.

Bicarbonate ions

As the cells metabolise they constantly produce CO_2 so that the PCO_2 of intracellular fluid is always greater than that of the blood in the tissue capillaries. This creates the pressure gradient for the removal of CO_2 from the tissues into the plasma. A small quantity will dissolve in the plasma to give carbonic acid. This is a reversible reaction:

$$CO_2 + H_2O \leftrightarrow H_2CO_3$$

An enzyme called **carbonic anhydrase** can catalyse (speed up) this reaction. Plasma contains little of this enzyme but the amount inside the red cell is much greater so that most of the CO_2 from the tissues diffuses through the plasma into the red cells. The rapid production of carbonic acid mops up the CO_2, keeping the red cell PCO_2 low. This ensures maintenance of the pressure gradient along which the CO_2 flows.

As is characteristic of acids, the carbonic acid in the red cell quickly ionises (dissociates) into hydrogen (H^{+}) and bicarbonate (HCO_3^-) ions, another reversible reaction:

$$CO_2 + H_2O \leftrightarrow H_2CO_3 \leftrightarrow H^+ + HCO_3^-$$

The chloride shift

HCO_3^- ions can readily pass out of the red cell into the plasma, unlike the H^+ ions, so that the HCO_3^- ions but not the H^+ ions can pass down a concentration gradient into the plasma. HCO_3^- ions are much more soluble in blood than CO_2. This movement of HCO_3^- ions out of the cell leaves the erythrocyte with a more positive electrical charge than the plasma and creates an electrical gradient down which chloride ions (Cl_2^-), the main plasma **anion** (anions are negatively charged ions and **cations** are positively charged ions), diffuse into the red cell to restore electrical neutrality. This is known as the **chloride shift**.

Hydrogen ions, carbon dioxide and the acid/base balance

Most of the accumulated H^+ ions inside the red cell become bound to the haemoglobin as reduced Hb as an affinity for them. This action of haemoglobin acts as a buffer which neutralises the released H^+ ions to prevent any rise in acidity within the red cell. The increased affinity for the uptake of CO_2 and H^+ ions that follows the removal of oxygen is called the **Haldane effect**. The Bohr effect and the Haldane effect work together to facilitate O_2 release and the uptake of CO_2 and H^+ ions by the red cells at tissue level. During exercise, much larger amounts of CO_2 are produced by the tissues but the increase in alveolar ventilation and in cardiac output ensure that arterial PCO_2 remains constant between 37 mmHg (4.9 kPa) and 43 mmHg (5.7 kPa).

The reactions are reversed once the blood reaches the lungs because of the reversed pressure gradients caused by the presence of atmospheric air in the alveoli. Here, CO_2 leaves the red cell to enter the plasma and cross into the alveoli and the freed H^+ ions combine with HCO_3^- ions to form H_2CO_3, which then separates into CO_2 and H_2O, generating more CO_2 to diffuse out to the alveoli. This reaction is also catalysed by carbonic anhydrase.

As the HCO_3^- ions within the red cell are used up to generate CO_2, there is a shift inside the red cell to a positive electrical charge and plasma HCO_3^- ions and Cl_2^- ions now move back into the cell to restore electrical neutrality once more. This is a main pathway through which acid is removed from the body to maintain the acid/base balance. About 200 ml/min are removed from the tissues and eliminated from the lungs. Now O_2 crosses from the alveoli into the plasma and then the red cell to bind to haemoglobin.

Because of the importance of fluid and electrolyte balance and the maintenance of pH, a full discussion of the role of the respiratory system in maintaining the pH is presented in Chapter 20.

CONTROL OF VENTILATION

Breathing, like the beating of the heart, must occur in a continuous rhythmic cycle in order to provide oxygen for the cells. The control of breathing is quite complex. The respiratory muscles, unlike cardiac muscle which has its intrinsic pacemaker, are skeletal muscles and must receive nervous stimulation from the brain to make them contract. In normal circumstances respiration is an involuntary act. The control of rhythmic breathing originates in the respiratory centre in the medulla.

The dorsal respiratory group

The pace-setting nucleus within the medulla oblongata is called the **inspiratory centre** or dorsal respiratory group (DRG). There is a second nucleus called the **expiratory centre** or ventral respiratory group but its function is not well understood. Two other centres higher in the brainstem in the pons which influence the respiratory centre are the **pneumotaxic centre**, which sends out inhibitory impulses to the DRG to prevent overinflation of the lungs, and the **apneustic centre**, which continuously stimulates the DRG to prolong inspiration. The apneustic centre is normally inhibited by the pneumotaxic centre. There is also a voluntary pathway of control by the cerebral cortex with descending pathways to the respiratory centre.

The respiratory cycle

Descending neurones from the respiratory centre terminate on the motor neurones controlling the respiratory muscles. As inspiration starts, there is a rapid increase in the number of nerve impulses from the DRG which travel along the phrenic and intercostal nerves to arrive at the respiratory muscles. The force of inspiration gradually increases and thoracic expansion occurs. At the end of inspiration the DRG becomes dormant and there is a sudden reduction in the number of impulses, resulting in relaxation of the respiratory muscles and passive elastic recoil of the thoracic cage and lungs. Inspiration lasts about 2 s and expiration about 3 s. This cycle is repeated about 12–18 times in a minute but the level of ventilation is continuously adapted to changes in bodily requirements or atmospheric conditions so that adequate oxygenation is maintained.

Factors influencing the rate and depth of breathing

Multiple factors are involved in the regulation of respiration. These include neural, mechanical and chemical events and are best summarised in a diagram (Fig. 18.6).

Voluntary control of breathing

Voluntary control of the rate and rhythm of respiration such as hyperventilation or breath holding is limited by the chemical stimuli that such efforts induce. Complex control of the respiratory system is necessary during speech and singing as well

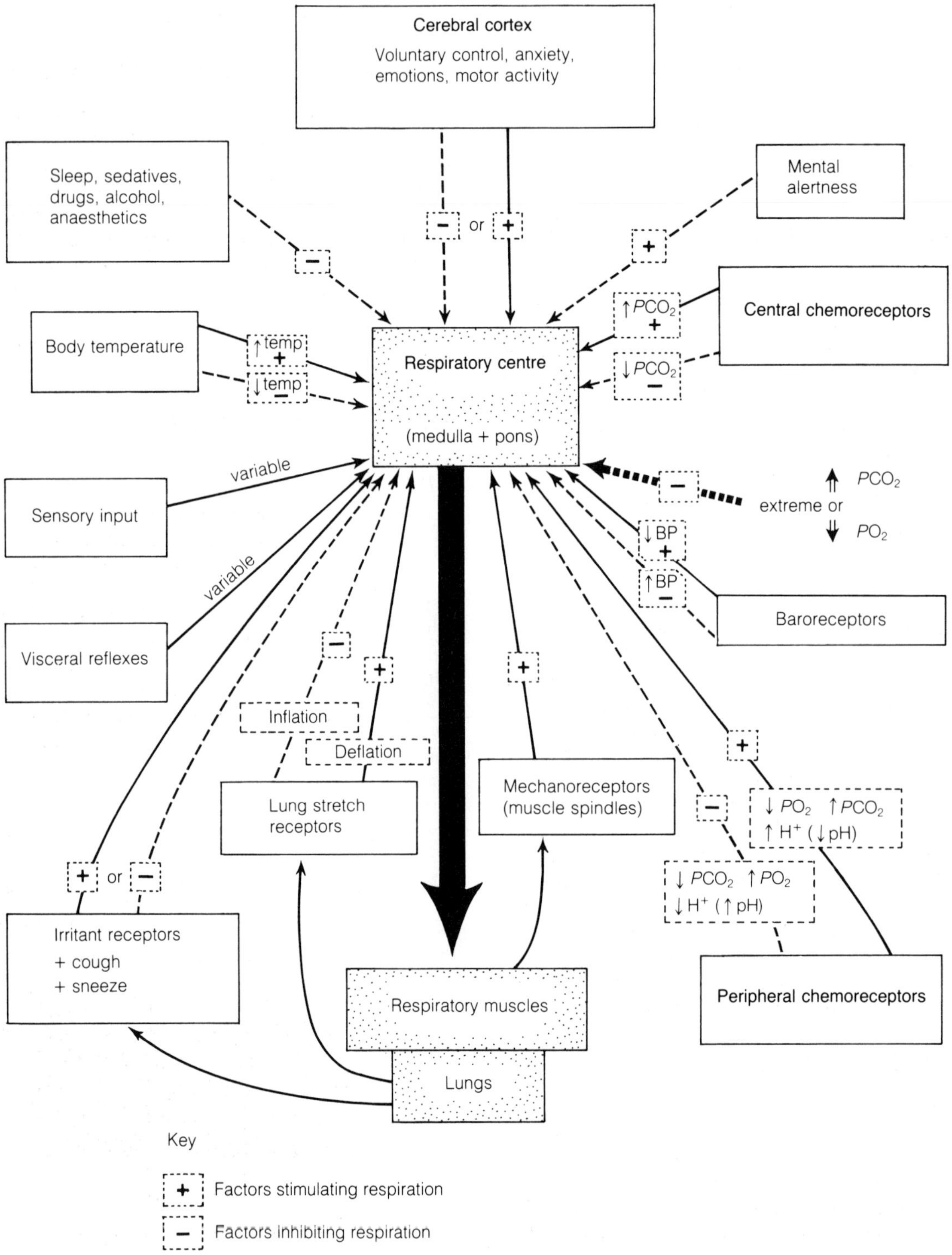

Figure 18.6 *Summary of factors controlling respiration (from Hinchliff SM, Montague SE, 1990, with permission).*

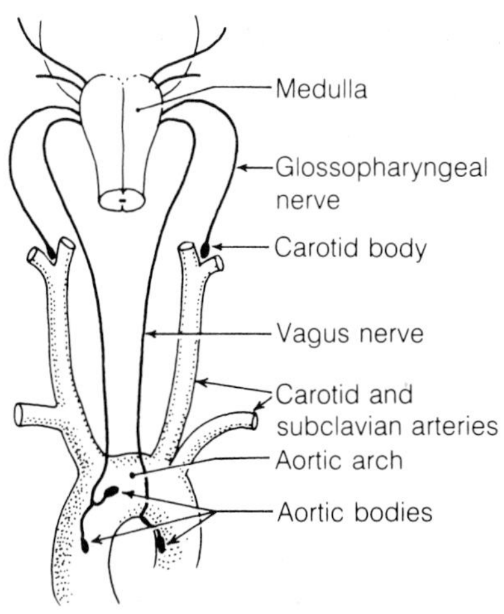

Figure 18.7 *Peripheral chemoreceptor system involved in the control of breathing (from Hinchliff SM, Montague SE, 1990, with permission).*

as playing a wind instrument. Laughing and crying also change respiratory patterns. When nerve impulses are sent to the vocal cords, simultaneous impulses are sent to the respiratory centre to control the flow of air between the vocal cords. Mental states influence respiratory rhythm with alertness and wakefulness having a stimulating effect and sleep, sedatives, alcohol and some anaesthetics having an inhibitory effect.

Chemoreceptor effects

Both peripheral and central chemoreceptors are able to respond to small changes in arterial PO_2 and PCO_2 to affect the rate and rhythm of respiration. **Peripheral chemoreceptors** are situated in the carotid bodies and other vascular structures around the aortic arch (Fig. 18.7). These receptors respond to chemical changes in the blood. They sense the levels of PO_2, PCO_2 and H^+ ions and relay the information to the respiratory centre.

The response to oxygen levels depends primarily on these peripheral chemoreceptors but the response to excessive levels of CO_2 (**hypercapnia**) depends on **central chemoreceptors** situated under the surface of the medulla. It is probable that with a rise in arterial PCO_2, carbon dioxide crosses the blood–brain barrier from the cerebral blood vessels into the cerebrospinal fluid (CSF). This bathes the central chemoreceptors. Once in the CSF, hydrogen ions are released and these stimulate the central chemoreceptors which send excitatory messages to the respiratory centre to increase the rate of respiration. A fall in PCO_2 will inhibit respiration.

The Hering–Breuer reflex

Stretch receptors in the visceral pleura and in the conducting passages of the lung are stimulated if the lungs are overinflated. Inhibitory impulses are sent by these receptors via the vagus nerve to the medullary inspiratory centre and these result in the termination of inspiration so that expiration can occur. The stretch receptors quieten down as the lungs recoil so that inspiration can begin again. This is called the **inflation** or Hering–Breuer reflex.

MATERNAL ADAPTATIONS TO PREGNANCY

Blackburn & Loper (1992) remind us that the respiratory system undergoes changes in pregnancy to meet the increased metabolic needs for oxygen of the altered maternal body and the fetoplacental unit (Fig. 18.8). The changes are brought about by hormonal and biochemical influences as well as the mechanical effect of the enlarging uterus.

Anatomical configuration of the chest

The muscles and cartilage of the thorax relax, creating anatomical changes in the shape of the chest cavity. These develop as pregnancy progresses and have implications for respiratory function (Fig. 18.9). The diaphragm becomes raised by a maximum of 4 cm and the transverse diameter of the rib cage is increased by 2 cm. The subcostal angle widens from the normal 68° to 103° in late pregnancy. There is a change from abdominal to thoracic breathing, the main work of respiration being carried out by increased diaphragmatic movement. Some of these changes occur in advance of the increasing size of the uterus.

Biochemical changes

Carbon dioxide

The tendency to overbreathe causes CO_2 to be washed out of the lungs so that the alveolar and arterial CO_2 concentration is lower than in the non-pregnant woman. This reduction in arterial PCO_2 from a norm of 35–40 mmHg (4.7–5.3 kPa) to a level of 30 mmHg (4 kPa) has been found in the luteal phase of each menstrual cycle before any embedding of a fertilised ovum is possible. It is the result of progesterone which is thought to stimulate the respiratory centres directly, causing an increased sensitivity to CO_2 with a lowered threshold (Blackburn & Loper 1992). Progesterone also causes an increase in carbonic

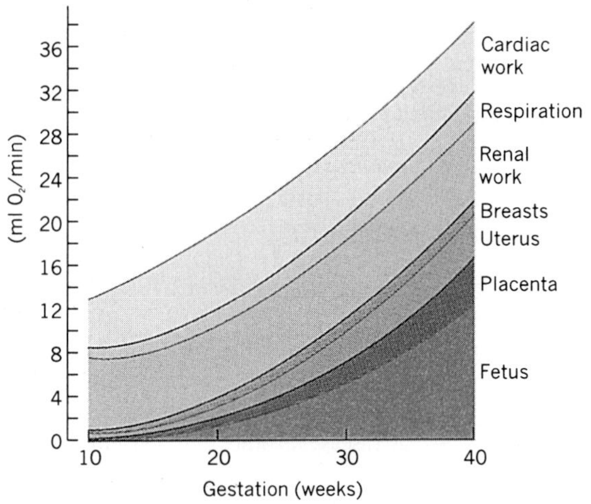

Figure 18.8 *Partition of the increased oxygen consumption in pregnancy among the organs concerned. (Reproduced with permission from de Swiet 1991.)*

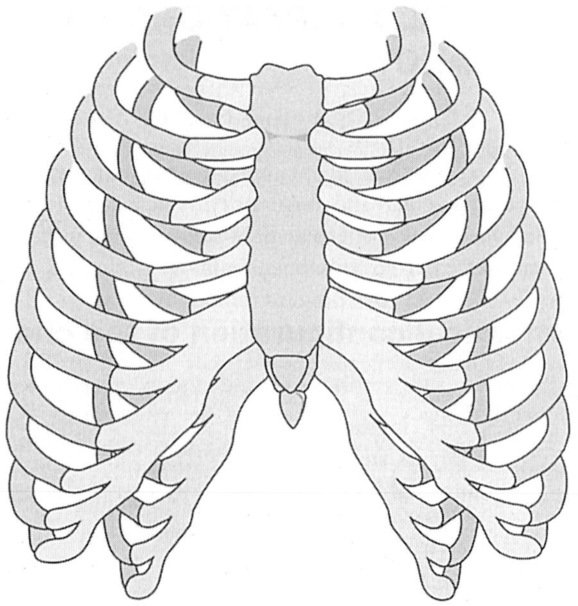

Figure 18.9 *The ribcage in pregnancy and the non-pregnancy state showing the increased subcostal angle, the increased transverse diameter and the raised diaphragm in pregnancy. (Reproduced with permission from de Swiet 1991.)*

anhydrase in the red cells which in turn facilitates CO_2 transfer, tending to decrease PCO_2 even without the presence of a change in ventilation (de Swiet 1991). The resulting slight respiratory alkalosis is essential to create the gas gradients for exchange across the placenta.

Progesterone may also lower resistance in the airway, leading to a greater inflow of air. By relaxing the smooth muscles of the bronchioles, prostaglandins, especially $PGF_{2\alpha}$, may also influence the smooth muscle in the lung tissue by acting as a bronchoconstrictor and PGE_1 and PGE_2 act as bronchodilators. Increases have been seen in PGFs throughout pregnancy and PGEs in the last trimester but their role is not clear.

Oxygen

The increased alveolar ventilation not only causes a decrease in PCO_2 but raises PO_2. However, this rise is only slight and has no effect on the oxygen-haemoglobin dissociation curve.

Respiratory parameters

The respiratory parameters are discussed by de Swiet (1991) and summarised below.

Pregnancy causes less stress to the respiratory system than to the cardiovascular system. Therefore women with respiratory disease are less likely to show deterioration in their condition than those with cardiac disease. Studies can be found to support and refute an increase in vital capacity during pregnancy. Because of this, de Swiet suggests that some but not all women have an increase in vital capacity during pregnancy. When changes have been found, they have commenced from midpregnancy and are in the order of 100–200 ml.

Studies are unanimous in confirming that inspiratory capacity increases by about 300 ml and this is progressive throughout pregnancy. Expiratory reserve volume reduces by 200 ml progressively from early pregnancy. Tidal volume rises throughout pregnancy from the normal 500 ml to about 700 ml, an increase of 40%. The resting pregnant woman increases her ventilation by deepening her respirations and not by breathing more frequently so that the minute ventilation rises by 40% in line with the tidal volume. Oxygen consumption increases by about 15% and alveolar ventilation is increased by 50%, resulting in a physiological change to overbreathing.

Postpartum changes

There is a rapid return to normal of respiration patterns and acid/base balance in the third stage of labour and early puerperium. This is initiated by the fall in progesterone levels following delivery of the placenta and the reduction in intra-abdominal pressure following delivery of the baby. A rise in PCO_2 is seen within 48 h of delivery. Overall, anatomical changes and ventilation parameters return to normal about 1–3 weeks following delivery (Blackburn & Loper 1992).

CLINICAL IMPLICATIONS

Dyspnoea

As discussed above, the resting pregnant woman increases her ventilation, oxygen consumption and minute ventilation and there is a physiological change to overbreathing. The major influence leading to the overbreathing is central respiratory control but there are alterations in the lung volumes due to the anatomical changes mentioned above. The woman may experience dyspnoea and giddiness and mention that she is short of breath. This is more likely to occur when she is sitting down rather than walking about and is not always related to exercise.

Smoking

In a literature review, Tuormaa (1995) has summarised the effects of tobacco smoking. Smoking is probably one of the most dangerous avoidable risks taken by people and it is essential that both men and women who are thinking about starting a family should stop smoking, both for the child's sake and ultimately for their own safety. About the only benefit associated with smoking in pregnancy is a reduced incidence of pregnancy-induced hypertension but the other risks to the fetus and to health outweigh this statistically reported benefit. A full discussion of the effects of smoking on human reproduction can be found in Chapter 7 where the following list is addressed in detail.

- Male and female infertility
- Reduced length of gestation
- Low birth weight
- Spontaneous abortions
- Increased perinatal mortality (stillbirths + neonatal deaths in the first week)
- Fetal malformations
- Reduced immunocompetence

Summary of main points

- During respiration, oxygen is taken from the atmosphere and transported around the body in the blood and carbon dioxide produced as metabolic waste by the cells is returned to the lungs and excreted into the air. The respiratory system consists of the airways from the nasal passages to the pharynx and larynx as well as the bronchi, bronchioles and alveoli of the lungs. The respiratory system is divided into the upper and lower airways at the level of the cricoid cartilage.
- There are about 300 million alveoli in the lungs, providing an enormous area for gas exchange. Cuboidal type II alveolar cells secrete pulmonary surfactant, a phospholipid that helps to keep the membrane moist and also maintains the patency of the alveolus.
- There are two phases to breathing: inspiration and expiration. Mechanical factors and neural factors are involved in the control of respiratory rate. Expiration is a passive process brought about by the relaxation and elastic recoil of the diaphragm and accessory muscles, if in use. Active expiration may occur when the need for gas exchange increases.
- Respiratory parameters include tidal volume, inspiratory reserve volume, expiratory reserve volume and residual volume. Respiratory capacities include total lung capacity, vital capacity, inspiratory capacity and functional residual capacity. The total volume of air exchanged with the atmosphere in one minute is called the minute volume or pulmonary ventilation. The volume of fresh air entering the alveoli each minute is called the alveolar ventilation.
- About 99% of oxygen in the blood is bound to haemoglobin. There is a small quantity of oxygen dissolved in the blood which helps determine the partial pressure of oxygen in the blood and maintains the pressure gradients.
- The relationship between haemoglobin saturation and PO_2 is called the oxygen dissociation curve. Several factors can influence the affinity of haemoglobin for oxygen. These include factors that move the oxygen dissociation curve to the right, enhancing oxygen unloading, and factors that shift the oxygen dissociation curve to the left.
- The control of rhythmic breathing originates in the respiratory centre in the medulla. Multiple factors are involved in the regulation of respiration, including neural, mechanical and chemical events. Hyperventilation or breath holding is limited by the chemical stimuli that such efforts induce. Both peripheral and central chemoreceptors are able to respond to small changes in arterial PO_2 and PCO_2 and affect the rate and rhythm of respiration.
- The respiratory system undergoes changes in pregnancy to meet the increased metabolic needs for oxygen of the altered maternal body and the fetoplacental unit. The changes are brought about by hormonal and biochemical influences as well as the mechanical effect of the enlarging uterus.
- The muscles and cartilage of the thorax relax, creating anatomical changes in the shape of the chest cavity which have implications for respiratory function. The diaphragm becomes raised by up to 4 cm and the transverse diameter of the rib cage is increased by 2 cm. The subcostal angle widens from the normal 68° to 103° in late pregnancy. There is a change from abdominal to thoracic breathing, with increased diaphragmatic movement.
- Pregnancy causes less stress to the respiratory system than to the cardiovascular system. Therefore women with respiratory disease are less likely to show deterioration in their condition than those with cardiac disease.
- Inspiratory capacity increases by about 300 ml progressively throughout pregnancy whilst expiratory reserve volume reduces by 200 ml. Tidal volume increases by 40% to about 700 ml. The resting pregnant woman increases her ventilation by deepening her respirations and not by breathing more often. Oxygen consumption increases by about 15% and alveolar ventilation is increased by 50%, resulting in a physiological change to overbreathing.
- The pregnant woman may be uncomfortable with dyspnoea and giddiness, which she may perceive as shortage of breath. This is more likely to occur when she is sitting down rather than walking about and is not always related to exercise.
- Smoking is probably one of the most dangerous avoidable risks taken by people and both men and women who are thinking about starting a family should stop smoking. It may lead to male and female infertility, reduced length of gestation, low birth weight, spontaneous abortions, increased perinatal mortality, fetal malformations and reduced immunocompetence.

References

Blackburn ST, Loper DL. 1992 Maternal, Fetal and Neonatal Physiology, A Clinical Perspective. WB Saunders, Philadelphia.

Hinchliff SM, Montague SE. 1990 Physiology for Nursing Practice. Baillière Tindall, London.

de Swiet M. 1991 The respiratory system. In Hytten F, Chamberlain G (eds) Clinical Physiology in Obstetrics, 2nd edn. Blackwell Scientific, Oxford, pp 83–100.

Marieb EN. 1992 Human Anatomy and Physiology. Benjamin/ Cummings Publishing, California.

Sherwood L. 1988 Human Physiology: From Cells to Systems. West Publishing,

Tuormaa TE. 1995 The Adverse Effects of Tobacco Smoking on Reproduction. Foresight, AB Academic Publishers, Tacoma, Washington.

Recommended reading

de Swiet M. 1991 The respiratory system. In Hytten F, Chamberlain G (eds) Clinical Physiology in Obstetrics, 2nd edn. Blackwell Scientific, Oxford pp 83–100.

Stocks J. 1996 Respiration. In Hinchliff SM, Montague SE, Watson R (eds) Physiology for Nursing Practice. Baillière Tindall, London.

Tuormaa TE. 1995 The Adverse Effects of Tobacco Smoking on Reproduction. Foresight, AB Academic Publishers, Tacoma, Washington.

Chapter 19 The renal tract

In this chapter

INTRODUCTION

This chapter is about the structure and function of the renal tract and how these change in pregnancy. Although the production of urine is discussed, fluid and electrolyte balance and the regulation of acid/base balance are discussed in the following chapter in an attempt to integrate the roles of the respiratory and renal systems. This should be of value to the reader interested in the interactions between systems and it may avoid turning backwards and forwards in the text to synthesise material. The role of renin and the angiotensin-aldosterone system and the control of blood pressure is discussed in Chapter 20.

KIDNEY FUNCTIONS

The kidneys play a major role in maintenance of homeostasis within the internal environment by their regulation of the volume and composition of the body fluids. Each day the kidneys filter large amounts of fluid from the bloodstream, ensuring that toxins, metabolic wastes and excess ions are excreted out of the body in urine. Marieb (1992) outlines the roles of the kidney other than the excretory function as:

- regulation of the volume and chemical make-up of the blood;
- maintenance of balance between water and salts, acids and bases;
- production of the enzyme renin which helps to regulate blood pressure and the hormone erythropoietin which stimulates red cell production in the bone marrow;
- conversion of vitamin D to its active form.

Also part of the renal system are the two ureters which convey urine to the urinary bladder where it is stored until it is voided through the urethra.

ANATOMY OF THE KIDNEY

The sources for this part of the chapter are useful reference books for students of anatomy and physiology and include Hinchliff et al (1996) and Marieb (1992).

The kidneys are paired, compact organs situated on either side of the vertebral column at the level of the 12th thoracic to the 3rd lumbar vertebrae. They are situated behind the peritoneum and are attached to the posterior abdominal wall by adipose tissue. An adult kidney is bean-shaped with a convex lateral surface and concave medial surface. A cleft in the medial surface is called the **hilum** and leads to a space within the kidney called the **renal sinus**. The hilum is the site of entry to or exit from structures which include the ureters, renal blood vessels, lymphatics and nerves. Each kidney weighs about 150 g and measures 12 cm long by 6 cm wide and 3 cm thick. The adrenal gland sits on top of the kidney.

Structure

Three layers of supporting tissue surround each kidney.

1 The **renal capsule** is closest to the kidney and is fibrous and transparent. This is a strong barrier that prevents infections in nearby regions spreading to the kidneys.
2 The **adipose capsule** is a middle layer of fatty tissue which helps hold the kidney in place and protects it from trauma.
3 The **renal fascia** is the outermost covering and is made of dense fibrous connective tissue which surrounds both kidney and adrenal gland and anchors them to surrounding structures.

Beneath the capsule lie three distinct regions: the outer **cortex**, the **medulla** and the inner **renal pelvis**. The cortex has a light granular appearance. The medulla is darker and reddish brown with cone-shaped masses of tissue called **medullary** or **renal pyramids**. The base of each pyramid is broad and faces the renal cortex whilst the pointed apex (**papilla**) projects into a minor calyx. Several minor calyces open into each of two or three major calyces which then open into the renal pelvis. The pyramids have a striped appearance because they consist of bundles of microscopic tubules. The renal columns are extensions of cortical tissue that separate the pyramids. Each medullary pyramid and its cap of cortical tissue is known as a **lobe** of the kidney and there are usually between eight and 18 lobes in a kidney.

The renal pelvis

The renal pelvis is a flat, funnel-shaped tube which is continuous with the ureter. There is a continuous flow of urine from the papillae into the calyces, on down the ureter to be stored in the urinary bladder. The walls of the calyces, pelvis and ureter contain smooth muscle which contracts in peristaltic movements to propel urine towards the bladder.

Microscopic structure of the kidney

Each kidney contains over 1 million nephrons which are the functional units of the kidney. A nephron consists of a tuft of blood vessel capillaries called the **glomerulus** associated with a renal tubule. The end of the tubule, called a **Bowman's capsule**, is enlarged and invaginated to hold the glomerulus. The outer or parietal layer of the Bowman's capsule is composed of simple squamous epithelium and has a purely structural function. The inner or visceral layer which clings to the glomerulus is made up of branching epithelial cells called **podocytes** which form part of the filtration membrane. The branches of the podocytes end in **pedicles** or foot processes. The clefts between the pedicles form filtration slits or slit pores.

The capillary endothelium of the glomerulus is porous which allows large quantities of solute-rich fluid to pass from the blood into the glomerular capsule. This fluid is called the **filtrate** and is processed by the renal tubules to form urine. A basement membrane divides the endothelium of the capillary from the epithelium lining the Bowman's capsule. The Bowman's capsule and its contained glomerulus is known as a **renal corpuscle** and is situated in the renal cortex. The structure comprising the

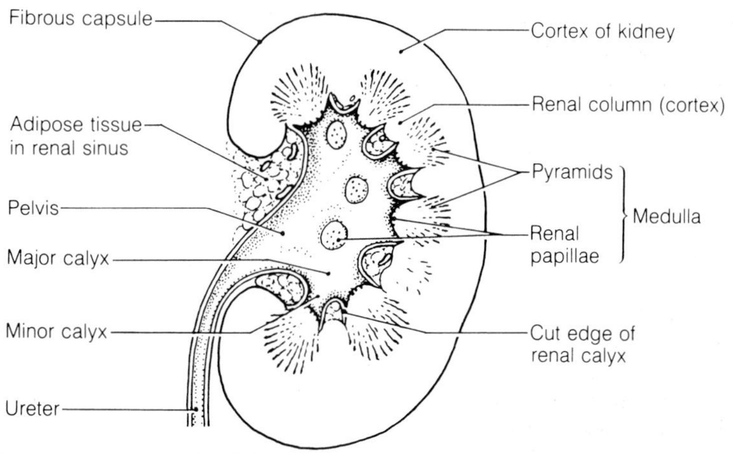

Figure 19.1 *Coronal section through a kidney (from Hinchliff SM, Montague SE, 1990, with permission).*

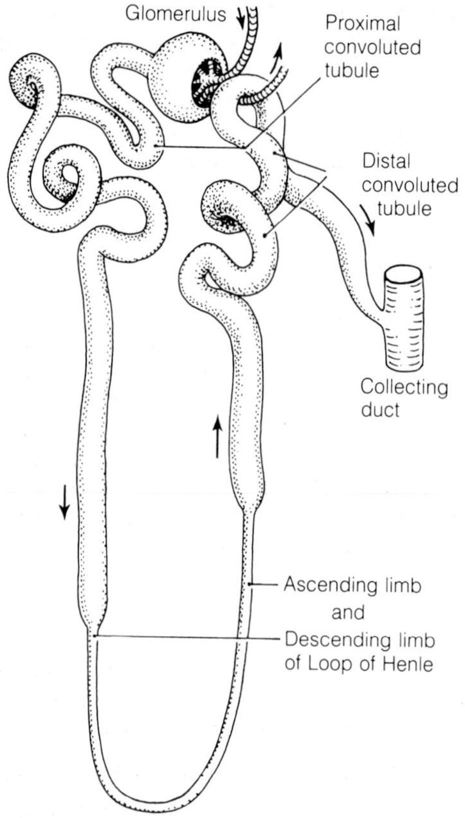

Figure 19.2 *Microanatomy of nephron (from Hinchliff SM, Montague SE, 1990, with permission).*

capillary endothelium, basement membrane and podocytic epithelium constitutes the selective filtration barrier.

The remainder of the renal tubule is about 3 cm long and can be divided into four anatomically distinct regions: the proximal convoluted tubule, the loop of Henle, the distal convoluted tubule and the collecting duct.

The **proximal convoluted tubule** extends about 16 mm through the cortex. This region of the tubule is lined by large columnar epithelial cells which have a brush border of microvilli on their internal surface for solute reabsorption.

The **loop of Henle** has a descending limb and an ascending limb. The descending limb extends from the proximal convoluted tubule, dips down into the medulla and makes a U turn, moving back into the cortex by the thicker walled ascending limb. In this loop the columnar cells are flatter and contain fewer microvilli on their luminal (side facing into the lumen) surfaces.

The **distal convoluted tubule**, continuous with the loop of Henle, is comparatively short, about 4–8 mm, and leads into the **collecting ducts** which fuse together as they approach the renal pelvis to form papillary ducts. These ducts open at the tips of the medullary papillae to discharge their urine into the calyces and renal pelvis. The first part of the distal tubule folds back to bring it nearer to the afferent arteriole to form the juxtaglomerular apparatus (see below).

Cortical and juxtamedullary nephrons

About 85% of the nephrons are called **cortical nephrons** because they are situated in the cortex except where their loops of Henle dip into the medulla. The remaining 15% of nephrons are different in structure and are called **juxtaglomerular nephrons**. They are located near to the cortex-medullary junction and their loops of Henle are found deep in the medulla. Their thin segments are more extensive than those of the cortical nephrons. The juxtamedullary nephrons have long thinwalled looping capillaries called the **vasa recta** running parallel with their loops of Henle.

Capillary beds of the nephron

Every nephron is closely associated with two capillary beds which form the microvasculature of the nephron. These are the glomerulus and the peritubular capillary bed. The glomerulus is unlike any other capillary bed in that it is fed and drained by arterioles. Glomeruli originate from afferent arterioles which arise from interlobular arteries which permeate the renal cortex and drain into efferent arterioles. The peritubular capillary bed consists of capillaries arising from the efferent arterioles draining the glomeruli. These capillaries cling closely to the renal tubules and empty into nearby venules. Just as the glomerular capillary bed is adapted for filtration, the peritubular bed is adapted for reabsorption. They are low-pressure porous capillaries. The additional vessels of the vasa recta play a part in reabsorption of salts.

The blood pressure within the glomerulus is very high for a capillary bed for two reasons:

1 arterioles are high-resistance vessels;
2 the afferent arteriole has a much larger diameter than the efferent arteriole.

This pressure forces fluids and solutes out of the blood in the glomerulus along its entire length into the Bowman's capsule. About 99% of this filtrate is reabsorbed into the blood in the peritubular capillary beds. As blood flows into the renal circulation it encounters high resistance first in the afferent and then in the efferent arterioles. Renal blood pressure declines from 95 mmHg in the renal arteries to 8 mmHg in the renal veins. The resistance of the afferent arterioles protects the kidney from large fluctuations in the systemic blood pressure. Resistance in the efferent arterioles maintains the high glomerular pressure and reduces the hydrostatic pressure in the peritubular arteries to facilitate reabsorption.

The juxtaglomerular apparatus

The juxtaglomerular apparatus is a region found in each nephron where the distal convoluted tubule lies against the afferent arteriole as it supplies the glomerulus. Where the two parts of the nephron touch, the cellular structures are modified. The afferent arteriolar wall contains juxtaglomerular (JG) cells. These are enlarged smooth muscle cells which contain granules filled with **renin**. They seem to be mechanoreceptors responding to the blood pressure in the afferent arterioles. The **macula densa** is a group of tall, closely packed distal tubule cells that act as chemoreceptors or osmoreceptors responding to sodium chloride concentration in the distal tubule. These two types of cell are important in the regulation of filtrate formation and systemic blood pressure.

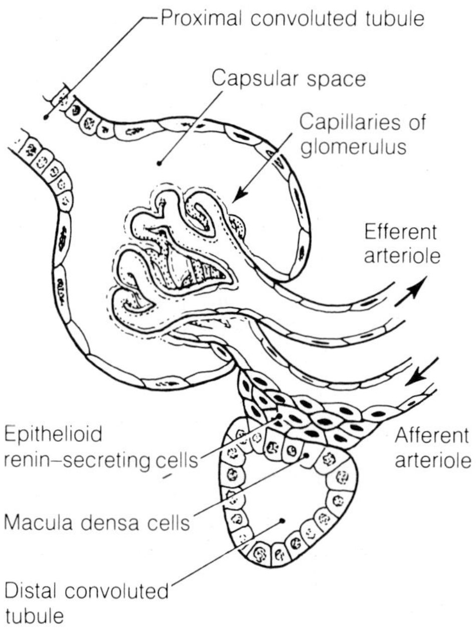

Figure 19.3 *The juxtaglomerular apparatus showing the macula densa. (Redrawn from Creager 1983.)*

Blood supply

About 25% of cardiac output is delivered to the kidneys each minute. This is a higher blood supply than any other tissue. The two renal arteries arise high up on the abdominal aorta and enter the hilum to divide in the renal tissue to form interlobar arteries between the pyramids. Arcuate arteries arise from these and give rise to interlobular arteries which branch to form the afferent arterioles supplying each glomerulus. Efferent arterioles emerge from the glomerulus and form a dense peri-tubular capillary network. Venous capillaries drain into interlobular, arcuate and interlobar veins and into the renal veins. The renal veins drain into the inferior vena cava which lies to the right of the vertebral column. Therefore, the left renal vein is twice as long as the right one.

Nerve supply

The kidneys are supplied by the autonomic nervous system. There is a rich supply of sympathetic fibres and a few parasympathetic fibres which supply the smooth muscle of the arterioles and the juxtaglomerular apparatus. Stimulation of these nerves causes vasoconstriction, reduced renal blood flow and glomerular filtration rate (GFR) and the release of renin from the juxtaglomerular apparatus. The kidneys also have some sensory nerve fibres which allow the sensation of pain to be perceived. These fibres are stimulated by distension of the renal capsule in such situations as bleeding, inflammation or obstruction by renal calculi. Ischaemia may also cause pain.

RENAL FUNCTION

The production of urine

In an adult about 180 litres of plasma are filtered every day and 99% of the filtrate is reabsorbed by the nephrons. This results in the production of about 1.5 litres of urine per day. Fluid intake, diet and extrarenal fluid losses will affect the amount of urine produced. Glomerular filtration is the first step in urine production. Prior to describing the physiology of glomerular filtration, some concepts to facilitate understanding will be briefly outlined.

Electrolytes

These substances are electrically charged solutes which dissociate into their constituent ions when placed in solution. Electrolytes are polarised into those carrying a positive charge (**cations**) and a negative charge (**anions**). They are located in both extracellular fluid (ECF) and intracellular fluid (ICF). In ECF sodium is the cation and chloride the main anion and in ICF potassium is the cation and protein the anion. Electrolytes are measured in milliequivalents per litre (mEq/l) which is the number of electrical charges per litre.

Diffusion

Diffusion is the movement of a solute molecule across a permeable membrane to a weaker solution down a concentration gradient. This movement depends on:

- the electrical potential across the membrane – cations are often repelled by positive charges in the membrane;
- the particle size – the smaller the particle, the more rapid the diffusion rate;
- lipid solubility – lipid-soluble substances are non-polar and pass easily through the cell membrane which is itself a lipid bilayer;
- water solubility – water-soluble particles tend to be polar and diffuse much more slowly

Osmosis

Osmosis is the movement of water down a concentration gradient across a semipermeable membrane from a high water content to a lower one. The membrane must be more permeable to water than to the solutes and there must be a greater concentration of solutes in the destination solution for water to move easily. Osmosis is directly related to hydrostatic pressure and solute concentration but not to particle size. For example, in the plasma the protein albumin is smaller but more concentrated than the protein globulin. Therefore, albumin exerts the greater osmotic force for drawing fluid back from the ECF into the intravascular compartment.

Osmolality is the concentration of molecules per weight of water measured in milliosmoles/kilogram. **Osmolarity** is the concentration of molecules in water, measured in milliosmoles/litre of water. The two terms are often used interchangeably.

Hydrostatic pressure

Hydrostatic pressure is the mechanical force of water pushing against cell membranes. In the vascular system it is generated by the blood pressure. In the capillaries a hydrostatic pressure of

25 mmHg is sufficient to push water across the capillary membrane into the extracellular space. It is partly balanced by **osmotic pressure**. The excess water moves into the lymph system.

The amount of hydrostatic pressure needed to oppose the osmotic pressure of the solution depends on:

- the type and thickness of the plasma membrane;
- the size of the molecules;
- the concentration of the molecules on the gradient;
- the solubility of the molecules.

An example would be the movement of water in the glomerulus of the kidney.

Tonicity is the effective osmolality of a solution. Solutions can be **isotonic**, with the same concentration of particles as the body fluids, **hypotonic**, with less concentration (will cause water to be pulled into the cells by osmosis), or **hypertonic** with more concentration of particles (will cause water to be pulled out of the cells).

Oncotic pressure is the overall osmotic effect of the plasma proteins, sometimes called colloid osmotic pressure.

pH and acid/base balance

Hydrogen ion concentration or pH is the negative logarithm of hydrogen ions in solution on a scale of 1 to 14. This means that from one pH unit to the next there is a 10-fold change in hydrogen ion concentration. It is negative because as hydrogen decreases, the pH value increases. Low pH values with more hydrogen ions result in an acid solution and high pH values with a low hydrogen ion concentration result in an alkaline solution. A pH of 7 is neutral and most body fluids, with the exception of acid gastric juices (pH 1–3) and urine (pH 5–6), are just alkaline with a pH between 7 and 8. Many pathological conditions disturb the acid/base balance.

Glomerular filtration

Filtration is described by Marieb (1992) as 'a passive, non-selective process in which fluids and solutes are forced through a membrane by hydrostatic pressure'. The passage of water and solutes across the filtration membrane of the glomerulus is similar to that in other capillary beds, moving down a pressure gradient. However, the glomerular filtration membrane is thousands of times more permeable to water and solutes and glomerular pressure is much higher than normal capillary blood pressure. There is a high net filtration pressure.

This results in the 180 litres of filtrate a day in contrast to the 4 litres a day formed by all other capillary beds combined. Unlike other capillary beds where water and solutes move back into the capillary as the balance of hydrostatic pressure changes, movement is one way only, from the capillary into the glomerulus. The **glomerular filtration rate** (GFR) is the volume of plasma filtered through the glomeruli in one minute and is normally 120 ml/min.

The filtration membrane of the glomerulus lies between the blood and the interior of the glomerular capsule. As described above, it is a porous membrane made up of three layers:

- the fenestrated capillary endothelium;
- the podocytic visceral membrane of the glomerular capsule;
- the intervening basement membrane.

The membrane allows free passage of water, solutes and small protein molecules (less than 3 nm in diameter) but larger molecules such as blood cells and larger protein molecules are prevented from passing through by the capillary pores. The basement membrane may also act as a selective molecular sieve. It is made up of anionic (negatively charged) glycoproteins and therefore repels filtrate anions and prevents their passage. Therefore the filtrate contains more cationic (positively charged) and uncharged molecules. The presence of the plasma proteins in the capillary provides the colloid osmotic pressure of the glomerular blood, limiting the loss of water to one-fifth of the plasma fluid.

Regulation of glomerular filtration

Intrinsic control by autoregulation

The kidney can control its own blood supply over a wide range of arterial blood pressure, from 80 to 180 mmHg. This intrinsic system is called **autoregulation** and depends on alterations in the diameter of the afferent and efferent arterioles in response to a systemic blood pressure change. Factors involved in autoregulation may include:

- the myogenic mechanism – the tendency of vascular smooth muscle to contract when stretched;
- a tubuloglomerular feedback mechanism directed by the macula densa cells and solute concentration;
- the renin-angiotensin mechanism and renal vasoconstriction (see below);
- prostaglandin E_2 and renal vasodilation.

Extrinsic control by sympathetic nervous system stimulation

When the body is stressed adrenaline is released into the blood from the adrenal medulla. This causes strong constriction of the afferent arterioles and inhibits filtrate formation. Blood can be shunted to the brain and muscles at the expense of the kidneys. The JG cells are also stimulated to release renin which activates angiotensin II to raise systemic blood pressure by generalised vasoconstriction. If there is a less intensive response afferent and efferent arterioles are constricted to the same extent. This restricts blood flow out of the glomerulus as well as into it and GFR declines only slightly.

Tubular reabsorption and secretion

During the second stage of urine production, the filtrate is greatly modified as it moves along the tubule. Most reabsorption occurs in the proximal tubule where two-thirds of the filtrate is removed. Prior to this modification filtrate is similar in every way to plasma except it does not contain blood cells and large protein molecules. Figure 19.4 shows regional specialisation in reabsorption and secretion by the nephron.

Vital solutes such as glucose, amino acids and electrolytes are reabsorbed together with water. They pass from the lumen of the nephron across the epithelial layer into the peritubular

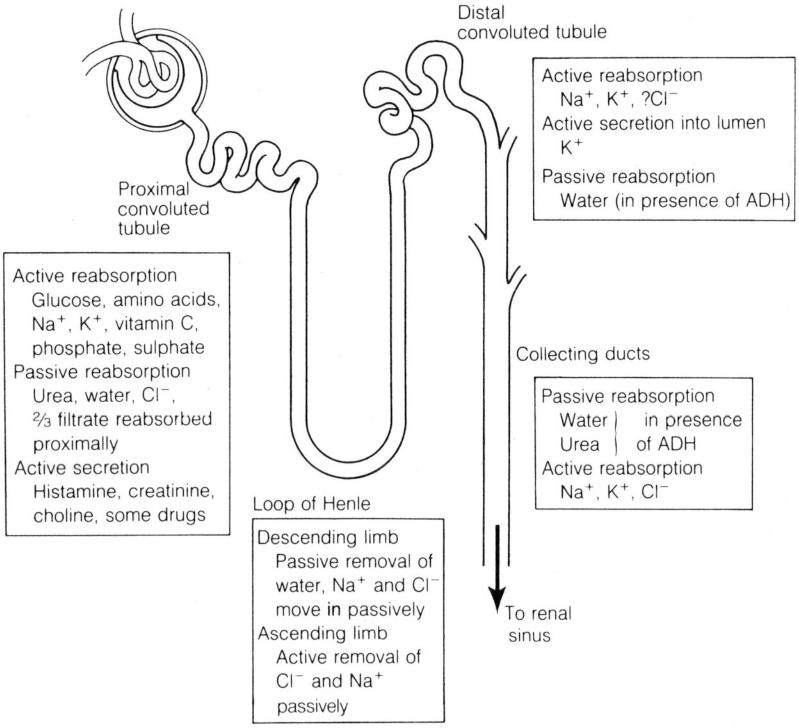

Figure 19.4 *Regional specialisation in reabsorption and secretion in the nephron. Throughout the nephron, exchange of Na^+ for H^+, HCO_3 reabsorption and NH_2 secretion occur (from Hinchliff SM, Montague SE, 1990, with permission).*

capillary network. A few substances are secreted into the filtrate from the peritubular capillaries. Mechanisms for the reabsorption from the nephron may be active or passive.

Transport mechanisms in the nephron

Active transfer

McClaren (1996) defines active transfer as 'the "uphill" movement of solutes against an unfavourable chemical or electrical gradient'. Solutes move from a low to a high chemical concentration or electrical potential. Energy in the form of adenosine triphosphate (ATP) is used. Sodium is actively transported bound to a carrier protein. About 80% of the energy is used in the transport of sodium ions. Substances actively reabsorbed include glucose, amino acids, lactate, vitamins and most ions. Many of these are cotransported bound to the sodium carrier complex (Marieb 1992). There is a transport maximum depending on the number of carriers available in the renal tubule. When the maximum is exceeded any surplus substance will be excreted in the urine. This is what happens in glycosuria.

Passive transfer

McClaren (1996) defines passive transfer as 'the movement of non-electrolytes and ions across cell membranes according to the chemical or electrical gradients that prevail'. Solutes could be said to move downhill from an area of high to low chemical concentration or electrical potential (see Chapter 2). No energy is directly used in passive transfer which includes diffusion, facilitated diffusion and osmosis.

Positively charged sodium ions are moved from the tubule to the peritubular capillaries and create an electrical gradient that favours the transfer of anions such as HCO_3^- and HCl^- so that electrical neutrality is restored in the plasma and filtrate. Sodium movement also establishes a strong osmotic gradient so that water moves from the lumen of the tubule into the peritubular capillaries. This movement of water out of the tubule increases the concentration of solutes in the filtrate and they begin to follow their concentration gradients out of the tubules. This movement of solutes after the solvent is called **solvent drag**.

Non-reabsorbed substances

Substances are not reabsorbed because:

- they lack carriers;
- they are not lipid soluble and cannot diffuse through cell membranes;
- they are too large to pass through the plasma membrane pores in the tubular cells.

These include the end products of protein and nucleic acid metabolism – urea, creatinine and uric acid. Urea is a small molecule and about 45% is reabsorbed but creatinine is not reabsorbed at all. It is therefore a useful substance to measure when assessing GFR and glomerular function.

Tubular secretion

Tubular secretion is an important mechanism in clearing the blood of unwanted substances. Urine is therefore composed of both filtered and secreted substances. Secreted substances include hydrogen ions, ammonia and drug metabolites. Also secreted into the tubules are drugs such as penicillin and undesirable substances that might have been reabsorbed such as urea or excess potassium ions.

Regulation of urine concentration and volume

The role of the kidney in maintaining fluid and electrolyte balance and regulating pH is discussed in detail in the following chapter. Briefly, an important function of the kidney is to keep the solute load of the body constant by regulating urine concentration and volume. This is accomplished by a function called the **countercurrent exchange**, which means that something flows in opposite directions through adjacent channels. In this case the loop of Henle and its adjacent blood vessels, the vasa recta, are involved.

The descending limb of the loop of Henle is quite impermeable to solutes and permeable to water. Water passes out of the filtrate into the interstitial fluid by osmosis along the course of the descending loop and the solute load becomes concentrated.

The ascending limb of the loop of Henle is impermeable to water and actively transports sodium into the surrounding interstitial fluid. The concentration of solutes in the filtrate as it enters the ascending limb is very high. Sodium is pumped out of the lumen into the interstitial fluid. The urine becomes more dilute and becomes hypotonic with respect to plasma.

The two loops are close enough to influence each other's activity. Water diffusing out of the descending limb produces the salty filtrate that the ascending limb uses to raise the osmolarity of the medullary interstitial fluid. The more salt the ascending limb extrudes, the saltier the filtrate in the descending limb becomes. This positive feedback mechanism is referred to as a **countercurrent multiplier**.

The collecting tubules add to the osmolality of the renal medulla by allowing urea to leak out into the interstitial space.

The vasa recta are freely permeable to both water and salt and provide another countercurrent exchange to regulate the content of the interstitial fluid whilst still maintaining the gradient established by the loop of Henle. Blood moving down the descending limb of the vasa recta gains solutes and loses water whilst in the ascending limb the blood loses solutes and gains water.

Formation of concentrated urine

Because water follows the osmotic gradients established by salt concentration, sodium and water balance are interrelated. Water balance is mainly regulated by antidiuretic hormone (ADH) from the posterior pituitary gland. The secretion of ADH is initiated by an increase in plasma osmolality, a decrease in circulating blood volume and a lowered blood pressure. If blood volume decreases volume receptors located in the right and left atria and in the thoracic vessels and baroreceptors in the aorta, pulmonary arteries and carotid sinus stimulate the release of ADH. The action of ADH is to increase the permeability of the renal tubular cells to water. Water absorption increases plasma volume and urine concentration is increased. This is called **facultative water reabsorption**. The amount of urine excreted is reduced and its concentration is increased.

The renin-angiotensin-aldosterone system

Sodium is regulated by aldosterone from the adrenal cortex. Sodium, along with its associated ions chloride and bicarbonate, regulates osmotic forces and therefore water balance. Sodium also works with potassium to maintain neurotransmission, regulates acid/base balance (via sodium bicarbonate) and participates in membrane reactions. The main anion in the ECF which neutralises the positive electrical charge of sodium is chloride. The transport of chloride is passive, following sodium, and concentrations of chloride vary inversely with concentrations of bicarbonate which competes for sodium binding.

Concentrations of sodium are maintained within a narrow range of 136–145 mEq/l primarily via renal tubular reabsorption. The average daily intake is 6 g but the need is only 500 mg. If sodium is taken in excess a combination of hormonal (aldosterone), neural and renal mechanisms work together via the renin-angiotensin system to control the balance (Fig. 19.5). Renin is produced by the juxtaglomerular apparatus in the kidney and stimulates production of the inactive blood peptide angiotensin I. This is converted into the active angiotensin II which acts as a hormone to stimulate the secretion of aldosterone and cause vasoconstriction.

Natriuretic hormone

The atria of the heart produce natriuretic hormone (ANH) which promotes urinary excretion of sodium by reducing tubular reabsorption. The excretion of sodium results in a diuresis. ANH is synthesised by the atrial myocytes and secreted into circulating blood by the coronary sinus. Increased right atrial pressure is the stimulus to hormone release. Increased circulating blood volume causes greater pressure on the atrial myocytes and the release of hormone seems to be directly related to the degree of mechanical load.

THE LOWER URINARY TRACT

The ureters

Anderson (1992) gives a good description of the lower urinary tract, taking into account the knowledge needed by those involved in caring for pregnant women. Much of the following information is based on her book. The two ureters are hollow muscular tubes. Urine secreted into the renal pelvis drains down through the ureters to be stored in the bladder. The muscle walls of the ureter undergo peristaltic movements to propel urine towards the bladder.

Structure

The walls of the ureters are composed of the following layers.

1 A lining layer of mucous membrane in longitudinal folds.
2 A fibrous tissue layer containing elastic fibres on which the epithelium rests.

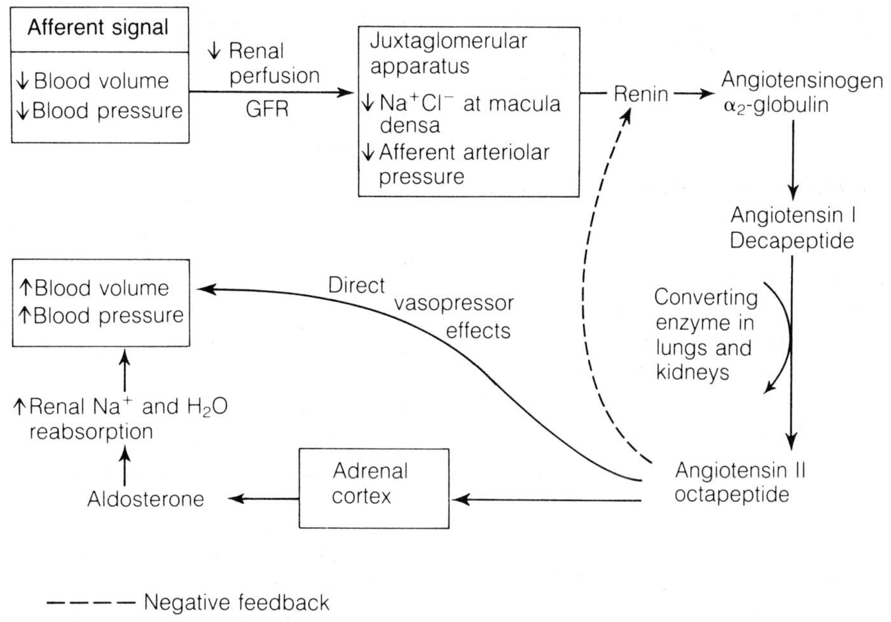

Figure 19.5 *The renin-aldosterone system (from Hinchliff SM, Montague SE, 1990, with permission).*

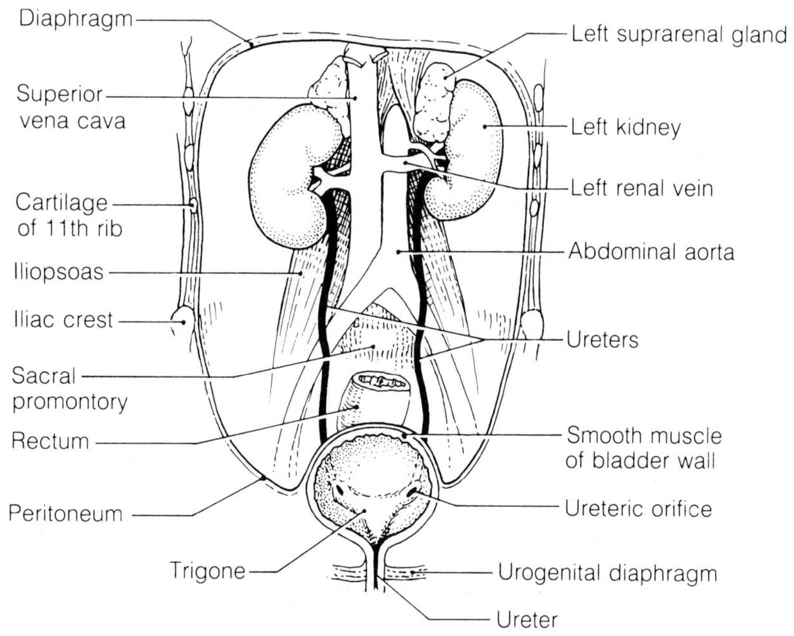

Figure 19.6 *Anatomy of the lower urinary tract (from Hinchliff SM, Montague SE, 1990, with permission).*

3 A smooth muscle layer consisting of three sets of fibres – a weak inner layer of longitudinal fibres, a middle layer of circular fibres and an outer well-defined longitudinal layer.
4 A coat of fibrous connective tissue.

Situation and size

The ureters lie outside and behind the peritoneum throughout their length. They extend from the renal pelvis to the posterior wall of the urinary bladder, crossing the pelvic brim anterior to the sacroiliac joints. The ureters run through the pelvic fascia and pass through special tunnels in the cardinal ligaments. They enter the posterior bladder wall in front of the cervix and run at an oblique angle for about 20 mm which prevents the back flow of urine. They open into the cavity of the bladder at the posterior lateral angles of the trigone. In an adult the ureter is about 30 cm long and 3 mm in diameter.

Blood supply, lymphatic drainage and nerve supply

Blood supply is from the common iliac, internal iliac, uterine and vesical arteries and drainage is by corresponding veins.

Lymphatic drainage is to the internal, external and common iliac nodes.

The nerve supply is via aortic, renal and hypogastric plexi.

The bladder

The bladder is a hollow, distensible muscular organ acting as a reservoir for the storage of urine. It is roughly pyramidal in shape when empty and lies in the pelvis when empty. It has a posterior base or **trigone** resting on the vagina and an anterior apex. The normal capacity of the full bladder is 500 ml. It then becomes globular and expands upwards and forwards into the abdomen.

The trigone of the bladder is triangular in shape and each of its sides measures 2.5 cm. The two ureteric orifices are situated on either side of the base of the triangle and the apex is formed by the internal meatus of the urethra. This region may be called the **bladder neck**.

Structure

The bladder walls are formed of the following structures.

1 A lining of transitional epithelium resting on a layer of **areolar tissue**. The lining, except for the trigone, is thrown into folds or **rugae** to allow it to distend. Over the trigone the epithelium is firmly bound to the muscle.
2 Three coats of smooth muscle, inner longitudinal, middle circular and outer longitudinal, called the **detrusor muscle**. This contracts to expel urine during micturition. Around the internal meatus the circular muscle is thickened to form the **internal sphincter** of the bladder which is in a state of sustained contraction except during micturition. In the trigone is a special arrangement of fibres which run between the ureteric openings, forming a band known as the **interureteric ridge**. The muscle fibres running from each ureteric opening to the urethral orifice are also raised into ridges.
3 The upper surface of the bladder is covered by peritoneum reflected off the uterus to form the **uterovesical pouch**. Its remaining surfaces are covered by visceral pelvic fascia.

Ligaments

There are five ligaments attached to the bladder.

- A fibrous band called the **urachus** runs from the apex of the bladder to the umbilicus.
- Two **lateral ligaments** pass from the bladder to the side walls of the pelvis.
- Two **pubovesical ligaments** attach the bladder neck anteriorly to the pubic bones. They form part of the pubocervical ligaments of the uterus.

Relations

- Anterior – the pubic bones are separated from the bladder by a space filled with fatty tissue called the cave of Retzius
- Posterior – the cervix and ureters
- Lateral – the lateral ligaments of the bladder and the side walls of the pelvis
- Superior – the body of the uterus and the intestines lying in the uterovesical pouch
- Inferior – the upper half of the anterior vaginal wall and the levator ani muscles.

Blood supply, lymphatic drainage and nerve supply

Blood supply is from the superior and inferior vesical arteries and drainage is by corresponding veins.

Lymphatic drainage is to the external iliac and obturator nodes.

The nerve supply is via sympathetic and parasympathetic fibres of the autonomic system.

The urethra

In the female the urethra is a narrow tube about 4 cm long passing from the internal meatus of the bladder to the vestibule where it opens externally. It runs embedded in the lower half of the anterior vaginal wall The internal sphincter surrounds it as it leaves the bladder. As it passes between the levator ani muscles it is enclosed by bands of striated muscle known as the **membranous sphincter** of the urethra which is under voluntary control.

Structure

The walls of the urethra consist of the following layers.

1 The lumen is lined by transitional epithelium in the upper half and squamous epithelium in the lower half thrown into small longitudinal folds. It is normally closed.
2 A layer of vascular connective tissue.
3 An inner longitudinal layer of smooth muscle.
4 An outer circular layer of smooth muscle.

Several small crypts open into the urethra at its lowest point. The two largest are **Skene's ducts** and correspond to the prostate gland in the male.

Blood supply, lymphatic drainage and nerve supply

Blood supply is from the inferior vesical and pudendal arteries and drainage is by corresponding veins.

Lymphatic drainage is to the internal iliac nodes.

The nerve supply to the internal sphincter is from the sympathetic system and the voluntary control of the membranous sphincter is achieved via sympathetic and parasympathetic fibres of the autonomic system.

The physiology of micturition

Micturition requires the coordination of autonomic and somatic nerves. Motor and sensory sympathetic and parasympathetic nerves pass to and from the bladder but the sympathetic fibres appear to play a minor role. When the bladder contains about 300 ml of urine stretch receptors are stimulated and sensory parasympathetic nerves convey sensations of fullness to the basal ganglia, reticular formation and cortical centres of the brain. The need to pass urine is perceived but can be voluntarily postponed until a suitable time. There is a centre for the reflex control of micturition in the 2nd to 4th sacral segments of the spinal cord. When the bladder contains 700 ml it may become impossible to avoid micturition.

Nerve impulses from the cerebral cortex increase parasympathetic activity and decrease sympathetic activity causing relaxation of the internal sphincter and contraction of the detrusor muscle. The external sphincter is relaxed, intra-abdominal pressure is raised and expulsion of urine occurs. Cortical control of micturition is learned in infancy and usually achieved at about 2 years of age.

MATERNAL ADAPTATIONS TO PREGNANCY

During pregnancy the renal system undergoes both structural and functional changes. Many of the structural changes are still present well into the postpartum period. Baylis & Davison (1991) stress that it is important to understand these changes in order to be aware of the possible effects of pregnancy on women with renal disease or hypertension or following renal transplant.

The main changes of pregnancy are sodium retention and increased extracellular volume. Parameters used to assess normal renal function become altered and alterations in renal function may be difficult to assess.

The antenatal period

Besides dealing with the increased intravascular and extracellular volume and metabolic waste products, the maternal kidneys must act as the 'primary excretory organ for fetal wastes' (Blackburn & Loper 1992). As in many of the physiological adaptations made by the woman's body during pregnancy, renal changes are related to the effects of progesterone on smooth muscle, pressure from the enlarging uterus and cardiovascular alterations such as increased cardiac output and increased blood volume.

Table 19.1 *Changes in the renal tract in pregnancy*

Organ	*Change*
Renal calyces, pelvis, ureters	Dilatation, elongation, increased muscle tone, decreased peristalsis
Bladder	Mucosa oedematous and hyperaemic, incompetence of vesico-ureteric sphincter, late pregnancy displacement
Renal blood flow	Increases 35–60%
Glomerular filtration rate	Increases 40–50%
Tubular function	Increased reabsorption of solutes Increased excretion of glucose, protein, amino acids, urea, uric acid, water-soluble vitamins, calcium, hydrogen ions, phosphorus Retention of sodium and water
Renin-angiotensin-aldosterone system	Increase in all components Resistance to pressor effects of angiotensin II

Structural changes – the kidneys and ureters

Kidney size

Kidney length increases by 1.5 cm mainly because of increased blood flow and vascular volume and also enlargement of the interstitial space. There is an increase in glomerular size but not in the number of cells and the microscopic structure of the kidney is the same in the pregnant and non-pregnant woman (Fig. 19.7).

Changes in the ureters

The most striking change is dilatation of the renal pelvis and ureters but there are also alterations in haemodynamics, glomerular filtration and tubular performance. The dilatation of

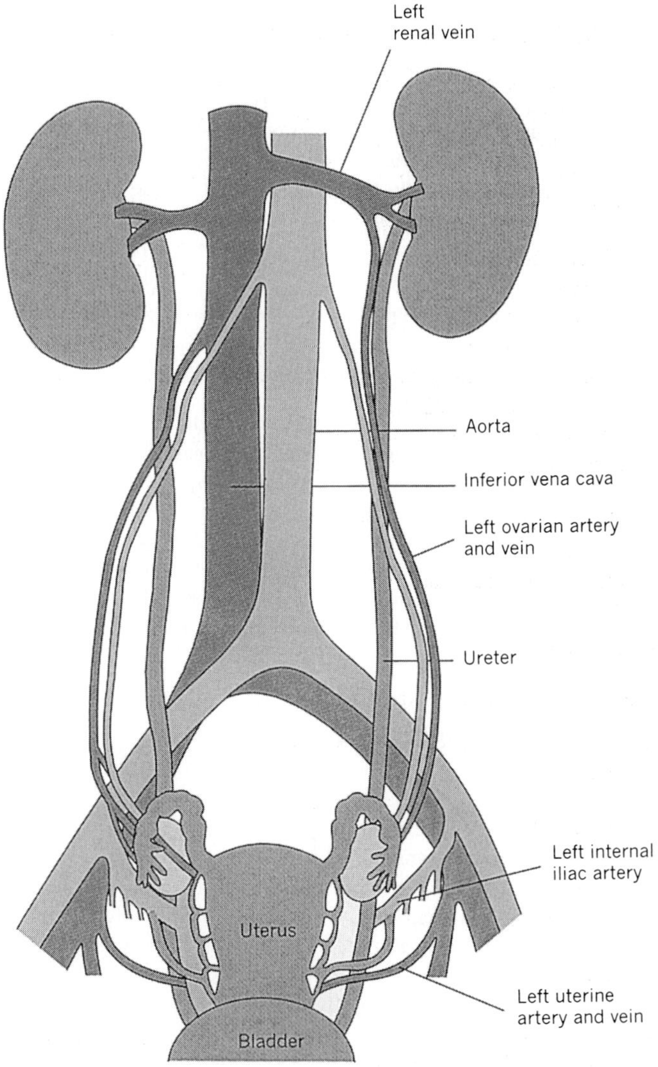

Figure 19.7 *Obstruction of the right ureter at the pelvic brim by an enlarged ovarian vein. Note that the ovarian vein enters the vena cava by several trunks and that the pelvic portion of the ureter is normal (from Hinchliff SM, Montague SE, 1990, with permission).*

the renal calyces, pelvis and ureters begins in the first trimester but becomes more prominent after 20 weeks. The changes can be referred to as physiological hydroureter and hydronephrosis (Blackburn & Loper 1992) and are mainly seen in the portion of the ureters above the pelvic brim.

The portion of the ureters below the pelvic brim does not usually enlarge. This may be because the connective tissue surrounding the ureters hypertrophies and prevents the hormonally induced dilatation. The diameter of the lumen of the ureter increases and there is hypertrophy of the smooth muscle of the ureters and an increase in muscle tone. There is no decrease in peristalsis (Marchant 1978). The ureters elongate and become more tortuous in the latter half of pregnancy and are also displaced laterally by the growing uterus. The ureters may hold up to 25 times more urine and contain as much as 300 ml. The changes greatly increase the risk of urinary tract infection.

Physiological hydroureter

The cause of physiological hydroureter is not understood but the main factor may be the external compression of the ureters against the pelvic brim by the growing uterus. Growing blood vessels such as the iliac arteries and venous plexi may also add to the compression effect. Dilatation is more prominent in primigravidae where the firmer abdominal wall does not permit the uterus to expand anteriorly. In 85% of women the right ureter is dilated more than the left, possibly because of dextrorotation of the growing uterus due to the presence of the sigmoid colon in the left quadrant of the pelvis. The increased flow of urine in pregnancy may result in a small amount of dilatation.

Structural changes – the bladder

Bladder capacity doubles by term to 1000 ml. Oestrogenic influences cause the trigone to become hyperplastic with muscle hypertrophy. The bladder mucosa becomes hyperaemic with an increase in size and tortuosity of blood vessels. The mucosa also becomes oedematous and is thus more vulnerable to trauma and infection. The decrease in bladder tone leads to incompetence of the vesicoureteric sphincters and there may be reflux of urine. This may be increased by the displacement of the bladder and of the terminal ureters.

Changes in renal physiology

Blood flow

It has been known since a paper by Bucht (1951) that there is a significant increase in renal blood flow of 35–60% by the end of the first trimester which then decreases slightly until the end of pregnancy. This is due to the increased blood volume and cardiac output as well as the decreased renal vascular resistance brought about by the relaxing effects of progesterone. There is vasodilation of the afferent and efferent glomerular capillaries.

Glomerular filtration

GFR increases 40–50% in pregnancy and the rise begins soon after conception and peaks at 9–16 weeks before stabilising. Values for GFR may reach more than 150 ml/min. The volume of urine produced in 24 h is 25% higher during pregnancy. A greater proportion of renal blood flow is filtered and this increases the excretion of glucose, protein, amino acids, water-soluble vitamins and hydrogen ions.

No single cause has been identified for the GFR increase in pregnancy but it is related to the increased renal blood flow. The decreased plasma oncotic pressure caused by the reduced concentration of plasma proteins due to haemodilution also increases GFR and there is involvement of hormones. Prolactin release from the pituitary gland has been found to induce changes in GFR in rats and is probably implicated in the human response to pregnancy. Prostaglandins may cause the renal vasodilation of pregnancy. Alterations in the renin-angiotensin-aldosterone system and in the role of antidiuretic hormone (Chapter 20) accommodate the increase in blood plasma volume and thus add to renal blood flow.

Tubular function

Glucose

The rise in GFR increases the amount of fluid and solutes present within the tubules by 50–100% so tubular reabsorption must increase to prevent the loss of sodium, chloride, glucose, potassium and water. However, tubular reabsorption rate and clearance may not accommodate the extra load and substances such as glucose and amino acids are excreted. Urinary glucose values may rise as much as 10-fold during pregnancy. There is a reduced ability of the tubules to reabsorb glucose in proportion to the amount in the filtrate (**fractional reabsorption**), possibly due to the changes in pregnancy steroid hormones (Baylis & Davison 1991) and glycosuria is a common occurrence in pregnancy. This is likely to be due to the increased plasma levels of oestrogen and progesterone and a similar effect is seen in some women taking the oral contraceptive pill.

Amino acids

Proteinuria is also more common during pregnancy with the extra excretion of amino acids. A value of 1+ on a protein dipstick is not abnormal and protein excretion of up to 300 mg/24 h can be accepted. Protein excretion does not correlate with the severity of renal disease and may not indicate progressive worsening of the disease. However, proteinuria associated with hypertension is serious and associated with increased risk to the woman and her fetus.

The postnatal period

During the postnatal period there is a rapid and sustained loss of sodium and a diuresis, especially on days 2–5. A normal urine output for a delivered woman may be up to 3000 ml with an individual voiding of 500–1000 ml at any one micturition. By the end of the first week urinary excretion of calcium, phosphate, vitamins, glucose and other solutes returns to normal but it may take up to 3 weeks to achieve normal fluid and electrolyte balance. Structural changes as described above may take up to 3 months to disappear although the structures will return to normal in 6–8 weeks in most women. It is important to remember this when women who have had renal problems in pregnancy are assessed following delivery.

Summary of main points

- The kidneys play a major role in maintenance of internal homeostasis by their regulation of the volume and composition of the body fluids. Kidneys regulate the volume and chemical make-up of the blood, maintain balance between water and electrolytes and produce renin and erythropoietin.
- The kidneys are situated on either side of the vertebral column at the level of the 12th thoracic to the 3rd lumbar vertebrae behind the peritoneum and are attached to the posterior abdominal wall by adipose tissue. They are surrounded by three layers of supporting tissue: the renal capsule, the adipose capsule and the renal fascia outermost. Beneath the capsule lie three distinct regions: the outer cortex, the medulla and the inner renal pelvis.
- Each kidney contains over 1 million nephrons. A nephron consists of a tuft of blood vessel capillaries called the glomerulus associated with a renal tubule. About 85% of the nephrons are cortical nephrons, situated in the cortex except where their loops of Henle dip into the medulla.
- The remaining 15% of nephrons are the juxtaglomerular nephrons. The juxtaglomerular apparatus is a region found in each nephron where the distal convoluted tubule lies against the afferent arteriole as it supplies the glomerulus.
- Every nephron is closely associated with two capillary beds which form the microvasculature of the nephron. These are the glomerulus and the peritubular capillary bed. About 25% of cardiac output is delivered to the kidneys each minute. This is a higher blood supply than any other tissue.
- The kidneys have a rich supply of sympathetic fibres and a few parasympathetic fibres supplying the smooth muscle of the arterioles and the juxtaglomerular apparatus. Stimulation of these nerves causes vasoconstriction, reduced renal blood flow and glomerular filtration rate and the release of renin from the juxtaglomerular apparatus. The kidneys also have some sensory nerve fibres which allow the sensation of pain to be perceived.
- In an adult about 180 litres of plasma are filtered every day and 99% of the filtrate is reabsorbed by the nephrons. This results in the production of about 1.5 litres of urine per day. Glomerular filtration is the first step in urine production.
- Electrolytes are electrically charged solutes which dissociate into their constituent ions when placed in solution. Electrolytes are polarised into cations and anions.
- Diffusion is the movement of a solute molecule across a permeable membrane to a weaker solution down a concentration gradient. Hydrostatic pressure is the mechanical force of water pushing against cell membranes. Osmosis is the movement of water down a concentration gradient across a semipermeable membrane from a high water content to a lower one. Osmolality is the concentration of molecules per weight of water in milliosmoles/kilogram. Osmolarity is the concentration of molecules/litre of water. Tonicity is the effective osmolality of a solution. Oncotic pressure (colloid osmotic pressure) is the overall osmotic effect of the plasma proteins.
- Hydrogen ion concentration or pH is the negative logarithm of hydrogen ions in solution on a scale of 1–14. From one pH unit to the next there is a 10-fold change in hydrogen ion concentration.
- Filtration is a passive, non-selective process in which fluids and solutes are forced through a membrane by hydrostatic pressure. The glomerular filtration rate is the volume of plasma filtered through the glomeruli in one minute and is normally 120 ml/min. The presence of the plasma proteins in the capillary provides the colloid osmotic pressure of the glomerular blood, limiting the loss of water to one-fifth of the plasma fluid into the tubules.
- The kidney can control its own blood supply over a wide range of arterial blood pressure. This intrinsic autoregulation system depends on alterations in the diameter of the afferent and efferent arterioles in response to a systemic blood pressure change.
- Extrinsic control is by sympathetic nervous system stimulation. When the body is stressed adrenaline is released into the blood from the adrenal medulla. This causes strong constriction of the afferent arterioles and inhibits filtrate formation.
- During the second stage of urine production the filtrate is greatly modified as it moves along the tubule. Most reabsorption occurs in the proximal tubule where two-thirds of the filtrate is removed. Vital solutes such as glucose, amino acids and electrolytes are reabsorbed together with water. They pass from the lumen of the nephron into the peritubular capillary network.
- Transport across the nephron may be active or passive. Substances are not reabsorbed because they lack carriers, they are not lipid soluble and cannot diffuse through cell membranes or they are too large to pass through the plasma membrane pores in the tubular cells. These include the end products of protein and nucleic acid metabolism.
- Tubular secretion is an important mechanism in clearing the blood of unwanted substances. Urine is therefore composed of both filtered and secreted substances. Secreted substances include hydrogen ions, ammonia and drug metabolites. The solute load of the body is kept constant by regulating urine concentration and volume.
- Because water follows the osmotic gradients established by salt concentration, sodium and water balance are interrelated. Water balance is mainly regulated by antidiuretic hormone. Sodium is regulated by aldosterone from the adrenal cortex. Sodium, along with its associated ions chloride and bicarbonate, regulates osmotic forces and therefore water balance. Concentrations of sodium are maintained within a narrow range primarily via renal tubular reabsorption. The atria of the heart produce natriuretic hormone (ANH) which promotes urinary excretion of sodium by reducing tubular reabsorption.
- Renin is produced by the juxtaglomerular apparatus in the kidney and stimulates production of the inactive blood peptide angiotensin I. This is converted into the active angiotensin II which acts as a hormone to stimulate the secretion of aldosterone and cause vasoconstriction.
- The two ureters are hollow muscular tubes. Urine secreted into the renal pelvis drains down through the ureters to be stored in the bladder. The muscle walls of the ureter undergo peristaltic movements to propel urine towards the bladder.
- The bladder is a hollow, distensible muscular organ acting as a reservoir for the storage of urine. It is roughly pyramidal in shape when empty and lies in the pelvis. It has a posterior base or trigone resting on the vagina and an anterior apex. The normal capacity of the full bladder is 500 ml. It then becomes globular and expands upwards and forwards into the abdomen.
- The trigone of the bladder is triangular in shape and each of its sides measures 2.5 cm. The two ureteric orifices are situated on either side of the base of the triangle and the apex is formed by the internal meatus of the urethra. This region may be called the bladder neck.
- In the female the urethra is a narrow tube about 4 cm long passing from the internal meatus of the bladder to the vestibule where it opens externally. It runs embedded in the lower half of the anterior vaginal wall. The internal sphincter surrounds it as it leaves the bladder. As it passes between the levator ani muscles it is enclosed by bands of striated muscle known as the membranous sphincter of the urethra which is under voluntary control.
- Micturition requires the coordination of autonomic and somatic nerves. Motor and sensory sympathetic and parasympathetic nerves pass to and from the bladder but the sympathetic fibres appear to play a minor role.

- During pregnancy the renal system undergoes structural and functional changes. Many of the structural changes are still present well into the postpartum period. The main functional changes are sodium retention and increased extracellular volume. Parameters used to assess normal renal function become altered and alterations in renal function may be difficult to assess.
- Kidney length increases by 1.5 cm because of increased blood flow and vascular volume and also enlargement of the interstitial space. There is an increase in glomerular size but not in the number of cells and the microscopic structure of the kidney does not change. There is dilatation of the renal pelvis and ureters but also alterations in haemodynamics, glomerular filtration and tubular performance. This begins in the first trimester but becomes more prominent after 20 weeks.
- The portion of the ureters below the pelvic brim does not usually enlarge. This may be because the connective tissue surrounding the ureters hypertrophies and prevents the hormonally induced dilatation. The diameter of the lumen of the ureter increases and there is hypertrophy of the smooth muscle of the ureters and an increase in muscle tone.
- The ureters elongate and become more tortuous in the latter half of pregnancy and are also displaced laterally by the growing uterus. The ureters may hold up to 25 times more urine and contain as much as 300 ml. The changes greatly increase the risk of urinary tract infection. The cause of physiological hydroureter is not understood but the main factor may be the external compression of the ureters against the pelvic brim by the growing uterus.
- Bladder capacity doubles by term to 1000 ml. Oestrogenic influences cause the trigone to become hyperplastic with muscle hypertrophy. The bladder mucosa becomes hyperaemic with an increase in size and tortuosity of blood vessels. The mucosa also becomes oedematous and is thus more vulnerable to trauma and infection.
- Renal blood flow increases by up to 60% by the end of the first trimester and then decreases slightly until the end of pregnancy. This is due to the increased blood volume and cardiac output as well as the decreased renal vascular resistance brought about by the relaxing effects of progesterone. GFR increases 50% in pregnancy, the rise beginning soon after conception and peaking at 9–16 weeks.
- Urinary glucose values may rise as much as 10-fold during pregnancy. There is reduced ability of the tubules to reabsorb glucose in proportion to the amount in the filtrate (fractional reabsorption) and glycosuria is a common occurrence in pregnancy.
- Proteinuria is also more common during pregnancy with the extra excretion of amino acids. Protein excretion does not correlate with the severity of renal disease and may not indicate progressive worsening of the disease. Proteinuria associated with hypertension is serious.
- During the postnatal period there is a rapid and sustained loss of sodium and a diuresis, especially on days 2–5. By the end of the first week urinary excretion of calcium, phosphate, vitamins, glucose and other solutes returns to normal but it may take up to 3 weeks to achieve normal fluid and electrolyte balance.
- Structural changes may take up to 3 months to disappear although the structures will return to normal in 6–8 weeks in most women. It is important to remember this when women who have had renal problems in pregnancy are assessed following delivery.

References

Anderson M. 1992 The Anatomy and Physiology of Obstetrics. Wolfe Publishing, London.

Baylis C, Davison J. 1991 The urinary system. In Hytten F, Chamberlain G (eds) Clinical Physiology in Obstetrics. Blackwell Scientific, Oxford, pp 245–302.

Blackburn ST, Loper DL. 1992 Maternal Fetal and Neonatal Physiology, A Clinical Perspective. WB Saunders, Philadelphia, pp 336–378.

Bucht H. 1951 Studies on renal function in man with special reference to glomerular filtration and renal plasma flow in pregnancy. Scandinavian Journal of Clinical and Laboratory Investigation, supplement 1.

Creager JG. 1983 Human Anatomy and Physiology. Wadsworth, Belmont, California.

Hinchliff SM, Montague SE. 1990 Physiology for Nursing Practice. Baillière Tindall, London.

Hinchliff SM, Montague SE, Watson R. 1996 Physiology for Nursing Practice. Baillière Tindall, London.

Marchant DJ. 1978 Alterations in anatomy and function of the urinary tract during pregnancy. Clinical Obstetrics and Gynaecology 21, 855.

Marieb EN. 1992 Human Anatomy and Physiology, 2nd edn. Benjamin/Cummings Publishing, California.

McClaren SM. 1996 Renal function. In Hinchliff SM, Montague SE, Watson R (eds) Physiology for Nursing Practice. Baillière Tindall, London, pp 582–617.

Recommended reading

Baylis C, Davison J. 1991 The urinary system. In Hytten F, Chamberlain G (eds) Clinical Physiology in Obstetrics. Blackwell Scientific, Oxford, pp 245–302.

Marchant DJ. 1978 Alterations in anatomy and function of the urinary tract during pregnancy. Clinical Obstetrics and Gynaecology 21, 855.

McClaren SM. 1996 Renal function. In Hinchliff SM, Montague SE, Watson R (eds). Physiology for Nursing Practice. Baillière Tindall, London, pp 582–617.

Chapter

20 Fluid, electrolyte and acid/base balance

In this chapter

INTRODUCTION

It is very important to understand that cell function depends on the maintenance of a stable environment. It is essential that the fluid and electrolyte, acid and base balances of the extracellular fluids are kept within a narrow range. For instance, changes in the composition of electrolytes can affect the electrical potentials of neurones and can move fluid from one compartment to another. Changes in pH can disrupt cellular enzyme systems. Cells also depend on a continuous supply of nutrients and the removal of metabolic wastes. Various organs are involved in coordinating this fluid balance and therefore this chapter will step outside individual systems and examine the integration of systems in the control of this extremely important aspect of life. The reader may wish to re-read Chapter 1, Basic Biochemistry, before proceeding.

FLUID AND ELECTROLYTES

Body water content

In an adult, water accounts for about 50% of the body mass although this ratio can vary depending on the age, sex and weight of individuals. Infants contain more water than older children because of their lower bone mass and body fat. Men contain more water than women because of the extra amount of adipose tissue and lower muscle mass of most women. Body fat leads to a reduction in water content as fat is the least hydrated of all body tissues so that obese people contain less water proportionate to their body weight. Older people have less water as their fat content is increased and their muscle content decreased. Also, as the kidney ages it is less able to concentrate urine so that more fluid is lost in urine. Other losses of body fluid can therefore be life threatening in the elderly.

Fluid compartments

There are three main compartments of the body where water can be found (Fig. 20.1). These are **intracellular fluid** (ICF), the fluid inside the cells, and extracellular fluid (ECF) which can be divided into **interstitial fluid**, the fluid between the cells, and **plasma**, the fluid inside the vascular system. Special types of ECF separate from interstitial fluid and plasma are lymph, transcellular fluid (secreted by cells), synovial, intestinal, cerebrospinal, sweat, urine, pleural, peritoneal, pericardial and introcular fluid. These are so similar in composition to ECF that they are usually considered part of it. The sum of all of the above is the **total body water** (TBW).

Composition of body fluids

Solutes: Electrolytes and non-electrolytes

Water is the universal solvent and contains a variety of solutes. Broadly speaking, these can be divided into electrolytes and non-electrolytes. The **non-electrolytes** have bonds that prevent them dissociating into their component particles in solution and therefore do not carry electrical charges. These are mainly organic molecules such as glucose, lipids, creatinine and urea. **Electrolytes** are chemical compounds that do dissociate into ions in water. They are said to **ionise** and are charged particles capable of conducting an electric current. Electrolytes include inorganic salts, both inorganic and organic acids and bases and some proteins.

All dissolved solutes contribute to the osmotic activity of a fluid but electrolytes have the greatest osmotic power because each molecule can dissociate into at least two ions. An example is sodium chloride (NaCl):

$$NaCl \rightarrow Na^{+} + Cl^{-} \quad (1)$$

Because water moves along osmotic gradients from areas of lesser osmolality to greater osmolality, electrolytes have the greatest ability to cause fluid shifts.

Differences in composition between intracellular and extracellular fluids

Each fluid compartment has its own pattern of electrolytes. Except for the high protein content of plasma, all extracellular compartments have a similar composition. Sodium is the most abundant ECF cation and chloride the anion. In the ICF potassium is the most abundant cation and phosphate (HPO_4^{2-}) its major anion. The concentrations of sodium in ECF and potassium in ICF balance, which reflects the activity of the **sodium pump** (see Chapter 2).

Movement of fluid between compartments

Water movement between plasma and interstitial fluid

The distribution of water and the movement of nutrients and waste products between the plasma in the capillary and the interstitial space occur because of changes in hydrostatic pressure and osmotic forces between the arterial and venous ends of the capillary network. The capillary membrane is semipermeable and allows interchange of fluids and solutes between the intravascular and interstitial fluid compartments.

The movement of fluid back and forth across the capillary wall is called **net filtration** (Starling's hypothesis). The major forces of filtration are within the capillary. Net filtration is the balance between forces favouring filtration, such as capillary hydrostatic pressure (blood pressure) and interstitial oncotic pressure, and forces opposing filtration, such as plasma oncotic pressure. As the plasma flows from the arterial to the venous end of the capillary, blood pressure falls, reducing the hydrostatic pressure. Oncotic pressure remains constant. At the arterial end of the capillary hydrostatic pressure exceeds oncotic pressure and fluid is forced out into the interstitial space. At the venous end of the capillary oncotic pressure exceeds hydrostatic pressure and fluid is drawn back into the capillary.

Water movement between ICF and ECF

This water movement between compartments is a function of osmosis. Water moves freely across cell membranes so that the osmolality of TBW is normally at equilibrium. The ICF balance is maintained by active transport of ions out of the cell and interstitial hydrostatic pressure. However, normally the interstitial forces are negligible because only a very small amount of plasma proteins cross the capillary membrane so that the major

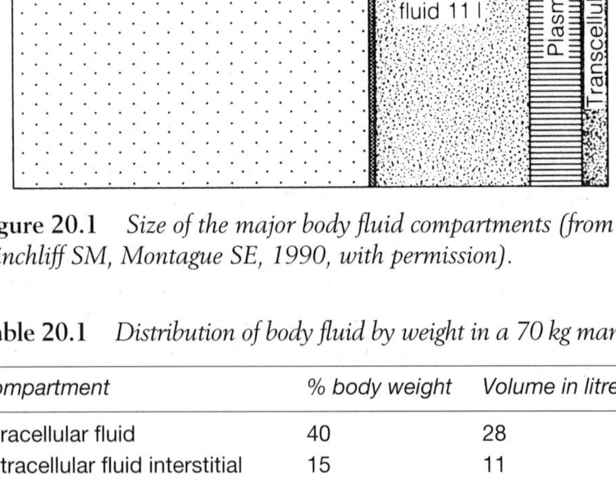

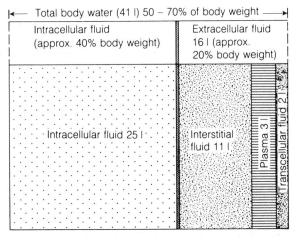

Figure 20.1 *Size of the major body fluid compartments (from Hinchliff SM, Montague SE, 1990, with permission).*

Table 20.1 *Distribution of body fluid by weight in a 70 kg man*

Compartment	% body weight	Volume in litres
Intracellular fluid	40	28
Extracellular fluid interstitial	15	11
Extracellular fluid intravascular	5	3
Total body water	60	42

Table 20.2 *Normal daily water losses and gains*

Intake	*Amount*	*Output*	*Amout (ml)*
Drinking	1400–1800	Urine	1400–1800
Water in food	700–1000	Faeces	100
Water of oxidation	300–400	Skin	300–500
		Lungs	600–800
Total	2400–3200		2400–3200

forces of filtration are within the capillary. Movements of respiratory gases, nutrients and wastes are unidirectional.

Water balance

Water intake must balance water loss and Table 20.2 demonstrates normal functions in an adult.

Regulation of water intake

Regulation of water intake is by the mechanism of thirst but it is poorly understood. A thirst centre in the hypothalamus responds to either a drop in plasma volume or an increase in plasma osmolarity. It is probable that the salivary glands, which obtain their fluid from the blood, produce less saliva and the resulting dry mouth makes us drink. Thirst is quenched as soon as we have taken on board the right amount of water, even before there has been time for it to affect blood volume.

Regulation of water output

Water is lost from the body in ways that cannot be avoided. These are the **obligatory water losses** and explain why we cannot survive long without drinking. They include the insensible loss of water from the lungs and via the skin. Because of the large amount of perspiration lost daily, especially in a hot climate, humans are of necessity a riverine species. That is to say that before the advent of piped water, most settlements were next to a river. Water in faeces must be added to the loss. There is an absolute minimum of 500 ml of urine per 24 hours that the kidneys must excrete even when the urine is concentrated to its maximum level possible.

Disorders of water balance

Oedema

Oedema is the accumulation of fluid within the interstitial space. It is a problem of fluid distribution and does not necessarily indicate excess intake. If fluid becomes sequestered (locked into) in a compartment oedema may be accompanied by signs of dehydration. It may be caused by factors that increase fluid flow out of the plasma or hinder its return. There are four major contributors to oedema.

- **Increased capillary hydrostatic pressure** may occur from venous obstruction such as in thrombophlebitis, hepatic obstruction, tight clothing or prolonged standing.
- **Reduced plasma oncotic pressure** follows the loss of plasma proteins found in renal failure, diminished production of plasma proteins found in liver disease or protein malnutrition.
- **Increased capillary membrane permeability** is usually associated with inflammatory or immune reactions. Burns, crush injuries, cancer and allergy also produce this effect.
- If the **lymphatic system is blocked** by infection or inflammation or lymphatic cancer or has had to be surgically removed in areas to prevent the spread of cancer, proteins and fluids accumulate in the interstitial spaces causing localised lymphoedema.

Clinical manifestations

Oedema may be generalised or localised. It is associated with weight gain, swelling of the tissues and puffiness. Clothing may feel tight. Movement may be limited and blood flow may be restricted. Wounds tend to heal more slowly and the risk of pressure sores and wound infections is increased. The sequestered fluid is not available for metabolic processes and dehydration may occur, for instance following burns. Hypovolaemic shock may occur. Treatment is tailored to fit the individual case and could include elevation of affected limbs, support stockings, avoiding prolonged standing, reducing salt intake and the prescribing of diuretics.

Electrolyte balance

Electrolytes include salts, acids and bases. Salts are the main electrolytes and are involved in many physiological processes. The four main electrolytes are sodium, potassium, calcium and magnesium. Salts are obtained from the food we eat and also, to a lesser extent, in our drinking water. Small amounts of salts may be released during metabolism. An example would be the release of phosphate during the breakdown of nucleic acids.

A major problem for humans is the love of salty food. This may be an acquired taste but could equally be an innate factor because of the need to replenish salts lost in perspiration. Salts are lost from the body in faeces and urine as well as in perspiration, as mentioned above. If we are depleted of salt our perspiration will be more dilute but even so, in hot weather a good deal of salt can be lost.

The role of sodium in fluid and electrolyte balance

Salts containing sodium account for at least 90% of solutes in the ECF. Regulating the balance between sodium intake and output is a major function of the kidneys. Sodium is the most abundant cation in the ECF and is the main cause of osmotic pressure. Sodium does not cross cell membranes very easily (Chapter 2) and therefore it is ideal for controlling the ECF volume and water distribution in the body. Water follows salt so that a change in sodium content will be followed by a change in water content of a fluid compartment. Blood volume and blood pressure are linked to sodium balance and there is a hormonal regulatory effect by the hormone aldosterone discussed more fully in Chapter 17.

Aldosterone

Aldosterone is produced by the cortical cells of the adrenal gland and its release is mediated by the production of renin by the juxtaglomerular apparatus of the kidney, as explained in the previous chapter. The renin-angiotensin-aldosterone system is discussed fully in Chapter 19. Briefly, renin catalyses a series of reactions leading to the activation of angiotensin II which causes aldosterone release. Normally, without the influence of aldosterone about 75% of the sodium in the renal filtrate is reabsorbed in the proximal tubules of the nephrons of the kidneys.

If aldosterone levels are high, most of the remaining sodium is reabsorbed in the distal tubules and collecting ducts. If the permeability of the tubules has been increased by antidiuretic hormone (ADH, also known as arginine vasopressin or AVP) water will passively follow the sodium. There will be sodium and water retention. When aldosterone release is inhibited, there will be little reabsorption of sodium beyond the proximal tubules. Urinary excretion of large amounts of sodium will always result in the excretion of large amounts of water. The effect of aldosterone is to allow large amounts of sodium free water to be excreted in times of sodium depletion. Like all hormones, aldosterone has a slow effect, taking hours or days to alter fluid compartments.

Other influences on fluid and electrolyte balance discussed in other chapters are the cardiovascular system baroreceptors, the regulation of ADH and the influence of atrial natriuretic factor. Oestrogens and glucocorticoids also play a part in enhancing tubular reabsorption of sodium.

Regulation of potassium balance

Potassium (K^+) is the main cation in ICF and is necessary for normal neuromuscular functioning and other processes such as protein synthesis. Potassium is quite toxic, especially to heart muscle. Both hyperkalaemia (excess potassium) and hypokalaemia (potassium depletion) can cause abnormalities of cardiac rhythm and even cardiac arrest. Potassium also acts as a part of the buffer system which controls the pH of body fluids. Shifts of hydrogen ions (H^+) into and out of cells are compensated by shifts of potassium (K^+) in the opposite direction to maintain cation balance.

Potassium balance is similar to sodium balance as it is maintained by renal mechanisms. However, whereas sodium loss or retention is controlled to meet the specific needs of the body, potassium loss is constant. Most potassium is reabsorbed by the proximal tubule but about 10–15% is lost in the urine despite any need changes in the body.

Tubular cell secretion of potassium

However, the amount of potassium secreted into the lumen of the tubule can be changed. When potassium levels in the ECF are low potassium leaves the cells. The kidneys then conserve potassium by reducing the amount secreted into the tubule. There are three factors which alter the rate and amount of potassium secretion: the intracellular potassium content of the tubule cells, aldosterone levels and the pH of the ECF.

Tubule cell potassium

If a high potassium load is taken on, there is an increase in potassium in the ECF and then in the ICF. This triggers the tubule cell to secrete potassium into the lumen of the proximal tubule of the nephron. A low potassium intake will have the reverse effect. Low ECF potassium levels result in low ICF potassium levels and the tubule cells reduce their secretion of potassium.

Aldosterone

Aldosterone helps to regulate potassium ions as well as sodium ions. To maintain electrolyte balance, there is a one-for-one exchange of Na^+ for K^+ in the collecting tubules of the kidney and for each Na^+ absorbed, a K^+ is secreted. Therefore as plasma sodium levels rise, potassium levels fall. The adrenal cortex is also sensitive to high levels of potassium and will react by releasing aldosterone.

pH of ECF

The excretion of both K^+ and H^+ is linked to the reabsorption of sodium ions. They are cotransported with sodium and compete for places. If the pH of blood begins to fall the secretion of H^+ ions increases and K^+ ions secretion falls.

Regulation of calcium balance

Almost all the calcium content of the body, 99%, is found in the bones. However, ionic calcium found in the ECF is extremely important 'for normal blood clotting, membrane permeability and secretory behaviour' (Marieb 1992). Calcium is like potassium and sodium in having a large effect on neuromuscular excitability – hypocalcaemia increases excitability and leads to muscle tetany whilst hypercalcaemia inhibits muscle cells and neurones and may lead to cardiac arrhythmias.

Calcium is extremely well regulated and is balanced by the interaction of two hormones: parathyroid hormone (PTH) and calcitonin. PTH is released by the parathyroid glands situated on the posterior aspect of the thyroid gland. Calcitonin is produced by the parafollicular cells of the thyroid gland.

PTH acts to release calcium from the bones into the blood. It also stimulates the small intestine to absorb calcium by causing the kidneys to transform vitamin D into its active form. Activated vitamin D is necessary for the intestinal absorption of calcium. PTH increases calcium reabsorption by the kidneys while at the same time there is a decrease in phosphate reabsorption. The release of PTH is stimulated by declining plasma levels of calcium.

Calcitonin encourages the deposition of calcium salts in bone tissue and inhibits bone reabsorption. Although it is an antagonist of PTH, its role in calcium homeostasis is small.

Regulation of magnesium balance

Magnesium is essential as an activator of coenzymes needed in carbohydrate and protein metabolism. It is also implicated in neuromuscular functioning. About 50% of it is in the skeleton and the remainder is found intracellularly in heart and skeletal muscle and in the liver. Although the mechanism of magnesium balance is not well understood, the renal tubules are probably involved.

Alterations in sodium, chloride and water balance

These mainly involve changes in tonicity and can be classified as isotonic, hypertonic and hypotonic (Table 20.3).

Table 20.3 *Changes in tonicity*

Tonicity	*Mechanism*
Isotonic (isoosmolar) imbalance	Gain or loss of ECF results in a concentration equivalent to a 0.9% NaCl solution (normal saline) with no shrinkage or swelling of cells
Hypertonic (hyperosmolar) imbalance	An imbalance with an ECF concentration greater than 0.9% salt solution due either to water loss or solute gain. Cells shrink as fluid moves out of them into the ECF
Hypotonic (hypoosmolar) imbalance	An imbalance with an ECF concentration of less than 0.9% salt solution due to either water gain or solute loss. Cells gain water from ECF and swell

Isotonic alterations

Depletion causes contraction of the ECF volume with weight loss, dry skin and mucous membranes, decreased urinary output and symptoms of hypovolaemia: rapid heart rate, flattened neck veins and normal or decreased blood pressure. **Excesses** are usually due to overadministration of intravenous fluids, hypersecretion of aldosterone or the effect of drugs such as cortisone. There will be weight gain and a decrease in haematocrit and plasma proteins. Neck veins distend and blood pressure increases. Increased capillary hydrostatic pressure results in tissue oedema. If the excess is severe enough pulmonary oedema and heart failure may be the consequence.

Hypertonic alterations

Hypertonicity may be due to excess sodium (**hypernatraemia**) or depleted water (**dehydration**). Hypernatraemia occurs when the serum sodium concentration exceeds 147 mEq/l. This is rarely due to dietary excess. Causes include inappropriate use of hypertonic saline solution such as the administration of sodium bicarbonate to correct acidosis. Medical conditions leading to hypernatraemia include hyperaldosteronism and Cushing's syndrome with oversecretion of adrenocorticotrophic hormone (ACTH).

Dehydration occurs mainly in people who cannot take in water by themselves. Pathological causes include water loss in fever, respiratory infections, diabetes insipidus, diabetes mellitus, profuse sweating and diarrhoea. Clinical manifestations include thirst, dry skin and mucous membranes, elevated temperature, weight loss and concentrated urine except in patients who have diabetes insipidus. Isotonic salt-free solutions such as 5% dextrose can be given in both hypernatraemia and water loss until the plasma serum concentration returns to normal. Plain water cannot be given as it would increase intracellular fluid and cause cell lysis.

Hypotonic alterations

The most common causes are sodium deficit (**hyponatraemia**) and water excess (**water intoxication**). Hyponatraemia develops when plasma sodium concentration falls below 135 mEq/l. It is rarely caused by low intake and may be caused by vomiting, diarrhoea, gastrointestinal suctioning and burns. Hyperglycaemia increases ECF osmolality and pulls fluid from the plasma into the tissues. Water excess may occur following overintake in thirsty people (**dilutional hyponatraemia**). Pathological conditions include reduced urinary output in oliguric renal failure, congestive cardiac failure and cirrhosis of the liver. Clinical manifestations include neurological symptoms such as lethargy, confusion, apprehension, nausea, headache, convulsions and coma. If symptoms are severe small doses of hypertonic saline can be given with caution. With dilutional hyponatraemia, oedema may develop. Sodium and water balances are calculated and appropriate intravenous solutions are given. Restriction of fluid may be necessary in dilutional hyponatraemia.

Box 20.1 Summary of hypertonicity and hypotonicity

Hypertonicity		
Sodium excess	Water normal	Hypervolaemia
Sodium normal	Water deficit	Hypernatraemia
Hypotonicity		
Sodium deficit	Water normal	Hypovolaemia
Sodium normal	Water deficit	Hypervolaemia

ACID/BASE BALANCE

Almost all biochemical reactions in the body are influenced by the pH of their fluid environment (Chapter 1). The acid/base balance of body fluids is crucial to many biochemical reactions. There is a slight difference in pH between fluid compartments. Arterial blood pH is normally 7.4, venous blood and interstitial fluid have a pH of 7.35 whilst inside the cell the pH is 7.0. The fall in pH is due to the presence of acid metabolites. **Alkalosis** is present when arterial blood pH is over 7.45 and **acidosis** when it falls below 7.35. This could be said to be a misuse of the term as even at 7.0, a fluid is not acidic but neutral.

The structure of proteins, particularly enzymes, is affected by small changes in pH and significant alterations could disrupt metabolic processes and result in death. The pH scale may soon be replaced and the hydrogen ion concentration expressed in nanomoles per litre (nmol/l). The hydrogen ion content of arterial blood in these units is 40 nmol/l.

Chemical buffers tie up excess acids and bases as a temporary measure but cannot excrete them from the body. The lungs can dispose of carbonic acid by excreting carbon dioxide. However, it is the kidneys that dispose of the **metabolic** or **fixed acids** generated by cellular metabolism. These include phosphoric and uric acid and ketone bodies, the causes of **metabolic acidosis**. Also, only the kidneys have the power to regulate blood levels of alkaline substances. The kidneys are therefore the main regulators of acid/base status and act slowly and steadily to regulate the large acid/base imbalances that occur due to diet, metabolism or disease. Their most important mechanisms are the regulation of hydrogen ions and the conservation or generation of bicarbonate ions.

The role of the kidney

Regulation of hydrogen ion secretion

The tubule cells and the cells of the collecting ducts appear to be able to respond directly to the pH of the ECF. They then alter their H^+ secretion as needed to restore balance. The secreted ions are obtained from the dissociation of carbonic acid H_2CO_3 (carbon dioxide + water) within the tubule cells and for each H^+ secreted into the lumen, one Na^+ is reabsorbed into the tubule cell from the filtrate. This maintains the electrochemical balance. The rate of H^+ secretion varies directly with CO_2 levels in the ECF. Because CO_2 levels in blood are directly associated with blood pH, the kidneys can respond to alterations in blood pH.

Conservation of filtered bicarbonate ions

Bicarbonate ions (HCO_3^-) are an important part of the carbonate buffer system. In order to maintain the **alkaline reserve** or available bicarbonate ions to act in the buffer system (see below), the kidneys must replenish stores of HCO_3^- as necessary. The tubule cells are almost impermeable to bicarbonate ions and cannot reabsorb them from the filtrate. However, they can shunt bicarbonate ions generated within them into the peritubular blood. Dissociation of one molecule of carbonic acid inside the tubule cell releases one HCO_3^- ion and one H^+ ion.

There is a one-to-one exchange of bicarbonate ions depending on the numbers of H^+ ions secreted by the tubule cells. For each filtered HCO_3^- ion that is lost from the body, another one is generated from the dissociation of carbonic acid in the tubule cells. When large amounts of H^+ are secreted equally large amounts of HCO_3^- enter the peritubular blood.

Respiratory regulation of hydrogen ions

Respiration and carbon dioxide transport have an important effect on the acid/base status (pH) of the body. Hydrogen ions are the most highly reactive cations in the body and it is the concentration of hydrogen ions that determines the acidity of blood and body fluids. The intake and production of hydrogen ions vary according to the diet, energy output, disease and some drugs. It is essential to buffer these ions in body fluids and excrete them from the body via the lungs and kidneys in order to maintain homeostasis.

These three mechanisms are brought into effect sequentially. Chemical buffers act within a fraction of a second and are the first line of defence against a change in pH. Respiratory rate is adjusted in 2–3 min. The kidneys are the most efficient regulator but may take hours to bring about a change in blood pH.

Excretion of hydrogen ions by the lungs

Any increase in PCO_2 and H^+ ion concentration with a consequent fall in pH will be sensed by the central and peripheral chemoreceptors and there will be a rapid rise in alveolar ventilation leading to a speeding up of the reaction:

$$H^+ + HCO_3^- \leftrightarrow H_2CO_3 \leftrightarrow CO_2 + H_2O \qquad (2)$$

This leads to the rapid excretion of excess CO_2 and H^+ ions. The reverse situation will occur with any decrease in PCO_2 and H^+ ion concentration with a consequent rise in pH leading to a decrease in respiratory effort. These two mechanisms form an efficient response to short-term chemical changes in blood. The main role in long-term control of pH and acid/base balance is played by the kidneys.

Chemical buffer systems

Buffers are systems which minimise changes in pH. Acids are proton donors releasing free H^+ ions into a solution. Bases are proton acceptors and mop up free H^+ ions from a solution. Chemical buffers minimise the changes in pH by binding to H^+ ions when there is a fall in pH, i.e. when the fluid is becoming more acidic, and releasing H^+ ions when pH rises, i.e. when the fluid is becoming more alkaline. There are three major buffer systems in the body which work together:

- the bicarbonate buffer system;
- the phosphate buffer system;
- the protein buffer system.

The bicarbonate buffer system

In a solution strong acids dissociate into their component molecules and release H^+ ions. In a similar manner strong alkalis dissociate to release hydroxyl (OH^-) ions. The bicarbonate buffer system is important in both ECF and ICF. It is a mixture of carbonic acid (H_2CO_3) and its salt sodium bicarbonate ($NaHCO_3$) in the same solution. Carbonic acid is a weak acid that does not dissociate to release H^+ ions in neutral or acidic solutions. However, in a buffered solution in the presence of a stronger acid such as hydrochloric acid, bicarbonate ions of the salt will tie up the H^+ ions released by the stronger acid to form more carbonic acid:

$$HCl + NaHCO_3 \rightarrow H_2CO_3 + NaCl \qquad (3)$$

In the same manner, if a strong base such as sodium hydroxide (NaOH) is added to a buffered solution, the weak base $NaHCO_3$ will not dissociate to release hydroxyl ions (OH^-) but the carbonic acid will be forced to dissociate and release H^+ ions to mop up the OH^- ions released by the strong alkali to form water (H_2O):

$$NaOH + H_2CO_3 \rightarrow NaHCO_3 + H_2O \qquad (4)$$

In either equation 3 or 4 the result will be to drive the pH of the solution back to a biologically acceptable level. Within cells where there is little sodium, potassium or magnesium is associated with the bicarbonate ion and acts as a buffer. The bicarbonate ion concentration in ECF is normally about 25 mEq/l. The concentration of carbonic acid is about one-twentieth of the bicarbonate. It is freely available from cellular respiration and is subject to respiratory control.

The phosphate buffer system

The phosphate buffer system is almost identical to the bicarbonate buffer system with the control of H^+ ions occurring in a similar manner. Phosphate ions (HPO_4) replace bicarbonate ions in the equations. It is a very effective buffer in ICF and in urine, where phosphate concentrations are high.

The protein buffer system

The most plentiful buffer in the body is the supply of proteins in plasma and within the cells. They hold at least three-quarters of the buffering power. Some amino acids have side groups called organic acid or **carboxyl groups** (COOH) which can release the H^+ ion if needed. Other amino acid side chains can accept hydrogen ions. An exposed NH_2 group can bind H^+ to form NH_3 or release it as needed. This type of molecule is said to be **amphoteric**. Haemoglobin in red cells is an excellent example of a protein that acts as an intracellular buffer.

Abnormalities of acid/base balance

- **Respiratory acidosis** is caused by any condition that impairs lung ventilation and gas exchange: rapid shallow breathing, narcotic or barbiturate overdose.
- **Metabolic acidosis** can be caused by severe diarrhoea, untreated diabetes mellitus, starvation and excess alcohol ingestion.
- **Respiratory alkalosis** is always caused by hyperventilation whatever the triggering factor.
- **Metabolic alkalosis** is caused by vomiting of acid gastric contents, some diuretics that cause salt loss or severe constipation.

The effects of acidosis and alkalosis

Severe acidosis will depress the central nervous system and the person will go into a coma, shortly followed by death if not corrected. Alkalosis overexcites the CNS resulting in muscle tetany, extreme nervousness and convulsions. Death may occur due to respiratory arrest.

Respiratory and renal compensation

If an acid/base imbalance occurs due to failure of either the lungs or kidneys, the other will try to compensate. Changes in respiratory rate and rhythm are usually easy to observe. In metabolic acidosis the respiratory rate and depth are increased due to stimulation of the respiratory centres by high levels of hydrogen ions. The respiratory system blows off as much carbon dioxide as it can to reduce blood pH. In respiratory acidosis the respiratory rate is normally depressed and is actually the cause of the acidosis. In metabolic alkalosis respiratory compensation involves slow, shallow breathing which allows carbon dioxide to accumulate in the blood.

MATERNAL ADAPTATIONS TO PREGNANCY

In order to meet the needs of the fetus and her own metabolic changes, a woman's body retains fluids and electrolytes. Renal processes are modified and a new balance is achieved, especially in sodium and water homeostasis (Blackburn & Loper 1992). This adaptation is achieved by the antidiuretic hormone (ADH) and the renin-angiotensin-aldosterone system.

Sodium

The increase in GFR brings about an increase of up to 50% in filtered sodium. Tubular reabsorption increases so that 99% of the filtered sodium is reabsorbed. Sodium retention is highest in the last 8 weeks of pregnancy when about 60% of the retained sodium is utilised by the fetus. The rest is distributed in maternal blood and ECF.

The maintenance of sodium retention during pregnancy is influenced by multiple factors. Besides ADH and the renin-angiotensin-aldosterone system, a decrease in plasma albumin, the vasodilation effects of prostaglandins and the effects of the pregnancy hormones, human placental lactogen (HPL) and oestrogen play their parts. Water accumulation is directly proportional to sodium retention.

Renin-aldosterone-angiotensin system

The increases in the components of the renin-angiotensin-aldosterone system and the decrease in response to the vasoconstrictor effects of angiotensin II are brought about by oestrogens, progesterone, prostaglandins and the alterations in sodium processing. Plasma renin activity increases by a factor of 4–10 times during the first trimester and remains elevated until delivery. Renin release is stimulated by oestrogens. Progesterone also has an effect by stimulating renal sodium loss which causes the release of renin and aldosterone.

Angiotensinogen levels double by 8 weeks and increase 3–5 times by 20 weeks (Blackburn & Loper 1992). This is due to the effect of oestrogen on the liver which manufactures the plasma protein. The plasma aldosterone level reaches a peak at 24 weeks of 2–5 times that in non-pregnant women. There is a second peak at 36 weeks when the aldosterone level can be 8–10 times that in the non-pregnant woman. Although angiotensin II rises during pregnancy blood pressure actually decreases because of the decreased peripheral vascular resistance.

Water

Pregnant women accumulate about 7 litres of fluid over the normal to meet the needs of the fetus and their own altered metabolism. About 75% of the weight gain in pregnancy is due to the accumulation of fluid in the ECF. Interstitial fluid increases by about 1.5 litres, beginning as early as 6 weeks and peaking at 30 weeks. This increase occurs despite decreases in plasma osmolality and colloid osmotic pressure which would normally lower the fluid in the intravascular compartment. The vasodilation brought about by oestrogen and progesterone, which enables the vascular system to accommodate more blood volume, is probably a major cause as the increased volume is retained without stimulating the production of ADH. Thirst and urine output remain in balance.

ADH

Early in pregnancy plasma osmolality decreases, in particular the decreased solute load. ADH secretion and its effect on reabsorption of water are similar in the pregnant and non-pregnant woman. During pregnancy the osmotic threshold is reset so that ADH release occurs at the lower plasma osmolality. As mentioned above, this allows the vascular tree to accommodate more fluid volume with a lower osmolarity due to the haemodilution of pregnancy. Human chorionic gonadotrophin may be the main influence on osmoregulation in pregnancy. Circulating HCG levels decrease the thresholds for thirst and also the secretion of ADH.

Acid/base regulation

The plasma hydrogen ion concentration decreases early in pregnancy and the change is sustained until term. This makes the blood slightly more alkaline with a pH change to 7.44 from a non-pregnant value of 7.4. Plasma bicarbonate concentration also decreases. This mild alkalaemia is thought to be respiratory in origin since women normally hyperventilate in pregnancy, reducing their arterial PCO_2. Renal bicarbonate reabsorption and H^+ excretion appear to be unchanged in pregnancy. The blood changes, especially the reduction in plasma CO_2 level, place the pregnant woman at a disadvantage if she develops significant metabolic acidosis such as in diabetic ketoacidosis or acute renal failure.

Potassium and calcium excretion

There is selective retention of potassium during pregnancy, most of which is utilised by the fetus. However, urinary calcium excretion increases. This may be to combat high levels of circulating 1,25-dihydroxyvitamin D (calcitriol) which increases the absorption of calcium in the intestines. Serum calcium levels are raised and renal calcium reabsorption is reduced.

The intrapartum period

During labour and delivery the renin-angiotensin-aldosterone systems of both mother and fetus are altered with an elevation of the components. Blackburn & Loper (1992) discuss the possibility that this mechanism assists uteroplacental blood flow during labour. The result is to cause fluid retention and labouring women who are given too much intravenous fluid, especially if it contains oxytocin which has an antidiuretic effect, may suffer from water intoxication. This produces symptoms of agitation and delirium in a few women although Millns (1991) says that most women will cope with 'overenthusiastic fluid administration in labour'. A full discussion of nutrition and fluid needs in labour will be given in Chapter 37.

The use of general anaesthesia is complicated by a decrease in GFR and sodium excretion and an increase in vasoconstriction. If the woman is stressed this effect may be increased. It is important to maintain accurate fluid balance recordings in labour and after a general anaesthetic.

The postnatal period

Renal blood flow and GFR return to normal by 6 weeks following delivery. Urinary excretion of electrolytes and glucose returns to normal after 1 week. There is a diuresis with loss of sodium and water until prepregnancy levels are reached by 21 days.

Summary of main points

- Cell function depends on the maintenance of a stable environment. The fluid and electrolyte, acid and base balance of the extracellular fluids must be kept within a narrow range. Cells depend on a continuous supply of nutrients and the removal of metabolic wastes.
- In an adult water accounts for about 50% of the body mass although this ratio can vary depending on the age, sex and weight of individuals. Water can be found in the intracellular fluid and extracellular fluid which can be divided into interstitial fluid and plasma. The sum of all the above is the total body water.
- Water is the universal solvent and contains a variety of solutes. Broadly speaking, these can be divided into electrolytes and non-electrolytes. Non-electrolytes have bonds that prevent them dissociating into their component particles in solution and do not carry electrical charges. Electrolytes include inorganic salts, both inorganic and organic acids and bases and some proteins.
- All dissolved solutes contribute to the osmotic activity of a fluid but electrolytes have the greatest osmotic power because each molecule can dissociate into at least two ions. Because water moves along osmotic gradients from areas of lesser osmolality to greater osmolality, electrolytes have the greatest ability to cause fluid shifts. Each fluid compartment has its own pattern of electrolytes.
- The distribution of water and the movement of nutrients and waste products between the plasma in the capillary and the interstitial space occurs because of changes in hydrostatic pressure and osmotic forces between the arterial and venous ends of the capillary network. The movement of fluid back and forth across the capillary wall is called net filtration.
- Water intake must balance water loss. Regulation of water intake is by the mechanism of thirst. Obligatory water losses include the insensible loss of water from the lungs and via the skin. Water in faeces must be added to the loss. There is an absolute minimum of 500 ml of urine per 24 hours that the kidneys must excrete.
- Oedema is the accumulation of fluid within the interstitial space. It is a problem of fluid distribution and does not necessarily indicate excess intake. Oedema may be generalised or localised. It is associated with weight gain, swelling and puffiness.
- Electrolytes include salts, acids and bases. Salts are the main electrolytes and are involved in many physiological processes. Salts are obtained from the food we eat and also, to a lesser extent, in our drinking water. Salts containing sodium account for at least 90% of solutes in the ECF. Regulating the balance between sodium intake and output is a major function of the kidneys.
- Influences on fluid and electrolyte balance include the cardiovascular system baroreceptors, the regulation of ADH and the influence of atrial natriuretic factor. Oestrogens and glucocorticoids also play a part in enhancing tubular reabsorption of sodium.
- Potassium is the main cation in ICF and is necessary for normal neuromuscular functioning and other processes such as protein synthesis. It also acts as part of the buffer system which controls the pH of body fluids. Potassium balance is maintained by renal

mechanisms. Sodium loss or retention is controlled to meet the specific needs of the body but potassium loss is constant.

- Aldosterone helps to regulate potassium ions as well as sodium ions and as plasma sodium levels rise, potassium levels fall. The excretion of both K^+ and H^+ is linked to the reabsorption of sodium ions. If the pH of blood begins to fall, the secretion of H^+ ions increases and K^+ ion secretion falls.
- Ionic calcium found in the ECF is extremely important for normal blood clotting, membrane permeability and secretory behaviour. Calcium is extremely well regulated by the interaction of two hormones: parathyroid hormone and calcitonin. Calcium has an important effect on neuromuscular excitability. Hypocalcaemia increases excitability, leading to muscle tetany, whilst hypercalcaemia may lead to cardiac arrhythmias.
- Magnesium is an activator of coenzymes needed in carbohydrate and protein metabolism. It is also implicated in neuromuscular functioning. About 50% of it is in the skeleton and the remainder is found inside cells in heart and skeletal muscle and in the liver. The mechanism of magnesium balance is not well understood, but the renal tubules are probably involved.
- Almost all biochemical reactions in the body are influenced by the pH of their fluid environment. There is a slight difference in pH between fluid compartments. The structure of proteins, particularly enzymes, is affected by small changes in pH and significant alterations could disrupt metabolic processes and result in death.
- Chemical buffers tie up excess acids and bases as a temporary measure but cannot excrete them from the body. The lungs can dispose of carbonic acid by excreting carbon dioxide but the kidneys dispose of the metabolic acids or fixed acids generated by cellular metabolism. Bicarbonate ions are important for the carbonate buffer system. To maintain the alkaline reserve or available bicarbonate ions to act in the buffer system, the kidneys must replenish stores of HCO_3^-.
- Respiration and carbon dioxide transport have an important effect on the acid/base status of the body. The concentration of hydrogen ions determines the acidity of blood and body fluids. It is essential to buffer these ions in body fluids and excrete them via the lungs and kidneys to maintain homeostasis. Chemical buffers act in less than a second and are the first line of defence against a change in pH. Respiratory rate is adjusted in 2–3 min. The kidneys are the most efficient regulator but may take hours to change the blood pH. There are three chemical buffer systems in the body which work together: the bicarbonate, the phosphate and the protein buffer systems.
- Respiratory acidosis is caused by any condition that impairs lung ventilation and gas exchange. Metabolic acidosis can be caused by severe diarrhoea, untreated diabetes mellitus, starvation or excess alcohol ingestion. Respiratory alkalosis is always caused by hyperventilation. Metabolic alkalosis is caused by vomiting of acid gastric contents, some diuretics that cause salt loss or severe constipation.
- Severe acidosis will depress the central nervous system and the person will go into a coma, shortly followed by death if not corrected. Alkalosis overexcites the CNS resulting in muscle tetany, extreme nervousness and convulsions. Death may occur due to respiratory arrest.
- To meet the needs of the fetus and her own metabolic changes, a woman's body retains fluids and electrolytes. Renal processes are modified and a new balance is achieved, especially in sodium and water. This adaptation is achieved by antidiuretic hormone and the renin-angiotensin-aldosterone system. Pregnant women accumulate about 7 litres more water and about 75% of the weight gain in pregnancy is due to the accumulation of ECF fluid. Interstitial fluid increases by about 1.5 litres.
- Early in pregnancy plasma osmolality decreases, in particular the decreased solute load. During pregnancy the osmotic threshold is reset so that ADH release occurs at the lower plasma osmolality. The hormone HCG may be the main influence on osmoregulation in pregnancy.
- The plasma hydrogen ion concentration decreases early in pregnancy and the change is sustained until term. This makes the blood slightly more alkaline. Plasma bicarbonate concentration also decreases. This mild alkalaemia may be respiratory in origin as pregnant women hyperventilate.
- There is selective retention of potassium during pregnancy, most of which is utilised by the fetus. However, urinary calcium excretion increases. This may be to combat high levels of circulating 1,25-dihydroxyvitamin D (calcitriol) which increases the absorption of calcium in the intestines. Serum calcium levels are raised and renal calcium reabsorption reduced.
- During labour and delivery the renin-angiotensin-aldosterone systems of both mother and fetus are altered with an elevation of the components. The result is to cause fluid retention and labouring women who are given too much intravenous fluid, especially if it contains oxytocin which has an antidiuretic effect, may suffer from water intoxication.
- The use of general anaesthesia is complicated by a decrease in GFR and sodium excretion and an increase in vasoconstriction. If the woman is stressed this effect may be increased. It is important to maintain accurate fluid balance recordings in labour and after a general anaesthetic.
- Renal blood flow and GFR return to normal by 6 weeks following delivery. Urinary excretion of electrolytes and glucose returns to normal after 1 week. There is a diuresis with loss of sodium and water until prepregnancy levels are reached by 21 days.

References

Blackburn ST, Loper DL. 1992 Maternal Fetal and Neonatal Physiology, A Clinical Perspective. WB Saunders, Philadelphia, pp 336–378.

Hinchliff SM, Montague SE. 1990 Physiology for Nursing Practice. Baillière Tindall, London.

Marieb EN. 1992 Human Anatomy and Physiology, 2nd edn. Benjamin/ Cummings Publishing, California.

Millns JP. 1991 Fluid balance in labour. Current Opinion in Obstetrics and Gynaecology 1, 35–40.

Recommended reading

Bayliss C, Davison J. 1991 The urinary system. In Hytten F, Chamberlain G. (eds), Clinical Physiology in Obstetrics. Blackwell Scientific, Oxford, pp 245–302.

Campbell MK. 1995 Biochemistry, 2nd edn. Saunders College Publishing, Philadelphia.

McClaren SM. 1996 Renal function. In Hinchliff SM, Montague SE, Watson R (eds) Physiology for Nursing Practice, 2nd edn. Baillière Tindall, London.

Millns JP. 1991 Fluid balance in labour. Current Opinion in Obstetrics and Gynaecology 1, 35–40.

Wood EJ, Myers A. 1991 Essential Chemistry for Biochemistry, 2nd edn. Biochemical Society, London.

Chapter 21 The gastrointestinal tract

In this chapter

INTRODUCTION

An adult consumes approximately 1 kg of solids and 1.2 kg of fluid daily (Hinchliff et al 1996). The organs of the digestive system can be described as those of the alimentary canal and those comprising the accessory digestive organs of teeth, tongue, salivary glands, liver, gallbladder and pancreas (Marieb 1992). The description of the anatomy and physiology of the non-pregnant human draws on Hinchliff et al (1996) and Marieb (1992). The alimentary canal is also called the gastrointestinal tract and will be discussed in this chapter, followed by significant changes in pregnancy. The accessory organs of salivary glands, liver, gallbladder and pancreas will be discussed fully in Chapter 22 and nutrition in Chapter 23.

ANATOMY OF THE GASTROINTESTINAL TRACT

The adult gastrointestinal (GI) tract is a continuous, coiled, fibromuscular tube of variable diameter about 4.5 metres long, open to the external environment at both ends and extending from the mouth to the anus. It varies in structure and function throughout its length. The organs of the GI tract are the mouth, pharynx, oesophagus, stomach, small intestine and large intestine (Fig. 21.1). For more detailed anatomy, readers are referred to one of the many textbooks which include anatomy, such as Marieb (1992). A brief description is given below.

The basic structure of the gastrointestinal tract is the same throughout its course. The wall of the tube consists in the main of four layers (Fig. 21.2).

- The **mucosal layer** is innermost and lines the tube. This layer is very variable along the length of the tube depending on the required function. Stratified epithelial cells line the lumen from which glands develop. There are also mucus-secreting cells throughout the epithelium. The turnover rate for the epithelial cells is high because of the amount of frictional damage. The epithelial cells are supported by a sheet of connective tissue called the **lamina propria** and beneath that is a thin layer of smooth muscle called the **muscularis mucosae**. The mucosal layer also contains patches of lymphoid tissue which defend the tract against microorganisms.
- The **submucosa** consists of loose connective tissue which supports blood vessels, lymphatics and nerves. The nerve fibres are called the **submucosal** or **Meissner's plexus**.
- The **muscularis layer** is formed of smooth involuntary muscle fibres, bound together in sheets called **fasciculi**. There are two sheets: an inner circular layer and an outer longitudinal layer. In the stomach there is an additional oblique layer. Between the two layers of muscle fibres is a network of nerve fibres called the **myenteric** or **Auerbach's plexus**. The muscle fibres respond rhythmically to stimulation by the autonomic nervous system and some hormones. They respond slowly and less forcefully than striated muscle fibres and their contractions are not as finely controlled.

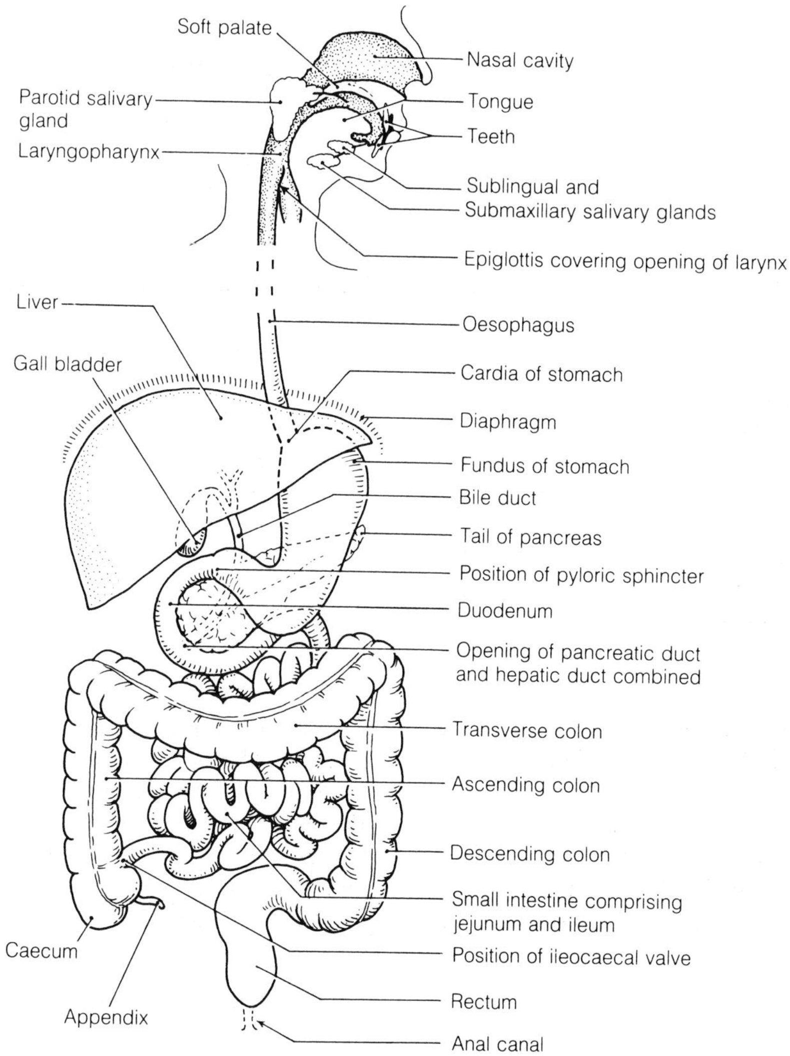

Figure 21.1 *Diagrammatic representation of the gastrointestinal tract (from Hinchliff SM, Montague SE, 1990, with permission).*

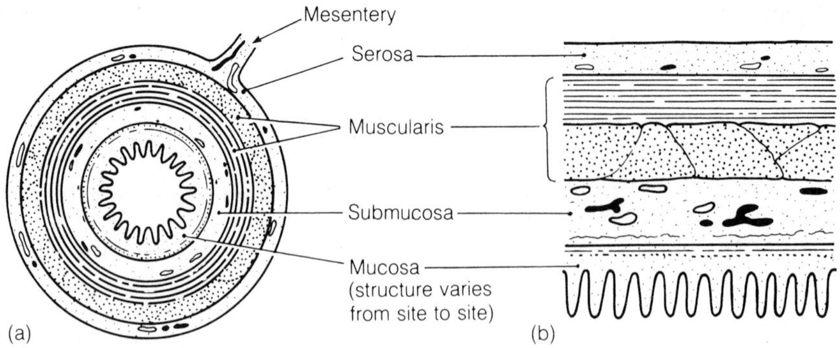

Figure 21.2 *Generalised structure of the gut wall. (a) Cross-section; (b) longitudinal section (from Hinchliff SM, Montague SE, 1990, with permission).*

- The **adventitia** or **serosa** (visceral peritoneum) is the outermost protective layer and is formed of connective tissue and squamous, serous epithelium. It is continuous with the mesentery of the abdominal cavity and supports blood vessels and nerves.

The peritoneum

Most of the digestive organs lie in the abdominopelvic cavity. All body cavities contain friction-reducing serous membranes and the peritoneum of the abdominopelvic cavity is the largest of these membranes. The visceral peritoneum covers the external surface of most of the digestive organs and is continuous with the parietal peritoneum that lines the walls of the abdominopelvic cavity. Between the two layers is the peritoneal cavity containing fluid secreted by the serous membranes.

The mesentery

Connecting the visceral and parietal layers of the peritoneum is a fused double layer of peritoneum called the mesentery. This supports the blood vessels, lymphatics and nerves to the digestive organs and helps support the organs. It also stores fat and is able to wall off areas of infection and inflammation to prevent the spread of peritonitis. Another fold of peritoneum, the **lesser omentum**, runs from the liver to the stomach. The **greater omentum** is a fold of peritoneum that hangs in front of the intestines and is reflected off the stomach. In most places the mesentery is attached to the posterior abdominal wall. The peritoneum surrounding the small intestine is shaped like a fan with the small intestine attached to its outer edge.

Blood supply

Branches of the abdominal aorta serve the digestive organs and the special hepatic portal circulation. These include the hepatic, splenic and left gastric branches of the coeliac trunk supplying the liver, spleen and stomach and the superior and inferior mesenteric arteries supplying the small and large intestines. The hepatic portal circulation collects nutrient-rich venous blood from the digestive organs and takes it to the liver, as discussed in Chapter 22.

CONTROL OF THE GASTROINTESTINAL TRACT

Autonomic nervous system

Nerve fibres from the autonomic nervous system (ANS) control the function of the gastrointestinal tract. The submucosal and myenteric nerve plexi are the local tracts. In the submucosal plexus parasympathetic nerve fibres synapse with ganglion cells present in small clusters in the submucosal tissue. Postganglionic fibres leave the ganglion cells and send impulses to the glands and smooth muscle of the tract. They are accompanied by some sympathetic fibres.

In the myenteric plexus parasympathetic nerve fibres synapse with ganglion cells which lie in large clusters between the circular and longitudinal fibres of the muscularis layer. Postganglionic fibres leave the ganglion cells and send impulses to the smooth muscle. Sympathetic fibres also supply this muscle. Both plexi run the length of the gut and receive both sympathetic and parasympathetic nerve fibres. The two plexi are connected and activity in one can affect the other. Stimulation at the upper end of the gastrointestinal tract can be transmitted to more distal parts; for instance, stimulation of gastric and intestinal enzyme secretion follows entry of food into the oesophagus.

Parasympathetic activity leads to an increase in both the motility and secretory functions of the tract and to relaxation of the gut sphincters. The vagus nerve, which is the 10th cranial nerve, is the source of parasympathetic supply to the oesophagus, stomach, pancreas, bile duct, small intestine and proximal colon. The parasympathetic supply to the distal colon is via the nervi erigentes from the sacral outflow.

Sympathetic activity leads to a decrease in blood supply to the gut with a decrease in secretions and in gut motility. There is contraction of the gut sphincters. As in other parts of the body, there are two types of catecholamine receptors in the gut: α and β_2 receptors (β_1 receptors are present only in cardiac muscle). Stimulation of α receptors causes contraction of the smooth muscle of the gastrointestinal tract whilst stimulation of the $\beta 2$ receptors causes relaxation.

Regulatory chemicals

Two chemicals produced by the tract help in neural regulation. These are substance P and serotonin.

- **Substance P** is a small peptide of only 11 amino acids which is found in high concentrations in the gut. It may be a chemical mediator (Wingerson 1980). It acts like a neurotransmitter and is referred to as a neuropeptide. It is involved in the conduction of pain impulses but brings about vasodilation and contraction of non-vascular smooth muscle.
- **Serotonin** (5-hydroxytryptamine or 5-HT) is synthesised in the myenteric plexus and may also act as an interneuronal transmitter substance.

FUNCTIONS OF THE GASTROINTESTINAL TRACT

The role of the gastrointestinal (alimentary) tract is to alter food so that it can be utilised by the body cells. Six processes can be described.

- Ingestion
- Propulsion
- Mastication
- Mechanical and chemical digestion
- Absorption
- Elimination of non-usable residues as faeces.

Ingestion and mastication

These two processes take place in the mouth. There food is mixed with saliva, broken into small pieces by the teeth and propelled backwards into the oesophagus by the tongue. The tongue allows us to taste food. On its superior surface are numerous peg-like projections called **papillae**. These contain most of the 10 000 taste buds which allow differentiation between the four taste modalities – sweet, sour, salty and bitter (Marieb 1992). All taste buds have the potential for recognising the four tastes although particular ones are associated with one taste. The four tastes result in different neural firing patterns which are interpreted in the cerebral cortex. Taste is aided by the sense of smell which sends impulses to the brain via the olfactory nerve. This is why any inflammation and hypersecretion of the nasal mucosa which may occur in pregnancy will result in a loss or alteration of taste.

Saliva

The salivary glands and the production of saliva are discussed more fully in the next chapter. The three pairs of salivary glands – the parotid, submaxillary and sublingual – produce 1.5 litres of saliva daily, consisting of 99% water and with a pH of 7.0. Saliva contains the digestive enzyme salivary (α) amylase which acts upon cooked starch to convert the polysaccharides into disaccharides. It facilitates the formation of a bolus of partly broken up food which is ready to swallow, once lubricated by salivary mucins. Saliva is produced in response to the cerebral perception of the thought, sight or smell of food or the presence of food in the mouth.

The ingested and masticated food is propelled down the oesophagus into the stomach for digestion of the food to continue. The process is called **deglutition**. The tongue contracts and presses the bolus of food against the hard palate in the roof of the mouth. It then arches backwards and the bolus of food is propelled into the oropharynx.

THE STOMACH

Chemical breakdown of food by the secretion of enzymes begins in the stomach and is completed in the small intestine. The stomach is 25 cm long and lies in the left side of the abdominal cavity partly hidden by the diaphragm and liver. It is continuous with the oesophagus above and the duodenum below. When empty, it is J shaped. Its mucosal layer has folds (**rugae**) which allow distension. The rugae are further folded, providing a large absorptive surface, and contain millions of deep **gastric pits** with microscopic gastric glands that produce gastric juice.

Functions of the stomach

- A reservoir for food
- Production of the intrinsic factor
- Gastric absorption
- A churn to mix food
- Secretion of mucus, hormones and gastric juice.

A reservoir for food

At rest the stomach's capacity is only 50 ml but receptive relaxation of the stomach wall musculature can allow distension by up to 1.5 litres. Under exceptional circumstances the stomach can hold 4 litres of content. The pyloric sphincter prevents an over-rapid transfer of food to the small intestine.

Production of the intrinsic factor

The intrinsic factor is a glycoprotein necessary for the absorption of vitamin B_{12} (cyanocobalamin) produced by the gastric parietal cells which also produce gastric acid. Intrinsic factor binds to vitamin B_{12} in the terminal ileum of the small intestine to form a complex which appears to bind to receptors in the wall of the ileum and is transferred into the blood. Vitamin B_{12} is required for the maintenance of healthy myelin sheaths around the nerves and also for the formation of red blood cells in the bone marrow. Lack of it may lead to megaloblastic anaemia. The resulting pernicious anaemia may lead to subacute combined degeneration of the spinal cord.

Gastric absorption

Food reaching the stomach is only partly broken down there and many of the molecules are still too large to be absorbed. There are also no carrier systems present in the gastric mucosa. Water and some drugs such as aspirin (acetylsalicylic acid), which is a weak acid, can be absorbed from the stomach. Absorption of aspirin lowers intracellular pH and may cause damage, leading to gastric irritation and bleeding.

A churn to mix food

The stomach converts food to a thick soup consistency by mixing it with gastric secretions. This also dilutes the food and makes it compatible with the extracellular fluid in the duodenum. The semiliquid formed by waves of peristalsis of the smooth muscle in the stomach wall is called **chyme**.

Secretion of mucus

Mucus is produced by the cells in the necks of the deep gastric glands in both the cardiac and pyloric sphincters. It adheres to the gastric mucosa to protect the stomach from being digested by the proteolytic gastric enzyme **pepsin**. The layer of mucus that protects the mucosa must be 1 mm thick.

Secretion of hormones

Enteroendocrine cells release a variety of hormones which diffuse into blood capillaries and are returned to the GI tract to influence digestive system target organs. These include gastrin, serotonin, cholecystokinin, somatostatin and endorphins. Histamine, produced by circulating mast cells and basophils, increases gastric acid secretion by binding to histamine receptors (H_2 receptors) on the gastric parietal cells.

Secretion of gastric juice

Two to three litres of gastric juice, which is a mixture of secretions from two types of cells present in the gastric pits (Fig. 21.3) but absent from the pylorus, are produced daily. The gastric pit cells are:

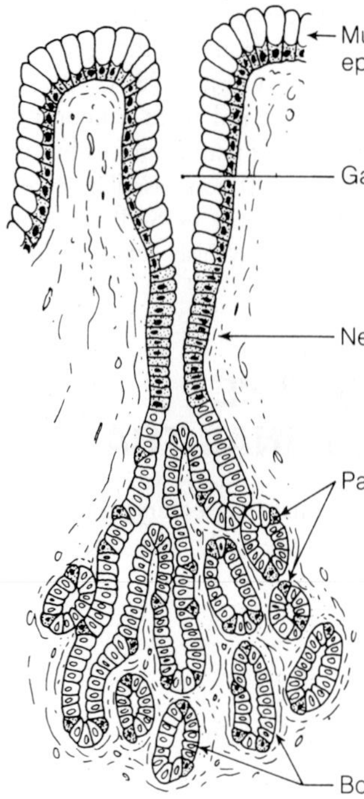

Figure 21.3 *Diagram of gastric pit (from Hinchliff SM, Montague SE, 1990, with permission).*

Table 21.1 *Hormones that aid digestion*

Hormone	*Stimulus*	*Target organ*	*Effect*
Gastrin	Presence of food in the stomach	Stomach Small intestine Ileocaecal valve Large intestine	Increased gastric gland secretions, most effect on HCl production Causes contraction of intestinal muscle Relaxes valve Stimulates mass movements
Serotonin	Food in stomach	Stomach	Contraction of stomach musculature
Histamine	Food in stomach	Stomach	Release of HCl
Somatostatin	Food in stomach Sympathetic nerve stimulus	Stomach Pancreas Small intestine Gallbladder	Inhibits gastric secretion, motility, emptying Inhibits secretion Inhibits GI blood flow and intestinal absorption Inhibits contraction and bile release
Intestinal gastrin	Acidic/partly digested food in duodenum	Stomach	Stimulates gastric glands and motility
Secretin	Acidic or irritant chyme, partially digested fats and proteins	Stomach Pancreas Liver	Inhibits gastric secretion and motility during gastric phase Increases bicarbonate-rich pancreatic juice and potentiates CCK action Increases bile output
CCK	Fatty chyme or partially digested proteins	Liver/ pancreas Gallbladder Sphincter of Oddi	Potentiates secretin's action Increases enzyme-rich output Stimulates contraction with expulsion of bile Relaxes to allow bile and pancreatic juice to enter duodenum
Gastric inhibitory peptide (GIP)	Fatty and/or glucose-containing chyme	Stomach	Inhibits gastric gland secretion and motility during gastric phase

- parietal or oxyntic cells which secrete hydrochloric acid (HCl) and the intrinsic factor;
- chief or zygomen cells which secrete the enzymes.

There are about a thousand million parietal cells in the gastric pits of an adult stomach. Hydrogen ions are secreted into the lumen of the stomach against a concentration gradient, probably by an active pump mechanism in the cell membrane. CO_2 diffuses into the parietal cells from arterial blood and combines with water to form H_2CO_3 (carbonic acid). Equal numbers of hydrogen ions formed by the dissociation of H_2CO_3 into hydrogen ions (H+), bicarbonate ions (HCO_3^-) and chloride ions are secreted into the lumen of the gastric pits. This forms HCl which is then diluted by water. Histamine or the hormone **gastrin** stimulates the secretion of HCl into the lumen of the stomach.

The functions of gastric acid are:

- inactivation of salivary amylase;
- bacteriostasis;
- alteration of the molecular structure of proteins to tenderise them;
- curdling of milk;
- conversion of pepsinogen to pepsin.

Children produce an enzyme called **renin** which acts on the milk protein casein and converts it into curds.

The chief cells produce a pepsinogen-rich secretion. When gastric pH is lower than 5.5 pepsinogen is converted into the active proteolytic enzyme pepsin by hydrochloric acid which converts proteins to polypeptides by breaking the bonds between specific amino acids. Once chyme leaves the stomach there is a change to an alkaline medium and pepsin's activity ceases.

Control of gastric juice secretion

There are both neural and hormonal aspects of control of gastric juice secretion.

Neural control

There are two phases in neural control although the two work interdependently. The **cephalic phase** is an anticipatory conditioned reflex to the sight, smell or thought of food mediated by the vagus nerve which stimulates both parietal and chief cells. The **gastric phase** is mediated by stretch and chemoreceptors. Stretch receptors in the stomach wall respond to distension by food. Chemoreceptors respond to the presence of protein molecules within the stomach. Impulses from these two types of receptor are sent to the submucosal plexus where they synapse with parasympathetic neurones. Excitatory impulses are then dispatched to the parietal cells.

Hormonal control

Although the neural influences described above are important, hormonal influences, especially gastrin, contribute most to the gastric phase of secretion. Throughout the gut regulatory hormones, called **peptides**, are active. Many of them are also found in the central nervous system and alternative names for them are neurohormones, neuropeptides or neurotransmitters. Gastrin is a term that refers to a group of similar hormones produced by the G cells in the lateral walls of the gastric glands in the antrum of the stomach. A small amount of gastrin is produced by the duodenal mucosa, sometimes referred to as a third or **intestinal phase** of gastric juice secretion. The production of gastrin is stimulated by meat, alcohol, tea, coffee and colas (Hinchliff et al 1996).

P cells throughout the gastrointestinal tract secrete **bombesin**, the gastrin-releasing peptide. Gastrin enters the gastric circulatory capillaries and the systemic circulation and when it reaches the stomach via the bloodstream it has the following actions.

- It stimulates the production of gastric acid by the parietal cells by the release of histamine.
- It has a minor role in stimulating the production of pepsinogen by the chief cells.
- It stimulates the growth of the gastric and intestinal mucosa.
- It causes enhanced contraction of the cardiac sphincter to prevent gastric reflux.
- It stimulates the secretion of insulin and glucagon in the pancreas.

Control of gastric motility

Increase of gastric motility

Stomach contractions empty the stomach and also compress, knead and mix the food with gastric juice to produce chyme. Waves of peristalsis pass from the cardiac sphincter to the pylorus about three times a minute. The more liquid parts of chyme pass through the pylorus into the small intestine whilst the more solid parts are sent back to the body of the stomach for further gastric mixing. The regulatory peptide **motilin**, produced by cells in the duodenum and jejunum in response to the entry of acid chyme, increases gastric motility.

Food remains in the stomach depending on its consistency and composition. Carbohydrates and liquids leave the stomach fastest followed by proteins and fats. The **enterogastric reflex** is initiated when the products of protein digestion together with the acid enter the duodenum, resulting in a slowing of gastric motility. Gastric emptying usually takes 4–5 h, during which the antrum, pylorus and duodenal cap contract in sequence. This is the gastric pump mechanism which results in squirts of chyme entering the duodenum.

Inhibition of gastric motility

When glucose and fats enter the duodenum a regulatory peptide – **gastric inhibitory peptide** (GIP) – is secreted by the K cells of the duodenal and jejunal mucosa. GIP, also known as glucose-dependent insulin-releasing peptide, decreases gastric secretion and motility and stimulates the secretion of insulin. **Vasoactive intestinal polypeptide** (VIP), produced in the D cells of the duodenum and colon, also inhibits gastric motility by acting as a smooth muscle relaxant. It also stimulates the intestinal secretion of electrolytes.

THE SMALL INTESTINE

Structure

The small intestine is a long coiled tube about 3–3.5 m long, extending from the pyloric sphincter to the ileocaecal valve. Its diameter is only 2.5 cm. It is the body's main digestive organ where food digestion is completed and absorption of nutrients and most of the water from the chyme takes place.

There are three sections of the small intestine.

- The C-shaped duodenum lies mainly behind the peritoneum. It is about 25 cm long and surrounds the head of the pancreas.
- The jejunum, 250 cm long, makes up about 40% of the remainder of the small intestine.
- The ileum, 360 cm long, makes up the other 60%, joining the large intestine at the ileocaecal valve. The jejunum has thicker walls and is more vascular whilst the ileum has fewer folds in its lumen. Protective lymph nodes called **Peyer's patches** are present in the ileum.

The duodenum

Salivary amylase begins the digestion of cooked starch into maltose and dextrins. Pepsin begins the breakdown of proteins into polypeptides. There is no secretion of enzymes by the duodenum although it does secrete hormones. The duodenum receives the secretions of the pancreas and liver via the pancreatic duct and common bile duct after they join together at the ampulla of Vater at the sphincter of Oddi. These secretions are alkaline with a pH of about 8 and produce a sharp change in pH from the acidity of the stomach to the alkalinity of the duodenum. Enzymes are pH sensitive and function within a narrow range. The first few centimetres of the duodenum are called the **duodenal cap**. The tissue is protected from the acid chyme by a large number of mucus-secreting **Brünner's glands**.

Pancreatic extrinsic secretions

The exocrine function of the pancreas is achieved by secretions from **acinar cells** and plays a major role in digestion. The production of the enzymes will be discussed more fully in Chapter 22. The enzymes are secreted into the pancreatic duct and the duodenum. The three proteolytic enzymes are:

- **trypsinogen**, which is in an inactive form to safeguard the gut from autodigestion;
- this is converted to **trypsin** by the enzyme enterokinase. Trypsin completes the breakdown of proteins to amino acids;
- **carboxypeptidase**, which acts on peptides.

Other enzymes are:

- pancreatic amylase, which converts starch to maltose;
- pancreatic lipase, which breaks down triglycerides to three fatty acids and glycerol;
- ribonuclease (RNAase), which breaks down RNA;
- deoxyribonuclease (DNAase), which acts on DNA to release free nucleotides.

Control of pancreatic juice secretion

The hormone **secretin** causes secretion of the watery component, rich in bicarbonate but low in enzymes. Another hormone, **cholecystokinin** (CCK), causes the release of the enzymes. Stimulation of pancreatic juice secretion can be divided into a cephalic phase, with vagal control brought about by the sight, smell or thought of food or the presence of food in the mouth, and a gastric phase stimulated by the release of gastrin (Fig. 21.5).

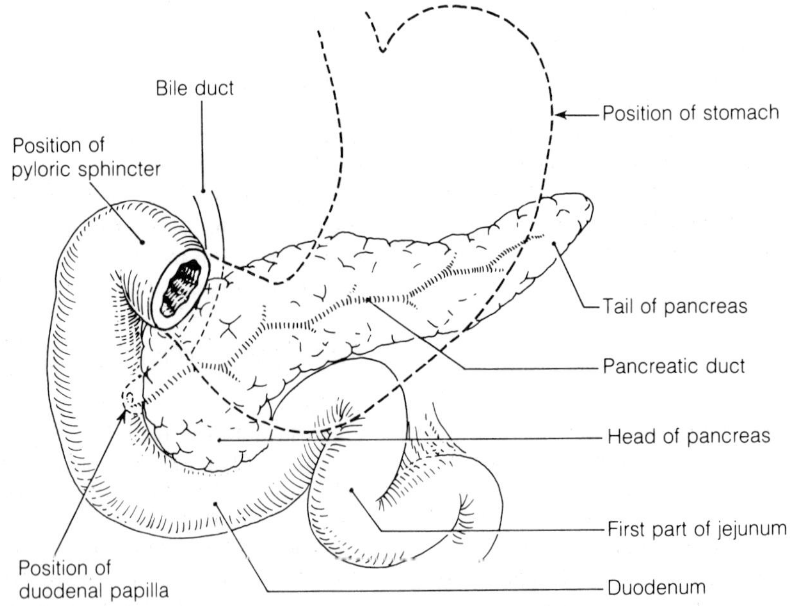

Figure 21.4 *The position of the pancreas (from Hinchliff SM, Montague SE, 1990, with permission).*

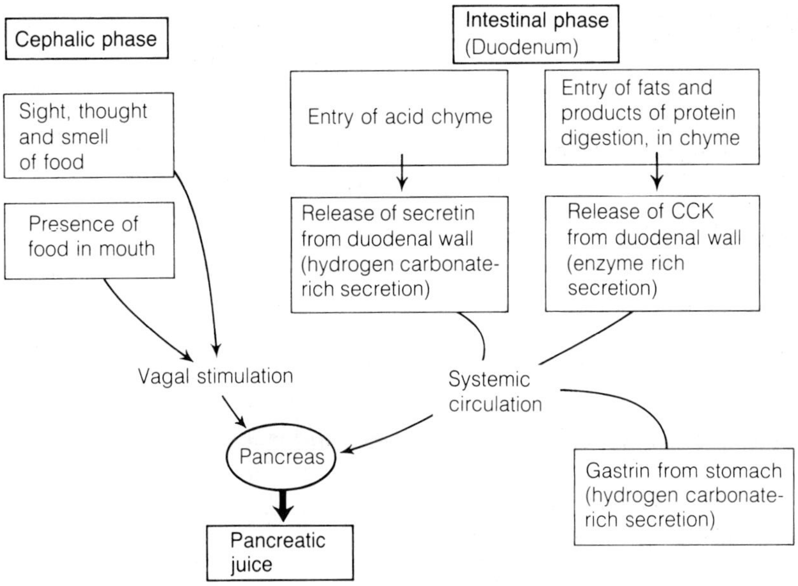

Figure 21.5 *Flow chart to illustrate pancreatic juice secretion (from Hinchliff SM, Montague SE, 1990, with permission).*

CCK causes:

- stimulation of enzyme-rich pancreatic secretion;
- augmentation of the activity of secretin;
- slowing of gastric emptying and inhibition of gastric secretion;
- stimulation of the secretion of enterokinase;
- stimulation of glucagon secretion;
- stimulation of intestinal motility;
- contraction of the gallbladder with the release of bile.

Bile

Bile is produced by the liver and stored in the gallbladder. It contains no digestive enzymes but emulsifies fats so that they, the fat-soluble vitamins and iron can be absorbed. Its production, content and function will be discussed more fully in the next chapter. The control of bile secretion also involves neural and hormonal factors. CCK is the major controller, causing contraction of the gallbladder and relaxation of the sphincter of Oddi. Once the gallbladder is empty, further flow of bile into the duodenum occurs directly from the liver. Vagus nerve stimulation will bring about a similar action. About 97% of bile salts are reabsorbed into the portal circulation and returned to the liver.

Intestinal juice

The process of digestion is completed by juices secreted by the duodenum and jejunum. This juice is rich in mucus, some of which comes from the Brünner's glands in the proximal duodenum. Most of the watery juice is secreted by **Lieberkühn's glands** in the jejunum and ileum. The nutrients are absorbed into the circulating blood through small finger-like projections in the surface of the small intestine called **villi**, which are covered by a layer of mucus to prevent autodigestion.

Intestinal enzymes

These enzymes are produced by enterocytes in the villi and break down food particles into their absorbable form. They are probably released from shed enterocytes. Proteins are broken down into amino acids while fats are in the form of fatty acids and glycerol. Carbohydrates are broken down into monosaccharides – glucose, fructose and galactose. The enzymes are:

- aminopeptidases, which act on peptides;
- dipeptidases, which act on dipeptides;
- maltase, which converts maltose to glucose;
- lactase, which converts lactose to glucose and galactose;
- sucrase, which converts sucrose into glucose and fructose.

The villi

The surface area of the small intestine is increased by visible folding of the mucosa and submucosa into **plicae circularis** (circular folds). The addition of villi and microvilli increases the surface area to 600 times that of a simple tube of the same size, giving a surface area of $200\ m^2$ (Hinchliff et al 1996). Between the villi are small pits called the **crypts of Lieberkühn** where the mucus-secreting glands are situated. Villi have an external covering of simple columnar epithelium continuous with the crypts (Fig. 21.6) and a central lacteal containing lymph which empties into the local lymphatic circulation. There is a capillary blood supply linked to both hepatic and portal veins.

Two other types of cell are associated with the villi. **Goblet cells** secreting mucus are situated mainly in the crypts while **enterocytes** are tall columnar cells involved in digestion and absorption. Enterocytes have many mitochondria to provide the energy for enzyme secretion and nutrient absorption. They have a high rate of mitosis and those at the tip of the villi are replaced every 30 h.

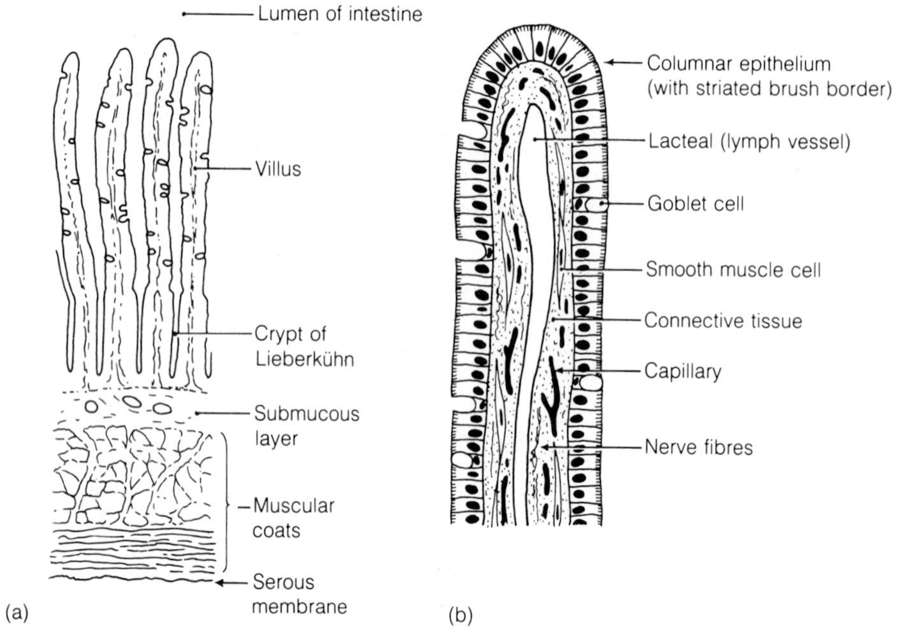

Figure 21.6 *(a) Villi in small intestine. (b) A single villus (from Hinchliff SM, Montague SE, 1990, with permission).*

A few smooth muscle cells are present in villi which contract to assist lymph drainage in the central lacteals. Lymphocytes and plasma cells are situated at intervals between the enterocytes. The plasma cells secrete IgA to protect the gut from pathogens.

There are also cells in the intestinal wall secreting 5-HT which may increase intestinal motility.

ABSORPTION

Eight to 9 litres of water and 1 kg of nutrients daily are absorbed across the gut wall. The transport of nutrients can be either active or passive. **Active transport** requires energy and is usually against a concentration gradient. Most such substances require carrier molecules, including vitamin B_{12}, iron, sodium ions, glucose, galactose and amino acids. Water follows passively along an osmotic gradient. **Passive transport** requires no energy, depending on the direction of concentration and electrical gradients. It includes water, lipids, drugs and some electrolytes and vitamins. Some substances pass passively across the gut wall membrane with the help of carrier molecules by **facilitated diffusion**.

Nutrients and minerals

Monosaccharides

About 500 g of monosaccharides is absorbed daily. Galactose and glucose pass into the villous capillaries and then to the hepatic portal vein. A high concentration of sodium ions on the surface of enterocytes facilitates the active transport of these molecules. Glucose and sodium ions share the same carrier molecule. Sodium concentration in the enterocyte is low so that sodium moves into the cell along a concentration gradient accompanied by glucose. Fructose has a different carrier molecule and its transport is not influenced by sodium.

Monosaccharides are transported to the liver where galactose and fructose are converted to glucose (Fig. 21.7). Some of the glucose is converted to glycogen (**glycogenesis**) under the influence of insulin. About 100 g of glucose is stored in the liver, sufficient to maintain blood glucose levels for 24 h. Some glycogen is stored in skeletal muscle to provide energy for muscle action. Any glucose surplus to the body's needs is converted by the liver into adipose tissue.

Blood glucose is maintained normally at a level of 3.5–5.5 mmol/l. When the glucose level falls, glycogen is broken down in the liver (**glycogenolysis**) to release glucose. This occurs under the influence of glucagon and adrenaline. Once glycogen stores in the liver are depleted the liver manufactures glucose from amino acids and glycerol (**gluconeogenesis**).

When circulating glucose arrives at the tissues it is taken up by the cells by facilitated diffusion under the influence of insulin. In the mitochondria of the cells glucose is oxidised to form energy in the **Krebs'** or **citric acid cycle**. The glucose is converted to pyruvic acid which, in turn, is converted to acetyl coenzyme A, usually referred to as **acetyl CoA**, a process requiring oxygen, i.e. aerobic. Acetyl CoA enters the Krebs' cycle to undergo changes mediated by enzymes. The energy storage molecules – adenosine triphosphate, water and carbon dioxide – are formed in the process of oxidation. If there is insufficient oxygen to convert pyruvic acid to acetyl CoA, lactic acid is formed.

Amino acids

In an adult approximately 200 g of amino acids is absorbed daily from the ileum, of which 50 g a day is needed to maintain nitrogen balance and to provide for tissue growth and repair. The mechanism for absorption of amino acids is not fully understood but may depend on whether the amino acid is acidic, basic or neutral. Sodium appears to facilitate the absorption of amino acids.

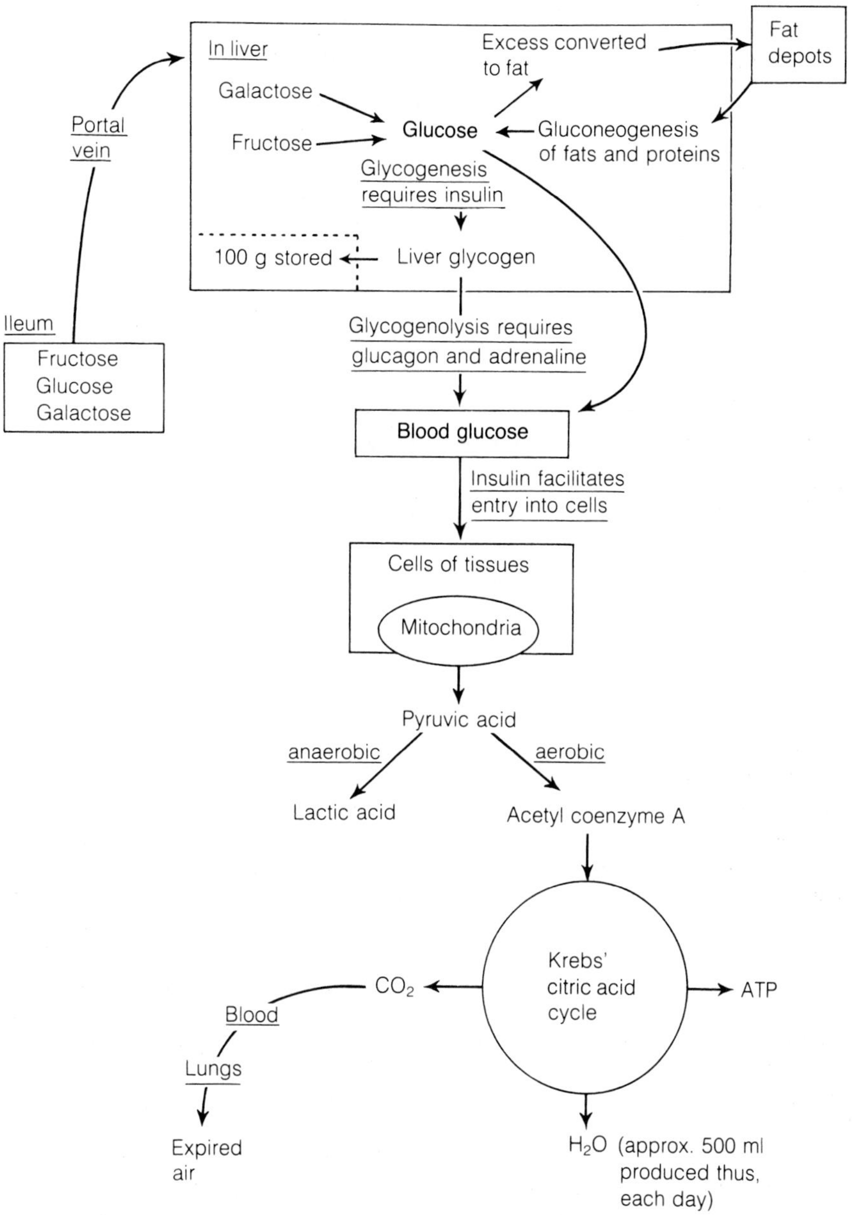

Figure 21.7 *Metabolic pathways for glucose (from Hinchliff SM, Montague SE, 1990, with permission).*

Amino acids cannot be stored by the body and are absorbed into the blood to enter a common circulating pool from which cells can remove them as necessary (Fig. 21.8). However, the liver can interconvert amino acids by utilising the eight essential amino acids to synthesise the non-essential amino acids. Any excess amino acids are broken down by the liver by a process of **deamination**. The nitrogen portion is converted into urea which enters the blood and is excreted by the kidney.

Fats

About 80 g of fat is absorbed daily, mainly in the duodenum. The contents of the micelles are discharged onto the microvilli and enter the enterocytes by passive diffusion. Short-chain fatty acids enter the capillary network and travel in the hepatic portal vein as free fatty acids. Longer chain fatty acids are resynthesised in the enterocyte to become triglycerides coated with a layer of lipoprotein, cholesterol and phospholipid. These complexes enter the central lacteals to form **chyle** which enters the lymphatic system and then the bloodstream. Faeces contain about 5% fat.

Bile salts, steroid hormones and cell membranes are formed from cholesterol. Cholesterol is found in the blood, mainly in combination with a protein carrier, as lipoproteins, of which there are three types:

- high-density lipoproteins (HDLs);
- low-density lipoproteins (LDLs);
- very low-density lipoproteins (VLDLs).

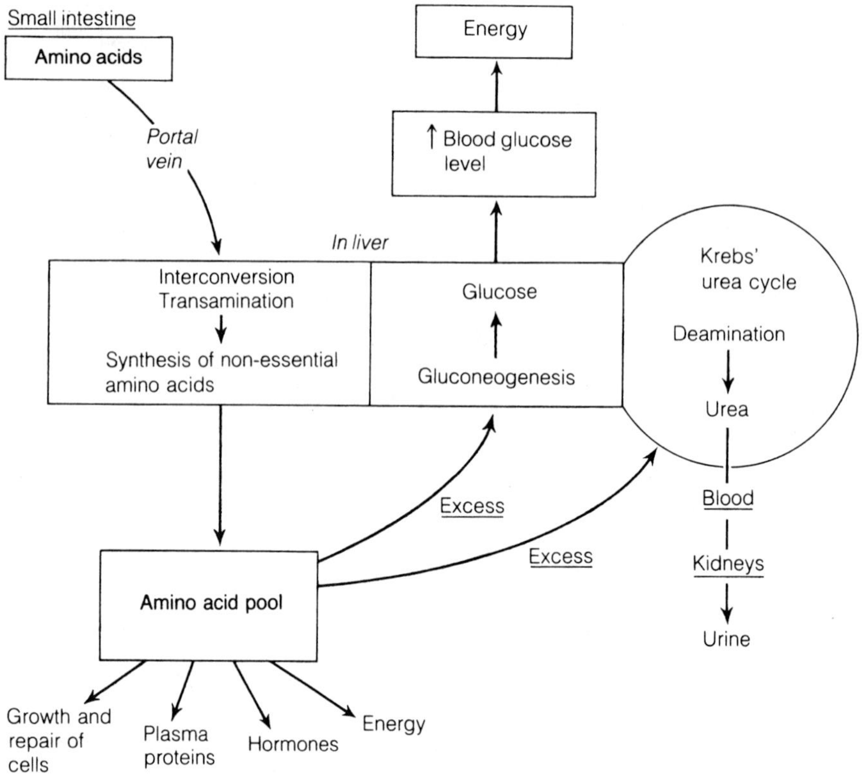

Figure 21.8 *Metabolic pathways for amino acids (from Hinchliff SM, Montague SE, 1990, with permission).*

Cholesterol is laid down as atheromatous plaques in arterial walls in the form of LDLs and VLDLs. A high ratio of HDLs to LDLs and VLDLs may offer protection against ischaemic heart disease. The ratio of HDLs to LDLs and VLDLs has been shown to be increased in vegetarians, in those whose fat intake is largely unsaturated and in those who take regular exercise. The ratio is reduced in those who smoke cigarettes.

Fat can be utilised by the body to form energy and any excess fat is stored as adipose tissue. When fat stores are needed for energy production they are mobilised under the influence of growth hormones or cortisol and taken to the liver where the triglycerides are broken down into free fatty acids and glycerol. The fatty acids are converted to acetyl CoA in the presence of oxygen and glucose and these enter the Krebs' citric acid cycle (Fig. 21.9). If no glucose is available acetyl CoA metabolism is deranged and the ketone bodies acetoacetic acid and β-hydroxybutyric acid accumulate in the blood. These can be oxidised to release energy but metabolic acidosis will occur.

Sodium, potassium and water

About 2 litres of fluid are ingested daily. A further 8–9 litres of fluid are added to the gut during the production of digestive juices. Only 50–200 ml is lost in the faeces, the rest being absorbed from both the small and large intestine at a rate of 200–400 ml per minute. The jejunum, ileum and colon actively reabsorb sodium ions which are followed passively by chloride and water. Some potassium is actively secreted into the gut and reabsorbed from the ileum and colon along a concentration gradient.

Vitamins

The water-soluble vitamins, with the exception of B_{12} which is absorbed as a complex with the intrinsic factor in the terminal ileum, are passively absorbed with water. The fat-soluble vitamins, A D E and K, enter the enterocytes in the micelles. Bile and lipase are necessary for their absorption.

Most calcium is absorbed in the upper part of the small intestine under the influence of parathyroid hormone and calcitonin. The active process is facilitated by vitamin D.

Iron

In developed countries about 15–20 mg of iron is ingested daily, mostly as ferric salts, but only 5–10% is absorbed into the blood. There is a daily loss of 1 mg a day from desquamation of the skin and in the faeces. Women lose about 25 mg each month during menstruation. Iron is more readily absorbed in the ferrous form and the ferric form is reduced to the ferrous form by gastric juice and vitamin C. Iron is actively absorbed in the upper part of the small intestine and is stored in the enterocytes when their cellular stores are low. The enterocytes discharge iron into the bloodstream when serum levels fall. Iron travels in the blood bound to **apoferritin**, known as **ferritin** when iron is bound to it. About 70% of iron in the body is in haemoglobin and 3% in myoglobin in muscle protein. The rest is stored in the liver as ferritin or **haemosiderin**.

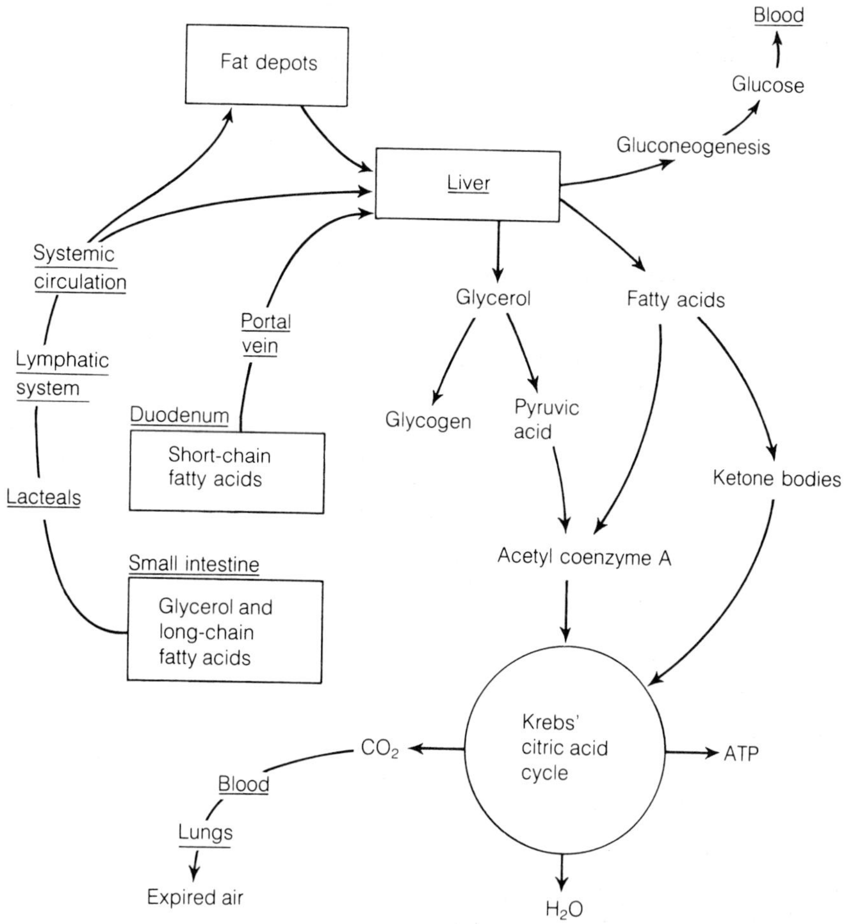

Figure 21.9 *Metabolic pathways for fats (from Hinchliff SM, Montague SE, 1990, with permission).*

THE LARGE INTESTINE

The adult large intestine is about 1.5 m long, consisting of the caecum, appendix, colon and rectum (Fig. 21.10). It has a diameter of 5–6 cm and can store large quantities of food residues. The large intestine has no villi and a much smaller internal surface than the small intestine. The colon differs from the generalised structure of the gastrointestinal tract as the longitudinal muscle bands are incomplete and the wall is gathered into three longitudinal bands, the **taenia coli**. These bands are shorter than the remaining colon so that the wall pouches outwards into **haustrations** (buckets) between the taeniae when the circular muscles contract. The filling and emptying of the haustrations help to mix the colonic contents. Patches of lymphoid tissue are scattered throughout the length of the large intestine, providing a protection against pathogens.

About 1 litre of porridge-like chyme enters the large intestine daily through the ileocaecal valve. This valve, normally closed because of back pressure from the colon's contents, opens in response to peristaltic waves. The caecum relaxes and the ileocaecal valve opens, a reflex called the **gastrocolic reflex**. The colonic peristalsis that follows fills the rectum with faeces, resulting in the urge to defaecate.

The **caecum**, a blind pouch between the ileocaecal valve and the colon, is about 7 cm long. Though involved in cellulose digestion in herbivores, it has no known function in humans. The **vermiform appendix**, a worm-like blind-ending sac projecting from the end of the caecum about the size of an adult's little finger, contains lymphoid tissue and enlarges in the presence of infection or inflammation (appendicitis). An enlarged appendix may rupture so that faecal material and bacteria enter the abdominal cavity, leading to peritonitis.

The colon

The large intestine is divided anatomically into three regions.

- The **ascending colon**, about 15 cm long, commences at the caecum and extends upwards on the right of the abdominal cavity as far as the lower border of the liver.
- The **transverse colon** begins at the hepatic flexure and traverses the abdominal cavity below the liver and stomach to the slightly higher splenic flexure.
- The **descending colon**, about 25 cm long, descends along the left side of the abdominal cavity. The sigmoid colon, about 4 cm long, is a continuation of the descending colon and empties into the rectum.

The large intestine has five functions.

1 Storage of unabsorbed food residues prior to defaecation. About 70% of food residue is excreted within 72 h of

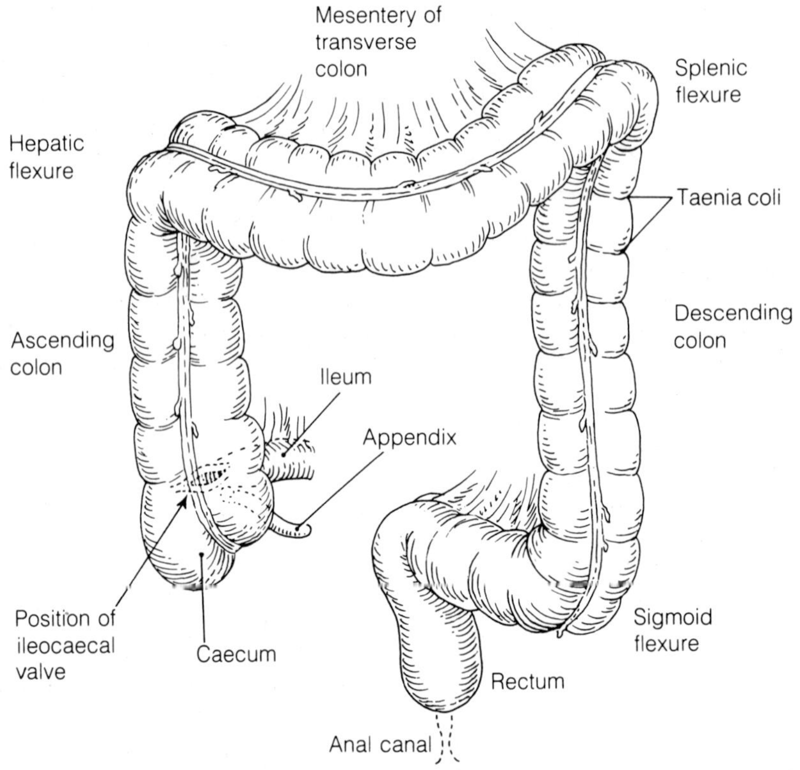

Figure 21.10 *The large intestine (from Hinchliff SM, Montague SE, 1990, with permission).*

ingestion but the remainder may stay in the colon for a week. Non-absorbable dietary fibre gives bulk to the faeces.

2 Absorption of water, electrolytes and some vitamins. Sodium is actively reabsorbed into the hepatic portal vein, followed passively by water and chloride. The amount of water reabsorbed depends on how long the residue remains in the colon. In constipation the residue may stay in the colon for several days, resulting in removal of most of the water.
3 Vitamin K and some B vitamins – thiamine, folic acid and riboflavin – are synthesised by commensal colonic bacteria. Bacterial fermentation of food residues results in the formation of flatus which consists of nitrogen, carbon dioxide, hydrogen, methane and hydrogen sulphide. Between 500 and 700 ml of flatus is produced daily depending on the type of food eaten; legumes lead to an increase in flatus production.
4 Secretion of mucus, which acts as a lubricant for elimination of faeces. The mucus contains bicarbonate which gives the contents of the colon a pH of 7.5–8.0.
5 Some potassium ions may also be secreted.

Movements of the colon

Contraction of the circular muscle fibres occurs about once every half hour. This causes **segmentation**, a non-propulsive movement in the colon which mixes the colonic contents and facilitates absorption. Peristalsis moves the faeces towards the rectum. Following meals there is an increase in colonic activity due to the gastrocolic reflex. Associated with the gastrocolic reflex is **mass movement**, which propels the faeces towards the rectum. The haustrations in the midcolon disappear and the tube becomes flattened and shortened by waves of rapid, powerful contractions, moving the colonic contents rapidly into the sigmoid colon.

The rectum

The rectum is a muscular tube about 15 cm long. It is capable of great distension but is usually empty until just before defaecation. The sudden distension of the rectal walls caused by filling of the rectum during mass movement brings about the urge to defaecate. The rectum opens to the exterior by the anal canal which has both internal and external sphincters.

The anal canal

The anal canal is about 3 cm long and begins where the rectum perforates the levator ani muscle of the pelvic floor. It has a sphincter at both ends. The **internal anal sphincter** is composed of smooth muscle fibres and is not under voluntary control. When nerve fibres from the sympathetic system are stimulated, the muscle fibres in the internal anal sphincter contract. Fibres from the parasympathetic system inhibit contractions and the sphincter relaxes. The **external anal sphincter** is made up of striated voluntary muscle and is supplied by fibres from the pudendal nerve. The sphincter is under conscious control from about 18 months of age. Damage to the sphincter or its nerve supply may occur in childbirth, resulting in incontinence of faeces.

The mucosa of the anal canal hangs in long ridges called **anal columns** and is made of stratified squamous epithelium. There are anal recesses between the columns which secrete mucus which aids in defaecation. Two superficial venous plexi called the haemorrhoidal veins are associated with the anal canal. These may become distended resulting in varicosities or haemorrhoids.

Defaecation

Afferent nerve impulses travel to the sacral spinal cord when faeces enter the rectum. Impulses then travel back from the spinal cord in a reflex arc to the terminal ileum and anal sphincter to allow defaecation. The cerebral cortex receives nerve messages which allow inhibition of the spinal reflex arc if it is not convenient to defaecate. Defaecation is usually assisted by voluntary effort which raises intraabdominal pressure. A deep breath is taken and expired against a closed glottis. This is called **Valsalva's manoeuvre**. The levator ani muscles contract and the pressure in the rectum is raised to about 200 mmHg (26 kPa). The anal sphincters relax and the contents of the rectum are expelled. During straining there is a sharp rise in blood pressure followed by a sudden fall.

Faeces

About 100–1250 g of faeces is eliminated each day, consisting of 30–50 g solids and 70–100 g water. The solid portion consists mainly of cellulose, shed epithelial cells, bacteria, some salts and stercobilin which gives it the brown colour. The characteristic odour is caused by bacterial breakdown of amines.

MATERNAL ADAPTATIONS TO PREGNANCY

Blackburn & Loper (1992) write: 'The gastrointestinal and hepatic systems during pregnancy are characterised by marked anatomic and physiologic alterations that are essential in supporting maternal and fetal nutrition'. Hytten (1991) states that 'Upsets of the gastrointestinal function are perhaps the commonest cause of complaint by pregnant women'. These minor disorders are discussed in Chapter 30.

The mouth

Pregnant women usually find they have an increased appetite, craving for certain foods, avoidance of others and pica, a craving for non-food substances. These alterations in nutrition habit may be a response to fetal needs. Progesterone is a known appetite stimulant as shown by changes in appetite during the menstrual cycle that closely follow the hormonal changes. During pregnancy alterations in the balance of oestrogen, progesterone, glucagon and insulin contribute to the changes in food intake.

The gums and teeth

The gums may become swollen and spongy and bleed easily. There is an increase in gingivitis and periodontal disease, caused by oedema rather than by an increased presence of irritant particles of food. The oedema is part of the generalised change in connective tissue ground substance and is due to the increase in circulating oestrogens. About 1 in 100 women will develop an **epulis** (pregnancy tumour), a friable growth or hyperplasia of the gum usually found on the palatal side of the maxillary gingiva. It may bleed or interfere with chewing and occasionally needs excising but will usually regress after delivery.

There is no consensus on whether pregnancy damages teeth although many women believe it does. Early studies carried out in the 1940s and mentioned by Hytten (1991) suggested that there was no demineralisation of the dentine of teeth during pregnancy. Blackburn & Loper (1992) add that fetal calcium needs are drawn from maternal body stores, not from teeth.

Saliva

Changes in the pH of saliva are debatable with some research finding an increase in pH whilst others found a decrease in pH. Blackburn & Loper (1992) state that saliva becomes more acid in pregnancy. **Ptyalism** or excess salivation may occur, especially in Afro-Caribbean women. Hytten (1991) suggests that the 1–2 litres produced is probably normal and that reluctance to swallow because of nausea is the major problem. If ptyalism becomes a major problem, ganglion-blocking drugs usually help.

The oesophagus

Heartburn during pregnancy is thought to be due to reflux oesophagitis which occurs because of reduced competence of the cardiac sphincter between the oesophagus and stomach. However, this may not be the only cause as acid reflux has been found to be present not only in those with heartburn but in four out of 10 people with no heartburn (Hey et al 1977). Displacement of the cardiac sphincter into the thorax (**hiatus hernia**) affects European women more than African women and heartburn occurred in 80% of European women and only 10% of African women. However, after studying the research, Hytten (1991) believes that if displacement of the sphincter does play a part in heartburn it is probably only a minor one. Sphincter strength is probably the main cause.

The stomach

Acid secretion

Gastric acid secretion has been found to be reduced during pregnancy, beginning early in pregnancy and increasing in late pregnancy. A related finding is that peptic ulceration is rare in pregnant women and in women who had prepregnancy ulcers, there was a clear remission but a return to symptoms by the 3rd month after delivery.

Emptying time

Gastric muscle tone and motility are reduced during pregnancy due to the effect of progesterone. However, low levels of circulating motilin have been found during pregnancy (Christofides et al 1982). The delay in emptying is probably due to the lower secretion rate of gastric juices. This results in prolonged digestion time for solid food although watery food is digested and passed on to the small intestine with little delay. Drinks containing high levels of glucose such as those administered in glucose tolerance tests have a high osmotic effect and gastric emptying is delayed in hyperosmotic foods. The reduced activity of the gastric muscle may exaggerate the effect and result in nausea. During labour, reduced stomach motility leads to delayed emptying and risk of acid aspiration.

The small intestine

There is no increase in the absorption of food even though the metabolism of pregnant women is anabolic. Any increased nutrition must come from increased intake. Iron and calcium appear to be absorbed more readily. However, Hytten (1991) discusses a case reported by Montgomery & Pincus (1955) where a young woman, following an ileostomy, demonstrated increased absorption of food during pregnancy whilst the number of daily stools decreased. The delay in passage of food through the gut was probably responsible for both phenomena.

The large intestine

Constipation is a common complaint as the colon shares in the general relaxation of smooth muscle found throughout the body. The constipation is made worse by the increased absorption of water in the colon. Increased flatulence may also occur.

Summary of main points

- The adult gastrointestinal tract is a continuous, coiled, fibromuscular tube of variable diameter about 4.5 metres long, open to the external environment at both ends and extending from the mouth to the anus. It consists of the mouth, pharynx, oesophagus, stomach, small intestine and large intestine. Most of the digestive organs lie in the abdominopelvic cavity.
- Body cavities contain friction-reducing serous membranes and the peritoneum of the abdominopelvic cavity is the largest. The visceral peritoneum covers the external surface of most of the digestive organs and is continuous with the parietal peritoneum that lines the walls of the abdominopelvic cavity. Between the two peritoneal layers is the peritoneal cavity containing fluid secreted by the serous membranes.
- Connecting the visceral and parietal layers of the peritoneum is a fused double layer of peritoneum called the mesentery, supporting blood vessels, lymphatics and nerves supplying the digestive organs and helping to support the organs. A fold of peritoneum, the lesser omentum, runs from the liver to the stomach. A fold of peritoneum that hangs in front of the intestines and is reflected off the stomach is called the greater omentum.
- Nerve fibres from the autonomic nervous system control the function of the gastrointestinal tract. Parasympathetic activity leads to an increase in both the motility and secretory functions of the tract and to relaxation of the gut sphincters. Sympathetic activity leads to a decrease in blood supply to the gut with a decrease in secretions and in gut motility.
- The role of the gastrointestinal tract is to process the food so that it can be utilised by the body cells. Six processes can be described: ingestion, propulsion, mastication, mechanical and chemical digestion and absorption and elimination of non-usable residues as faeces.
- Saliva contains the digestive enzyme salivary (α) amylase which acts upon cooked starch to convert polysaccharides into disaccharides. Digestion of food begins in the stomach and is completed in the small intestine. It involves break down of ingested food by the secretion of enzymes. The stomach also produces the intrinsic factor, histamine and gastric juice.
- There may be a thousand million parietal cells in the gastric pits of an adult stomach. Hydrogen ions are secreted into the lumen of the stomach against a concentration gradient. Histamine or the hormone gastrin stimulates the secretion of HCl into the lumen of the stomach. Gastric acid inactivates salivary amylase, is bacteriostatic, alters the molecular structure of proteins to tenderise them, curdles milk and converts pepsinogen to pepsin.
- The chief cells of the stomach produce a pepsinogen-rich secretion. When gastric pH is lower than 5.5 pepsinogen is converted into pepsin by hydrochloric acid. Pepsin converts proteins to polypeptides. Once chyme leaves the stomach there is a change to an alkaline medium and pepsin's activity ceases.
- There are both neural and hormonal aspects of control of gastric juice secretion. There are two phases in the neural control. The cephalic phase is an anticipatory conditioned reflex mediated by the vagus nerve to stimulate both parietal and chief cells. The gastric phase is mediated by stretch and chemoreceptors responding to the presence of food within the stomach.
- Hormonal influences contribute most to the gastric phase of secretion. Gastrin is produced by the G cells in the lateral walls of the gastric glands in the antrum of the stomach in response to the presence of food. P cells secrete bombesin which causes gastrin to enter the gastric circulatory capillaries and the systemic circulation. The regulatory peptide motilin increases gastric motility.
- When glucose and fats enter the duodenum a regulatory peptide – gastric inhibitory peptide (GIP) – is secreted by the K cells of the duodenal and jejunal mucosa. This decreases gastric secretion and motility and stimulates the secretion of insulin. Vasoactive intestinal polypeptide from the D cells of the duodenum and colon acts as a smooth muscle relaxant, inhibiting gastric motility.
- There are three sections of the small intestine: the duodenum, the jejunum and the ileum. Protective lymph nodes called Peyer's patches are present in the ileum. The digestion of food is completed and absorption of nutrients and most of the water takes place in the small intestine.
- The duodenum secretes no enzymes but receives the secretions of the pancreas and liver via the pancreatic duct and common bile duct. These secretions are alkaline with a pH of about 8. The first few centimetres of the duodenum are called the duodenal cap. As the acid chyme is received here the tissue is protected by a large number of mucus-secreting Brünner's glands.
- Pancreatic digestive enzymes are secreted into the duodenum. Pancreatic juice contains three proteolytic enzymes: trypsinogen, trypsin and carboxypeptidase. Other pancreatic enzymes are pancreatic amylase, ribonuclease and deoxyribonuclease. Secretin causes the secretion of a watery component rich in bicarbonate but low in enzymes. Cholecystokinin (CCK) causes the release of enzymes.
- Bile contains no digestive enzymes but emulsifies fats so that they, the fat-soluble vitamins and iron can be absorbed. CCK is the major controller of bile release, causing contraction of the gallbladder and relaxation of the sphincter of Oddi.
- The process of digestion is completed by juices secreted by the duodenum and jejunum. The basic nutrients are then absorbed into the circulating blood through intestinal villi. Intestinal enzymes

produced by enterocytes in the villi break down food particles into their absorbable form.

- About 500 g of monosaccharides is absorbed daily and transported to the liver where galactose and fructose are converted to glucose. Some of the glucose is converted to glycogen under the influence of insulin. At least 50 g a day of amino acids is needed to maintain nitrogen balance and to provide for growth and repair of tissues. About 80 g of fat is absorbed daily, mainly in the duodenum.
- About 2 litres of fluid are ingested daily. A further 8–9 litres of fluid are added to the gut during the production of digestive juices. Only 50–200 ml is lost in the faeces, the rest being absorbed from both the small and large intestine at a rate of 200–400 ml per minute. The jejunum, ileum and colon actively reabsorb sodium ions, followed passively by chloride and water. Potassium is actively secreted into the gut and is usually reabsorbed from the ileum and colon along a concentration gradient.
- The water-soluble vitamins, with the exception of B_{12} which is absorbed as a complex with the intrinsic factor in the terminal ileum, are passively absorbed with water. The fat-soluble vitamins, A D E and K, enter the enterocytes in the micelles. Bile and lipase are necessary for their absorption.
- Most calcium is absorbed in the upper part of the small intestine under the influence of parathyroid hormone and calcitonin. The active process is facilitated by vitamin D. Calcium absorption is facilitated by lactose and proteins and inhibited by oxalates and phytic acid found in cereals and rhubarb and phosphate.
- About 15–20 mg of iron is ingested daily but only 5–10% is absorbed. There is a daily loss of 1 mg a day from desquamation of the skin and in the faeces and women lose about 25 mg each month during menstruation. Iron is actively absorbed in the upper part of the small intestine, stored in the enterocytes and discharged into the bloodstream when serum iron levels fall.
- The large intestine is about 1.5 m long in an adult and consists of the caecum, appendix, colon and rectum. It can store large quantities of food residues. The longitudinal muscle bands are gathered into three taeniae coli which are shorter than the remaining colon. The wall pouches outwards into haustrations between the taeniae when the circular muscles contract. About 1 litre of porridge-like chyme enters the large intestine daily. The gastrocolic reflex and colonic peristalsis fill the rectum with faeces, resulting in the urge to defaecate.
- The colon also absorbs most of the remaining water and electrolytes, synthesises vitamin K and some B vitamins, and secretes mucus which contains bicarbonate and acts as a lubricant for elimination of faeces. It may also secrete some potassium ions.
- The rectum is usually empty until just before defaecation and sudden distension results in the urge to defaecate. The rectum opens to the exterior by the anal canal. Afferent nerve impulses travel to the sacral spinal cord when faeces enter the rectum. If there is no barrier to defaecation nerve impulses travel back from the spinal cord to the terminal ileum and the anal sphincter and defaecation will occur. Impulses also travel to the cerebral cortex which can inhibit the spinal reflex. About 100–150 g of faeces is eliminated each day.
- Pregnant women usually find they have an increased appetite and food consumption, craving for certain foods and avoidance of others. Pica is a craving for non-food substances. These alterations in nutrition habit may be a response to fetal needs. Progesterone is a known appetite stimulant. During pregnancy alterations in the balance of oestrogen, progesterone, glucagon and insulin contribute to the changes in food intake.
- The gums may become swollen and spongy in pregnancy and bleed easily. There is an increase in gingivitis and periodontal disease, caused by oedema rather than by an increased presence of irritant particles of food. There is no consensus on whether pregnancy damages teeth.
- Gastric acid secretion has been found to be reduced during pregnancy, beginning early in pregnancy and increasing in late pregnancy, and peptic ulceration is rare in pregnant women.
- Gastric muscle tone and motility are reduced during pregnancy due to the effect of progesterone. The delay in emptying may also be due to the lower secretion of gastric juices, resulting in prolonged digestion time for solid food. Watery food is digested and passed on to the small intestine with little delay.
- The generalised relaxation of the gut is generally thought to be due to the high levels of circulating progesterone. However, low levels of circulating motilin have been found during pregnancy. During labour this sluggishness of the stomach's action leads to delayed emptying and a risk of acid aspiration.
- There is no increase in the absorption of food even though the metabolism of pregnant women is anabolic. Any increased nutrition must come from increased intake. Iron and calcium appear to be absorbed more readily. Constipation is a common complaint as the colon shares in the general relaxation of smooth muscle found throughout the body.

References

Blackburn ST, Loper DL. 1992 Maternal, Fetal and Neonatal Physiology, A Clinical Perspective. WB Saunders, Philadelphia.

Christofides ND, Ghatei MA, Bloom SR, Borberg C, Gillmer MDG. 1982 Decreased plasma motilin concentrations in pregnancy. British Medical Journal 285, 1453.

Hey VMF, Cowley DJ, Ganguli PC, Skinner LD, Ostick DG, Sharp DS. 1977 Gastrooesophageal reflux in late pregnancy. Anaesthesia 32, 372.

Hinchliff SM, Montague SE. 1990 Physiology for Nursing Practice. Baillière Tindall, London.

Hinchliff SM, Montague SE, Watson R. (eds) 1996 Physiology for Nursing Practice, 2nd edn. Baillière Tindall, London.

Hytten F. 1991 The alimentary system. In Hytten F, Chamberlain G (eds) Clinical Physiology in Obstetrics, 2nd edn. Blackwell Scientific, Oxford, pp 137–149.

Marieb EN. 1992 Human Anatomy and Physiology, 2nd edn. Benjamin/Cummings California

Montgomery TL, Pincus IJ. 1955 A nutritional problem in pregnancy resulting from extensive resection of the small bowel. American Journal of Obstetrics and Gynecology 69, 865.

Wingerson L. 1980 Gut feeling about peptides. New Scientist 85(1208) 16–18.

Recommended reading

Christofides ND, Ghatei MA, Bloom SR, Borberg C, Gillmer MDG. 1982 Decreased plasma motilin concentrations in pregnancy. British Medical Journal 285, 1453.

Hytten F. 1990 The alimentary system in pregnancy. Midwifery 6, 201–204.

Hytten F. 1991 The alimentary system. In Hytten F, Chamberlain G (eds) Clinical Physiology in Obstetrics, 2nd edn. Blackwell Scientific, Oxford, pp 137–149.

Chapter 22 The accessory digestive organs

In this chapter

INTRODUCTION

The alimentary system contains not only the gastrointestinal tract discussed in the previous chapter but associated and accessory organs. It is a rather artificial divide to separate out these accessory organs as their function is integrated into the system. However, the sheer complexity of the physiology may be better understood by this format. For instance, the salivary glands, the pancreas and the liver contribute to the process of digestion. The role of the liver in detoxification of drugs and ingested substances and the limitations to the protective role of the placenta are also discussed.

THE SALIVARY GLANDS

Three pairs of salivary glands produce the saliva that aids speech, chewing and swallowing: the parotid, submaxillary and sublingual glands. The **parotid glands** are the largest pair and are situated by the angle of the jaw. These glands produce a watery solution forming 25% of the daily saliva secretion. The **submaxillary glands** lie below the upper jaw and produce a thicker saliva which forms 70% of the total daily output. The **sublingual glands** lie under the tongue on the floor of the mouth and produce only 5% of the daily output. Their solution is rich in mucin which gives the saliva its sticky feel. Each day 1.5 litres of saliva is produced, consisting of 99% water with a pH of 7.0.

The functions of saliva

- It cleanses the mouth. It contains lysozyme which has an antiseptic action and the immunoglobulin IgA as a defence against microorganisms.
- It provides oral comfort, reducing friction and allowing speech.
- It ensures that food is in solution so that the taste buds can recognise the contained chemicals.

- It facilitates the formation of a bolus of partly broken-up food ready to swallow. The mucins present in saliva help to mould and lubricate the bolus.
- It contains a digestive enzyme, salivary (α) amylase (formerly know as ptyalin), which acts upon cooked starch to convert the polysaccharides into disaccharides.

Control of saliva production

The flow of saliva depends on parasympathetic supply from the facial nerve (7th cranial nerve) and glossopharyngeal nerve (9th cranial nerve). Parasympathetic stimulation produces copious watery secretions whilst sympathetic activity produces a sparse viscid secretion and the dry mouth most of us experience when we are nervous or following the administration of atropine or hyoscine which block receptor sites for the neurotransmitter acetylcholine (Hinchliff et al 1996).

The salivary nuclei are situated in the reticular formation in the floor of the 4th ventricle. Saliva is produced as a conditioned reflex in response to the cerebral perception of the thought, sight or smell of food. The presence of food in the mouth will also lead to saliva production – an unconditioned reflex where the impulse created by the physical presence of food in the mouth directly stimulates the salivary nuclei without the cerebral cortex being involved.

The ingested and masticated food must be propelled down the oesophagus into the stomach before the next stage, digestion of the food, can continue. The process is called **deglutition**. The tongue contracts and presses the bolus of food against the hard palate in the roof of the mouth. It then arches backwards and the bolus of food is propelled into the oropharynx. The food then enters the oesophagus and the process becomes involuntary due to the swallowing reflex which has its source in impulses located in the medulla.

THE PANCREAS

The pancreas, a gland lying just below the stomach, has both endocrine and exocrine functions It is a soft friable pink gland, 'tadpole' shaped, with a head surrounded by the C-shaped loop of the duodenum and a tail which extends towards the right side of the abdomen. Most of the pancreas is retroperitoneal. Through the centre of the pancreas runs the **pancreatic duct** which fuses with the common bile duct just before it enters the duodenum at the hepatopancreatic ampulla.

Exocrine functions of the pancreas

Within the pancreas are the **acini** which are clusters of cells surrounding small ducts. These provide the exocrine function and play a major role in digestion. The cells form and store **zygomen granules** which consist of a wide range of digestive enzymes that act on all nutrients. The enzymes are secreted into the pancreatic duct and then into the duodenum.

Pancreatic juice

The pancreatic enzymes were briefly mentioned in Chapter 21. About 1.5–2 litres of pancreatic juice are secreted daily with a pH of 8–8.4. A mixture of two types of secretions is produced: a copious watery solution and a scanty solution rich in enzymes. The profuse watery solution contains the ions hydrogen carbonate (bicarbonate), sodium, potassium, calcium, magnesium, chloride, sulphate and phosphate and some albumin and globulin proteins. The enzyme-rich secretion contains the following three proteolytic enzymes whose activity is summarised in Figure 22.1.

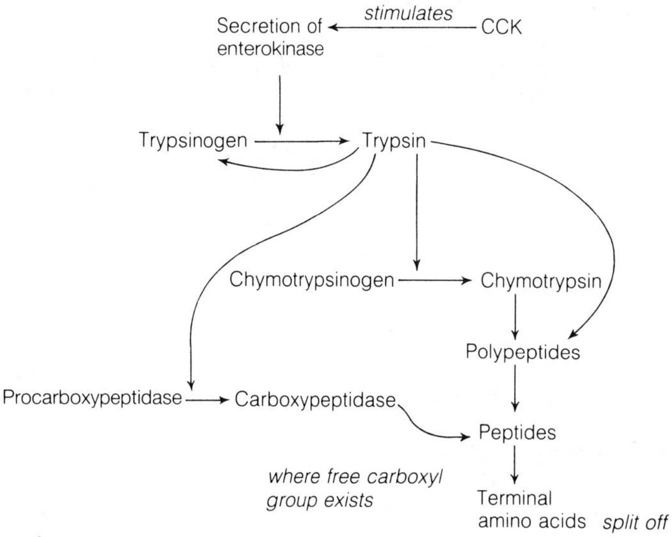

Figure 22.1 *Summary of activity of the pancreatic proteolytic enzymes (from Hinchliff SM, Montague SE, 1990, with permission).*

- **Trypsinogen**, which is in an inactive form to safeguard the gut from autodigestion.
- This is converted to **trypsin** by the enzyme enterokinase. Trypsin completes the breakdown of proteins to amino acids.
- **Carboxypeptidase**, which acts on peptides.

Other enzymes are:

- pancreatic amylase, which converts starch to maltose;
- pancreatic lipase, which breaks down triglycerides to three fatty acids and glycerol;
- ribonuclease (RNAase), which breaks down RNA;
- deoxyribonuclease (DNAase), which acts on DNA to release free nucleotides.

Control of pancreatic juice secretion

The hormones secretin and cholecystokinin were mentioned in Chapter 21. Secretin is produced by the S cells in the duodenum and upper jejunum when acid chyme enters the duodenum. This enters the venous systemic circulation and arrives back at the pancreas via the pancreatic artery. Its presence results in the secretion of the watery component which is rich in bicarbonate but low in enzymes.

Cholecystokinin (CCK), secreted by the columnar cells of the duodenum and jejunum in response to the presence of the products of protein and fat digestion, also circulates to return to the pancreas via the pancreatic artery. Its presence causes the release of the enzyme-rich secretion. It has many important functions.

Table 22.1 *The effects of insulin on foods*

On glucose	*On fat*	*On protein*	*On electrolytes*
Stimulates glucose utilisation Stimulates glycogen synthesis Inhibits glycogen breakdown Inhibits gluconeogenesis	Stimulates fatty acid and triglyceride synthesis Inhibits triglyceride breakdown	Stimulates the incorporation of amino acids into protein molecules	Stimulates the entry of potassium into cells

- Stimulation of the enzyme-rich pancreatic secretion.
- Augmentation of the activity of secretin.
- The slowing of gastric emptying and inhibition of gastric secretion.
- Stimulation of the secretion of enterokinase.
- Stimulation of glucagon secretion.
- Stimulation of motility of the small intestine and colon.
- Contraction of the gallbladder with the release of bile.

Endocrine function of the pancreas

Scattered among the acini are the **islets of Langerhans** that can be called mini-endocrine glands (Marieb 1992). About 1% of the pancreas consists of the islet cells. There are two types of cells: the α cells synthesise glucagon and a more numerous population of cells; the β cells produce insulin. The normal human pancreas produces about 40 IU of insulin in 24 h. The δ cells produce somatostatin which acts to suppress islet cell hormone production. A hormone called **amylin** appears to be an insulin antagonist (Marieb 1992).

Glucagon

Glucagon is a short polypeptide of 29 amino acids and is a strong hyperglycaemic agent. Marieb (1992) writes that one molecule of glucagon causes the release of 100 million molecules of glucose into the blood. Glucagon acts mainly in the liver to promote:

- glycogenolysis (the breakdown of glycogen to glucose);
- lypolysis;
- gluconeogenesis (the formation of glucose from fatty acids and amino acids).

The liver releases the glucose into the bloodstream, raising the blood sugar level. There is a fall in serum amino acid levels as the liver then takes up amino acids to synthesise new glucose molecules.

α cell secretion of glucagon is stimulated mainly by falling blood sugar levels. Increasing amino acid levels also stimulate glucagon release. Glucagon release is suppressed by increasing blood sugar levels and by somatostatin.

Insulin

Insulin is also a small polypeptide and consists of 51 amino acids. It begins as the middle part of a larger polypeptide chain called **proinsulin**. Enzymes cut amino acid bonds to release the functional hormone just before the insulin is secreted from the β cell. Insulin affects the metabolism of fats and protein as well as glucose.

Production of insulin

Insulin production is stimulated by glucose, amino acids and fatty acids in blood and hyperglycaemic agents such as glucagon, adrenaline, growth hormone, thyroxine or glucocorticoids. It is inhibited by somatostatin. Insulin binds firmly to a receptor site on the cell membrane and appears to modify cellular activity without entering the cell. The presence of calcium is necessary for its functioning (Boore 1996). A high-carbohydrate diet leads to increased tissue sensitivity to insulin and Turner & Williamson (1982) suggested that this may be due to a rise in the number of insulin receptors in the cell walls.

The role of insulin at cellular level

Insulin assists the entry of glucose into muscle cells, connective tissue cells and white blood cells but not into liver, kidney and brain cells, which have easy access to glucose regardless of insulin (Marieb 1992). Insulin counters any metabolic activity that would increase plasma glucose levels such as glycogenolysis and gluconeogenesis. These last effects are probably due to insulin inhibition of glucagon. Once glucose has entered the cells, insulin triggers enzyme activity which:

- catalyses the oxidation of glucose to produce ATP;
- joins glucose molecules together to form glycogen;
- converts glucose to fat, particularly in adipose tissue.

These processes will be considered in more detail in Chapter 23.

THE LIVER AND GALLBLADDER

The liver, which is one of the accessory organs and is associated with the small intestine, is one of the body's most important organs. Whilst it has many metabolic roles which will be discussed in the next chapter, its only digestive function is to secrete bile which it stores in the gallbladder and discharges into the duodenum. Bile acts on fats to emulsify it, i.e. to break it up into tiny particles so that it is more accessible to digestive enzymes.

Anatomy

The liver is a very large gland and weighs on average 1.4 kg. It is located in the abdominal cavity under the diaphragm, extending more to the right of the midline than the left, obscuring the stomach (Fig. 22.2). It lies totally protected by the rib cage. The liver has four lobes (Fig. 22.3):

1 the right lobe, which is the largest;
2 the smaller left lobe;

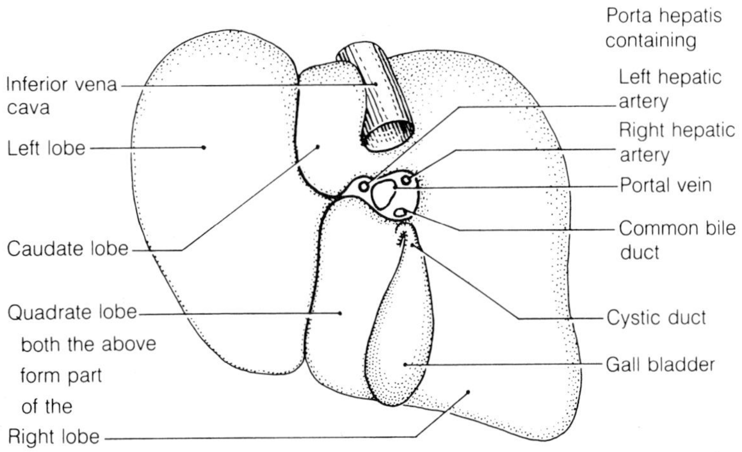

Figure 22.2 *The inferior surface of the liver showing the position of the four lobes (from Hinchliff SM, Montague SE, 1990, with permission).*

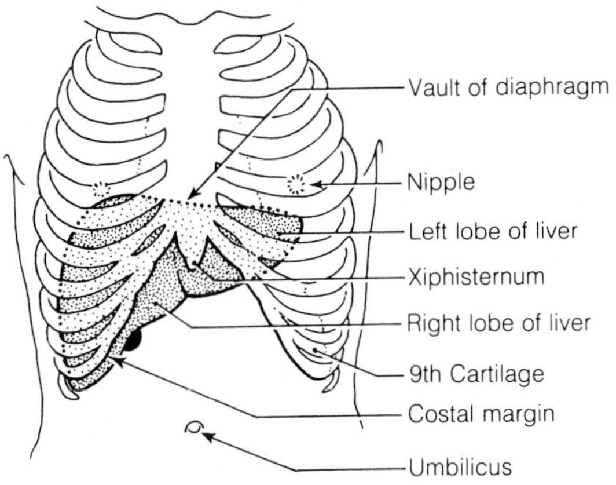

Figure 22.3 *The position of the liver in relation to the rib cage (from Hinchliff SM, Montague SE, 1990, with permission).*

3 the caudate lobe which is the posterior lobe;
4 the quadrate lobe which lies inferior to the left lobe.

The right lobe is the largest and is separated from the left lobe by a deep fissure. The right and left lobes are also separated by the **falciform ligament**, a cord of mesentery which suspends the liver from the diaphragm and the anterior abdominal wall. A fibrous remnant of the left umbilical vein, called the **ligamentum teres**, runs along the free edge of the falciform ligament. The superior aspect of the liver or bare area is fused to the diaphragm whilst the remainder of the organ is enclosed in visceral peritoneum. The lesser omentum anchors the liver to the lesser curvature of the stomach.

Microscopic anatomy

The liver is composed of small units called liver lobules. Lobules are small hexagonal cylinders consisting of plates of **hepatocytes** (epithelial liver cells). The hepatocytes produce bile, process bloodborne nutrients and play an important role in detoxification (see below). The hepatocytes radiate outwards from a central vein running along the longitudinal axis of the lobule. At each of the six corners of a lobule is a **portal triad**. The three structures present in the triad (Fig. 22.4) are:

1 a branch of the hepatic artery supplying arterial blood to the liver;
2 a branch of the hepatic portal vein (Fig. 22.5) carrying nutrient-rich blood from the digestive tract;
3 a bile duct.

The hepatic artery and the hepatic portal vein enter the liver at the **porta hepatis**. Between the hepatocyte plates are enlarged capillaries called **sinusoids**. Blood percolates through the sinusoids from both the hepatic artery and the hepatic portal vein and is collected up into the central veins. Inside the sinusoids are the **Kupffer cells**, hepatic macrophages which remove debris such as worn-out blood cells and bacteria from the blood.

Digestive functions

The liver produces bile and also enzymes which are able to detoxify many noxious substances which arrive at the organ via the bloodstream.

The production of bile

Bile produced by the hepatocytes flows into tiny channels called **bile canaliculi** and enters the bile duct branches in the portal triads. Collectively the hepatocytes produce as much as 1000 ml of bile daily or more if a fatty meal is taken. Blood and bile flow in opposite directions in the liver lobules (Fig. 22.6). The bile flows into the hepatic duct and, if needed by the digestive system, flows into the duodenum. If no bile is needed the sphincter of Oddi is tightly closed and bile flows through the cystic duct to be stored in the gallbladder (Fig. 22.7).

The gallbladder is a thinwalled muscular bag about 10 cm long which is situated in a fossa on the inferior surface of the right lobe of the liver. It stores secreted bile and concentrates it by absorbing water and ions. When empty, its walls are thrown into rugae to allow for distension. When the muscular wall contracts, bile is ejected into the cystic duct which leads to the common bile duct. It is covered with visceral peritoneum.

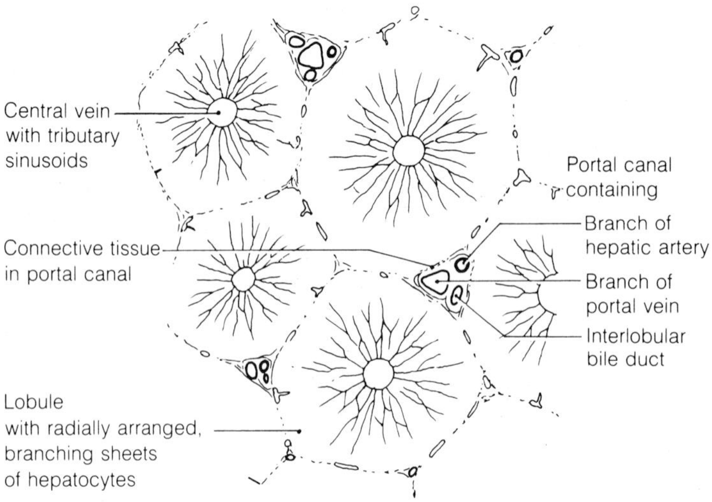

Figure 22.4 *The main features of the portal vein (from Hinchliff SM, Montague SE, 1990, with permission).*

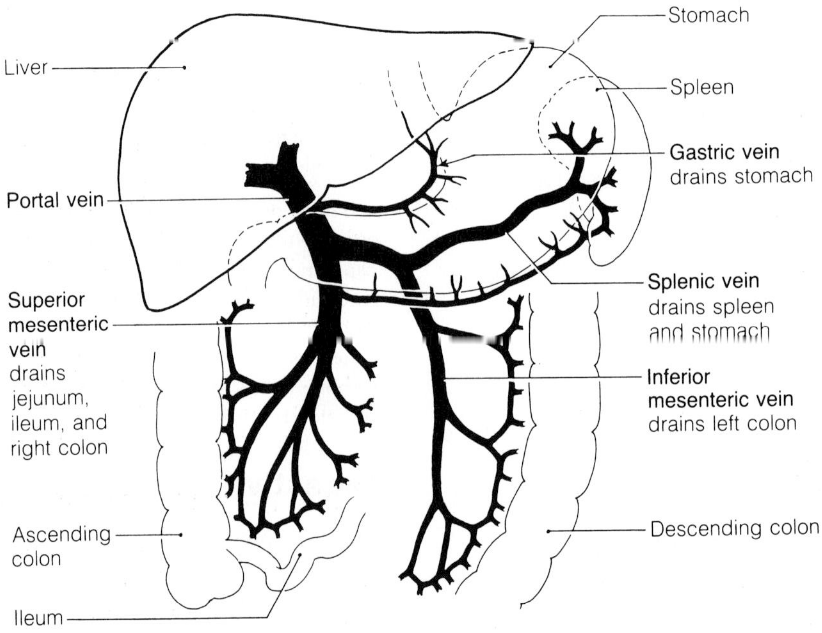

Figure 22.5 *The general features of the liver lobules at low magnification, showing the portal triad (from Hinchliff SM, Montague SE, 1990, with permission).*

Bile contains no digestive enzymes and its chief role in digestion is to emulsify fats so that they and the fat-soluble vitamins and iron can be absorbed. Bile is a viscous fluid coloured greeny-yellow to brown. It contains 97% water, 0.7% bile salts, mucin and bicarbonate. Also present in bile are fatty acids, lecithin, inorganic salts, alkaline phosphatase and the excretory products of steroid-based hormones. Bile is alkaline with a pH of 7.8–8.0.

Bile salts

Bile salts are formed from the steroids cholic and deoxycholic acid, manufactured in the liver from cholesterol. In the liver cholic acid is **conjugated** (joined together with the elimination of water) with the amino acids taurine and glycine to form taurocholic acid and glycocholic acid. The bile acids form salts with sodium and potassium which are in solution in the bile.

The functions of the bile salts are to:

- deodorise faeces;
- activate lipase and proteolytic enzymes in the duodenum;
- reduce the surface tension of fat droplets which helps to emulsify them.

Bile salts combine with lipids, lecithin and cholesterol to form micelles which are water soluble and allow fat to be absorbed more easily. If bile salts are absent about 25% of ingested fat will be lost in the stools. These stools will be bulky and have an offensive odour.

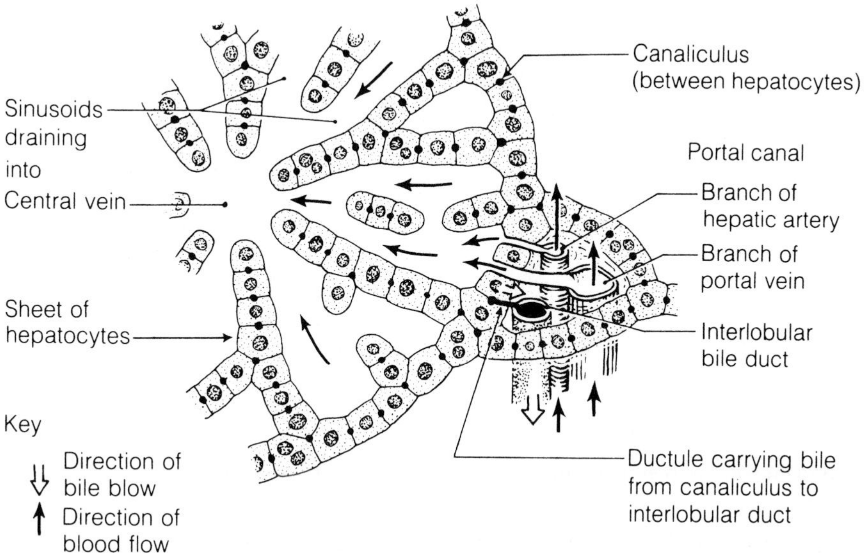

Figure 22.6 *The flow of blood and bile within the liver lobule (from Hinchliff SM, Montague SE, 1990, with permission).*

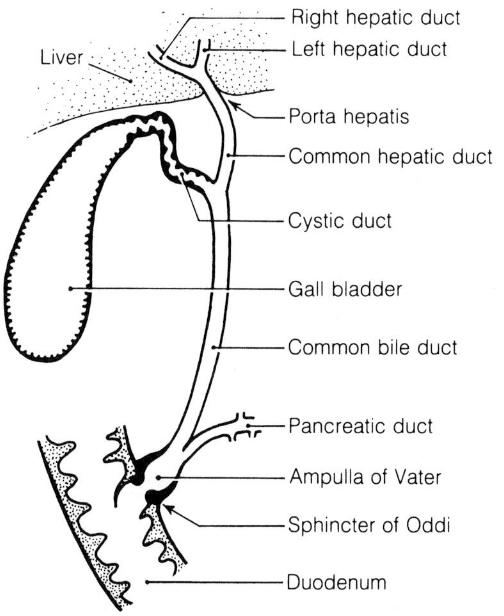

Figure 22.7 *The drainage of bile from the liver to the intestine (the biliary tract) (from Hinchliff SM, Montague SE, 1990, with permission).*

Bile pigments

The pigments make up 0.2% of the composition of bile. They are produced from the breakdown of red blood cells and are mainly bilirubin with a small amount of biliverdin. The pigments are taken to the liver bound to plasma albumin where they are conjugated with glucuronic acid in the presence of the enzyme glucuronic transferase. This forms the water-soluble bilirubin diglucuronide which enters bile to give it the golden colour. In the gut stercobilinogen is formed and, following conversion by bacterial action, is excreted as stercobilin. Some stercobilinogen is absorbed by the bloodstream and is then excreted as urobilinogen by the kidneys.

Control of bile secretion

As with other secretions into the gastrointestinal tract, the control of bile secretion involves neural and hormonal factors. CCK is the major controller, causing contraction of the gallbladder and relaxation of the sphincter of Oddi. Once the gallbladder has emptied its contents, further flow of bile into the duodenum occurs directly from the liver. Vagus nerve stimulation will bring about a similar action. About 97% of bile salts are reabsorbed into the portal circulation following their passage through the intestine and returned to the liver. This is called the **enterohepatic circulation of bile salts**. The production of bile by the liver depends on the blood level of bile salts. High blood levels stimulate the liver cells to secrete more bile.

Detoxification of ingested material

A second important function of the liver is the detoxification of ingested substances. Systems have evolved to protect humans from ingested poisons found especially in plants (see Chapter 7). This involves detoxification by enzyme systems and subsequent excretion of the byproducts by the liver. Any alteration in liver or kidney function may reduce the ability of the body to handle harmful chemicals. Many drugs are simply purified naturally occurring chemicals and even those synthesised in the laboratory will have similar chemical structures to naturally occurring substances.

The role of the liver in metabolism

The liver processes nearly every type of nutrient absorbed from the digestive tract. It also plays a major part in controlling plasma cholesterol levels. The hepatocytes carry out at least 500 metabolic functions. It would take a textbook devoted to the topic to begin to explore all the functions of the liver. That is why the liver is such an important organ. Major metabolic roles include:

- packaging fatty acids into forms that can be stored and transported;

- synthesising plasma proteins;
- formation of non-essential amino acids;
- converting ammonia, resulting from deamination of amino acids, to urea for excretion;
- storing glucose as glycogen;
- regulating blood sugar level by glycogenolysis and gluconeogenesis;
- storing vitamins;
- conserving iron from the breakdown of red blood cells;
- detoxifying substances such as alcohol or drugs.

ABSORPTION, DISTRIBUTION AND FATE OF DRUGS

Much of the content of this section is developed from Rang & Dale (1991). There are two main ways of describing how drugs are handled by the body. **Pharmacokinetics** is concerned with the way the body handles drugs and **pharmacodynamics** is concerned with the effect drugs have on the body function. Drugs are often given to patients to support a failing system or organ. Examples are the administration of insulin in diabetes mellitus when the pancreas is unable to make sufficient or any insulin of its own or the use of antibiotics to support the immune system in bacterial invasion. Drugs may also be used to control a function; for example, the administration of the contraceptive pill to control reproductive function. Drugs usually have the following attributes. They:

- bind to protein targets;
- exert chemical influences on one or more cellular components;
- may affect one or more tissues;
- may have agonist or antagonist effects.

The protein targets of drugs may be enzymes in metabolic reactions, carrier molecules on cell membranes, receptor molecules on cell membranes or ion channels in cell membranes.

Drug disposition

Drug disposition is the process of drug molecules behaviour in the body. There are four stages:

1. absorption from the site of administration;
2. distribution within the body;
3. metabolic alteration;
4. excretion from the body.

Absorption

Absorption is the passage of a drug from the site of administration into the plasma. Except for some topical applications and some inhaled substances, most drugs must enter the plasma to travel to target tissues. Drugs are absorbed at different rates from different sites and some may be unsuitable for some routes.

Distribution within the body (translocation)

There are two main phases in drug distribution. The first is **bulk flow transfer** which is the transport of drugs around the body by the circulatory system. Some drugs may be transported freely in solution but many are carried around the blood attached to a carrier molecule such as plasma albumin. At cellular level, **diffusional transfer** describes the carriage of drugs into the cells in a specific tissue. Diffusional transfer may be by:

- diffusion through the lipid cell membrane;
- diffusion through aqueous pores which traverse the lipid membrane;
- combination with a carrier molecule to ferry the drug across the membrane;
- pinocytosis to engulf the substance.

There is controversy over whether aqueous pores exist and, if they do, they are probably too small to allow entry of most molecules. Pinocytosis, where a piece of cell membrane surrounds the substance and draws it into the cell, concerns large biological molecules only.

Diffusion through the lipid membrane

This is one of the most important pharmacokinetic characteristics of a drug. Fat-soluble drugs diffuse across capillary walls and through cell membranes easily. Other determinants of diffusion include the pH of body fluids (acids and alkalis neutralise each other to precipitate a salt and water) and ionisation (drugs that are strongly ionised are not lipid soluble and may not be able to enter cells unaided).

Carrier mediation

Many drugs have specialised transport mechanisms to regulate entry and exit from cells. This usually involves a carrier molecule incorporated into the cell membrane. In facilitated diffusion, energy is not needed but in active transport the cell must use energy. Some pharmaceutical effects are the result of interference with the function of carrier proteins.

Drug metabolism in the liver

Drugs pass through the liver several times whilst they are in the circulation. Metabolic alteration of drug molecules involves two kinds of biochemical reactions brought about by liver enzymes. **Phase 1 reactions**, which may result in a more active or toxic metabolite of the drug, involve:

- oxidation – adding oxygen or removing hydrogen;
- reduction – adding hydrogen or removing oxygen;
- hydrolysis – splitting of the molecule into separate parts by water.

Phase 2 reactions involve conjugation by liver enzymes which results in a water-soluble inactive product ready for excretion.

Excretion of drugs

Drugs are mainly excreted by the kidney but may also be excreted in expired air, perspiration, faeces and breast milk. In pregnancy they may cross the placental barrier to the fetus. In the kidney there are three processes for excretion of drugs:

1 **glomerular filtration** – if drugs are free in the plasma, i.e. not bound to plasma proteins and if their molecular weight is below 20 000;
2 **active tubular secretion/reabsorption** – independent carrier systems are present in the cells of the proximal tubule for non-lipid soluble drugs or ionised drugs, one for acids and one for bases;
3 **passive diffusion across the tubular epithelium** – diffusion of lipid-soluble drugs occurs across the tubular and capillary cell membranes in the distal tubule and collecting tubule.

Drugs that are hydrophilic and poorly lipid soluble such as antibiotics do not enter cells readily. They have a lower density volume and are readily excreted by the kidney. Lipid-soluble drugs are readily reabsorbed in the renal tubule and need breaking down to water-soluble byproducts, usually in the liver, in order to be excreted.

MATERNAL ADAPTATIONS TO PREGNANCY

The pancreas

Although there is a slight decrease in serum amylase and lipase, this seems to have no significance. Much more significant are the alterations in glucose metabolism because of increasing insulin resistance. This may be enough to precipitate diabetes mellitus in susceptible women. Glucose metabolism will be discussed in Chapter 23 and diabetes in pregnancy in Chapter 35.

The gallbladder

Progesterone affects the muscle of the gallbladder wall so that its volume is increased and its emptying rate is decreased. There is an increased fasting volume which is probably due to decreased water absorption by the mucosa of the gallbladder. This change is due to reduced activity of the cell wall sodium pump which is a function of the increased circulating oestrogens. Alterations in gallbladder tone also lead to a retention of bile salts which may lead to pruritus (Blackburn & Loper 1992). Hytten (1991) states that it is widely accepted that pregnancy predisposes to gallstones but that there is little empirical evidence to support the belief.

The liver

Liver size and liver blood flow seem to be unchanged in pregnancy and no histological changes have been seen in pregnancy (Reynolds 1991). However, the liver is displaced superiorly, posteriorly and anteriorly by the growing uterus as pregnancy progresses. Although there is no change in blood flow to the liver there may be a reduction in the proportion of cardiac output to the liver of about 30% (Blackburn & Loper 1992).

There is an alteration in the production of plasma proteins, bilirubin, serum enzymes and serum lipids by the liver. Some changes arise from the presence of oestrogen and some from haemodilution. The changes reduce liver function and make normal testing of liver function less useful.

Hytten (1991) describes a reversible disturbance of liver function in pregnancy in women who are otherwise healthy. A small proportion of women taking the contraceptive pill show the same effect. There will be jaundice, histologically dilated bile canaliculi and increased bile viscosity. Increased phagocytosis by the Kupffer cells under the stimulus of oestrogen has been seen in primate studies and may occur in humans. Storage and mobilisation of liver glycogen may occur more rapidly because of the 50% increase in glomerular filtration rate.

PHARMACOKINETICS AND PREGNANCY

Health professionals who prescribe drugs must consider the likelihood of a woman being pregnant. Drugs taken in early pregnancy may be teratogenic, a prime example being the tragedy of thalidomide in the 1960s. Drugs given in late pregnancy may cause behavioural anomalies in children. Many women are unaware of the danger of taking over-the-counter drugs. Taking drugs in pregnancy may be essential for some women and their life and the life of the fetus may be endangered if the drugs are discontinued even though the drugs may be involved in causing abnormalities in the fetus. A good example would be epilepsy which may cause oral deformities.

Modification of pharmacokinetics

Ingestion

Many knowledgeable women will not comply with taking medicines in pregnancy. Nausea and vomiting may cause rejection of the drug.

Absorption

Most drugs are taken orally and are absorbed by the stomach and small intestine. Gastric motility is reduced throughout pregnancy and especially in labour. This slows down absorption of some drugs but may increase absorption of others. Most common drugs show little change from normal. Taking antacid preparations will lead to reduced absorption of some drugs.

Distribution

Increased extracellular fluid and body fat may alter the compartmental distribution of drugs. The fetus is considered to be a compartment and although probably resistant to bolus doses, may be at risk in long-term drug therapy of some chemicals.

Protein binding

Many drugs circulate around the body bound to plasma proteins, especially albumin which is reduced in pregnancy. There is an increase in some specific proteins such as transferrin and thyroid-binding hormone. Some drugs which bind to α-1 acid glycoprotein are more likely to cross the placenta.

Elimination

Drugs that act within the central nervous system or within cells are lipid soluble and cannot be effectively excreted without conjugation to water-soluble by products in the liver. Drugs excreted by the renal tubules will be excreted by the kidney.

The placenta and fetus

Almost all drug reactions carried out by the liver have been identified in placental tissue. However, no studies have been carried out in vivo. This means we cannot trust the placenta to protect the fetus from the effect of drugs. The main trophoblastic layer in the placenta is a syncytium and covered by a continuous lipid membrane. This membrane acts in a similar way to the blood – brain barrier so that lipid substances of low molecular weight (below 1000) can readily diffuse across the membrane. Water-soluble molecules of up to 100 MW can also diffuse easily but charged ionic molecules cannot pass unless they are bound to a carrier protein. This means that drugs that affect the central nervous system will readily cross the placental barrier.

Other drugs such as barbiturates, non-steroidal antiinflammatory agents, warfarin and anticonvulsants are weak acids whilst narcotics, local anaesthetics, β-blockers or β-stimulants are weak bases. These act as non-ionic substances and will cross the placental barrier slowly. Polar drugs such as the penicillins and cephalosporins are transferred so slowly that the fetus has no problem eliminating the drugs faster than they are transferred. Heparin is a large molecule and cannot cross the placenta. The fetus and neonate have a much reduced ability to handle drugs because of immaturity of liver enzyme systems.

Maternal elimination of polar non-lipid drugs is much faster during pregnancy as these are excreted by the kidney. This means that the dose requirements of some drugs such as anticonvulsants may rise during pregnancy. Some of these drugs cannot cross the placental barrier whilst others are excreted rapidly by the fetus and pose no problem. Some drugs, such as anticonvulsants, build up slowly in the fetus and may cause malformations. Maternal breakdown of lipid-soluble drugs is slower in pregnancy and these drugs readily cross the placenta into fetal tissues and may be excreted very slowly.

Summary of main points

- Three pairs of salivary glands produce saliva which aids speech, chewing and swallowing. Saliva contains lysozyme and immunoglobulin IgA as defence against microorganisms. A digestive enzyme, salivary (α) amylase acts upon cooked starch to convert polysaccharides into disaccharides.
- The flow of saliva depends on stimulation which produces copious watery secretions. Sympathetic activity produces a sparse viscid secretion and a dry mouth. Saliva is produced as a conditioned reflex when the salivary nuclei are stimulated in response to the perception of the thought, sight or smell of food. The presence of food in the mouth directly stimulates the salivary nuclei without the cerebral cortex being involved.
- The pancreas has both endocrine and exocrine functions. Within the pancreas the acini cells surrounding small ducts form and store zygomen granules which consist of a wide range of digestive enzymes that act on all nutrients. The pancreas produces 1.5–2 litres of alkaline pancreatic juice daily which is a mixture of two types of secretions: a copious watery solution containing ions and a scanty solution rich in three proteolytic enzymes – trypsinogen, trypsin and carboxypeptidase. Other pancreatic enzymes are amylase, lipase, ribonuclease and deoxyribonuclease.
- Secretin causes the secretion of the watery component. Cholecystokinin stimulates secretion of enzyme-rich pancreatic juice, augments the activity of secretin, slows gastric emptying, inhibits gastric secretion, stimulates secretion of enterokinase and glucagon, stimulates motility of the small intestine and colon and causes contraction of the gallbladder to release bile. Pancreatic juice secretion is divided into a cephalic phase, in response to food stimuli, and a gastric phase stimulated by the release of gastrin.
- About 1% of the pancreas consists of the islet of Langerhans cells. The α cells synthesise glucagon and the more numerous β cells produce insulin. The δ cells produce somatostatin which acts to suppress islet cell hormone production.
- Glucagon acts in the liver to promote glycogenolysis, lypolysis and gluconeogenesis. Insulin stimulates glucose utilisation, glycogen synthesis, inhibition of glycogen breakdown and inhibition of gluconeogenesis. It causes stimulation of fatty acid and triglyceride synthesis and inhibition of triglyceride breakdown. It leads to the incorporation of amino acids into protein molecules and stimulates the entry of potassium into cells. Insulin assists the entry of glucose into muscle, connective tissue and white blood cells, but not liver, kidney and brain cells.
- The liver is composed of small units called liver lobules consisting of plates of hepatocytes radiating outwards from a central vein. The hepatocytes produce bile, process bloodborne nutrients and play an important role in detoxification. At each of the six corners of a lobule is a portal triad containing a branch of the hepatic artery supplying arterial blood to the liver, a branch of the hepatic portal vein carrying nutrient-rich blood from the digestive tract and a bile duct
- Bile produced by the hepatocytes flows into tiny channels called bile canaliculi and enters the bile duct branches in the portal triads. The bile flows into the hepatic duct and if needed by the digestive system, flows into the duodenum. If no bile is needed the sphincter of Oddi is tightly closed and bile flows through the cystic duct to be stored in the gallbladder.
- Bile salts manufactured in the liver from cholesterol deodorise faeces, activate lipase and proteolytic enzymes in the duodenum and reduce the surface tension of fat droplets which helps to emulsify them. Bile pigments are produced from the breakdown of red blood cells and are mainly bilirubin with a small amount of biliverdin.
- The control of bile secretion involves neural and hormonal factors. CCK is the major controller, causing contraction of the gallbladder and relaxation of the sphincter of Oddi. High blood levels of bile salts stimulate the liver cells to secrete more bile.
- The liver detoxifies ingested substances by enzyme systems and excretes the byproducts. The liver processes nearly every type of nutrient absorbed from the digestive tract. Pharmacokinetics is concerned with the way the body handles drugs and pharmacodynamics is concerned with the effect drugs have on the body function.
- Drug disposition is the process of drug molecule behaviour in the body. There are four stages: absorption from the site of adminis-

tration, distribution, metabolic alteration and excretion. Drugs pass through the liver several times whilst they are in the circulation. Metabolic alteration of drug molecules involves two kinds of biochemical reactions brought about by liver enzymes.

- Drugs are mainly excreted by the kidney but may be excreted in expired air, perspiration, faeces and breast milk. In pregnancy they may cross the placental barrier to the fetus. Drugs that are water soluble do not enter cells readily and are excreted by the kidney. Lipid-soluble drugs are readily reabsorbed in the renal tubule and need conjugating in the liver to be excreted.
- Liver size and liver blood flow seem to be unchanged in pregnancy and no histological changes have been found. The liver is displaced by the growing uterus as pregnancy progresses. The production of plasma proteins, bilirubin, serum enzymes and serum lipids is altered in pregnancy. There is a reversible disturbance of liver function in pregnancy in women who are otherwise healthy. There will be jaundice, histologically dilated bile canaliculi and increased bile viscosity.
- Taking drugs in pregnancy may be essential for some women and their life and the life of the fetus may be endangered if the drugs are discontinued even though the drugs may be involved in causing abnormalities in the fetus.
- Most drugs are taken orally and are absorbed by the stomach and small intestine. Gastric motility is reduced throughout pregnancy and especially in labour. This slows down absorption of some drugs but may increase absorption of others. Most common drugs show little change from normal.
- Increased extracellular fluid and body fat may alter the compartmental distribution of drugs. The fetus is considered to be a compartment and although probably resistant to bolus doses, may be at risk in long-term drug therapy of some chemicals.
- Many drugs circulate around the body bound to plasma proteins, especially albumin which is reduced in pregnancy. There is an increase in some specific proteins such as transferrin and thyroid-binding hormone. Some drugs are likely to cross the placenta.
- Almost all drug reactions carried out by the liver have been identified in placental tissue. This means we cannot trust the placenta to protect the fetus from the effect of drugs. The fetus and neonate have a reduced ability to handle drugs because of immaturity of liver enzyme systems.
- Maternal elimination of polar non-lipid drugs is much faster during pregnancy as these are excreted by the kidney. This means that the dose requirements of some drugs, such as anticonvulsants, may rise during pregnancy. Maternal breakdown of lipid-soluble drugs is slower in pregnancy and these drugs readily cross the placenta into fetal tissues and may be excreted very slowly.

References

Blackburn ST, Loper DL. 1992 Maternal, Fetal and Neonatal Physiology, A Clinical Perspective. WB Saunders, Philadelphia.

Boore JRP. 1996 Endocrine function. In Hinchliff SM, Montague SE, Watson R (eds) Physiology for Nursing Practice, 2nd edn. Baillière Tindall, London.

Hinchliff SM, Montague SE. 1990 Physiology for Nursing Practice. Baillière Tindall, London.

Hinchliff SM, Montague SE, Watson R. (eds) 1996 Physiology for Nursing Practice, 2nd edn. Baillière Tindall, London.

Hytten F. 1991 The alimentary system. In Hytten F, Chamberlain G (eds) Clinical Physiology in Obstetrics, 2nd edn. Blackwell Scientific, Oxford, pp 137–149.

Marieb EN. 1992 Human Anatomy and Physiology, 2nd edn. Benjamin/Cummings Publishing, California.

Rang HP, Dale MM. 1991 Pharmacology. Churchill Livingstone, Edinburgh.

Reynolds F. 1991 Pharmacokinetics. In Hytten F, Chamberlain G (eds) Clinical Physiology in Obstetrics, 2nd edn. Blackwell Scientific, Oxford, pp 224–241.

Turner RC, Williamson DH. 1982 Control of metabolism and alterations in diabetes. In O'Riorden JLH (ed) Recent Advances in Endocrinology and Metabolism III. Churchill Livingstone, Edinburgh.

Recommended reading

Boore JRP. 1996 Endocrine function. In Hinchliff SM, Montague SE, Watson R (eds) Physiology for Nursing Practice, 2nd edn. Baillière Tindall, London, pp 202–244.

Hytten F. 1991 The alimentary system. In Hytten F, Chamberlain G (eds) Clinical Physiology in Obstetrics, 2nd edn. Blackwell Scientific, Oxford, pp 137–149.

Rang HP, Dale MM. 1991 Pharmacology. Churchill Livingstone, Edinburgh.

Reynolds F. 1991 Pharmacokinetics. In Hytten F, Chamberlain G (eds) Clinical Physiology in Obstetrics, 2nd edn. Blackwell Scientific, Oxford, pp 224–241.

Chapter

23 Nutrition and metabolism

In this chapter

NUTRITION

This section considers the need for various nutrients, their destination and metabolism at cellular level. Nutrients are utilised by the body for tissue growth, maintenance and repair. They can be divided into six categories: the three major nutrients are **carbohydrates**, **lipids** and **proteins**, **vitamins** and **minerals** are required in small amounts and **water** is usually considered as a food because of its role as a solvent. Most foods provide a combination of nutrients and water makes up 60% of the volume of food intake.

There are hundreds of molecules involved in maintaining good health. Many cells, especially those in the liver, can convert one type of food molecule to another but there are about 50 essential nutrients which cannot be manufactured by the body cells and therefore must be provided in the diet if the body is to synthesise the remainder (Marieb 1992).

Food groups

There are four food groups which must be eaten in order to provide a balanced diet.

- Grains
- Fruits and vegetables
- Meat and fish
- Milk (dairy) products

Tiran (1997) adds a 5th group – fats and sugary foods. These can be arranged in a pyramid showing the quantities in relation to the health benefits of consumption (Fig. 23.1). The three major nutrients, vitamins and minerals will be discussed below.

Carbohydrates

Most of the carbohydrate we eat comes from plants but a small amount is found as lactose in milk and glycogen in meats. The polysaccharide starch is found in grains, legumes such as peas

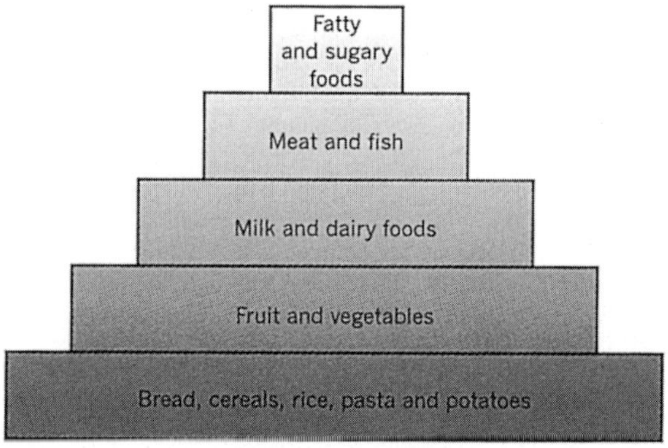

Figure 23.1 *The 'good food guide', showing the five main groups of food (from Sweet B, 1997, with permission).*

and root vegetables whilst the sugars, monosaccharides and polysaccharides, are found in fruits. Cellulose is a form of plant carbohydrate that the human digestive system cannot process. It provides roughage to increase the bulk of faeces, thus facilitating defaecation.

Lipids

The most common source of lipids is neutral fats in the form of triglycerides or triacylglycerols. Meat and dairy products contain saturated fats whilst unsaturated fats are found in seeds, nuts and most vegetable oils. Fats are also ingested as cholesterol found in egg yolk, meats and dairy products. All fats except for cholesterol are converted to fatty acids and triglycerides. The liver cannot synthesise linoleic acid, which is a component of lecithin, so that it is an essential component of the diet. This fatty acid and others are found in vegetable oil.

Fats are essential for many of the body's functions.

- The absorption of the fat-soluble vitamins.
- Triglycerides provide the major fuel for energy for hepatocytes and skeletal muscle. Phospholipids are a component of the myelin sheaths that surround larger nerves as well as all cell membranes.
- Fatty deposits act as protective cushions for the eye and kidney.
- They provide an insulating layer under the skin.
- Some regulatory molecules called prostaglandins are formed from linoleic acid and play a role in smooth muscle contraction and inflammatory responses.

Proteins

The best source of essential amino acids is found in animal products. Eggs, meat and milk proteins are complete proteins that meet all the body's requirements for essential amino acids. Proteins found in legumes, nuts and cereals are nutritionally incomplete and are low in one or more of the essential amino acids. Strict vegetarians can obtain all the essential amino acids by varying their diet carefully. For instance, cereals and legumes contain all the essential amino acids when taken together. An example of such a meal is West Indian rice and peas.

Proteins include important structural molecules such as muscle protein, collagen and elastin in connective tissue and keratin in skin. Proteins also function as hormones, enzymes and transport molecules such as haemoglobin. Amino acids can be used to synthesise proteins or can be converted to glucose to provide energy. These uses depend on:

- the concurrent presence within the cell of all the amino acids needed to manufacture a protein;
- adequacy of calorie intake in the form of carbohydrates and fats for energy production;
- nitrogen balance which is the balance between protein synthesis and protein breakdown;
- the influences of hormones – anabolic hormones such as growth hormone and the sex hormones stimulate tissue growth whilst the glucocorticoids produced in stress enhance protein breakdown and the conversion of amino acids to glucose.

The amount of protein needed in the diet is influenced by age, size, metabolic rate and nitrogen balance. There is a recommended intake of 0.8 g per kg body weight in non-obese individuals. This is equivalent to 2 ounces of fish or meat and a glass of milk daily. Meat eaters in the developed countries eat far in excess of the daily requirement whilst some people in the developing countries rarely eat meat.

Vitamins

Vitamins are organic compounds needed in small amounts for growth and health (Marieb 1992). They mainly function as coenzymes to assist in the catalysis of chemical processes in the body. The human body is unable to synthesise most vitamins with the exception of vitamin K and some of the B vitamins. Some vitamins are fat soluble, such as A, D, E and K, and are absorbed bound to digested lipids. The water-soluble vitamins, such as most of the B complex and vitamin C, are absorbed with water from the gastrointestinal tract. A normal varied diet should provide all the vitamins. Excessive intake can create as many health problems as insufficient intake. The following paragraphs outline the chemical nature of the vitamins, the source of vitamins, their use in the body and the results of deficiency.

Fat-soluble vitamins

Vitamin A – retinol

Vitamin A is stored in the liver, is easily oxidised and destroyed rapidly by light. The recommended daily dose (RDA) should not be exceeded in pregnancy (DHSS 1990) and pregnant women should avoid liver and liver products.

Sources

Vitamin A is found in fish liver oils, egg yolk, liver and fortified milk and margarine and in deep yellow and deep green leafy vegetables. It is formed in the body from the provitamin **carotene** in the intestine, liver and kidneys.

Importance in body

Needed for synthesis of photoreceptor pigments, stability of cell membranes, skin and mucous membranes, tooth and bone development, reproduction. Absorption from the diet is impeded by alcohol, coffee and vitamin D deficiency.

Deficiency

May cause anaemias, blindness, skin disorders, tooth decay and gastrointestinal disorders. Birth defects have occurred in women taking supplements or eating excessive amounts such as in liver. It is thought that retinol is a teratogenic agent (Ranjan 1991).

Vitamin D – antirachitic factor

Vitamin D is a sterol stored in liver and skin and stable to heat and light. Routine supplementation of vitamin D in pregnancy is not recommended. Theoretically, dark-skinned immigrants to Britain or those who avoid dairy produce may be prone to deficiency.

Sources

It is produced in skin by irradiation with ultraviolet light and modified to the active form in the liver. Vitamin D is found in fish liver oils, egg yolk, liver and fortified milk. Laxatives and antacids may inhibit absorption from the gut.

Importance in body

Acts as a hormone to increase calcium blood levels and is essential for bones and teeth. It is also needed for renal, cardiac and nervous system functions and is involved in blood clotting.

Deficiency

Deficiency causes poor mineralisation of bones and teeth such as rickets in children and osteomalacia in adults. There may be poor muscle tone, restlessness and irritability.

Vitamin E – antisterility factor

Compounds called tocopherols (approximate meaning: to bring forth children). It is chemically related to sex hormones, stored in muscle and adipose tissue and is heat and light resistant. It is an antioxidant, unstable in oxygen.

Sources

Vitamin E is found in vegetable oils, margarine, whole grains and dark green leafy vegetables. It is destroyed by food processing, rancid fats and oils and inorganic iron. Absorption is reduced by the contraceptive pill.

Importance in body

It is required in many body functions, including reproduction. It may assist in holding the ageing process at bay.

Deficiency

Deficiency may result in spontaneous abortion, preterm labour and stillbirth.

Vitamin K – coagulation vitamin

A quinone with small amounts stored in the liver. Heat resistant but destroyed by acids, alkalis, light and oxidising agents.

Sources

Vitamin K is synthesised by coliform bacteria in the large intestine. Food sources include leafy green vegetables and pork liver. Vitamin K production by the bacteria is antagonised by anticoagulant drugs and by antibiotics.

Importance in body

It is essential for the formation of clotting proteins and some other proteins in the liver.

Deficiency

Deficiency is rare in normal health but easy bruising and bleeding occur due to prolonged clotting time.

Water-soluble vitamins

Vitamin C – ascorbic acid

Vitamin C is a 6-carbon crystalline substance derived from glucose. Unlike other primates, humans cannot synthesise vitamin C and must take it in with food. It is rapidly destroyed by heat, light and alkalis.

Sources

Vitamin C is found in fruits and vegetables, particularly in citrus fruits, strawberries, tomatoes and fresh potatoes. Some drugs, such as aspirin, anticoagulants, antibiotics, diuretics, cortisone, the contraceptive pill and antidepressants, may interfere with absorption, as may pollution, industrial toxins, overcooking or poor food storage (Tiran 1997).

Importance in body

It is essential for the health of all cells in all systems. It facilitates the absorption of iron and the metabolism of amino acids.

Deficiency

Deficiency can cause poor resistance to bacterial infections, anaemia, bruising and haemorrhage, oedema, poor digestion and gum disease. This combination of symptoms, if severe, is called scurvy.

Vitamin B_1 – thiamin

This member of the B group vitamins is an antioxidant which is rapidly destroyed by heat. A small amount can be stored while excess is eliminated in urine.

Sources

Vitamin B_1 is found in lean meat, liver, eggs, whole grains, nuts, leafy green vegetables and legumes. Its absorption will be reduced by alcohol, coffee, food additives and overcooking.

Importance in body

It helps to maintain healthy nerves, cardiac muscle and digestive tract and forms part of an enzyme which acts in carbohydrate metabolism (the transformation of pyruvic acid to acetyl CoA).

Deficiency

Deficiency causes the disease beri-beri with gastrointestinal disturbance, peripheral nerve disorders, cramping of calf muscles and numbness of feet. There may be enlargement of the heart with tachycardia. The full-blown disease is rarely seen in developed countries.

Vitamin B_2 – riboflavin

This member of the B group vitamins is similar in structure to ribose sugar. A small amount can be stored while excess is eliminated in urine.

Sources

Vitamin B_2 is found in lean meat, yeast, liver, eggs, whole grains, nuts, meats and legumes. Its absorption is reduced by the contraceptive pill and antibiotics.

Importance in body

It forms part of enzymes which help to metabolise fats, carbohydrates and proteins.

Deficiency

Deficiency causes the disease pellagra with listlessness, headache, weight loss, loss of appetite and later, soreness and redness of the lips and tongue, vomiting and diarrhoea and skin ulceration. Neurological symptoms may also occur. This disease is rarely seen in developed countries.

Vitamin B_3 – niacin (nicotinamide)

This member of the B group vitamins is a simple, stable organic compound. A small amount can be stored and daily intake is desirable. Excess is eliminated in urine.

Sources

Vitamin B_3 is found in any protein food. It can easily be synthesised in the body from the amino acid tryptophan. Its absorption is reduced by alcohol, coffee, antibiotics and antitubercular drugs.

Importance in body

It forms part of enzymes which help to metabolise fats, carbohydrates and proteins.

Deficiency

Deficiency causes the disease pellagra (see Vitamin B_2 above).

Vitamin B6 – pyridoxine

This member of the B group vitamins occurs in free and phosphorylated forms in the body. It is stable to heat and acids but destroyed by alkalis and light. Body stores are limited and excess is eliminated in urine.

Sources

Vitamin B_6 is found in meat and fish. Limited amounts are found in potatoes and tomatoes. Its absorption is reduced by antibiotics and antitubercular drugs as well as the contraceptive pill.

Importance in body

It forms part of enzymes which help to metabolise proteins, for glycogenolysis and for the formation of antibodies and haemoglobin.

Deficiency

Deficiency causes convulsions, irritability, vomiting and abdominal pain in infants and dermatitis and depression in adults.

Vitamin B_{12} – cyanocobalamin

This member of the B group vitamins is complex and contains cobalt. It is stable to heat but inactivated by acids and alkalis.

Sources

Vitamin B_{12} is found in meat, fish, eggs and butter. It is not found in any vegetable or fruit. Its absorption is reduced by aspirin and the contraceptive pill.

Importance in body

It is the intrinsic factor necessary for the transportation of iron across the intestinal membrane. It is stored in the liver with stores sufficient to last 3–5 years in normal health. It is also involved in enzymes forming DNA in the bone marrow. In its absence, erythrocytes do not divide.

Deficiency

Deficiency causes pernicious anaemia. Women who are strict vegetarians are at risk.

Folic acid

This is a crystalline mineral which is stable in heat but easily oxidised in acidic solutions. It is stored mainly in the liver.

Sources

Folic acid is found in liver, yeast, eggs, whole grain and deep green vegetables and nuts. It is also synthesised in the gut by enteric bacteria. Absorption is hindered by alcohol and folic acid antagonists such as anticonvulsants, aspirin and sulphonamides.

Importance in body

It is essential for the formation of red blood cells. It is necessary for the health of the nervous system and in the development of the fetus.

Deficiency

Folic acid is needed for the production of the red cell membranes and in deficiency megaloblastic anaemia occurs. An increased incidence of fetuses with neural tube defects occurs in women who are deficient in folic acid (see Chapter 15).

Minerals

The body requires adequate supplies of seven minerals and traces of about 12 others. The seven are calcium, phosphorus, potassium, sulphur, sodium, chloride and magnesium. Minerals constitute about 4% of the body's weight. Most are found in solution in body fluids or are bound to organic molecules such as iron in the formation of haemoglobin. Calcium and phosphorus are found in bone, adding strength to the structure, and they make up three-quarters of the amount. These are discussed in Chapter 24. Iron is discussed in Chapter 16 and sodium and potassium in Chapter 20.

REGULATION OF FOOD INTAKE

When energy intake and energy output are balanced, body weight remains stable. If intake exceeds output, weight is gained. If output exceeds intake, weight is lost. There appear to be body mechanisms that control intake and enable most people to maintain a steady weight. However, no such regulator has been found. Current theories, according to Marieb (1992), involve four factors:

- nutrient signals related to body energy stores;
- hormones;
- body temperature;
- psychological factors.

METABOLISM

Nutrients are involved in a great many processes within the cells. These biochemical reactions are known collectively as metabolism. Metabolic processes are either **anabolic**, in which molecules are built up, or **catabolic**, which involves the breakdown of complex substances to simpler ones. There are three major stages involved in metabolism:

Box 23.1 The Ob gene

In 1995 Friedman and his team at Rockefeller University in New York (see Cohen 1996), researching a gene called Ob which produces a hormone called **leptin**, found that a strain of overweight mice with insufficient leptin in their blood became obese. Leptin seemed to be involved in the regulation of the balance between fat stored and fat excreted in mice. Obese mice given leptin quickly reduced to normal weight (Gibbs 1996). The findings created much interest because of the prevalence of obesity in Western societies.

Cohen (1996) reported that Comings, a geneticist at the City of Hope National Medical Center in Duarte, California, and his team recruited 211 people of various weights and ages for a study into obesity. They found that although the Ob gene was present in humans it was not strongly related to obesity. Also, unlike the rats, obese humans seemed to have too much leptin rather than too little. A minority of the volunteers carried abnormally short Ob genes but not in the part of the gene that codes for leptin. The abnormality seemed to be in the part of the gene coding for the rate at which leptin is produced.

There was a statistical correlation between having two copies of the shortened Ob gene and excess weight in women between the ages of 26 and 30. However, the most significant finding in humans having two copies of the short Ob gene was seen in the psychological profile questionnaire. There was a correlation with depression, regardless of the sex and age of the person. This shortened gene has also been found in alcoholics and it is thought that it may be related to predisposition to addiction. People with the two Ob genes may need to eat more to obtain the same satisfaction as slimmer people. This field of research still has much to discover but may be of value in understanding and managing obesity in the future.

- **stage 1** is digestion, discussed in Chapter 22;
- **stage 2** occurs in the cytoplasm where the nutrients delivered to the cells are involved in either anabolic processes, with incorporation into cellular molecules, or catabolic processes, being broken down to pyruvic acid and acetyl CoA;
- **stage 3** is almost entirely catabolic and is the production of adenosine triphosphate (ATP) in cellular respiration.

Nutritional states

There are two nutritional states: the **absorptive** state when nutrients are being eaten and absorbed by the digestive tract and the **postabsorptive** state when the GI tract is empty and energy requirements are met by breakdown of body stores. The absorptive state lasts for about 4 h after a reasonable meal has been eaten. If three meals are eaten in the day there is a balance between the two states, each occupying about half of a 24 h period. Insulin directs the events of the absorptive state, mainly by its control of blood glucose levels.

The body can be maintained in the postabsorptive state for days or weeks in a famine or during illness as long as sufficient water is taken. Glucose is made generally available to cells via the bloodstream by glycogenolysis in the liver. Muscle glycogen cannot be broken down to glucose because it lacks the enzymes. It is partly oxidised to pyruvic acid or, in anaerobic conditions, to lactic acid. These substances enter the blood and are converted to glucose by the liver. The hormone glucagon is released when blood sugars become too low. Glucagon targets the liver and adipose tissue to enable glucose to be released into the blood.

ATP synthesis

As a student, the author was fascinated by the concept of the storage of energy from food as ATP. Energy is stored in carbon-hydrogen bonds in ingested food but the body cells cannot use energy in this form. They must convert it into the high-energy phosphate bonds of ATP (Sherwood 1989). ATP consists of adenosine with three phosphate groups attached. When a bond between adenosine (one of the nucleotides) and one of the phosphate groups is split, large amounts of energy are released and adenosine diphosphate + an inorganic phosphate molecule (P_1) is formed. Some of the energy produced is in the form of heat and helps to maintain the temperature of the body.
This can be written as:

Splitting by hydrolysis

$$ATP \rightarrow ADP + P_1 + \text{energy}$$

Carbohydrate metabolism

The Krebs or tricarboxylic acid or citric acid cycle

When glucose in the circulating blood arrives at the tissues it is taken up by the cells by facilitated diffusion under the influence of insulin. Glucose is taken to the mitochondria of the cells where it is oxidised to form energy in the Krebs cycle (Figs 23.2 and 23.3). No less than nine reactions are involved when glucose, which is a 6-carbon molecule, is broken down into two 3-carbon molecules of pyruvic acid, a process called **glycolysis**.

Pyruvic acid is broken down further to a 2-carbon molecule called **acetic acid** and the released carbon atom forms carbon dioxide by combining with oxygen. The acetic acid now combines with coenzyme A (a derivative of a B complex vitamin, pantothenic acid) to form the enzyme acetyl CoA. Acetyl CoA enters the Krebs cycle to undergo changes mediated by enzymes. ATP, water and carbon dioxide are formed in the process of oxidation.

The Krebs citric acid cycle consists of a series of eight separate biochemical reactions. This cycle of reactions is like one revolution of a wheel with acetyl CoA sitting at the top. Each glucose molecule produces two pyruvic acid molecules and allows two turns of the cycle. As well as carbon dioxide produced when the excess carbon atoms unite with oxygen, excess hydrogen atoms need to be disposed of. Two hydrogen carrier molecules, nicotinamide adenine dinucleotide (NAD) and flavine adenine dinucleotide (FAD), perform this function. The transfer of the hydrogen atoms converts the compounds into NADH and $FADH_2$ respectively.

Cellular respiration

Aerobic cellular respiration

Only six molecules of ATP are produced for each turn of the Krebs cycle – two from glycolysis and four from the cycle itself.

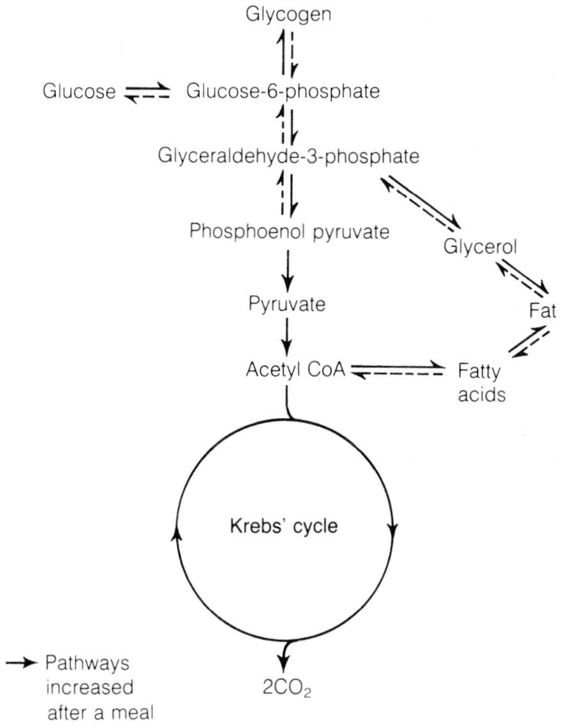

Figure 23.2 *A summary of glucose metabolism after a meal (from Hinchliff SM, Montague SE, 1990, with permission).*

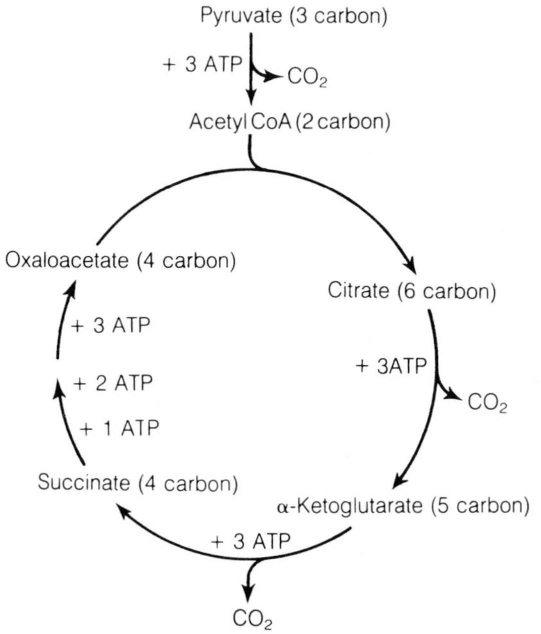

Energy released:

from pyruvate	15 ATP
from 2 × pyruvate formed from 1 glucose molecule	30 ATP
from glycolysis of 1 glucose molecule to 2 × pyruvate	8 ATP
Total from aerobic metabolism of 1 glucose molecule	38 ATP

Figure 23.3 *A summary of the Krebs cycle (from Hinchliff SM, Montague SE, 1990, with permission).*

The main role of the cycle is to prepare the hydrogen acceptors for entry into the electron transport chain (respiratory chain) in the inner mitochondrial membrane. This entry leads to the main bulk of ATP being produced as energy is released from the hydrogen atoms. The electron transfer molecules are proteins bound to metallic atoms. Most are brightly coloured iron-containing pigments called **cytochromes**. They are arranged in a specific order on the inner membrane which allows high-energy electrons to pass through a chain of reactions, resulting in a lowering of the energy levels with each step. At the end of this chain, the electrons are passed to the final electron acceptor which is inspired oxygen.

The stepwise release of energy during this progression through the electron transport chain is used to pump protons into the intermembrane space. This creates an electrochemical proton gradient across the inner membrane of the mitochondrion which temporarily stores the energy. Protons flow back across the membrane through the enzyme ATP synthetase, providing the electrical energy to attach a phosphate group to ADP to create a further 32 ATP molecules for each glucose molecule processed.

The total production of ATP for one turn of the cycle is therefore 38 molecules. NAD and FAD are released to capture more hydrogen and begin the energy transfer again. The hydrogen atoms contain electrons that exist at high energy levels. This process, which uses oxygen and phosphate, is called **oxidative phosphorylation** or aerobic respiration (Marieb 1992).

Anaerobic cellular respiration

If there is no oxygen available, a few molecules of ATP are synthesised during glycolysis but the process cannot proceed further. Only two molecules of ATP are available for each glucose molecule. This is called **substrate-level phosphorylation** (Marieb 1992). The energy remains trapped in the molecules of pyruvic acid and lactic acid is formed (anaerobic respiration), creating an oxygen debt as extra oxygen will be needed to remove the lactic acid.

ATP is produced more rapidly from glycolysis during anaerobic respiration and is useful for short bursts (20–30 s) of strenuous muscle activity. Most of the lactic acid diffuses out of the muscles into the bloodstream to create metabolic acidosis (Sherwood 1989). When oxygen becomes available the lactic acid is gradually reconverted to pyruvic acid and fed into the Krebs cycle.

Lipid metabolism

Fats are the body's most concentrated source of energy. The energy obtained from fat breakdown or **lypolysis** is twice that obtained from the metabolism of glucose or protein, providing 9 kcal per g in contrast to only 4 kcal per g of the other two nutrients. About 80 g of fat is absorbed daily, mainly in the duodenum. Any excess fat is stored as adipose tissue in subcutaneous and retroperitoneal tissue. When fat stores are needed for energy production, they are mobilised from the stores under the influence of growth hormones or cortisol. They are taken to the liver where the triglycerides are broken down into free fatty acids and glycerol which are released into the blood for use by the cells.

The glycerol is converted to one of the intermediate products of glycolysis called **glyceraldehyde phosphate** and is thus assimilated into the energy-releasing process. Further oxidation of the fatty acids releases the 2-carbon acetic acid which is fused to coenzyme A to form acetyl CoA which then enters the Krebs cycle. Fatty acids cannot be used for gluconeogenesis because they enter the cycle beyond the pyruvic acid stage when the changes are irreversible.

The fatty acids are converted to acetyl CoA in the presence of oxygen and glucose and these enter the Krebs citric acid cycle. If no glucose is available, such as in starvation or diabetes mellitus, acetyl CoA accumulates and the liver converts the molecules to ketone bodies, i.e. **acetoacetic acid** and **β-hydroxybutyric acid**, which accumulate in the blood. These can be oxidised to release energy but metabolic acidosis will occur.

Cholesterol

Bile salts, steroid hormones and cell membranes are formed from cholesterol. Cholesterol is found in the blood, mainly in combination with a protein carrier, as lipoproteins, of which there are three types:

- high-density lipoproteins (HDLs);
- low-density lipoproteins (LDLs);
- very low-density lipoproteins (VLDLs).

It is also thought that cholesterol is laid down as atheromatous plaques in arterial walls in the form of LDLs and VLDLs. A high ratio of HDLs to LDLs and VLDLs may offer protection against ischaemic heart disease. The ratio of HDLs to LDLs and VLDLs has been shown to be increased in vegetarians, people whose fat intake is largely unsaturated and those who take regular exercise but reduced in smokers.

Amino acid metabolism

At least 50 g a day is needed to maintain nitrogen balance and to provide for growth and repair of tissues. Amino acids cannot be stored by the body. However, the liver can interconvert amino acids by utilising the eight essential amino acids to synthesise the non-essential amino acids. Any excess amino acids are broken down by the liver by a process of deamination. The nitrogen portion is converted into urea which enters the blood and is excreted by the kidney.

Proteins are needed by the body for the following functions.

- Development, growth and the formation of new cells.
- Manufacture of enzymes, hormones and antibodies.
- The transport molecules such as haemoglobin.
- Plasma proteins which act as buffers to maintain acid/base balance.
- The control of osmotic pressure between body fluid compartments.
- Amino acids can be used in gluconeogenesis once glucose stores are depleted.

Metabolic rate and body heat production

The metabolic rate of the body is its energy use per time unit, usually calculated per hour. The basal metabolic rate (BMR) can be calculated by taking measurements during the postabsorptive state with the person at rest in a thermoneutral environment that requires no energy expenditure to maintain body warmth. The BMR is reported as the number of kilocalories needed to maintain normal body functions. In general, the younger the person, the higher the BMR. Males have a higher BMR than females because of the ratio of metabolically active muscle to the metabolically sluggish fatty tissue.

The total metabolic rate (TMR) is the rate of kilocalorie consumption that is needed for all activities. Even slight increases in muscle work can cause remarkable leaps in metabolic rate and heat production. Ingestion of food also increases the metabolic rate. This is called **dietary** or **food-induced thermogenesis**. The extra use of energy is probably due to the activity of the liver as nutrient absorption is carried out.

Regulation of body temperature

Humans are **homeothermic**, that is, they are warm blooded. The maintenance of body temperature depends on the balance between heat production and heat loss. The body temperature of humans is usually maintained within a range of 36.1–37.8°C independently of external environment or internal heat production. Body temperature rarely varies during the day by more than 1°C and is usually lowest in the early morning and highest in the afternoon or early evening. This temperature is optimum for enzyme activity.

A raise in body temperature increases enzyme activity and most adults will have convulsions when their temperature reaches 41°C and die if their temperature exceeds 43°C. Temperature varies slightly depending on where in the body it is recorded. The body's core (organs within the body's cavities) has the highest temperature and the shell (heat loss surface of the skin) has the lowest temperature. Rectal temperature is nearer the core than oral temperature. The hypothalamus is the major heat-regulating centre. It receives input from both peripheral thermoreceptors in the skin and central thermoreceptors in the core. Like a thermostat, the hypothalamus responds to any heat change by initiating heat promotion or heat loss mechanisms.

Radiation is the loss of heat as infrared waves from a warm object into a cooler environment. Normally about half of the heat produced by the body is lost as radiation. **Conduction** is the transfer of heat between objects in direct contact with each other. **Convection** is the transfer of heat to the environment caused by the heat rising and displacing cooler air in a continuous process. **Evaporation** is the escape of water from the surface of the body as gas. Water absorbs much of the surface heat which accompanies the evaporating gas.

Box 23.2 Body temperature – balance between loss and gain

Heat production	Heat loss
Ingestion of foods	Radiation
Basic metabolic rate	Conduction
Muscular activity and shivering	Convection
External temperature	Evaporation

Heat-promoting mechanisms include:

- vasoconstriction of cutaneous skin vessels mediated by the sympathetic nervous system;
- an increase in metabolic rate mediated by adrenaline and thyroxine;
- shivering;
- enhancement of thyroxine release;
- taking up a position that reduces heat loss from body surfaces, such as the fetal position.

Heat loss mechanisms include:

- vasodilation of cutaneous blood vessels by inhibition of the vasomotor nerve supply;
- sweating;
- seeking a cooler environment;
- maintaining an open body posture to maximise evaporation from limbs and body trunk skin surfaces.

MATERNAL ADAPTATIONS TO PREGNANCY

Nutrition

Tiran (1997) reminds us that there has been much recent research into the effects of poor nutrition on the fetus. There is a relationship between poor intake of essential nutrients and a higher than normal perinatal morbidity and mortality. Fetal growth may be compromised with an increase in preterm delivery and a decrease in weight for gestational age. Luke (1994) suggests this may be due to low placental weight. The implications of low birth weight in the causation of diabetes mellitus and hypertension have been postulated by Barker (1992). The importance of diet in preconception care is discussed in Chapter 7.

Specific requirements of pregnancy

There is a need for more nutrients to supply the increase in maternal tissue, such as the growth of the uterus and breasts, and to meet the needs of the fetus. The estimated extra need in pregnancy is about 250 kcal/day. It is probable that this could be met by reducing energy expenditure without increasing intake.

Protein

Proteins are needed for many functions in the body during normal health and are required in larger quantities in pregnancy (Tiran 1997). The quality of protein intake depends on both the type and quantity of food eaten and the conditions under which it is eaten. For example, if the total energy supplied by the diet is so low that gluconeogenesis utilises amino acids to provide energy, the ability to construct new tissue will be reduced. The average pregnant woman in Britain will need an extra 8.5 g of dietary protein daily (Hytten 1991).

However, Kramer (1997) concluded that there appears to be no long-term benefit to the babies when mothers significantly increase their protein intake above normal. This is probably because most women in developed countries eat far more protein than is needed for health. Protein supplements have been known to impair fetal growth. It may be important to discuss protein intake with vegetarian or vegan mothers to ensure that the full range of essential amino acids is taken.

Carbohydrates and lipids

Apart from the brain which is obligated to use glucose for energy, most tissues can and will use fats for the provision of energy. There is little need to increase either glucose or fats for energy but the absorption of fat-soluble vitamins must be considered when advising women about diet in pregnancy. There may also be a need to increase unsaturated fats as the placenta can synthesise polysaturated fats for fetal needs. As Hytten (1991) reminds us, it is essential that women eat sufficient non-protein energy-providing foods to avoid the use of amino acids for energy production. There may therefore be a need to increase the daily intake of fats and carbohydrates. However, if the reader remembers that this could be achieved by eating two extra slices of bread or one Mars bar, sensible advice can be given.

Vitamins

There is seldom a need to add vitamin supplements to the diet of normal healthy women. However, in women with restricted dietary intake or those with gastrointestinal surgery, especially ileostomy, supplementation may be necessary. In particular, it is important to remember the role of folic acid in the prevention of neural tube defects. There has been an effort to add folic acid to basic foods to ensure compliance with intake, especially prior to conception.

Iron supplementation is discussed in detail in Chapter 16.

Metabolism

Metabolic processes in the pregnant woman are closely linked with the function of various endocrine glands. Many of these metabolic adjustments occur early in pregnancy when the fetus is too small to make large demands on the mother's nutrient consumption. Some of the changes are mediated by a resetting of the hypothalamus and the woman's metabolism changes totally during pregnancy. There is a rise in BMR of 80 kcal/24 h during pregnancy, with energy requirements being at their highest in the middle 20 weeks. Some of the changes, for instance glucose metabolism, would be considered pathological in the non-pregnant state (Hytten 1991).

Similarly, Blackburn & Loper (1992) state that there are major alterations in metabolism during pregnancy. The changes allow the woman to provide adequate nutrients to support fetal growth and development. There is also a need to store energy to meet the increased physiological demands of pregnancy and labour. In some women the metabolic changes will result in ill health, for example the exacerbation or precipitation of diabetes mellitus.

During pregnancy the fetus and placenta have a major influence on maternal metabolism because of the hormones they produce. Maternal metabolism is influenced by HPL, oestrogen and progesterone and there is a major alteration in glucose metabolism mediated by antagonism of insulin. This is why pregnancy is said to be diabetogenic. Lipid and protein metabolism are also affected.

Carbohydrates

Blood glucose levels are generally between 10% and 20% lower than in the non-pregnant state. This decrease leads to lower insulin levels in the postabsorptive state and a tendency towards ketosis. As pregnancy progresses there is less peripheral use of glucose by the mother because of increasing insulin antagonism (blockage of uptake by the cells). Glucose therefore becomes more readily available to the fetus.

Insulin resistance is thought to be due to a decrease in sensitivity of tissue cell receptors resulting from the effects of HPL, progesterone and cortisol. The most potent of the insulin antagonists is HPL. In response, the β islet cells in the pancreas undergo hyperplasia and hypertrophy to produce increased insulin during meals. The results of changes in the above hormones are listed briefly below.

- Progesterone also helps to increase insulin secretion, decreases peripheral insulin usage and increases insulin levels after meals.
- Oestrogen increases the level of plasma cortisol which is an insulin antagonist, stimulates β cell hyperplasia and enhances peripheral glucose usage.
- Cortisol depletes hepatic glycogen stores and increases hepatic glucose production.
- HPL correlates with fetal and placental weight so that it increases in the plasma as pregnancy progresses and is higher in multiple pregnancy. A few of its functions are to antagonise insulin to cause hyperglycaemia and make glucose available for the placenta to take up. It increases the synthesis and availability of lipids which can be utilised by the woman as an alternative fuel to glucose.

Proteins

There are decreased serum amino acid and protein levels in pregnancy because of the placental uptake, increased insulin levels and hepatic use of amino acids for gluconeogenesis. There may be a biphasic pattern in humans, as has been found in animals. In the first half of pregnancy protein storage increases and during the second half of pregnancy protein breakdown occurs to provide amino acids for the fetus and energy for the mother.

Lipids

Every aspect of lipid metabolism changes in pregnancy. During the first two trimesters triglyceride synthesis and fat storage increase (**lipogenesis**), mediated by the increase in insulin production and enhanced by progesterone. The pregnant woman usually increases her daily intake by 200 calories and reduces energy output. There is an overall store of 3.5 kg in normal pregnancy (Hytten 1991). The balance between lipogenesis and lipolysis is maintained as there is an increase in lipolysis.

During the 3rd trimester lipolysis increases further, probably due to the increase in HPL. There is accelerated ketogenesis in the liver due to increased oxidation of free fatty acids for conversion into energy. Fats are therefore acting as an alternative source of energy so that the mother can conserve glucose for the fetus. At the same time in the last trimester, when glucose transfer to the fetus is maximal, there is decreased lipogenesis in adipose tissue and the balance is tipped in the direction of lypolysis (Blackburn & Loper 1992, Hytten 1991). As pregnancy progresses, there is a serial increase in blood cholesterol unrelated to diet until a plateau is reached for the last few weeks before delivery. Serum phospholipids also rise in a similar way to cholesterol.

Insulin

As mentioned above, insulin usage undergoes a major change. Maternal insulin levels double by the 3rd trimester. However, there is increased tissue resistance to the effects of insulin, making it more difficult for the cells to take up the molecules of insulin, most profoundly in the liver cells, muscles and adipose tissue. If the pregnant woman is unable to produce more insulin in response to the antagonistic effects of HPL, progesterone and cortisol, she may develop gestational diabetes. Women who are already diabetic develop problems. Diabetes mellitus in pregnancy is discussed in Chapter 35.

Changes in the absorptive and postabsorptive states

During the absorptive state ingested nutrients are digested and absorbed by the gastrointestinal tract. The absorptive state in pregnancy is characterised by relative hyperinsulinaemia and hyperglycaemia due to reduced liver uptake. There is also hypertriglyceridaemia and increased lipogensis due to the conversion of glucose to fat for storage. Gluconeogenesis and circulating free fatty acids are decreased.

In the postabsorptive or fasting state energy has to be supplied from the body stores. Most of this comes from the catabolism of fat. Fat and protein synthesis are decreased and catabolism exceeds anabolism. The central nervous system has no alternative but to carry on using available glucose but other organs move to production of energy from lipids. Triglycerides are broken down and fed into the Krebs cycle with the production of ketone bodies (described above). If these accumulate, ketoacidosis will occur.

Summary of main points

- There are hundreds of molecules involved in maintaining good health. Many cells, especially in the liver, can convert one type of food molecule to another but there are about 50 essential nutrients which cannot be manufactured by the body cells and must be provided in the diet.
- Four food groups provide a balanced diet – grains, fruits and vegetables, meat and fish and milk products. Most carbohydrate comes from plants but a small amount is found as lactose in milk and

glycogen in meats. The most common source of lipids is neutral fats in the form of triglycerides or triacylglycerols. Meat and dairy products contain saturated fats whilst unsaturated fats are found in seeds, nuts and most vegetable oils. Fats are also ingested as cholesterol.

- The best source of essential amino acids is found in animal products. Proteins have many important functions and are found also in legumes. Nuts and cereals are nutritionally incomplete and are low in one or more of the essential amino acids. Strict vegetarians can obtain all the essential amino acids by varying their diet carefully.
- Vitamins may be fat soluble or water soluble. Their main role is to function as coenzymes to assist in the catalysis of chemical processes in the body. The human body is unable to synthesise most vitamins with the exception of vitamin K and some of the B vitamins. The body requires adequate supplies of seven minerals and traces of about 12 others. The seven are calcium, phosphorus, potassium, sulphur, sodium, chloride and magnesium.
- When energy intake and energy output are balanced, body weight remains stable. There appear to be body mechanisms that control intake and enable most people to maintain a steady weight. However, no such regulator has been found. Current theories of obesity involve nutrient signals related to body energy stores, hormones, body temperature and psychological factors.
- A gene called Ob which produces a hormone called leptin seemed to be involved in the regulation of the balance of fat stored and excreted in mice. The Ob gene has been found in humans but does not appear to be strongly related to obesity. There is a statistical correlation between having two copies of the shortened Ob gene and excess weight in women between the ages of 26 and 30.
- Metabolic processes are either anabolic, in which molecules are built up, or catabolic, which involves the breakdown of complex substances to simpler ones. There are two nutritional states: the absorptive state when nutrients are eaten and absorbed by the digestive tract and the postabsorptive state when the GI tract is empty and energy requirements are met by breakdown of body stores.
- Body cells must convert ingested food into the high-energy phosphate bonds of ATP which consists of adenosine with three phosphate groups attached. When glucose arrives at the tissues it is taken up by the cells by facilitated diffusion under the influence of insulin. Glucose is taken to the mitochondria where it is oxidised to form energy in the Krebs cycle.
- Cellular respiration may be aerobic or anaerobic. Many more molecules of ATP are formed from aerobic respiration than anaerobic respiration. Fats are the body's most concentrated source of energy. The energy obtained from lypolysis is twice that obtained from the metabolism of glucose or protein, providing 9 kcal per g in contrast to only 4 kcal per g of the other two nutrients.
- Excess fat is stored as adipose tissue. When fat is needed for energy production it is mobilised from the stores under the influence of growth hormones or cortisol, taken to the liver and broken down into free fatty acids and glycerol which are released into the blood for use by cells.
- Cholesterol is found in the blood in combination with a protein carrier as lipoproteins, of which there are three types: high-density lipoproteins (HDLs), low-density lipoproteins (LDLs) and very low-density lipoproteins (VLDLs). The ratio of HDLs to LDLs and VLDLs is increased in vegetarians, in those whose fat intake is largely unsaturated and those who take regular exercise but reduced in cigarette smokers.
- At least 50 g of protein a day is needed to maintain nitrogen balance and to provide for growth and repair of tissues. Amino acids cannot be stored by the body but the liver can interconvert amino acids by utilising the eight essential amino acids to synthesise the non-essential amino acids.
- The basal metabolic rate is the rate needed to maintain the body at rest with no energy expenditure to maintain body warmth. Even slight increases in muscle work can cause remarkable leaps in metabolic rate and heat production. Ingestion of food also increases the metabolic rate.
- Humans are homeothermic and the maintenance of body temperature depends on the balance between heat production and heat loss. The hypothalamus is the major heat-regulating centre and receives input from both peripheral thermoreceptors in the skin and central thermoreceptors in the core. Heat is lost by radiation, conduction, convection and evaporation brought about by vasodilation of cutaneous blood vessels, sweating, seeking a cooler environment and maintaining an open body posture.
- Heat is produced and conserved by vasoconstriction of cutaneous skin vessels, an increase in metabolic rate, shivering, enhanced thyroxine release and adopting a position that reduces heat loss from body surfaces, such as the fetal position.
- There is a relationship between poor intake of essential nutrients and a higher than normal perinatal morbidity and mortality. Fetal growth may be compromised with an increase in preterm delivery and a decrease in weight for gestational age, possibly due to low placental weight.
- There is a need for more nutrients to supply the increase in maternal tissue and to meet the needs of the fetus although reducing energy expenditure without increased intake may be sufficient. Proteins are required in larger quantities but there is little need to increase either glucose or fats. In women with restricted dietary intake or those with gastrointestinal surgery, especially ileostomy, vitamin supplementation may be necessary. Folic acid deficiency is implicated in the causation of neural tube defects.
- Metabolic processes in the pregnant woman are closely linked with the function of endocrine glands. There are changes in carbohydrate, lipid and protein metabolism. Some of the changes, for instance glucose metabolism, would be considered pathological in the non-pregnant state. During pregnancy, the fetus and placenta have a major influence on maternal metabolism because of the hormones they produce. Maternal metabolism is influenced by HPL, oestrogen and progesterone.
- As pregnancy progresses there is less peripheral use of glucose by the mother because of increasing insulin antagonism. Glucose becomes more readily available to the fetus. Insulin resistance is thought to be due to a decrease in sensitivity of tissue cell receptors resulting from the effects of HPL, progesterone and cortisol.
- There are decreased serum amino acid and protein levels in pregnancy because of the placental uptake, increased insulin levels and hepatic use of amino acids for gluconeogenesis. There may be a biphasic pattern. In the first half of pregnancy protein storage increases and during the second half protein breakdown occurs to provide amino acids for the fetus and energy for the mother.
- During the first two trimesters fat storage increases due to raised insulin production and progesterone. There is an overall store of 3.5 kg. During the 3rd trimester lipolysis increases due to the rise in HPL. Fats act as an alternative source of energy to conserve glucose for the fetus.
- Maternal insulin levels double by the 3rd trimester but there is increased tissue resistance to the effects of insulin, making it more difficult for the cells to take it up. If the pregnant woman cannot produce more insulin in response to the antagonistic effects of HPL, progesterone and cortisol, she may develop gestational diabetes. Women who are already diabetic develop problems.
- The central nervous system can only use available glucose but other organs move to production of energy from lipids. Triglycerides are broken down and fed into the Krebs cycle with the production of ketone bodies. If these accumulate, ketoacidosis will occur.

References

Barker DJP. (ed) 1992 Fetal and Infant Origins of Adult Disease. BMJ Books, London.

Blackburn ST, Loper DL. 1992 Maternal, Fetal and Neonatal Physiology, A Clinical Perspective. WB Saunders, Philadelphia.

Cohen P. 1996 In the mood to overeat. New Scientist 151 (2051) 18.

DHSS. 1990 Vitamin A and pregnancy. PL/C (90) 10 and 11. DHSS, London.

Gibbs WW. 1996 Gaining on fat. Scientific American 275(2) 70–76.

Hinchliff SM, Montague SE. 1990 Physiology for Nursing Practice. Baillière Tindall, London.

Hytten F. 1991 The alimentary system. In Hytten F, Chamberlain G (eds) Clinical Physiology in Obstetrics, 2nd edn. Blackwell Scientific, Oxford, pp 137–149.

Kramer MS. 1997 Balanced protein/energy supplementation in pregnancy. In Neilson JP, Crowther CA, Hodnett ED, Hofmeyr GJ, Keirse MJNC (eds) Pregnancy and Childbirth module of the Cochrane Database of Systematic Reviews, the Cochrane Library. Update Software, Oxford.

Luke B. 1994 Nutrition during pregnancy. Current Opinion in Obstetrics and Gynaecology 6(5), 402–407.

Marieb EN. 1992 Human Anatomy and Physiology, 2nd edn. Benjamin/ Cummings Publishing California

Ranjan V. 1991 Vitamin A and birth defects. Professional Care of Mother and Child 1(1), 3–4.

Sherwood L. 1989 Human Physiology – From Cells to Systems. West Publishing, Maine.

Sweet B. 1997 Mayes' Midwifery. Baillière Tindall, London.

Tiran D. 1997 Maternal Nutrition. In Sweet BR with Tiran D (eds) Mayes Midwifery, 12th edn. Baillière Tindall, London, pp 185–195.

Recommended reading

Bradley SG with Bennett N. 1995 Preparation for Pregnancy, An Essential Guide, Argyll publishing, Argyll.

Clark NAC, Fisk NM. 1994 Minimal compliance with the Department of Health recommendation for routine folate prophylaxis to prevent neural tube defects. British Journal of Obstetrics and Gynaecology 101(8), 709–710.

Enkin M, Keirse MJNC, Renfrew M, Neilson J. 1995 A Guide to Effective Care in Pregnancy and Childbirth, 2nd edn. Oxford University Press, Oxford pp 26–33.

Hytten F. 1990 Nutritional requirements in pregnancy. What happens if they are not met? Midwifery 6(3), 140–145.

Reeves J. 1992 Pregnancy and fasting during Ramadan. British Medical Journal 304(6830), 843–844.

Smithells RW, Sheppard S, Schorar CJ et al. 1981 Apparent prevention of neural tube defects by periconceptual vitamin supplementation. Archives of Disease in Childhood 56, 911–918.

Wald N, Sneddon J, Densem J et al. 1991 Prevention of neural tube defects: results of the Medical Research Council vitamin study. Lancet 338, 1331–1337.

Chapter
24 The nature of bone, the female pelvis and fetal skull

In this chapter

INTRODUCTION

The successful outcome of childbearing depends on the relationship between the size and shape of the maternal pelvis and the fetal skull. The evolution of **bipedalism** (walking on two legs) and the large size of the human brain have increased the risk to both mother and fetus. This chapter looks at the nature of bone and calcium and phosphorus metabolism. It will concentrate on general structure and function of bone. However, a detailed description of the bones of the pelvis and of the fetal skull will be given.

THE NATURE OF BONE

Functions

Bone is a connective tissue which contains deposits of calcium and phosphorus. It performs important functions for the body including support and protection of the soft organs, movement by acting as anchorage for muscles and levers, storage of fat but mainly of minerals such as calcium and phosphorus and smaller amounts of potassium, sulphur, magnesium and copper, and blood cell formation.

Structure

Bone consists of three basic components: an organic matrix of **collagen** known as **osteoid**, a mineral matrix of calcium and phosphorus, and bone cells which include osteoblasts, osteoclasts, osteocytes and fibroblasts. Calcium, the commonest mineral in the body, is found mainly in the bones and teeth. Calcium and phosphorus are present in the skeleton as crystals of **hydroxyapatite** with a chemical formula $3Ca_3\ (PO_4)_2\ Ca(OH)_2$. These crystals are attached to collagen fibres resulting in the typical hardness of bone. Bone is continuously remodelled by bone cells with calcium and phosphorus slowly exchanged between bone and the extracellular fluid (ECF).

Bone can be divided into **compact** or lamellar bone and **spongy** bone (trabecular, cancellous bone). Compact bone forms the outer rim or cortex of all bones and consists of units called **osteons** or **Haversian systems**. There is a central Haversian canal oriented to the long axis of the bone. Bone is a living tissue and these canals carry nerves, blood vessels and lymphatic vessels. Around the central canal are concentric hollow tubes of bone known as a **lamella**. Lamellae have small concavities at their junctions called **lacunae** containing the spider-shaped osteocytes. Hair-like canals called **canaliculi** connect the lacunae to each other and to the central canal, linking all the osteocytes in an osteon together for exchange of nutrients and removal of waste products. Some osteons are newly formed and others are remnants in the process of being removed. Spongy bone contains far fewer Haversian systems and is made up of a lattice of **trabeculae** with red or fatty bone marrow filling the cavities (Figs 24.1 and 24.2).

Periosteum and endosteum

Most bones have a tough outer covering of fibrous connective tissue, the **periosteum**, which does not cover the articular surfaces of joints. It transmits blood vessels and acts as an attachment surface for ligaments and muscles. It is supplied abundantly with nerve fibres. Beneath this is a layer of **osteoblasts**. Lining the marrow cavity of a bone is a fine layer of tissue called the **endosteum** containing the osteoblasts and osteoclasts and their precursor cells.

Bone cells

Osteoblasts

Osteoblasts are present on all bone surfaces in single layers next to the unmineralised osteoid of newly forming bone. Osteoblasts may be differentiated from haemopoietic stem cells and are uniform in size, linked to each other by the fine cytoplasmic processes. Osteoblasts synthesise and secrete the constituents and promote mineralisation of the organic matrix.

Osteocytes

Osteocytes are derived from osteoblasts that have become trapped in lacunae. The osteocytes maintain the bone matrix and if they die the surrounding matrix is resorbed.

Osteoclasts

Osteoclasts resorb bone and are found in numbers on or near surfaces undergoing erosion. They may have developed separately to the osteoblasts and derive from mononuclear phagocytic cells. They vary a great deal in size and in nuclear form and are very mobile. Osteoclasts contain a large number of enzymes which can remove both the organic and mineral matrix.

Calcium and phosphorus metabolism

The skeleton contains 99% of the calcium and 85% of the phosphorus present in the body. The small amount of calcium found in body fluids and cells plays a very important part in the metabolic processes of the body and needs to be maintained within narrow limits. Phosphorus is also crucial to body function (Boore 1996, Reeve 1991). The normal plasma concentration of calcium is 2.10–2.70 mmol/l and of phosphate 0.70–1.40 mmol/l.

Functions of calcium

Calcium is present in the ECF in two forms, about half bound to the proteins albumin and globulin and half in ionised form. The ionised form Ca^{2+} is important in many cell activities, including:

- nerve and muscle function;
- hormonal actions;
- blood clotting;
- cell motility;
- acting as a secondary messenger between environmental stimulus and cell function by modulation of enzyme response function when bound to the protein **calmodulin**.

Functions of phosphorus

In the form of phosphates, phosphorus plays a large role in cell function:

- as a component of nucleic acids;
- regulating energy storage as adenosine triphosphate (ATP).

Hormonal control of calcium and phosphorus metabolism

Three hormones are involved in the control of calcium and phosphorus metabolism, mainly by maintaining the concentration of calcium in ECF. These are **parathyroid hormone** (PTH), **vitamin D** and **calcitonin**. Plasma inorganic phosphate is

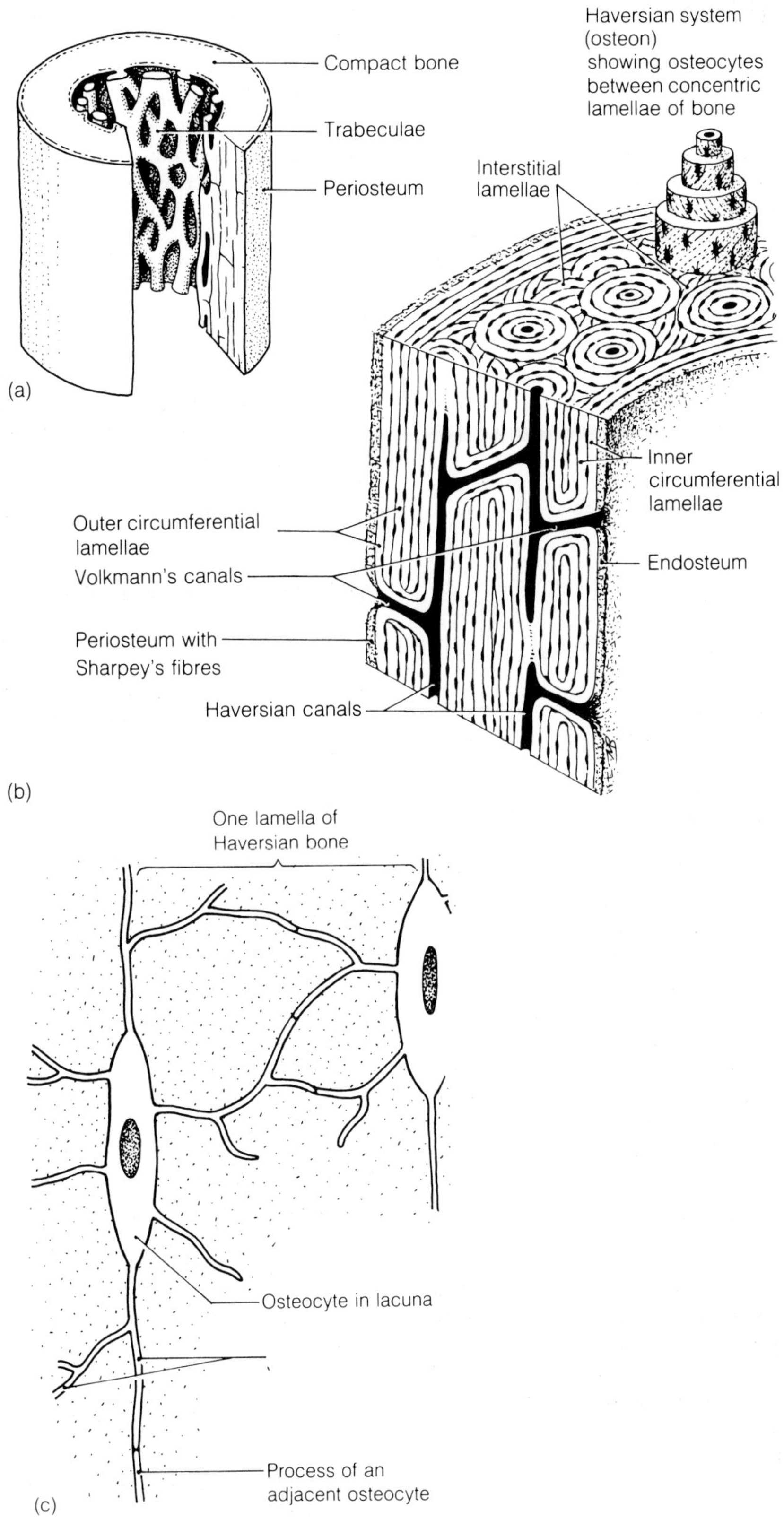

Figure 24.1 *Structure of compact bone (from Hinchliff SM, Montague SE, 1990, with permission).*

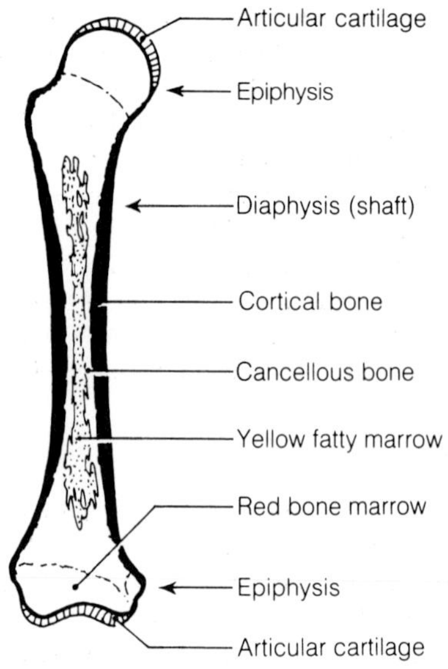

Figure 24.2 *Anatomical features of a long bone (from Hinchliff SM, Montague SE, 1990, with permission).*

more loosely controlled than calcium. If there is no change in the amount of calcium in the skeleton, ECF calcium level depends on the balance between calcium absorption in the gut and its excretion in urine and faeces. About 50% of the calcium in the blood passing through the capillaries of bone is exchanged in a single passage and about 300 mmol of calcium is involved in the exchange of calcium between blood and bone every day.

Parathyroid hormone

Four parathyroid glands embedded in the thyroid gland secrete PTH. The main effects of this hormone are to increase the concentration of Ca^{2+} in the ECF and to depress plasma phosphate concentration by acting on bone and kidneys. PTH increases osteocyte reabsorption of bone with a rapid release of calcium and phosphorus into the ECF. Calcium reabsorption in the kidney tubules is increased but the excretion of phosphate is also increased, resulting in a rise in the plasma level of calcium and a fall in phosphate level. PTH activity is directly related to ECF calcium concentration. When the level of calcium rises PTH production falls, resulting in calcium deposition in bone and vice versa.

Vitamin D

The D vitamins are a group of steroid substances formed from **ergosterol** in plants and **7-dehydrocholesterol** in animals. Ultraviolet radiation modifies these to **ergocalciferol** (vitamin D_2) and **cholecalciferol** (vitamin D_3). Humans can either ingest vitamin D from plant and animal sources or manufacture it by the action of sunlight on the skin to form cholecalciferol. Whichever the source, vitamin D is transported to the liver bound to a plasma protein and stored there as **25-dihydroxycholecalciferol**. The active form, called **1,25-dihydroxycholecalciferol**, is produced by the kidney in response to PTH stimulation and is released into the circulation to be transported to its target organs of intestine, bone and kidneys. Its overall effect is to increase the concentration of calcium in the ECF. In the upper small intestine, vitamin D enters the cells and causes increased calcium and phosphate absorption. In the kidney, calcium and phosphate reabsorption are increased but the phosphate reabsorption is masked by the effect of PTH increasing its excretion. Calcium is released from bone into the ECF. Hypocalcaemia increases the secretion of PTH which in turn increases the production of active vitamin D by the kidney. Once the level of plasma calcium has returned to normal, the secretion of PTH decreases and the level of active vitamin D secretion falls.

Calcitonin

Calcitonin is secreted by the **parafollicular cells** (clear cells or C cells) of the thyroid gland. Its main effect is opposite to that of parathyroid hormone, causing a fall in plasma concentration of calcium and phosphate. This hormone may play an important part in the regulation of skeletal growth in children but appears to have no major role in adults other than pregnant women. The secretion of calcitonin is directly related to plasma calcium concentration.

THE PELVIC GIRDLE

Aiello & Dean (1990) state that the pelvic girdle is for attachment of the lower limbs and for support of the pelvic and to some extent abdominal organs. The continuous bony basin is important in an upright posture as it transmits the weight of the trunk to the legs and it is necessary for the sacroiliac joints to be strong and stable. Compared to other primates, the human pelvis is short, squat and basin shaped. Trevathen (1987) discusses the human pelvis in relation to childbearing, stating that the size, shape and rigidity of the pelvic girdle are related directly to the bipedal method of locomotion.

Morgan (1990) reminds us that the mammalian spine is highly efficient and developed for walking on four legs. In quadrupeds the abdominal organs are suspended from a single horizontal arch. This single arch is still present in the human neonate but when babies learn to sit up their spines develop a forward curve near the top of the spine. When they learn to stand their spines develop a second forward curve near the base. The adult curved spine is essential for maintenance of an upright posture.

The evolving changes in the pelvic shape place constraints on the baby's head size, limiting the gestation length and resulting in a very immature baby (Morgan 1990). This feature is referred to as **altricial** and is seen in mammals and birds who give birth to litters which are hidden in a den or nest. The gynaecoid pelvis is adapted for giving birth to a comparatively large-headed baby but mechanisms are necessary to facilitate the descent of the head through the pelvis, including passive alterations in the position of the fetus and moulding of the skull bones.

Bones

Although diagrams and text can illustrate the features of the pelvis, there is no substitute for handling a life-sized model of the pelvis. The reader is strongly encouraged to do so repeatedly. The knowledge is for clinical application and familiarity with the shape and size of the pelvis may enable life-saving decisions to be made. Whenever vaginal examinations are carried out relevant features must be identified in vivo.

The bony ring of the pelvis is made up of four irregularly shaped bones, two **innominate bones** forming the lateral and anterior walls and the **sacrum** and **coccyx** forming the posterior wall. Each innominate bone consists of three fused bones: the **ilium**, **ischium** and **pubis**. The three bones were formed as cartilage in the fetus and their ossification centres fuse at puberty. Ossification in the pelvis is not completed until about 25 years of age. The description of these three bones given below is mirrored to the left and right of the pelvis.

The ilium

The ilium has an upper flat plate of bone and forms part of the **acetabulum** below (Figs 24.3 and 24.4). The external part of the plate of bone is curved and has a roughened surface for attachment of the gluteal muscles which form the buttocks while the inner surface forms the **iliac fossa** which is smooth and concave. The iliacus muscle, which forms a platform on which the abdominal organs rest, originates from this surface. The upper ridge of the ilium is called the **iliac crest** and is shaped like a letter S. The muscles of the abdominal wall have attachments to this surface.

At the anterior end of the iliac crest is the **anterior superior iliac spine**, which can be identified under the skin, and at the posterior end is the **posterior superior iliac spine**, which is marked externally by a dimple at the level of the 2nd sacral vertebra. Two **inferior iliac spines**, anterior and posterior, can be found below the superior spines. The lower margin of the ilium forms two-fifths of the acetabulum where it fuses with the ischium and pubis. Behind the acetabulum, the ilium forms the **greater sciatic notch** through which the nerves from the sacral plexus pass. Above the greater sciatic notch is the area of ilium which articulates with the sacrum at the **sacroiliac joint**.

The ischium

The ischium forms the lowest aspect of the innominate bone. The upper part forms two-fifths of the acetabulum where it fuses with the ilium and ischium. Below the acetabulum, a thick buttress of bone called the **ischial tuberosity** takes the weight of the seated body. The hamstring muscles in the thigh arise from this bone. Passing upwards and inwards from the ischial tuberosity, a shaft of ischium meets the **inferior ramus** of the pubis to form the **pubic arch**. The ischium also forms the lower

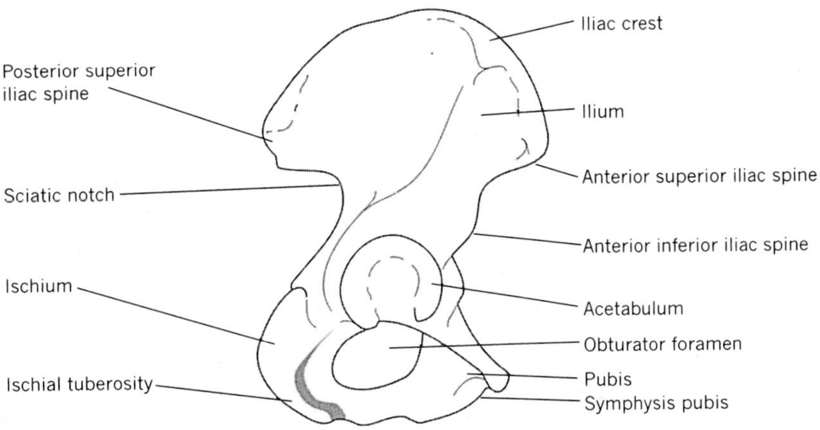

Figure 24.3 *The outer or lateral surface of the right innominate bone (from Sweet B, 1997, with permission).*

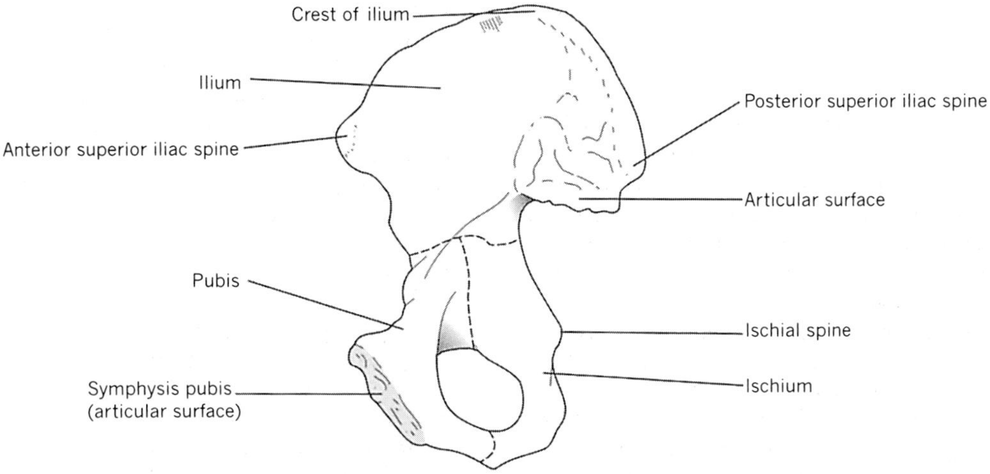

Figure 24.4 *The inner or medial surface of the right innominate bone (from Sweet B, 1997, with permission).*

boundary of the **obturator foramen**, a large opening in the lower part of each innominate bone below the acetabula. On its internal surface, protruding from its posterior edge and about 5 cm above the tuberosity is a protuberance called the **ischial spine**, an important landmark to be found on vaginal examination. The ischial spine separates the greater sciatic notch from the lesser sciatic notch.

The pubis

This square bone forms the anterior aspect of the innominate bone. The two pubic bones articulate medially to form the joint called the **symphysis pubis**. Laterally the superior ramus of the pubic bone passes to the acetabulum and forms one-fifth of this structure. The superior ramus also forms the upper boundary of the obturator foramen. The inferior ramus passes downwards and outwards to join the ischium and form the pubic arch. The upper surface of the pubis forms the **pubic crest** which ends laterally in the **pubic tubercle**.

The sacrum

The sacrum is a shield-shaped mass of bone formed from five fused sacral vertebrae (Fig. 24.5). It articulates with the two innominate bones at the sacroiliac joints. The anterior surface is smooth and concave both from above downwards and from side to side. This curvature is called the **hollow of the sacrum**. The first sacral vertebra overhangs the sacral hollow and the central point of this projection is called the **sacral promontory**. Through the centre of the bone, the sacral and coccygeal nerves pass through the **sacral canal**.

Four pairs of **foramina** (openings) are present anteriorly between the five fused sacral vertebrae where the sacral nerves exit to form the **sacral plexus**. Posteriorly, eight small foramina are present through which posterior branches of the sacral nerves exit to supply the skin of the buttocks and the muscles of the lower part of the back. On its upper surface a smooth oval area forms an articular surface for the 5th lumbar vertebra to form the **lumbosacral joint**. Lateral masses of bone on either side of the sacrum are known as the **wings of the sacrum** or **sacral alae**.

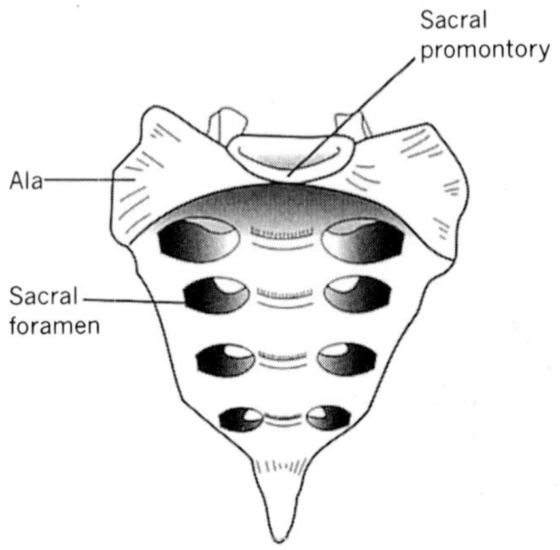

Figure 24.5 *The sacrum (from Sweet B, 1997, with permission).*

The coccyx

This small bone is triangular in shape with its base uppermost. It is formed of four fused coccygeal vertebrae. The first coccygeal vertebra articulates with the lower end of the sacrum at the **sacrococcygeal joint**. The rudimentary vertebrae forming the rest of the coccyx are smooth on their inner surface and support the rectum. The external anal sphincter is attached to the lowest point.

Joints

There are four joints – two sacroiliac joints, one symphysis pubis and one sacrococcygeal joint.

The sacroiliac joints

These are **synovial** joints with the usual formation of a joint cavity filled with synovial fluid, a capsule formed of synovial membrane and tough external supporting ligaments. Special features include a very small joint cavity and very strong posterior ligaments which transmit the weight of the trunk, head and arms to the legs. Movement at these joints is normally slight but they increase in range during pregnancy when the ligaments become softened under the influence of the hormone **relaxin**.

The symphysis pubis

This joint consists of an oval disc of fibrocartilage about 4 cm long lying between the bodies of the two pubic bones. The joint is reinforced by ligaments crossing from one pubic bone to the other.

The sacrococcygeal joint

This small joint lies between the sacrum and coccyx. There is sometimes a small synovial joint cavity present. Slight movement can occur backwards and forwards and the backwards movement is greatly increased as the baby's head passes through the pelvis in the second stage of labour.

Ligaments

Besides the ligaments supporting each of the pelvic joints, there are three other pairs of ligaments.

The **sacrotuberous ligament** crosses from the posterior superior iliac spine and the lateral borders of the sacrum and coccyx to the ischial tuberosity. It bridges the greater and lesser sciatic notches.

The **sacrospinous ligament** passes in front of the sacrotuberous ligament from the side of the sacrum and coccyx, crosses the greater sciatic notch and is attached to the ischial spine.

The **inguinal ligament** (Poupart's ligament) runs from the anterior superior iliac spine to the pubic tubercle and forms the groin.

Regions

There is a clear line of bone separating the upper flare of the iliac fossae from the basin-shaped part of the pelvis. This line of bone is called the **pelvic brim**. The area above this is called the **false pelvis** and is of no consequence in childbearing whilst below the brim is the **true pelvis** with a cavity and outlet through which the fetus must pass in order to be born.

The pelvic brim

Landmarks are identifiable on the pelvic brim or inlet and it is important to be aware of these as measurements are made between them. In the normal gynaecoid (female) pelvis the brim is oval in shape with the anteroposterior diameter reduced by the sacral promontory (Fig. 24.6). Starting at the centre of the sacral promontory and tracing the brim round to the symphysis pubis, the landmarks are:

- the sacral promontory;
- the sacral ala;
- the upper border of the sacroiliac joint;
- the iliopectineal line;
- the iliopectineal eminence;
- the inner upper border of the superior pubic ramus;
- the inner upper border of the body of the pubis;
- the upper inner border of the symphysis pubis.

If a piece of paper was placed across the landmarks a flat surface would be formed. This imaginary flat surface is called a **plane** and the concept can also be applied to the cavity and outlet. The **diameters** of the pelvis which will be described are measured from the landmarks across the planes.

The cavity of the pelvis

The cavity is that part of the pelvis between the brim and the outlet. It is a curved canal with a short anterior surface measuring 4.5 cm, formed by the inner aspect of the pubic bones and symphysis pubis, and a longer posterior surface measuring 12 cm formed by the hollow of the sacrum. The lateral walls are formed from the greater sciatic notch, the inner surface of part of the ilium, the body of the ischium and the obturator foramen. The plane of the pelvic cavity is taken from the midpoint of the symphysis pubis anteriorly to the junction of the 2nd and 3rd sacral vertebrae posteriorly.

The outlet of the pelvis

It is traditional to describe two pelvic outlets – the anatomical and obstetric outlets. The anatomical outlet is traced from the lower border of the symphysis pubis along the pubic arch to the inner border of the ischial tuberosity and along the sacro-tuberous ligament to the tip of the coccyx. It is of no value in labour as it is not a flat surface but the lower border of the pelvis and varies in size during labour because of the range of backwards tilting of the coccyx in different women. Therefore a more useful landmark is the obstetric outlet which is the constricted lower portion of the true pelvis. The structures making up the obstetric outlet are:

- the lower border of the symphysis pubis;
- a line passing along the pubis, obturator foramen and ischium to the ischial spine;
- the sacrospinous ligament;
- the lower border of the sacrum.

The plane of the outlet is the imaginary flat surface between these structures. It is occupied by the muscles of the pelvic floor (Chapter 25)

Dimensions (diameters)

Measurements are taken of the planes of the pelvic brim, cavity and outlet using the landmarks described above. These are taken in three directions – anteroposterior, oblique and transverse. The measurements given are the average measurements of a gynaecoid pelvis.

The brim

The **anteroposterior diameter** is the smallest diameter of the

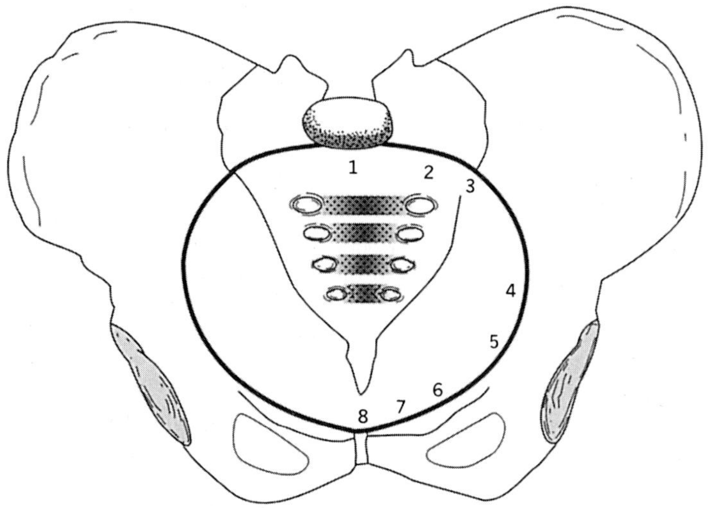

Figure 24.6 *The pelvic brim. 1, sacral promontory; 2, sacral ala; 3, sacroiliac joint; 4, iliopectineal line; 5, iliopectineal eminence; 6, superior pubic ramus; 7, body of pubic bone; 8, symphysis pubis (from Sweet B, 1997, with permission).*

Table 24.1 *Pelvic measurements in centimetres*

	Anteroposterior	*Oblique*	*Transverse*
Brim	11 cm	12 cm	13 cm
Cavity	12 cm	12 cm	12 cm
Outlet	13 cm	12 cm	11cm

brim and can be measured from the uppermost part of the symphysis pubis to the sacral promontory and is called the **anatomical conjugate**, which measures 12 cm. However, as discussed above, this does not measure the available space for accommodating the fetal head. If the measurement is taken from the upper inner border of the symphysis pubis, which is about 1.25 cm lower, to the sacral promontory the measurement is 11 cm and this is known as the **obstetric conjugate**. Both of these two measurements can be referred to as the **true conjugate**. A more important anteroposterior measurement is the **diagonal conjugate** which is measured by vaginal examination during a pelvic assessment. It is taken from the lower border of the symphysis pubis to the sacral promontory and measures about 13 cm. If this diameter is measured the obstetric conjugate can be calculated by subtracting 2 cm.

The two **oblique diameters** are taken from one sacroiliac joint to the opposite iliopectineal eminence. They are named left and right after the corresponding sacroiliac joint. All the oblique diameters throughout the pelvis are 12 cm.

- The **transverse diameter** is taken between points on the two iliopectineal lines that are farthest apart and measures 13 cm. However, the descending colon passes near to the left sacroiliac joint and may limit the space available for passage of the fetus.
- The **sacrocotyloid diameter** is also measured at the brim and is taken from the sacral promontory to the iliopectineal eminence. This measures about 9.5 cm and is important if the fetus is presenting with the occiput posteriorly. The parietal eminences may become caught in this diameter, causing the head to extend.

The cavity

The cavity is considered to be circular in diameter and the measurements taken through the plane of the cavity are all 12 cm.

The obstetric outlet

The outlet is diamond shaped with its longest diameter in the anteroposterior direction. This is measured from the lower border of the symphysis pubis to the sacrococcygeal joint and is 13 cm.

The oblique diameter has no fixed points but is between the obturator foramen and the opposite sacrospinous ligament. It is 12 cm.

The transverse diameter is measured between the two ischial spines. It is the smallest diameter and measures 11 cm.

The planes of the pelvis and pelvic inclination

When a human being stands up the pelvic basin is tilted in relation to the horizontal. This concept can be checked if the reader stands facing and pressed up against a vertical surface. The two points of the pelvis which touch the vertical surface will be the pubic bones and the anterior superior iliac spines. The brim is tilted so that the plane of the brim forms an angle of 60° to the horizontal. The plane of the cavity forms an angle of 30° and that of the outlet 15° (Fig. 24.7).

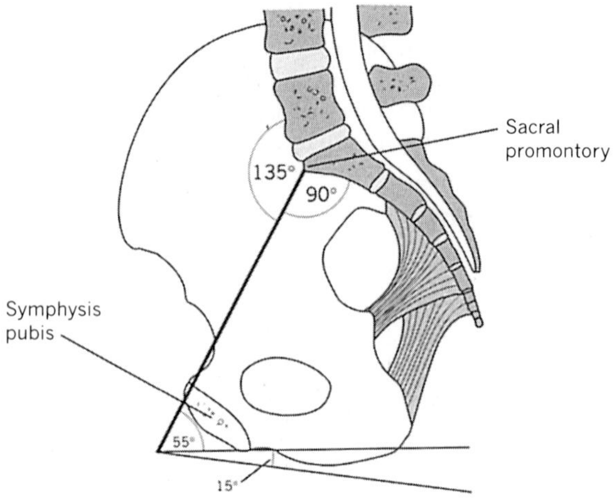

Figure 24.7 *The pelvis, showing the degrees of inclination. Inclination of the pelvic brim to the horizontal, 55°; inclination of pelvic outlet to the horizontal, 15°; angle of pelvic inclination, 135°; inclination of the sacrum, 90° (from Sweet B, 1997, with permission).*

The subpubic angle of the pubic arch is important in childbearing because it indicates the adequacy of the pelvic size. It measures 90° in the typical gynaecoid pelvis. Other angles measuring 90° are the sacral angle between the plane of the brim and the anterior surface of the first sacral vertebra and the greater sciatic notch.

Axes of the pelvic canal

If imaginary lines are drawn at right angles through the planes of the pelvis, axes will be created. If these lines are joined together a curve can be traced because each plane is at a different angle

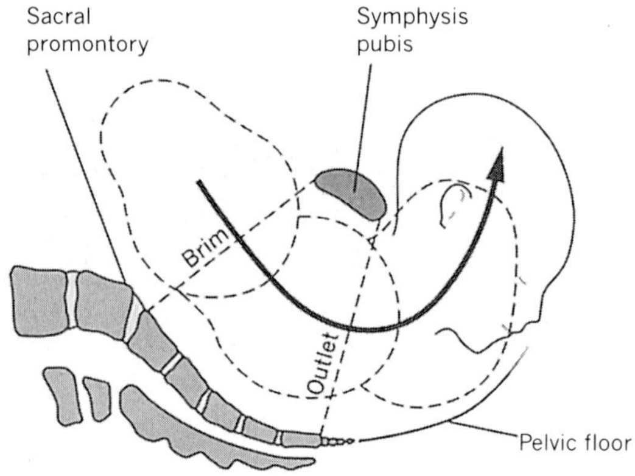

Figure 24.8 *The axis of the birth canal (from Sweet B, 1997, with permission).*

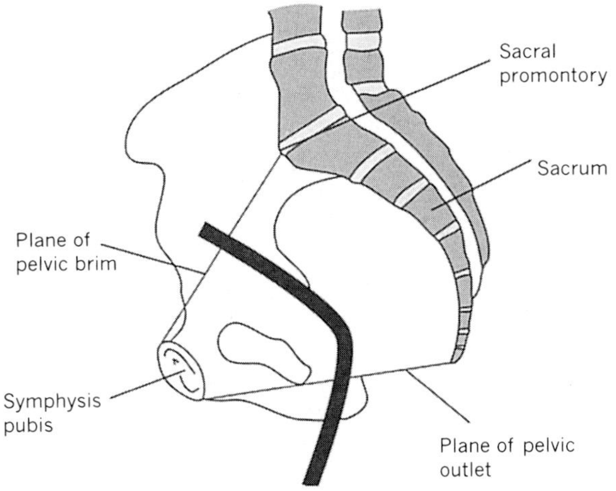

Figure 24.9 *The curve of the birth canal (from Sweet B, 1997, with permission).*

to the horizon. This is called the curve of Carus and the fetus must pass through it during birth. This is unique to the human and is the price paid for our upright posture as it makes delivery of the fetus more difficult. Instead of an easy journey through a relatively large, straight pelvic canal the fetus must be moved passively to overcome the changing curves and diameters (Figs 24.8 and 24.9).

Basic types of pelvis

There are four basic types of pelvis described according to the shape of the brim and other features (Fig. 24.10). These are **gynaecoid**, **android**, **anthropoid** and **platypelloid**. However, many pelves cannot be classified so easily and may contain features of different types. It is now considered that the size of the pelvis in relation to the fetus that must pass through it is more important than a slight abnormality of shape and there is a saying that the fetal head is the best pelvimeter.

The gynaecoid pelvis

This is the ideal female pelvis. Its main features are a rounded brim, large forepelvis (that portion in front of the widest transverse diameter, a transverse diameter that bisects the anteroposterior diameter), parallel side walls, a shallow cavity, blunt ischial spines, a wide sciatic notch and a pubic angle of 90°. It is associated with women of average height and shoe size of 4 or over.

The android pelvis

The name android suggests that the pelvis has male features. Its brim is more heart shaped with a narrow forepelvis and a widest transverse diameter set towards the back. The side walls converge and the sacrum is straight, making the cavity funnel shaped. The ischial spines are prominent and the subpubic angle and the angle of the greater sciatic notch are less than 90°. Women with this type of pelvis may present with recognisable features. They may be of short stature, heavily built and have a tendency to be hirsute. There may be occipitoposterior position of the head at the commencement of labour and this type of pelvis is the least suitable for childbearing as it becomes narrower as the fetus descends (Fig. 24.11).

The anthropoid pelvis

This pelvis has a long oval brim with the anteroposterior diameter greater than the transverse, as is found in other primates; hence the name anthropoid or ape-like. This results from a reduction in the transverse diameter but the pelvis is generally large all over. The side walls diverge and the sacrum is long and deeply concave. There may be a sixth sacral vertebra present, especially in tall African women. This is called a **high assimilation pelvis**. The ischial spines are not prominent and the angle of the greater sciatic notch is wide whilst the subpubic angle may be normal or wide. Although the fetus may present with the occiput anterior the pelvis is so large that the baby may descend and deliver still in this position.

The platypelloid pelvis

This pelvis is flat with a reduced anteroposterior diameter. It is usually referred to as kidney shaped. The side walls diverge, the sacrum is flat and the cavity shallow (Fig. 24.12). The ischial spines are blunt and the sciatic notch and subpubic angle are wide. The fetal head may have difficulty negotiating the brim, a feature that will be discussed later, but once through the brim there should be no further difficulty.

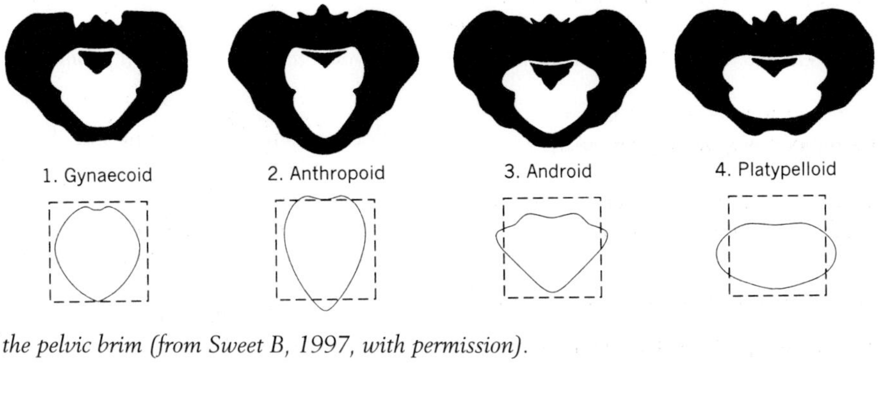

Figure 24.10 *Shapes of the pelvic brim (from Sweet B, 1997, with permission).*

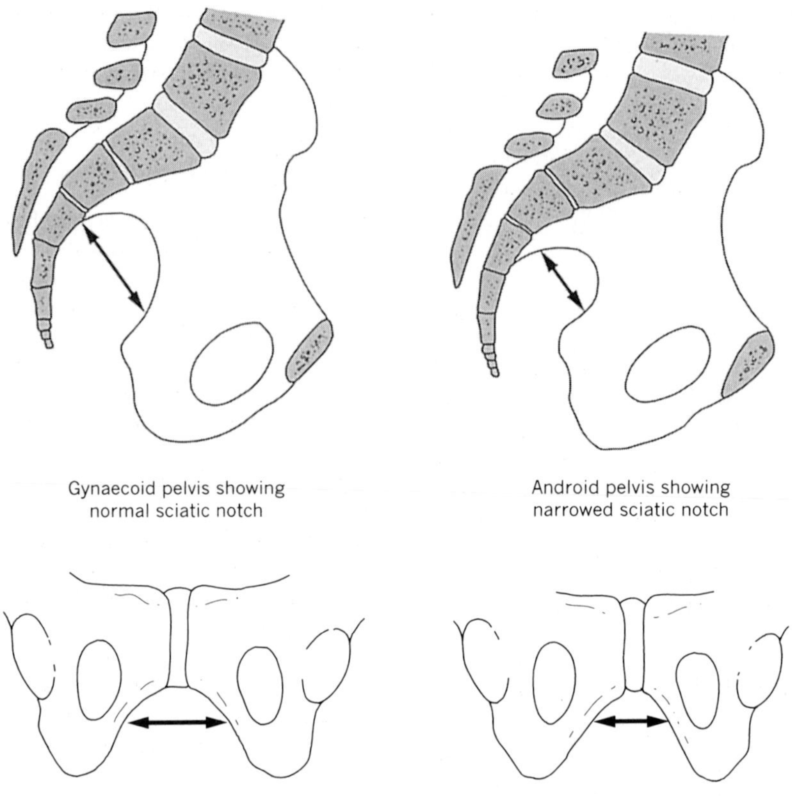

Figure 24.11 *Comparison between a normal (gynaecoid) pelvis and an android pelvis. An android pelvis has a narrower outlet because of the narrow sciatic notch and pubic arch (from Sweet B, 1997, with permission).*

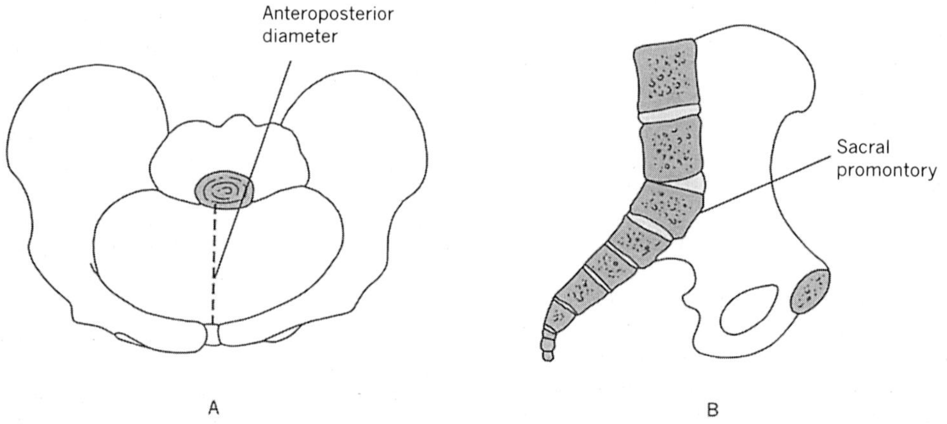

Figure 24.12 *A rachitic flat pelvis. (a) Reduced anteroposterior diameter; widened and irregular transverse diameter. (b) Sacral promontory pushed forwards and downwards; sacrum pushed backwards (from Sweet B, 1997, with permission).*

MATERNAL ADAPTATIONS TO PREGNANCY

Calcium and phosphorus metabolism

Maternal calcium metabolism is altered to meet fetal needs for calcium and phosphorus to enable skeletal growth and development. The amount and efficiency of calcium absorption by the intestinal cells are increased because of increased parathyroid hormone (PTH) and active vitamin D. The total extra calcium by term is about 25–30 g, most of which is used for fetal bone formation (Blackburn & Loper 1992). Fetal plasma calcium level exceeds that of the mother, suggesting that the mineral is actively transported across the placenta. The hormones PTH and calcitonin cannot pass across the placenta so that the fetus must manufacture his own. The placenta can transfer vitamin D to the fetus and can also synthesise vitamin D.

During pregnancy maternal calcium, phosphate and magnesium levels fall due to the increased production of PTH, calcitonin and vitamin D. These changes occur under the influence of oestrogen and HPL. Calcium metabolism is related to the changes in ECF volume, renal function and fetal needs.

Calcium

Calcium levels begin to fall soon after fertilisation and reach their lowest levels at about 30 weeks of pregnancy. Whilst serum calcium total may fall by 5%, Blackburn & Loper (1992) report that most investigators have found a slight but non-significant fall in the level of ionised calcium. Although there may be an increase in calcium storage in preparation for lactation, extra dietary calcium does not appear to enhance bone density. Any increase in bone calcium due to HPL is counter-balanced by the effect of oestrogen, causing a decrease in reabsorption. Oestrogen increases PTH which enhances intestinal calcium absorption and reduces renal calcium losses.

Phosphorus and magnesium

Serum inorganic phosphate levels and magnesium levels fall slightly until 30 weeks of pregnancy and return to non-pregnant levels by term. These changes are related to haemodilution.

Control of calcium metabolism pregnancy

Parathyroid hormone

There is parathyroid gland hyperplasia during pregnancy which accounts for the increase in PTH. This may be hormonally caused but may also be due to the small but constant reduction in serum calcium stimulating an increase in PTH and thus hyperplasia of the glands in response to the extra work required of them. The rise in PTH increases release of calcium from bone and the availability of calcium for transfer to the fetus. It also counteracts the influence of other factors that would decrease calcium in maternal ECF.

Vitamin D

Levels of active vitamin D (1,25-dihydroxycholecalciferol) show a small rise by 10 weeks of pregnancy although staying within recognised normal limits. They rise above the normal limit in the last few weeks of pregnancy. Intestinal absorption of vitamin D is enhanced throughout pregnancy. Elevated amounts of vitamin D are necessary to ensure both maternal and fetal demands for calcium are met.

Calcitonin

During pregnancy calcitonin levels rise. This is thought to counteract the action of the increased PTH to protect the mother from excessive loss of calcium and increase the intestinal and renal actions to provide calcium for the fetus.

The effects of relaxin

During pregnancy the corpus luteum of the maternal ovary and the placenta secrete specific hormones that alter the function of nearly every system in the body. Oestrogen and progesterone are the best known of these hormones but there is a hormone called relaxin which is produced mainly by the corpus luteum although there is probably some production by the decidua and the amnion (Klopper 1991).

Relaxin has a similar biochemical structure to insulin. It is a small peptide, probably acting as a growth-controlling hormone, which affects collagen and appears to be a potent stimulator of uterine growth in pregnancy. Relaxin may also contribute to fetal growth. It is involved in the softening and effacement of the cervix and in the onset of labour. During pregnancy it plays a major role in restraining uterine muscle contractability. With progesterone, it also causes relaxation of the ligaments and muscles, reaching its maximum effect in the last few weeks of pregnancy.

Softening of the symphysis pubis and sacroiliac joints of the pelvis leads to instability of the pelvic girdle. The sacrococcygeal joint also softens, allowing extra backward movement. These changes facilitate engagement of the presenting part in late pregnancy, especially in primigravidae with firm abdominal wall muscles, and delivery by increasing the pelvic diameters. Some women develop a rolling gait and as the pregnancy progresses, the weight and position of the uterus change the centre of gravity. The woman leans backwards to compensate, exaggerating the normal lumbar curve.

CLINICAL IMPLICATIONS

Maternal calcium and phosphorus intake

It is recommended that pregnant women increase their calcium and phosphorus intake from 800 mg/day to 1200 mg/day. Supplementation may be needed by pregnant adolescents or by women in groups where dietary insufficiency is suspected. Adequate vitamin D is essential to ensure absorption and 400 IU/day is recommended. Supplementation is recommended if dietary intake is poor or there is poor exposure to sunlight. Milk is an excellent source of calcium, phosphorus and vitamin D and women who cannot drink milk can be encouraged to take cheese, yoghurt, sardines, whole grain foods or green leafy vegetables.

Some foods, such as those which contain excessive fats, phytates (found in many vegetables) and oxalates, interfere with the absorption of calcium by forming insoluble calcium salts within the intestine, which are excreted. High sodium intake may also interfere with calcium absorption. Although phosphorus is essential during pregnancy, high intake levels limit calcium absorption whilst high plasma phosphorus levels increase the urinary excretion of calcium. Processed meats, snack foods and cola drinks all have high phosphorus but low calcium levels (Blackburn & Loper 1992)

Leg cramps

Women may suffer from intense sudden cramping pains in the calf muscles, especially during the 3rd trimester of pregnancy.

These tend to occur in bed and may awaken the woman. Lowered serum ionised calcium and increased phosphates are thought to be responsible for the muscle contractions. Respiratory alkalosis may precipitate muscle spasm. A possible alternative cause of leg pain that must be eliminated is thrombophlebitis. Cramps may be prevented by reducing milk and processed food intake (reducing phosphate intake) and performing stretching exercises before retiring. Jimenez (1994) suggests that taking calcium salts that are free of phosphates or taking the antacid aluminium hydroxide may prevent phosphorus absorption and correct the balance.

Restless leg syndrome

This disorder is seen in about 10–15% of pregnant women and occurs usually about 15 minutes after going to bed (Blackburn & Loper 1992). There is a burning, twitching feeling in the lower leg and the more the wish to fidget is resisted, the worse the sensation becomes. The cause of this syndrome, either in pregnancy or in non-pregnant women and men, is unknown. Iron and/or folic acid deficiency have been implicated and replacement therapy has helped. Circulatory problems may also be involved. Walking about and the application of a cold compress may relieve symptoms.

Rickets and osteomalacia

Turton et al (1977) linked lower calcium concentrations in pregnant Asian women and lower neonatal plasma calcium levels in their babies with marginal vitamin D shortage. Osteomalacia is a condition of malabsorption of calcium brought about by a deficiency in vitamin D caused by low intake but sometimes combined with decreased exposure to sunlight. The bones are poorly ossified and soft and become deformed. In childhood the condition is called rickets and in adults osteomalacia. Distortion of the pelvis may occur, leading to severe problems in childbirth. Both rickets and osteomalacia are more common in the Asian population in Britain (Dunnigan et al 1982).

Spinal cord injury

Paraplegic or quadriplegic women can have a successful outcome to their pregnancy. Although there are dangers of urinary tract infections, constipation and pressure sores, most of these problems can be avoided. Uterine contractions in labour are mainly independent of neurological control and labour should progress normally. Pain may be perceived if the spinal lesion is below T10 (see Chapter 38). Delivery of the baby may need to be assisted if the control of expulsive muscles is lost.

THE FETAL SKULL

The shape and size of the human pelvis create birthing difficulties not found in other primates (Morgan 1994). This is further compounded by the large human brain. In general, the larger the primate (monkeys and apes), the smaller its brain as a proportion of its body weight (Walker & Shipman 1996). At birth the average human baby weighs 3300 g, of which its brain constitutes about 385 g and continues to grow at fetal rates for the next 20 months to reach 1000 g. Brain growth now becomes slower than the rest of the body, achieving its average adult size of 1400 g (Jones et al 1992). In contrast, a newborn gorilla weighs 2000 g and has a correspondingly smaller brain of 225 g, already half the adult size of 450 g after a gestation only 6 days shorter than the human pregnancy. Gorillas have very easy births (Morgan 1994).

To overcome the tight fit between the human pelvis and the fetal skull, the following evolutionary changes have developed.

- Birth whilst the fetus is very immature.
- Continuation of fetal rate of brain growth after delivery.
- Flexion of the head on the neck so that the narrowest diameters pass through the pelvis.
- Moulding of the skull to change the shape (but not the size) from globular to cylindrical.

Because of this pattern of brain growth, the baby remains very dependent on its parents for a long time but the continued growth of the brain during childhood allows time for complex social skills to be learned. In contrast to the gorilla, where behaviour is largely 'hard wired' into the genes, behaviour in the human is more dependent on the influence of the environment, allowing creativity in response to novel situations (Bogin 1988).

Anatomy

The fetal skull is ovoid in shape and the bones can be divided into the vault, the face and the base. The vault extends from the orbital ridges to the base of the occiput and contains the brain, which sits in the bones forming the base of the skull. The fetal skull differs from the adult skull in its proportions as the vault is large in relation to the face (Sweet 1997). For the purposes of measurement and to describe the degree of flexion and extension in the different presentations, the fetal skull is divided into regions of face, brow, vertex and occiput (Fig. 24.13).

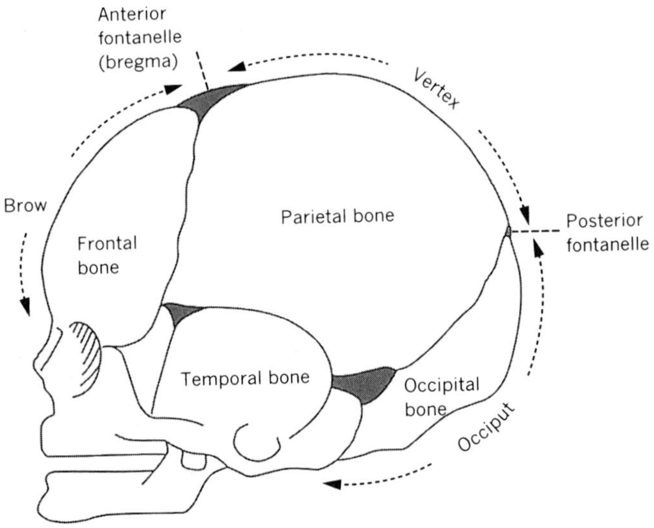

Figure 24.13 *The bones, fontanelles and regions of the fetal skull (from Sweet B, 1997, with permission).*

- The **face** extends from the chin to the orbital ridges.
- The **brow or sinciput** is the area of the two frontal bones extending from the orbital ridges to the anterior fontanelle.
- The **vertex** is bounded by the anterior fontanelle, the posterior fontanelle and the two parietal eminences.
- The **occiput** is the area over the occipital bone extending from the posterior fontanelle to the nape of the neck.

The face and base of the skull are laid down in cartilage and are almost completely ossified by birth. The vault of the fetal skull is composed of flat bones which develop from membrane. Ossification centres within the membrane lay down bone around them. The ossification centre of each bone is visible on the ossified bone (Bennett & Brown 1996).

Bones – the vault

Five main bones make up the vault with two others helping to form the lateral walls – the squamous (flattened) parts of the temporal bones. Each bone is named for the lobe of the brain lying beneath it (Anderson 1992).

- Two frontal bones from ossification centres indicated by the frontal bosses.
- Two parietal bones from ossification centres indicated by the parietal eminences.
- Two squamous portions of the temporal bones.
- One occipital bone from an ossification centre indicated by the occipital protuberance.

The process of ossification is incomplete at birth so that membranous sutures remain between the bones and membranous fontanelles where two or more sutures meet. These areas of membrane facilitate moulding of the fetal skull during birth. They also provide landmarks on the skull for identification during vaginal examination (Fig. 24.14).

The sutures

- The **frontal** suture lies between the two frontal bones.
- The **sagittal** suture runs from the anterior to the posterior fontanelle uniting the two parietal bones.
- The **lambdoidal** suture (after its resemblance to the Greek letter lambda – λ) lies between the posterior edges of the parietal bones and the occipital bone.
- The **coronal** suture separates the posterior edges of the two frontal bones from the anterior edges of the two parietal bones.

The fontanelles

There are two main fontanelles. The **anterior** fontanelle or **bregma** is roughly diamond shaped and is formed at the junction of four sutures – the frontal, parietal and two halves of the coronal sutures. It measures 2.5 cm across by 3 cm long and is not fully closed by ossification until 18 months of age.

The **posterior** fontanelle or **lambda** is much smaller and triangular in shape, formed at the junction of three sutures – the sagittal suture and the two halves of the lambdoidal suture. It closes by the 6th week after birth.

Besides these two main fontanelles, four minor fontanelles form in the side walls of the vault. These are the two temporal fontanelles at the ends of the coronal suture and two mastoid fontanelles at the ends of the lambdoidal suture. These are not of any significance in childbearing (Anderson 1992).

Bones – the base

The fused bones of the base of the skull are perforated by the foramen magnum which allows passage of the spinal cord leading from the brain.

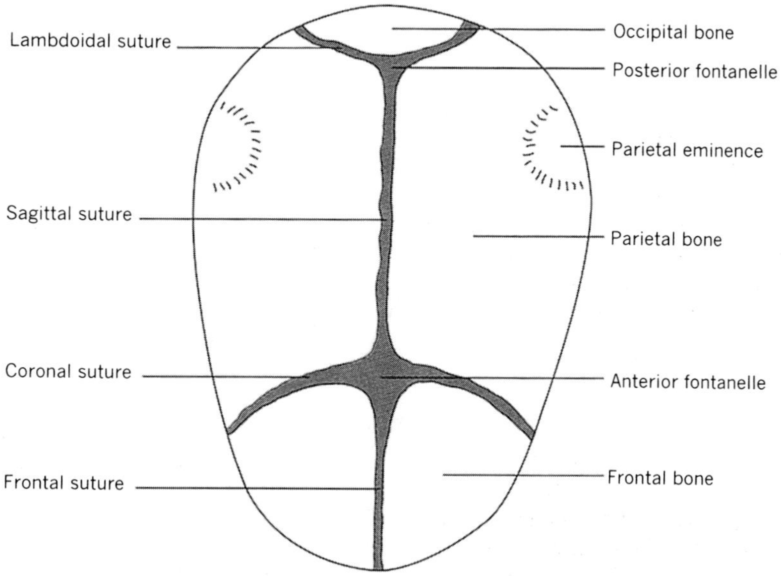

Figure 24.14 *The fetal skull, showing the bones, fontanelles and sutures (from Sweet B, 1997, with permission).*

Diameters

Measurements of the skull are used to assess its size in relation to the maternal pelvis. Longitudinal diameters are taken between key landmarks so that the diameters presenting at the pelvis in different degrees of flexion or extension of the head on the neck can be estimated (Figs 24.15 and 24.16).

- **Suboccipitobregmatic** is measured from the nape of the neck to the centre of the anterior fontanelle. It is 9.5 cm and presents when the head is fully flexed.
- **Suboccipitofrontal** is measured from the nape of the neck to the centre of the frontal suture. It is 10 cm and presents when the head is almost completely flexed.
- **Occipitofrontal** is measured from the glabella (bridge of the nose) to the occipital protuberance. It is 11.5 cm and presents when the head is deflexed in an occipitoposterior position.
- **Mentovertical** is measured from the point of the chin to the highest point of the vertex. It is 13.5 cm and presents when the head is midway between flexion and extension in a brow presentation.
- **Submentovertical** is measured from the junction of the chin with the neck to the highest point on the vertex. It is 11.5 cm and presents when the head is not fully extended in a face presentation.
- **Submentobregmatic** is measured from the junction of the chin with the neck. It is 9.5 cm and presents when the head is fully extended in a face presentation.

Transverse diameters are also taken

- The **biparietal**, measured between the parietal eminences. It measures 9.5 cm and is the widest transverse diameter of the skull.
- The **bitemporal**, measured between the widest aspects of the coronal suture. It is 8 cm.

Circumferences of the skull are:

- **suboccipitobregmatic** – 33 cm. Presents when the head is well flexed. The head engages, fits well onto the cervix and labour should be easy;
- **occipitofrontal** – 35 cm. Presents when the head is deflexed. Engagement is delayed, the membranes may rupture early and labour may be difficult;
- **mentovertical** – 39 cm. Presents when the head is fully extended. The head cannot descend into the pelvis and labour is obstructed.

Moulding

Moulding of the fetal skull results in a change in shape but not size of the vault brought about by the pressures of the pelvis and pelvic floor during labour. The diameters which are compressed reduce in size by at least 0.5 cm whilst those at right angles to them are elongated. The skull changes shape from ovoid to cylindrical to facilitate passage through the cylindrical birth canal. The sutures and fontanelles allow overlap of the bones of the vault in a typical way:

- the frontal bones are pushed under the anterior edge of the parietal bones;
- the occipital bone is pushed under the posterior part of the parietal bones;
- the medial edge of the leading parietal bone is pushed under the other parietal bone.

Moulding is abnormal if it involves wrong diameters (Fig. 24.17), with a risk of intracranial damage if it is extreme.

Caput succedaneum

During labour and especially after rupture of the membranes, the fetal head is pressed against the ring of the dilating cervix. In

Table 24.2 *Involvement of diameters of the fetal skull in moulding*

Presentation	*Diameters decreased*	*Diameters increased*
Vertex presentation	Suboccipitobregmatic Biparietal	Mentovertical
Brow presentation	Mentovertical Biparietal	Suboccipitobregmatic
Face presentation	Submentobregmatic Biparietal	Occipitofrontal
Occipitoposterior position	Occipitofrontal Biparietal	Submentobregmatic

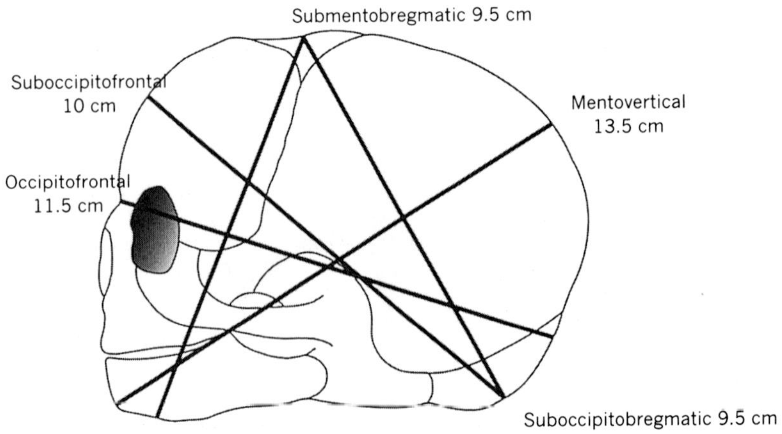

Figure 24.15 *The diameters of the fetal skull (from Sweet B, 1997, with permission).*

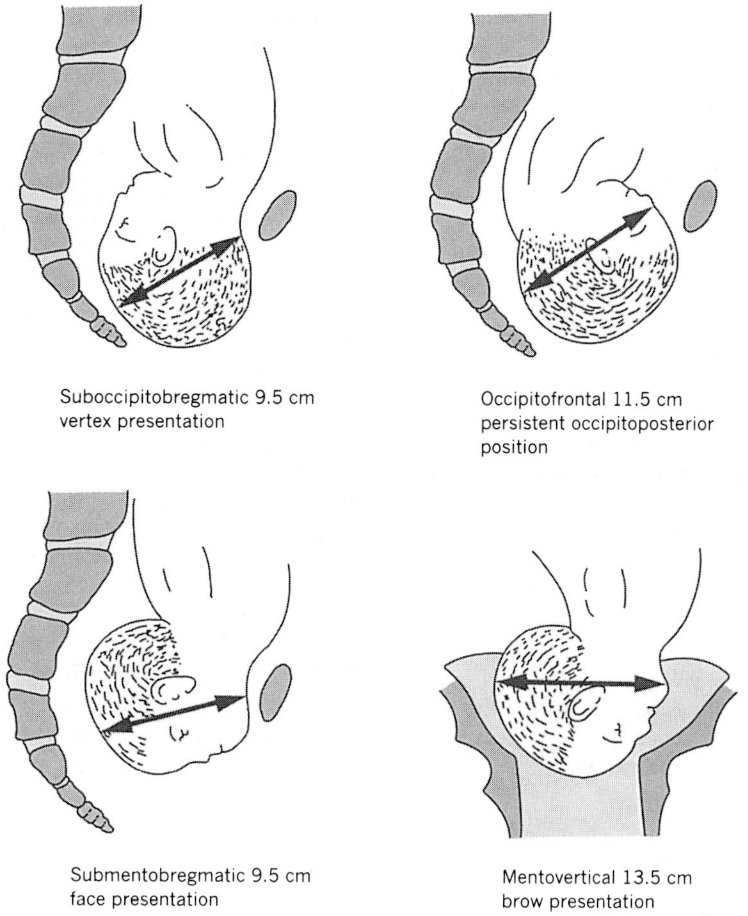

Figure 24.16 *The diameters of the fetal head in relation to the maternal pelvis (from Sweet B, 1997, with permission).*

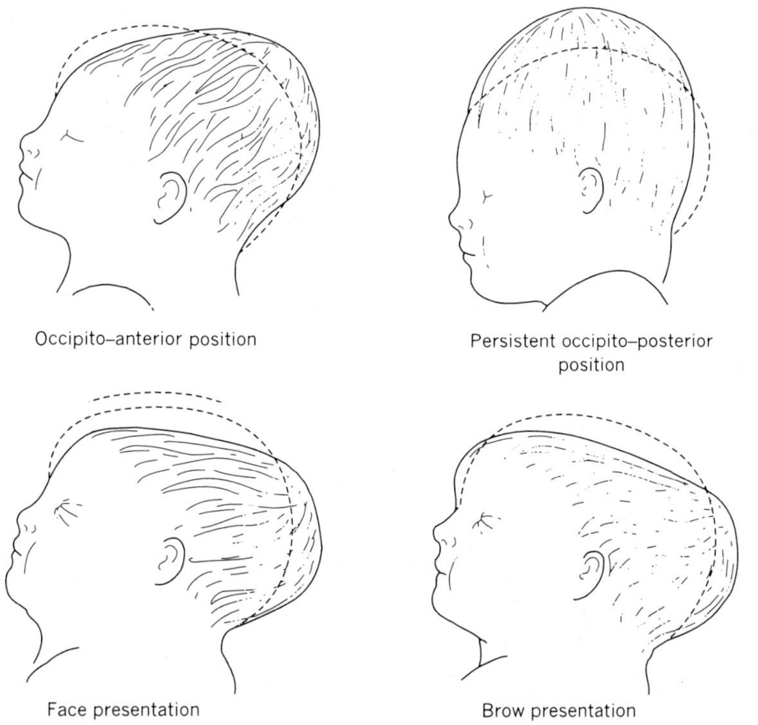

Figure 24.17 *Moulding of the fetal head (from Sweet B, 1997, with permission).*

cephalic presentations venous return in the scalp circulation is impeded and oedema forms in the loose tissues. This is called a caput succedaneum and varies in size with the length and difficulty of the delivery. Caput forms on the leading parietal bone, which is the left one when the occiput is to the right and vice versa. It forms on the anterior part if the position is occipitoanterior and on the posterior part of the parietal bone if the position is occipitoposterior.

External structures

The scalp of the fetal skull consists of five layers. From the inside out, these are:

1. the **pericranium**, which covers the outer surface of the bones and is firmly attached to the edges of the bones. Bleeding may occur between the bone and the pericranium to form a swelling called a **cephalhaematoma**. The size of the haematoma is limited to that of the bone over which it forms because of the attachment of the pericranium to the bony edges;
2. a loose layer of **areolar tissue** permitting limited movement of the scalp over the skull;
3. a layer of tendon known as the **galea** attached to the frontalis muscle anteriorly and the occipitalis muscle posteriorly;
4. a layer of **subcutaneous tissue** containing blood vessels and hair follicles. This is the part of the scalp affected by the caput succedaneum (Fig. 24.18);
5. the skin.

Internal structures

The meninges

The brain is surrounded by three membranes. From the inside, these are the **pia mater**. which is closely applied to the surface of the brain, the **arachnoid mater**, which contains cerebrospinal fluid, and the outer, tough **dura mater**.

The dura mater covers the outer surface of the brain and dips down to form compartments (Fig. 24.19). There are two main folds of the dura mater. The **falx cerebri** is a double fold forming a partition between the two cerebral hemispheres. It is attached to the skull following the line of the frontal and sagittal sinuses from the root of the nose to the internal aspect of the occipital protuberance. Its lower edge is unattached and is sickle shaped.

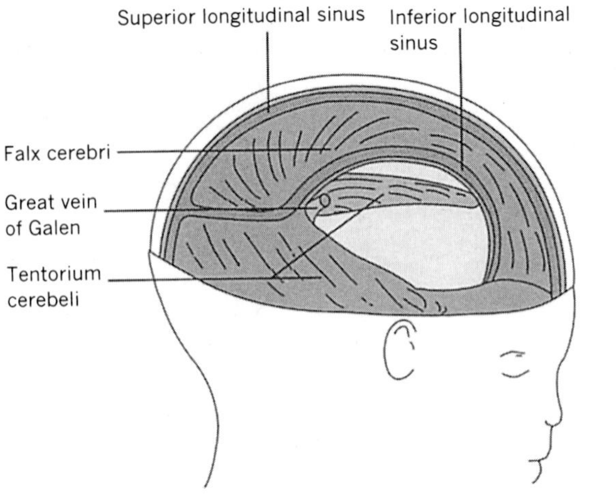

Figure 24.19 *Internal structures of the fetal skull (from Sweet B, 1997, with permission).*

The **tentorium cerebelli** lies horizontally, separating the cerebrum from the cerebellum. It is at right angles to the falx cerebri and is horseshoe shaped. Each side of the horseshoe is attached laterally to the sphenoid bone and along the inner surface of the petrous portion of the temporal bone. It meets the falx at the internal occipital protuberance. The brainstem passes in front of the junction of the two folds of dura mater.

Blood supply of the brain

The arterial blood supply is via two internal carotid arteries and two vertebral arteries. The internal carotid arteries give off pairs of anterior, middle and posterior cerebral arteries. Each vertebral artery gives off a branch which supplies the cerebellum and medulla oblongata before uniting with its partner to form the basilar artery. The basilar artery gives off two pairs of arteries to the cerebellum and upper brainstem before dividing into two terminal branches that link up with the ends of the internal carotids. One-quarter of the population maintain three cerebral arteries on both sides of the brain whilst in the majority of people the vertebral arteries take over the

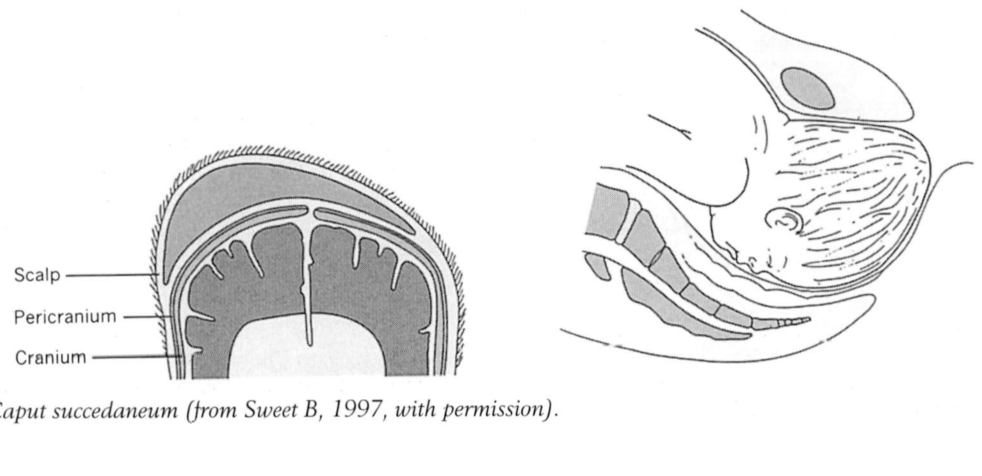

Figure 24.18 *Caput succedaneum (from Sweet B, 1997, with permission).*

posterior cerebral arteries. These intercommunicating arteries at the base of the brain are known as the **circle of Willis** (Fig. 24.20).

The venous drainage is by channels in the dural folds called sinuses.

- The superior longitudinal (or sagittal) sinus runs along the upper border of the falx cerebri.
- The inferior longitudinal (or sagittal) sinus runs along the lower border of the falx cerebri.
- The straight sinus is a continuation of the inferior longitudinal sinus which runs posteriorly to join the superior longitudinal sinus.
- The great vein of Galen joins the straight sinus at the junction with the inferior venous sinus.
- From the confluence of sinuses, the lateral sinuses pass along the line of attachment of the tentorium cerebelli and emerge from the skull to become the internal jugular veins of the neck.

When moulding is severe, rapid or in the wrong direction these membranes and sinuses may be torn, especially at the junction of the two folds of dura. The tentorium is most likely to be damaged and bleeding involves the great vein of Galen, the straight sinus and the inferior longitudinal sinus.

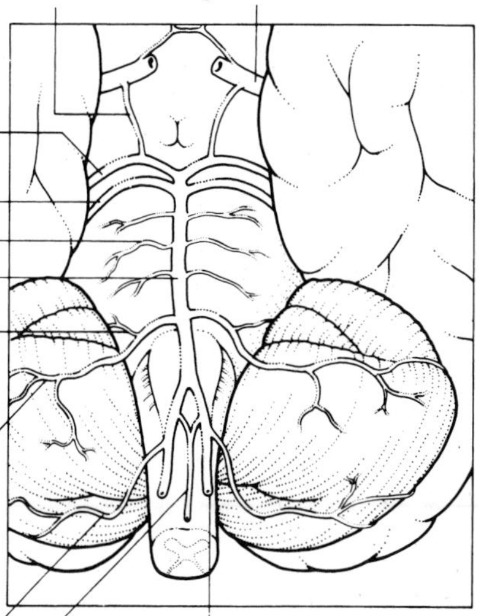

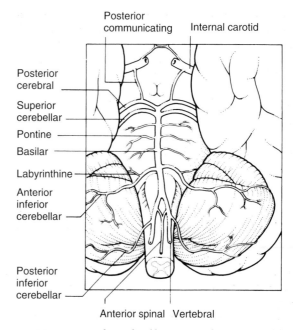

Figure 24.20 *Arterial supply of brainstem (from Fitzgerald MJT, 1996, with permission).*

Summary of main points

- Bone is a connective tissue which contains deposits of calcium and phosphorus and performs important functions for the body. It consists of three basic components: an organic matrix of collagen known as osteoid, a mineral matrix of calcium and phosphorus and bone cells. Bone can be divided into compact or lamellar bone and spongy bone.
- Most bones have a tough outer covering called the periosteum. Lining the marrow cavity of a bone is a fine layer of tissue called the endosteum which contains the osteoblasts, osteoclasts and their precursor cells. Osteoblasts synthesise and secrete the constituents of and promote mineralisation of the matrix. Osteocytes maintain the bone matrix. Osteoclasts contain a large number of enzymes which can remove both the organic and mineral matrix.
- The skeleton contains 99% of the calcium and 85% of the phosphorus present in the body. Three hormones are involved in the control of calcium and phosphorus metabolism: parathyroid hormone (PTH), vitamin D and calcitonin.
- The pelvic girdle is for attachment of the lower limbs and for support of the pelvic abdominal organs. The size, shape and rigidity of the pelvic girdle are related to bipedal locomotion. The curved spine is essential for maintaining an upright posture. The gynaecoid pelvis is adapted for giving birth to a baby with a comparatively large head.
- The bony ring of the pelvis is made up of four irregularly shaped bones: two innominate bones forming the lateral and anterior walls and the sacrum and coccyx forming the posterior wall. Each innominate bone consists of three fused bones: the ilium, ischium and pubis. There are four joints – one symphysis pubis, two sacroiliac joints and one sacrococcygeal joint. Besides the ligaments supporting each of the pelvic joints, there are three other pairs of ligaments: the sacrotuberous ligament, the sacrospinous ligament and the inguinal ligament.
- A line of bone called the pelvic brim separates the upper flare of the iliac fossae from the basin-shaped part of the pelvis. The area above this is called the false pelvis whilst below the brim is the true pelvis forming the birth canal with a cavity and outlet.
- If a piece of paper was placed across the landmarks a flat surface would be formed called a plane and the concept can also be applied to the cavity and outlet. Measurements are taken of the planes of the pelvic brim, cavity and outlet in three directions: anteroposterior, oblique and transverse.
- When a person stands up the pelvic basin is tilted in relation to the horizontal. Imaginary lines drawn at right angles through the planes of the pelvis and joined together form a curve that the fetus must pass through during birth – the curve of Carus. There are four basic types of pelvis described, gynaecoid, android, anthropoid and platypelloid.
- Maternal calcium metabolism alters to meet fetal needs for calcium and phosphorus to enable skeletal growth and development. Serum calcium levels begin to fall soon after fertilisation and reach their lowest levels at about 30 weeks of pregnancy. Serum inorganic phosphate levels and magnesium levels fall slightly until 30 weeks of pregnancy and return to non-pregnant levels by term. Pregnant women should increase their calcium and phosphorus intake. Adequate vitamin D is essential to ensure absorption. Some foods which contain excessive fats, phytates and oxalates interfere with the absorption of calcium.
- Pregnancy problems include intense cramping pain in the calf muscles, restless leg syndrome and backache. Serious problems are rickets, osteomalacia and spinal cord injury.
- The fetal skull is ovoid in shape and the bones can be divided into the vault, the face and the base. The face and base of the skull are laid down in cartilage and are almost completely ossified by birth. The vault of the fetal skull is composed of flat bones which develop from membrane.
- For the purposes of measurement and to describe the degree of flexion and extension in the different presentations, the fetal skull is divided into regions of face, brow, vertex and occiput. The process of ossification is incomplete at birth so that membranous sutures remain between the bones and membranous fontanelles where two or more sutures meet. Measurements of the skull are used to assess

its size in relation to the maternal pelvis.

- Moulding of the fetal skull results in a change in shape but not size of the vault brought about by the pressures of the pelvis and pelvic floor during labour. The diameters which are compressed reduce in size by at least 0.5 cm whilst those at right angles to them are elongated. Moulding is abnormal if it involves wrong diameters, is extreme or too rapid.
- The brain is surrounded by three meninges: the pia mater, the arachnoid mater and the dura mater. The dura mater covers the outer surface of the brain and dips down to form compartments. There are two main folds of the dura mater: the falx cerebri and the tentorium cerebelli.
- The arterial blood supply to the brain is via two internal carotid arteries and two vertebral arteries. The internal carotid arteries give off pairs of anterior, middle and posterior cerebral arteries. The intercommunicating arteries at the base of the brain are known as the circle of Willis. The venous drainage is by channels in the dural folds called sinuses.

References

Aiello L, Dean C. 1990 An Introduction to Human Evolutionary Anatomy. Academic Press, New York.

Anderson M. 1992 The Anatomy and Physiology of Obstetrics. Wolfe Publishing, London.

Bennett VR, Brown LK. (Eds) 1996 Myles Textbook for Midwives, 12th edn. Churchill Livingstone, Edinburgh, pp 57–64.

Blackburn ST, Loper DL. 1992 Maternal, Fetal and Neonatal Physiology, A Clinical Perspective. WB Saunders, Philadelphia.

Bogin B. 1988 Patterns of Human Growth. Cambridge University Press, Cambridge.

Boore JRP. 1996 Endocrine function. In Hinchliff SM, Montague SE, Watson R (Eds) Physiology for Nursing Practice. Baillière Tindall, London, pp 202–244.

Davis DC. 1996 The discomforts of pregnancy, Journal of Obstetric, Gynecologic and Neonatal Nursing 25, 73–80.

Dunnigan MG, MicIntosh WB, Ford JA, Roberson I. 1982 Acquired disorders in vitamin D metabolism. In Heath D, Marx SJ (eds) Calcium Disorders. Butterworths, London.

Fitzgerald MJT. 1996 Neuroanatomy. Saunders, Philadelphia.

Hinchliff SM, Montague SE. 1990 Physiology for Nursing Practice. Baillière Tindall, London.

Jimenez S. 1994 If you can't get comfortable. Childbirth 11(1), 37–40.

Jones S, Martin M, Pilbeam D. 1992 The Cambridge Encyclopedia of Human Evolution. Cambridge University Press, Cambridge.

Klopper A. 1991 The ovary. In Hytten F, Chamberlain G (eds) Clinical Physiology in Obstetrics, Blackwell Scientific, Oxford, pp 377–389.

Morgan E. 1990 The Scars of Evolution. Penguin, Harmondsworth.

Morgan E. 1994 The Descent of the Child. Souvenir Press, London.

Reeve J. 1991 Calcium metabolism. In Hytten F, Chamberlain G (Eds) Clinical Physiology in Obstetrics. Blackwell Scientific, Oxford, pp 213–223.

Sweet BR. 1997 The fetal skull. In Sweet BR with Tiran D (Eds) Mayes Midwifery, 12th edn. Baillière Tindall, London, p 116.

Trevathen W. 1987 Human Birth: An Evolutionary Perspective. Aldine de Gruyter, New York.

Turton CWG, Stanley P, Stamp TCB, Maxwell JD. 1977 Altered vitamin D metabolism in pregnancy. Lancet I, 222.

Walker A, Shipman P. 1996 The Wisdom of the Bones. Weidenfeld and Nicolson.

Recommended reading

Bogin B. 1988 Patterns of Human Growth. Cambridge University Press, Cambridge.

Davis DC, 1996 The discomforts of pregnancy, Journal of Obstetric, Gynecologic and Neonatal Nursing 25, 73–80.

Morgan E. 1990 The Scars of Evolution. Penguin, Harmondsworth.

Morgan E. 1994 The Descent of the Child. Souvenir Press, London.

Morgan E. 1997 The Aquatic Ape Hypothesis. Souvenir Press, London.

Reeve J. 1991 Calcium metabolism. In Hytten F, Chamberlain G (eds) Clinical Physiology in Obstetrics. Blackwell Scientific, Oxford, pp 213–223.

Chapter 25 Muscle – the pelvic floor and the uterus

In this chapter

INTRODUCTION

This chapter will describe the nature of muscle but not individual muscles except for the pelvic floor and uterus. Anatomy and physiology texts are useful additional reading if more detail on other muscle systems is required.

If bones form the framework of the body then muscles form the cladding. Muscle makes up almost half of the body's mass and is the tissue that enables movement to occur. It transforms the chemical energy in adenosine triphosphate into mechanical energy. There are three basic muscle types: skeletal muscle that allows movement of the whole body by exerting force on the skeleton, smooth muscle found in the walls of the hollow viscera of the gastrointestinal, genitourinary and respiratory tracts and the specialised cardiac muscle.

All muscle cells are elongated and therefore referred to as **fibres** and they all contain two kinds of protein filaments – **actin** and **myosin**. Muscles have four functions: they produce movement, maintain posture, stabilise joints and generate heat (Marieb 1992). They have four properties: excitability which is the ability to receive and respond to a stimulus, contractility or the ability to shorten when stimulated, extensibility or the ability to be stretched or extended beyond the resting length and elasticity or the ability of muscle to recoil back to its resting length (Marieb 1992).

SKELETAL MUSCLE

Skeletal muscles are attached to and cover the bony skeleton. The longest muscle fibres are found in skeletal muscle and the fibres have obvious bands or striations, hence the term **striated muscle**. Another term used for skeletal muscle is **voluntary**, as this is the only muscle type under voluntary control. Skeletal muscle can contract rapidly but tires easily and must be rested after short bursts of activity. Each skeletal muscle is a discrete organ made up of multiple muscle fibres. Other tissues are also found in the individual muscle such as connective tissue, blood vessels and nerve fibres. Muscle fibres are gathered into functional units by a network of fibrous connective tissue (Fig. 25.1). This connective tissue condenses to become the tendons which form the muscular origins and insertions onto bone.

The activity of skeletal muscle depends on its rich blood and nerve supply. Whilst the other muscle types can contract without nerve stimulation, each skeletal muscle fibre is supplied with a nerve ending. The blood supply is essential to deliver the large amounts of oxygen and nutrients and remove equally large amounts of metabolic waste. The smaller blood vessels are long and winding which permits the changes in muscle length to occur.

Microscopic anatomy of a skeletal muscle fibre

Skeletal muscle fibres are long cylindrical cells which taper at both ends (McClaren 1996). The plasma membrane is called the **sarcolemma** and there are multiple oval nuclei arranged just below the surface. Muscle cells are enormously large, normally ranging between 1 and 40 mm, but some may reach 300 mm (one foot) in length. Their diameter ranges from 10 to 100 μm. The presence of multiple nuclei indicates that each muscle fibre is a **syncytium** (fusion of many cells) formed during embryonic development. The cytoplasm in muscle cells is called **sarcoplasm** and the endoplasmic reticulum is referred to as **sarcoplasmic reticulum**. The sarcoplasm contains large amounts of stored glycogen and a unique oxygen-binding protein called **myoglobin** similar to haemoglobin.

Myofibrils

Each muscle fibre contains a large number of rod-like myofibrils extending the full length of the cell and parallel to each other. Myofibrils are densely packed and form 80% of the cellular content. Mitochondria, the energy-producing organelles, and other organelles are packed in between the myofibrils. Myofibrils are the contractile elements of the cells and each myofibril consists of smaller contractile units called **sarcomeres**. Several sarcomeres are arranged along each myofibril.

Myofibrils appear to be made of alternate dark or **A bands** and light or **I bands**, giving the characteristic striped appearance under the light microscope. The bands are given their names because of how they refract (bend) polarised light (light waves with a definite direction). The A in A bands stands for **anisotropic** (tropic means pertaining to a turn), meaning that their ability to refract light depends on its angle. The I in I bands stands for **isotropic**, meaning that they refract light whatever its angle (Lang 1990, Marieb 1992).

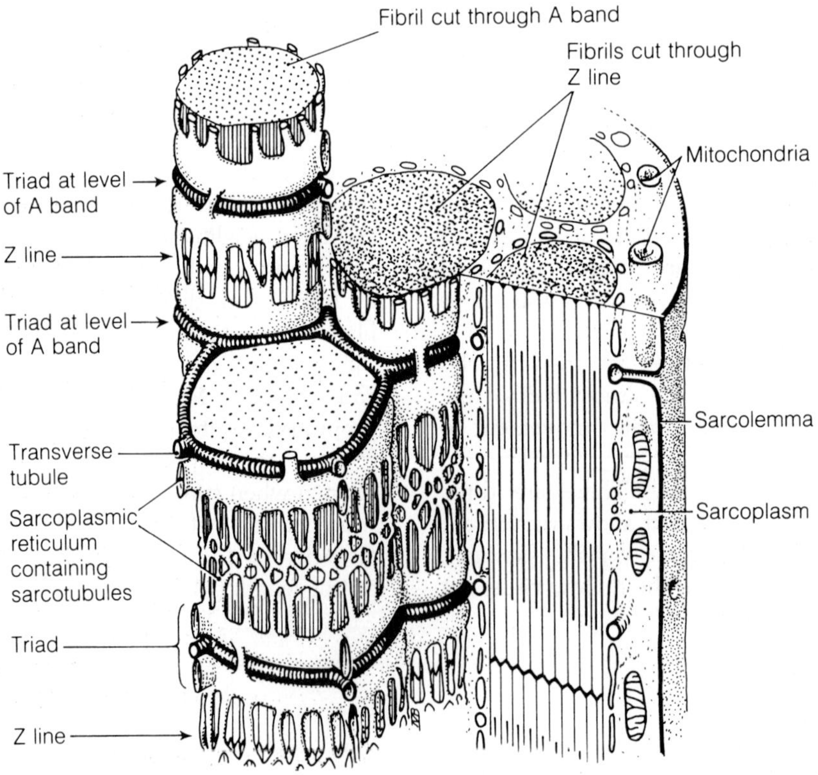

Figure 25.1 *Intracellular tubular systems (from Hinchliff SM, Montague SE, 1990, with permission).*

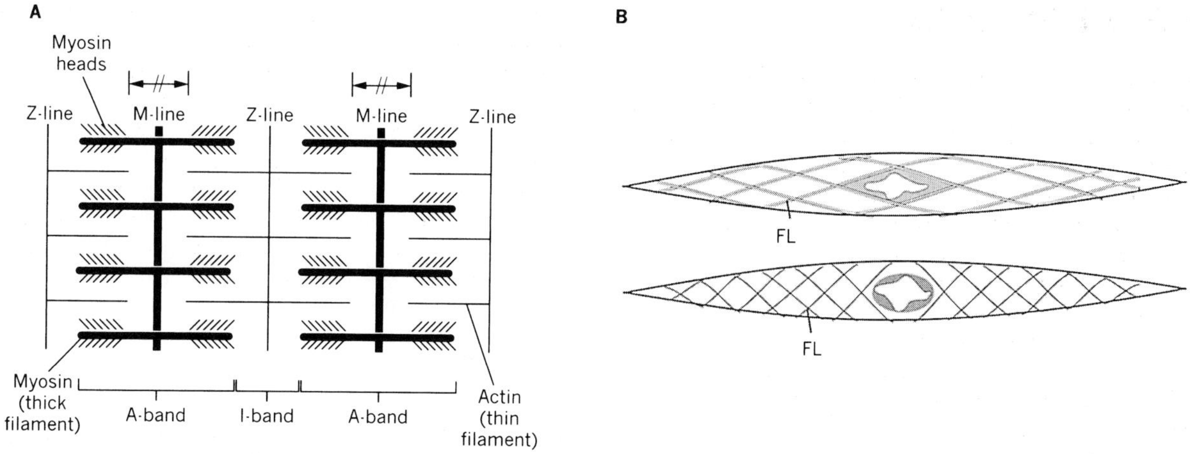

Figure 25.2 *(a) Striated and (b) smooth fibres. A, actin; M, myosin; FL, filaments. (Reproduced with permission from Huszar & Roberts 1982.)*

The A band is interrupted in its midsection by the highly refractive **H zone** (H stands for helle, which means bright). Each H zone is bisected by a dark line called the **M line**. The I bands also have a midline interruption called the **Z line** (Figs 25.1 and 25.2). A sarcomere is the region of a myofibril that extends from one Z line to the next. Brief explanations of the other features are given below.

- The Z line is a flat protein sheet that forms a point of attachment for the thin filaments.
- The H zone is only visible in relaxed muscle when the thick filaments are not overlapped by the thin filaments.
- The M line in the centre of the H zone appears darker because it is slightly thicker due to the presence of fine strands that connect adjacent thick filaments together.

The higher magnifying power of the electron microscope shows that the A-bands are formed of the thick filaments of myosin (Fig. 25.3). The thin filaments are formed of three different proteins: **actin**, **troponin** and **tropomyosin** run the length of the I-band overlapping the thick filaments (Fig. 25.4). In an intact muscle fibre the bands are aligned horizontally across the width of the cell. Each myosin molecule has a rod-like tail or axis and two globular heads or crossbridges which interact with special sites on the thin filaments. Each thick filament within a sarcomere contains about 200 myosin molecules.

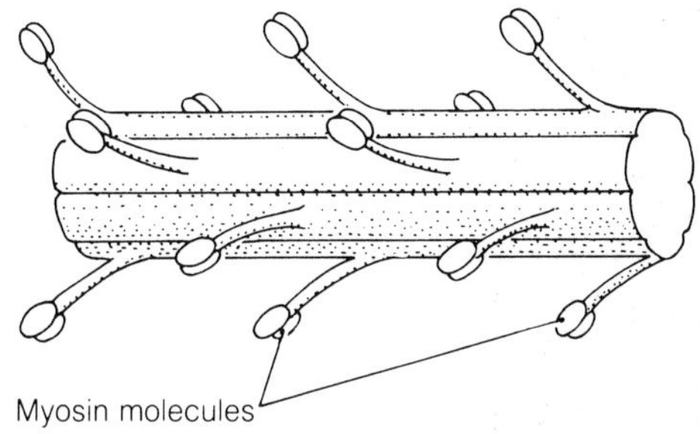

Figure 25.3 *Structure of a thick filament (from Hinchliff SM, Montague SE, 1990, with permission).*

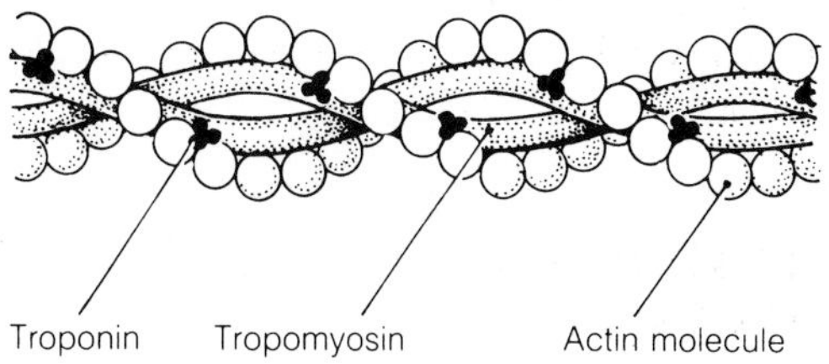

Figure 25.4 *Structure of a thin filament (from Hinchliff SM, Montague SE, 1990, with permission).*

The thin filaments are mainly composed of actin. Subunits called **globular** or **G actin** bear the active sites to which the myosin crossbridges attach themselves during muscle contraction. The backbone of each actin molecule is formed by two strands of **fibrous** or **F actin** arranged in a helical structure. Regulatory proteins include tropomyosin which spirals around the F actin to stiffen it. In resting muscle the orientation of the tropomyosin blocks the myosin-binding sites on the actin molecules, preventing the formation of crossbridges. Troponin actually consists of three polypeptides. One binds to actin and another to tropomyosin helping to position it on the actin, while the third binds calcium.

Intracellular tubular systems

The muscle cell is penetrated by two tubular systems (see Fig. 25.1) both ending near the A–I band junctions. One tubular system is called the **transverse** or **T system** extending from the cell exterior into the sarcoplasm where they branch and terminate. The other is the **internal system** formed by fine tubules called **sarcotubules** of the sarcoplasmic reticulum which end in terminal sacs called the **terminal cysternae**. Both systems play a key role in muscle contraction. T tubules conduct electrical stimuli deep within the muscle cell to the sarcomeres and the sarcoplasmic reticulum regulates the calcium ions.

Muscle contraction

There are several theories of how muscle fibres contract but

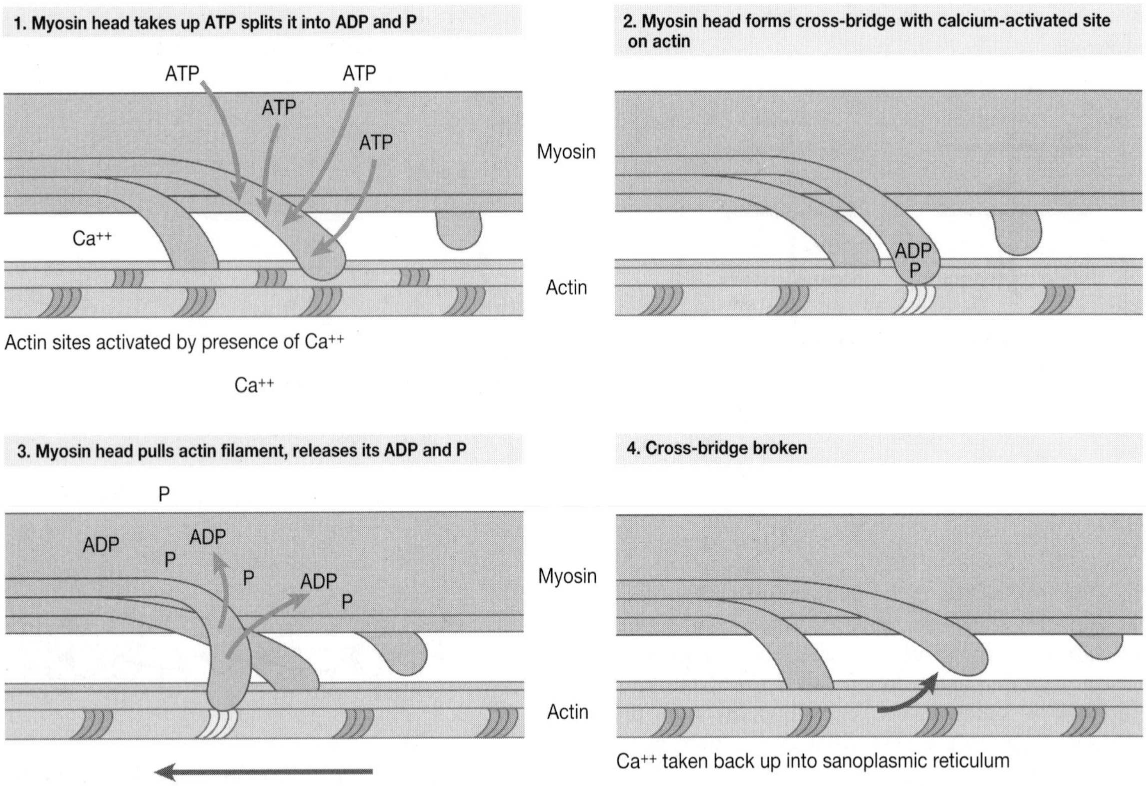

Figure 25.5 *Diagrammatic representation of the sliding-filament theory showing how the thick filaments of skeletal muscle move relative to one another as crossbridges are formed and broken (from Hinchliff SM, Montague SE, Watson R, 1996, with permission).*

most evidence supports the **sliding filament theory**. This explains that during contraction, the thin filaments slide past the thick ones to increase the amount of overlap, with the thin filaments penetrating more deeply into the central region of the A band. This is brought about by the crossbridges of the sarcomeres acting simultaneously as a ratchet to pull the thin filaments towards the centre of the sarcomeres, resulting in shortening of the muscle cell. The myosin heads are said to walk up the actin filaments step by step from one binding site to the next (Fig. 25.5). This requires the presence of calcium which binds to the troponin to form a complex. This changes the configuration of tropomyosin to move it away from the myosin-binding sites. As calcium is removed by the sarcoplasmic reticulum, the contraction comes to an end and the muscle cell relaxes.

Regulation of contraction

Skeletal muscles contract in response to nerve stimulation which results in an **action potential** being sent along the sarcolemma. This electrical event results in a rise in intracellular calcium ion levels that triggers off the contraction. The axon of a lower motor neurone (see Chapter 26) branches profusely as it enters the muscle and each mound-shaped unmyelinated axonal terminal forms a junction with a single muscle fibre, approximately in the middle of the cell. This is called a neuromuscular junction or **motor endplate** (Fig. 25.6). The plasma membrane of the axonal ending does not actually touch the muscle fibre; between them there is a small fluid-filled extracellular space called the **synaptic cleft**. The action potential must be transmitted across this space and this happens by the release of the neurotransmitter substance **acetylcholine** (ACh) from small membranous sacs in the axon terminal called **synaptic vesicles**.

When a nerve impulse reaches the end of an axon, **voltage-regulated calcium channels** open and calcium flows in from the ECF. The entry of the calcium causes some of the synaptic vesicles to fuse with the plasma membrane and release the ACh into the synaptic cleft. This process is called **exocytosis**. ACh diffuses across the synaptic cleft and attaches itself to ACh receptors on the sarcolemma. All plasma membranes are polarised with a voltage gradient (membrane potential) across the membrane. The inside of the cell is negative. This attachment of ACh molecules opens chemically regulated ion gates. The positively charged ion sodium passes from its higher concentration in the ECF fluid down a gradient into the cell, leading to a slight decrease in the negative potential. This event, called **depolarisation**, allows a muscle cell action potential to be generated and to pass in all directions across the sarcolemma.

Repolarisation of the sarcolemma follows the wave of the muscle action potential when sodium channels close and potassium channels open. Potassium rapidly diffuses out of the cell into the ECF down a gradient to restore the negativity inside the cell. The normal ionic balance of sodium and potassium is restored during the refractory period when the muscle cannot respond to stimuli. After the release of ACh and its binding to the ACh receptors, it is quickly destroyed by the enzyme **acetylcholinesterase**. This prevents the muscle contraction lasting longer than the stimulus requires.

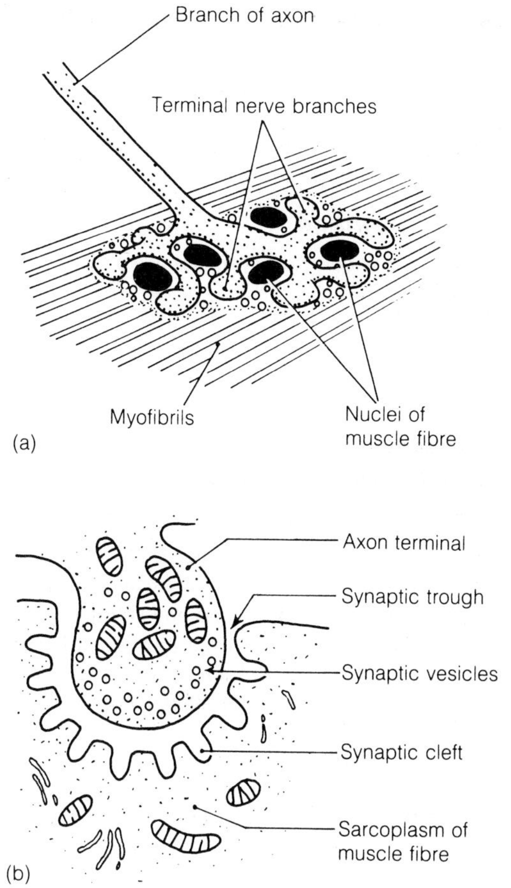

Figure 25.6 *The neuromuscular junction (from Hinchliff SM, Montague SE, Watson R, 1996, with permission).*

Excitation-contraction coupling

This is the process whereby the generation of an action potential is followed by activation of the contractile machinery in the myofibrils. It involves the exposure of the binding sites on the actin to allow the formation of crossbridges. Energy released from ATP is used to fuel the muscle contraction. As action potentials continue to arrive, the process is repeated many times, allowing sustained muscle contraction. Calcium ions are continuously released and taken up by troponin. This also requires energy from ATP. However, muscles store very little ATP and the supply is soon exhausted, in about 6 s! If contraction is to continue, ATP must be regenerated. This can occur in three ways:

- by the interaction of ADP with creatine phosphate;
- by aerobic respiration;
- by lactic acid fermentation.

The pelvic floor

The bony pelvis provides protection to the pelvic organs whilst the pelvic floor holds them in situ. The pelvic floor is formed by the soft tissues that fill the outlet of the pelvis (Bennett & Brown 1996). It is a gutter shaped skeletal muscle diaphragm situated in the bony pelvic outlet, higher posteriorly than anteriorly (Fig. 25.7). It is perforated by three canals in the female, anteriorly to posteriorly, the **urethral meatus**, **vagina** and **rectum** (Bennett & Brown 1996, Marieb 1992). It consists of six layers of tissue from the inside outwards (Anderson 1992):

- pelvic peritoneum;
- visceral layer of pelvic fascia thickened to form pelvic ligaments which support the uterus;
- deep muscles encased in fascia;
- superficial muscles encased in fascia;
- subcutaneous fat;
- skin.

Superficial muscles

These muscles lie external to the deep muscles and provide additional strength, a little like the webbing beneath the cushion on some chairs. They consist of:

- the transverse perinei;
- the bulbocavernosus;
- the ischiocavernosus;

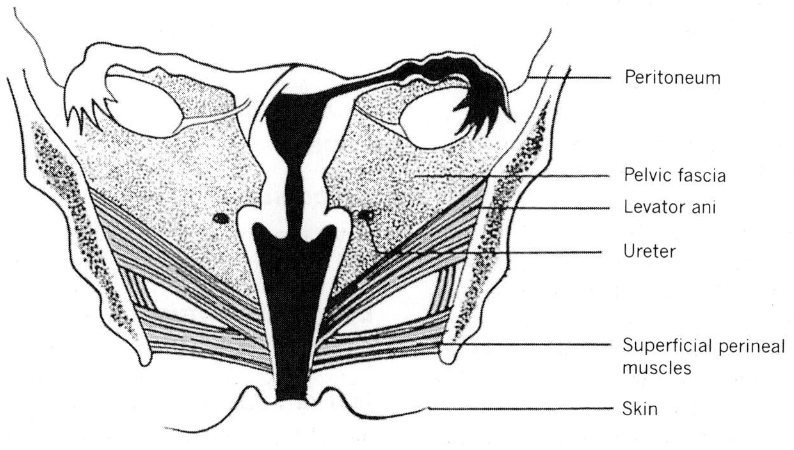

Figure 25.7 *The layers of the pelvic floor (from Sweet B, 1997, with permission).*

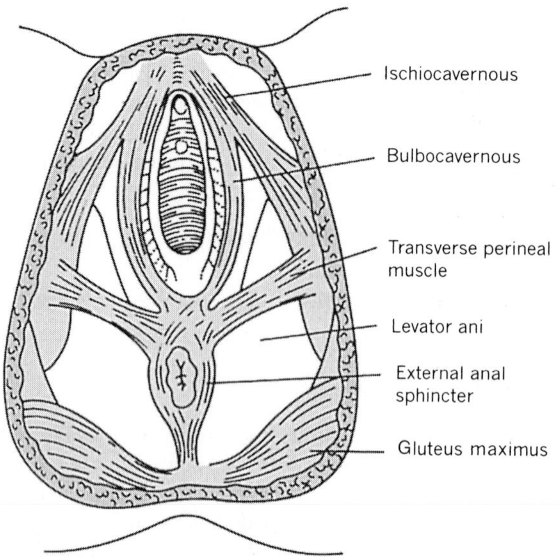

Figure 25.8 *The perineal muscles (from Sweet B, 1997, with permission).*

- the external anal sphincter;
- the external urethral meatus, sometimes called the membranous sphincter (Fig. 25.8).

The transverse perinei

One muscle arises from the inner surface of each ischial tuberosity of the pelvis and passes transversely to meet its fellow inserting into the perineal body. Some fibres pass posteriorly to blend with the anal sphincter.

The bulbocavernosus

This arises in the centre of the perineum and fibres pass on either side of the vagina and urethra, encircling them both, to insert into the body (**corpus**) of the clitoris. This muscle is responsible for erection of the clitoris and contraction of the vaginal walls.

The ischiocavernosus

A muscle runs from each ischial tuberosity to the clitoris and fibres interweave with the membranous sphincter of the urethra.

External anal sphincter

This is a circle of muscle surrounding the anus formed by merging of muscle fibres from deep and superficial layers.

External urinary meatus

This is a weak and not too important muscle.

These muscles do not form a continuous sheet and there are gaps filled with other tissues. Anteriorly is the **triangular ligament** bounded by the ischiocavernosus and the transverse perinei. It consists of two layers of fascia. Where the triangular ligaments stretch across the pubic arch, they help to support the bladder neck. Posteriorly, the gap is filled with fat and is bounded by the gluteus maximus muscle, the sacrotuberous ligament and the transverse perinei. This area is known as the **ischiorectal fossa**.

Blood supply, lymphatic drainage and nerve supply

Blood supply

Arterial supply is by branches of the two internal iliac arteries and drainage is by corresponding veins.

Lymphatic drainage

Lymph drainage is widespread both laterally and medially.

Nerve supply

The pelvic floor muscles are under voluntary control. The nerve supply is by branches of the pudendal nerve via the sacral plexus.

Deep pelvic floor muscles

These are situated above the superficial muscles and are about 5 cm deep. They insert around the coccyx and are therefore collectively known as the coccygeus muscles (Fig. 25.9). These are *vital* to the control of bladder and bowel function.

Three pairs of muscles arise from the inner border of the pubis and from the white line of fascia (arcus tendineus fasciae) extending from the ischial spine to the body of the pubis.

The pubococcygeus

Arises from the inner border of the body of the pubis and from the white line of fascia. It sweeps posteriorly in three bands.

- A central band surrounds the urethra.
- Some fibres form a U-shaped loop around the vagina and insert into the lateral and posterior vaginal walls in the perineum.
- Others loop around the anus and insert into the lateral and posterior walls of the anal canal and the coccyx.

The ischiococcygeus

These arise from each ischial spine and insert into the upper edge of the coccyx and lower border of the sacrum. They help to stabilise the sacroiliac and sacrococcygeal joints of the pelvis.

The iliococcygeus

Arise from the inner border of the white line of fascia on the iliac bone and also from the ischial spines and run to the coccyx, some crossing over in the perineal body.

Blood supply, lymphatic drainage and nerve supply

Blood supply

Arterial supply is by branches of the two internal iliac arteries and drainage by corresponding veins.

Lymphatic drainage

Lymphatic drainage is widespread both laterally and medially.

Nerve supply

The pelvic floor muscles are under voluntary control. The nerve supply is by branches of the pudendal nerve via the sacral plexus.

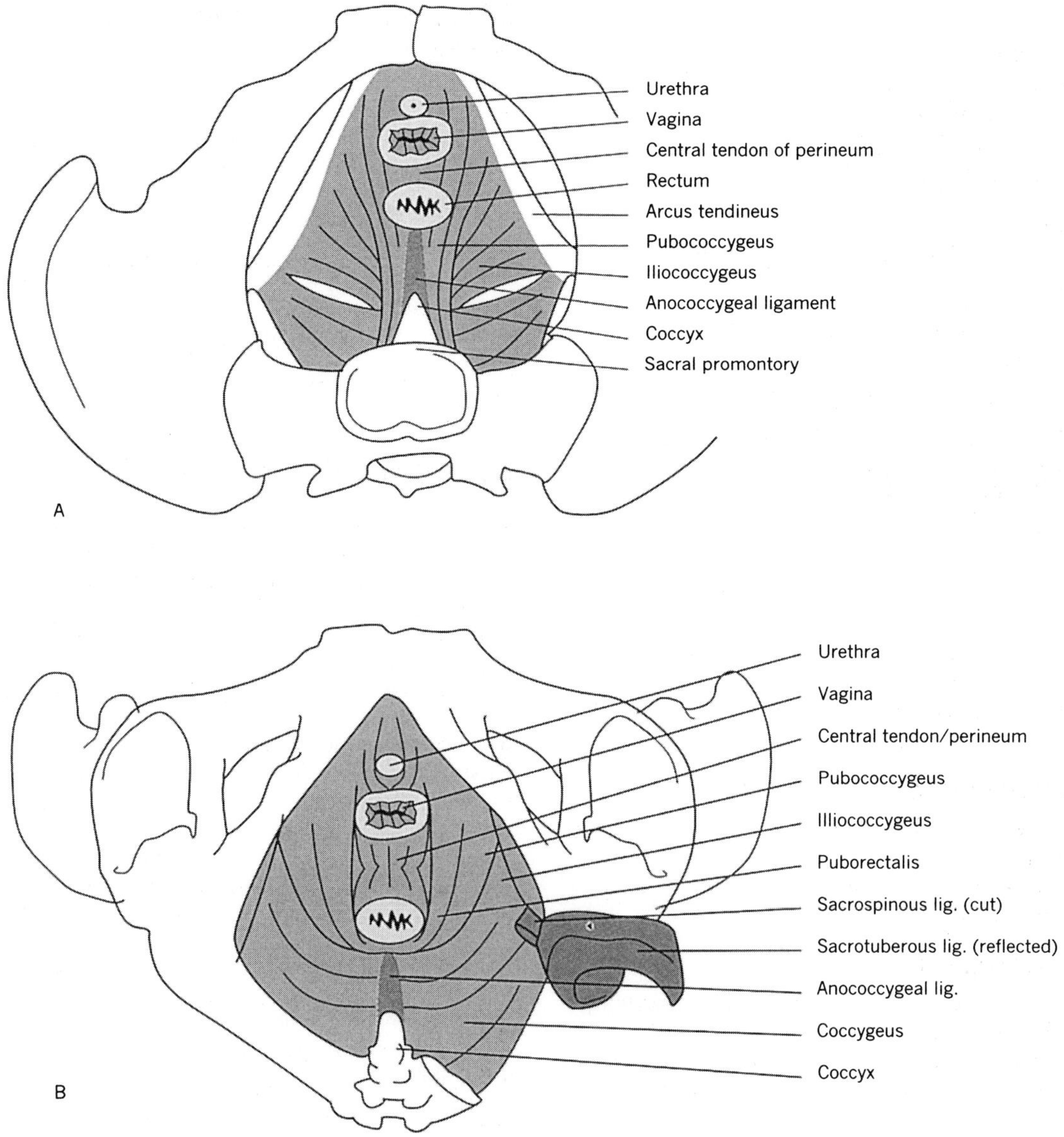

Figure 25.9 *Muscles of the pelvic diaphragm. (a) Superior view (b) Inferior view. (Reproduced with permission from Gabbe et al 1991.)*

The **perineal body** is a 'wedge-shaped mass of muscular and fibrous tissue' (Sweet 1997) that lies between the vaginal and anal canals with its apex uppermost and is the central point of the pelvic floor. Both the superficial and deep pelvic floor muscles are involved in its structure. Each side of the triangular shape measures about 3.5 cm.

Functions

Effective functioning is dependent on the integrity of the muscle fibres and maintenance of muscle tone. The pelvic floor may become traumatised in childbirth. The pelvic floor has the following functions.

- Supports the pelvic organs.
- Maintains intraabdominal pressure.
- Defaecation and micturition.
- Expulsion of the fetus in childbirth.

Clinical implications

Uterovaginal prolapse

Prolapse of the pelvic organs, with the possibility of urinary and faecal incontinence, may cause women much anxiety, embarrassment and discomfort. Symptoms may occur with ageing due to loss of muscle tone and withdrawal of oestrogen, prolonged immobility due to muscle atrophy and congenital weakness of the muscles. However, the problems are most often related to childbearing and damage to the pelvic floor during childbirth may lead to long-term problems. These include uterine prolapse which is downward displacement of the uterus to varying degrees. It is now rare to see **procidentia**, which is total prolapse of the uterus outside the body.

Vaginal prolapse – anterior wall

A **cystocoele** is a herniation of the bladder which may present with bladder irritation or a feeling of a lump in the vagina. This is often symptomless but, if large, may lead to collection of residual urine, infection and pyelonephritis. A **urethrocoele** is a displacement of the urethra with loss of the acute angle between it and the bladder. This angle helps to maintain continence so the result may be urinary stress incontinence which is the involuntary loss of small amounts of urine during coughing, sneezing or any other activity that increases intra-abdominal pressure.

Vaginal prolapse – posterior wall

A **rectocoele** is a prolapse of the posterior middle vaginal wall which allows herniation of the rectum. As in the cystocoele, this may be symptomless unless very large when faeces become lodged in the herniated sac and defaecation is difficult unless digital pressure is applied on the vaginal side of the sac. An **enterocoele** is a herniation higher in the vagina and on examination will not be palpable per vaginam.

Dyspareunia (painful sexual intercourse)

This may occur if the degree of prolapse is sufficient.

Treatment

Treatment is usually by surgical repair. In a few women, such as those who refuse surgery or are too ill or frail, insertion of a ring pessary may be the treatment of choice (Llewellyn-Jones 1990).

Prevention of prolapse

A midwife can minimise the risk by careful practice.

- Avoid pushing by the woman until full cervical dilatation is achieved.
- Prevent obstetricians from delivering the baby before full dilatation of the cervix.
- Ensure that the second stage is not prolonged with no obvious progress.
- Avoid fundal pressure to deliver the placenta.
- Ensure careful repair of any perineal trauma.
- Ensure early ambulation of the woman and pelvic floor exercises in the puerperium.

The role of the pelvic floor in labour will be discussed in Chapter 37 on the physiology of the second labour.

SMOOTH MUSCLE

Smooth muscle is **non-striated** and **involuntary** and is often referred to as **visceral muscle** (Marieb 1992). The contractions of this type of muscle are slow and sustained. The fibres of smooth muscle are small, spindle-shaped cells with a central nucleus. They have no striations and have a large surface area, allowing calcium ions to enter the cells easily. In smooth muscle there are many fewer myosin fibres than actin fibres and the myosin heads are arranged along the length of the myosin fibre so that each myosin fibre is attached to many actin fibres.

The fibres are arranged in a spiral around the muscle cell and can change their lengths much more than skeletal muscle fibres. The fibres are arranged in two (or more) sheets, usually at right angles to each other. For instance, in the body of the uterus there are three layers: outer longitudinal, middle oblique and inner circular. In the cervix of the uterus the muscle fibres are mainly circular with a few longitudinal and there is no oblique sheet of fibres.

There are no clear neuromuscular junctions in smooth muscle. The innervating fibres have bulbous varicosities and release their neurotransmitter substance directly onto many fibres. This allows a slow, synchronised contraction of the whole muscle sheet. Action potentials are transmitted from cell to cell until the whole sheet is contracting. Some fibres act as **pacemaker cells** to set the contractile pace for the whole sheet. In the uterus it is thought that such fibres are beneath the cornua so that the fundus dominates. Both the rate and intensity of smooth muscle contraction can be modified by neural and chemical stimuli.

Calcium triggers the onset of contractions and ATP provides the energy. Contraction in smooth muscle is slow, sustained and resistant to fatigue. Smooth muscle fibres take 30 times longer to contract and relax than skeletal muscle. The same muscle tension can be maintained for long periods at less than 1% of the energy cost in skeletal muscle. Smooth muscle tone in many parts of the body is maintained continuously with low energy expenditure and often by anaerobic ATP production.

Special features of smooth muscle include:

- a less vigorous contractile response to being stretched so that distension of a hollow organ can occur without provoking expulsive contractions;
- an ability to change more in length and create more tension than skeletal muscle;
- an ability to divide – hyperplasia;
- the secretion of the connective tissue proteins collagen and elastin.

Uterine muscle during pregnancy

The uterus must grow to accommodate the developing fetus and placenta and the muscle fibres must become more compliant to prevent the expulsion of the conceptus. Smooth muscle fibres can divide, a feature called **hyperplasia**. In the uterus smooth fibres undergo hyperplasia in early pregnancy and this occurs under the influence of oestrogen and independently of fetal growth. If the fetus embeds outside the uterus (**ectopic gestation**), this early growth of the uterus would still occur.

The main part of uterine growth is due to **hypertrophy** (increase in size) in response to various stimuli. Steer (1991) says that the growth of the fetus with stretch of the uterus acts as a powerful stimulator of growth, promoting synthesis of the contractile proteins of the myometrium. By 3–4 months the uterine wall has thickened from 10 to 25 mm but thins 5 to

10 mm by term (Blackburn & Loper 1992) although Hytten & Leitch (1971) suggest the increase in muscle tissue and weight could be continuous throughout pregnancy. By term the uterus has grown from its normal size of 7.5 cm in length, 5 cm in width and 2.5 cm in depth to 30 cm long, 22.5 cm wide and 20 cm deep. The weight of the uterus increases 20-fold from 50 g to 1000 g.

Uterine growth

The height of the uterine fundus is used to measure fetal growth during pregnancy with the umbilicus and xiphisternum being useful landmarks.

Uterine growth is expected to follow a predicted rate but it is better to use it as an indicator in the first 20 weeks of pregnancy. Uterine size is less reliable as a predictor of gestational age as pregnancy progresses. The uterine fundus reaches the xiphisternum and its maximum height at 36 weeks, after which the fetal presenting part enters the pelvis and the uterus becomes broader and the fundus lower (Thomson 1996). This is generally known by lay people as 'lightening'.

By 12 weeks the uterus has risen out of the pelvis and becomes an abdominal organ. It is no longer anteverted and anteflexed. As it becomes upright it often inclines to and rotates to the right. This may be because the space in the left side of the pelvic cavity is occupied by the colon. This is known as **right obliquity of the uterus** and increases as pregnancy progresses. At this time the conceptus fills the uterine cavity and the isthmus opens out. The fundus of the uterus can be palpated just above the symphysis pubis.

The uterus also changes in shape and position as pregnancy progresses in order to accommodate the growing fetus. Following implantation, the embedded blastocyst does not require much space but the upper part of the uterus begins to enlarge due to the influence of oestrogen and becomes globular until about 20 weeks and then pear shaped or cylindrical until term. The lower part of the uterus consisting of the isthmus elongates from its original 7 mm until about 10 weeks of pregnancy when it measures 25 mm. This is the beginning of the differentiation of the lower uterine segment (LUS). By 30 weeks it is possible to identify the LUS as that part of the uterus lying below the reflection of the uterovesical fold of peritoneum and above the internal os of the cervix. By 36 weeks, softening of the tissues of the pelvic floor, formation of the LUS and lightening occur.

Hormonal influences on the uterus in pregnancy

Hormones, in particular the interaction between oestrogen and progesterone initially from the corpus luteum and then synthesised by the placenta, have a growth-promoting effect and increase uterine muscle compliance. Each fibre increases in diameter by a factor of 3 and in length by 10 by term. Oestrogen promotes growth of the muscle fibres and progesterone maintains the quiescence of the myometrium by blocking the excitation and conduction mechanisms of the muscle cells.

Actions of oestrogen and progesterone on target cells

The hormone probably enters the target cell by passive diffusion across the cell membrane and then binds to specific receptor proteins present in the cellular cytoplasm. The complex formed between the steroid and the receptor is transferred to the nucleus where gene function is regulated. The hormone oestradiol stimulates RNA synthesis. The RNA is transferred to the cytoplasm where it is responsible for the synthesis of new protein. The role of progesterone has not been researched as thoroughly but it may be responsible for increasing membrane resting potential in pregnancy so that muscle fibre contractions are less likely to occur, reducing conduction of electrical activity between cells and preventing synchronised contraction of myometrial cells.

The uterus at term

The uterus at term is generally described as having two main structural compartments: the upper uterine segment (UUS) formed of the body and fundus and the lower uterine segment (LUS) formed of the isthmus and cervix. However, the uterus cannot be simply divided in this way as there is a gradual fall in the smooth muscle content from the fundus to the cervix although the isthmus has a lower muscle content than the UUS which correlates with function during labour. The muscle content of the cervix is estimated to be 10% and the functional significance of this cervical muscle is not understood. Nor is the physiology of the cervix or the pathophysiology, for example in incompetent cervix.

The decidua

During pregnancy the endometrium becomes thicker, richer and more vascular in the upper part of the body of the uterus and the fundus, the normal site for implantation. It is then known as the decidua, a name chosen because, like deciduous trees, it is shed at the end of pregnancy. The decidua is thinner and less vascular in the lower pole of the uterus. It provides a glycogen-rich environment for the blastocyst until the placenta is able to fulfil its functions. As the zygote embeds the following changes occur in the endometrium due to increased progesterone production by the corpus luteum (Anderson 1992).

1. The endometrium hypertrophies to become 6–8 mm in thickness.
2. The stroma becomes more vascular and oedematous and the functional layer becomes organised into two distinct areas.
3. The stroma cells enlarge and become more closely packed together to form the compact layer. They are now known as **decidual cells** and become polygonal in shape because of the pressure they exert on each other.
4. The tubular glands become dilated and more tortuous in their deeper parts and the lumen becomes packed with secretion. This dilatation below the compact layer gives the stroma a cavernous spongy appearance so it is known as the spongy or cavernous layer.
5. The basal layer remains unchanged.

The myometrium

During pregnancy the muscle fibres, which are not very organised in the non-pregnant uterus, become more differentiated and organised in order to fulfil their roles in labour (Figs 25.10 and 25.11). As mentioned above, smooth muscle fibres are arranged in two or more sheets at right angles to each other. In the body of the uterus there are three layers – an outer **longitudinal** layer which will contract and retract during labour and a middle **oblique** layer which is involved in expulsion of the fetus but forms a network around blood vessels in order to achieve haemostasis after delivery of the placenta. The inner **circular** layer is more evident around the cornua and in the lower uterine segment and cervix. It is involved in distension of the lower segment and dilatation of the cervix during labour. The muscle cells are grouped into bundles with thin sheets of connective tissue including collagen, elastic fibres, fibroblasts and mast cells between the bundles. Around the bundles of smooth muscle cells are fibroblasts, blood and lymphatic vessels and nerve cells.

The perimetrium

This layer of peritoneum does not cover the lower uterine segment but is deflected over the bladder anteriorly to form the uterovesical pouch and over the rectum posteriorly to form the pouch of Douglas. This loosely applied layer allows for unrestricted growth of the uterus during pregnancy.

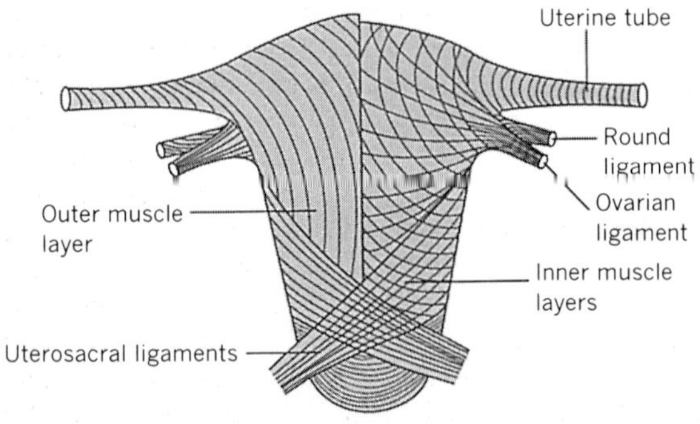

Figure 25.10 *The outer and inner layers of uterine muscle (from Sweet B, 1997, with permission).*

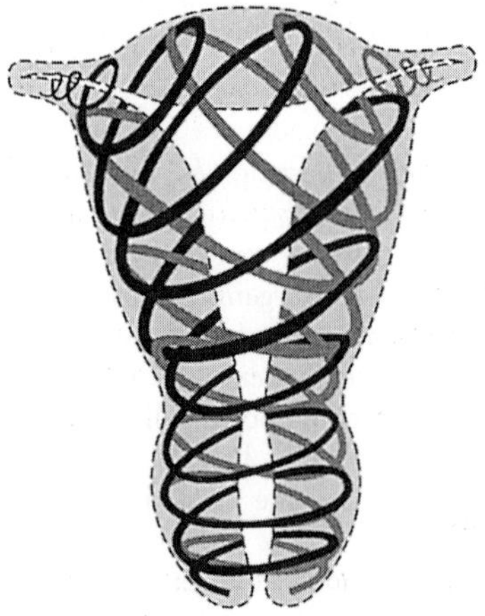

Figure 25.11 *The spiral arrangement of the uterine muscle fibres (from Sweet B, 1997, with permission).*

Cervical changes

In line with the gradual build-up of uterine activity in pregnancy, changes take place in the cervix. It changes from a firm structure to a soft elastic tissue that can dilate up to 10 cm during labour (Steer 1991). During pregnancy the cervix increases in mass, water content and vascularity (Blackburn & Loper 1992). It remains 2.5 cm long throughout pregnancy until effacement begins (Thomson 1996). Early in pregnancy cervical softening occurs and some opening of the external os is detectable from 24 weeks and of the internal os in about one-third of primigravidae by 32 weeks (Steer 1991). **Effacement** or shortening of the cervix and its gradual inclusion in the LUS occurs in the last few weeks of pregnancy. These changes are seen only in the human cervix; the cervices of most other animals that have been studied remain closed until the onset of parturition (Steer 1991).

The changes involve degradation of the collagen content by enzymes such as collagenase and elastase (Dobson 1988). Changes also occur in the proteoglycans, a ground substance matrix which attracts water, and smooth muscle fibres which become more stretchable (Blackburn & Loper 1992). Oestrogen causes increased vascularity and the cervix appears purple when viewed through a speculum (Thomson 1996).

Myometrial contractions have little effect on the ripening of the cervix which usually occurs prior to the onset of labour. Hormonal control of cervical ripening may involve multiple changes in oestrogen, progesterone, relaxin and prostaglandins and seems to correlate well with a gradual rise in circulating oestrogens. PGE_2 and $PGF_{2\alpha}$ have a localised action on cervical softening independently of uterine activity and PGE_2 is used to improve the cervical state prior to induction of labour (Blackburn & Loper 1992). However, there is much variation from woman to woman in the cervical changes outlined above. Labour may begin in some women when the cervix is long, firm, uneffaced and undilated and in others the cervix may be soft, effaced and partly dilated for some weeks prior to the onset of labour.

The cervix also acts as an efficient barrier to infection. Under the influence of progesterone the mucus secreted by the endocervical cells becomes thicker and more viscous. It forms a cervical plug called the **operculum** which prevents ascending infection (Thomson 1996).

Uterine blood flow

Increased vessel diameter and lowered resistance causes an increase in uterine blood flow during pregnancy. Prostacyclin (PGI_2) is produced by the pregnant and non-pregnant myometrium as well as by the placental blood vessels and acts as a potent vasodilator that inhibits platelet aggregation and also protects the vascular epithelium. It is therefore important in maintaining blood flow to the placenta and to the uterus during labour. Unlike other prostaglandins, PGI_2 has little effect on uterine contractility.

Innervation of the human uterus

The uterus is innervated by both sympathetic and parasympathetic fibres of the autonomic branch of the nervous system. In comparison with other smooth muscle cells, the uterus is poorly innervated with a low density of nerves to smooth muscle. The physiological result of the innervation of the uterus is unknown as labour will occur even if complete spinal transection is present. It is probable that central nervous system connections are not essential to the onset and progress of labour.

Sympathetic fibres

Preganglionic fibres leave the spinal cord and enter a chain of ganglia running alongside the spinal column from T-1 to L-5 vertebrae. In the ganglia they synapse with postganglionic fibres that synapse with the target organ. The uterus is unusual as the preganglionic fibres leaving T10–12 run directly to the uterus to synapse there with the postganglionic fibres. Preganglionic fibres release acetylcholine into the synapse from their endings and postganglionic fibres release noradrenaline onto the target organ from their terminals.

There are two types of adrenergic receptors in target organs: α receptors which are normally excitatory and β fibres which are normally inhibitory. There are two types of beta receptors: β_1 and β_2. β receptors are cardiospecific and are excitatory whilst β_2 receptors are present in the uterus and are inhibitory. Drugs such as salbutamol and ritodrine inhibit uterine contractions in preterm labour but will excite cardiac muscle, causing a rise in pulse rate leading to increased cardiac output and blood pressure. The β-blocking agent propranolol will enhance uterine activity.

Parasympathetic fibres

The parasympathetic innervation to the pelvis is through the sacral outflow from S-2, 3 and 4. The preganglionic fibres end in or near the target organs and synapse with short postganglionic fibres. The neurotransmitter substance in both pre- and postganglionic fibres is acetylcholine. The fibres innervating the uterus synapse in two nerve plexi on either side of the pouch of Douglas. These are the **paracervical plexi** (Lee Frankenhauser's plexi).

Vaginal changes in pregnancy

Oestrogen produces changes in both the muscle layer and the epithelium. There is hypertrophy of the muscle layer and changes in the surrounding connective tissue make the vagina more elastic, allowing it to distend during the second stage of labour. There is a marked desquamation of the superficial cells of the epithelium, giving rise to an increased amount of normal vaginal discharge, called **leucorrhoea** because of its white colour.

The epithelial cells also have an increased glycogen content and interaction with Doderlein's bacillus produces a more acid environment which adds to the protection against many micro-organisms. Unfortunately, this means an increased susceptibility to the organism *Candida albicans* which causes moniliasis or thrush. There is increased vascularity and the vagina appears reddish purple in colour, a change referred to as **Jacqemenier's sign**. The increased vascularity of the pelvic organs gives rise to another sign of pregnancy called **Osiander's sign** which is increased pulsation in the lateral vaginal fornices.

Uterine activity in pregnancy

As in skeletal muscle, myosin-containing thick filaments interact with the actin-containing thin filaments and the energy source is from adenosine triphosphate (ATP). There are no clear neuromuscular junctions in smooth muscle and innervating neurones release their neurotransmitter substance directly onto many fibres, resulting in a change in intracellular calcium concentration and allowing a slow, synchronised contraction of the whole muscle sheet.

Calcium is a key ion in the contraction process and mainly comes from the ECF where its concentration is 10 000 times that of the myometrial cell. At rest the cell membrane does not allow calcium to enter the cell but after a contraction calcium enters the cell through ion channels. Action potentials are transmitted from cell to cell until the whole sheet is contracting. The uterus at term appears to have enhanced communication between cells and the action potential can spread across the entire uterus in 2–3 s.

The role of pacemakers

Some fibres may act as pacemaker cells to set the contractile pace for the whole sheet. Specific pacemaker cells have not yet been identified and it used to be thought that fibres beneath the cornua of the uterus acted as pacemakers so that the fundus dominates. Investigations do not support this theory and although it is likely that cells near the cornua may initiate contractions, it is now thought that any myometrial cell would have this property (Garfield et al 1988). Both the rate and intensity of smooth muscle contraction can be modified by neural and chemical stimuli. Contraction in smooth muscle is slow, sustained and resistant to fatigue. The action potential is conducted from the cell membrane down the sarcoplasmic reticulum so that there is a rapid release of calcium deep in the cell.

In pregnancy, uterine activity gradually evolves, being seen as early as 7 weeks with high frequency, about two contractions a minute, but very low intensity of about 1–1.5 kPa (Steer 1991). This continues until about 20 weeks when uterine contractions increase in both frequency and amplitude until term. The main increase occurs in the last 8 weeks of pregnancy. This is thought to be facilitated by the development of gap junctions within the myometrium where the plasma membranes of adjacent cells are closely applied which act as areas of low resistance so that conduction of electrical impulses can spread rapidly from one cell to another. They are important in the spread of action potentials and the development of the coordinated uterine activity that is seen in efficient labour.

Gap junctions

The appearance of gap junctions seems to depend on changes in the levels of oestrogen, progesterone and prostaglandins occurring in late pregnancy. Garfield et al (1979) proposed that the absence of gap junctions may be important for the maintenance of pregnancy and their appearance may be necessary to allow the development of effective uterine contractions in labour. Low-frequency but high-pressure Braxton-Hicks contractions are perceived by the mother. They may be as strong as labour contractions but are not painful and the cervix does not dilate.

Sensitivity to oxytocin and prostaglandins

Sensitivity to oxytocin is dependent on both gestational age and the level of spontaneous uterine activity. Up to about 30 weeks the uterus is very insensitive to oxytocin and it is necessary to give very high infusion rates of oxytocin in order to stimulate uterine activity (up to 128 mU/min). After 30 weeks the uterus will respond to much smaller concentrations of oxytocin of 8 mU/min and by 40 weeks as little as 4 mU/min will cause uterine activity similar to that seen in spontaneous labour. In contrast to this variable response, prostaglandins E_2 and $F_{2\alpha}$ will induce uterine contractions at any gestational age. Prostaglandins therefore are probably the final mediator of uterine contractions.

Summary of main points

- Muscle makes up almost half of the body's mass and is the tissue that enables movement to occur by transforming chemical energy from adenosine triphosphate into mechanical energy. All muscle cells are elongated and contain two kinds of protein filaments: actin and myosin.
- There are three basic muscle types: skeletal muscle that allows movement of the whole body by exerting force on the skeleton, smooth muscle found in the walls of the hollow viscera of the gastrointestinal, genitourinary and respiratory tracts and the specialised cardiac muscle. Muscles have four functions: they produce movement, maintain posture, stabilise joints and generate heat. They have four properties: excitability, contractility, extensibility and elasticity.
- Skeletal muscles are attached to and cover the bony skeleton. The fibres have obvious bands or striations. Skeletal muscle contracts rapidly but tires easily and must be rested after short bursts of activity. Activity depends on a rich blood supply which is essential for the delivery of large amounts of oxygen and nutrients and the removal of equally large amounts of metabolic waste.
- Skeletal muscle fibres are long cylindrical cells which taper at both ends. They are enormously large and some may reach 300 mm (one foot) in length. Their diameter ranges from 10 to 100 µm. Each muscle fibre is a syncytium formed during embryonic development. It contains a large number of rod-like myofibrils extending the full length of the cell and parallel to each other.
- Mitochondria and other organelles are packed in between the myofibrils which are the contractile elements of the cells and each myofibril consists of smaller contractile units called sarcomeres. Myofibrils appear to be made of alternate dark or A bands and light or I bands, giving the characteristic striped appearance under the light microscope. The A band is interrupted in its midsection by the highly refractive H zone which is bisected by a dark line called the M line. The I bands have a midline interruption called the Z line.
- The A bands are formed of the thick filaments of myosin. The thin filaments are mainly composed of actin and are formed of three different proteins: actin, troponin and tropomyosin. Each myosin molecule has a rod-like tail or axis and two globular heads or cross bridges which interact with special sites on the thin filaments.
- The muscle cell is penetrated by two tubular systems, both ending near the A–I band junctions. The transverse or T system extends from the cell exterior into the sarcoplasm where it branches and terminates. The internal system is formed by fine tubules called sarcotubules of the sarcoplasmic reticulum, which end in terminal sacs called the terminal cysternae.
- The sliding filament theory of muscle action is most commonly supported. Skeletal muscles contract in response to nerve stimulation which results in an action potential being sent along the sarcolemma. This electrical event results in a rise in intracellular calcium ion levels that triggers off the contraction.
- Excitation-contraction coupling is the process whereby the generation of an action potential is followed by activation of the contractile machinery in the myofibrils. It involves the exposure of the binding sites on the actin to allow the formation of crossbridges. Energy released from ATP is used to fuel the muscle contraction.
- The pelvic floor is formed by the soft tissues that fill the outlet of the pelvis. It is a gutter shaped skeletal muscle diaphragm situated in the bony pelvic outlet, higher posteriorly than anteriorly. It is perforated by three canals in the female, anteriorly to posteriorly, the urethral meatus, vagina and rectum.
- The superficial muscles lie external to the deep muscles and provide additional strength, a little like the webbing beneath the cushion on some chairs. Deep pelvic floor muscles are situated above the superficial muscles. Each inserts around the coccyx and they are collectively known as the coccygeus muscles, vital for the control of bladder and bowel function.
- The perineal body is a wedge-shaped mass of muscular and fibrous tissue that lies between the vaginal and anal canals with its apex uppermost and is the central point of the pelvic floor. Both the superficial and deep pelvic floor muscles are involved in its structure.
- Effective functioning of the pelvic floor depends on the integrity of the muscle fibres and maintenance of muscle tone. The pelvic floor may become traumatised in childbirth. It supports the pelvic organs, maintains intraabdominal pressure and enables defaecation, micturition and expulsion of the fetus in childbirth.
- Prolapse of the pelvic organs, with the possibility of urinary and faecal incontinence, may cause women much anxiety, embarrassment and discomfort. Symptoms may occur with prolonged immobility and congenital weakness of the muscles. The conditions are most often related to childbearing and include uterine prolapse, cystocoele, urethrocoele and rectocoele. Treatment is usually by surgical repair.
- A midwife can minimise the risk of prolapse by careful management of labour, ensuring prompt repair of any perineal trauma and encouraging early ambulation of the woman and pelvic floor exercises in the puerperium.
- Smooth muscle is non-striated and involuntary and is referred to as visceral muscle. Its contractions are slow and sustained. The fibres of smooth muscle are small, spindle-shaped cells with a central nucleus. They have a large surface area, allowing calcium ions to enter the cells easily. There are many fewer myosin fibres than actin fibres and the myosin heads are arranged along the length of the myosin fibre so that each myosin fibre is attached to many actin fibres.
- There are no clear neuromuscular junctions in smooth muscle. The innervating fibres release their neurotransmitter substance directly onto many fibres, allowing slow, synchronised contraction of the whole muscle sheet. Smooth muscle fibres take 30 times longer to contract and relax than skeletal muscle.
- Special features of smooth muscle include a less vigorous contractile response to being stretched so that distension of a hollow organ can occur without provoking expulsive contractions, an ability to change

more in length and width than skeletal muscle, an ability to divide and secretion of the connective tissue proteins collagen and elastin.

- In the uterus smooth fibres undergo hyperplasia in early pregnancy but the main part of uterine growth is due to hypertrophy. By term the uterus has grown to 30 cm long, 22.5 cm wide and 20 cm deep and weighs 1000 g. Uterine size is best as an indicator of fetal age in the first 20 weeks of pregnancy. It is less reliable as a predictor of gestational age as pregnancy progresses.
- The uterus at term is generally described as having two main structural compartments: the upper uterine segment formed of the body and fundus and the lower uterine segment formed of the isthmus and cervix.
- During pregnancy the endometrium becomes thicker, richer and more vascular in the upper part of the body of the uterus and the fundus, the normal site for implantation. It is then known as the decidua which is thinner and less vascular in the lower pole of the uterus.
- The smooth muscle fibres of the myometrium are arranged in two (or more) sheets, usually at right angles to each other. In the body of the uterus there are three layers: outer longitudinal, middle oblique and inner circular, mainly found in the lower uterine segment.
- Changes in the cervix include an increase in mass, water content and vascularity. It remains 2.5 cm long until effacement begins in the last few weeks of pregnancy. Under the influence of progesterone endocervical cell mucus thickens and becomes more viscous, forming the operculum which prevents ascending infection.
- Under the influence of oestrogen the muscle layer in the vagina hypertrophies and the surrounding connective tissue becomes more elastic, allowing the vagina to distend during the second stage of labour. Increased desquamation of the superficial cells of the epithelium leads to leucorrhoea. The epithelial cells have an increased glycogen content and interaction with Doderlein's bacillus produces a more acid environment, protecting against microorganisms.
- Some fibres may act as pacemaker cells to set the contractile pace for the whole muscle sheet. Sensitivity to oxytocin and prostaglandins depends on gestational age and the level of spontaneous uterine activity. Prostaglandins are probably the final mediator of uterine contractions.

References

Anderson M. 1992 The Anatomy and Physiology of Obstetrics. Wolfe Publishing, London.

Bennett VR, Brown LK. 1996 The reproductive organs. In Bennett VR, Brown LK (eds) Myles Textbook for Midwives, 12th edn. Churchill Livingstone, Edinburgh, pp 13–32.

Blackburn ST, Loper DL. 1992 Maternal, Fetal and Neonatal Physiology, A Clinical Perspective. WB Saunders, Philadelphia.

Dobson H. 1988 Softening and dilation of the human cervix. Oxford Review of Reproductive Biology 19, 491.

Gabbe SG, Niebyl JR, Simpson JL. (eds) 1991 Obstetrics: Normal and Problem Pregnancies. Churchill Livingstone, New York, pp. 6–7.

Garfield RE, Blennerhassett MG, Miller SM. 1988 Control of myometrial contractility: role and regularity of gap junctions. Oxford Review of Reproductive Biology 19, 436.

Hinchliff SM, Montague SE, 1990 Physiology for nursing practice. Baillière Tindalle, London.

Hinchliff SM, Montague SE, Watson R, 1996, Physiology for nursing practice. Baillière Tindalle, London.

Huszar and Roberts. 1982 Biochemistry and pharmacology of the myometrium and labour: regulation at the cellular and molecular levels. American Journal of Obstetrics and Gynecology 142(2), 225–237.

Hytten FE, Leitch I. 1971 The Physiology of Human Pregnancy, 2nd edn. Blackwell Scientific, Oxford.

Lang R. 1990 Energy for movement – muscle function. S325, Book 1, Biochemistry and Cell Biology. Open University Press, Buckingham.

Llewellyn-Jones D. 1990 Fundamentals of Obstetrics and Gynaecology: Volume 2 Gynaecology, 5th edn. Faber and Faber, London.

Marieb EN. 1992 Human Anatomy and Physiology, 2nd edn. Benjamin/ Cummings Publishing, California.

McClaren SM. 1996 Skeletal muscles. In Hinchliff SM, Montague SE, Watson R (eds) Physiology for Nursing Practice, 2nd edn. Baillière Tindall, London, pp 261–283.

Steer PJ. 1991 The genital system. In Hytten F, Chamberlain G (eds) Clinical Physiology in Obstetrics, 2nd edn. Blackwell Scientific, Oxford, pp 245–302.

Sweet BR. 1997 The pelvic floor and its injuries. In Sweet BR with Tiran D (eds) Mayes Midwifery, 12th edn. Baillière Tindall, London, pp 444–454.

Thomson V. 1996 Psychological and physiological changes in pregnancy. In Bennett VR, Brown LK (eds) Myles Textbook for Midwives, 12th edn. Churchill Livingstone, Edinburgh, pp 94–105.

Recommended reading

Blackburn ST, Loper DL. 1992 Maternal, Fetal and Neonatal Physiology, A Clinical Perspective. WB Saunders, Philadelphia.

Dobson H. 1988 Softening and dilation of the human cervix. Oxford Review of Reproductive Biology 19, 491.

Garfield RE, Blennerhassett MG, Miller SM. 1988 Control of myometrial contractility: role and regularity of gap junctions. Oxford Review of Reproductive Biology 19, 436.

Marieb EN. 1992 Human Anatomy and Physiology, 2nd edn. Benjamin/ Cummings Publishing, California

Sweet BR 1997 The pelvic floor and its injuries. In Sweet BR with Tiran D (eds) Mayes Midwifery, 12th edn. Baillière Tindall, London, pp 444–454.

Chapter 26

The central nervous system

In this chapter

INTRODUCTION

The ability to respond appropriately to environmental change depends on rapid communication. This is achieved by two systems in the body: the nervous system and the endocrine system.

The nervous system communicates by the rapid transmission of electrical signals. The endocrine glands secrete hormones into the bloodstream which modify the working of target organs. Normal functioning of the nervous and endocrine systems is critical for the maintenance of homeostasis in pregnancy, as it is in the non-pregnant population.

'The nervous system is the master controlling and communicating system of the body; every thought, action and emotion reflects its activity' (Marieb 1992). It is only possible to give a brief outline of this immensely complex system and to elaborate on some of the important aspects such as pain perception. Even within this plan, the nervous system will be examined in two chapters. This chapter will concentrate on tissues and the central nervous system while Chapter 27 will consider the peripheral and autonomic nervous systems and neural integration.

The development of the nervous system is outlined in Chapter 8. Detailed anatomy will only be given if needed to clarify the physiology. Anyone wishing to deepen their knowledge further should read Marieb (1992) or Hinchliff et al (1996). Neuroanatomy is presented in an easily readable form in Fitzgerald (1992).

ORGANISATION OF THE NERVOUS SYSTEM

The central nervous system (CNS) consists of the brain and spinal cord. It has an integrating function and receives messages from and sends messages via the **peripheral nervous system** (PNS) to all parts of the body. That part of the PNS that controls the viscera is called the **autonomic nervous system** (ANS). It innervates the smooth muscle and glands of the viscera and cardiac muscle. The ANS can be subdivided into two distinct parts: the **sympathetic nervous system** and **parasympathetic nervous system**. There are also the **sensory organs** such as the eyes and ears which feed information about the environment back to the brain.

NEUROANATOMY

Nervous tissue is made of two cell types: the **neurones** (Fig. 26.1) and a group of cell types collectively known as **neuroglia**.

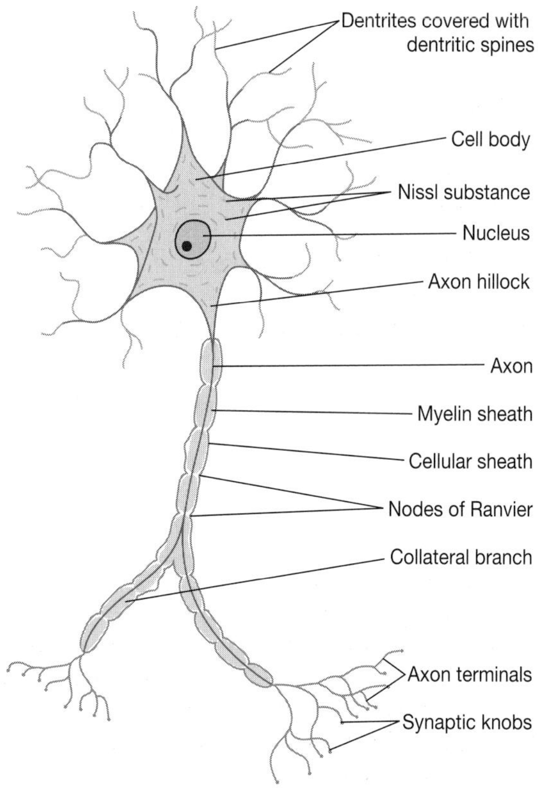

Figure 26.1 *Structure of a whole nerve fibre (from Hinchliff SM, Montague SE, Watson R, 1996, with permission).*

The tissue is supplied by blood vessels and supported by connective tissue.

Neurones

The structural units of the nervous system are the neurones. These specialised cells have the following characteristics.

- Processes called axons and dendrites communicate with other cells.
- Conduction of messages by nerve impulses from one part of the body to another.
- They are extremely long lived.
- They cannot undergo mitosis and divide.
- They have a very high metabolic rate and need continuous glucose and oxygen.
- They cannot survive for more than a few minutes without oxygen.

Dendrites are the short, diffusely branching extensions which receive messages from other cells at synapses. Each cell has only one **axon** arising from the **axon hillock** on the cell body. This slender elongated process is the same diameter along its length and some axons can be over a metre long, such as those travelling from the spine to the foot. Axons may give off branches called axon **collaterals** and usually have terminal branches ending in **synaptic knobs** or **boutons**. Axons contain **microtubules** and **microfilaments** for the transport of substances to the cell body (**anterograde**) and from the cell body (**retrograde**).

Axons are responsible for conducting messages by electrical nerve impulses to the terminal bouton and by chemicals known as **neurotransmitters** (NT) which are secreted in the soma and sent along to be stored in the terminal bouton. Neurotransmitters can excite or inhibit other neurones by attaching to receptors in their plasma membrane.

Myelin sheaths

Larger nerve fibres are covered in a white fatty segmented covering called the **myelin sheath**. Myelin protects and insulates fibres and increases the rate of impulse transmission; messages can be transmitted up to 100 times more rapidly than via unmyelinated fibres (Fig. 26.2). Myelin sheaths in the PNS are formed by the **Schwann cells** which wrap themselves around the axon. As the Schwann cell protoplasm is squeezed out of the cell, the axon remains wrapped in a multilayered membrane. The external portion of this is called the **neurolemma** or Schwann sheath. Adjacent Schwann cells along the axon do not touch and the gaps between them, which occur at regular intervals, are called the **nodes of Ranvier**. Axon collaterals can only emerge at these nodes.

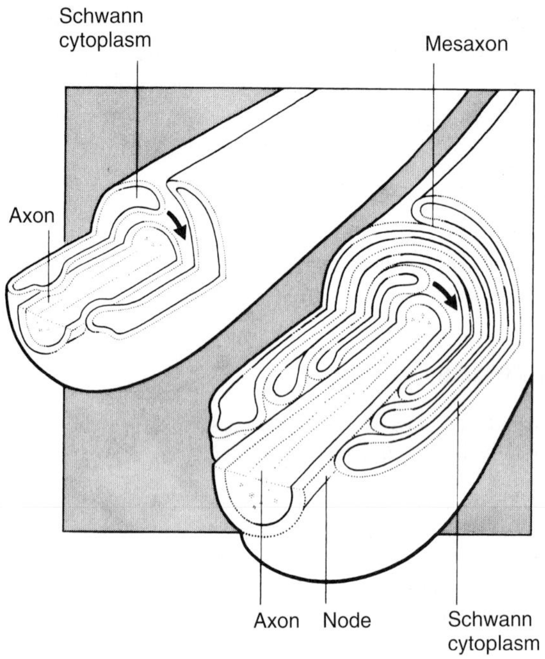

Figure 26.2 *Myelination in peripheral nervous system. Arrows indicate movement of flange of Schwann cytoplasm (from Fitzgerald MJT, 1996, with permission).*

The myelin sheaths in the central nervous system are produced by cells called **oligodendrocytes** which are described below. Myelinated fibres form the white matter in the brain and spinal cord and the cell bodies form the grey matter. Cell bodies are outside the white matter in the brain and inside the white matter in the spinal cord.

Classification of neurones

- **Motor neurones** have cell bodies mainly in the CNS carrying impulses to control effector organs such as muscles or glands.
- **Sensory neurones** have cell bodies located in the sensory ganglia outside the CNS. Their dendritic branches are often very long, gathering impulses from the periphery of the body such as the ends of the toes and fingers.
- **Association neurones**, often called **interneurones**, carry signals between motor and sensory neurones in complex networks.

Neuroglia

Neuroglial cells provide support and protection for the neurones. They outnumber neurones in a ratio of 10:1. There may be 10 000 million neurones in the brain so that the number of neuroglial cells is enormous. These cells are subdivided according to size, shape and function.

- **Astrocytes** are star-shaped cells with long, fine processes arising from their cell body. Astrocytes have one process against a neurone and other processes close to capillary walls.
- **Oligodendrocytes** in the CNS and Schwann cells in the PNS are smaller than astrocytes and have fewer processes. They form the myelin sheaths around nerve fibres.

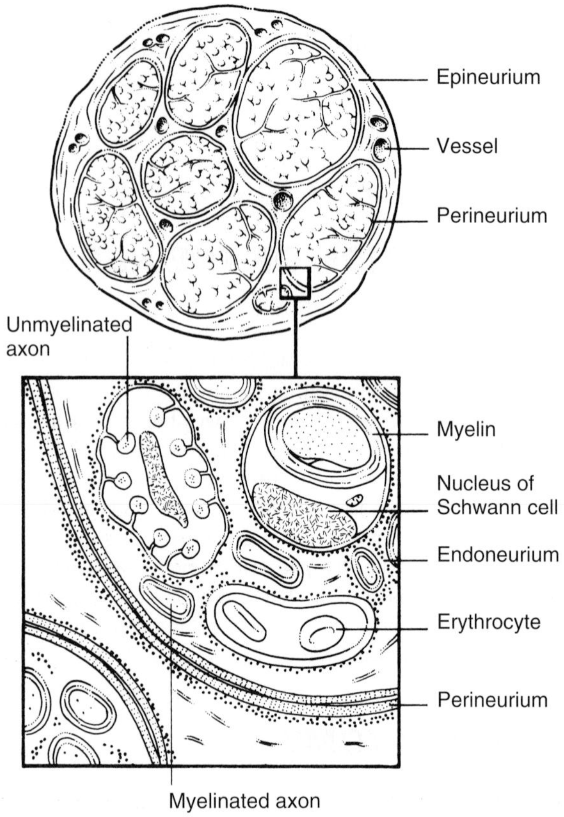

Figure 26.3 *Transverse section of a nerve trunk. (a) Light microscopy; (b) electron microscopy (from Fitzgerald MJT, 1996, with permission).*

- **Ependyma** form a continuous layer of cells lining the ventricles of the brain and central canal of the spinal cord. They help to produce the cerebrospinal fluid.
- **Microglia** are small cells which are part of the immune system, acting as macrophages.

The structure of a nerve

The axons from single neurones are bound together to form nerves (Fig. 26.3). Nerves often contain **afferent** fibres (to the CNS), **efferent** fibres (from the CNS) or both. Those with both types of fibres are referred to as **mixed nerves**. Each separate nerve fibre is embedded in a fibrous connective tissue sheath called the **endoneurium**. These are bound in groups by a connective tissue sheath called the **perineurium** and the complete nerve is surrounded by the **epineurium**. Each nerve has an arterial blood supply and venous drainage.

NEUROPHYSIOLOGY

The nerve impulse

Both nerve fibres and muscle fibres conduct electrochemical signals and are called **excitable tissues**. When a neurone is stimulated, an electrical impulse is sent along the length of its axon (Fig. 26.4). The human body is electrically neutral, i.e.

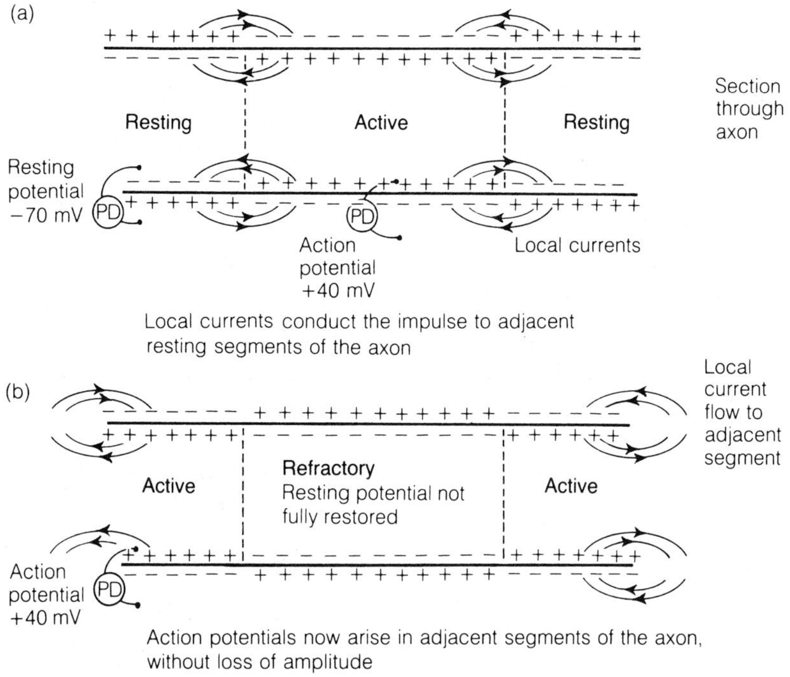

Figure 26.4 *Propagation of an action potential along a nerve fibre (from Hinchliff SM, Montague SE, 1990, with permission).*

positive and negative charges are equal. Potential electrical energy is called **voltage** which is measured in volts (V) or millivolts (mV). The flow of electricity from one point to another is called a **current**. Substances that hinder the flow are said to provide **resistance**. Ions, which are electrically charged particles, provide the currents, usually flowing through an aqueous solution across a plasma membrane. Plasma membranes are studded with proteinous ion channels.

Polarisation

When a membrane is resting its potential is polarised, i.e. the inside of the cell has a different electrical potential from the outside of the cell. The **resting potential** of neurones averages −70 mV. This is maintained by the distribution and relative concentration of negative and positive ions. Inside the cell the positive ion is potassium and the negative ion is protein. Outside in the interstitial fluid, the positive ion is sodium and the negative ion is chloride.

The role of sodium ions

When the cell is stimulated, sodium channels open in the membrane and sodium ions rush into the cell. This changes the membrane potential to +40 mV, a process called **depolarisation**. This is what is meant by the action potential which proceeds down the axon in a wave. The action potential is the sum of all negative and positive charges stimulating the cell. Behind the wave the cell pumps three sodium ions out in exchange for two potassium ions. The membrane potential falls to −90 mV (**hyperpolarisation**) and then recovers.

Depolarisation increases the chance of a nerve impulse being generated but hyperpolarisation decreases it. The period of hyperpolarisation is known as the **refractory period**, during which the cell cannot generate an action potential. Firing of a neurone is an all-or-nothing phenomenon and the potential must reach a threshold before firing will occur. Strong stimuli will result in more impulses being generated rather than stronger impulses.

Saltatory conduction of the impulse

Nerve fibres can be classified according to their speeds of conduction of the action potential. The larger the nerve, the more rapidly it can conduct its impulses. Myelinated nerves can conduct nerve impulses more rapidly than unmyelinated nerves. The myelin sheath increases the electrical resistance of a nerve but it is more leaky at the nodes of Ranvier. The electrical current flows smoothly along each section of the sheath between nodes of Ranvier and it is only necessary to generate an action potential at the nodes. The impulse seems to jump from node to node. In a non-myelinated nerve, new action potentials have to be generated across each adjacent section of the nerve membrane. This is called **saltatory conduction** (Fig. 26.5).

Classification of nerves by speed of impulse conduction

- **Group A fibres** are all myelinated and can conduct impulses up to 120 metres per second (m/s). Group A fibres are further subdivided into α, β, γ and δ fibres.
- **Group B fibres** are also myelinated. They are all preganglionic fibres of the autonomic nervous system (see below).
- **Group C fibres** are non-myelinated and conduct impulses as slowly as 1 m/s.

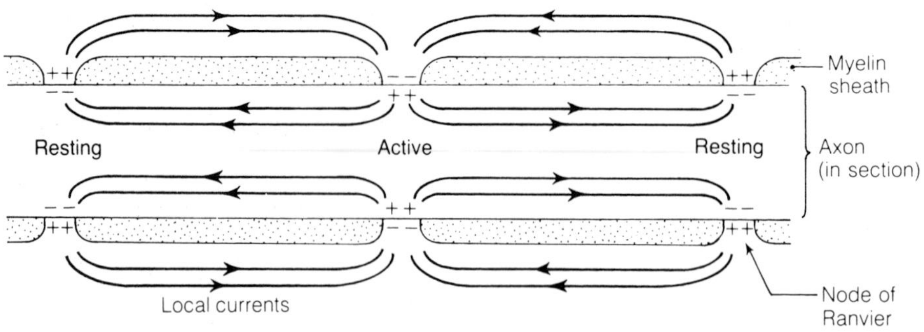

Figure 26.5 *Saltatory conduction in a myelinated nerve fibre. Local currents conduct the impulse from node to node. The action potential is regenerated at each node of Ranvier (from Hinchliff SM, Montague SE, 1990, with permission).*

The synapse

Synapses are junctions between the terminal bouton of the axon and its target tissue, which may be a neurone cell body, a gland or a muscle (Fig. 26.6). Between the neurone and its target cell, the **synaptic cleft** is a fluid-filled space into which neurotransmitters are released from the **presynaptic membrane**. These open and shut ion channels in the **postsynaptic membrane**. The electrical message of the action potential is conducted across the gap to enable the impulse to be transferred. This is a reversible change and the neurotransmitter is removed in one of three ways.

- Enzymes which degrade the NT are released into the synaptic cleft.
- The NT is retaken up by the presynaptic membrane.
- The NT diffuses away from the synapse.

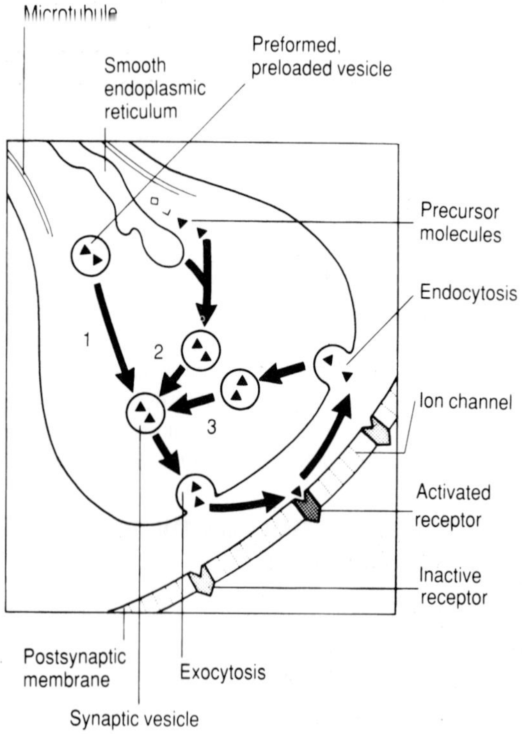

Figure 26.6 *Diagram to show origin and fate of synaptic vesicle and transmitter–receptor binding (from Fitzgerald MJT, 1996, with permission).*

Neurotransmitters

Neurotransmitters are molecules which help neurones to communicate messages and regulate body activities and states (Marieb 1992). They are classified according to chemical structure and are synthesised by the body with the help of enzymes.

Acetylcholine

Acetylcholine (ACh) was the first neurotransmitter to be identified. It is easy to study because it is the NT released at neuromuscular junctions and is accessible. ACh is synthesised and stored within synaptic vesicles in the presence of the enzyme choline acetyltransferase. Acetic acid is bound to coenzyme A to form acetyl CoA. This is then combined with choline and the coenzyme is released.

$$\text{Acetyl CoA} + \text{choline} \xrightarrow{\text{Choline acetyl transferase}} \text{ACh} + \text{CoA}$$

The released ACh binds to the postsynaptic membrane and is then degraded to acetic acid and choline by the enzyme acetylcholinesterase (AChE). The released choline is captured by the presynaptic membrane and used to synthesise more ACh. ACh is also released by some neurones of the ANS and is found in the CNS.

The biogenic amines

The biogenic amines include the **catecholamines**, such as dopamine, noradrenaline and adrenaline, and the **indolamines**, serotonin (5-hydroxytriptamine or 5-HT) and histamine. The catecholamines are synthesised from the amino acid tyrosine in a common pathway. Neurones produce only the enzymes which control the steps necessary to produce the NT they need. The common pathway for the synthesis of the catecholamines is as follows:

Tyrosine → L-dopa → Dopamine → Noradrenaline → Adrenaline

These NTs are widely distributed in the brain where they are involved in emotional behaviour and regulation of the body clock. The catecholamines, especially noradrenaline, are also released by some motor neurones of the ANS. Serotonin is also synthesised from tyrosine but via a different pathway. Histamine is synthesised from the amino acid histidine.

Amino acids

The most important amino acids involved in neurotransmission are γ-aminobutyric acid (GABA) and glutamate.

Peptides

The neuropeptides are strings of amino acids which produce diverse effects. These include the endorphins and encephalins that will be discussed in full in chapter 38.

THE BRAIN

During the course of evolution there has been an increasing tendency to elaboration of the brain, reaching its greatest complexity in humans. This process is referred to as **cephalisation**. Development of the brain is outlined in Chapter 8. The average brain weighs about 1500 g and is slightly heavier in men than women. It is the complexity of the wiring that determines the power of the brain, not its size.

Although the brain is described as a single organ (Figs 26.7 and 26.8), it is more easily understood if an analogy is made with the gastrointestinal system with individual parts performing their discrete functions.

The brain can be subdivided into four main parts (Marieb 1992).

1 The cerebral hemispheres
2 The diencephalon, made up of the thalamus and hypothalamus
3 The brainstem, made up of midbrain, pons and medulla
4 The cerebellum

The cerebral hemispheres

The two cerebral hemispheres form the uppermost part of the brain. Together, they form 85% of the total weight of the brain and sit like an umbrella over the diencephalon and brainstem. The neurones are organised with their cell bodies outermost forming the **grey matter** or **cortex** (outer rind) and their fibres innermost forming the **white matter**. The cortex is thrown into elevated ridges called **gyri**, separated by shallow grooves called **sulci**. This vastly increases the surface area of the cortex. The deepest of these grooves are called **fissures** and are the same in everyone, forming important landmarks in the brain. A midline longitudinal fissure called the **midsagittal fissure** separates the two cerebral hemispheres and the **transverse fissure** separates the cerebral hemispheres from the **cerebellum**. Where neurone cell bodies are gathered into a functioning group, the term **nucleus** is used.

Each hemisphere is divided into six main lobes. Four of these have the same names as the bones under which they lie: the **frontal**, **parietal**, **occipital** and **temporal** lobes. The other two lobes are buried in the hemispheres. These are the **insula**, revealed if the frontal and temporal lobes are eased apart, and the **limbic** lobe, which can be seen if the brain is divided along the midsagittal fissure.

The cerebral cortex

The cerebral cortex can also be divided into primary projection areas, consisting of the **primary sensory area** which receives stimuli from the periphery of the body and the **primary motor area** sending out impulses that control the periphery and

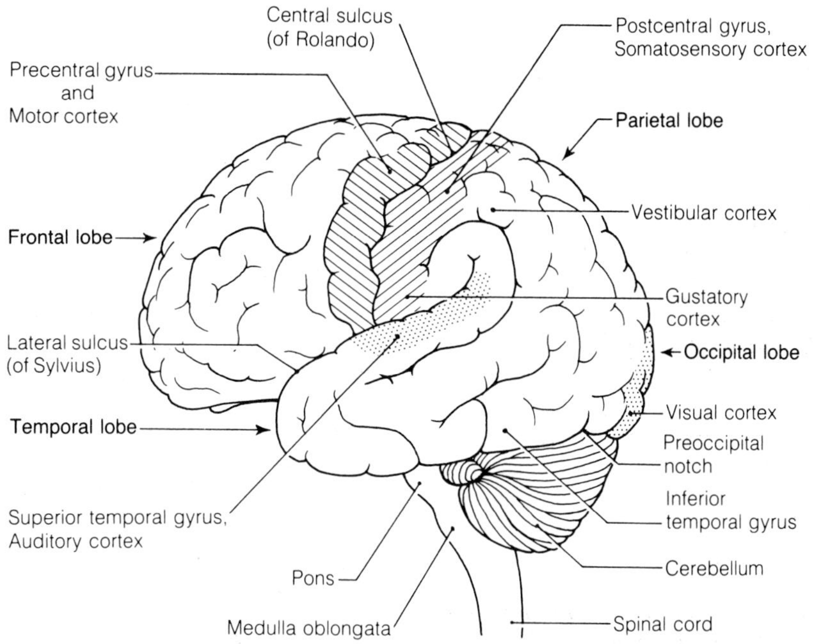

Figure 26.7 *Lateral aspect of the human brain (from Hinchliff SM, Montague SE, 1990, with permission).*

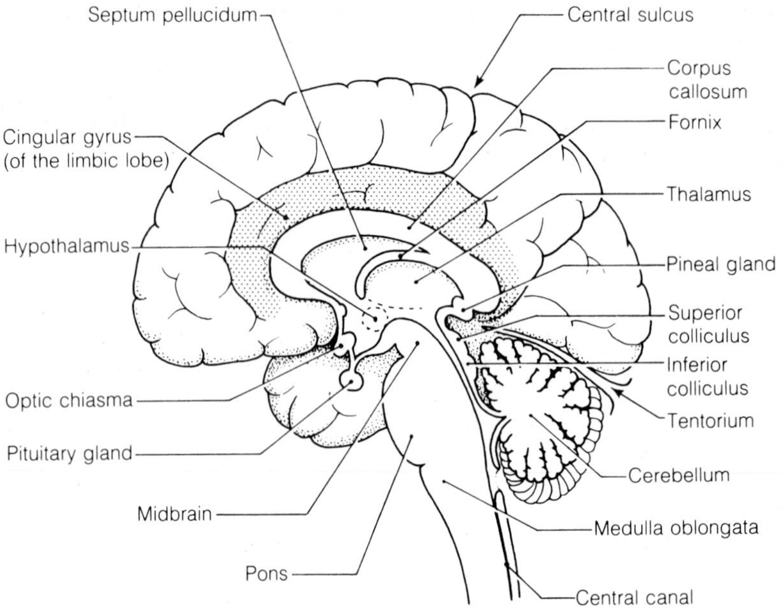

Figure 26.8 *Medial aspect of the human brain (from Hinchliff SM, Montague SE, 1990, with permission).*

association areas. Sensory areas are posterior to the central sulcus as they are posterior in the spinal columns. The motor areas are anterior to the central sulcus and in the spinal column.

The association areas integrate diverse information to allow appropriate actions to be taken. These include the **prefrontal cortex**, occupying the most anterior part of the frontal lobes and concerned with intellect, the **diffuse gnostic area**, contributing memory of sensation and emotional response, and the **language areas**, usually in the left hemisphere. There is insufficient space here to discuss brain lateralisation and the reader is referred to an excellent book by Springer & Deutsch (1989). The concept of lateralisation in mothers and babies is discussed in Chapter 57.

Prefrontal cortex

The prefrontal cortex is concerned with higher mental functions such as abstract thinking, decision making, social behaviour and anticipating the effects of actions. It links with the cortex on the same side of the brain (**ipsilateral**), the cortex of the opposite side of the brain (**contralateral**), the thalamus and the hypothalamus.

Sensory cortex

Nerve fibres from the thalamus project to the sensory areas of the cerebral cortex. It is essential that nerves coming into the spinal cord from the periphery of the body maintain their somatotropic organisation so that a representation of the body is faithfully organised in the sensory cortex. The size of the sensory cortex area given over to receiving input from a body part depends on the degree of innervation of that part. This results in a rather peculiarly shaped homunculus represented upside down in the sensory cortex. Those parts of us that are most sensitive, such as the tongue, lips, fingers and toes, are well represented.

The control of movement

Motor cortex

Movement of the body by the skeletal muscles is controlled by input from the nervous system. Motor control can be divided into three neural systems (Allan et al 1990). These are:

- the **pyramidal system**, a fast and usually direct descending pathway from the cortex;
- the **extrapyramidal system** with multiple synapses involving many brain structures, the basal ganglia being the most important;
- the **cerebellum**.

Traditionally the above order has represented the relative importance of the system to motor control. Recently, research has shown that the extrapyramidal system is much more involved and the intention to act is developed by the integration of widespread neuronal impulses. The motor cortex is involved at the end of the integration and development of intent. It is organised in a similar way to the sensory cortex. The efferent fibres from the motor cortex project to the basal ganglia, the thalamus, the red nucleus, the lateral reticular formation and the spinal cord in a topographically organised manner.

The extrapyramidal system

The basal ganglia

The basal ganglia consist of three large nuclei which lie lateral to the thalamus. These are the **globus pallidus**, the **putamen** and the **caudate nucleus**. Motor activity is strongly influenced by the basal ganglia which constitute the main extrapyramidal control. The caudate nucleus and the putamen are referred to as the **corpus striatum**, which is the largest subcortical mass of cells in the brain. The caudate nucleus has a tail which sweeps under the lateral ventricle to merge with the amygdala.

The red nucleus

The red nucleus is found between the substantia nigra and the aqueduct of Sylvius. It is an oval-shaped structure involved in the control of limb flexion.

The cerebellum

This large brain structure lies beneath the occipital lobes and is separated from them by a fold of dura mater called the **tentorium cerebelli** (see Chapter 24). The cerebellum is bilaterally symmetrical with a midline structure called the **vermis** separating the two parts. There are no interhemispheric nerve fibres so that messages are not relayed between the two halves. The cerebellum is involved in monitoring the strength and execution of movements and therefore motor coordination. It is able to do this because of incoming sensory stimuli. Its function is entirely inhibitory in nature and the neurotransmitter is the inhibitory γ-aminobutyric acid (GABA).

The limbic system

The limbic system consists of nuclei and fibres located on the medial aspect of each cerebral hemisphere. Its structures encircle the upper part of the brainstem, hence its name, as *limbus* means a ring. It includes the cingulate gyrus, the parahippocampal gyrus, the hippocampus, the amygdala, the hypothalamus, part of the thalamus, the insula and the septum. It is closely related to the reticular formation.

Its function is concerned with emotional (**affective**) feelings and responds to a wide variety of environmental stimuli. The limbic system interacts with higher brain centres and therefore there is a close relationship between cognition and emotion. All the 'Trekkies' out there should wonder what has happened to the limbic system of Mr Spock to dampen down his emotional reactions and leave his logical mind standing alone!

The cingulate gyrus

The cingulate gyrus involves part of the cortex and part of the limbic system. A bundle of fibres form a neural network interconnecting parts of the limbic lobe. The cingulate gyrus receives fibres from the parahippocampal gyrus, the temporal lobe, the thalamus and visual and tactile areas of the cortex. Its function is the emotional interpretation of pain and vision.

The hippocampus

This is part of the limbic cortex and is situated in the temporal lobe. It has a complex three-dimensional trumpet shape and is called 'Ammon's horn'. The hippocampus communicates with the neocortex, the thalamus and other subcortical regions. Its functions include memory, learning, spatial awareness and cognitive mapping.

The amygdala

The amygdala is involved in emotion. It consists of a paired set of nuclei next to the lateral ventricles in the temporal lobes of the brain. It is a focal point between incoming sensory systems and outgoing effector systems responsible for emotion. Lesion studies suggest a different role for each nucleus. The right seems to be involved in the strength of emotion and in negative emotions, the left in unemotional response and positive emotions.

The hypothalamus

This structure occupies the side walls and floor of the third ventricle and is involved in homeostasis and survival. It contains centres involved in the regulation of food intake, water intake, sleep/wake cycles, sexual behaviour and defence against attack. The hypothalamus controls the output of anterior pituitary hormones by producing releasing and inhibiting factors. It secretes the posterior pituitary hormones directly.

The thalamus

The thalami are a pair of organs joined in the midline. They are at the centre of the brain and could be said to act like a traffic conductor. The thalami contain multiple nuclei, each with a specific function including hearing, vision, memory, cognition, judgement and mood. There are multiple projections to the cortex and the thalami are continuous with the reticular formation.

The insula

The insula lies deep in the brain and its function is poorly understood. It is covered by the frontal, parietal and temporal lobes and continuous with the anterior temporal cortex, the entorrhinal cortex and the amygdala. The insula is involved in olfaction, taste and autonomic reflexes.

The septum

The connections of the septum lie central to the brain. Fibres are received from the amygdala, olfactory tract, hippocampus and brainstem. Fibres from the septum connect with the hypothalamus, brainstem and hippocampus. The functions of the septum are sensations of pleasure, well-being and appetites that will stimulate those feelings. It is also involved in memory.

The reticular formation

The reticular formation is a phylogenetically (evolutionary) old part of the brain, sometimes called the reptilian brain. It extends through the medulla, pons and midbrain. It is closely related to the olfactory and limbic parts of the brain. In humans it is responsible for automatic and reflex activities. It has loosely clustered neurones with long, branching dendrites. Its fibres run in three main columns: the main column, which is the midline raphe, the medial nuclear group and the lateral nuclear group. The fibres of the activating system make multiple synapses throughout the brainstem. This aspect of the reticular formation is called the **reticular activating system** (RAS) and is involved in the level of consciousness and alertness and the sleep/wake cycle.

Other reticular formation neurones are involved in the motor system and act with the cerebellum to maintain muscle tone and produce coordinated skeletal muscle contractions. Reticular formation neurones also form the autonomic centres of the medulla and thus help to regulate visceral muscle action.

The medulla oblongata

The medulla is the conical-shaped lowest part of the brainstem blending into the spinal cord at the level of the foramen magnum in the base of the skull. The central canal of the spinal cord broadens out in the medulla to form the fourth ventricle. The role of the medulla is as an autonomic reflex centre, maintaining homeostasis. Its nuclei include the cardiac centre, the vasomotor centre, the respiratory centre and nuclei that control vomiting, swallowing, coughing and sneezing.

The pons

The pons is a bulbous structure between the medulla and the midbrain. It forms part of the anterior wall of the third ventricle. It is a bridge formed of nerve fibres running between the spinal cord and the higher brain centres.

ALTERATIONS IN CONSCIOUSNESS

Conscious awareness allows the nervous system to undertake deliberate interaction with the environment. The neural processes that underlie altered states of consciousness, even the normal sleep/wake cycles, are not well understood. Dark and light cycles are known to play a role in the sleep/wake cycle. Waterhouse (1991) is an expert on circadian rhythms and how the body clock works. He wrote that, left to its own devices i.e. to free wheel, the body clock will complete its cycle in a period of about, but not exactly, 24 h. However, in our everyday life the cycle is driven by environmental cues called ***zeitgeibers*** which synchronise the clock with the 24 h solar cycle. *Zeitgeibers* include light, social activity and diet.

The sleep/wake cycle

Sleep is a complex phenomenon and involves many physiological processes (Allan et al 1996). The pattern of sleep has been studied by measuring the electrical activity of the brain by means of an **electroencephalogram** (EEG). Normal sleep consists of two types; non-rapid eye movement (NREM) and rapid eye movement (REM) sleep.

NREM sleep

NREM sleep can be divided into four stages:

1. a transitional phase lasting 1–7 min when the person is relaxed but with the eyes closed;
2. light sleep when dreaming may commence and the person becomes difficult to arouse;
3. moderately deep sleep which occurs about 20 min after falling asleep and the person is very relaxed. Blood pressure and body temperature are falling;
4. deep sleep.

REM sleep

REM sleep is characterised by depression of muscle tone except for rapid movements of the eyes. The sleeper's respiratory and pulse rates increase and dreaming occurs. There is a typical pattern in a normal 8-h sleep. The sleeper passes through stages 1–4 and then through stages 3 and 2. REM sleep now occurs. This cycle is repeated about every 90 min, about 3–5 times throughout the sleep experience. REM sleep increases from 10 min to a final period of 50 min.

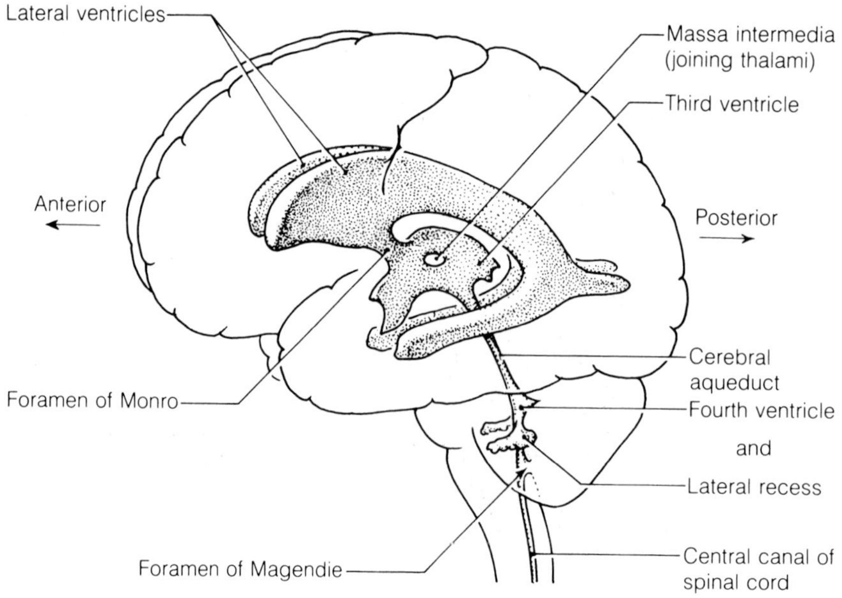

Figure 26.9 *The ventricular system of the brain, lateral view (from Hinchliff SM, Montague SE, 1990, with permission).*

The reason why humans sleep is not known. Behaviourists such as Carlsson (1991) theorise that sleep may have two purposes. It may be restorative, a necessary part of replenishing energy and restoring tissues, or it may be a protective measure to ensure safety for a daytime species by limiting activity during the hours of darkness. REM sleep may allow the integration of the day's events into long-term memory, promoting learning, species-typical reprogramming or brain development. Carlsson (1991) gives a full description of sleep which includes descriptions of the EEG patterns found in different states of consciousness. He also explores the theories of why we sleep and the effects of sleep deprivation.

PROTECTION OF THE BRAIN

The ventricles

There are four fluid-filled ventricles that help to cushion and protect the brain (Fig. 26.9): the two lateral ventricles and the third and fourth ventricles. The ventricles are continuous with each other and with the central canal of the spinal cord via the aqueduct of Sylvius. The hollow chambers are filled with cerebrospinal fluid (CSF) and lined by ependymal cells. There are three apertures in the wall of the fourth ventricle connecting the ventricles to the fluid-filled subarachnoid space surrounding the brain.

Choroid plexi, which are tufts of capillaries, hang from the roof of each ventricle and form the CSF. CSF moves freely through the ventricles and into the central canal of the spinal cord (Fig. 26.10). Most of the CSF enters the subarachnoid space. CSF bathes the outer surfaces of the brain and cord and returns in the blood via arachnoid villi to the dural sinuses. Anything causing obstruction to the flow will result in CSF accumulating in the ventricles and putting pressure on the brain. In a neonate the skull bones are not fused and a collection of fluid in the ventricles will cause enlargement of the skull, a condition known as **hydrocephalus** (see Chapter 15).

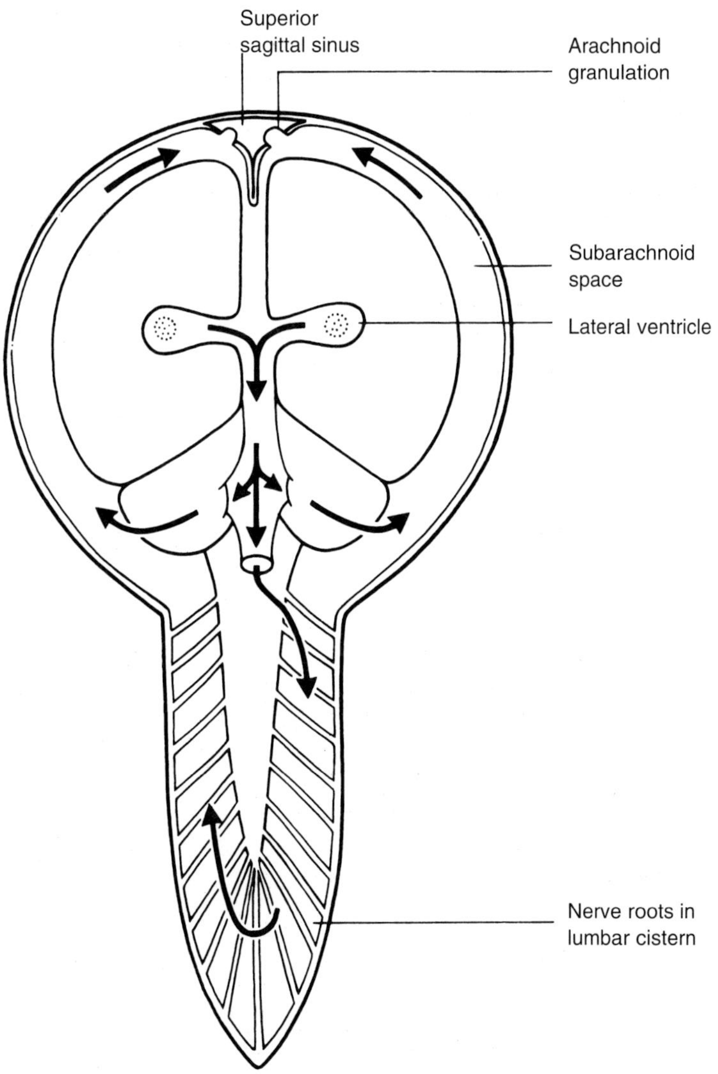

Figure 26.10 *Circulation of cerebrospinal fluid (from Fitzgerald MJT, 1996, with permission).*

The meninges

The meninges are three membranes made of connective tissue that cover and protect the brain and spinal cord, protect blood vessels and enclose venous sinuses and contain CSF. They are the pia, arachnoid and dura maters.

The **pia mater** is very delicate and has many tiny blood vessels. It clings tightly to the surface of the brain, following every convolution. The **arachnoid mater** forms a loose brain covering and is attached to the pia mater by thread-like arachnoid extensions which cross the subarachnoid space which is filled with CSF. The knob-like extensions of the arachnoid, called **arachnoid villi**, protrude through the dura mater into the dural sinuses which carry venous blood. The **dura mater** is the double-layered membrane that lines the skull with its periosteal layer and is reflected onto the surface of the brain as the meningeal layer. In places the dura extends inwards to form septa that anchor the brain to the skull and limit movement. These include:

- the **falx cerebri** which runs vertically in the sagittal plane of the skull;
- the **falx cerebelli**, another small vertical septum in the sagittal plane that runs along the vermis of the cerebellum;
- the **tentorium cerebelli** which is a horizontal fold of dura extending into the transverse fissure between the cerebral hemispheres and the cerebellum.

The blood–brain barrier

The blood–brain barrier is a protective mechanism to ensure that the brain's internal environment remains stable. In other body regions extracellular concentrations of hormones, amino acids, ions and other substances are in constant flux, especially after eating or taking exercise. If the brain were exposed to these variations, neurones could fire uncontrollably as many of the substances can act as neurotransmitters, especially potassium. Bloodborne substances within the brain's capillaries are separated from the extracellular space and the neurones by:

- a continuous endothelial capillary wall with tight junctions;
- a thick basal lamina surrounding the external face of the capillary;
- the bulbous feet of astrocytes clinging to the capillaries. The astrocytes signal the capillaries to maintain their tight junctions.

It is a selective barrier so that substances needed by the brain, such as glucose, amino acids and some electrolytes, can cross by facilitated diffusion. Drugs and toxic chemicals are kept within the capillary network.

THE CRANIAL NERVES

Twelve pairs of cranial nerves are associated with the brain and pass through foramina in the skull. The first two pairs originate from the forebrain but the rest have their origins in the brainstem. All but the vagus nerve target structures in the head and neck. Briefly, the cranial nerves are as follows.

I Olfactory, concerned with the sense of smell
II Optic, which is the nerve concerned with vision
III Oculomotor, which moves four of the extrinsic muscles of the eye
IV Trochlear, which also innervates an extrinsic muscle of the eye
V Trigeminal, supplying facial sensory fibres and motor fibres for chewing muscles
VI Abducens, which controls the extrinsic muscle that turns the eyeball laterally
VII Facial, innervating the muscles of facial expression
VIII Vestibulocochlear, the sensory nerve for hearing and balance
IX Glossopharyngeal, which innervates the tongue and pharynx
X Vagus, which innervates thoracic and abdominal viscera
XI Accessory, helping the vagus nerve
XII Hypoglossal, which innervates the tongue-moving muscle

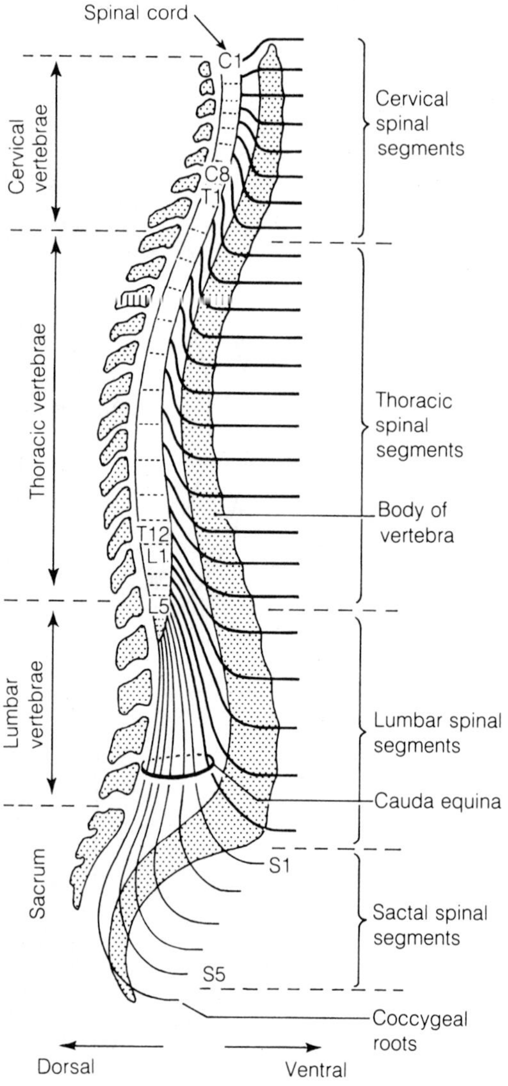

Figure 26.11 *The relationship between the spinal cord and the vertebral column (from Hinchliff SM, Montague SE, 1990, with permission).*

THE SPINAL CORD

Knowledge of spinal cord anatomy is important to those caring for childbearing women because of the use of **epidural analgesia**. Details of the nerve supply to the uterus and the route for epidural anaesthesia in labour are given in Chapter 38. The spinal cord is enclosed within the vertebral column and extends from the foramen magnum of the skull to the level of the first lumbar vertebra (Chapter 9). The cord is about 42 cm long and 1.8 cm thick and carries ascending and descending nerve pathways (Fig. 26.11). There are enlargements of the spinal cord in the cervical and lumbosacral regions where the nerves supplying the limbs arise.

The spinal column is protected by bone, cerebrospinal fluid and meninges. The dura mater here is a single layer only and is not attached to the bony walls of the vertebral column. Between the bones and the dural sheath is the large epidural space filled with fat and blood vessels. The subarachnoid space, between the pia and arachnoid maters, is filled with CSF. The dura and arachnoid meningeal membranes extend well beyond the end of the spinal cord to the 2nd sacral vertebra.

The spinal nerves

Thirty-one pairs of spinal nerves arise from the cord by paired roots and leave the vertebral column by the intervertebral foramina to target specific areas of the body. The spinal cord is segmented and each segment is defined by a pair of spinal nerves. Each spinal nerve conducts sensory information from a specific body area. These areas are called **dermatomes** and are shown in Figure 26.12.

Inferiorly the spinal cord ends in a cone-shaped structure, the **conus medullaris**, and nerve roots fan outwards and downwards to exit through relevant vertebrae. This collection of nerve roots is called the **cauda equinae** because it looks a little like a horse's tail. There is a fibrous extension of the pia called the **filum terminale** extending downwards to attach to the posterior surface of the coccyx.

A cross-section of the anatomy of the spinal cord

The grey matter and the spinal roots

The grey matter of the cord consists of neuronal cell bodies, their unmyelinated process and neuroglia. It is central to the white matter and looks like a letter H. There are two posterior or dorsal horns which contain interneurones and two anterior or ventral horns which house the nerve cell bodies of the somatic motor neurones (Fig. 26.13).

The ventral roots of the spinal cord contain the axons of the somatic motor neurones on their way to the skeletal muscles. Small lateral horns are columns of grey matter found in the thoracic and upper lumbar segments of the cord. These carry the neurones of the autonomic motor system. Their axons also leave via the ventral roots. Afferent fibres of the peripheral sensory nerves form the dorsal roots of the spinal cord. The cell bodies of these nerves are found in the dorsal root ganglion, an

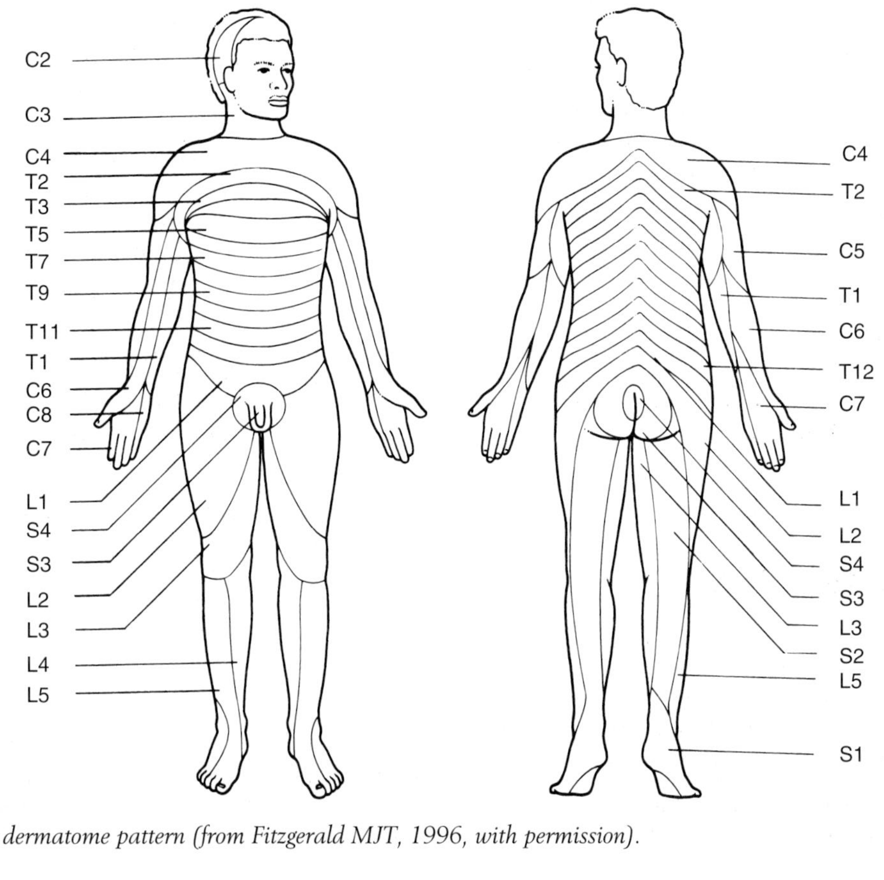

Figure 26.12 *Adult dermatome pattern (from Fitzgerald MJT, 1996, with permission).*

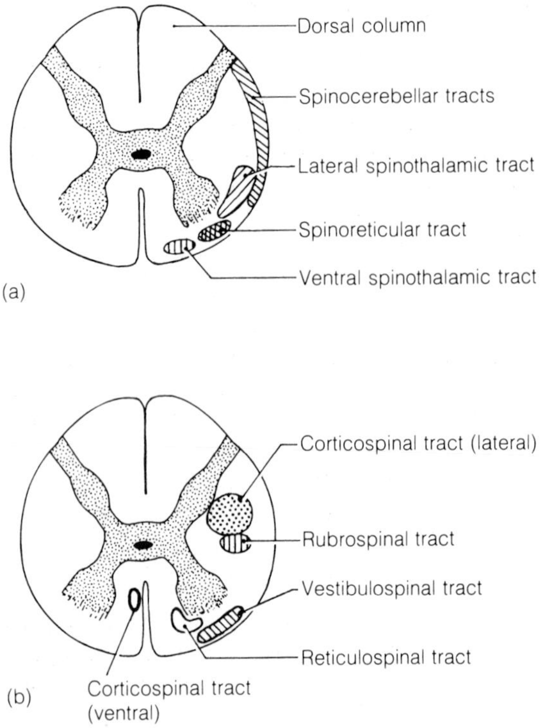

Figure 26.13 *Major nerve tracts of the spinal cord. (a) Ascending nerve tracts. (b) Descending nerve tracts (from Hinchliff SM, Montague SE, 1990, with permission).*

enlargement of the dorsal root. The dorsal and ventral roots are very short and fuse laterally to form the spinal nerves.

The white matter

The white matter of the spinal cord is composed of myelinated and unmyelinated nerve fibres running in three directions:

1 ascending tracts of sensory inputs going to the higher centres;
2 descending tracts of motor outputs coming from the brain;
3 across from one side of the spinal cord to the other (**commissural fibres**).

The white matter on each side of the cord is divided into three white columns: the posterior, lateral and anterior **funiculi**. These spinal tracts connect the periphery of the body to the brain. There are some generalisations that can be made (Marieb 1992).

- Most pathways cross from one side to the other of the spinal column. This is called **decussation**.
- Most consist of a chain of two or three neurones contributing to successive tracts of the pathway.
- Most show **somatotopy**, reflecting an orderly mapping of the body.
- All pathways and tracts are paired right and left.

Ascending sensory pathways

Ascending pathways take sensory impulses upwards to the brain through small chains of neurones. These are called first-, second- and third-order neurones. Incoming information is transmitted to the brain for conscious interpretation by six main pathways.

- The **fasciculus cuneatus** and **fasciculus gracilis** in the posterior funiculus, also known as the dorsal white column, transmit information from fine touch receptors and joint proprioceptors. These tracts decussate in the medulla. The pathway is called the dorsal column–medial lemniscal pathway.
- The **lateral** and **anterior spinothalamic tracts** convey information about pain, temperature, deep pressure and coarse touch. These tracts decussate in the cord. As pain management is central to the success of labour, detail on pain transmission, including the gate theory (Melzack & Wall 1991), is given in Chapter 36.
- The **anterior** and **posterior spinocerebellar tracts** convey information from the proprioceptors to the cerebellum and do not contribute to conscious sensation.

MATERNAL ADAPTATIONS TO PREGNANCY

The function of the central nervous system and brain is complex and covers all activities from basic reflex actions to detailed cognitive and emotional changes. Discussion of the higher brain functions enters the realm of physiological psychology. Blackburn & Loper (1992) highlight the complexity of the system and include the following list of changes, many due to the altered output from the endocrine system.

- Musculoskeletal discomforts
- Sleep disturbances
- Alterations in sensation
- The experience of pain

Neurohormonal control of reproduction is described in Chapter 3, musculoskeletal changes are discussed in Chapters 24 and 25 and pain is discussed in full in Chapter 38. The complex issue of maternal–child interaction is considered in Chapter 57. Neurological problems in pregnancy, including epilepsy and carpal tunnel syndrome, are discussed in Chapter 34.

The CNS

Many of the hormones of pregnancy affect the central nervous system. However, these effects are not as well understood as the effect of hormones on other systems. The effects of the hormones on the sensory systems are better documented. In January 1997 a team led by anaesthetist Anita Holdcroft described to a meeting of the Psychological Society findings from magnetic resonance imaging in a small group of 10 healthy women (Moore 1997). Women often report that their cognitive ability alters for the worse in pregnancy, with difficulty in concentration and poor memory top of the list. The author's daughter calculated the change to be 'worth a reduction of at least 10 points on the IQ scale'.

Holdcroft and her team believe that women's brains shrink during pregnancy and return to normal following delivery. This is believed to be brought about by changes in the volume of individual cells and not by a reduction of cell numbers. Holdcroft hypothesised that the shrinkage of the brain and the reduction in cognitive abilities could be linked but much more research needs to be carried out. The pituitary gland showed the opposite effect, increasing in pregnancy and returning to normal after delivery.

Sleep

Sleep patterns change during pregnancy and in the postpartum period. From about 25 weeks the pregnant woman experiences more REM sleep. This decreases to non-pregnant levels by term. There is a corresponding decrease in NREM sleep when the body undertakes tissue repair and recovers from fatigue (Blackburn & Loper 1992). This returns to normal immediately after delivery. During the first trimester sleep time and napping both increase but later night wakening occurs because of the minor disorders of nocturia, dyspnoea, heartburn, nasal congestion, muscle aches and anxiety.

Alterations in sensation

Changes in the ear, nose and larynx occur because of the changes in fluid dynamics and vascular permeability. This is related to the increase in circulating oestrogen. Congestion and hyperaemia of the nasal mucosa cause nasal stuffiness and rhinorrhoea. Blocked ears and ear stuffiness may also occur. Loss of sleep may accompany the nasal congestion. The vascular congestion may lead to nose bleeds. Similar laryngeal changes may result in voice changes or persistent cough.

The perceptions of smell and taste are closely related. A reduction in the sense of smell may lead to altered taste sensations and a change in food preference. Alterations in taste perception may be a factor in nausea and food aversions, especially for foods that taste bitter in pregnancy. Profet (1992) believes these alterations in perception are protective as bitter foods in nature are often poisonous or teratogenic.

Summary of main points

- The nervous system communicates by the rapid transmission of electrical signals. The endocrine glands secrete hormones into the bloodstream which modify the working of target organs. The central nervous system consists of the brain and spinal cord. It has an integrating function and receives messages from and sends messages via the peripheral nervous system to all parts of the body.
- The part of the PNS that controls the viscera is called the autonomic nervous system. It innervates the smooth muscle and glands of the viscera and cardiac muscle and is subdivided into two distinct parts: the sympathetic and parasympathetic nervous system.
- Nervous tissue is made of two cell types: neurones, the structural units of the nervous system, and a group of cell types collectively known as neuroglia. Neurones have axons and dendrites which communicate with other cells and conduct messages by nerve impulses. They are extremely long-lived, cannot undergo mitosis and divide and have a very high metabolic rate, needing continuous glucose and oxygen.
- Axons are responsible for conducting messages by electrical nerve impulses along to the terminal bouton and by chemicals known as neurotransmitters secreted in the soma and sent along to be stored in the terminal bouton. Larger nerve fibres are covered in a white fatty segmented covering called the myelin sheath which protects and insulates fibres and increases the rate of impulse transmission; messages can be transmitted up to 100 times more rapidly than via unmyelinated fibres.
- Neuroglial cells provide support and protection for the neurones. They outnumber neurones in a ratio of 10:1. Neuroglial cells are subdivided into astrocytes, oligodendrocytes, ependyma and microglia.
- The axons from single neurones are bound together to form nerves. Nerves often contain afferent fibres or efferent fibres or both. Those with both types of fibres are referred to as mixed nerves.
- Both nerve fibres and muscle fibres conduct electrochemical signals and are called excitable tissues. Nerve electrical activity is maintained by the distribution and relative concentration of negative and positive ions. Inside the cell the positive ion is potassium and the negative ion is protein. Outside in the interstitial fluid, the positive ion is sodium and the negative ion is chloride.
- Nerve fibres can be classified according to their speeds of conduction of the action potential. The larger the nerve, the more rapidly it can conduct its impulses. Myelinated nerves can conduct nerve impulses more rapidly by saltatory conduction.
- Synapses are junctions between the terminal bouton of the axon and its target tissue which may be a nerone cell body, a gland or a muscle. Between the neurone and its target cell, the synaptic cleft is a fluid-filled space into which neurotransmitters are released from the presynaptic membrane.
- The average brain weighs about 1500 g and is slightly heavier in men than women. It is the complexity of the wiring that determines the power of the brain, not its size. The brain can be subdivided into the cerebral hemispheres, the diencephalon, made up of the thalamus and hypothalamus, the brainstem, made up of midbrain, pons and medulla, and the cerebellum.
- The two cerebral hemispheres form the uppermost part of the brain. The neurones have their cell bodies outermost, forming the grey matter or cortex, and their fibres innermost, forming the white matter. The cortex is thrown into elevated gyri separated by shallow sulci to increase the surface area of the cortex. Each hemisphere is divided into six main lobes: the frontal, parietal, occipital and temporal lobes and the buried insula and limbic lobe.
- The cerebral cortex is also divided into primary projection areas, consisting of the primary sensory area, receiving stimuli from the periphery of the body, and the primary motor area, sending out impulses that control the periphery, and the association areas. Sensory areas are posterior to the central sulcus and motor areas are anterior to the central sulcus and in the spinal column. The prefrontal cortex is concerned with higher mental functions such as abstract thinking, decision making, social behaviour and anticipating the effects of actions.
- Nerve fibres from the thalamus project to the sensory areas of the cerebral cortex. It is essential that nerves coming into the spinal cord from the periphery of the body maintain their somatotopic organisation so that a representation of the body is faithfully organised in the sensory cortex.
- Movement of the body by the skeletal muscles is controlled by input from the nervous system. Motor control can be divided into three neural systems: the pyramidal system, the extrapyramidal system and the cerebellum.
- The limbic system structures encircle the upper part of the brainstem and are closely related to the reticular formation. They include the cingulate gyrus, the parahippocampal gyrus, the hippocampus, the amygdala, the hypothalamus, part of the thalamus, the insula and the septum: Limbic system function is concerned with emotional feelings and the limbic system interacts with higher brain centres so that there is a close relationship between cognition and emotion.

- The cingulate gyrus functions in the emotional interpretation of pain and vision. The hippocampus functions include memory, learning, spatial awareness and cognitive mapping. The amygdala is involved in emotion. The right nucleus of the amygdala seems to be involved in the strength and negativity of emotions, the left in unemotional response and positive emotions.
- The hypothalamus is involved in homeostasis and survival. Its centres are involved in regulation of food intake, water intake, sleep/wake cycles, sexual behaviour and defence. It controls the output of anterior pituitary hormones by producing releasing and inhibiting factors but secretes posterior pituitary hormones directly.
- The thalami are a pair of organs joined in the midline at the centre of the brain whose functions include hearing, vision, memory, cognition, judgement and mood. They are continuous with the reticular formation.
- The insula is continuous with the anterior temporal cortex, the entorrhinal cortex and the amygdala. It is involved in olfaction, taste and autonomic reflexes. The functions of the septum are sensations of pleasure, well-being and appetites that will stimulate those feelings and memory.
- The reticular formation extends through the medulla, pons and midbrain. It is closely related to the olfactory and limbic parts of the brain. In humans it is responsible for automatic and reflex activities. The fibres of the reticular activating system are involved in the level of consciousness and alertness and the sleep/wake cycle. Other reticular formation neurones act with the cerebellum to maintain muscle tone and produce coordinated skeletal muscle contractions.
- Reticular formation neurones form the autonomic centres of the medulla, an autonomic reflex centre maintaining homeostasis. Its nuclei include the cardiac centre, the vasomotor centre, the respiratory centre and others that control vomiting, swallowing, coughing and sneezing.
- The pons is a bulbous structure between the medulla and the midbrain forming part of the anterior wall of the third ventricle. It is a bridge formed of nerve fibres running between the spinal cord and the higher brain centres.
- Conscious awareness allows the nervous system to interact with the environment. Behaviourists theorise that sleep may have two purposes. It may be restorative or it may be a protective measure to ensure safety for a daytime species by limiting activity during darkness. REM sleep may allow the integration of the day's events into long-term memory.
- The four fluid-filled ventricles are continuous with each other and with the central canal of the spinal cord via the aqueduct of Sylvius. The hollow chambers are filled with cerebrospinal fluid and lined by ependymal cells. Choroid plexi hang from the roof of each ventricle and form the cerebrospinal fluid.
- The meninges are three membranes made of connective tissue that cover and protect the brain and spinal cord, protect blood vessels and enclose venous sinuses and contain CSF. They are the pia, arachnoid and dura maters. In places the dura extends inwards to form septa that anchor the brain to the skull. These include the falx cerebri, the falx cerebelli and the tentorium cerebelli.
- The blood–brain barrier is a protective mechanism to ensure that the brain's internal environment remains stable. It is selective so that substances needed by the brain, such as glucose, amino acids and some electrolytes, can cross by facilitated diffusion. Drugs and toxic chemicals are kept within the capillary network.
- Twelve pairs of cranial nerves are associated with the brain and pass through foramina in the skull. The first two pairs originate from the forebrain but the rest have their origins in the brainstem. All but the vagus nerve target structures in the head and neck.
- The spinal cord is enclosed within the vertebral column and extends from the foramen magnum of the skull to the level of the first lumbar vertebra. The cord carries ascending and descending nerve pathways. There are enlargements of the spinal cord in the cervical and lumbosacral regions where the nerves supplying the limbs arise.
- The cord is protected by bone, cerebrospinal fluid and meninges. Between the bones and the dural sheath is the large epidural space filled with fat and blood vessels. The subarachnoid space is filled with CSF. The dura and arachnoid membranes extend beyond the end of the spinal cord to the 2nd sacral vertebra.
- Thirty-one pairs of spinal nerves arise from the segmented spinal cord by paired roots and leave the vertebral column by the intervertebral foramina to target specific areas of the body. Each segment is defined by a pair of spinal nerves. Each spinal nerve conducts sensory information from a specific body area called a dermatome.
- Inferiorly the spinal cord ends in a cone-shaped structure, the conus medullaris, and nerve roots fan outwards and downwards to exit through relevant vertebrae. This collection of nerve roots is called the cauda equinae. The filum terminale extends downwards to attach to the posterior surface of the coccyx.
- The grey matter of the cord consists of neuronal cell bodies, their unmyelinated process and neuroglia. It is central to the white matter and looks like a letter H. There are two posterior or dorsal horns and two anterior or ventral horns.
- The white matter of the spinal cord is composed of myelinated and unmyelinated nerve fibres running in three directions: ascending tracts, descending tracts and across from one side of the spinal cord to the other. The white matter on each side of the cord is divided into three white columns – the posterior, lateral and anterior funiculi – which connect the periphery of the body to the brain.
- The following changes occur in pregnancy: musculoskeletal discomforts, sleep disturbances, alterations in sensation and the experience of pain. Women often report that their cognitive ability alters for the worse in pregnancy, with difficulty in concentration and poor memory top of the list. Women's brains may shrink during pregnancy and return to normal following delivery. The pituitary gland increases in pregnancy and returns to normal after delivery.
- Sleep patterns change during pregnancy and in the postpartum period. During the first trimester sleep time and napping both increase but later in pregnancy night wakening occurs because of the minor disorders of nocturia, dyspnoea, heartburn, nasal congestion, muscle aches and anxiety.
- Congestion and hyperaemia of the nasal mucosa cause nasal stuffiness and rhinorrhoea. Blocked ears and ear stuffiness may also occur. Loss of sleep may accompany the nasal congestion, sometimes leading to nose bleeds. Laryngeal changes may result in voice changes or persistent cough.
- A reduction in the sense of smell may lead to altered taste sensations and a change in food preference. Alterations in taste perception may lead to nausea and food aversions, especially for foods that taste bitter. These may be protective against the ingestion of teratogenic foods.

References

Allan D, Nie V, Hunter M. 1996 Control and co-ordination. In Hinchliff SM, Montague SE, Watson R (eds) Physiology for Nursing Practice, 2nd edn. Baillière Tindall, London.
Blackburn ST, Loper DL. 1992 Maternal, Fetal and Neonatal Physiology, A Clinical Perspective. WB Saunders, Philadelphia.
Carlsson NR. 1991 Physiology of Behaviour, 4th edn. Allyn and Bacon, London.
Fitzgerald MJT. 1996 Neuroanatomy. Saunders, Philadelphia.
Hinchliff SM, Montague SE. 1990 Physiology for Nursing Practice. Baillière Tindall, London.
Hinchliff SM, Montague SE, Watson R. 1996 Physiology for Nursing Practice. Baillière Tindall, London.
Marieb EN. 1992 Human Anatomy and Physiology, 2nd edn. Benjamin/ Cummings Publishing, California.
Melzack R, Wall P. 1988 The Challenge of Pain. Penguin, Harmondsworth.
Moore P. 1997 Pregnant women get that shrinking feeling. New Scientist 153(2066) 5.
Profet M. 1992 Pregnancy sickness as adaptation: a deterrent to maternal ingestion of teratogens. In Barkow J, Cosmides L, Tooby J (eds) The Adapted Mind: Evolutionary Psychology and the Generation of Culture. Oxford University Press, New York, pp 327–365.
Springer SP, Deutsch G. 1989 Left Brain, Right Brain, 3rd edn. WH Freeman, New York.
Waterhouse J. 1991 Light dawns on the body clock. New Scientist 132(1797) 30–34.

Recommended reading

Carlsson NR. 1991 Physiology of Behaviour, 4th edn. Allyn and Bacon, London.
Fitzgerald MJT. 1992 Neuroanatomy: Basic and Clinical, 2nd edn. Baillière Tindall, London.
Hinchliff SM, Montague SE, Watson R. 1996 Physiology for Nursing Practice, 2nd edn. Baillière Tindall, London.
Wills C. 1995 The Runaway Brain. Flamingo, London.
Gazzaniga MS. 1992 Nature's Mind. Penguin, Harmondsworth.
Greenfield S. (ed) 1996 The Human Mind Explained. Cassell, London.

Chapter

27 The peripheral and autonomic nervous systems

In this chapter

THE PERIPHERAL NERVOUS SYSTEM

The purpose of the peripheral nervous system (PNS) is to detect changes in the external or internal environment of the body, code it into nerve impulses by sensory receptors and pass the information back to the central nervous system so that appropriate action can be instituted. Not all the messages are passed back to the brain. Some may influence reflex actions at the level of the spinal cord or brainstem. The PNS therefore includes all the neural structures outside the brain and spinal cord, i.e. the sensory receptors, peripheral nerves and associated ganglia and efferent motor endings.

Ascending sensory tracts

Categories of sensation

Neurologists divide sensation into two groups: conscious and unconscious (Fitzgerald 1992). Conscious sensation or **exteroception** involves messages from the outside world which are perceived in the cerebral cortex. They may be sensations perceived by the body surface receptors, called **somatic receptors**, or by the special sense receptors called **telereceptors**. Another form of conscious sensation is that transmitted to the cortex by **proprioceptors** in the locomotor system and the labyrinth of the inner ear. They inform the brain of position when stationary (position sense) and during movement (kinaesthetic sense).

Unconscious sensation can also be divided into two kinds. **Unconscious proprioception** has its effect in the cerebellum and involves messages received through spinocerebellar pathways and the brainstem. The messages are essential for smooth motor coordination. **Enteroception** refers to unconscious signals involved in visceral reflexes.

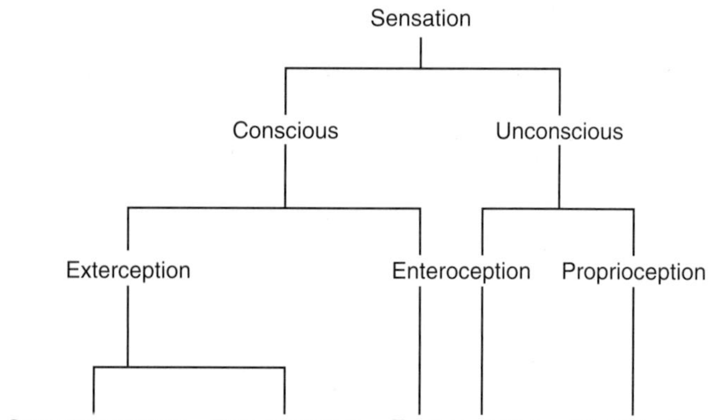

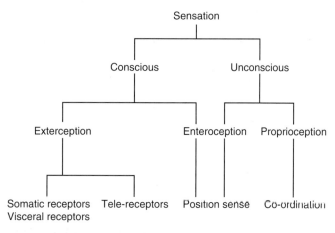

Figure 27.1 *Categories of sensation.*

Somatic sensory perception

Two major pathways are involved in somatic perception sensations: the posterior column-medial lemniscal pathway and the spinothalamic pathway (Fig. 27.2). Both pathways have common features (Fitzgerald 1992).

- They contain first-order, second-order and third-order sensory neurones.
- The cell bodies of the first-order neurones are in the posterior root ganglia.
- The cell bodies of the second-order neurones are on the same side of the CNS grey matter as the first-order neurones.
- Second-order axons cross the midline to ascend and terminate in the thalamus.
- The third-order neurones project to the somatosensory cortex.
- Both pathways are somatotopic, that is, they represent the body parts in an orderly fashion up to the sensory cortex.
- The pathways can be modulated, either inhibited or enhanced, by other neurones.

The posterior column-medial lemniscal pathway

The first-order nerve fibres enter the dorsal columns without synapsing. They are usually large A fibres with conduction velocities of about 70 m/s. As nerve fibres from higher levels in the cord are added, they take up lateral positions so that the higher the level of origin, the more lateral the position of the fibre in the column. The fibres of the cell bodies of second-order neurones at the level of the brainstem cross the midline to projec to the thalamus. This crossing over is the reason why one side of the brain controls the opposite or contralateral side of the body. Cells in the sensory relay nucleus of the thalamus are third-order neurones and project their fibres to the somatosensory cortex.

The spinothalamic tract

The dorsal root fibres of this pathway tend to be the smaller A-δ or unmyelinated C fibres with slow conduction velocity. The dorsal root fibres enter the spinal cord and may ascend or descend a few segments of the cord before synapsing with cells of the dorsal horn in the **substantia gelatinosa** (Fig. 27.3). The dorsal horn cell second-order fibres ascend or descend a few segments before crossing over the midline to ascend in the spinothalamic tract. These fibres terminate on third-order neurones in the thalamus, which themselves synapse on the cells of the sensory cortex. The role of the substantia gelatinosa in the

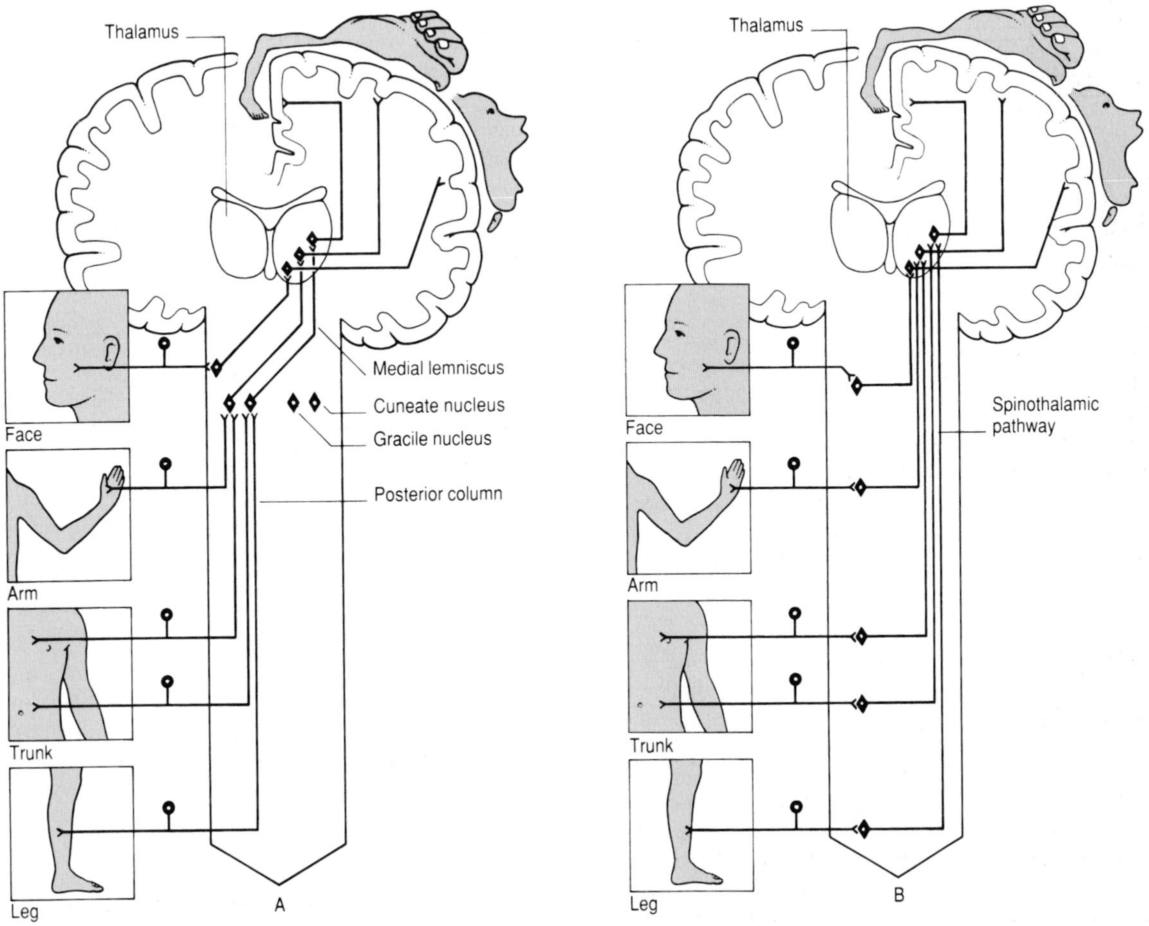

Figure 27.2 *Basic plans of: (a) posterior column-medial lemniscal pathway; (b) spinothalamic pathway (from Fitzgerald MJT, 1996, with permission).*

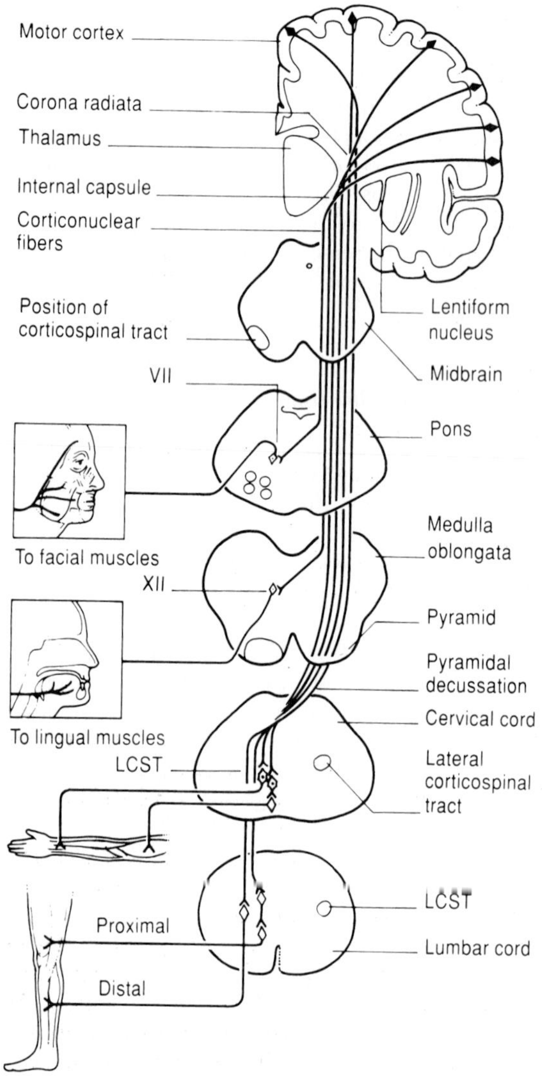

Figure 27.3 *Corticospinal tract viewed from the front. At spinal cord level, only the lateral corticospinal tract is shown. LCST, lateral corticospinal tract; VII, nucleus of facial nerve; XII, hypoglossal nucleus (from Fitzgerald MJT, 1996, with permission).*

gate control theory of perception of pain will be discussed in Chapter 38.

Somatosensory receptors

Sensory receptors are mostly adapted nerve fibre endings that respond to changes in the environment. They can be classified by structure or function. Those sensory afferent nerves arising from the body are grouped together as the somatosensory system and include sensation from the skin, muscles, joints or viscera. The special senses are associated with organs in the head: vision, hearing, balance, taste and smell. The special senses will not be considered in this book and anatomical and physiological aspects of vision and hearing can be found in Fitzgerald (1992) whilst Carlsson (1991) places the senses in the context of psychology.

Types of somatosensory receptors

- **Mechanoreceptors** – respond to touch, pressure, vibrations and stretch, such as the proprioceptors in joints and muscles
- **Thermoreceptors** – respond to temperature change
- **Photoreceptors** – respond to light
- **Chemoreceptors** – respond to smell, taste and changes in blood chemistry
- **Nociceptors** – respond to damage by causing pain

For a detailed explanation of general sensory receptors, the reader is referred to Marieb (1992). Nearly all receptors will function as nociceptors if overstimulated. Because of this feature and its relevance to the management of labour, the perception and response to pain will be described separately in detail in Chapter 38.

Descending motor pathways

The descending tracts carry efferent messages from the brain down the spinal cord and are divided into two groups.

1. The **pyramidal** or **corticospinal tracts** (Fig. 27.3) are the major motor pathways involved with voluntary movement. They synapse with interneurones or directly with the anterior horn neurones. The pyramidal tracts decussate in the medulla and their fibres are arranged somatotopically (Fig. 27.4).
2. The other group used to be called the extrapyramidal fibres but are now thought to have independent functions, so are referred to separately. They are the **rubrospinal**, **vestibulospinal** and **tectospinal tracts** originating in the different subcortical motor nuclei of the brainstem.

The neurones of the motor cortex are called the **pyramidal cells** because of the shape of their cell bodies. They are referred to as the **upper motor neurones**. The **anterior horn neurones**, whose axons leave the cord to innervate the skeletal muscles, are called the **lower motor neurones**. Damage to one or the other of these neuronal pathways will cause different symptoms.

REFLEX ACTIVITY

A reflex is a rapid, predictable, unlearned, involuntary response to a stimulus. Many of the control systems of the body come into this category. Some reflex activity is protective, such as the rapid removal of a body part from a noxious stimulus like heat. Other reflexes occur without any awareness of change such as those that control visceral activities. There can be learned reflexes that come from practice or repetition: for instance, the way that driving a car becomes automatic. In fact, many reflex actions are modifiable by learning and conscious effort.

The reflex arc

'Reflexes occur over specific neural paths called reflex arcs' (Marieb 1992). Reflex arcs (Fig. 27.5) have five main components.

1. The receptor at the site where the stimulus occurs.
2. The sensory neurone taking the message to the CNS.

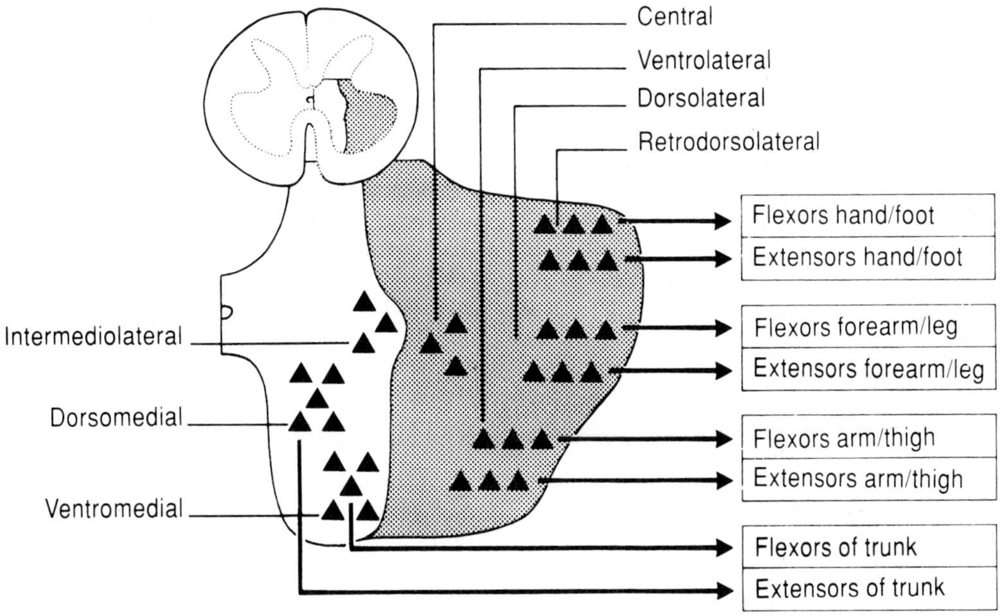

Figure 27.4 *Cell columns in the anterior grey horn of the spinal cord: somatotopic organisation (from Fitzgerald MJT, 1996, with permission).*

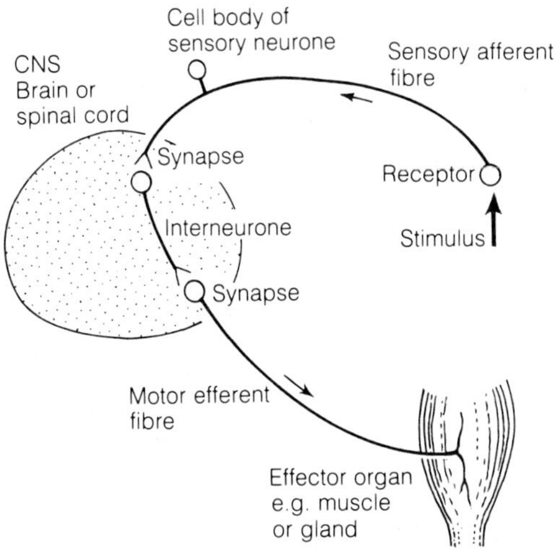

Figure 27.5 *The component structures of a reflex arc (from Hinchliff SM, Montague SE, 1990, with permission).*

3 The integration centre within the CNS which may only be a single synapse or may involve a chain of interneurones.
4 The motor neurone which conducts efferent impulses from the integration centre to an effector organ.
5 The effector, which may be a gland or a muscle fibre which acts to complete the reflex action. Reflexes may be somatic or autonomic. Somatic reflexes can be tested to confirm normal neural function at any age.

Spinal reflexes

Many spinal reflexes occur with little or no brain input.

- **Stretch** and **deep tendon reflexes**, where the messages from the proprioceptors in the muscles and joints are transmitted to the cerebellum and cerebral cortex. These allow normal muscle tone and activity to be maintained.
- The **flexor reflex**, which causes automatic withdrawal of the body from a painful stimulus.
- The **crossed extensor reflex** consists of an ipsilateral withdrawal reflex and a contralateral extensor reflex. These are extremely important in maintaining balance.
- **Superficial reflexes** can be elicited by gentle stroking of the body. The best known is the plantar reflex, with incurling of the toes occurring in response to stroking the sole of the foot. Babinski's reflex, with extension of the toes, occurs in infants less than a year old. The abdominal reflex occurs when the skin on one side of the trunk is stroked. Reflex contraction of the abdominal muscles at or below the umbilicus will cause reflex contraction of the abdominal muscles, moving the umbilicus towards the stimulated side.

THE AUTONOMIC NERVOUS SYSTEM

The autonomic nervous system or ANS is responsible for maintaining the stability of the body's internal environment. Motor neurones of the ANS innervate smooth muscle, cardiac muscle and glands, making adjustments to alter function in response to messages from the viscera sent to the central nervous system (CNS). Changes in the systems brought about by the ANS include making adjustments to:

- shunting of blood to the needy areas;
- the heart rate;
- the blood pressure;
- the respiratory rate;
- body temperature;
- stomach secretions.

Marieb (1992) reminds us of the alternative names for the ANS: the involuntary nervous system, signifying its unconscious control, and the general visceral motor system, describing its effects. There are differences between the somatic and autonomic nervous systems in their pathways and neurotransmitters. The ANS is divided into two arms: the **sympathetic system** (Fig. 27.6), which prepares the body for emergency action, and the **parasympathetic system** (Fig. 27.7), which has a calming effect and allows general body maintenance to occur and also the conservation of energy. The two systems counterbalance each other.

Pathways in the ANS

The motor unit of the ANS is a two-neurone chain. The first neurone is called the **preganglionic neurone**. Its cell body is found in the brain or spinal column. It synapses with the second motor or **postganglionic neurone**, which has its cell body in the autonomic ganglion outside the CNS. The postganglionic neurone extends to the target tissue.

Preganglionic neurones are thin and lightly myelinated whilst postganglionic fibres are even thinner and unmyelinated. Both pre- and postganglionic fibres may run with somatic nerves in spinal or cranial nerves.

The role of the two divisions

Although the following explanations outline the extremes of function, it is important to remember that there is usually a dynamic interaction between the two systems aimed at maximising homeostasis. The parasympathetic division is active when the systems are unstressed. It has been called the 'resting and digesting' system and is concerned with digestion and elimination of waste. Blood pressure, heart rate and respiratory rate are low and digestion is occurring. The skin is warm as the skeletal muscles do not require extra blood supply. The eye pupils are constricted and the eye lenses are adjusted for close vision.

The sympathetic division is sometimes referred to as the 'fight or flight' system. It is activated if we are excited or find ourselves in a threatening situation. The heart rate increases, there is rapid breathing, a cold sweaty skin and dilated eye pupils. Visceral blood vessels are constricted and digestion ceases. Blood is shunted to the heart and skeletal muscles and the liver

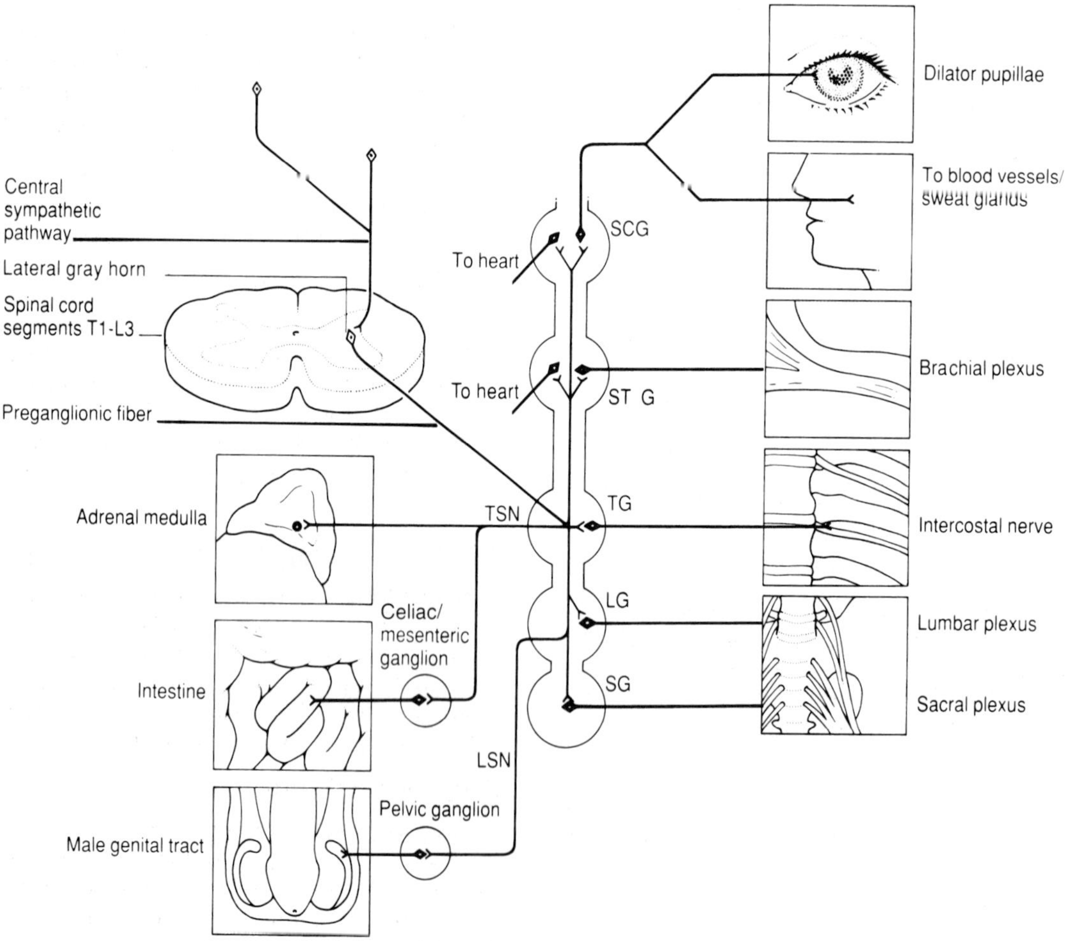

Figure 27.6 *General plan of the sympathetic system. Ganglionic neurones and postganglionic fibres are shown in red. LG, lumbar ganglia; LSN, lumbar splanchnic nerve; SCG, superior cervical ganglion; SG, sacral ganglia; ST.G, stellate ganglion; TG, thoracic ganglia; TSN, thoracic splanchnic nerve (from Fitzgerald MJT, 1996, with permission).*

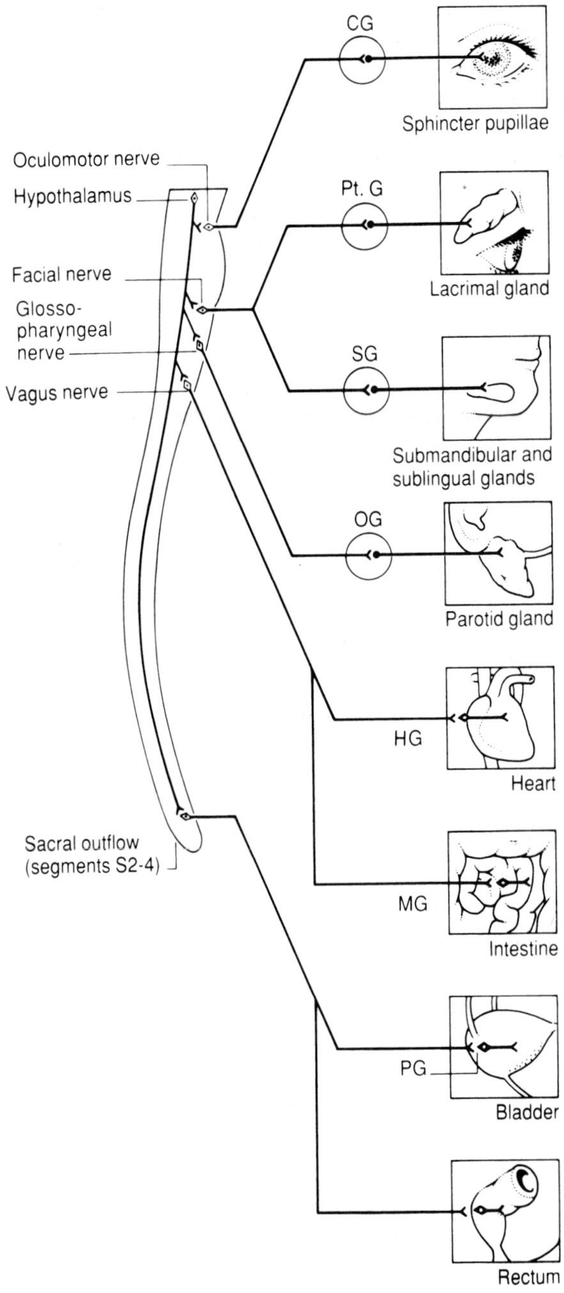

Figure 27.7 *General plan of the parasympathetic system. Ganglionic neurones and postganglionic fibres are shown in red. CG, ciliary ganglion; HG, heart ganglia; MG, myenteric ganglia; OG, otic ganglion; PG, pterygopalatine ganglion; SG, submandibular ganglion (from Fitzgerald MJT, 1996, with permission).*

releases glucose into the blood so that the cells are provided with energy.

Anatomy

Differences between the two divisions

- Parasympathetic fibres emerge from the brain and sacral spinal cord (craniosacral division) whilst the sympathetic fibres originate from the thoracolumbar region of the spinal cord.
- The parasympathetic division has long preganglionic and short postganglionic fibres. The sympathetic division has short preganglionic and long postganglionic fibres.
- Parasympathetic ganglia are located in terminal ganglia within or close to the visceral target organs. Sympathetic ganglia lie close to the spinal cord.

Parasympathetic division

The cranial outflow

The cranial parasympathetic preganglionic fibres run in the oculomotor, facial, glossopharyngeal and vagus nerves.

- The oculomotor nerve parasympathetic fibres innervate smooth muscle within the eyes, causing the pupils to constrict and the lenses of the eyes to shorten and thicken so that focus is aimed at near objects.
- The facial nerve parasympathetic fibres stimulate the large glands in the head such as the nasal and lacrimal glands and the submandibular and sublingual salivary glands.
- The glossopharyngeal parasympathetic nerve fibres activate the parotid salivary glands.
- The vagus nerve parasympathetic activity accounts for 90% of all the preganglionic parasympathetic nerve activity. Fibres from the two vagus nerves serve almost every organ in the thoracic and abdominal cavities. The preganglionic axons synapse on intramural (within the walls) ganglia of the target organs. Thoracic organs receiving innervation are the heart, lungs and oesophagus. Abdominal organs receiving innervation are the liver, stomach, small intestine, kidneys, pancreas and the proximal half of the large intestine.

The sacral outflow

The sacral outflow arises from neurones in the lateral grey matter of the sacral spinal cord segments S2–S4. The axons of these neurones run in the ventral roots of the spinal cord and branch off to form the splanchnic nerves. Most fibres synapse in intramural ganglia in the distal half of the large intestine, the urinary bladder, the ureters and reproductive organs such as the uterus.

Sympathetic division

The sympathetic division is much more complex, partly because it innervates more organs. Sympathetic activity tends to inhibit the activity of visceral organs, some body wall structures, such as sweat glands, and smooth muscles, such as the hair-raising muscles (**erector pili**). Also all arteries and veins, superficial and deep, are innervated by sympathetic fibres.

Preganglionic fibres

The preganglionic fibres arise from cell bodies of neurones located in thoracic and lumbar spinal cord segments from T1 to L2 which is why it is named the **thoracolumbar division**. The presence of these preganglionic sympathetic neurones produces the **lateral horns** (visceral motor horns) of the spinal cord, found in these sections. The fibres leave the spinal cord via the ventral root and pass through a myelinated **white ramus communicans** to enter the appropriate **paravertebral (chain) ganglion** which forms part of the sympathetic trunk or chain. Two sympathetic trunks flank the vertebral column, one on each side. They look like glistening strands of white beads (Marieb 1992). The fibres arising from the thoracolumbar region normally innervate 23 ganglia running from neck to pelvis:

- three cervical;
- 11 thoracic;
- four lumbar;
- four sacral;
- one coccygeal.

A preganglionic fibre reaching a paravertebral ganglion may:

- synapse with a postganglionic neurone in the same ganglion;
- ascend or descend within the sympathetic chain to synapse in another ganglion.

Fibres from T5 to L2 pass through the ganglion and emerge without synapsing.

These latter fibres help form the **splanchnic nerves** – thoracic, lumbar and sacral – which contribute to a number of plexi such as the abdominal aortic plexus, the coeliac plexus, the superior and inferior mesenteric plexi and the hypogastric plexi. Postganglionic fibres fan out from these plexi to their target organs. The lumbar and sacral nerves send most of their fibres to the inferior mesenteric and hypogastric ganglia from where postganglionic fibres supply the distal half of the large intestine, the urinary bladder, the ureters and reproductive organs such as the uterus.

Postganglionic fibres

From the synapse, postganglionic axons join the spinal nerves by non-myelinated branches called **grey rami communicantes**. They are then distributed to the sweat glands and smooth muscle of the hair roots and blood vessels.

Some postganglionic fibres travelling in the thoracic splanchnic nerves synapse with the adrenal medullary cells and are stimulated to produce adrenaline (**epinephrine**) and noradrenaline (**norepinephrine**) into the blood.

Visceral sensory neurones

Although the ANS is considered to be a motor system there are sensory neurones, mainly visceral pain afferents, in autonomic nerves. These travel along the same pathways as somatic pain fibres. Pain perception is referred to the somatic area of the specific dermatome. For example, the pain of a heart attack is felt in the chest and along the medial aspect of the left arm.

Table 27.1 *Segmental sympathetic supply to the organs*

Organ	*Spinal cord segment*
Head and neck + heart	T1 – T5
Bronchi and lungs	T2 – T4
Upper limb	T2 – T5
Oesophagus	T5 – T6
Stomach, spleen and pancreas	T6 – T10
Liver	T7 – T9
Small intestine	T9 – T10
Kidney and reproductive organs	T10 – L1
Lower limb	T10 – L2
Large intestine, bladder and ureter	T11 – L2

Physiology

Sherwood (1988) wrote that 'an autonomic nerve pathway consists of a two-neuron chain, with the terminal neurotransmitter differing between the sympathetic and parasympathetic nerves'. The major neurotransmitters of the ANS are acetylcholine (ACh) and noradrenaline (NA). ACh is released by all preganglionic axons and by the postganglionic axons of the parasympathetic system. ACh-releasing fibres are called **cholinergic** fibres. Most sympathetic postganglionic fibres release NA and are called **adrenergic** fibres. The exceptions to the above rule are sympathetic postganglionic fibres innervating sweat glands, some skeletal muscle blood vessels and the external genitalia, which release ACh. ACh and NA do not consistently produce excitation or inhibition on their target tissues. The response of visceral effectors depends on the type of receptor to which the NTs attach. There are at least two receptors for both NTs.

Cholinergic receptors

The two types of ACh-binding receptors are named for the drugs which bind to them and mimic ACh's effects. They are nicotinic receptors, to which nicotine binds, and muscarinic receptors (muscarine is a mushroom poison).

Nicotinic receptors are found on:

- motor endplates of skeletal muscle cells (somatic targets);
- all postganglionic neurones, both sympathetic and parasympathetic;
- the hormone-producing cells of the adrenal medulla.

The effect of ACh binding to nicotinic receptors is always excitatory.

Muscarinic receptors are found on all cells stimulated by postganglionic cholinergic fibres targeted by the parasympathetic system and a few sympathetic targets such as the sweat glands and some blood vessels of skeletal muscles. The effect of ACh binding to muscarinic receptors may be excitatory or inhibitory, depending on the target organ.

Adrenergic receptors

There are two major classes of adrenergic receptors: α and β. In general, NA binding to α receptors is excitatory whilst binding to β receptors is inhibitory. There are notable and medically important exceptions. Binding of NA to β receptors of cardiac muscle induces vigorous activity in the heart. This is due to both α and β receptors having subclasses (α_1 and α_2, β_1 and β_2). A detailed overview of these receptor subclasses is found in Marieb (1992).

Interactions of the autonomic divisions

Most visceral organs receive innervation from both sympathetic and parasympathetic fibres. They are said to receive **dual innervation**. If, as normal, both divisions are partially active a dynamic antagonism is present that allows precise control of visceral activity. Antagon-istic effects are more easily seen on the activity of the heart, respiration and gastrointestinal organs, as discussed, i.e. the 'fight or flight' versus the 'rest and digest' modes.

Sympathetic and parasympathetic tone

The sympathetic division is the major actor in controlling blood pressure, even at rest. The vascular system is innervated by sympathetic fibres. The partial constriction of blood vessels to maintain sympathetic or vasomotor tone is under the control of the sympathetic division. If blood flow needs increasing sympathetic impulses increase, vessels constrict and blood pressure rises. If blood pressure needs decreasing impulses decrease, smooth muscle relaxes and the vessels dilate.

The heart, however, along with the gastrointestinal tract and urinary tract, is dominated by parasympathetic effects. The smooth muscles of these organs exhibit parasympathetic tone. The sympathetic division overrides this parasympathetic tone in times of stress.

Cooperative efforts

This is best seen during sexual intercourse. The parasympathetic division causes dilatation of the blood vessels of the external genitalia and results in erection of the penis and clitoris. Sympathetic stimulation then results in the rhythmic contractions that result in ejaculation in men and reflex rhythmic contractions of the pelvic floor in women.

Effects unique to the sympathetic division

Some physiological functions are not under parasympathetic influences and are controlled totally by the sympathetic division. These include:

- control of the adrenal medulla;
- the sweat glands;
- the erector pili muscles;
- the production of renin by the kidney;
- thermoregulatory response to heat;
- mobilisation of glucose and fats to be used as fuel.

Control of autonomic functioning

Several levels in the CNS contribute to the regulation of the ANS. These include controls in the spinal cord, brainstem, hypothalamus and cerebral cortex.

Brainstem controls

The most direct influence seems to be via the reticular formation. Most sensory impulses that cause the autonomic reflexes arrive in the brainstem via afferents from the vagus nerve. Centres in the medulla that are influenced include the cardiac, vasomotor, respiratory and those controlling gastrointestinal activities. Control of micturition and defaecation are reflexes that can be overcome by conscious control.

Hypothalamic controls

The hypothalamus is the main integration centre for the ANS. Medial and anterior hypothalamic regions appear to direct parasympathetic activities whilst the posterior and lateral areas direct sympathetic functions. The route of influence is:

Hypothalamus → Reticular formation → Preganglionic ANS motor neurones

The hypothalamus is central to homeostasis. It coordinates heart activity, blood pressure, body temperature, water balance, endocrine activity, emotional states such as rage or pleasure and biological drives such as hunger and thirst. It can influence and be influenced by the higher cortical centres.

Cortical controls

There is growing knowledge and interest in the effect of the higher brain centres on regulation of the autonomic system. This is an expanding research area and includes such behaviours as meditation, biofeedback, neuropsychoimmunity and psychosomatic illness. The effect of stress on the immune system will be discussed in Chapter 29.

MATERNAL ADAPTATIONS TO PREGNANCY

Changes in the functioning of the peripheral and autonomic nervous systems are related to changes in the endocrine system during pregnancy and the relevant neurohormonal reflexes such as that involved in lactation will be discussed in their relevant chapters. The role of the sympathetic nervous system in the stress response is an important consideration for uterine muscle activity and cervical dilatation in labour. Disorders of the peripheral nervous system are mentioned in Chapter 34.

Summary of main points

- The peripheral nervous system detects changes in the external or internal environment of the body, codes it into nerve impulses by sensory receptors and passes the information back to the central nervous system so that appropriate action can be instituted. It includes all the neural structures outside the brain and spinal cord.
- The dorsal columns are large bundles of first-order nerve fibres consisting of ascending fibres of the dorsal root. The fibres immediately enter the dorsal columns without synapsing. They are usually large A fibres arranged somatotopically.
- The fibres cross the midline to synapse with cell bodies of second-order neurones in brainstem nuclei at the level of the medulla which project second-order fibres to the thalamus. This crossing over is the reason why one side of the brain controls the opposite or contralateral side of the body. Cells in the sensory relay nucleus of

the thalamus are third-order neurones and project their fibres to the sensory area of the cerebral cortex.

- The dorsal root fibres of the spinothalamic tract tend to be the smaller A-δ or unmyelinated C fibres with slow conduction velocity. They ascend or descend a few segments before crossing over the midline to ascend in the spinothalamic tract and terminate on third-order neurones in the thalamus. The fibres of these third-order neurones synapse on the cells of the sensory cortex.
- The descending tracts carry efferent messages from the brain down the spinal cord and are divided into pyramidal or corticospinal tracts and the extrapyramidal fibres. The pyramidal cells of the motor cortex are referred to as the upper motor neurones. The anterior horn neurones, whose axons leave the cord to innervate the skeletal muscles, are called the lower motor neurones.
- Sensory receptors are mostly adapted nerve fibre endings which respond to changes in the environment. Sensory afferent nerves arising from the body are grouped together as the somatosensory system and include sensation from the skin, muscles, joints or viscera.
- Some involuntary reflex activity is protective, such as the rapid removal of a body part from a noxious stimulus like heat. Other reflexes occur without any awareness of change. Reflexes occur over specific neural paths called reflex arcs and may be somatic or autonomic. Many spinal reflexes occur with little or no brain input.
- The autonomic nervous system or ANS is responsible for maintaining the stability of the body's internal environment. Motor neurones of the ANS innervate smooth muscle, cardiac muscle and glands, making adjustments to alter function in response to messages from the viscera sent to the central nervous system.
- The ANS is divided into two arms: the sympathetic system, which prepares the body for emergency action, and the parasympathetic system, which has a calming effect and allows general body maintenance to occur and also the conservation of energy. There is usually a dynamic interaction between the two divisions of the ANS aimed at maximising homeostasis.
- The parasympathetic division is active when the systems are unstressed and can be called the 'resting and digesting' system, concerned with digestion and elimination of waste. The sympathetic division is sometimes referred to as the 'fight or flight' system and is activated in threatening situations.
- Parasympathetic fibres emerge from the brain (cranial outflow) and sacral spinal cord (craniosacral division) whilst the sympathetic fibres originate from the thoracolumbar region of the spinal cord (sacral outflow).
- The sympathetic division is complex, partly because it innervates more organs. Sympathetic activity tends to inhibit the activity of visceral organs. Sympathetic fibres innervate some body wall structures such as sweat glands and smooth muscle erector pili. All arteries and veins are innervated by sympathetic fibres.
- The lumbar and sacral nerves send most of their fibres to the inferior mesenteric and hypogastric ganglia from where postganglionic fibres supply the distal half of the large intestine, the urinary bladder, the ureters and reproductive organs such as the uterus. Some postganglionic fibres travelling in the thoracic splanchnic nerves synapse with the adrenal medullary cells and are stimulated to produce adrenaline and noradrenaline into the blood.
- Although the ANS is considered to be a motor system there are sensory neurones, mainly visceral pain afferents, in autonomic nerves. These travel along the same pathways as somatic pain fibres.
- The neurotransmitters of the ANS are acetylcholine and noradrenaline. ACh is released by all preganglionic axons and by the postganglionic axons of the parasympathetic system. ACh-releasing fibres are called cholinergic fibres. Most sympathetic postganglionic fibres are adrenergic fibres releasing NA. Exceptions are sympathetic postganglionic fibres innervating sweat glands, some skeletal muscle blood vessels and the external genitalia, which release ACh.
- Most visceral organs receive innervation from both sympathetic and parasympathetic fibres. If both divisions are partially active, a dynamic antagonism is present that allows precise control of visceral activity.
- The sympathetic division is the major actor in controlling blood pressure, even at rest. The vascular system is innervated by sympathetic fibres. The partial constriction of blood vessels to maintain sympathetic or vasomotor tone is under the control of the sympathetic division. The heart, the gastrointestinal tract and urinary tract are dominated by parasympathetic effects.
- Some physiological functions are not under parasympathetic influences and are controlled totally by the sympathetic division. Several levels in the CNS contribute to the regulation of the ANS. These include controls in the spinal cord, brainstem, hypothalamus and cerebral cortex.

References

Allan D, Nie V, Hunter M. 1996 Control and co-ordination. In Hinchliff SM, Montague SE, Watson R (eds) Physiology for Nursing Practice, 2nd edn. Baillière Tindall, London.

Carlsson NR. 1991 Physiology of Behaviour, 4th edn. Allyn and Bacon, London.

Fitzgerald MJT. 1992 Neuroanatomy, Basic and Clinical, 2nd edn. Baillière Tindall, London.

Hinchliff SM, Montague SE. 1990 Physiology for Nursing Practice. Baillière Tindall, London.

Marieb EN. 1992 Human Anatomy and Physiology, 2nd edn. Benjamin/Cummings Publishing, California

Sherwood L. 1988 Human Physiology: From Cells to Systems. West Publishing, Maine

Recommended reading

Clarke M. 1996 The autonomic nervous system. In Hinchliff SM, Montague SE, Watson R. 1996 Physiology for Nursing Practice, 2nd edn. Baillière Tindall, London.

Fitzgerald MJT. 1992 Neuroanatomy, Basic and Clinical, 2nd edn. Baillière Tindall, London.

Chapter 28 The endocrine system

In this chapter

INTRODUCTION

The nervous system can be thought of as the rapid controller of the body, able to respond to immediate needs brought about by interaction with the environment. In contrast, the endocrine system provides a much slower control by modifying cell function and body metabolism. The two systems are closely related with many of the endocrine glands originating from the same embryonic layer as the nervous system. In particular, the **hypothalamus** provides a major link between the nervous and endocrine systems.

The endocrine system uses hormones produced by **ductless glands** that empty their products directly into the bloodstream or lymphatic circulation. The released hormones are carried round the bloodstream until they reach a target tissue. The hormones may also act locally in the gland, either on adjacent cells or on the cell of origin. Glands are small organs and are widely scattered around the body. This chapter covers the hormone-producing endocrine glands. Exocrine glands pass their products, which are not classified as hormones, into a body cavity or onto the surface of the skin. Typically, the hormone-secreting cells in a gland are arranged in cords and branching networks to maximise the contact between the cells and the capillaries that receive the secretions (Marieb 1992).

For continuity, endocrine system adaptations to pregnancy will be discussed directly after the anatomy and physiology of each gland.

OVERVIEW OF THE ENDOCRINE SYSTEM

The hypothalamus

The hypothalamus is the major controller of endocrine gland function and, as was seen in the previous two chapters, has wider links with other parts of the nervous system. The hypothalamus can therefore be considered as a **neuroendocrine organ**. Releasing and inhibiting hormones produced by the hypothalamus influence the production of hormones by the anterior pituitary gland (see below).

The endocrine glands

The endocrine glands include the pituitary, thyroid, parathyroid, adrenal, pineal, and thymus glands. These organs will be discussed below. Other organs contain hormone-producing tissue as part of their structure, including the pancreas and the ovaries and testes. The structure and function of the pancreas has been discussed in Chapter 22 and the ovary and testes are discussed in Chapters 3 and 4 respectively. The placenta, which produces hormones that affect the maternal body, is covered in Chapter 11.

The functions of the endocrine glands include reproduction, growth and development, mobilisation of body defences against stress, maintenance of fluid and electrolyte balance, nutrient content in the blood, regulation of cellular metabolism and energy balance. Tissue or organ responses to the hormones may take only a few seconds or may take days and are more prolonged than changes induced by the nervous system.

HORMONES

Marieb (1992) defines hormones as 'chemical substances, secreted by cells into the extracellular fluids, that regulate the metabolic function of other cells in the body'. They can be classified into two groups of molecules: the main group of amino acid-based molecules and a smaller group of steroid hormones. The amino acid-based hormones vary in their complexity from simple derivatives such as thyroxine to more complex peptides to the very complex macromolecules. All the steroid hormones are synthesised from cholesterol and include the gonadal hormones and the adrenocortical hormones.

Eicosanoids

It is possible to talk of a third type of molecule that may influence cell activity locally. These are the eicosanoids which are formed from the essential fatty acid arachidonic acid. This group of compounds includes the prostaglandins, biologically active lipids found in nearly all cell membranes. These molecules are not hormones and do not appear to circulate in the blood to influence distant tissues but act locally on adjacent cells (Boore 1996). Prostaglandins will be discussed in Chapter 36.

Target cells

All hormones are secreted into the capillaries passing through the endocrine gland and circulate to nearly all tissues but a particular hormone can only influence cells with specific protein receptors in their plasma membranes. Some hormones can only influence a few tissues; for example, adrenocorticotrophic hormone (ACTH) can only affect certain cells of the adrenal cortex, whilst others such as thyroxine are essential for the metabolism of all cells.

The half-life of a hormone is the time taken for half of it to be removed from the plasma (Boore 1996). The catecholamines and insulin are transported in the plasma in the free state and have very short half-lives. Hormones such as thyroxine and the corticosteroids are transported in the blood bound to specific carrier proteins and have a much longer half-life.

Hormone–receptor binding is a first step to target cell interaction. The extent of cellular activity then depends on:

- blood levels of the hormone;
- the relative numbers of receptors on the target cells;
- the affinity of the receptor for the hormone.

Target cells may make more receptors in response to high levels of hormone. This is called **upregulation**. Other cells may be desensitised to high levels of hormones so that they respond less vigorously, possibly by loss of receptors, a function called **down-regulation**. Hormones may also influence receptors responsive to other hormones. For example, progesterone causes a loss of oestrogen receptors, acting as an oestrogen **antagonist**, but oestrogen causes an increase in the number of progesterone receptors so that the cells have an enhanced ability to respond to progesterone.

Mechanisms of hormone action

The effects of hormones are brought about by either increasing or decreasing cell activity. A hormone stimulus usually produces one or more of the following changes (Marieb 1992):

- changes in cell membrane permeability and/or electrical potential;
- protein or regulatory molecule (e.g. enzymes) synthesis;
- enzyme activation or deactivation;
- induction of secretory activity;
- stimulation of mitotic cell division.

The effects of hormone action may be brought about by the formation of intracellular second messengers or direct DNA activation by the hormone.

Second and third messengers

Very few of the amino acid-based hormones can penetrate cell membranes and have to exert their influence through intracellular second messengers. These are generated in response to hormone–receptor binding. **Cyclic AMP** is the second messenger that has been studied most. When a hormone or first messenger binds to a receptor which is coupled with the membrane-bound enzyme **adenylate cyclase**, it uses an intermediary called a **G protein** to pass the signal to the adenylate cyclase. The enzyme is activated and catalyses the conversion of ATP to cyclic AMP.

Cyclic AMP then initiates a cascade of chemical reactions set off by activation of enzymes called **protein kinases**, which results in the correct cellular response. Cyclic AMP is rapidly degraded by the enzyme **phosphodiesterase** so that its action only persists briefly and cellular activity can be ended as necessary.

Other amino acid-based hormones involve a third messenger, calcium, in their pathway. Calcium acts either directly by altering the activity of specific enzymes or indirectly by binding to an intracellular protein called **calmodulin**. Eicosanoids may also involve cyclic AMP in their function.

Direct gene activation

The lipid-soluble steroid hormones and the small amino acid hormone thyroxine can diffuse easily into their target cells. They bind directly to a receptor probably located in the cell nucleus. The activated hormone–receptor complex interacts with nuclear chromatin and the hormone binds to a DNA-associated receptor protein. This interaction switches on DNA transcription of RNA and the specific protein molecule is produced. The protein products trigger the metabolic activity that the hormone induces.

Control of hormone release

The synthesis and release of hormones depend on a system of negative feedback or feedback inhibition. The hormone secretion is triggered by an internal or external stimulus. Hormone levels in the blood rise until they reach the required level and then further hormone release is inhibited. This acts to maintain blood levels within a narrow range. The stimuli that induce hormone release may be hormonal, humoral or neural.

Hormonal stimuli

The anterior pituitary gland produces multiple hormones whose release is regulated by releasing and inhibiting hormones produced by the hypothalamus. Some of these anterior pituitary hormones in turn induce other glands to secrete their hormones. The rise in blood levels of the hormones produced by the final target glands inhibits the release of anterior pituitary hormones.

Humoral stimuli

Changing blood levels of ions and nutrients may affect hormone release. For example, the production of parathyroid hormone (PTH) by the parathyroid gland is prompted by decreasing blood calcium levels. Other such hormones are **calcitonin**, produced by the thyroid gland, **insulin**, produced by the pancreatic islet cells, and **aldosterone** from the adrenal cortex.

Neural stimuli

In a few cases hormones are released in response to neural stimuli. This type of release is seen in the sympathetic nervous system stimulation of the release of catecholamines adrenaline and noradrenaline in response to stress.

THE PITUITARY GLAND

The pituitary gland (or **hypophysis**) is a small ovoid gland weighing about 500 mg. It is situated in the **sella turcica** (hypophyseal fossa) of the sphenoid bone. It has a stalk called the **infundibulum** which passes through an opening in the dura mater to connect the pituitary gland to the hypothalamus. The pituitary gland has two major lobes: the posterior lobe or **neurohypophysis** is made of nerve fibres and neuroglia and is derived from a downward growth of the hypothalamus. It does not make its own hormones but acts as a storage unit, releasing hypothalamic hormones. The anterior lobe or **adenohypophysis** is composed of glandular tissue and manufactures and releases its own hormones.

The gland has an extremely rich blood supply derived from the internal carotid artery via superior and inferior hypophyseal branches. Venous drainage is by short vessels which emerge from the gland and drain into the dural venous sinuses. The need for a rich blood supply makes the gland vulnerable to loss of blood, such as occurs in haemorrhage. This is particularly so in pregnancy, as will be discussed later.

The pituitary-hypothalamic axis

Running through the infundibulum is a nerve bundle called the **hypothalamic-hypophyseal tract** (Fig. 28.1). The tract neurones

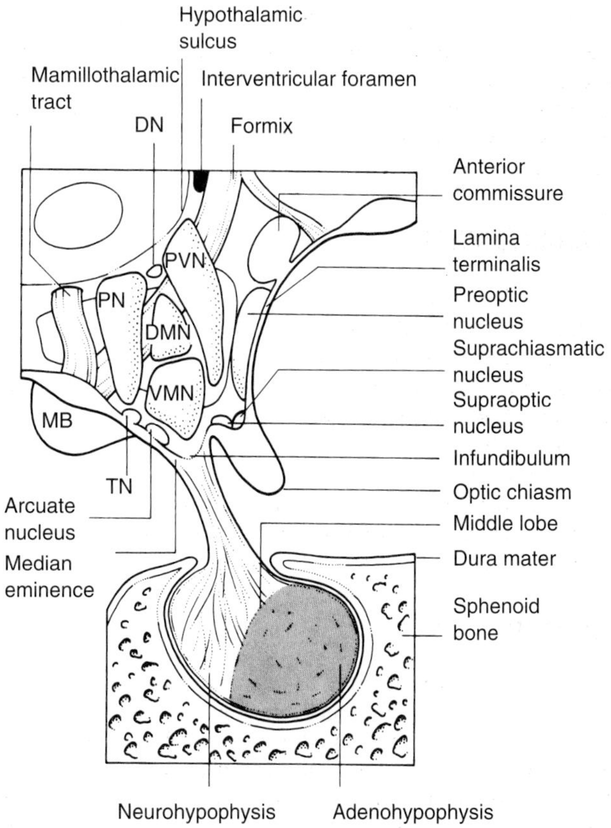

Figure 28.1 *Hypothalamic nuclei and hypophysis, viewed from the right side. DN, dorsal nucleus; DMN, dorsomedial nucleus; MB, mamillary body; PN, posterior nucleus; PVN, periventricular nucleus; TN, tuberomamillary nucleus; VMN, ventromedial nucleus (from Fitzgerald MJT, 1996, with permission).*

are situated in two nuclei in the hypothalamus and secrete two neurohormones. These are **oxytocin**, made by the paraventricular nuclear neurones, and **antidiuretic hormone** secreted by the supraoptic nuclear neurones. These hormones are transported along the axons to their terminals in the posterior lobe. In contrast, there is no direct neural connection between the anterior lobe of the pituitary gland and the hypothalamus. There is a vascular connection, the hypophyseal portal system, which carries the releasing and inhibiting hormones secreted by the ventral hypothalamus to the anterior pituitary gland. All these regulatory hypothalamic hormones are amino acid derivatives.

Anterior pituitary hormones

The anterior lobe of the pituitary gland has been called the master endocrine gland because many of its hormones regulate the hormone production of other glands. However, as we have seen, it in turn is controlled by the hypothalamus. There are six anterior pituitary hormones. Four of them regulate the hormonal functioning of other glands:

- thyroid-stimulating hormone (TSH);
- adrenocorticotrophic hormone (ACTH);
- follicle-stimulating hormone (FSH);
- luteinising hormone (LH).

The other two hormones have their influences on non-endocrine targets:

- growth hormone (GH);
- prolactin (PRL).

These hormones all utilise the second messenger system.

In addition to the above six hormones, there is a very large molecule called **proopiomelanocortin** (POMC) found in the anterior pituitary. POMC is a **prohormone**, a precursor molecule that is split into hormones by the action of enzymes. It is the source of ACTH, two natural opiates (an enkephalin and β-endorphin) and melanocyte-stimulating hormone (MSH). Growth hormone, prolactin and the posterior pituitary hormones will be discussed below whilst the trophic hormones will be considered with the glands they influence.

Growth hormone

Growth hormone (GH) stimulates most body cells to grow in size and divide. However, its major targets are the bones and skeletal muscles. GH is an anabolic hormone which stimulates protein synthesis. It facilitates the use of fats for fuel and conserves glucose. Although the second messenger system influencing the action of GH has not yet been fully identified, GH is known to be mediated indirectly by somatomedins which are growth-promoting proteins produced by the liver. It is possible that the kidneys and muscles also produce somatomedins.

Regulation of GH secretion

Two hypothalamic hormones with antagonistic effects regulate the production of GH. These are GH-releasing hormone (GHRH) and GH-inhibiting hormone (GHIH), which is also called **somatostatin**. Somatostatin has other functions and has far-reaching effects. It blocks the release of several of the anterior pituitary hormones and inhibits release of nearly all the gastrointestinal and pancreatic secretions.

GH has a diurnal cycle with the highest levels occurring during evening sleep. The total amount secreted daily declines with age. Hypersecretion of GH in childhood results in **gigantism** and the person may reach a height of 2.4 m (8 feet). After the closure of the epiphyseal plates and cessation of longitudinal bone growth, enlargement of bony areas of the hands, feet and face occurs, a condition known as **acromegaly**. Hyposecretion of GH in children leads to **pituitary dwarfism**. Such people have normal body proportions but a maximum height of 1.2 m (4 feet).

Prolactin

Prolactin (PRL) is a protein hormone similar to GH. Its only known effect in humans is the stimulation of milk production by the breasts (**lactation**). PRL is controlled by hypothalamic production of PRL-releasing hormone (PRH) and PRL-inhibiting hormone (PIH). PIH has been identified as the neurotransmitter dopamine (DA), which predominates in men and non-lactating women. PRL levels are influenced by oestrogen.

Low oestrogen stimulates PRH release and prolactin is secreted. The release of PRL just before a menstrual period accounts for premenstrual breast swelling and tenderness but the stimulation is so brief that no milk is produced. The role of PRL in lactation will be discussed fully in Chapter 54. Hypersecretion of prolactin will cause inappropriate lactation, called **galactorrhoea**, which is seen in both sexes, mostly due to a tumour of the anterior pituitary gland. Women will have amenorrhoea and men become **impotent**.

Posterior pituitary hormones

Oxytocin

Oxytocin is a strong stimulator of uterine action. Its synthesis and release are only important in childbirth and in nursing women and its role will be discussed in detail in the appropriate chapters on labour and on lactation.

Antidiuretic hormone (ADH)

ADH is a chemical substance that inhibits or prevents urine formation. It targets the renal tubules which respond to the stimulus by reabsorbing more water. Less urine is produced and a rise in blood volume occurs. Neurones in the hypothalamus called **osmoreceptors** monitor the solute concentration in blood and if too much solute is detected, as in heavy perspiration or inadequate fluid intake, the osmoreceptors send excitatory messages to the ADH-secreting neurones in the hypothalamus.

ADH release is also stimulated by pain, low blood pressure and drugs such as nicotine, morphine and barbiturates. In trauma conditions, such as heavy blood loss, enormous amounts of ADH are released. This high level has a pressor effect on blood vessels, causing vasoconstriction which results in a rise in systemic blood pressure. It is for that reason that ADH is sometimes referred to as **vasopressin**.

ADH inhibition is caused by ingestion of alcohol so that a diuresis occurs. This accounts for the thirst and dry mouth the following morning! Drinking large amounts of water will also suppress ADH release. Diuretic drugs are used in some conditions such as congestive cardiac failure to antagonise ADH and bring about large losses of fluid in urine. A rare disorder resulting in inadequate release of ADH is **diabetes insipidus**. The most common cause is trauma to the hypothalamus. This results in excessive urination and a balancing thirst but can be life threatening if the individual cannot regulate their fluid intake, such as in coma.

Changes in the hypothalamus and pituitary during pregnancy

Research indicates that a functioning pituitary gland is not essential for the maintenance of pregnancy once conception has occurred; for example, women whose pituitary gland was removed after 12 weeks of pregnancy have delivered healthy babies (Jacobs 1991). However, there are changes in both structure and function of the gland during a normal pregnancy. These changes underlie the process of lactation.

Structure

Autopsies have shown that the normal pituitary gland in non-pregnant women is about 20% heavier than in men. During pregnancy, its weight increases by 30% in first pregnancies and 50% in subsequent pregnancies, almost entirely due to changes in the anterior lobe. This is caused by an increase in the number of the elongated prolactin-secreting cells, known as **lactotrophs**. At the same time, the number of GH-producing cells falls. The number of cells is paralleled by blood levels of the two hormones.

During pregnancy the hormones produced by the feto-placental unit have a great influence on the pituitary gland. The pattern of hormone production by the anterior pituitary changes again in the puerperium to accommodate the need to lactate. This role will be discussed in detail in Chapter 54.

Changes in the relative production of anterior pituitary hormones

The secretion of the gonadotrophins follicle-stimulating hormone and luteinising hormone is inhibited during pregnancy, mediated by the placental hormones. This may be due to the presence of human chorionic gonadotrophin. However, the presence of hyperprolactinaemia of pregnancy also contributes to the fall in gonadotrophic secretion. The secretion of growth hormone is also inhibited in pregnancy. The number of GH-producing cells is reduced, probably due to the presence of human placental lactogen. Growth hormone secretion returns to normal within a few weeks of delivery.

ACTH plasma concentrations rise progressively during pregnancy. This is associated with a doubling of plasma cortisol. Normally a rise in plasma cortisol would suppress ACTH production but the normal feedback mechanism appears to be lost during pregnancy. The placenta may contribute to the increase in plasma ACTH. The myometrium and decidua convert cortisone to cortisol, resulting in a local cortisol concentration of nine times normal. This may contribute to the immunological protection of the fetus.

Thyrotrophin secretion is difficult to measure but the hormone may be reduced in the first trimester, returning to normal for the remainder of pregnancy.

Sheehan's syndrome

The enlargement of the anterior pituitary gland is presumed to need an increased oxygen supply carried to it by an augmented circulation. Sheehan & Stanfield (1961) found that this unique blood supply to the pituitary gland makes it vulnerable to a reduction in arterial blood supply due to vasospasm of the superior hypophyseal artery, leading to necrosis of the gland and swelling. As the increase in pituitary size already reduces the room in the pituitary fossa, swelling would further constrict the blood supply. Both the need for extra oxygen and extra sensitivity of the hypophyseal artery to vasospasm may explain why the pituitary gland is more readily damaged in pregnancy than in the non-pregnant population (Jacobs 1991).

Sheehan's syndrome or anterior pituitary necrosis is a rare condition associated with severe and prolonged obstetric shock (Jacobs 1991, Lindsay 1997, Sleep 1996). The usual cause is severe haemorrhage during labour, resulting in postpartum hypopituitarism. The symptoms and signs are caused by loss of the anterior pituitary hormones. The earliest sign is failure to lactate due to prolactin deficiency, followed by amenorrhoea due to deficiency of the gonadotrophic hormones. The activity of the thyroid and adrenal glands gradually diminishes and the woman becomes lethargic and feels cold. Her hair and skin become coarser and she suffers loss of libido. The genitalia and breasts atrophy. Adequate and prompt treatment of obstetric shock will prevent the syndrome developing (Sleep 1996). If the diagnosis is not made, the woman may die. Treatment is by replacement of affected hormones.

Posterior pituitary hormone secretion

Oxytocin is released by the pituitary gland during the final stages of labour due to the stretching of the lower genital tract, a phenomenon called **Ferguson's reflex**. It is also secreted during the puerperium as a response to suckling (Jacobs 1991). These two aspects of oxytocin production are discussed in detail in the relevant chapters.

ADH production and its effect on the renal tubules are similar in pregnant and non-pregnant women. However, the osmoreceptors are reset to accommodate the extra blood volume associated with pregnancy (Blackburn & Loper 1992).

THE THYROID GLAND

The thyroid gland lies in the neck in front of the trachea and just below the larynx. It has two lateral lobes joined by a medial isthmus and is shaped rather like a butterfly. It is the largest endocrine gland in the body and is very well supplied with blood via the superior and inferior thyroid arteries. The thyroid gland consists of hollow spherical structures called **follicles**. Each follicle is lined by cuboidal epithelial cells, the follicle cells, which produce a glycoprotein called **thyroglobulin**.

The lumen of a follicle stores an amber-coloured sticky material which consists of thyroglobulin molecules attached to iodine. This material gives rise to two thyroid hormones – **thyroxine** or T_4 and **triiodothyronine** or T_3. Another group of cells called the parafollicular cells are situated in the follicular epithelium. These produce the hormone **calcitonin** which is discussed in Chapter 24.

Thyroid hormones

Thyroxine is the major hormone and the follicle cells secrete more of it than triiodothyronine. The structure of the two hormones is very similar. Each is made from two tyrosine molecules linked together. The difference is that thyroxine binds four iodine atoms, which is why it is called T_4, and triiodothyronine binds three iodine atoms, hence T_3. Most of the T_3 is formed in the target tissues by enzymatic removal of an iodine group from T_4, which may be a prohormone. Triiodothyronine appears to be the active form. Thyroid hormone affects nearly every cell in the body. The exceptions are the tissues of the brain, spleen, testes, uterus and the thyroid gland.

Functions

1 Thyroid hormones stimulate enzymes concerned with the oxidation of glucose. They increase basal metabolic rate and therefore oxygen consumption and body heat production. This production of heat is known as the hormone's **calorigenic effect**.
2 Thyroid hormones also stimulate an increase in the number of adrenergic receptors in blood vessels and therefore have an important role in maintaining blood pressure.
3 Thyroid hormones regulate tissue growth and development, essential for normal skeletal and nervous system development.

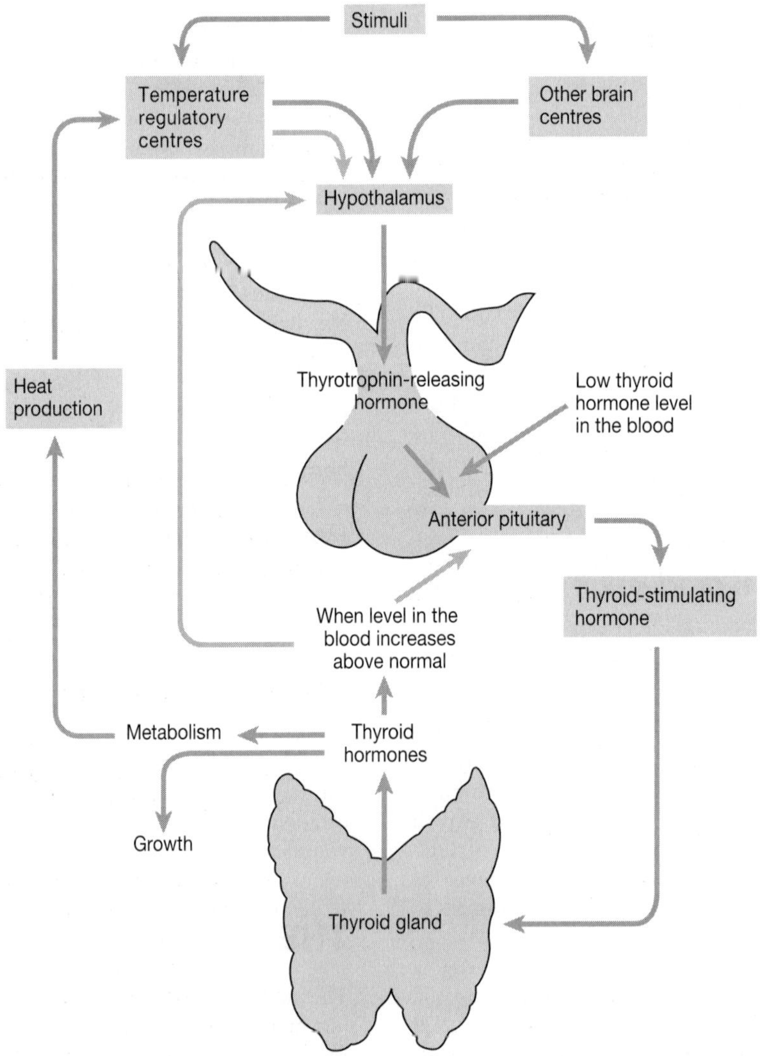

Figure 28.2 *Regulation of thyroid hormone secretion; yellow arrow indicate inhibition (from Hinchliff SM, Montague SE, Watson R, 1996, with permission).*

Secretion

The fetus begins to secrete thyroid hormones from about the 12th week of gestation. The iodine required for the manufacture of the thyroid hormones is obtained from the diet and about 1.2 mmol are required daily. The cells of the thyroid gland have a great affinity for iodine and remove it from the bloodstream. The iodine is then concentrated in the gland in combination with the thyroglobulin. If two iodine atoms are attached to a tyrosine molecule diiodotyrosine (DIT) is produced. The attachment of one iodine to a tyrosine produces monoiodotyrosine (MIT).

A coupling of DIT + DIT within the thyroglobulin molecule forms T_4 while coupling of a DIT + MIT forms T_3. Enzymes split the thyroid hormones off from the thyroglobulin molecule. The hormones are secreted into adjacent blood capillaries to circulate around the body bound to plasma proteins, especially thyroxine-binding globulin. Less than 1% of the hormones remain free in the blood and it is this free hormone that is available for stimulation of the tissues. Both T_3 and T_4 bind to tissues but T_3 is 10 times more active. Thyroid hormones are broken down in the tissues and some of the freed iodine is returned to the thyroid gland to be reused whilst some is excreted from the body.

Regulation of thyroid secretion

Regulation of thyroid hormone secretion is by a negative feedback loop from T_3 so that blood levels are maintained within a narrow limit. Thyrotrophin-releasing hormone (TRH) from the hypothalamus influences the secretion of thyroid-stimulating hormone (TSH) from the anterior pituitary gland (Fig. 28.2). TSH stimulates the secretion of the thyroid hormones by increasing the production of cyclic AMP in the thyroid cells, enhancing the cellular activity.

Changes in the thyroid gland during pregnancy

Thyroid function remains normal during pregnancy although some women exhibit some of the signs associated with an overactive thyroid gland including thyroid hyperplasia or goitre. Blackburn & Loper (1992) refer to this as **euthyroid hyperthyroxinaemia**. During pregnancy, a balance is achieved by alterations in the metabolism of iodine. Renal iodide clearance doubles, plasma inorganic iodide falls and thyroid clearance of iodine trebles. The absolute uptake of iodine remains within normal limits (Ramsay 1991).

There are significant alterations in plasma concentrations of the thyroid hormones and of thyroid-binding globulin (TBG) during pregnancy. It is probable that these changes are influenced mainly by oestrogen and human chorionic gonadotrophin (Blackburn & Loper 1992). Some of the changes which support the alterations in carbohydrate, protein and lipid metabolism found in pregnancy are as follows.

1. Under the influence of oestrogen, the liver synthesises up to 100% more TBG from 12 week gestation.
2. The ability of the TBG to bind thyroxine doubles.
3. T_3 and T_4 peak at about 12 weeks gestation.
4. Increased thyroid-stimulating hormone activity seems to be stimulated by HCG.
5. Basal metabolic rate increases by 25% from about 4 months.

Table 28.1 *Major effects of thyroid hormones on tissues*

System affected	*Physiological effects promoted*
Basal metabolic rate	Oxygen consumption and BMR, enhances effects of catecholamines
Nutrient metabolism	Glucose usage, mobilises fats, essential for protein synthesis, enhances liver secretion of cholesterol.
Nervous system	Normal development of the NS in infants and children, necessary for normal functioning in adults
Cardiovascular system	Normal cardiac functioning
Muscular system	Normal development, tone and function of muscles
Skeletal system	Normal growth and maturation of the skeleton
Gastrointestinal system	Normal GI motility and tone and increases secretion of gastric juices
Reproductive system	Normal female reproduction and lactation
Integumentary system	Normal secretory activity of the skin and also hydration

The above alterations have been linked with nausea and vomiting in early pregnancy. The changes revert to normal in the puerperium but it may take up to 12 weeks for them to be completely reversed.

Disorders of the thyroid gland are considered in Chapter 35.

THE ADRENAL GLANDS

The two adrenal glands each weigh about 4 g and are situated on top of each kidney. They are pyramid shaped and enclosed in a fibrous capsule and a cushion of fat. The name 'suprarenal gland' is sometimes used. The adrenal glands are actually, structurally and functionally, two endocrine glands, each producing its own hormones. The inner medulla is derived from the neural crest as an outgrowth of nervous tissue and is functionally part of the sympathetic nervous system. The outer cortex surrounds the medulla and forms the bulk of each gland and is derived from embryonic mesoderm similar to the ovary and testis.

The adrenal cortex

The steroid hormones, collectively called the **corticosteroids**, are synthesised from cholesterol in a multistep pathway. The cortex consists of large cells full of lipid arranged in three concentric regions.

1. The outer **zona glomerulosa** produces the **mineralocorticoids** which help control the amount of minerals and water in the blood.
2. The middle layer, called the **zona fasciculata**, secretes the **glucocorticoids** which are involved in the control of metabolic processes.
3. The inner-most zone, called the **zona reticularis**, produces glucocorticoids and small amounts of the sex hormones or **gonadocorticoids**.

The steroid hormones act on the nucleus of the cell. They stimulate the formation of messenger RNA (mRNA) leading to the production of enzymes that modify cell function (Boore 1996).

Mineralocorticoids

Mineralocorticoids regulate the amount of electrolytes and water in extracellular fluid. In particular, they affect the sodium and potassium concentrations. **Aldosterone** makes up more than 95% of the total output and is the most potent of the mineralocorticoids. The function of aldosterone is to regulate sodium balance. It targets the distal tubules of the kidneys and stimulates reabsorption of sodium ions from the urine and returns them to the bloodstream. Aldosterone is also involved in sodium reabsorption from perspiration, saliva and gastric juice. Potassium, hydrogen, bicarbonate and chloride ions are coupled to sodium regulation and water follows sodium passively.

Four mechanisms help to regulate its secretion (Fig. 28.3).

1. **The renin – angiotensin mechanism**. Renin is secreted into the circulation by the kidney juxtaglomerular apparatus. Renin acts on angiotensinogen, an inert plasma protein produced by the liver to release angiotensin I. Enzymes convert this to angiotensin II which triggers the release of aldosterone from the adrenal cortex.
2. **Plasma concentrations of sodium and potassium ions**. Rising levels of potassium ions in the blood, low levels of sodium in the blood,
3. **ACTH from the anterior pituitary** normally has little effect on aldosterone production but in severe stress the hypothalamus releases corticotrophin-releasing hormone (CRH) which steps up ACTH production, leading to an increased rate of aldosterone production. This increases blood volume and blood pressure, facilitating the delivery of oxygen and nutrients to the tissues. Decreasing blood volume and blood pressure stimulate aldosterone secretion.
4. **Plasma concentrations of atrial natriuretic factor**, secreted by the heart when the blood pressure rises, modify the effects of the renin-angiotensin system. Its effects are inhibitory and it blocks renin and aldosterone secretion. This will decrease blood pressure by allowing sodium and water to leave the body in urine.

Glucocorticoids

Glucocorticoids, which include cortisol (hydrocortisone), cortisone and corticosterone, have an effect on the metabolism of most body cells. About 75% of cortisol circulates in the blood bound to corticosteroid-binding globulin (CBG), another 15% is loosely bound to albumin and the remaining metabolically

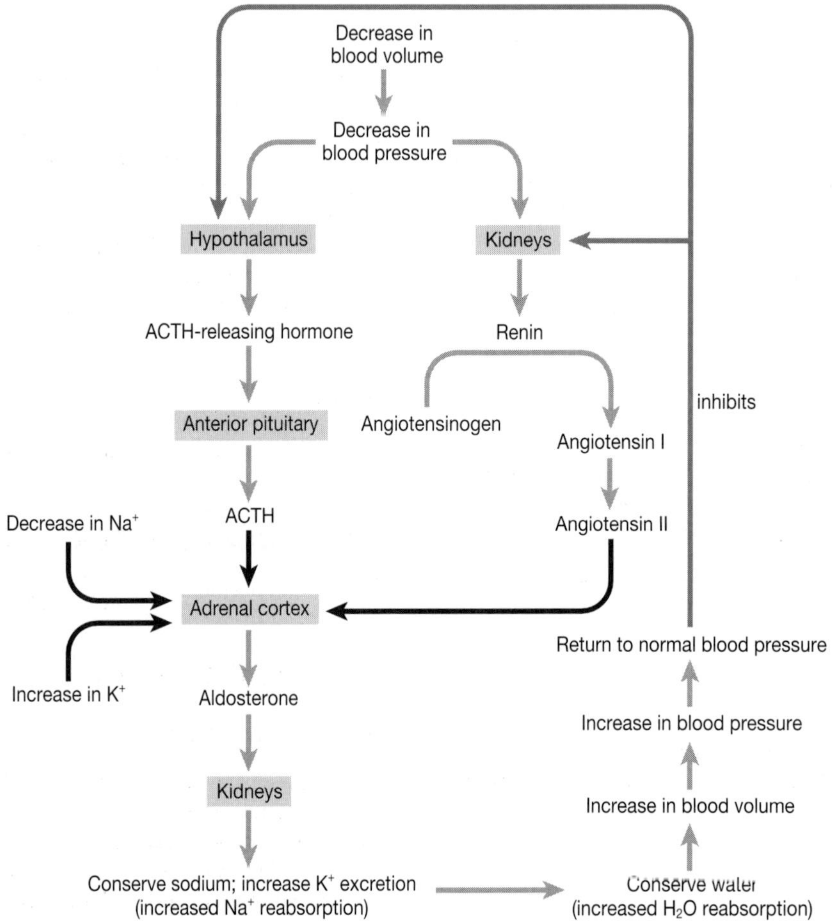

Figure 28.3 *Regulation of aldosterone secretion (from Hinchliff SM, Montague SE, Watson R, 1996, with permission).*

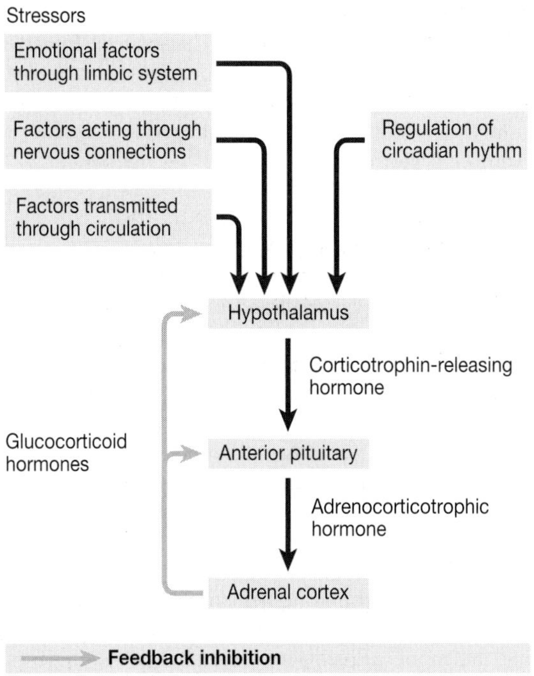

Figure 28.4 *Regulation of glucocorticoid secretion (Sweet B, 1997, with permission).*

active 10% is free. Their role is to convert the intermittent intake of food into a steady level of sugar in the plasma. They also maintain blood level by preventing the shift of water into tissue cells. In severe stress due to haemorrhage, infection, physical trauma or emotional distress, the output of glucocorticoids rises dramatically to help the body through the crisis. Only cortisol is secreted in significant amounts in humans (Marieb 1992).

The control of glucocorticoid secretion is by feedback mechanism (Fig. 28.4). CRH from the hypothalamus causes ACTH release by the anterior pituitary gland. This causes the release of cortisol. The functions of cortisol are:

1 the stimulation of gluconeogenesis;
2 the mobilisation of fatty acids;
3 the breakdown of proteins for repair of tissues or enzyme manufacture;
4 the enhancement of the vasoconstrictive effects of noradrenaline;
5 an increase in blood pressure and circulatory efficiency.

High levels of glucocorticoids will:

- depress cartilage and bone formation;
- inhibit the inflammatory response;
- depress the activity of the immune system;
- cause changes in cardiovascular, neural and gastrointestinal function.

Gonadocorticoids

The main gonadocorticoids are androgens, testosterone being the most common. Small amounts of oestrogen and progesterone are also secreted. In adult women, adrenal androgens are thought to be responsible for libido. Adrenal oestrogens may replace ovarian oestrogens at the menopause.

The adrenal medulla

The hormone-producing cells in the adrenal medulla are the **chromaffin cells**, arranged in clusters around capillaries and sinusoids. The two main hormones produced are adrenaline (**epinephrine**) and noradrenaline (**norepinephrine**), known collectively as the **catecholamines**. About 80% of hormone production is adrenaline. They are formed from the amino acid tyrosine. During short-term stress the sympathetic nervous system is stimulated, so that blood sugar levels rise and blood vessels constrict. The heart beats faster and blood pressure rises. Blood is diverted to the brain and muscles.

Sympathetic nerve endings stimulate the adrenal medulla to reinforce and prolong the 'fight or flight' response. Adrenaline is the more potent stimulator of heart and metabolic activity whilst noradrenaline has the greater effect on peripheral vasoconstriction and blood pressure. Catecholamines produce short-term responses, unlike the cortical hormones.

Changes in the adrenal gland during pregnancy

Cortisol

ACTH levels rise progressively in pregnancy but still remain in the range for non-pregnant women. There is also a steady rise in plasma cortisol due to a doubling of CBG (Ramsay 1991). An increase in free plasma cortisol also occurs, with a loss of diurnal variation so that there is greater tissue exposure, especially in late pregnancy. It has been suggested that some of the features of pregnancy giving a Cushingoid appearance (see below), such as striae gravidarum, impaired carbohydrate tolerance and hypertension, are due to the excess cortisol. Cortisol production is increased in labour, probably due to the stress response.

Aldosterone

There is an increase in renin substrate due to the increase in circulating oestrogens. Excretion of sodium and chloride is stepped up in response to the presence of progesterone (Ramsay 1991). Alterations in the renin-angiotensin mechanisms lead to increased aldosterone production which enhances the reabsorption of sodium to maintain balance (Thomson 1996).

Adrenal disorders in pregnancy

Addison's disease

Addison's disease is caused by inadequate secretion of the adrenal cortical hormones with a deficit in both glucocorticoids and mineralocorticoids. Symptoms include falling plasma sodium and glucose levels, a rise in serum potassium levels, skin hyperpigmentation and weight loss. Severe dehydration and hypotension are common. The main cause is now autoimmune destruction of the adrenal cortex and it often occurs combined with other autoimmune endocrine disorders such as Grave's disease. In pregnancy, the condition is treated by 20 mg oral hydrocortisone in the morning and 10 mg at night. In an acute episode intravenous hydrocortisone is necessary.

Cushing's disease

Cushing's disease is caused by excessive levels of corticosteroids. It is extremely rare and is seldom found associated with pregnancy because amenorrhoea and anovulation are usually present. The cause is often pituitary or adrenal carcinoma. As mentioned above, some normal pregnancy features mimic Cushing's disease but unless other signs such as a moon face, hirsutism, acne and proximal myopathy are present, it is unlikely to be true Cushing's disease. In the rare cases seen, fetal loss has been 25% and preterm delivery occurred in up to 50%.

Congenital adrenal hyperplasia

Congenital adrenal hyperplasia (see Chapter 15) occurs in about one in 7500 births. Women who remain undiagnosed tend to be hirsute and infertile. Girls treated in childhood and adolescence have a fertility rate of 64%. Because of the masculinisation of the pelvis, cephalopelvic disproportion is a serious problem.

Phaeochromocytoma

A phaeochromocytoma is a tumour of the adrenal medulla. It is often diagnosed as preeclampsia or essential hypertension. Its symptoms include intermittent or sustained hypertension, postural hypotension, sweating, palpitations and tachycardia, anxiety, nausea and vomiting. The tumour and symptoms can be treated medically until the fetus is viable when surgical removal of the tumour is carried out.

THE PINEAL GLAND

The pineal gland is very small and hangs from the floor of the 3rd ventricle. It is composed of neuroglial cells and secretory cells called **pinealocytes**. Calcium salts are deposited between the pinealocytes. These salts are radiopaque so that the gland is opaque to X-rays, allowing it to be used as a landmark. The secretion of its major hormone, **melatonin**, waxes and wanes in a diurnal cycle, being highest during the night and lowest about noon.

In animals melatonin is concerned with reproduction. Changing periods of light and dark noted by the visual system affect gonadal size and mating behaviour. In humans melatonin acts on the hypothalamus to inhibit release of gonadotrophin-releasing hormone. Precocious sexual development is thus inhibited in childhood. Melatonin levels are also involved in biorhythmic variations involving day/night cycles such as temperature, sleep and appetite.

Summary of main points

- The endocrine system uses hormones produced by ductless glands that empty their products directly into the bloodstream or lymphatic circulation. The hormones are carried round the bloodstream until they reach a target tissue.
- The hypothalamus is the major controller of endocrine gland function and has wider links with other parts of the nervous system. It can therefore be considered as a neuroendocrine organ. Releasing and inhibiting hormones produced by the hypothalamus influence the production of hormones by the anterior pituitary gland.
- The endocrine glands include the pituitary, thyroid, parathyroid, adrenal, pineal and thymus glands. Other organs which contain hormone-producing tissue are the pancreas, ovaries and testes. The placenta is a fetal organ producing hormones that affect the maternal body.
- The functions of the endocrine glands include reproduction, growth and development, mobilisation of body defences against stress, maintenance of fluid and electrolyte balance, nutrient content in the blood, regulation of cellular metabolism and energy balance.
- Hormones are chemical substances secreted by cells into the extracellular fluids that regulate the metabolic function of other cells in the body. They can be classified into two groups: amino acid-based molecules and a smaller group of steroid hormones. A third type of molecule that may influence cell activity locally are the eicosanoids, which include the prostaglandins.
- Hormone–receptor binding is a first step to target cell interaction. The extent of cellular activity depends on blood levels of the hormone, the relative numbers of target cell receptors and the affinity of the receptor for the hormone. Target cells may make more receptors in response to high levels of hormone. This is called upregulation. Other cells may be desensitised to high levels of hormones, responding less vigorously, possibly by receptor loss. This is called downregulation.
- The synthesis and release of hormones depends on a system of negative feedback or feedback inhibition. The hormone secretion is triggered by an internal or external stimulus. Hormone levels in the blood rise until they reach the required level and then further hormone release is inhibited.
- The pituitary gland has two major lobes. The posterior lobe is made of nerve fibres and neuroglia. It is derived from a downward growth of the hypothalamus. It does not make its own hormones but acts as a storage unit, releasing hypothalamic hormones. The anterior lobe is composed of glandular tissue and manufactures and releases its own hormones.
- Running through the infundibulum is a nerve bundle called the hypothalamic-hypophyseal tract. The tract neurones secrete two neurohormones: oxytocin and antidiuretic hormone. These are transported along the axons to the posterior lobe of the pituitary gland.
- There are six anterior pituitary hormones. Four of them regulate the hormonal functioning of other glands: thyroid-stimulating hormone, adrenocorticotrophic hormone, follicle-stimulating hormone and luteinising hormone. The other two hormones have their influences on non-endocrine targets: growth hormone and prolactin.
- GH stimulates body cells to grow in size and divide by stimulating protein synthesis. Its major targets are the bones and skeletal muscles. It facilitates the use of fats for fuel and conserves glucose. GH is known to be mediated indirectly by somatomedins and has a diurnal cycle with the highest levels occurring during evening sleep.
- Prolactin stimulates the production of milk by the breasts. It is controlled by hypothalamic production of PRL-releasing hormone and PRL-inhibiting hormone (dopamine).

- Oxytocin is released by the posterior pituitary gland. It stimulates uterine action in labour and is involved in milk ejection. ADH is also released by the posterior pituitary gland and inhibits or prevents urine formation, leading to a rise in blood volume. It targets the renal tubules which respond to the stimulus by reabsorbing more water.
- Changes in structure and function of the pituitary gland during pregnancy underlie lactation. During pregnancy its weight increases by 30% in first pregnancies and 50% in subsequent pregnancies, almost entirely due to changes in the anterior lobe. This is caused by an increase in the number of the elongated prolactin-secreting cells known as lactotrophs. At the same time the number of GH-producing cells falls.
- During pregnancy the hormones produced by the fetoplacental unit have a great influence on the pituitary gland. The pattern of hormone production by the anterior pituitary changes in the puerperium to accommodate lactation. The secretion of gonadotrophins, follicle-stimulating hormone and luteinising hormone is inhibited during pregnancy.
- ACTH plasma concentrations rise progressively during pregnancy. This is associated with a doubling of plasma cortisol. Normally, a rise in plasma cortisol would suppress ACTH production but the usual feedback mechanism appears to be lost during pregnancy. The placenta may contribute to the increase in plasma ACTH.
- The myometrium and decidua convert cortisone to cortisol, resulting in a local cortisol concentration of nine times normal. This may contribute to immunological protection of the fetus.
- The enlargement of the anterior pituitary gland is presumed to need an increased oxygen supply carried to it by an augmented circulation. The pituitary gland is vulnerable to a reduction in arterial blood supply due to vasospasm of the superior hypophyseal artery. Both the need for extra oxygen and extra sensitivity of the hypophyseal artery to vasospasm may explain why the pituitary gland is more readily damaged in pregnancy, resulting in Sheehan's syndrome. Adequate and prompt treatment of obstetric shock will prevent the syndrome developing.
- Antidiuretic hormone production and its effect on the renal tubules are similar in pregnant and non-pregnant women. However, the osmoreceptors are reset to accommodate the extra blood volume associated with pregnancy.
- The thyroid gland consists of hollow spherical structures called follicles which produce thyroglobulin. The lumen of a follicle stores an amber-coloured sticky material which consists of thyroglobulin molecules attached to iodine. This gives rise to two thyroid hormones – thyroxine or T_4 and triiodothyronine or T_3. The parafollicular cells produce calcitonin.
- Thyroid hormones stimulate enzymes concerned with the oxidation of glucose. They increase basal metabolic rate, oxygen consumption and body heat production. Thyroid hormones regulate tissue growth and development and are essential for normal skeletal and nervous system development. Thyroid function remains normal during pregnancy although some women exhibit some of the signs associated with an overactive thyroid gland, including goitre.
- There are significant alterations in plasma concentrations of the thyroid hormones and of thyroid-binding globulin during pregnancy. These changes are probably influenced by oestrogen and human chorionic gonadotrophin and support the alterations in metabolism found in pregnancy. The alterations have been linked with nausea and vomiting in early pregnancy.
- The adrenal glands consist of two endocrine glands, the cortex and medulla, each producing its own hormones. Corticosteroids are synthesised from cholesterol in the cortex. The outer zona glomerulosa produces the mineralocorticoids while the middle layer called the zona fasciculata secretes the glucocorticoids. The innermost zone called the zona reticularis produces glucocorticoids and small amounts of gonadocorticoids.
- Mineralocorticoids regulate the amount of electrolytes and water in extracellular fluid. In particular, they affect the sodium and potassium concentrations. Aldosterone makes up more than 95% of the total output. The function of aldosterone is to regulate sodium balance.
- Glucocorticoids, cortisol, cortisone and corticosterone, have an effect on the metabolism of most body cells. Their role is to convert the intermittent intake of food into a steady level of sugar in the plasma. They also maintain blood level by preventing the shift of water into tissue cells. In severe stress the output of glucocorticoids rises dramatically to help the body through the crisis.
- The main gonadocorticoids are androgens, testosterone being the most common. Small amounts of oestrogen and progesterone are also secreted. In women, adrenal androgens are thought to be responsible for libido. Adrenal oestrogens may replace ovarian oestrogens at the menopause.
- Chromaffin cells are arranged in clusters around capillaries and sinusoids in the medulla. They produce the catecholamines adrenaline and noradrenaline. Sympathetic nerve endings stimulate the adrenal medulla to reinforce and prolong the 'fight or flight' response. Adrenaline is the more potent stimulator of heart and metabolic activity whilst noradrenaline has the greater effect on peripheral vasoconstriction and blood pressure.
- ACTH levels rise progressively in pregnancy but still remain in the range for non-pregnant women. There is also a steady rise in plasma cortisol due to a doubling of CBG. Some of the features of pregnancy give a Cushingoid appearance with striae gravidarum, impaired carbohydrate tolerance and hypertension due to the excess cortisol.
- Alterations in the renin-angiotensin mechanisms lead to increased aldosterone production which enhances the reabsorption of sodium to maintain balance.
- Addison's disease is caused by inadequate secretion of the adrenal cortical hormones with a deficit in both glucocorticoids and mineralocorticoids. The main cause is autoimmune destruction of the adrenal cortex. In pregnancy the condition is treated by 20 mg oral hydrocortisone in the morning and 10 mg at night. In an acute episode, intravenous hydrocortisone is necessary.
- Cushing's disease is caused by excessive levels of corticosteroids. It is extremely rare and is seldom found associated with pregnancy because amenorrhoea and anovulation are usually present. In the cases seen, fetal loss has been 25% and preterm delivery occurred in up to 50%.
- Congenital adrenal hyperplasia occurs in about one in 7500 births. Women who remain undiagnosed tend to be hirsute and infertile. Girls treated in childhood and adolescence have a fertility rate of 64%. Masculinisation of the pelvis leads to cephalopelvic disproportion.
- A phaeochromocytoma is a tumour of the adrenal medulla. It is often diagnosed as preeclampsia or essential hypertension. Its symptoms include hypertension, postural hypotension, sweating, palpitations and tachycardia, anxiety, nausea and vomiting. The tumour is treated medically until after delivery when it is removed surgically.
- The pineal gland is composed of neuroglial cells and secretory cells called pinealocytes. Its major secretion is the hormone melatonin which waxes and wanes in a diurnal cycle, being highest during the night and lowest about noon. In humans melatonin acts on the hypothalamus to inhibit release of gonadotrophin-releasing hormone. Melatonin levels are also involved in biorhythmic variations involving day/night cycles such as temperature, sleep, appetite.

References

Blackburn ST, Loper DL. 1992 Maternal, Fetal and Neonatal Physiology A Clinical Perspective. WB Saunders, Philadelphia.

Boore JRP. 1996 Endocrine function. In Hinchliff SM, Montague SE, Watson R (eds) Physiology for Nursing Practice, 2nd edn. Baillière Tindall, London, pp 202–244.

Fitzgerald MJT. 1996 Neuroanatomy. Saunders, Philadelphia.

Hinchliff SM, Montague SE, Watson R. 1996 Physiology for Nursing Practice. Baillière Tindall, London.

Jacobs HS. 1991 The hypothalamus and pituitary gland. In Hytten F, Chamberlain G (eds) Clinical Physiology in Obstetrics, 2nd edn. Blackwell Scientific, Oxford, pp 345–356.

Lindsay P. 1997 Bleeding in pregnancy. In Sweet BR with Tiran D (eds) Mayes Midwifery, 12th edn. Baillière Tindall, London, pp 511–532.

Marieb EN. 1992 Human Anatomy and Physiology, 2nd edn. Benjamin/Cummings Publishing California.

Ramsay ID. 1991 The thyroid gland. In Hytten F, Chamberlain G (eds) Clinical Physiology in Obstetrics, 2nd edn. Blackwell Scientific, Oxford.

Sheehan HL, Stanfield JP. 1961 The pathogenesis of postpartum necrosis of the anterior lobe of the pituitary gland. Acta Endocrinologica 37,479.

Sleep J. 1996 Complications of the third stage of labour. In Bennett VR, Brown LK (eds) Myles Textbook for Midwives, 12th edn. Churchill Livingstone, Edinburgh, pp 462–476.

Sweet B 1997 Mayes' Midwifery. Baillière Tindall, London.

Thomson V. 1996 Psychological and physiological changes of pregnancy. In Bennett VR, Brown LK. 1996 Myles Textbook for Midwives, 12th edn. Churchill Livingstone, Edinburgh, pp 94–105.

Recommended reading

Greenspan FS. 1991 Basic Clinical Endocrinology. Lange Medical, East Norwalk, CT.

Jacobs HS. 1991 The hypothalamus and pituitary gland. In Hytten F, Chamberlain G (eds) Clinical Physiology in Obstetrics, 2nd edn. Blackwell Scientific, Oxford, pp 345–356.

Ramsay ID. 1991 The thyroid gland. In Hytten F, Chamberlain G (eds) Clinical Physiology in Obstetrics, 2nd edn. Blackwell Scientific, Oxford.

Chapter 29 The immune system

In this chapter

INTRODUCTION

The immune system plays an enormous part in the protection of the individual from environmental factors such as microorganisms, irritants and abnormal cells. **Pathogenic** microbes such as viruses, bacteria and fungi are constantly mounting invasions of the body both on its surface and internally. Larger organisms such as worms and flukes are **parasitic**, living by tapping into the metabolic processes of other organisms. There are also many microorganisms in soil, water, air, food and on the body that do not cause disease in the healthy person but may threaten life if the immune system is defective. The immune system protects against the pathogen by mounting an **immune response**.

In developed countries such as Britain and the United States of America, infection is no longer a major cause of mortality, accounting for under 2% of deaths. However, new problems arise, including the bacterial response to antibiotics of developing new resistant strains such as methicillin-resistant *Staphylococcus aureus* and the organism that causes tuberculosis. Global travel makes the transfer of deadly diseases much more rapid. Davey (1989) mentions that as many as 20 million children per year may die of diarrhoeal diseases world wide.

CELLS OF THE IMMUNE SYSTEM

The white blood cells or **leucocytes** (WBCs) are protective against bacteria, viruses, parasites, toxins and tumour cells. There are normally about 4–11 × 10^9/l). Most of the body's white cells are in the tissues which is the reason for the wide variation in the normal blood count as cells can enter and leave the circulation from hour to hour by **diapedesis**.

Types of leucocyte

Several types of leucocyte are distinguished by their shape, appearance and function. Granulocytes (polymorphonuclear leucocytes) are subdivided into neutrophils, eosinophils and basophils. These cells contain granules which carry substances in their cytoplasm that can fight infection. They are 10–14 μm in diameter and have a lobed nucleus. They are divided into three groups by the size of their granules. All these cells are **phagocytic**, engulfing and destroying foreign proteins directly. Natural killer cells are a specialised type of large granular lymphocyte. Agranulocytes, which include lymphocytes and monocytes, do not contain visible cytoplasmic granules.

Granulocytes

Neutrophils contain granules of varying sizes that stain violet because their granules take up both acidic red dyes and basic blue dyes. They are the most common type of leucocyte, accounting for more than 50% of all white cells, and they have the most lobular nucleus. Neutrophils are chemically attracted to sites of inflammation and will ingest and destroy bacteria and some fungi.

Eosinophils have large granules which are stained red by acidic dyes. They make up about 1–4% of the white cell population. Their most important role is to attack parasitic worms by surrounding them and releasing enzymes from their granules onto the parasite's surface to digest it from the outside. Eosinophils also deal with allergy attacks by destroying antigen–antibody complexes.

Basophils have large granules that take up a basic dye and stain blue-black. These are the rarest of the white cells, accounting for only 0.5%. Their large granules contain histamine, an inflammatory substance that acts as a vasodilator and draws other white blood cells to the site of inflammation. Cells similar to basophils present in connective tissue are called **mast cells**. Both types of cell release histamine when they bind to immunoglobulin E.

Production of granulocytes

Granulocytes arise from **myeloid precursor cells** in the red bone marrow. The process takes about 14 days but can be considerably reduced if cells are urgently needed, such as in an infection. For every granulocyte in the circulation, there may be more than 50 in bone marrow. During granulopoiesis there is progressive condensation and lobulation of the nucleus, loss of organelles and development of the granules in the cell cytoplasm. Within 7 h of reaching the circulation, half the granulocytes will have left to meet tissue needs and will not return. They normally survive about 5 days. Dead cells are eliminated from the body in faeces and respiratory secretions and form the pus at infection sites.

Natural killer cells (NK cells) are large specialised granular lymphocytes present in blood and lymph which destroy cancer cells and virus-infected body cells. Unlike other lymphocytes which can only recognise and react to specific virus-infected or tumour cells, NK cells can react against any such cell by recognising surface changes.

Agranulocytes

Lymphocytes are involved in immunity and produced in the bone marrow. They are round cells with large round nuclei and are the second most common type of leucocyte. Immature cells migrate to the thymus and other lymphoid tissue to divide and mature. Large numbers exist in the body but most are found in lymphoid tissue. They can be subdivided into small and large lymphocytes.

There are two types of lymphocytes: T and B. T cells mature in the thymus gland, are involved in cell-mediated immune responses and form 80% of the lymphocytes present in blood. B cells are involved in humoral immunity and produce antibodies. Lymphocytes recirculate between blood and lymph.

Monocytes are large cells produced in the bone marrow. Mature cells spend about 30 h in the blood and then migrate to the tissues where they develop into phagocytic macrophages. Macrophages are also involved in regulating the immune response by activating B and T lymphocytes.

Production of lymphocytes

Lymphocytes originate in the red bone marrow and some cells leave the bone marrow in an immature state to become **immunocompetent**, i.e. able to recognise foreign antigens and bind to them by migrating to the thymus gland where they become T cells. They are selected so that they will not attack **self-antigens** present on the surface of the individual's own cells. B cells are so called because they were first identified in the bursa of Fabricius in birds, a pocket of lymphatic tissue associated with the digestive tract.

DIVISIONS OF THE IMMUNE SYSTEM

Marieb (1992) calls the immune system a 'functional system rather than an organ system' because its main work is carried out by enormous numbers of individual cells. Three lines of defence can be distinguished in the immune system.

1 The surface barriers such as skin and mucous membranes.
2 The inflammatory response.
3 Specific (acquired, adaptive) immunity.

The first two are non-specific and the third is a specific response to a particular foreign protein.

There are also many chemical messenger molecules involved in the control of immunity. The cells and molecules that make up the immune response work together through a finely balanced network of interactions to produce a diverse response,

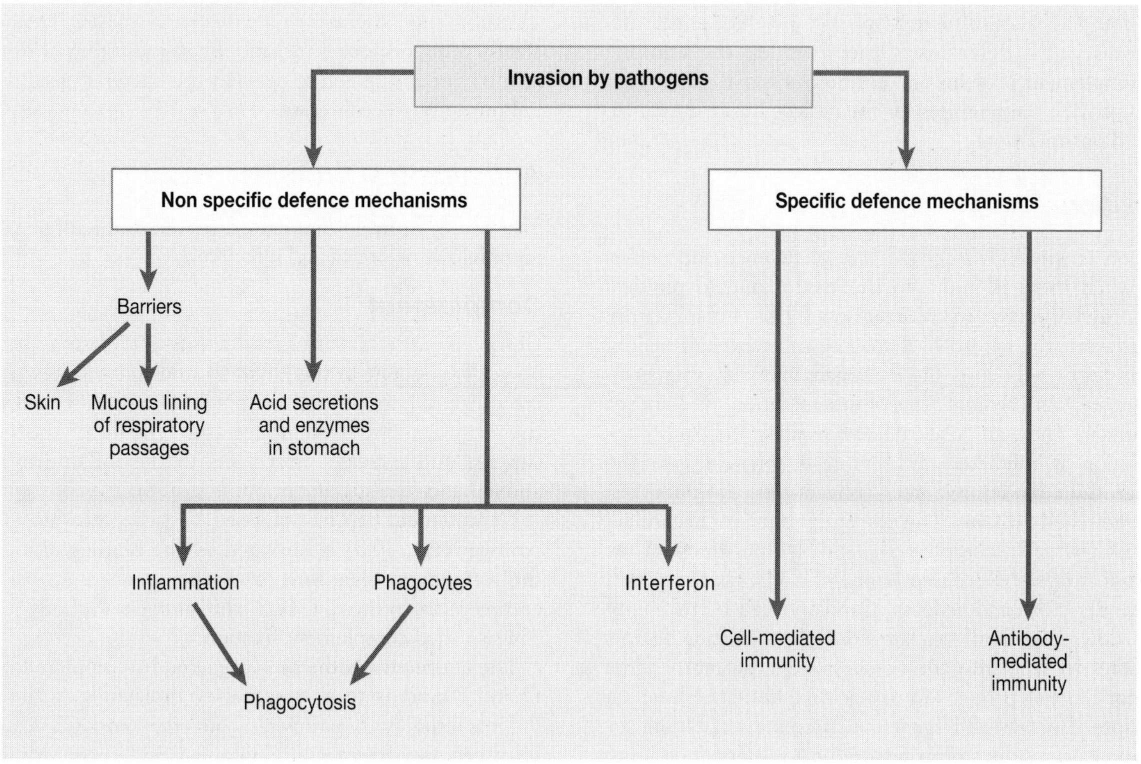

Figure 29.1 *Summary of specific and non-specific defence mechanisms. Non-specific mechanisms prevent entry of many pathogens and act rapidly to destroy those that manage to cross the barriers. Specific defence mechanisms take longer to mobilise but they are highly effective in destroying invaders (from Hinchliff SM, Montague SE, Watson R, 1996, with permission).*

either destroying the invading organism or reducing its harmful effects.

It is usual to divide the immune system into two groups of actions although there is a high level of interdependence between the two categories (Fig. 29.1). The first is **non-specific (innate) immunity** that can immediately protect the body from all foreign substances. The second is called **specific (acquired, adaptive) immunity** that acts against a particular invader but needs to be primed by the presence of the invader and therefore takes time to develop.

Non-specific defences

These can be divided into surface barriers such as the skin and mucous membranes, which are the body's first line of defence, and cellular and chemical defences.

Surface barriers include:

- a thickly keratinised unbroken skin;
- intact mucous membranes lining the organs;
- acidic secretions such as in the vagina, gastric juices and urine;
- sticky mucus to trap organisms;
- ciliated cells that can sweep particles towards the outside;
- the presence of lysozyme, an enzyme that destroys bacteria, in saliva and tears.

If the intact surfaces are breached other non-specific mechanisms are triggered into action. These are the cellular and chemical defences.

Phagocytes

In most cases, phagocytic cells (Fig. 29.2) will be involved. These are amoeba-like and travel through tissue spaces in search of invading organisms or other debris which they engulf and destroy. The main phagocytic cells are the **macrophages** (giant eaters). Neutrophils become phagocytic if an infection is present. Macrophages are long-lived cells but neutrophils are destroyed during phagocytosis. Both cells destroy microbes by

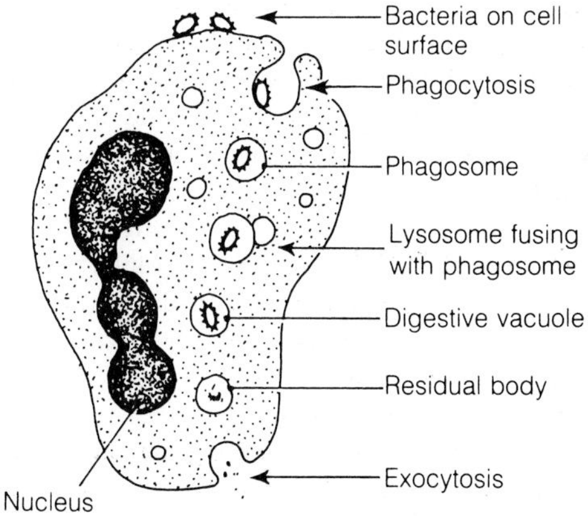

Figure 29.2 *Diagram of a neutrophil undergoing phagocytosis (from Hinchliff SM, Montague SE, 1990, with permission).*

producing free radicals and neutrophils also produce antibiotic-like chemicals called **defensins**. Other parts of the immune system – **complement proteins** and **antibodies** – coat the foreign particles to provide binding sites for the phagocytes to attach to. This is called **opsonisation**.

Inflammation

Inflammation is the body's second line of defence and comes into play when there is injury to the tissues due to physical trauma or invasion by microorganisms. The inflammatory response prevents the spread of damaging substances to nearby tissues, disposes of cell debris and pathogens and allows repair to begin. There are four **cardinal signs** of inflammation, well known to most humans! These are heat, redness, swelling and pain.

Inflammation is mediated by chemicals released into the extracellular fluid by injured cells, phagocytes, lymphocytes, mast cells and blood proteins. The most important are histamine, kinins, prostaglandins, complement and lymphokines. They cause vasodilation of localised small blood vessels which accounts for the heat and redness. Capillary wall permeability increases, allowing a fluid exudate containing clotting factors and antibodies to seep into the tissue spaces, causing oedema and swelling. Clotting proteins form a gel-like fibrin mesh which limits the spread of harmful agents and forms a scaffolding for tissue repair. Pain results from pressure on local nerve endings, release of bacterial toxins, lack of cellular nutrition and the effects of prostaglandins and kinins. Loss of function may occur, forcing the person to rest the injured part to aid healing.

The damaged area is invaded by phagocytes and an immune response is triggered with antibody formation. Rapid release of neutrophils by the bone marrow is caused by leucocyte-inducing factors so that four times as many neutrophils may be in the bloodstream after a few hours. These cells are attracted to the injury site by chemicals called **chemotactic agents**. Once there, they cling to the capillary walls (**margination** or **pavementing**) and squeeze through them (**diapedesis**) to the site, where they devour bacteria, toxins and dead tissue. Monocytes, which are immature macrophages, now enter the tissue, swell and mature. Macrophages are central to many functions of the immune system.

If the infection is severe pus may be produced, which is a mixture of dead neutrophils, living and dead pathogens and damaged tissue cells. If this becomes walled off by collagen fibres, an abscess forms. Some bacteria, like the tuberculosis bacillus, are resistant to digestion by macrophages because they are protected by a waxy outer coat. They can live inside the macrophage. Infectious **granulomas** develop which have a central core of infected macrophages surrounded by uninfected macrophages and an outer fibrous capsule. The person carries the pathogens without becoming ill until his resistance to infection is reduced when the bacteria can break out and cause disease.

Fever

Fever is an elevation of the body temperature in response to chemicals called **pyrogens** secreted by macrophages. High fevers are dangerous because they inactivate enzymes and disrupt cellular metabolic processes but mild to moderate fevers are helpful to the body. Fever increases the metabolic rate of tissue, speeding up defensive actions and aiding repair. Other antibacterial responses include the sequestering of iron and zinc in the liver and spleen to prevent the bacteria using these essential nutrients to proliferate.

Antimicrobial proteins

The two most important categories of antimicrobial proteins are complement proteins and interferon.

Complement

Complement is a system of about 20 plasma proteins that normally circulate in the blood in an inactive state. The proteins are called C1 to C9 and factors B, D and P. The activation of the complement system releases chemical mediators that support and increase most parts of the inflammatory process and enhance the specific immune system.

Complement can be activated by two pathways. The **classic pathway** (Fig. 29.3) is activated by the binding of antibodies to the offending organisms and the attachment of the first complement protein C1 to the antigen-antibody complexes. This is called **complement fixation**.

The **alternative pathway** is triggered by complement factors B, D and P binding to polysaccharide molecules on the surface of the bacteria. Both pathways converge onto C3, causing it to split into two fragments, C3a and C3b. An orderly cascade of complement protein activation occurs and C3b binds to the target cell's surface, resulting in the insertion of a group of complement proteins called the **membrane attack complex** (MAC) into the bacterial cell wall. This forms a hole, allowing solutes to leak from the cell, and the cell is **lysed** (destroyed).

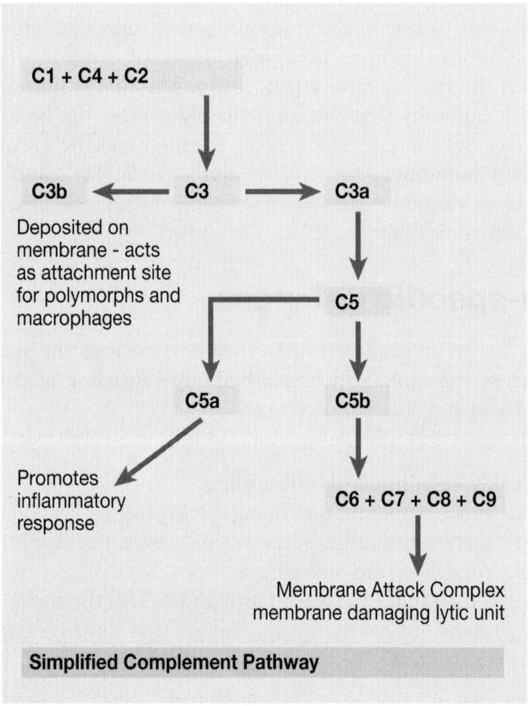

Figure 29.3 *Simplified complement pathway (from Hinchliff SM, Montague SE, Watson R, 1996, with permission).*

Interferons

Interferons are small proteins which can act against a variety of intracellular viruses. They diffuse to nearby cells and stimulate them to produce proteins that inhibit viral replication. They are host species specific and there are α, produced by most white cells, and γ-interferons, also known as immune interferons, produced by lymphocytes. Interferons can also activate macrophages and γ-interferons mobilise NK cells.

SPECIFIC DEFENCES – THE IMMUNE SYSTEM

Tissues of the lymphatic system

The lymphatic system is divided into primary lymphoid organs, such as the bone marrow and thymus gland where the B cells and T cells differentiate and mature, and the peripheral lymphoid system where they spend most of their active lives (Fig. 29.4). The peripheral lymphoid system includes encapsulated organs such as the spleen, tonsils and lymph nodes. Unencapsulated lymphoid tissue is found in the gut, lungs and urogenital tract where many types of white cells are densely packed in (Davey 1989).

Lymph nodes

The immune response takes place in the lymphatic system. Lymph nodes (Fig. 29.5) are encapsulated glands about the size of a broad bean which filter the lymph. The gland mainly consists of a network of reticular cells in which lymphocytes are embedded. There are two distinct regions: the outer cortex and the inner medulla. Macrophages are found throughout the gland but are concentrated in the medulla. B cells are concentrated in primary follicles in the cortex of the nodes. Cells at the centre of the follicle actively divide whilst those at the periphery of the follicle produce antibodies. T cells are found in the paracortical area.

Macrophages tend to be fixed in the lymphoid organs whereas lymphocytes also circulate throughout the body. T cells account for 65–85% of bloodborne lymphocytes. Lymph capillaries pick up pathogens and other foreign proteins so that the presence of immune cells in lymph nodes is very protective. For instance, lymphocytes and macrophages in the tonsils combat organisms that invade the nasal and oral cavities.

Some other lymphoid organs

The spleen

The spleen, the largest lymphoid organ, is located on the left side of the body just below the diaphragm. It is composed of venous sinuses and reticular connective tissue forming the **red pulp** where its main function, the removal of ageing and defective red cells, cellular debris and microorganisms from the blood, takes place. There are areas of reticular fibres with attached lymphocytes called the white pulp which provide sites for the proliferation of lymphocytes and for the immune response. The spleen stores the products from broken-down red

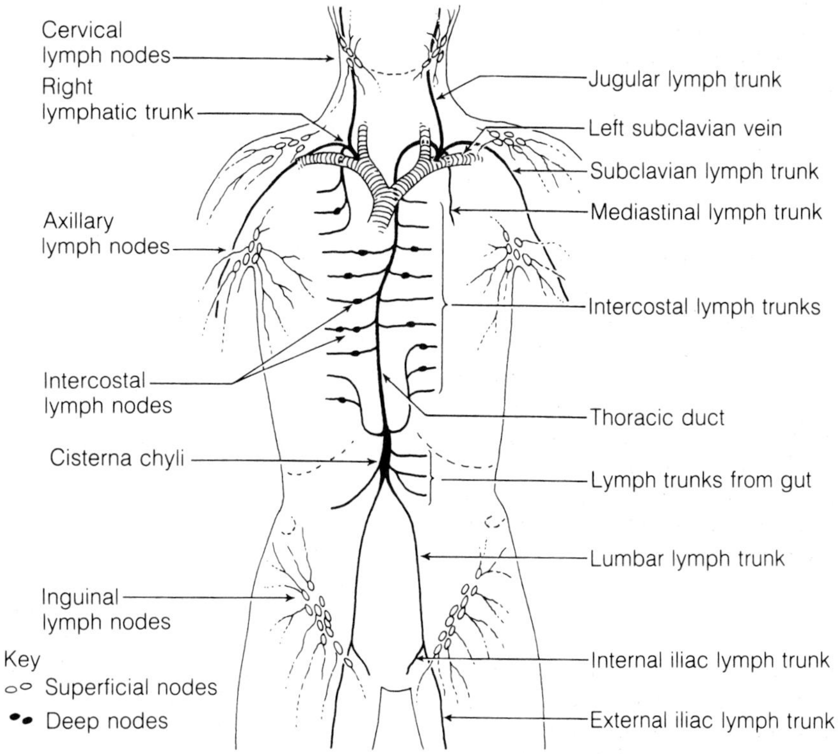

Figure 29.4 *General arrangement of the lymphatic system (from Hinchliff SM, Montague SE, 1990, with permission).*

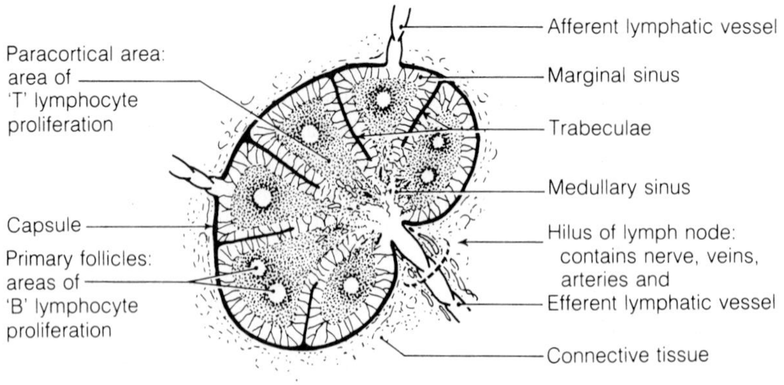

Figure 29.5 *Section through a lymph gland (from Hinchliff SM, Montague SE, 1990, with permission).*

cells for future use and stores blood platelets. During fetal life it is a site of red cell production.

The thymus gland

This bilobed gland is more active in the early years of life. It is found in the mediastinum of the thorax and during adolescence it decreases in size and starts to atrophy. Its structure is similar to that of the lymph node, with lymphocytes densely packed in the medullary areas. It is involved in the differentiation of the T lymphocytes.

Lymphatic vessels

An extensive network of lymphatic vessels similar to the vascular system runs throughout the body, connecting tissues to the lymphoid organs. Lymphatic capillaries are like blood capillaries but the endothelial cells of their walls do not lie on a basement membrane. They join up to make larger lymphatic vessels which contain smooth muscles in their walls and have one-way valves. There is no equivalent organ to the heart but the flow of lymph is ensured by skeletal muscle contraction and negative intrathoracic pressure. Unlike veins, lymphatic vessels contract rhythmically to help the lymph flow (Hinchliff 1996).

Lymph

Lymph originates as plasma which leaks from the blood capillaries. It transports water and small molecules and contains proteins which enter the capillary lumen between the endothelial cells. Fluids and solutes enter the lymphatic capillaries along their length and dietary fat is absorbed as triglycerides from the villi of the small intestine.

Up to 4 l of lymph accumulates over 24 h and is returned to the blood. Lymph enters lymph nodes by afferent vessels and leaves via an efferent vessel. Lymph is returned to the blood via the large veins in the neck through two ducts. The **thoracic duct**, which arises anterior to the second lumbar vertebra as an enlarged sac called the **cisterna chyli**, drains the lower limbs, digestive system, the left arm and left side of the thorax, neck and head. The smaller **right lymphatic duct** accepts lymph from the right arm and right side of thorax neck and head.

Functioning of the immune response

Researchers have identified three important aspects of the immune response.

1 It is antigen specific: the response is directed against particular pathogens or foreign substances.
2 It is systemic, with the response not being restricted to the initial site of infection.
3 It has memory and once it has recognised an antigen as foreign, it will respond by producing antibodies to subsequent invasion by the same molecule.

Immunity could be divided into two types. **Humoral immunity** or antibody-mediated immunity is provided by the presence of antibodies in the body fluids (humors). When the lymphocytes attack the invader directly the process is called cellular immunity or **cell-mediated immunity** (Fig. 29.6). The three cell types involved in the immune response are B lymphocytes or B cells, which are involved in antibody production and are responsible for the humoral-mediated immunity, T lymphocytes, which do not produce antibodies and are involved in cell-mediated immunity, and macrophages which support the two sets of lymphocytes.

Macrophages are at the centre of the immune response. They present bits of antigens in their cell surfaces to the T cells so that they can recognise them as foreign. Macrophages also secrete substances that activate T cells which in turn secrete chemicals that activate macrophages to become phagocytic and to secrete bactericidal chemicals.

The humoral immune response

Antigens

The first encounter between an invading antigen and an immunocompetent lymphocyte commonly takes place in the spleen or in a lymph node but it may happen in any lymphoid tissue (Marieb 1992). This involves the activation of a B cell and the collaboration of T cells which is the body's third line of defence, providing protection targeted at specific foreign antigens which are macromolecules such as proteins, nucleic acids, some lipids and large polysaccharides not usually present in the body and therefore non-self. A small area on an antigen

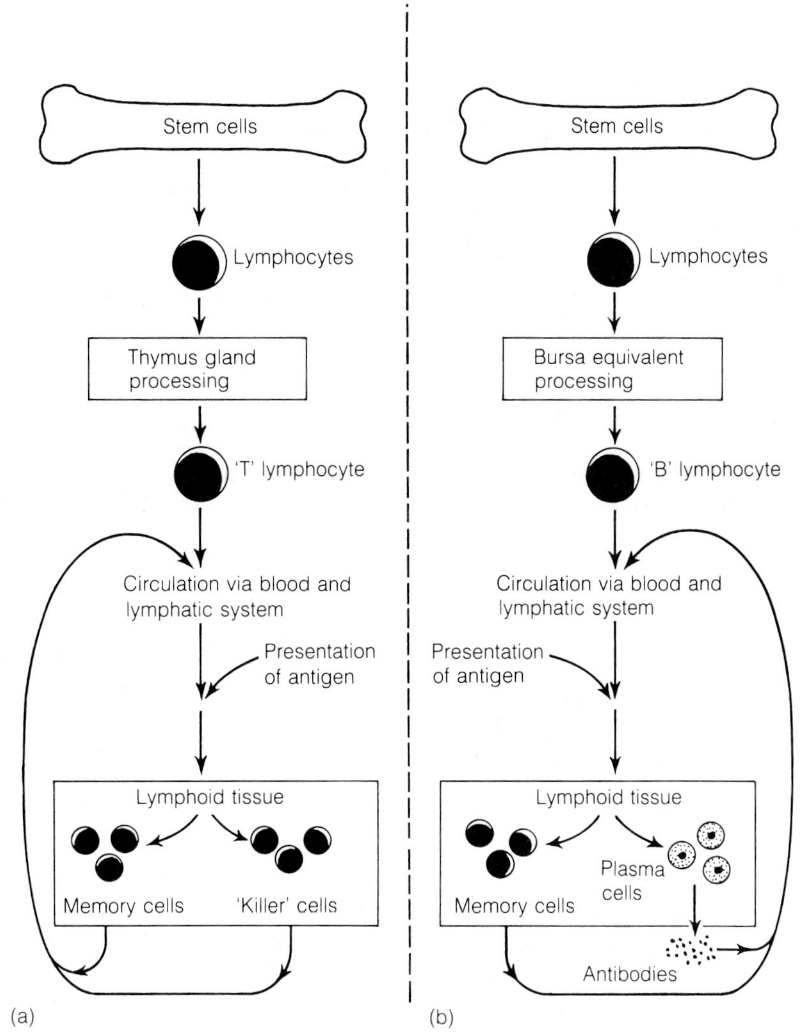

Figure 29.6 *Summary of the development of (a) the cell-mediated immune system, and (b) the humoral immune system (from Hinchliff SM, Montague SE, 1990, with permission).*

called the **epitope** is recognised by a small area on a receptor, present in the B lymphocyte cell membrane, called the **antigen-binding site**. Pollen grains and microorganisms are the strongest antigens.

Normally small molecules such as peptides, nucleotides and hormones are not immunogenic but if they link up with the body's proteins, they cause allergies. Such molecules are called **haptens** and include drugs such as penicillin, detergents, plant products and many industrial pollutants. The defence system responds to the complex by the production of antibodies.

Clonal selection

The binding of the antigen and the lymphocyte stimulates the B cell to divide rapidly, forming a **clone** of identical cells able to recognise that antigen. As the response is so specific, a huge variety of lymphocytes must be available to recognise the enormous number of antigens met throughout life. This response to a particular antigen by a specific lymphocyte which has receptors that can bind to it is called clonal selection.

Most of these clone cells differentiate into plasma cells which secrete antibody molecules at about 2000 per second for about 5 days before the cell dies. Antibodies circulate around the body in blood and lymph where they bind to antigen molecules and present them for destruction to phagocytes. This **primary immune response** occurs the first time the body meets the antigen. There is a lag of about 3–6 days as the B cells proliferate and form plasma cells. Plasma antibody levels then begin to rise, reaching a peak at 10 days.

Immunological memory

Those clone cells that do not differentiate into plasma cells become long-lived **memory cells** able to mount a rapid humoral response if the antigen is encountered at a later date. If a person is reexposed to a particular antigen, a **secondary immune response** occurs that is faster, more prolonged and more effective because the memory cells are already in place and produce a new clone of plasma cells within hours. They produce sufficient antibodies to reach peak levels within 2 days.

Antibodies

Antibodies are also called **immunoglobulins** (Igs) and are present in the blood as the protein γ-globulin (Fig. 29.7). These soluble proteins are secreted by the activated B cell and the cloned plasma cells. Antibodies are grouped into five classes, each with a specific function. There is a basic antibody structure made of four polypeptide chains linked together by disulphide bonds. Two identical heavy chains are made up of about 400 amino acids. Two identical light chains are about half as long. The heavy chains are hinged about halfway along their length. There are two types of light chains, λ and κ, whose structures differ slightly. The chains form a Y-shaped molecule called an **antibody monomer**.

Each of the four chains is made up of different regions joined together. Each has a variable (V) region which is different from antibody to antibody and forms the binding site at one end and a much larger constant (C) region with the amino acid sequence being the same for all antibodies in a particular class. Between the V and C sections of the light chains is a region of amino acids called the joining (J) region. In the heavy chains, there is an additional region between the J and V sections called the diversity (D) region.

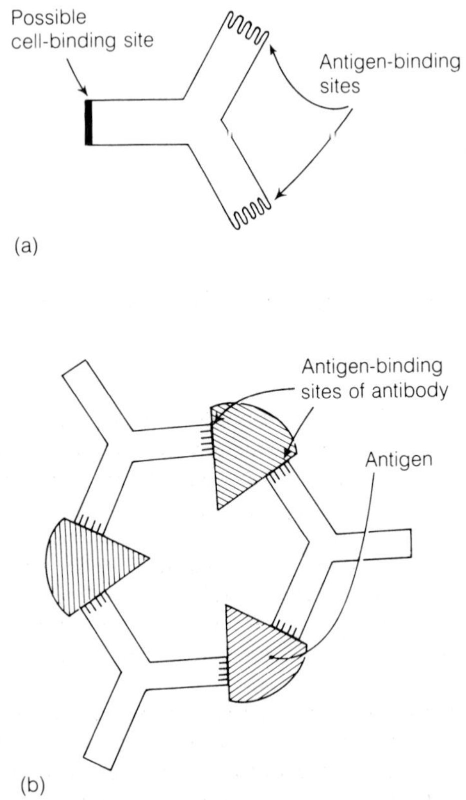

Figure 29.7 *Schematic diagram (a) to represent the structure of a simple (IgG type) antibody, and (b) to illustrate the way in which this bivalent structure enables antigens to be clumped together (from Hinchliff SM, Montague SE, 1990, with permission).*

Generation of antibody diversity

A relatively small number of immunoglobulin genes are recombined in individual B cells as they mature so that each mature B cell contains a unique antibody molecule. The genes are found on different chromosomes so that the chains are made separately and recombined as antibody monomers inside the cell.

Antibody classes

The five classes of immunoglobulin are given Greek alphabet names depending on their heavy chain structure and are referred to as Ig + the English alphabet letter.

Gamma = γ – IgG

This is produced in large quantities in the secondary response and diffuses most easily through blood vessel walls. It is the major class of antibody found in tissue fluids. It can cross the placenta to protect the fetus and is found in colostrum and breast milk to protect the infant.

Alpha = α – IgA

The main function of IgA is to protect the exposed surfaces of the body, in particular against bacteria and fungi. It is found in the mucus secretions of the mucous membranes lining the organs and in watery secretions such as tears, saliva and perspiration. The antibody monomers are combined in IgA to make a dimer (2) giving it a valency (number of binding sites) of 4.

Mu = μ – IgM

This immunoglobulin is found mainly in serum and is the first and most abundant antibody to be secreted during the primary response. It is found in the serum as a pentamer (5), taking the shape of a star and having a valency of 10, making it a large molecule. This allows it to bind to many antigens and causes them to agglutinate so that they are more easily recognised by the phagocytes.

Delta = δ – IgD

This molecule is almost always found attached to B cells and may be important in their activation.

Box 29.1 Gene recombination

The concept of immunoglobulin gene recombination can best be understood by thinking about Lego bricks. If a box held five bricks of each of the five colours (red, black, blue, yellow and white) and these could be combined in any order from all one colour through to five different colours, spend a few moments thinking about how many combinations of five bricks could be achieved! There are over 300 different genes for V κ light regions and five genes for J light regions, giving 1500 possible combinations of just the κ light chains! In the heavy chains there are 100 V genes, 30 D genes and four J genes, giving 100 × 30 × 4 = 12 000. As the light and heavy chains are combined separately from each other, this gives 18 million different possible antibody configurations.

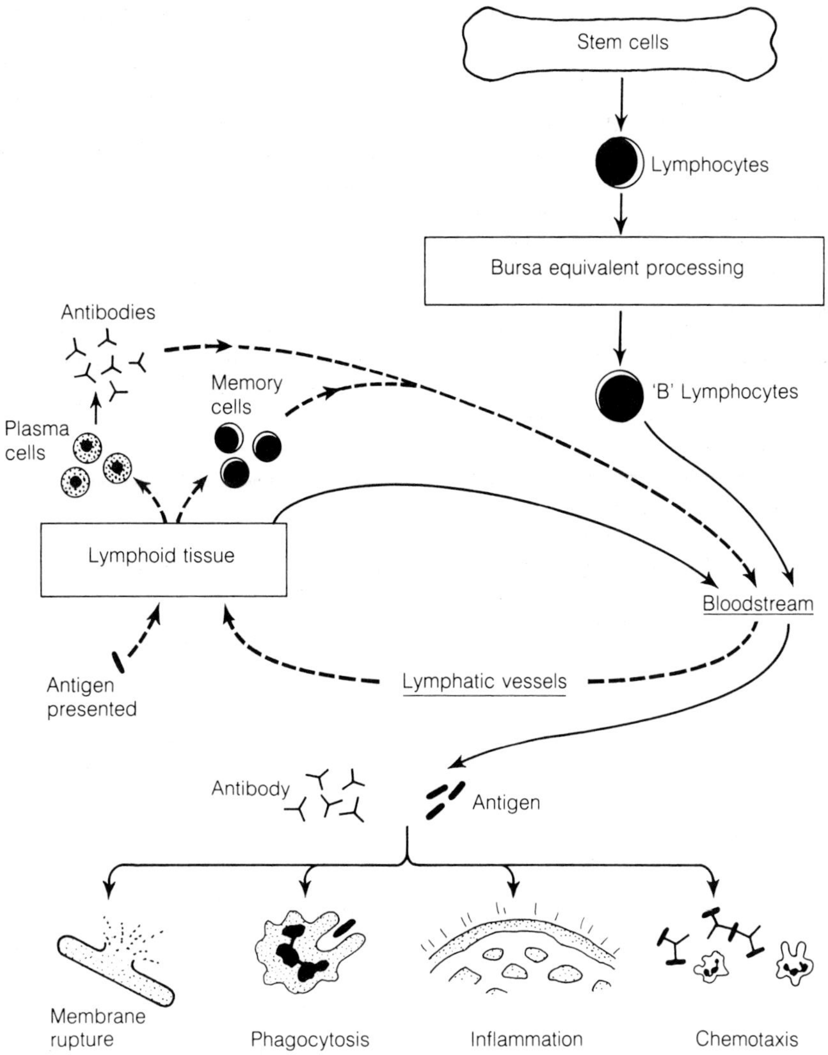

Figure 29.8 *Diagram to summarise the formation and protective function of the humoral immune system (from Hinchliff SM, Montague SE, 1990, with permission).*

Epsilon = ϵ – IgE

This molecule evolved to precipitate inflammatory reactions around parasites. It is seldom found free but is mainly bound by its constant region to the surface of basophils and mast cells found in skin, lungs and mucous membranes. These antibodies are likely to be synthesised in response to inhaled antigens. When an antigen binds to an IgE antibody, the cell degranulates, causing an acute inflammatory reaction. IgE is especially implicated in allergy or hypersensitivity reactions.

Antibody functioning

Antibodies do not destroy antigens directly but inactivate them and tag them for other parts of the immune system to destroy. They form antigen–antibody (immune) complexes with antigens. The destruction of the antigen-bearing molecules is accomplished by mechanisms including complement fixation, neutralisation, agglutination and precipitation. The first two of these are most important.

Complement fixation is the main protection against cellular antigens such as bacteria. When antibodies bind to the target cell their shape changes and this exposes complement-binding sites on their constant regions which trigger the complement cascade.

Neutralisation is a simple mechanism where antibodies block specific sites on viruses or chemicals secreted by bacteria called **exotoxins**, preventing them from binding to tissue cells and causing injury. Phagocytes then destroy the resulting immune complexes.

Agglutination or clumping together of cell-bound antigens occurs because antibodies have more than one binding site and molecules have more than one antigenic site. Large lattices are formed by the crosslinkage of immune complexes (remember blood typing).

Precipitation is a similar mechanism where soluble molecules are crosslinked into large complexes that settle out of solution. The large complexes caused by agglutination or precipitation become a target for engulfing by phagocytes.

Active and passive humoral immunity

Active immunity

Immunity to infectious diseases can be naturally acquired when a person's B cells produce antibodies against a bacterium or virus during an infection. However, the symptoms of the disease may cause serious illness or even death. Edward Jenner noticed that people who caught cowpox were unaffected by smallpox. In 1796 he inoculated young James Phipps with liquid from a pustule on the hand of Sarah Nelmes, a milkmaid who had cowpox. He then inoculated James with pus from a smallpox sufferer and James did not develop the disease. This technique is now used on a massive scale; the artificial protection of a person against infectious diseases by raising antibodies (Kedzierski 1992). The word vaccine derives from this first experiment (the Latin for a cow is *vacca*). Most vaccines contain dead or **attenuated** (weakened) pathogens which actively challenge the immune system without producing symptoms.

Passive immunity

Just as active immunity can be naturally or artificially acquired, so can passive immunity. The antibodies are not actively produced by a person's immune system but are obtained from another source. Protection against disease is limited to the survival time of the passively acquired antibodies which is at most 2–3 weeks. Naturally occurring passive immunity is acquired by the fetus from the mother with the transfer of IgG across the placenta and by the breastfed baby because of the presence of antibodies in breast milk. Injection of immune serum such as γ-globulin can offer passive immunity to a person needing short-term protection from a pathogen with which they have been in contact, such as hepatitis.

Cell-mediated immune response

T lymphocytes form the basis for cellular immunity. They are much more complex than B cells in their classification and function. There are three major groups of T cells: **cytotoxic** (killer cells), **helper** and **suppressor** T cells (Fig. 29.9). T cells are also classified according to which of two glycoproteins is present on the cell surface. These are the **CD4** and **CD8 surface receptor molecules** (CD means cluster of differentiation). Generally, helper T cells have CD4 proteins and are also known as T4 cells, especially in the HIV and AIDS literature, and the

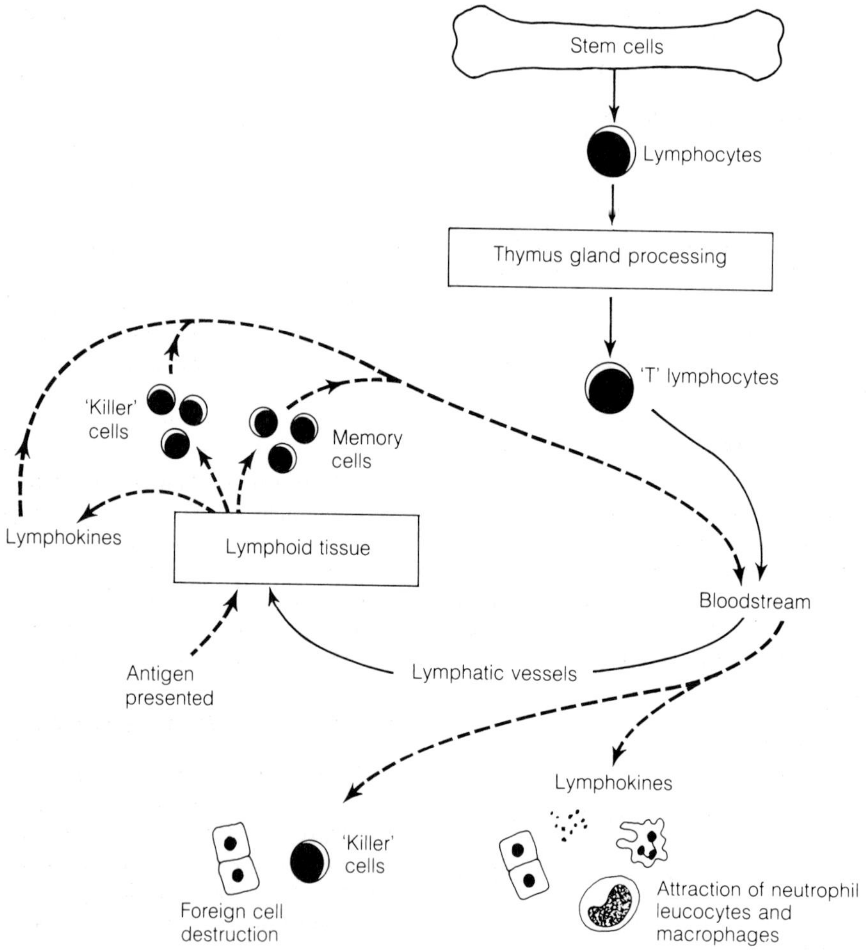

Figure 29.9 *Diagram to summarise the formation and protective function of the cell-mediated immune system (from Hinchliff SM, Montague SE, 1990, with permission).*

cytotocic and suppressor T cells have CD8 (T8) molecules on their surfaces.

Cytotoxic T cells act mainly against virus-infected cells but can kill cells invaded by certain bacteria such as the tubercle bacillus. Helper T cells chemically or directly stimulate the proliferation of other T cells and B cells by releasing a lymphokine called **interleukin 2**. Suppressor T cells release lymphokines that inhibit the activity of the activated B and T cells. This ensures that the immune response is brought to an end after the successful destruction of an antigen.

T cell response

There is a response by T cells as well as B cells to an antigen infection. B cells react with free antigens found in body fluids to form antigen–antibody complexes but T cells cannot recognise free antigens. They can only react to fragments of antigens attached to or displayed on the surface of the body cells. Most of the T cell activity (by cytotoxic T cells) is a direct attack on body cells infected by microorganisms, abnormal or cancerous cells or transplanted tissue.

The cells of the immune system are mutually supportive and release chemicals called **cytokines** (from cells) to stimulate each other. When activated T cells release such chemicals, they are known as **lymphokines** (from lymphocytes). Lymphokines enhance the activity of the cells in the immune system including the T cells themselves, B cells and macrophages. Macrophages release chemicals called **monokines** which stimulate T cells.

Differentiation of T cells – the major histocompatibility complex (MHC)

In order for T cells to be selected so that cloning can occur, there must be a double recognition of antiself (the antigen) and self. Every body cell has surface proteins that identify it as self. Proteins are coded for by the genes of the major histocompatibility complex (MHC) and provide the basis of human uniqueness as it is possible to combine them in millions of ways. Tissue transplants from one person to another are difficult as it is unlikely that two people will have identical MHC proteins unless they are identical twins.

There are two main classes of MHC protein important for T cell activation (Engelhard 1994). These are MHC class I and MHC class II. MHC I proteins are present on most body cells to enable self recognition but MHC II proteins are found only on the surfaces of mature B cells, macrophages and some T cells. MHC proteins act as the self part of the self–antiself complex which can activate the T cells. They are shaped like a hammock so that the antigenic fragment to be displayed sits inside them. If an antigen is sufficiently similar to self proteins, the T cells will not be able to recognise them.

Helper and cytotoxic T cells prefer different classes of MHC protein, a phenomenon called **MHC restriction**.

- Helper T cells bind only to complexes including MHC II proteins on the surfaces of macrophages.
- Cytotoxic T cells are activated by complexes with MHC I proteins on any body cell.

T cells crawl over other cells searching for antigens, a process called **immunologic surveillance**. When the T cell is activated by binding to the self–antiself complex, it enlarges and forms a clone. As with B cells, this is the primary response and some are left as memory cells.

The brain's immune system

White cells secrete substances capable of killing neurones. They are prevented from entering the brain by the blood–brain barrier and can only escape into the brain if the blood vessels are damaged (Streit & Kincaid-Colton 1995). Microglia metamorphose into a phagocytic state and behave like macrophages. Disturbed regulation of these cells has recently been implicated in neural disorders such as Alzheimer's disease and multiple sclerosis. These are the cells that HIV attacks in the brain and their activation is implicated in the development of AIDS dementia.

MATERNAL ADAPTATIONS TO PREGNANCY

The immune system in the pregnant woman alters so that she becomes to some extent immunocompromised (Blackburn & Loper 1992). The fetus is antigenically unique, as are all humans, and scientists wonder why the fetus is not rejected as foreign tissue by the mother's immune system. There are alterations to both primary and secondary host defence mechanisms in pregnancy. Although helping to protect the fetus, they may increase the severity of maternal infections and influence the progress of autoimmune diseases.

White cell count

The total white cell count rises in pregnancy, beginning at 2 months, mainly due to an increase in neutrophils. The neutrophil count rises in the menstrual cycle at the time of the oestrogen peak and continues to rise if fertilisation of the ovum occurs. A peak is reached at 30 weeks and a plateau maintained until delivery. There is a further rise in labour and the count returns to normal by the 6th postnatal day. Circulating oestrogen is probably the cause of the extra neutrophil production. There is a decrease in the number of natural killer cells, which may protect the placental trophoblast from destruction. There is a slight rise in eosinophils in relation to the increased white cell count but a sharp fall in circulating eosinophils occurs during labour. They are absent at delivery, returning to normal by the 3rd postnatal day. The basophil and monocyte counts appear to remain unchanged.

Cell-mediated immunity

Although the lymphocyte count remains unchanged in pregnancy there is profound depression of cell-mediated immunity. Oestrogen may increase the number of glycoproteins on the cell surface, leading to impaired response to stimuli. Human chorionic gonadotrophin from the placenta and prolactin from the anterior pituitary are known to suppress lymphocyte function. The depression of cell-mediated immunity is essential to the survival of the fetus but may increase susceptibility to viral infections. There is little if any change in humoral-mediated immunity. Levels of IgG become lower as pregnancy progresses. This may be due to haemodilution or the transfer of IgG across to the fetus.

THE IMMUNOLOGY OF IMPLANTATION AND PLACENTATION

The fetoplacental unit can be considered as an allograft, i.e. foreign tissue from the same species (Blackburn & Loper 1992). The fetus is separated from its mother by the placental barrier keeping the two circulatory systems separate. Paternal antigens are expressed on fetal cells as early as the eight-cell stage. This may mean that there are major antigenic differences between the mother and fetus. Any theory of maternal immune tolerance of the fetus must explain why the normal mechanisms of graft rejection do not occur. Normally, activated T cells would accumulate in a graft and cytotoxic activity would be directed against the graft tissue, resulting in its rejection and destruction. The alterations in the woman's immune system during pregnancy are insufficient to prevent the rejection of the fetus so other explanations have been sought. At the time of writing there is no consensus on the non-rejection of the fetus.

Blackburn & Loper (1992) summarise the theories of non-rejection as follows:

1 formation of blocking antibodies;
2 reduced antigenicity of the trophoblast;
3 production of immunosuppressor cells or factors by the fetus;
4 suppression of maternal immune system by hormonal or other factors such as the pregnancy-associated plasma proteins (PAPPS);
5 intrinsic alterations in the maternal immune system.

Stirrat (1991) examines the potentially immunoprotective elements using the following format:

1 the maternal uterus, in particular the endometrium and decidua;
2 the placenta with reference to the trophoblast;
3 the maternal immune response;
4 the fetal immune response.

The following paragraphs will attempt to summarise some of the findings by using Stirrat's headings.

The maternal uterus

It has been postulated that the uterus is an immunologically privileged site (IPS). This is probably not so and it is necessary to look at the specific role the endometrium/decidua plays. During pregnancy, the epithelial cells lining the endometrial glands have an absent or reduced expression of MHC I antigens. MHC II molecules are found in endometrial gland tissues. Bulmer et al (1986) suggested that steroid hormones in pregnancy may alter gene expression in the uteroplacental tissues. This may be important for the control of trophoblast invasion of maternal tissues.

Suppression of the immune response

Bulmer et al (1986) also discussed the presence of small endometrial granulocytes that may be related to NK cells. Stirrat mentions that Lala et al (1987) suggested that these granulocytes may release chemicals that suppress the activation of cytotoxic T cells. One of the chemicals has been found to be a prostaglandin – PGE_2. Other cells with leucocyte ability to present antigens are scattered throughout the decidua and these are most numerous at the implantation site. These may also produce suppressor factors.

The role of the placenta

MHC antigens

The role of the trophoblast at the fetomaternal interface may be important in protecting the fetus from the maternal immune system. Studies have shown that neither the villous cytotrophoblast nor the syncytiotrophoblast express MHC I antigens. Extravillous trophoblast cells express an unusual type of MHC I molecule which does not seem to be involved in immunological reactions. Therefore, it is unlikely that trophoblastic cells can initiate an attack or be the target for MHC-restricted T cells. Studies also indicate that there are no MHC II antigens expressed on any trophoblast cells, so it is unlikely that this tissue can initiate a classic immune reaction.

Other antigens

A system of antigens called trophoblast-lymphocyte cross-reactive (TLX) antigens may help to modify the immune reaction or maternal antibodies against these antigens have been found. They may act by downregulation of the complement system. Villous trophoblast cells also contain another complement regulatory protein called decay accelerating factor (DAF).

Maternal immune responses

It used to be thought that the immune system of a pregnant woman was unable to effect a response during pregnancy but this is not so, as discussed above. A brief summary of current findings discusses the role of the maternal immune system in relation to fetal and paternally derived antigens.

Sensitisation to trophoblast

IgG and IgM antibodies have been detected against the trophoblastic antigens other than MHC and TLX antigens The IgM response, as would be expected, falls to background levels by the 10th week but IgG is found throughout pregnancy. They are not found in every pregnancy and have no known role.

Sensitisation to paternally derived MHC antigens

Antipaternal antibodies are common but not universal in pregnancy. They appear by about 12 weeks and decline, only to increase again after delivery, and are present in 15% of first pregnancies and 60% of subsequent pregnancies. These antibodies are directed against both class I and II MHC antigens and may act by blocking stimulation of the B cell immune reaction. Mechanisms probably exist that block the recognition phase of the T cell response of cell-mediated immunity.

The fetal immune response

The human fetus begins to develop cell-mediated and humoral immunity from about 12 weeks. IgM antibody responses dominate and the fetus produces IgG and IgA with difficulty. Protection of the fetus from transplacental infection is therefore passive and due to maternal transfer of IgG. A high concentration of suppressor T cells has been seen which may help to develop self tolerance in the immune system. They may also destroy any maternal lymphocytes that cross into the fetal circulation.

Both maternal and fetoplacental mechanisms help prevent fetal rejection during pregnancy.

The immunology of breast milk

During the first week following delivery, colostrum and breast milk contain enormous quantities of immunoglobulin capable of reacting against many microorganisms. Bacteria that may cause gastroenteritis in the neonate, particularly Gram-negative coliform bacteria, are especially protected against. After the first week, IgA predominates. A wider discussion on the antiinfective benefits of breastfeeding will be given in Chapter 54.

CLINICAL IMPLICATIONS

Autoimmune disorders

Depending on the disorder, there may be improvement, deterioration or no change in the status of autoimmune disorders during pregnancy. The pathology of autoimmune disorders is thought to involve impairment of T cell suppressor activity, resulting in hyperactive B lymphocytes. These produce autoantibodies targeted against the body's own tissues and form immune complexes with the self antigens. The immune complexes activate the complement system, mediating phagocytosis and an inflammatory response (Blackburn & Loper 1992).

The changes in the immune system in pregnancy are exactly opposite to the above events so that in theory women with autoimmune disorders should experience relief from their symptoms. Most women with rheumatoid arthritis improve during pregnancy. However, women with systemic lupus erythematosus (SLE), particularly those who have renal involvement, will have an exacerbation of their condition. SLE is also associated with an increase in stillbirth, abortion, preterm birth and intrauterine growth retardation. This is possibly due to an immunoglobulin which binds to prothrombin-activating complexes, resulting in thrombosis in the spiral arteries of the uterus with placental abruption.

Maternal antibodies and the fetus

Maternal IgG is actively transported across the placenta by a carrier protein attached to a trophoblast surface receptor and protects the fetus from infectious diseases against which the mother has developed antibodies. However, dangerous IgG antibodies, such as those that develop in Rh incompatibility, can also cross the placenta.

The fetus of a woman with autoimmune disease may develop transient autoimmune symptoms. In Graves' disease, a thyroid-stimulating immunoglobulin passes across the placenta and may cause neonatal hyperthyroidism. Myasthenia gravis is associated with an antibody against acetylcholine receptors, resulting in profound muscle weakness. These antibodies can cross the placenta to produce transient myasthenia gravis in about 15% of neonates.

Pregnancy-induced hypertension (PIH) and the HELPP syndrome

The presence of antibodies to human vascular endothelial cells has been reported in many women with PIH and the HELLP syndrome. Blackburn & Loper (1992) write that some believe that the HELLP syndrome is a severe form of preeclampsia whilst others believe it is a different disorder and a specific form of pregnancy-induced immune syndrome (see Chapter 32).

Summary of main points

- The immune system plays an enormous part in the protection of the individual from environmental factors such as microorganisms, irritants and abnormal cells. Leucocytes are protective against bacteria, viruses, parasites, toxins and tumour cells. Most of the body's white cells are in the tissues and enter and leave the circulation from hour to hour by diapedesis.
- Several types of white cell can be distinguished by their shape, appearance and function. Granulocytes can be subdivided into neutrophils, eosinophils and basophils. Natural killer cells are a specialised type of large granular lymphocyte. Agranulocytes include lymphocytes and monocytes.
- Chemical messenger molecules are involved in the control of immunity. The cells and molecules that make up the immune response work together through a finely balanced network of interactions to produce a diverse response to either destroy the invading organism or reduce its harmful effects.
- The immune system can be divided into two groups of actions although there is a high level of interdependence between them. These are non-specific immunity, which immediately protects the body from all foreign substances, and specific immunity that acts against a particular invader but takes time to develop.
- Non-specific defences, including surface barriers such as the skin and mucous membranes, are the body's first line of defence. If the intact surfaces are breached other non-specific mechanisms are triggered into action. These are the cellular and chemical defences. In most cases there will be involvement of the phagocytic cells which engulf and destroy pathogens.
- Inflammation is the body's second line of defence and comes into

play when there is injury to the tissues. This response prevents the spread of damaging substances to nearby tissues, disposes of cell debris and pathogens and allows repair to begin. There are four cardinal signs of inflammation: heat, redness, swelling and pain.

- Fever occurs in response to pyrogens secreted by macrophages. High fevers inactivate enzymes and disrupt cellular metabolic processes but mild fevers are helpful to the body. Fever speeds up the metabolic rate of tissue, accelerating defensive actions and aiding repair. Other antibacterial responses include the sequestering of iron and zinc in the liver and spleen to prevent the bacteria from proliferating.
- The lymphatic system can be divided into the primary lymphoid organs, such as the bone marrow and thymus gland where the B cells and T cells differentiate and mature, and the peripheral lymphoid system, where they spend most of their active lives. The latter includes encapsulated organs such as the spleen, tonsils and lymph nodes and unencapsulated lymphoid tissue found in the gut, lungs and urogenital tract where white cells of many types are densely packed.
- There are two distinct regions in a lymph node: the outer cortex and the inner medulla. Macrophages are found throughout the gland but are concentrated in the medulla. B cells are concentrated in primary follicles in the cortex of the nodes. Cells at the centre of the follicle actively divide whilst those at the periphery of the follicle produce antibodies. T cells are found in the paracortical area.
- Lymph capillaries pick up pathogens and other foreign proteins so that the presence of immune cells in lymph nodes is very protective. Lymph transports water and small molecules and contains proteins, fluids, solutes and dietary fat. About 2–4 litres of lymph accumulates over 24 h and is returned to the blood via the large veins in the neck through the thoracic duct.
- The spleen's main function is the removal of ageing and defective red cells, cellular debris and microorganisms from the blood. There are also sites for the proliferation of lymphocytes. The thymus gland is more active in the early years of life and during adolescence it decreases in size and starts to atrophy. It is involved in the differentiation of T lymphocytes.
- Immunity could be divided into two types. Humoral or antibody-mediated immunity is provided by the presence of antibodies in the body fluids. When the lymphocytes attack the invader directly, the process is called cellular or cell-mediated immunity. The three main cell types involved in the immune response are B lymphocytes, T lymphocytes and macrophages.
- Macrophages are the cells at the centre of the immune response. They present antigens to the T cells for recognition by engulfing the foreign particles and presenting pieces on their cell surfaces. Macrophages secrete substances that activate T cells. T cells in turn secrete chemicals that activate macrophages to become phagocytic and secrete bactericidal chemicals.
- The immune response is the body's third line of defence, providing adaptive protection targeted at antigens recognised as non-self. The antigen has a small area called the epitope which is recognised by a small area on a receptor in the B lymphocyte cell membrane, called the antigen-binding site.
- Normally small molecules such as peptides are not immunogenic. If they link up with the body's own proteins they cause allergies. Molecules that do this are referred to as haptens and include penicillin and industrial pollutants. The defence system responds by producing antibodies.
- The binding of the antigen and the lymphocyte stimulates the B cell to divide rapidly to form a clone of identical cells all able to recognise that specific antigen. Most clone cells differentiate into plasma cells secreting antibodies at about 2000 per second for 5 days before the cell dies. This is the primary immune response. Clone cells that do not differentiate into plasma cells become long-lived memory cells able to mount a rapid secondary response if the antigen is encountered again.
- Antibodies are grouped into five classes, each with a specific function. These are IgG, IgA, IgM, IgD and IgE. Antibodies do not destroy antigens directly but inactivate them and tag them for other parts of the immune system to destroy. Mechanisms that complete the destruction of the antigen-bearing molecules include complement fixation, neutralisation, agglutination and precipitation.
- Immunity to infectious diseases can be naturally acquired when a person's B cells produce antibodies against a bacterium or virus during an infection. However, the symptoms of the disease will develop and in some cases death may result. Most vaccines contain dead or attenuated pathogens which actively challenge the immune system without producing symptoms.
- Just as active immunity can be naturally or artificially acquired, so can passive immunity. The antibodies are not actively produced by a person's immune system but are obtained from another source. Protection against disease is limited to the survival time of the passively acquired antibodies which is at most 2–3 weeks.
- Naturally occurring passive immunity is acquired by the fetus from the mother with the transfer of IgG across the placenta and by the breastfed baby because of the presence of antibodies in breast milk. Injection of immune serum such as γ-globulin can offer passive immunity.
- T lymphocytes confer cellular immunity. Cytotoxic T cells act against virus-infected cells but can kill cells invaded by certain bacteria. Helper T cells chemically or directly stimulate the proliferation of other T and B cells by releasing interleukin 2. Suppressor T cells release lymphokines that inhibit the activity of the activated B and T cells. T cells cannot recognise free antigens and react to antigenic fragments displayed on the surface of the body cells.
- The cells of the immune system are mutually supportive and release chemicals called cytokines to stimulate each other. Activated T cells release lymphokines which enhance the activity of the cells in the immune system, including themselves. Macrophages release chemicals called monokines which stimulate T cells.
- Every body cell has surface proteins that identify it as self, coded for by the genes of the major histocompatibility complex which is the basis of human uniqueness. It is difficult to transplant tissue from one person to another as it is unlikely that two people would have identical cell surface MHC proteins unless they were identical twins.
- There are two main classes of MHC protein important for T cell activation. MHC I proteins are present on most body cells, enabling self recognition, but MHC II proteins are found only on the surfaces of mature B cells, macrophages and some T cells. Helper T cells bind only to complexes which include MHC II proteins on the surfaces of macrophages. Cytotoxic T cells are activated by complexes with MHC I proteins on any body cell.
- Microglia in the brain become phagocytic and behave like macrophages. Disturbed regulation of these cells has been implicated in neural disorders such as Alzheimer's disease and multiple sclerosis. HIV attacks microglia and their activation is implicated in AIDS dementia.
- The immune system in the pregnant woman alters so that she becomes immunocompromised. The fetus is antigenically unique and it is not understood why the fetus is not rejected as foreign tissue by the maternal immune system. Alterations to both primary and secondary host defence mechanisms in pregnancy help to protect the fetus but may increase the severity of maternal infections and influence the progress of autoimmune diseases.
- Although the lymphocyte count remains unchanged in pregnancy with no alteration in circulating T cells and B cells there is profound depression of cell-mediated immunity which is essential to the fetal survival but may increase susceptibility to viral infections. There seems to be no impairment to immunoglobulin production or to humorally mediated immunity. Levels of IgG become lower as pregnancy progresses, possibly due to haemodilution or to the transfer of IgG to the fetus.

- The fetus is separated from its mother by the placental barrier. It inherits its MHC protein molecules and other tissue types from both its mother and father and paternal antigens are expressed on fetal cells as early as the eight-cell stage. Although there may be major antigenic differences between the mother and fetus, the feto-placental unit is tolerated by the maternal immune system for as long as necessary.
- Some of the better hypotheses on the non-rejection of the fetus are: formation of blocking antibodies, reduced antigenicity of the trophoblast, production of immunosuppressor cells or factors by the fetus, suppression of maternal immune system by hormonal or other factors and intrinsic alterations in the maternal immune system.
- During the first week following delivery, colostrum and breast milk contain enormous quantities of immunoglobulin capable of reacting against many microorganisms. Bacteria that may cause gastroenteritis in the neonate, particularly Gram-negative coliform bacteria, are especially protected against. After the first week IgA predominates.
- There may be improvement, deterioration or no change in the status of autoimmune disorders during pregnancy. The pathology of autoimmune disorders may involve impairment of T cell suppressor activity resulting in hyperactive B lymphocytes. The changes in the immune system in pregnancy are exactly opposite to the above events so that in theory women with autoimmune disorders should experience relief from their symptoms.
- Maternal IgG is actively transported across the placenta and can protect the fetus from infectious diseases against which the mother has developed antibodies. However, dangerous IgG antibodies, such as those that develop in Rh incompatibility, can also cross the placenta.
- Modern research suggests an immunological role in the cause of PIH.

References

Blackburn ST, Loper DL. 1992 Maternal, Fetal and Neonatal Physiology, A Clinical Perspective. WB Saunders, Philadephia.

Bulmer JN, Wells M, Bharra K, Johnson PM 1986 Immunohistological characterisation of endometrial gland epithelium and extravillous trophoblast in third trimester human placental bed tissues. British Journal of Obstetrics and Gynaecology 93, 823.

Davey B. 1989 Immunology. S325 Book 5, Biochemistry and Cell Biology. Open University Press, Buckingham.

Engelhard VH. 1994 How cells process antigens. Scientific American 270(2), 44–51.

Hinchliff SM, Montague SE. 1990 Physiology for Nursing Practice. Baillière Tindall, London.

Hinchliff SM. 1996 Innate defences. In Hinchliff SM, Montague SE, Watson R (eds) Physiology for Nursing Practice. Baillière Tindall, London, pp 621–653.

Kedzierski M. 1992 Vaccines and immunisation. New Scientist 133(1811) (suppl), 1–4.

Lala PK, Kearns M, Parhar RS. 1987 Immunology of the decidual tissue. In Gill TJ, Wegmann TG, Nisbet-Brown E (Eds) Immunoregulation and Fetal Survival. Oxford University Press, Oxford, cited in Stirrat G 1991 The Immune system. In Hytten F, Chamberlain G (Eds) Clinical Physiology in Obstetrics. Blackwell Scientific Press, Oxford.

Marieb EN. 1992 Human Anatomy and Physiology. Benjamin/Cummings Publishing California.

Stirrat G, 1991 The immune system. In Hytten F, Chamberlain G (Eds) Clinical Physiology in Obstetrics. Blackwell Scientific Press, Oxford, 101–136.

Streit WJ, Kincaid-Colton CA. 1995 The brain's immune system. Scientific American 38–43.

Recommended reading

Bulmer JN, Wells M, Bharra K, Johnson PM. 1986 Immunohistological characterisation of endometrial gland epithelium and extravillous trophoblast in third trimester human placental bed tissues. British Journal of Obstetrics and Gynaecology 93, 823.

Hinchliff SM. 1996 Innate defences. In Hinchliff SM, Montague SE, Watson R (Eds) Physiology for Nursing Practice, Baillière Tindall, London, pp 621–653.

Engelhard VH. 1994 How cells process antigens. Scientific American 270(2), 44–51.

Kedzierski M. 1992 Vaccines and immunisation. New Scientist 133(1811) (suppl), 1–4.

Streit WJ, Kincaid-Colton CA. 1995 The brain's immune system. Scientific American, 273(5), 38–43.

Section

2C

PREGNANCY – THE PROBLEMS

Section contents

Although pregnancy is a normal physiological function some women may develop illnesses independently of their pregnancy. Some minor health problems accompany many pregnancies but are not life threatening. These are discussed in chapter 30. Some long-term health problems such as diabetes mellitus are influenced greatly by the pregnancy and, perhaps the most widespread danger to pregnant women, pregnancy itself may precipitate a hypertensive condition in up to 10% of women. The remainder of Section 2C, chapters 31 to 35, discusses pathophysiological states relevant to the pregnant woman. Chapter 31 examines the possible causes and management of bleeding in pregnancy. Chapters 32 to 35 utilise a systems approach and each disorder is discussed in depth with its management in terms of diagnosis and physical treatment outlined.

Chapter 30 Minor disorders of pregnancy

In this chapter

INTRODUCTION

During pregnancy women suffer inconvenient but not life-threatening symptoms referred to collectively as the minor disorders of pregnancy or, as in a paper by Davis (1996), the discomforts of pregnancy. Jamieson (1996) gives a timely reminder that to the woman experiencing them either singly or, more likely, in combination, they are anything but minor. Also, a minor disorder may suddenly become a much more serious illness. For these two reasons it is essential for the midwife or doctor caring for women to pay attention to these symptoms and to offer safe and sensible advice on their alleviation.

MAINTENANCE OF PREGNANCY

Maternal physiological recognition of pregnancy begins with the presence of the blastocyst in the uterine cavity. The development of the embryo and placentation are described elsewhere.

The maintenance of the corpus luteum of pregnancy has been ascribed to the production of human chorionic gonadotrophin (HCG) by the cells of the trophoblast as they invade the endometrium. This is secreted into maternal blood and taken to the ovary where it augments the action of luteinising hormone from the anterior pituitary gland. It can be identified in blood early after embedding and before the first missed period and is excreted in urine to form the basis of the widely available and highly efficient immunological pregnancy tests. There is no ovulation and the endocrine production is changed to maintain the pregnancy. The role of the corpus luteum is to maintain the pregnancy by secreting steroid hormones, mainly progesterone, until the placenta can take over the major role about 50–60 days after the last menstrual period.

The corpus luteum continues to secrete progesterone until term. Another mechanism important in maintaining early pregnancy is the suppression of prostaglandin concentration in decidual tissue. Prostaglandin concentrations in early pregnancy are lower than those measured in the endometrium during the menstrual cycle. It is possible that prostaglandin production is inhibited by a glycoprotein called **lipocortin**. The hormone **relaxin**, a small polypeptide, seems to be produced by the corpus luteum in early and late pregnancy. It inhibits myometrial activity and may play a role in the maintenance of early pregnancy (Fig. 30.1).

Overview of the changes in pregnancy

Great changes occur in the major systems in pregnancy. The cardiovascular and haematological systems are particularly

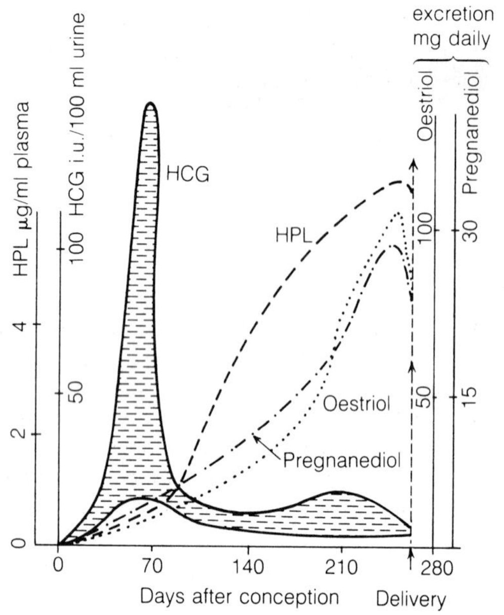

Figure 30.1 *Changes in hormone levels during pregnancy (HCG, human chorionic gonadotrophin; HPL, human placental lactogen) (from Hinchliff SM, Montague SE, 1990, with permission).*

affected but changes also involve all the other systems. This chapter describes minor problems resulting from the adaptation of the maternal body to provide a safe environment for the fetus.

MINOR DISORDERS OF PREGNANCY

Minor disorders of pregnancy are not life threatening but cause discomfort and distress to many women. The incidence, aetiology and midwifery management of minor pregnancy problems will be discussed below. Jamieson (1996) attributes the causes of the disorders to four categories: hormonal changes, accommodation changes, metabolic changes and postural changes. The hormonal changes are responsible for many of these irritating symptoms. In particular, the effect of progesterone on the smooth muscle and connective tissue of the body plays a large part in their causation. Davis (1996) divides the disorders into the trimester in which they are most likely to occur. The list is impressive but some of the disorders may be present throughout pregnancy, especially those associated with psychological well-being.

Disorders by trimester

- **1st trimester (0–14 weeks)** Breast tenderness, morning sickness, increased urinary frequency, fatigue
- **2nd trimester (15–28 weeks)** Fainting/dizziness
- **3rd trimester (29 weeks until delivery)** Slight nausea, increased urinary frequency
- **2nd and 3rd trimesters only** Constipation, heartburn, dyspnoea, varicose veins, ankle oedema, excessive weight gain, leg cramps, restless leg syndrome, carpal tunnel syndrome, increased vaginal discharge

Throughout pregnancy

- **Physical changes** Skin changes, backache, ligament pain, headache, stuffy nose, bleeding gums
- **Emotional changes** Mood swings, changing body image, depression, fearfulness, increased sensitivity, indecisiveness, alterations in libido

The digestive system

Nausea and vomiting

Incidence

This troublesome complaint begins early in pregnancy at the 4th week and persists usually until about week 12 in most sufferers, with a few continuing to have symptoms until the 16th week. Although commonly referred to as morning sickness, many women feel nauseous and may vomit at any time of day. Nausea and vomiting affects between 50% and 88% of women sufficiently to disrupt their day (O'Brien & Naber 1992). A few women will develop severe vomiting, known as **hyperemesis gravidarum**, which is life threatening to the woman and is discussed in Chapter 34.

Aetiology

The aetiology of nausea and vomiting is not fully understood and it may be that a combination of physical and emotional factors is involved. However, this period of time is close to the peak presence of HCG which may be a trigger. Oestrogen and progesterone may also be involved. Blackburn & Loper (1992) have found studies using a placebo to suppress nausea and vomiting that support a psychological component. This may be a simplistic concept of the manner in which the mind and body work in unison.

Alterations in thyroid function have been linked with nausea and vomiting in early pregnancy (Mori et al 1988). The severity of morning sickness has been correlated with the increased amount of free T_4 and decreased TSH. There is a link between altered thyroid gland function and nausea and excessive vomiting in pregnancy (Lao et al 1988).

An interesting theory put forward by Profet (1992) is derived from evolutionary theory. Profet believes morning sickness is adaptive and nausea and food aversions are there to minimise the exposure of the fetus to toxins during the period of organogenesis. Women are inclined to eat bland food without strong odours and flavours. This avoids the ingestion of spicy foods and plant toxins produced by bacterial and fungal decomposition. She supports this theory with one statistical observation that women who have no pregnancy nausea are more likely to miscarry. Nesse & Williams (1995) comment that if this is correct, pregnancy nausea is unlikely to be unique to humans.

Management

Non-pharmacological measures are safest and usually sufficient to combat nausea in pregnancy as there have been anxieties about the safety of antiemetic drugs. Light snacks instead of large meals and carbohydrate snacks at bedtime and before rising can prevent the hypoglycaemia that appears to be involved in the cause. The avoidance of iron supplements is advisable. Ginger capsules and ginger root tea have been found to combat nausea and vomiting in some diseases but Davis (1996) warns that the safety of this substance taken in quantity has not been established. If vomiting persists or becomes severe a medical practitioner should be consulted.

Heartburn

Incidence

Heartburn (**reflux oesophagitis**) is a burning sensation felt behind the sternum caused by reflux of acid gastric contents into the oesophagus. It is most problematic after 30 weeks of pregnancy, increasing in intensity until term and disappearing after delivery. Various studies have reported an incidence of 30–70% of women at some time in their pregnancy with 25% complaining of symptoms daily in the latter half of pregnancy (Blackburn & Loper 1992).

Aetiology

There are multiple factors involved in the cause of heartburn in pregnancy. The main factor is the relaxing effect of progesterone on the smooth muscle of the cardiac sphincter between the stomach and the oesophagus. In the non-pregnant woman sphincter tone increases in response to increased intragastric pressure as a protective measure to prevent reflux. This is greatly diminished in pregnancy. Pressure from the growing uterus increases the intragastric pressure and flattening of the diaphragm distorts the shape of the stomach and decreases the angle at the gastrojejunal junction. The incidence of heartburn is also increased by a higher frequency of development of hiatus hernia, affecting 15–20% of women after 7 months of pregnancy.

Management

Reflux can be prevented by not bending over when doing housework, such as cleaning the bath. Sleeping in a more upright position by using additional pillows can help at night. Small, frequent, bland meals low in spices and the avoidance of foods that may lower sphincter pressure, such as chocolate, coffee and alcohol, may be helpful. An antacid, such as a combination of aluminium and magnesium hydroxide, may be taken after meals and at bedtime under medical supervision.

Ptyalism

This disorder is excess salivation and is the equivalent of morning sickness. It is more common in women with an Afro-Caribbean background. In some cases the woman must continuously wipe saliva from her mouth with a tissue. The author's West Indian friends tell her it is referred to as 'spitting' and is a sign of pregnancy. If severe, it may lead to loss of fluids and electrolytes and dehydration. Similar advice as for morning sickness may help. It may also accompany heartburn.

Pica

This is the medical term for the craving for foods or substances such as coal. There is a belief that the craving occurs because of the fetus's need for certain minerals. Hormones and metabolic changes have also been implicated. Some substances, if eaten in excess, may be dangerous for the fetus so the person caring for the pregnant woman needs to know and to give advice if necessary.

Constipation

Incidence

There is a saying that each country has its problem organ and explains minor day-to-day illness as a malfunction of this organ. The French blame their livers and the British blame their colons and probably take more aperients than many nationalities. Constipation is a very common and troublesome disorder of pregnancy and may lead to the development of haemorrhoids which in turn may increase constipation because of a fear of pain.

Aetiology

The increased production of progesterone in pregnancy causes relaxation and reduced peristalsis in the smooth muscle of the digestive tract. This increases the transit time of food through the gut. The gut is also displaced upwards and outwards by the growing uterus. Faulty diet and disregarding the need to defaecate add to the problem. Oral iron therapy is also implicated by some women.

Management

Advice should be given to pregnant women as soon as they have had their pregnancies confirmed to avoid the situation if possible. It is necessary to ensure that they have an adequate fluid intake, maintain regular bowel habits and take in enough roughage in the form of fruits, vegetables and grains. Exercise is also useful. A stool softener or mild laxative can be helpful as an adjunct to the above advice.

The cardiovascular system

Fainting

Fainting and dizziness occur when insufficient blood and its oxygen reach the brain. As in many of these discomforts of pregnancy, the effect of progesterone on smooth muscle increases the incidence of fainting, although the expansion in circulating blood volume partly compensates. Standing erect for long periods and increasing vasodilation by being too warm may precipitate a faint. Later in pregnancy a woman may feel faint if she lies on her back and the weight of the uterus compressing the inferior vena cava prevents venous return to the heart, thus reducing cardiac output. This is called **supine hypotension syndrome**. It is easily prevented or reversed by avoiding the total supine position or turning a woman quickly onto her side if she begins to feel faint.

Varicosities

Varicosities are caused by the relaxing effect of progesterone on the smooth muscle of the walls of the veins. The circulation in the lower limbs becomes sluggish and the veins dilate, reducing the efficiency of the valves. The situation is made worse by the pressure of the growing uterus causing pelvic congestion and poor venous return. Varicose veins may occur in the legs, the anus (as haemorrhoids) and the vulva.

Varicose veins of the leg can be prevented by avoiding prolonged standing or sitting and exercising the leg muscles. Sitting with the legs elevated may help and support stockings can be put on before rising or after resting with the legs elevated.

Haemorrhoids are caused by the relaxing effect of progesterone on the veins of the anus, the reduction of venous return by the growing uterus and the incidence of constipation. Haemorrhoids can be helped by the prevention and treatment of constipation. If needed, topical applications can be suggested and medical advice sought. As the haemorrhoids often disappear after delivery and because of the alteration in venous tone, surgery would not be performed in pregnancy.

Vulval varicosities, whilst rare, are very painful. A sanitary pad or sometimes a panty girdle may give support. Care must be taken during delivery as there is a risk of haemorrhage from the distended veins, especially if cut during an episiotomy.

The musculoskeletal system

Backache

Incidence and aetiology

Davis (1996) reports that at least 50% of women experience backache in pregnancy. It is essential to differentiate the cause of back pain so that appropriate treatment can be obtained. Ostgaard et al (1991) state that some of the contributing factors are postural changes resulting in lumbar lordosis with overstretched abdominal muscles and strained back muscles. There is also the relaxing effect of progesterone on the pelvic ligaments, allowing movement of the symphysis pubis and lumbosacral joints. They also write that relaxin may affect the intervertebral joints, making them unstable as they try to support the increased weight of pregnancy. Davis (1996) mentions that Brooks et al (1990) hypothesise that demineralisation of bone may play its part in causing hip and back pain in late pregnancy. Mild backache may present at the beginning of labour whilst pain in the flank may indicate a urinary tract infection.

Assessment will include:

- location, extent, onset, duration, nature and degree of pain
- any other symptoms
- relationship to activities
- self treatment strategies.

Management

Once the more worrying causes of backache are excluded, the woman can be advised on back care to minimise pain. Brayshaw (1996) gives the following advice.

Sitting

She should choose a comfortable chair which supports both back and thighs when sitting. She should sit well back and it may be necessary to place a small cushion behind the lumbar spine.

Standing

The woman should stand tall with her tummy and buttocks tucked in. Weight should be evenly distributed on both legs and a low shoe heel should be worn.

Lying

Equal pressure on all parts of the body should be ensured by a good mattress. Women should avoid lying on their backs because of the risk of supine hypotension and diminished blood flow to the uterus. Lying on the side with sufficient pillows to be comfortable is best. Care should be taken when changing from lying down to avoid strain on back and abdominal muscles. The arms should be used to push up into a sitting or kneeling position. This advice should be heeded by those giving care. The author has seen many a doctor turn away to write up notes following examination, leaving the woman to struggle upright on the narrow high couch!

Work

Lifting or dragging heavy objects should be avoided and women should discuss the best position for managing their work both in business and at home.

Two other muscle discomforts of pregnancy, restless leg syndrome and cramp, are discussed in Chapter 24 as calcium metabolism may be implicated in their cause.

The nervous system

Carpal tunnel syndrome

Women who develop carpal tunnel syndrome complain of numbness and tingling, often called pins and needles, in their fingers and hands. This is most likely to be present in the morning but can occur at any time of day. The cause is fluid retention and swelling of connective tissue which compresses the median nerve as it runs through the carpal tunnel in the wrist. It may be necessary for the woman to wear a splint at night and elevate the hand. Occasionally diuretics may be prescribed by the doctor.

Fatigue

Incidence

Reeve (1991) reported on an exploratory study on fatigue in early pregnancy and found that the symptom of fatigue necessitated changes in the daily routine of 70% of the sample of 30 women. The women had reduced the amount of housework they did and reported an increased need for sleep. They reported that they had begun to experience fatigue within 4 weeks of the first missed menstrual period and that the symptom continued into the 2nd trimester of pregnancy.

Aetiology

Fatigue was associated with the younger women in the above sample and correlated positively with nausea. Davis (1996) refers to Lee & DeJoseph (1992) in her summary of the aetiology of fatigue. Associated factors include poor nutrition, anaemia, slowed circulation and sleep disturbances caused by urinary frequency, leg cramps, breathing problems and vomiting. Jamieson (1996) considers the effect of nausea and vomiting associated with fatigue on the well-being of women in early pregnancy.

Management

The management of fatigue in pregnancy includes attending to all the possible associated factors. Carers should ensure that women take a balanced diet, are involved in moderate exercise and are able to relax. Dealing with sleeplessness is part of the care. Adjusting the phosphorus content may decrease the likelihood of leg cramps.

Emotional changes

Emotional changes in pregnancy include mood swings, changing body image, depression, fearfulness, increased sensitivity, indecisiveness and alterations in libido with either increased or decreased sexual activity. Davis (1996) briefly discusses these changes which are complex and involve the personality type of the woman, her knowledge base, her response to physical symptoms and fears and anxieties about the outcome of pregnancy as well as psychological and social factors.

Many authors, such as Oakley and Kitzinger, have written extremely good books on these aspects of pregnancy and it remains for this author to remind readers that many physical symptoms may have their origin in emotional states. These include palpitations, breathlessness, headache, lack of appetite, nausea and vomiting and loss of weight, to mention a few. It is sensible to consider the woman as a whole person, body and mind together, when planning care or diagnosing problems.

Genitourinary system

Frequency of micturition

Urinary frequency affects women most in the first and 3rd trimesters, mainly because of pressure on the bladder from the growing uterus. During the 2nd trimester the uterus is displaced upwards over the pelvic brim and the incidence of frequency is lower.

There is also the enhanced reabsorption of sodium and water which increases the need to pass urine through the night, called **nocturia**. During the day the excess water is trapped in the lower extremities because of venous stasis. When the woman lies down at night pressure on the large veins is reduced, there is increased cardiac return, cardiac output and renal blood flow with a subsequent increase in urinary output.

Small lifestyle changes can reduce nocturia.

- Restrict fluids in the evening by increasing the fluid intake earlier in the day.
- Limit the intake of natural diuretics such as caffeine.
- Lie down in the left lateral recumbent position during the evening to encourage a diuresis.

Leucorrhoea

There is an increase in white, non-irritant vaginal discharge in pregnancy. Once the possibility of vaginal moniliasis or trichomonal infection has been excluded, simple personal hygiene will ensure comfort for the woman. Wearing cotton pants and avoiding tights will also increase comfort.

Summary of main points

- Maternal physiological recognition of pregnancy begins with the presence of the blastocyst in the uterine cavity. The corpus luteum of pregnancy is maintained by trophoblastic HCG. There is no ovulation and the endocrine production is changed to maintain the pregnancy. The corpus luteum continues to secrete progesterone until term.
- During pregnancy women suffer minor disorders of pregnancy. A minor disorder may suddenly become a much more serious illness. The causes of the disorders are hormonal, accommodation, metabolic and postural changes.
- Minor disorders include breast tenderness, morning sickness, increased urinary frequency, leg cramps, restless leg syndrome, carpal tunnel syndrome, increased fatigue, fainting/dizziness, constipation, heartburn, dyspnoea, varicose veins, haemorrhoids, ankle oedema, vaginal discharge, skin changes, backache, ligament pain, headache, stuffy nose, bleeding gums, mood swings, changing body image, depression, increased sensitivity, indecisiveness and alterations in libido.

References

Blackburn ST, Loper DL. 1992 Maternal, Fetal and Neonatal Physiology, A Clinical Perspective. WB Saunders, Philadelphia.

Brayshaw E. 1996 Special exercises for pregnancy, labour and the puerperium. In Bennett VR, Brown LK (eds) Myles Textbook for Midwives, 12th edn. Churchill Livingstone, Edinburgh, pp 648–659.

Brooks GG, Thomas BV, Wood MJ. 1990 Hip pain in late pregnancy. Journal of Reproductive Medicine 35, 969–970.

Davis DC. 1996 The discomforts of pregnancy. Journal of Obstetric, Gynecologic and Neonatal Nursing 25(1) 73–81.

Hinchliff SM, Montague SE. 1990 Physiology for Nursing Practice. Baillière Tindall, London.

Jamieson L. 1996 Minor disorders of pregnancy. In Bennett VR, Brown LK (eds) Myles Textbook for Midwives, 12th edn. Churchill Livingstone, Edinburgh, pp 117–122.

Lao T, Chin R, Mak Y, Panesar N. 1988 Plasma zinc concentration and thyroid function in hyperemetic pregnancies. Acta Obstetrica et Gynaecologica Scandinavica 677, 599–604.

Lee KA, DeJoseph JF. 1992 Sleep disturbances, vitality and fatigue among a select group of employed childbearing women. Birth 19, 208–213.

Mori M, Amino N, Tamaki H et al. 1988 Morning sickness and thyroid function in normal pregnancy. Obstetrics and Gynaecology 72(3,1), 355–359.

Nesse RM, Williams GC. 1995 Evolution and Healing. Weidenfeld and Nicolson, London.

O'Brien B, Naber S. 1992 Nausea and vomiting during pregnancy: effects on the

quality of women's life. Birth 19, 138–143.
Ostgaard HC, Andersson GB, Karlson K. 1991 Prevalence of back pain in pregnancy. Spine 16, 549–552.
Profet M. 1992 Pregnancy sickness as adaptations: a deterrant to maternal ingestion to toxins In Barkow JH et al (eds) The Adapted Mind. Oxford University Press, New York, pp 327–365.
Reeve J. 1991 Calcium metabolism. In Hytten F, Chamberlain G (eds) Clinical Physiology in Obstetrics, 2nd edn. Blackwell Scientific, Oxford, pp 213–223.

Recommended reading

Davis DC. 1996 The discomforts of pregnancy. Journal of Obstetric, Gynecologic and Neonatal Nursing 25(1), 73–81.
Lee KA, DeJoseph JF. 1992 Sleep disturbances, vitality and fatigue among a select group of employed childbearing women. Birth 19, 208–213.
Mori M, Amino N, Tamaki H et al. 1988 Morning sickness and thyroid function in normal pregnancy. Obstetrics and Gynaecology 72(3,1), 355–359.
O'Brien B, Naber S. 1992 Nausea and vomiting during pregnancy: effects on the quality of women's life. Birth 19, 138–143.
Ostgaard HC, Andersson GB, Karlson K. 1991 Prevalence of back pain in pregnancy. Spine 16, 549–552.

Chapter 31 Bleeding in pregnancy

In this chapter

BLEEDING IN EARLY PREGNANCY

Any bleeding from the genital tract during pregnancy is abnormal and all women who bleed should be seen by a doctor. Barron (1995) wrote that bleeding from the genital tract may be considered in two groups: bleeding before or after the 24th week of pregnancy, an arbitrary cut-off point of fetal viability. Lindsay (1997) lists the causes of bleeding prior to the 24th week as implantation bleeding, abortion, ectopic pregnancy, cervical lesions and vaginitis.

Bleeding from trophoblastic disease with hydatidiform mole and choriocarcinoma is another possible cause of bleeding in early pregnancy. Axelsen et al (1995) examined the characteristics of bleeding during pregnancy. They found that the overall incidence was 19%, with the median being 8 weeks. Duration of bleeding was about 2 days and there was usually only one episode. Two-thirds of the women had no abdominal pain accompanying the bleeding and only one in five women was admitted to hospital.

Implantation bleeding

As the trophoblast cells erode the maternal endometrium during embedding a small amount of bleeding may occur. The bleeding is bright red and occurs about 8–12 days after fertilisation which is just before the next menstrual period is due. The woman may give this date as the first day of her last menstrual period and the expected date of delivery will be calculated wrongly.

Abortion

Spontaneous abortion is a serious cause of bleeding in early pregnancy and is fairly common. Human reproduction is not very efficient and it has been estimated that 45% of conceptions may be lost before the 20th week (Arias 1993). However, most of them are lost before implantation and only a quarter of them are clinically recognised as abortions. The risk of a recognisable spontaneous abortion is about 15% in women with no previous pregnancy loss and 19% for repeated abortion in women with no living children. If two consecutive pregnancies are lost in spontaneous abortion, the risk rises to 35% and to 47% after three consecutive abortions (Arias 1993). The aetiology of abortion is shown in Table 31.1.

About 80% will occur before 12 weeks gestation, classified as early abortions, and the rest will occur between 13 and 24 weeks and are referred to as late abortions. There is a clinical reason for differentiating abortions into early and late. The majority of early abortions are due to anembryonic pregnancies or blighted ova whilst those with a formed fetus present usually occur after 13 weeks. Anembryonic abortions are suggestive of genetic faults whilst the development of a fetus suggests the possibility of many causes.

Classification of spontaneous abortion

Spontaneous abortions may be classified as threatened,

Table 31.1 *Aetiology of abortion*

Cause	*Percentage of total*
Genetic abnormalities – mainly chromosomal abnormalities arising during meiosis of ovum or sperm	50–60
Endocrine abnormalities – progesterone deficiency, thyroid deficiency, diabetes, increased androgens, elevated luteinising hormone as in polycystic ovary	10–15
Chorioamniotic separations – there may be bleeding beneath the chorion or between the amnion and chorion	5–10
Incompetent cervix – usually the result of cervical trauma	8–15
Infections – usually ascending but occasionally due to systemic microbial infections such as rubella, *Listeria*, toxoplasmosis, *Chlamydia*	3–5
Abnormal placentation – failure of the trophoblastic invasion of the spiral arteries	5–15
Immunological abnormalities – may be the cause of repeated spontaneous abortions and have recognisable serum antibodies	3–5
Uterine anatomic abnormalities – caused mainly by failure of the Mullerian ducts to unite in the embryonic stage, resulting in septate uterus. A fibroid uterus may also cause abortion	1–3
Unknown reasons	<5

inevitable, missed, recurrent or septic (Fig. 31.1). A brief description of each type follows.

Threatened abortion

In threatened abortion bleeding may occur. It may be painless or there may be lower abdominal pain or backache. There is usually no cervical dilatation. Ultrasound may be used to ensure the presence of a living fetus and the treatment is bed rest. If the bleeding becomes heavy the pregnancy may be proceeding to inevitable abortion.

Inevitable abortion

Inevitable abortion is accompanied by cervical dilatation. The bleeding is more severe and may result in maternal collapse. The gestation sac separates from the uterine wall and the uterus contracts to expel it. This results in pain similar to that experienced in labour. If the gestation sac is completely expelled the term used is **complete abortion**. If part, usually the placental tissue, is retained this is termed an **incomplete abortion**. Any products of conception should be retained for inspection by the doctor to ascertain whether the abortion is complete or incomplete.

If the abortion is complete and the condition of the woman is good all that is required at that time is ergometrine 0.5 mg or syntometrine 1 ml. If the abortion is incomplete or the woman has lost a lot of blood she is transferred to hospital by a paramedic team and ambulance. The paramedics can resuscitate her if necessary. The retained products of conception must be removed under general anaesthetic and a blood transfusion carried out if necessary.

Missed abortion

Missed abortion may also be called carneous mole, blood mole or fleshy mole. A threatened abortion occurs, bleeding between the gestation sac and the endometrium takes place and the embryo dies. The uterus does not grow but there may be no bleeding so that the woman thinks her pregnancy is continuing. There is usually a brownish discharge. Gradually the signs of pregnancy disappear. Diagnosis by ultrasound is made and the woman should be admitted for evacuation of the uterus. A suction curette may be used or oral mifepristone (RU46) may be used. If the uterus is larger than 13 weeks a combination of vaginal prostaglandins and intravenous syntocinon will be used. Although the uterus would eventually expel the mole there is a risk of disseminated intravascular coagulation.

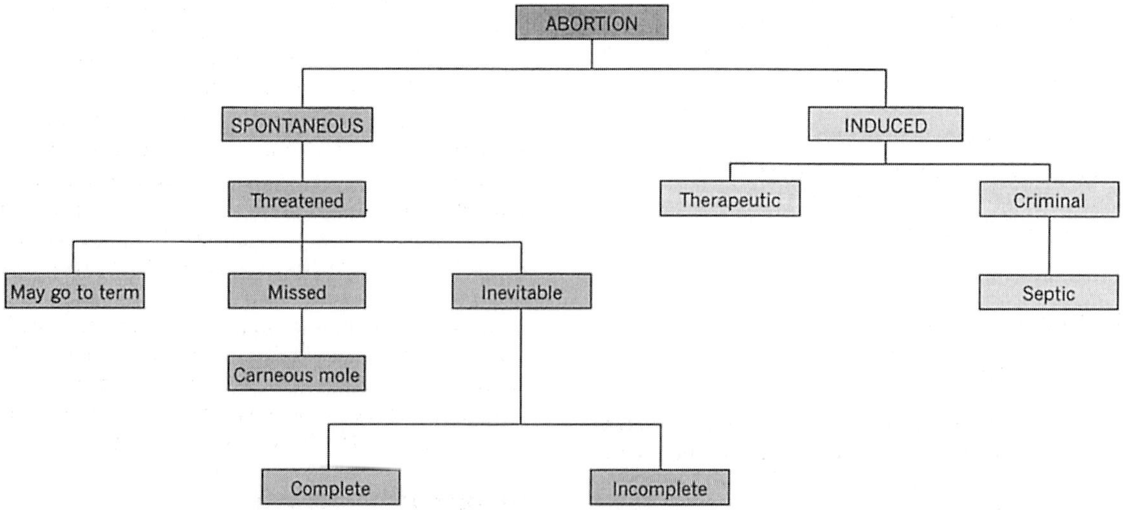

Figure 31.1 *The classification of abortion (from Sweet B, 1997, with permission).*

Recurrent abortion

The term recurrent abortion is used if three or more consecutive abortions occur. The cause is usually the same in all the recurrences.

In women who have recurrent abortions investigations to ascertain the cause are made. Treatment will then vary depending on the cause. For instance, if the cause is immunological and the woman is found to have none of the blocking antibodies that normally protect the fetus, she may be injected with paternal or donor lymphocytes before pregnancy. However, this treatment is still controversial as the theory of alloimmune rejection of the fetus by the mother's immune system is difficult to support (Arias 1993).

Therapeutic abortion

Abortions may be induced in unwanted pregnancies. Therapeutic abortions have been available in the United Kingdom since 1967 but there are other countries where the procedure is illegal. The lack of an abortion law leads to the risk of women seeking illegal abortions, often carried out in unfavourable conditions by unskilled practitioners, including the woman herself. The methods used to evacuate the uterus are those described under the heading of missed abortion:

- mifepristone (RU486);
- suction evacuation;
- menstrual evacuation if the woman's menstrual period is late;
- prostaglandin administration.

The older methods of intraamniotic saline and hysterotomy are rarely used.

Septic abortion

Sepsis may follow any type of abortion, spontaneous or therapeutic. The term septic abortion is used in such cases. This is a serious condition and is potentially fatal. Septicaemia, endotoxic shock and disseminated intravascular coagulation may follow. Liver and renal damage may also occur. Pelvic infection may lead to the formation of adhesions, salpingitis and infertility. Sepsis may also occur in any invasive uterine operation such as chorionic villus sampling or amniocentesis.

A woman with sepsis will be ill with a raised temperature and pulse, headache, nausea and general malaise. The uterus may be tender and there may be an offensive vaginal discharge. Typically the organisms responsible are *Staphylococcus aureus, Clostridium welchii, Escherichia coli, Klebsiella* and occasionally the haemolytic streptococcus group A. Antibiotics may need to be given intravenously. These are started before any surgical intervention is made (Lindsay 1997).

Trophoblastic disease

Hydatidiform mole

Hydatidiform mole is a benign neoplastic disease, an abnormal growth of the trophoblast where the chorionic villi proliferate, become avascular and are filled with fluid (Fig. 31.2). The decidual spaces become obliterated and maternal blood cannot circulate (Kelly 1996). The mole has the appearance of a creamy white bunch of grapes which may be up to 1 cm in diameter (Lindsay 1997). This degeneration of the chorionic villi in early pregnancy is usually accompanied by the death and reabsorption of the fetus because of the lack of oxygen and nutrients. The mole enlarges rapidly to fill the whole uterus which is larger than the period of gestation indicates. **Partial moles** may occur where there is a fetus and areas of normal villi with patchy areas of cystic villi. Partial moles are rarely followed by malignant change whereas this may occur in up to 10% of complete moles.

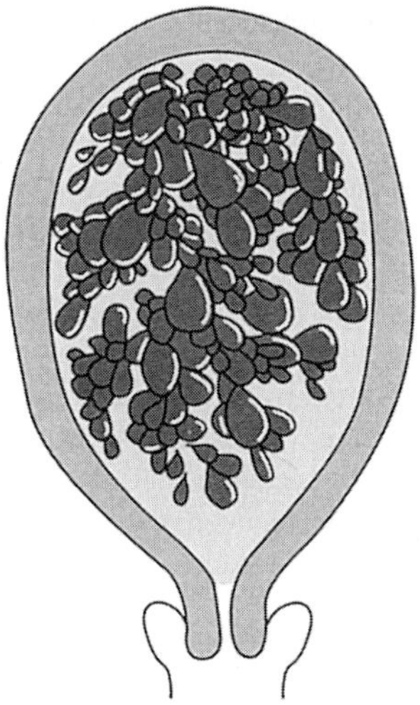

Figure 31.2 *A hydatidiform mole (from Sweet B, 1997, with permission).*

Aetiology

In the United Kingdom hydatidiform mole occurs in one in 1000 pregnancies. It is more common in:

- women under 15 or over 50;
- multiparous women;
- women who smoke;
- those who have a previous history of hydatidiform mole.

The condition has been reported to vary in geographical distribution, being four times as common in Asia as in Europe and the USA (Llewellyn-Jones 1990). The incidence doubled in the United Kingdom between 1973 and 1983.

Genetic and biochemical markers have shown that over 90% of complete hydatidiform moles are derived entirely from paternal genes. It may be that the sperm enters an ovum which has lost its nucleus. The haploid sperm duplicates its chromosomes and the sperm must be an X-bearing one giving a 23X complement, as 46YY is non-viable. Therefore, moles are 46XX in their karyotype. In about 10% of cases two sperm may penetrate the anuclear ovum, one X-bearer and one Y-bearer, to give a karyotype of 46XY (Llewellyn-Jones 1990). This heterozygous diploid fertilisation is associated with an increased risk of malignancy. The karyotype of a partial mole is usually triploid, either 69XXX or 69XXY (Blackburn & Loper 1992).

Signs and symptoms

- Intermittent vaginal bleeding may occur from about the 12th

week of pregnancy and there may be heavy bleeding when the mole begins to abort.
- The pregnancy may be complicated by early onset of preeclampsia and hyperemesis gravidarum.
- On examination the uterus is found to be large for dates and no fetal parts will be palpated in a complete mole, nor will a fetal heart be heard.
- There may be mild signs of thyrotoxicosis due to the action of HCG which is similar to TSH.
- Diagnosis is confirmed by ultrasound scan, which will show a snowstorm effect of multiple vesicles. Urinary or serum HCG is very high, exceeding that of a multiple pregnancy. Molar pregnancies have been detected through the triple screening for Down's syndrome.

Management

Immediately diagnosis is confirmed the uterus must be emptied by suction curettage. If the mole has begun to abort the process can be accelerated by syntocinon infusion or prostaglandins. Once the mole has aborted the uterus is carefully curetted as any remaining placental tissue may lead to the development of a choriocarcinoma.

Following the emergency treatment careful observation must be continued for one year to ensure that there is no progression to choriocarcinoma. β HCG levels are monitored fortnightly for 2 months then monthly for a year. Serum assays are more accurate but it is easier to obtain urinary assays. Persistently high HCG levels indicate that the mole is still growing and the woman is at risk of malignant trophoblastic disease. Women who have had hydatidiform moles must avoid a further pregnancy until the follow-up programme is completed. Hormonal contraception should be avoided as it increases the chance of developing malignant disease.

Choriocarcinoma

Between 5% and 10% of women may go on to develop malignant trophoblastic disease or choriocarcinoma. The incidence of malignancy is one in 10 following a hydatidiform mole, one in 5000 following a spontaneous abortion and one in 50 000 following a normal pregnancy. The malignancy begins within 6 months of molar expulsion (Llewellyn-Jones 1990). The tumour is very invasive and treatment must be commenced immediately following diagnosis. There are two forms of the disease:

1 malignancy confined to the uterus (**invasive mole**);
2 malignancy with extrauterine spread (**choriocarcinoma**).

Diagnosis

- The test for HCG will be strongly positive, as in a pregnancy.
- Vaginal bleeding may recur.
- Serum concentrations of the hormone **inhibin** may be significantly elevated.
- There is an increase in pain.
- Local invasion and metastases to the lungs, liver and brain will occur unless treatment is vigorous.

Treatment

Choriocarcinoma responds very well to chemotherapy. The administration of cytotoxic drugs such as methotrexate, etoposide and actinomycin-D will provide a cure in almost every case. The problem of toxicity is as for every use of cytotoxic drugs, with malaise, stomatitis, pharyngitis, diarrhoea, leucopenia and alopecia. Follow-up treatment continues for 1 year with the avoidance of pregnancy or the hormonal contraceptive.

Ectopic pregnancy

An ectopic pregnancy is when the fertilised ovum implants outside the uterine cavity. In 95% of cases the site of implantation is the uterine tube, a **tubal pregnancy**. More rarely, the implantation site may be the ovary, the cervical canal or the abdominal cavity. Ectopic pregnancy is a serious condition and is the major cause of maternal death before 20 weeks of pregnancy. The incidence of ectopic pregnancy varies from one in 28 in the West Indies to one in 150 whilst the overall incidence has tripled since 1970 (Blackburn & Loper 1992). However, these figures may not reflect an absolute rise in incidence as diagnosis may now be made more often because of the use of ultrasound. It is possible that up to 50% of ectopic pregnancies abort spontaneously or are resorbed. Abdominal pregnancy is much commoner in African countries than elsewhere.

Tubal pregnancy

The rise in incidence of tubal pregnancies is thought to be due to the increase in sexually transmitted diseases, the use of the oral contraceptive pill and the intrauterine device and the delay in starting a family until later in reproductive life. Any condition that delays the transport of the zygote along the uterine tube may lead to a tubal pregnancy (Fig. 31.3). This may be due to malformation of the tubes but is more likely to be due to tubal scarring and the loss of cilia due to pelvic infection. Once the zona pellucida is shed at about the 4th day following fertilisation, implantation can occur. If the ovum is fertilised just before the onset of menstruation the zygote may be delayed by the backflow of menstrual blood (Llewellyn-Jones 1990). The right and left uterine tubes are affected equally.

Risk factors for tubal pregnancy include:

- an older woman;
- women of low gravidity or parity;

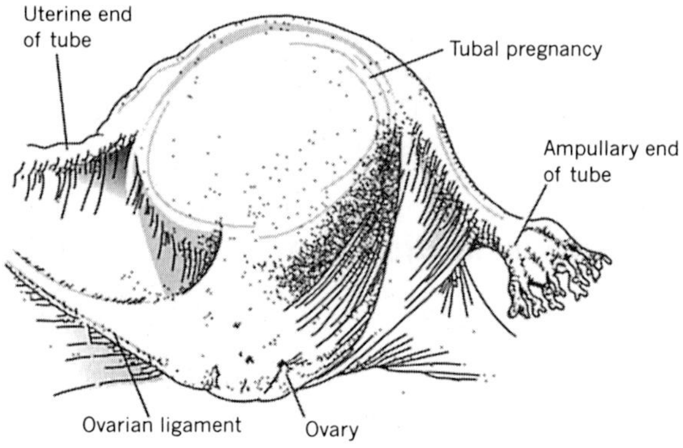

Figure 31.3 *Tubal pregnancy (from Sweet B, 1997, with permission).*

- previous tubal pregnancy;
- tubal surgery;
- salpingitis;
- intrauterine contraceptive device;
- hormonal stimulation of ovulation;
- in vitro fertilisation and embryo transplant;
- tubal endometriosis;
- pelvic inflammatory disease (PID);
- pelvic or abdominal surgery;
- progestogen-only pill (interferes with the action of the cilia).

Pathophysiology

Implantation occurs in:

- the fimbriated part of the tube – 17%;
- the ampulla – 55%;
- the isthmus – 25%;
- the ovary – 0.5%;
- the abdominal cavity – 0.1%.

The hormones produced by the corpus luteum and the trophoblast influence uterine growth and the formation of a decidua. The outcome varies depending on where in the tube implantation occurs, its ability to distend and the size of blood vessel eroded. If the pregnancy occurs in the fimbriated end or the ampulla the conceptus may continue to grow until 10 weeks. The gestation sac may be expelled into the abdominal cavity as a tubal abortion (Fig. 31.4). Blood clot may be organised around the separated sac to form a tubal mole which may remain in the uterine tube or be expelled from the fimbriated end as a tubal abortion. Tubal rupture (Fig. 31.5) may lead to devastating haemorrhage. The most severe haemorrhage occurs if the zygote implants at the level of the isthmus where the mucosa is thinner and the blood vessels larger. Tubal rupture is likely to occur between the 5th and 7th weeks of pregnancy.

Diagnosis

The condition may be subacute with most of the signs but without the shock and collapse present with the classic acute picture. Because of the dangerous nature of the condition it should always be suspected in women of childbearing age, especially if there is a history of amenorrhoea or previous salpingitis. Llewellyn-Jones (1990) gives the following likely signs:

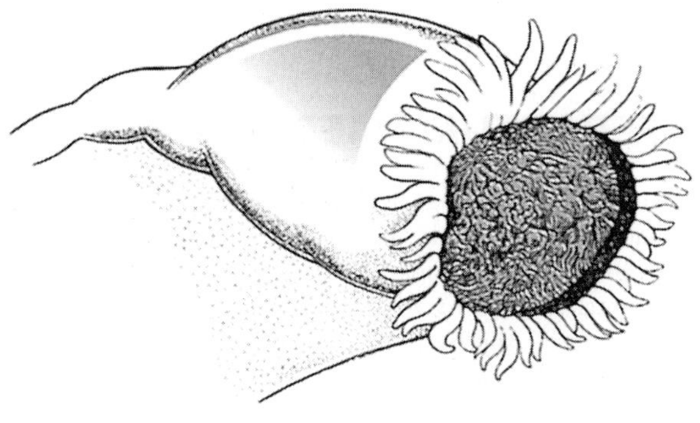

Figure 31.4 *Tubal abortion (from Sweet B, 1997, with permission).*

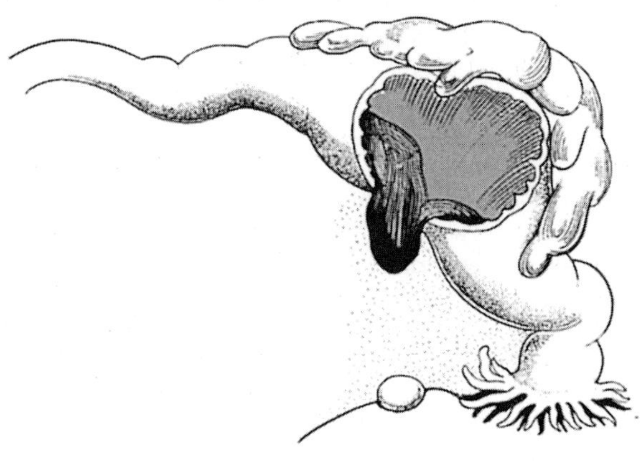

Figure 31.5 *Rupture of the uterine tube (from Sweet B, 1997, with permission).*

- abdominal pain – 90%;
- amenorrhoea – 80%;
- brownish vaginal bleeding – 70%;
- adnexal tenderness – 80%;
- adnexal mass – 80%;
- abdominal tenderness – 50%.

Delay in diagnosis may be fatal as the clinical picture is similar to PID or threatened abortion.

- The woman will give a history of early pregnancy signs.
- The uterus will have enlarged but feel soft.
- Abdominal pain may occur as the tube distends and uterine bleeding may be present as the endometrium begins to degenerate.
- The abdomen is tender and may be distended.
- Blood may track up towards the diaphragm and result in referred pain at the shoulder tip.
- The woman may appear pale, complain of nausea and collapse.
- Severe pain may be felt during pelvic examination, especially if the cervix is moved.
- A mass may be felt in the adnexa on one or other side of the uterus.
- Hormonal assay will find progesterone levels to be low and HCG levels may be low or falling.
- Ultrasound scanning may show fluid or a mass in the pelvic cavity and absence of an intrauterine pregnancy.

Management

The condition is an obstetric emergency. An intravenous line is commenced immediately to combat hypovolaemia and blood is taken for crossmatching. Morphine or pethidine may be given to counteract the pain. As soon as possible the woman is taken to theatre for a laparoscopic **salpingectomy** (removal of uterine tube), even if she has collapsed. Bleeding is heavy and can only be stopped surgically.

Prognosis

About 40% of women may never become pregnant following an ectopic pregnancy. About 75% of these women avoid pregnancy voluntarily and 25% are infertile. The risk of a 2nd ectopic pregnancy is 10% as compared with only 0.4% in other women (Llewellyn-Jones 1990).

Abdominal pregnancy

This is a rare occurrence which may be primary or secondary to tubal abortion. The zygote attaches itself to the abdominal organs and the fetus develops outside the uterine cavity. The condition is sometimes suspected by a persistent abnormal lie and sometimes is diagnosed by ultrasound scan. The fetus may suffer from intrauterine growth retardation. Delivery is by laparotomy and the placenta is left in situ to be reabsorbed. Because of the absence of the unique oblique muscle fibres of the uterus there is nothing to control bleeding. In the past the fetus would die and occasionally become calcified. This is called a **lithopaedion** and such calcified remains have been found inside the abdominal cavities of women when their graves are disturbed.

BLEEDING FROM ASSOCIATED CONDITIONS

The following conditions may cause bleeding in pregnancy but are not caused by the pregnancy. They can occur at any time during the pregnancy.

Cervical polyps

Cervical polyps are benign growths which are bright red, fleshy and attached by a pedicle. They usually originate in the cervical canal and can be seen on speculum examination. Polyps may have been present before the onset of pregnancy but bleed during pregnancy because of the increased blood supply. They can be removed during pregnancy by torsion but bleeding may be heavy.

Cervical erosion

Cervical erosion (**eversion, ectropion**) forms when the columnar epithelium lining the cervical canal proliferates because of the influence of the pregnancy hormones. Columnar epithelium secretes mucin and the woman may complain of profuse vaginal discharge. This may be bloodstained because of rupture of capillaries, especially following sexual intercourse. The epithelium should recede after delivery but if it persists, treatment by diathermy or cryosurgery can be given.

Carcinoma of the cervix

Carcinoma of the cervix is rarely seen in pregnancy (Lindsay 1997) and although a serious complication, there is no evidence that pregnancy causes it to become more rapidly invasive (Kelly 1996). **Cellular dysplasia** (abnormal growth of cells) and **nuclear dyskaryosis** (abnormal chromosomes) are associated with infection with the human papillomavirus (HPV) types 6, 16 and 18 and between 10% and 30% of women have been affected by age 30 (Llewellyn-Jones 1990). HPV is transmissible and is a cause of genital warts. About 60% of the partners of women with HPV infection of the cervix have penile infection. HPV virus acts with a coagent to cause carcinoma of the cervix. Clinical findings may show **cervical intraepithelial neoplasia** (CIN) or **invasive carcinoma of the cervix**.

Cervical intraepithelial neoplasia

The equipment needed for taking a cervical smear is:

- a slide;
- a vaginal speculum;
- an Ayres spatula;
- a spray-on fixative.

The technique should only be carried out by a trained person. Cervical cytology may show normal cells, mild, moderate or severe dysplasia or carcinoma in situ. When carried out in the antenatal period, one in 200 mothers has abnormal cell changes. If these are consistent with CIN a repeat Papanicolau smear is taken and the cervix is assessed by colposcopy. A small cervical biopsy may be carried out. If the tissue is precancerous, treatment can be deferred until after delivery.

Invasive carcinoma of the cervix

Invasive carcinoma of the cervix occurs in about one in 5000 women of childbearing age. It is an aggressive cancer and may progress rapidly. The cervix feels hard and nodular and bleeds when touched. Decisions about treatment should be discussed with each woman and will depend on the degree of invasion and the duration of pregnancy. The maturity and survival of the fetus must be weighed against the risk to the woman. It is likely that if the pregnancy is allowed to continue caesarean section will be carried out and followed by radical hysterectomy with excision of pelvic nodes. The increased vascularity of the genitalia during pregnancy will lead to a greater blood loss and need for transfusion. Radiotherapy may also be needed.

Vaginitis

Occasionally the use of vaginal deodorants may lead to inflammation and bleeding from the vaginal epithelium. Infections such as *Candida albicans* or *Trichomonas vaginalis* are more likely causes of vaginitis which may be accompanied by slight bleeding. Following culture of the organism the correct antibiotic should be given.

ANTEPARTUM HAEMORRHAGE

Antepartum haemorrhage is bleeding after the 24th week of pregnancy and before the birth of the baby. Bleeding during labour can be called **intrapartum haemorrhage**. Bleeding is from the placental site and may be severe enough to cause the death of the woman or the fetus. The two main types of antepartum haemorrhage are **placenta praevia**, where the bleeding occurs from a placenta implanted wholly or partly in the lower uterine segment, and **placental abruption**, where there is premature separation of a normally situated placenta.

Placenta praevia

Normally the chorionic villi surround the whole embryo but later degenerate under the decidua capsularis to form the chorion laeve. The fetus grows to fill the uterine cavity and the decidua capsularis fuses with the decidual vera by about 4 months. If the chorionic villi near the lower pole of the uterus fail to degenerate as the decidua capsularis fuses with the decidua vera, the area will become part of the placenta, encroaching on the lower uterine segment (Blackburn & Loper 1992).

The incidence of placenta praevia ranges between 0.5% and 1% at term, rising to 2% in grandmultiparity (Mabie 1992). Although a low-lying placenta may be detected on routine ultrasound scanning in early pregnancy, it may be detected in as many as 25% of pregnancies in the 2nd trimester. Growth of the lower segment in later pregnancy appears to remove the placental site away from the internal os. In the later weeks of pregnancy sheering stresses may detach the placenta from the uterine wall, resulting in haemorrhage. When the placenta is found to be covering the internal os in early pregnancy the woman is most at risk of haemorrhage (Sanderson & Milton 1991) and the earlier the first episode of bleeding, the worse the prognosis (Arias 1993).

Classification

The standard classification of placenta praevia is shown below although in practice such precision between types I–III is not always possible (Fig. 31.6). The use of ultrasound has improved the diagnosis and allows prognosis of outcome (Arias 1993).

- **Type I** The placenta lies mainly in the upper uterine segment but encroaches on the lower segment.
- **Type II** The placenta reaches to the edge of the internal os.
- **Type III** The placenta covers the internal os when it is closed but not completely when it is dilated.
- **Type IV** The placenta completely covers the internal os.

> Vaginal examination is an extremely dangerous procedure in placenta praevia and must never be carried out unless in theatre with the ability to perform an immediate caesarean section.

Aetiology

In most cases of placenta praevia no specific cause can be assigned. However, the following conditions are associated with its presence.

Conditions which may damage the endometrium and myometrium

- Previous caesarean section (Hershkowitz et al 1995, Khouri and Sultan 1994, Obed & Adequole 1996, Taylor et al 1994)
- Previous placenta praevia
- Previous uterine curettage (Rose & Chapman 1986)
- Spontaneous abortion
- Endometriosis
- Multiparity
- Closely spaced pregnancies

Maternal health

- Age (Zhang & Savitz 1993)

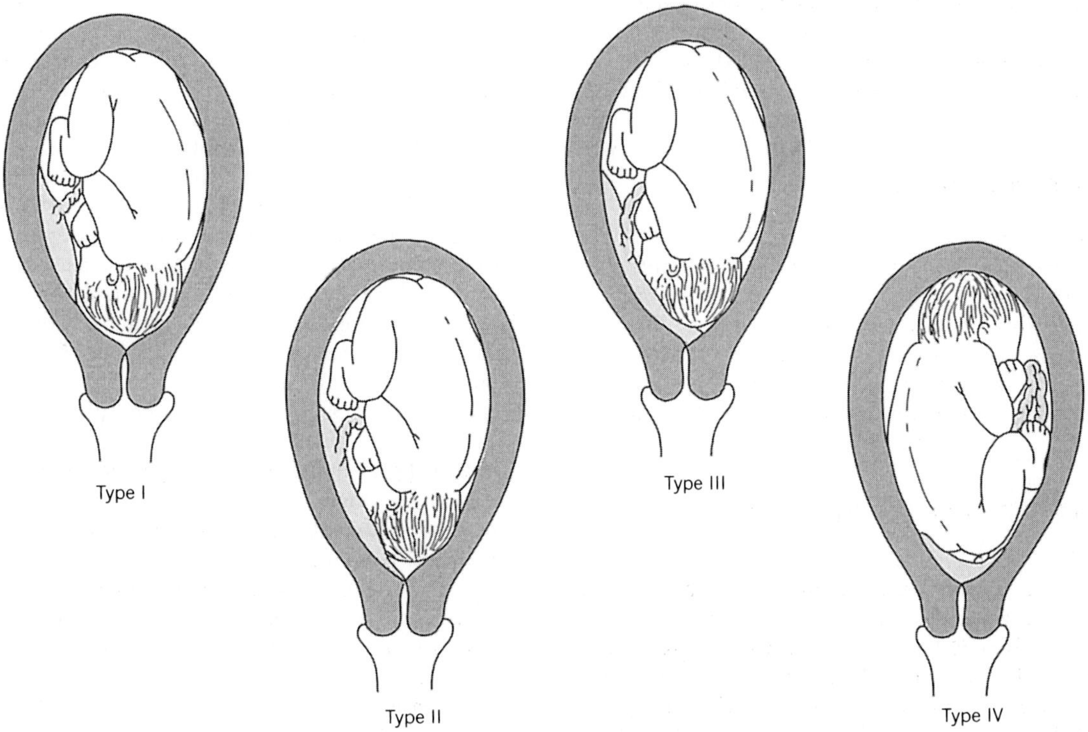

Figure 31.6 *Placenta praevia, types I to IV (from Sweet B, 1997, with permission).*

- Anaemia
- Smoking, possibly due to enlargement of the placenta as a response to hypoxia (Andres 1996, Chelmow et al 1996, Lilja 1995)

Fetoplacental causes

- Multiple pregnancy, as the larger placental site is more likely to encroach on the lower segment
- Congenital malformations
- Presence of a male fetus (Jacobovits & Zuibek 1989)
- Placental abnormality such as bipartite placenta and placenta membranacea (diffusa).

Signs and symptoms

In units where early ultrasound scanning is routine, at-risk women will be identified. Women with low-lying placentae should be rescanned at about 30 weeks gestation. If the placenta is still considered to be low-lying, placenta praevia should be diagnosed and subsequent care modified. Other indications occur because the placenta occupies space in the lower uterine segment and include:

- malpresentations of the fetus;
- non-engagement of the presenting part;
- the presence of a loud maternal pulse originating in the placental bed below the umbilicus.

The bleeding

In 98% of cases painless fresh recurrent vaginal bleeding occurs after 24 weeks, due to stretching of the lower uterine segment and detachment of the placenta, although it may occur earlier. The placenta is in the lower part of the uterus and blood escapes easily. The first episode of bleeding usually stops after a few hours and is rarely dangerous. Subsequent episodes of bleeding due to increased development of the lower uterine segment and further detachment of the placenta tend to become worse and may need a blood transfusion. Torrential maternal haemorrhage may occur at any time, especially if labour commences and the cervix begins to dilate.

The fetus may be compromised if maternal bleeding is severe enough to reduce the uterine blood supply. The placenta may be torn and fetal bleeding occur.

Management

Rankin (1996) writes that 'The management of placenta praevia depends on:

- the amount of bleeding;
- the condition of the mother and fetus;
- the location of the placenta;
- the stage of pregnancy.'

It may be conservative or active.

Any woman bleeding in her own home should be transferred to hospital by ambulance. She should be encouraged to lie down and her condition assessed. Blood pressure and pulse should be recorded and signs of shock looked for. The amount of blood lost should be estimated. If she has a rising pulse rate, falling blood pressure and the pallor, sweating and restlessness associated with hypovolaemic shock, a paramedical team will resuscitate her prior to transferring her to hospital.

On admission

In hospital the woman is placed in bed and given a full examination.
On general examination:

- there may be a history of spotting or small blood losses;
- observations of maternal pulse and blood pressure should correspond with the blood loss;
- her temperature should be normal.

On abdominal examination:

- the uterus should feel soft and should not be tender;
- the size will correspond to the period of gestation;
- there may be a malpresentation, an unstable lie and a high presenting part;
- usually the fetus is in good condition with a fetal heart of normal rate and rhythm.

Blood is taken for crossmatching and at least two units placed on standby. Haemoglobin level and Kleihauer estimation should be measured if the woman is rhesus negative. An intravenous infusion of Hartmann's solution is commenced if bleeding is persistent. Blood loss is estimated and the woman remains on bed rest until the bleeding ceases.

Conservative management

If bleeding is slight to moderate and occurs before the 38th week of pregnancy and both maternal and fetal conditions are satisfactory, conservative treatment is commenced. The aim is to maintain the pregnancy until 38 weeks to avoid prematurity. When bleeding ceases the obstetrician may carry out a speculum examination of the cervix to exclude incidental bleeding.

Ultrasound examination is used to identify the placental site and if this is found to be normal, the woman is allowed home. If placenta praevia is diagnosed the woman will be advised to remain in hospital to reduce any risk of severe bleeding in the absence of immediate medical help. Fetal growth will be monitored and any women who are rhesus negative will receive anti-D γ-globulin after each episode of bleeding.

A study by Love & Wallace (1996) highlights an alternative viewpoint. These authors reviewed the outcome of 58 pregnancies complicated by placenta praevia in Edinburgh. Of these women, 42 (72%) had one or more episodes of bleeding. Repeated episodes of bleeding did not affect the outcomes of pregnancy. Both diagnosis and delivery occurred earlier in the women who bled and delivery by caesarean section was more common in these women. Only three women required emergency delivery because of bleeding. They concluded that as the clinical outcome of placenta praevia is so variable in both women who have no bleeding and those who bleed, outpatient management is safe and appropriate.

Delivery

If no serious haemorrhage occurs the fetus is delivered at 38 weeks. If placental location is not clear, an examination under general anaesthetic in theatre should be made. The surgical team should be ready to carry out an immediate caesarean section. The obstetrician performs a gentle vaginal examination through the fornices. If the placenta is felt a caesarean section is carried out. If the placenta is not palpable the cervical os is examined and if no placenta is felt the membranes will be swept and ruptured. An oxytocin infusion will be commenced.

Vaginal delivery should be possible in type 1 placenta praevia although many clinicians believe caesarean section should be carried out in all cases of placenta praevia. Enkin et al (1996) list the hazards of vaginal delivery as:

- profuse maternal haemorrhage;
- malpresentation;
- cord accidents;
- placental separation;
- fetal haemorrhage;
- dystocia if the placenta is situated posteriorly.

Active management

This is more likely to be needed in the last 2 weeks of pregnancy. If bleeding is severe or continuous or there is a deterioration in maternal or fetal condition or if labour has commenced, the woman's condition is stabilised and an emergency caesarean section is carried out. Blood must be crossmatched but it may be necessary to give the woman a transfusion of O-negative blood in a dire emergency. Anterior situation of the placenta can complicate the surgery as it underlies the site of normal surgical incision. Even if the fetus has died caesarean section will be needed in types III and IV to prevent torrential maternal haemorrhage and death.

Third stage

The lack of oblique fibres in the lower uterine segment may encourage bleeding and postpartum haemorrhage may occur. **Placenta accreta** is often associated with placenta praevia as the thin decidua over the lower uterine segment increases the likelihood of myometrial invasion. Hysterectomy may be required to control haemorrhage and save life.

Placental abruption (abruptio placentae)

Placental abruption is bleeding due to the separation of a normally situated placenta (Fig. 31.7). It can also be called **accidental haemorrhage** and may occur at any stage in pregnancy or labour. It occurs in about 1% of all deliveries and bleeding occurs into the decidua basalis. A haematoma is formed which separates the placenta from the maternal vascular system and the fetus is deprived of oxygen and nutrients. Most maternal complications arise from hypovolaemia. The haemorrhage may be secondary to degenerative changes in the arteries supplying the intervillous spaces (Blackburn & Loper 1992). The fetus is lost in up to 35% of cases (Arias 1993).

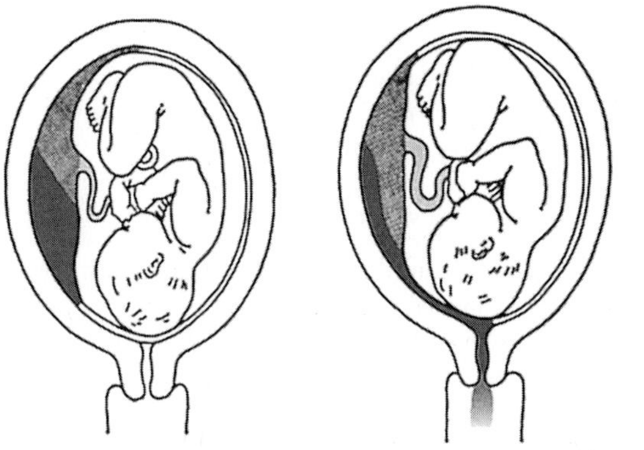

Figure 31.7 *Abruptio placentae (from Sweet B, 1997, with permission).*

Causes

In the majority of cases bleeding is slight and no cause may be found. The following risk factors are associated with this serious complication of pregnancy.

- Hypertensive states – essential hypertension or preeclampsia is present in 50% of severe cases (Arias 1993)
- Sudden decompression of the uterus as when membranes rupture in polyhydramnios
- Preterm, prelabour rupture of the membranes (Ananth et al 1996, Major et al 1995)
- Previous history of placental abruption (Ananth et al 1996)
- Trauma as in a fall or road traffic accident
- Smoking (Andres 1996, Spinillo et al 1994)
- Illegal drug abuse such as cocaine (Hoskins et al 1991)

Previously accepted causes such as short cord, uterine anomalies, inferior vena caval occlusion and dietary folate deficiency are probably not significant (Arias 1993).

The bleeding

The bleeding is from the maternal venous sinuses and may be revealed, partly revealed or concealed (Fig. 31.8) and is darker than that seen in placenta praevia because of the time taken to trickle out of the vagina. Vaginal bleeding is present in 78% of cases (Arias 1993). Some experts believe that the magnitude of

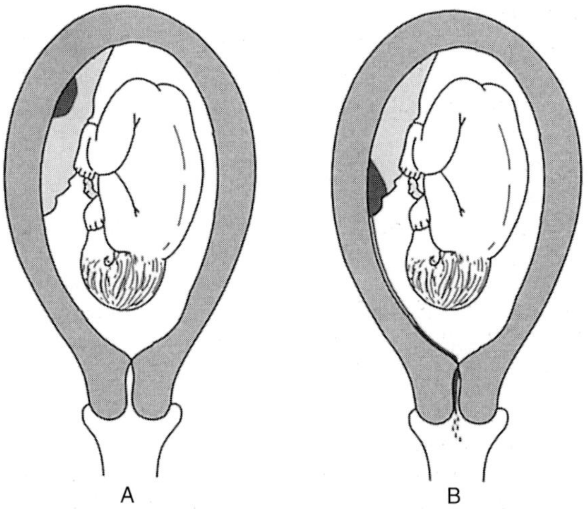

Figure 31.8 *(a) Concealed abruptio placentae. (b) Revealed abruptio placentae (from Sweet B, 1997, with permission).*

placental separation is determined at the outset and that no further separation occurs. Others believe that abruption causes progressive placental separation.

Revealed bleeding occurs when the site of placental detachment is at the margin. The blood trickles down between the membranes and decidua and escapes per vaginam. The condition of the woman is directly related to the observed blood loss.

Partially revealed bleeding occurs when some of the blood remains in the uterus. The bleeding may exceed that which is visibly lost and the degree of shock may be greater than expected.

Concealed bleeding occurs when the site of detachment is near to the centre of the site of placental attachment. Blood cannot escape and a large retroplacental clot forms. Extravasated blood may also infiltrate the full thickness myometrium, a condition known as **Couvelaire uterus**. The uterus appears bruised and oedematous (Rankin 1996). There may be no vaginal blood loss and pain and shock are usually severe.

Depending on the amount of placental separation and blood lost, either revealed or concealed, placental abruption may be mild, moderate or severe (Lindsay 1997). This corresponds closely to the suggested grading system of grades I–III proposed by Sher (1978). **Grade I** includes cases where the diagnosis of placental abruption is made retrospectively. The retroplacental clot is usually between 150 ml and 500 ml. The fetus is rarely at risk. **Grade II** corresponds to cases where signs of placental abruption are present and the fetus is alive. The retroplacental clot is usually 15–500 ml but 27% have a clot larger than 500 ml. Fetal distress is present and vaginal delivery is associated with perinatal death. **Grade III** is present when the fetus has died. There may also be coagulopathy. Most maternal deaths occur in this latter group and it is important to monitor cardiovascular and renal status closely to ensure a good maternal outcome.

Management

When bleeding is slight and there is no effect on maternal or fetal condition, it may be difficult to differentiate the cause of bleeding, especially if there is no sign of hypertension. Because of the risk of placenta praevia the woman is treated as if that condition is present until it is excluded by ultrasound scan. It is important to remember that the presence of a cervical lesion does not exclude bleeding of placental site origin (Lindsay 1997). If the placenta is localised in the upper uterine segment, the bleeding stops and the condition of mother and fetus is satisfactory, the woman may go home.

Moderate or severe placental abruption is usually easy to diagnose and is an obstetric emergency. The woman is resuscitated if necessary and an intravenous infusion commenced. Morphine 15–20 mg may be ordered to relieve pain and shock and the woman is then transferred to hospital. The aim is to restore blood loss and deliver the baby as quickly as possible to avoid complications such as renal failure and bloodclotting defects.

Blood is taken for grouping and crossmatching and it is wise to have at least six units standing by. Checks should be made on haemoglobin estimation, platelet count, urea and electrolytes, clotting studies and fibrin degradation products. Central venous pressure is monitored to avoid under- or overtransfusion. The woman's blood pressure, pulse and respiratory rate are monitored frequently and a Foley's urinary catheter inserted to observe urinary output and allow urine to be tested.

The only way to stop the bleeding is to empty the uterus. Vaginal delivery may be achieved if the fetus has died or is in a good enough condition to allow the time. The membranes are ruptured and an oxytocic infusion is commenced. Caesarean section will be carried out if the fetus is alive but in poor condition. Postpartum haemorrhage is likely due to the poor ability of the uterine muscle to contract when it is infiltrated by blood so intravenous ergometrine 0.5 mg is given and the oxytocic infusion continued for some hours following delivery.

Table 31.2 *The main features of bleeding in abruptio placentae*

	Mild	*Moderate*	*Severe*
Blood loss	Slight	Heavy	Exceeds 1 litre
Uterus on abdominal examination	Soft, not tender	Firm and tender	Hard (woody) and tender, backache if the placenta is posterior
Pain	None or mild	Quite severe	Severe
Shock	No sign	Tachycardia, hypotension	Extreme shock
Fetus	Fetal heart normal	Signs of fetal distress	Fetal heart absent

> The amount of bleeding per vaginam is no guide to the degree of placental separation.

Complications

Blood coagulation disorders

Damage to tissue causes the release of **thromboplastins** from the cells. In normal circumstances thromboplastin activates the clotting mechanism and fibrinogen is converted to fibrin, forming a clot to seal any broken blood vessels. This clot is later dispersed by plasmin releasing fibrin degradation products (FDPs). The tissue damage in placental abruption is so severe that there is a massive release of thromboplastin into the circulation. Widespread clotting occurs within the vascular tree, a condition called **disseminated intravascular coagulation** (DIC). DIC will affect about 13% of women (Arias 1993). The microthrombi produced occlude small blood vessels which results in ischaemic damage in organs (Lindsay 1997). The damaged tissue then releases more thromboplastins and a vicious circle commences.

- Damage to the kidney results in reduced urinary output and may result in anuria.
- The liver may be damaged leading to jaundice.
- Damage to the lungs may result in dyspnoea and cyanosis.
- Brain involvement may result in convulsions or coma.
- The retina may be affected and cause blindness.
- If the pituitary gland is damaged Sheehan's syndrome may occur.

In the end platelets and clotting factors are depleted and no further coagulation can occur. Bleeding begins from puncture wound sites, mucous membranes, petechiae develop in the skin and there will be uncontrollable uterine bleeding. Specific tests for coagulation failure are:

- partial thromboplastin time (normal = 35–45 s);
- prothrombin time (normal = 10–14 s);
- thrombin time (normal = 10–15 s);
- fibrinogen levels (normal = 2.5–4 g/l);
- fibrin degradation products;
- whole blood film and platelet count.

> Transfusions of fresh frozen plasma, packed cells and platelets will be needed.

Other complications

The complications of acute renal failure, Sheehan's syndrome, postpartum haemorrhage, infection, anaemia and mental disturbances are discussed in relevant chapters. Women who have had a placental abruption have a higher risk of complications such as spontaneous abortion or repeated abruption in later pregnancies.

Marginal placental separation

Women with vaginal bleeding in the 3rd trimester, with no evidence of placenta praevia, placental abruption or cervical lesion, have probably had a marginal placental separation or marginal sinus bleeding (Arias 1993). Placental examination may show old clot attached to the placental margins. Some women may have more than one episode of this type of bleeding. There is no evidence of placental separation on ultrasound scan.

Vasa praevia

This is an unusual cause of bleeding in pregnancy where the blood lost is fetal. It is associated with velamentous insertion of the umbilical cord where one of the fetal vessels crosses the membranes between the presenting part of the fetus and the internal os of the uterus. The vessel may be torn when the membranes rupture and fetal bleeding may be severe. There is a high incidence of perinatal mortality with this condition.

It is possible to diagnose the condition by feeling a pulsating vessel on examination and Doppler ultrasound has been used. If the condition is suspected during a vaginal examination the membranes are left intact and the fetus delivered by emergency caesarean section. If the woman is in the 2nd stage of labour rapid delivery is made by forceps. Any sudden vaginal bleeding accompanied by fetal distress following rupture of the membranes should alert the practitioner and the blood should be tested for fetal cells. Although this sounds sensible the reality is that there may be no time and the fetus should be delivered immediately. A blood transfusion may be needed to restore the baby's blood volume. Healy & Wood (1989) found a much higher incidence of velamentous cord insertion following IVF pregnancies.

Summary of main points

- Any bleeding from the genital tract during pregnancy is abnormal and all women who bleed should be seen by a doctor. The causes of bleeding prior to the 24th week of pregnancy are implantation bleeding, abortion, ectopic pregnancy, cervical lesions, vaginitis and bleeding from trophoblastic disease with hydatidiform mole and choriocarcinoma.
- Spontaneous abortion is a fairly common serious cause of bleeding in early pregnancy. The risk is about 15% in women with no previous pregnancy loss, 19% for a repeated abortion in women with no living children and increases with the number of previous abortions, with 80% occurring before 12 weeks gestation. The most frequent causes are genetic abnormalities, maternal endocrine abnormalities, infections, abnormal placentation and cervical incompetence.
- Inevitable abortion is accompanied by cervical dilatation. The bleeding is severe and may result in maternal collapse. The gestation sac separates from the uterine wall and the uterus contracts to expel it. If the gestation sac is completely expelled the term used is complete abortion. If part is retained, it is an incomplete abortion. In women who have recurrent abortions investigations to ascertain the cause are made in order to plan treatment.
- Abortions may be induced in unwanted pregnancies. Sepsis may follow any type of abortion. The term septic abortion is used in such cases. This is a serious condition and is potentially fatal. Antibiotics are commenced before surgical intervention is undertaken.
- Hydatidiform mole is a proliferative growth of trophoblast. The mole looks like creamy white grapes and there is no fetus. It enlarges rapidly to fill the uterus. Genetic and biochemical markers have shown that most hydatidiform moles are derived from paternal genes. The uterus must be emptied by suction curettage.
- Following the emergency treatment careful observation must be continued for 1 year to ensure that there is no progression to choriocarcinoma. Between 5% and 10% of women may go on to develop choriocarcinoma which responds well to chemotherapy.
- An ectopic pregnancy is when the fertilised ovum implants outside the uterine cavity. In 95% of cases the site of implantation is the uterine tube. The incidence of ectopic pregnancy has tripled since 1970 possibly due to the increase in sexually transmitted diseases, the use of the oral contraceptive pill and the intrauterine device and the delay in starting a family.
- Ectopic pregnancy may be subacute with most of the signs but without the shock and collapse present with the classic acute picture. Tubal rupture is an obstetric emergency. As soon as possible the woman is taken to theatre for a laparoscopic salpingectomy. Bleeding is heavy and can only be stopped surgically.
- Cervical polyps, vaginitis, cervical erosion and carcinoma of the cervix may cause associated bleeding and require treatment in pregnancy.
- Antepartum haemorrhage is bleeding after the 24th week of pregnancy and before the birth of the baby. Bleeding is from the placental site and may be severe enough to cause the death of the woman or the fetus. The two main types of antepartum haemorrhage are placenta praevia and placental abruption.
- In placenta praevia sheering stresses during the later weeks of pregnancy may detach the placenta from the uterine wall, resulting in haemorrhage. In units where early ultrasound scanning is routine, at-risk women will be identified. If the placenta is still considered to be low-lying at 30 weeks, placenta praevia should be diagnosed and subsequent care modified. In 98% of cases painless fresh recurrent vaginal bleeding occurs.

- Placental abruption is bleeding due to the separation of a normally situated placenta. Risk factors include hypertensive states, sudden decompression of the uterus, preterm, prelabour rupture of the membranes, previous history of placental abruption, trauma, smoking and abuse of cocaine. The bleeding is from the maternal venous sinuses and may be revealed, partly revealed or concealed.
- When bleeding is slight and there is no effect on maternal or fetal condition it may be difficult to differentiate the cause of bleeding, especially if there is no sign of hypertension.
- Moderate or severe placental abruption is easy to diagnose and is an obstetric emergency. The aim is to restore blood loss and deliver the baby as quickly as possible to avoid renal failure and bloodclotting defects. The only way to stop the bleeding is to empty the uterus. Vaginal delivery may be achieved if the fetus has died or is in a good enough condition to allow the time. Caesarean section will be carried out if the fetus is alive but in poor condition.
- In vasa praevia the blood lost is fetal. It is associated with velamentous insertion of the umbilical cord. The vessel may be torn when the membranes rupture and fetal bleeding may be severe. There is a high incidence of perinatal mortality with this condition.

References

Ananth CV, Savitz DA, Williams MA. 1996 Placental abruption and its association with hypertension and prolonged rupture of the membranes: a methodologic review and meta-analysis. Obstetrics and Gynecology 88(2), 309–318.

Andres RL. 1996 The association of cigarette smoking with placenta previa and abruptio placentae. Seminars in Perinatology 20(2), 154–159.

Arias F. 1993 Practical Guide to High Risk Pregnancy and Delivery, 2nd edn. Mosby Year Book, Chicago.

Axelsen SM, Hendriksen TB, Hedegaard M et al. 1995 Characteristics of vaginal bleeding in early pregnancy. European Journal of Obstetrics and Gynecology and Reproductive Biology 63(2), 131–134.

Barron S. 1995 Bleeding in pregnancy. In Chamberlain G (ed) Turnbull's Obstetrics. Churchill Livingstone, Edinburgh.

Blackburn ST, Loper DL. 1992 Maternal, Fetal and Neonatal Physiology, A Clinical Perspective. WB Saunders, Philadelphia.

Chelmow D, Andrew E, Baker ER. 1996 Maternal cigarette smoking and placenta previa. Obstetrics and Gynecology 87(5), 703–706.

Enkin M, Keirse MJNC, Renfrew M and Neilson J 1996 A Guide to Effective Care in Pregnancy and Childbirth, Oxford University Press: 137–140.

Healy D, Wood C. 1989 Extracorporeal fertilisation (IVF). In Turnbull A, Chamberlain G (eds) Obstetrics. Churchill Livingstone, Edinburgh

Hershkowitz R, Frazer D, Mazor M et al. 1995 One or multiple previous caesarean sections are associated with similar increased frequency of placenta previa. European Journal of Obstetrics and Gynecology and Reproductive Biology 62, 185–188.

Hoskins IA, Friedman DM, Frieden FJ et al. 1991 Relationship between antepartum cocaine abuse, abnormal umbilical artery Doppler velocimetry and placental abruption. Obstetrics and Gynecology 78(2), 279–282.

Jacobovits A, Zuibek L. 1989 Sex ratio and placenta praevia. Acta Obstetrica et Gynaecologica Scandinavica 68, 503–505.

Kelly S. 1996 Disorders caused by pregnancy. In Bennett VR, Brown LK (eds) Myles Textbook for Midwives, 12th edn. Churchill Livingstone, Edinburgh, pp 306–319.

Khouri JA, Sultan MG. 1994 Previous caesarean section and the rising incidence of placenta praevia and placenta accreta. Journal of Obstetrics and Gynecology 14(1), 14–16.

Lilja GMC. 1995 Placenta previa, smoking and recurrence. Acta Obstetrica et Gynaecologica Scandinavica 74(5), 341–345.

Lindsay P. 1997 Bleeding in pregnancy. In Sweet BS with Tiran D (eds) Mayes Midwifery 12th edn. Baillière Tindall, London, pp 511–532.

Llewellyn-Jones D 1990 Fundamentals of Obstetrics and Gynaecology, Gynaecology, (5th edn) London, Faber and Faber.

Love CDB, Wallace EM. 1996 Pregnancies complicated by placenta praevia: what is appropriate management? British Journal of Obstetrics and Gynaecology 103(9), 864–867.

Mabie W. 1992 Placenta praevia. Clinical Perinatology 19(2), 425–435.

Major CA, de Vaciana M, Lewis DF et al. 1995 Preterm premature rupture of the membranes and abruptio placentae: is there an association between these pregnancy complications? American Journal of Obstetrics and Gynecology 172(2,1), 672–676.

Obed JY, Adequole IF. 1996 Placenta praevia: a late sequela of previous lower segment caesarean scars, as manifest in subsequent pregnancies. Journal of Obstetrics and Gynaecology of Eastern and Central Africa 12(1), 15–17.

Rankin S. 1996 Disorders of pregnancy. In Bennett VR, Brown LK (eds) Myles Textbook for Midwives, 12th edn. Churchill Livingstone, Edinburgh, pp 320–334.

Rose GL, Chapman MG. 1986 Aetiological factors in placenta praevia – a case-controlled study. British Journal of Obstetrics and Gynaecology 93(6), 586–588.

Sanderson DA, Milton PJD. 1991 The effectiveness of ultrasound screening at 18–20 weeks gestational age for prediction of placenta praevia. Journal of Obstetrics and Gynaecology 11(5), 320–323.

Sher G. 1978 A rational basis for the management of abruptio placentae. Journal of Reproductive Medicine, 21: 123–129.

Spinillo A, Capuzzo E, Colonna L et al. 1994 Factors associated with abruptio placentae in preterm deliveries. Acta Obstetrica et Gynaecologica Scandinavica 73(4), 307–312.

Sweet B. 1997 Mayes' Midwifery. Baillière Tindall, London.

Taylor VM, Kramer MD, Vaughan TL et al, 1994 Placenta previa and prior cesarean delivery: how strong is the association? Obstetrics and Gynecology, 84(1): 55–57.

Zhang J, Savitz DA. 1993 Maternal age and placenta previa: a population-based case-control study. American Journal of Obstetrics and Gynecology 168(2), 641–645.

Recommended reading

Ananth CV, Savitz DA, Williams MA. 1996 Placental abruption and its association with hypertension and prolonged rupture of the membranes: a methodologic review and meta-analysis. Obstetrics and Gynecology 88(2), 309–318.

Axelsen SM, Hendriksen TB, Hedegaard M et al. 1995 Characteristics of vaginal bleeding in early pregnancy. European Journal of Obstetrics and Gynecology and Reproductive Biology 63(2), 131–134.

Love CDB, Wallace EM. 1996 Pregnancies complicated by placenta praevia: what is appropriate management? British Journal of Obstetrics and Gynaecology 103(9), 864–867.

Sanderson DA, Milton PJD. 1991 The effectiveness of ultrasound screening at 18–20 weeks gestational age for prediction of placenta praevia. Journal of Obstetrics and Gynaecology 11(5), 320–323.

Spinillo A, Capuzzo E, Colonna L et al. 1994 Factors associated with abruptio placentae in preterm deliveries. Acta Obstetrica et Gynaecologica Scandinavica 73(4), 307–312.

Chapter

32 Cardiac and hypertensive disorders

In this chapter

INTRODUCTION

According to Chamberlain (1991), pregnant women are generally young and fit and rarely have chronic medical conditions. However, caring for those who do requires a consideration of how the disease might affect pregnancy and how pregnancy might affect the disease. Heart disease in pregnancy is serious (de Swiet 1989) and may lead to maternal death (DoH 1996). The most dangerous cardiac lesions are those that involve pulmonary hypertension such as **primary pulmonary hypertension** and **Eisenmenger's syndrome** where there is a congenital right-to-left shunt of blood in the heart – either a ventricular septal defect or a patent ductus arteriosus – with pulmonary hypertension. Other dangerous cardiac conditions include **Marfan's syndrome** which is an autosomal dominant disorder of connective tissue where aortic dilatation is present. Rupture of the aorta may occur in late pregnancy or in labour.

Maternal mortality when pulmonary hypertension is present may be as high as 50% (Blackburn & Loper 1992). However, Chamberlain (1991) states that most heart disease in childbearing women is still rheumatic in origin despite the reduction in rheumatic fever in the British population. The most common lesion was **rheumatic mitral stenosis** with the most common complication being **pulmonary oedema** occurring in late pregnancy or immediately after delivery.

THE INCIDENCE OF CARDIAC DISORDERS IN PREGNANCY

Lloyd & Lewis (1996) report a fall in the overall incidence in pregnancies complicated by cardiac disease in Europe and North America due to the much lower incidence of rheumatic heart disease. There is a changing pattern of heart disease with more women surviving congenital heart anomalies and the number of women developing coronary artery disease is on the increase. However, in parts of the world rheumatic heart disease is still the most common problem and should be considered when caring for recent immigrants.

It is important to know the changes in the cardiovascular system, outlined below and discussed in Chapter 16, in order to understand the detrimental effects of a pregnancy on the health of a woman with diagnosed heart disease. The changes that occur in the cardiovascular system in pregnancy which begin early and reach their maximum at about 30 weeks and are then maintained until term (de Swiet 1991) are outlined below for easy reference.

- An increase in cardiac output by 40%
- An increase in blood volume up to 50%
- A decrease in total peripheral resistance

Risk factors

Each of the changes in the cardiovascular system in pregnancy involves increased cardiac work (Arias 1993). In some women their combined effect may exceed the ability of the heart to function and congestive cardiac failure with pulmonary oedema may occur or, more rarely, sudden death. Arias (1993) discusses periods during pregnancy when the danger of cardiac decompensation is higher. The first period is between 12 and 32 weeks when the haemodynamic changes are increasing towards their maximum, with the most critical time being between 28 and 32 weeks.

The second dangerous period is during labour and delivery. During labour every uterine contraction injects blood from the uteroplacental circulation into the maternal bloodstream. This temporarily increases the cardiac output by 15–20% and the continuous demand on the heart might precipitate heart failure. Pushing during the 2nd stage of labour increases the risk further by reducing venous return. Another danger period is immediately after delivery with the sudden injection of 300–500 ml of blood into the maternal circulation. Congestive heart failure is frequent at this time.

Finally, 4–5 days following delivery is a danger period with possible thrombus formation and pulmonary embolism.

Main types of cardiac disorder

Rheumatic heart disease

The main effect of this disease is to cause valvular lesions. Mitral and aortic incompetence may be improved during pregnancy because of the lower pressure within the arterial tree. However, there is a risk of endocarditis. Mitral stenosis, which requires an increase in left atrial pressure to push blood into the left ventricle, will require an even greater effort in pregnancy. The left atrium may fail and pulmonary oedema may develop.

Congenital heart disease

Atrial or ventricular septal defect and patent ductus arteriosus are the most likely uncorrected defects to be seen in pregnancy. All these allow communication between right and left sides of the heart and main arteries. The woman's well-being will depend on the amount of blood flowing in the correct direction. When the hydrostatic pressure gradients are normal there is likely to be no problem as blood will flow from high- to low-pressure areas. For example, blood is more likely to flow from the left ventricle to the aorta, where pressure is low, than across a ventricular septal defect into the right ventricle, where pressure is higher than in the aorta.

The problem arises when pulmonary vascular resistance forces blood to flow from the right to left ventricle instead of into the pulmonary artery. The addition to the systemic circulation of deoxygenated blood leads to poor oxygenation of the tissues and cyanosis. Preeclampsia will increase the risk of this and so may the 3rd stage of labour, when there is a sudden return of up to 500 ml of blood to the circulation.

Eisenmenger's syndrome with pulmonary hypertension has a high risk of maternal mortality, up to 50%. Another major defect likely to have been surgically treated in childhood is **Fallot's tetralogy** where the four defects are pulmonary stenosis, ventricular septal defect, an aorta that overrides the septum and right ventricular hypertrophy.

Any of these structural defects will predispose to bacterial endocarditis and thromboemboli. Fetal growth and survival will depend on how well the compromised maternal cardiovascular system can compensate for the changes in pregnancy. Artificial replacement of heart valves is now more common, mainly of the mitral or aortic valves.

Diagnosis

The woman may already be aware of her disease and may have sought preconception advice. Occasionally the midwife may suspect a problem during history taking. The presence of breathlessness, fatigue and orthopnoea may suggest left heart failure whilst weight gain, dependant oedema, swollen ankles and palpitations suggest right heart failure Any of these symptoms may occur in a normal pregnancy but not usually early on. If symptoms are sufficient to cause the woman anxiety or are reported as having been present before the onset of pregnancy in a woman with no previous history, a cardiologist must be consulted.

Assessment

Assessment will be made jointly by the cardiologist and obstetrician so that counselling and decision taking can be considered. If a termination of pregnancy is the decision, it needs to be carried out in the first trimester as after 16 weeks, continuing with the pregnancy may be the safer option.

New York Heart Association Classification

It is traditional to use the New York Heart Association classification to describe the severity of heart disease but in practice this has little predictive value of the effect of pregnancy on the disease process.

1 No symptoms during ordinary physical activity
2 Symptoms during ordinary physical activity
3 Symptoms during mild physical activity
4 Symptoms at rest.

Management

Pregnant women with heart disease will achieve the safest outcome if continuity of care is provided by one obstetrician and one cardiologist. If care of the woman is to be successful, not only physical care but social and psychological aspects need to be considered from first appointment to final postnatal visit. The major maternal complications which must be avoided if possible are:

- bacterial endocarditis;
- thromboemboli;
- cyanosis;
- heart failure.

Measures to prevent the onset of heart failure include, as appropriate, bed rest and dietary salt restriction. Occasionally diuretics may help. The major concern about the use of diuretics is the reduction in plasma volume because of its association with fetal growth. Digoxin may be used to improve the contractility of the heart and prevent the development of ventricular tachycardia. Heart failure may occur if the following factors are present:

- urinary tract infection;
- respiratory infection;
- hypertension;
- anaemia;
- multiple pregnancy;
- obesity;
- physical work both inside the house and at work;
- smoking.

Prevention of the above complications is preferable to curing them if they occur.

Fetal outcome

Perinatal mortality used to be high for women with heart disease but improvements in the care of the mother have greatly reduced this. However, fetal death may still occur in women with cyanotic heart conditions. If the mother has congenital heart disease there is an increased risk of the baby having a congenital cardiovascular anomaly (Arias 1993, Chamberlain 1991). Fetal growth retardation and preterm labour are common in women with heart disease, probably because of compromised uteroplacental circulation. Obviously the severity of these last effects will depend on the degree of functional impairment of the heart and the severity of tissue hypoxia.

SPECIFIC ASPECTS OF CARE

Intrapartum care

Only aspects of care in labour specific to the needs of women with cardiac disease will be discussed. There are many good sources for care in normal labour to add to this information to enhance the mother's comfort and safety. This method will be followed in all discussions on medical problems complicating childbearing.

Admission and first stage

If possible the labour should be spontaneous in onset with a vaginal delivery. The use of intravenous fluids will lead to an increase in circulating blood volume which may result in pulmonary oedema. If it is necessary to induce labour, prostaglandin pessaries are advocated. The anaesthetist and cardiologist should be informed of the admission. Blood should be crossmatched and oxygen and adult resuscitation equipment should be available. The heart may be monitored by ECG. Some advise antibiotic prophylaxis because of the risk of bacterial endocarditis.

Position

It is important to remember that pregnant women are at greater risk of aortocaval compression with reduced venous return, cardiac output and hypotension if cared for in the supine position. This could compromise the safety of mother and fetus. Women should be cared for in a position they find comfortable. The lithotomy position, where the legs are placed higher than the trunk, is extremely dangerous and could result in sudden heart failure.

Pain relief

It is often stated that women with heart disease have rapid uncomplicated labours. Epidural analgesia may be the pain relief of choice, as long as the woman is not on anticoagulant therapy, as it reduces pain and stress, decreases cardiac output, causes peripheral vasodilation and decreases venous return, thus reducing the risk of pulmonary oedema.

Second stage

This stage should be kept short and without exertion. Prolonged pushing with breath holding, e.g. the Valsalva manoeuvre, should be avoided as it results in rapid changes in haemodynamics which may provoke heart failure. Several short pushes with an open mouth are better. Some doctors may prefer to perform an elective forceps delivery and some advocate avoiding the supine position and conducting the delivery with the woman lying in the left lateral position.

Third stage

Some medical practitioners prefer to avoid the use of oxytocic drugs, especially if the woman is in heart failure. Ergometrine should be avoided as it causes rapid contraction of the uterus and the sudden return of up to 500 ml of blood to the circulation but syntocinon may be used in order to prevent haemorrhage. If haemorrhage occurs, syntocinon infusion accompanied by a diuretic such as intravenous frusemide should be given to prevent pulmonary oedema.

Postnatal care

The risk of cardiac failure with pulmonary oedema is greatest in the early puerperium. Signs include tachycardia, cyanosis, oedema and distension of the liver. If pulmonary oedema occurs, acute dyspnoea with frothy sputum and haemoptysis will ensue. Management includes alleviating anxiety and the woman is nursed in a supported sitting position. Occasionally venesection may be used to reduce venous congestion and relieve the pressure on the right side of the heart.

Drug treatment

Drugs will be administered to relieve anxiety and pain and to aid vasodilation. Morphine 15–20 mg can be used but it may cause neonatal respiratory depression if given in labour. A diuretic such as frusemide will relieve oedema and a bronchodilator such as aminophylline will relieve dyspnoea. If there are cardiac dysrhythmias, digoxin will correct them. Oxygen and prophylactic antibiotics may be given.

Anticoagulant therapy

Another complication is the risk of developing thromboemboli, especially in women with artificial heart valves. Anticoagulants may be given to avoid this. There is a choice of drug. Oral warfarin can be given but crosses the placenta. It is known to be teratogenic if given in the first trimester and may cause fetal and neonatal haemorrhage. Subcutaneous heparin is not passed to the fetus but may not be as effective in preventing thromboemboli. Each doctor will have a preferred regime.

Chamberlain (1991) suggests a regime of warfarin throughout pregnancy until about 2 weeks before expected delivery, when it should be replaced by heparin. However, if emergency delivery is needed so that warfarin cannot be discontinued, there may be a problem. Arias (1993) suggests substituting heparin for the duration of the pregnancy because of the risks of teratogenicity and fetal haemorrhage. Also, coagulation returns to normal 4–6 h after discontinuation of heparin whilst although the effects of warfarin can be reversed in the mother by giving fresh frozen plasma, it may take 1–2 weeks to reverse its anticoagulation effects in the fetus. Risks of long-term (more than 6 months) heparin administration are thrombocytopenia and osteoporosis. Although warfarin appears in breast milk there is no evidence that it harms the baby. Prothrombin times must be monitored whilst the woman is taking warfarin.

HYPERTENSION IN PREGNANCY

Hypertension which develops for the first time in the 2nd half of pregnancy and is caused by the pregnancy is common. There are other hypertensive conditions occurring in pregnancy which may be wrongly diagnosed, such as essential hypertension, phaeochromocytoma (adrenal tumour) and renal disease. The main consideration in this section of the chapter is hypertension which develops in pregnancy and returns to normal after delivery but a brief consideration of essential hypertension is given. Renal problems and adrenal problems are discussed elsewhere in the book.

Terminology

There is a problem with terminology that can cause confusion in the minds of students and sometimes researchers (Wallenburg 1989). Kelly (1996) states that terms are often used interchangeably. She gives the following definitions:

> **Pregnancy-induced hypertension** is a condition specific to pregnancy that occurs mainly after the 28th week and disappears following delivery. **Preeclampsia** is similar but more severe and is also associated with proteinuria of more than 500 mg/l/24 h (Broughton Pipkin 1995). As its name implies, it may lead on to **eclampsia**, a very serious state in which generalised convulsions occur.

Some researchers have questioned whether pregnancy-induced hypertension (PIH) and preeclampsia (PE) may be two separate disease processes but Broughton Pipkin (1995) believes that PE is a more severe form of PIH characterised by proteinuria, thrombocytopenia and failing renal and hepatic function.

Classification

Pregnancy-induced hypertension is a multisystem disorder which may result in maternal and fetal morbidity and mortality. Although the disease process is progressive, it is possible to classify PIH into mild, moderate and severe by the diastolic blood pressure and the onset of other signs and symptoms. This is of benefit when considering the likely outcomes and making decisions on the management. There are various classifications and the following one (Chamberlain 1992) is useful.

- **Mild PIH** is diagnosed if the woman has a diastolic blood pressure of more than 90 mmHg after the 20th week of pregnancy with no raised blood pressure beforehand and no proteinuria.
- **Moderate preeclampsia** involves a rise in diastolic blood pressure to over 100 mmHg after the 20th week of pregnancy with no raised blood pressure beforehand and no proteinuria.
- **Severe preeclampsia** is diagnosed when the diastolic blood pressure exceeds 90 mmHg after the 20th week of pregnancy with any degree of proteinuria.
- **Oedema** may or may not be present depending on the degree of kidney involvement.

Incidence

More than one in 10 women develop PIH although it is possible that some cases, especially in multiparous women, are being misdiagnosed. Arias (1993) reports that whilst 75% of primigravidae who had kidney biopsy showed the typical endothelial changes, only one in 10 of the multigravidae did and there is good reason to suspect chronic renal disease in every multigravid woman until tests prove otherwise. The above statement is supported by Broughton Pipkin (1995) who says that as parity increases, a diagnosis of PIH or preeclampsia is increasingly likely to be erroneous and underlying renal disease is more likely to be present. This supports the theory that preeclampsia is mainly a disease of primigravidae.

An interesting finding is that PIH may occur in a multiparous woman in a first pregnancy by another partner. There is also evidence that in a prolonged sexual relationship women develop an immune response to sperm and are therefore immunologically protected in later pregnancies (Robillard et al 1994). Women who are already hypertensive may have preeclampsia superimposed on the existing condition.

Significance

Thinking in terms of evolutionary medicine, PIH occurs in so many pregnancies that it is likely to be of benefit to the fetus and is a compensatory mechanism to increase uteroplacental perfusion. In support of this theory, hypertension developing in late pregnancy with no other symptoms is not associated with adverse fetal outcome and has been associated with bigger than average babies. However, preeclampsia has remained high on the list of causes of maternal death and also leads to fetal loss. A major problem is that PIH can really only be diagnosed in retrospect by a postdelivery return to normal blood pressure (Hearnshaw 1996). There is also a difficulty in predicting which woman is likely to progress to the more serious condition so that it is better to use the term preeclampsia as a reminder of the possible sudden increase in severity which can occur.

Pathogenesis

The cause of PIH is still not completely certain. There is a genetic predisposition, women being more likely to develop the disorder if their mothers did. In normal pregnancy the spiral arterial walls are invaded by trophoblast and are transformed into large tortuous channels that carry large amounts of blood to the intervillous space. This has occurred by 22 weeks and leads to a fall in peripheral resistance. These uterine vessels are also resistant to vasomotor substances. Bewley (1997) refers to the latest theory of causation which suggests there is a maladaptation of the maternal circulatory system to the trophoblast. In women with preeclampsia, there is inadequate invasion of the spiral arterioles by trophoblastic cells so that decreased uteroplacental perfusion occurs.

This disruption of normal placentation possibly leads to altered endothelial cell function, generalised vasoconstriction, reduced tissue perfusion and multiple organ damage. The spiral arterioles remain sensitive to circulating pressor agents, in particular angiotensin II. The vasomotor tone depends on the relative influences of **prostacyclin**, a potent vasodilator and protector against angiotensin II, and **thromboxane**, a vasoconstrictor. The reduced volume of trophoblast in the spiral arterioles leads to an underproduction of prostacyclin and a relative overproduction of thromboxane which encourages vasospasm of the spiral arteries. The damaged endothelium of the spiral arteries undergoes acute atherosclerosis, thus narrowing the lumen, which causes a rise in blood pressure to overcome the increased resistance.

Cardiovascular changes

Broughton Pipkin (1995) writes that the **cardiac index**, which is the ratio of cardiac output to body surface area, is reduced by 22% in established preeclampsia while systemic vascular resistance is raised. This raised systemic resistance is not due to the action of the sympathetic nervous system. Associated with vasoconstriction is a reduced plasma volume and haemoconcentration and usually, but not inevitably, oedema develops. Coagulation abnormalities occur in a few patients with severe disease. This has been called the **HELLP syndrome** (Weinstein 1982) and consists of Haemolytic anaemia, Elevated Liver enzymes and Low Platelet count.

Morphological changes

As has already been pointed out, preeclampsia is a multisystem disorder. There are two common features: arteriolar vasoconstriction and disseminated intravascular coagulation (DIC). These lead to changes in the kidney, liver and placental bed (Bewley 1997). The changes in the kidney are only distinguishable from acute glomerulonephritis by electron microscopy. Narrowing of the capillary lumen by vasospasm is made worse by the presence of fibrinous material deposited between the endothelial cells and the basement membrane as the disease progresses. In glomerulonephritis, the narrowing is caused by swelling of the basement membrane. The same fibrinous deposit has been found in the liver of patients with preeclampsia. In severe cases intracapsular haemorrhages and necrosis occur. Oedema of the liver cells may produce epigastric pain. Impaired liver function may occur and jaundice become significant.

The vessels supplying the placental bed may become constricted and the reduction in uterine blood flow and vascular lesions in the placenta may result in separation of the placenta – placental abruption. Reduced blood flow through the maternal capillaries in the placental villi may result in the placental tissue becoming ischaemic and infarctions may occur. These changes have grave implications for fetal growth and survival. The release of thromboplastin into the maternal circulation which results in DIC is probably from the damaged placental tissue. The brain becomes oedematous with the development of headache and visual disturbances. Thrombosis and necrosis of the blood vessel walls may result in a cerebrovascular accident, a main cause of death. Lung congestion may impair oxygenation and cyanosis occurs.

Prediction

As the disease process may already be quite extensive when the signs and symptoms become obvious, there have been many studies aimed at predicting in early pregnancy which women will develop the disorder. To be of use, a test must be non-invasive to mother and fetus, be easy to perform and have a hig
predictive value. None has been found to be very succes
Conde-Agudelo et al (1994) assessed the rollover test
MAP readings, angiotensin II sensitivity and ma
methods and concluded that angiotensin II sensiti
best predictor but not of value in the clir
Currently there is no test that fulfils all th
adequate screening method. Therefore vigil
of early signs must be maintained by thos
care.

Management

Rest

Kelly (1996) writes that the aims of care are to provide rest and tranquillity, to monitor the disease and give care and treatment to prevent it worsening and to prolong the pregnancy until the fetus is mature enough to survive. Women with mild PIH can be asked to rest at home but if the disease is moderate to severe or worsening, the mother will be admitted to hospital where bed rest is central to the management (Chamberlain 1992). Resting in a sitting position or on the side will improve uterine blood flow and prevent aortocaval compression with reduced venous return. Whilst strict bed rest may not always be necessary, it will improve renal circulation, facilitate kidney filtration and reduce oedema by producing a diuresis. Blood pressure is usually reduced by bed rest.

Drugs

Low-dose aspirin of 60–150 mg inhibits thromboxane production but the multicentre Collaborative Low-dose Aspirin Study in Pregnancy (CLASP 1994) did not show sufficient effect to be of use prophylactically in the prevention of preeclampsia. However, there may be a place for its use in women with a history of severe preeclampsia if the drug therapy is commenced early in the 2nd trimester.

Antihypertensive drugs such as **methyldopa** help to protect the woman's circulation, in particular against the risk of cerebrovascular accident, but have no effect on the progression of the disease or on fetal growth. They may allow the pregnancy to continue until the fetus is more mature but should probably be used only in women whose hypertension increases despite bed rest.

β-adrenoreceptor antagonists which lower cardiac output by reducing heart rate and stroke volume, **labetalol** being the most common, may give better control and are preferentially used by some doctors. However, they may impair maternal and fetal circulation, especially as stroke volume has already been impaired by reduced blood volume. They are probably best used in essential hypertension without preeclampsia. As atenolol has been associated with fetal growth retardation, it is not recommended for use before the 3rd trimester.

Calcium channel blockers such as **nifedipine** have been used in trials to try to achieve vasodilation (Lopez-Jaramillo et al 1990). There is a significant rise in intracellular free calcium in preeclampsia with urinary calcium excretion falling in direct proportion to the severity of the condition.

Diuretics are contraindicated in preeclampsia because there is already a low plasma volume. The balance between tissue fluid and intravascular fluid would not be altered.

Observations

The purpose of taking and recording observations is to ensure that the treatment is safeguarding the health of mother and fetus.

Maternal observations

Maternal observations should include urinalysis for protein, fluid intake and output, the presence and level of oedema, blood pressure and abdominal examination for pain and tenderness. Plasma urate concentrations are the only useful biochemical indicator of deterioration and severe disease is present if platelet counts begin to fall.

Fetal observations

Fetal observations will include heart rate and rhythm, activity charts and serial ultrasonic assessments of growth. Doppler measurements of blood velocity in the placental bed and umbilical arteries are useful. Any signs of impending eclampsia may necessitate rapid delivery. It is essential to prevent the onset of convulsions which are life threatening to both mother and fetus.

The following signs should be reported to the medical team.

- A sharp rise in blood pressure
- Diminishing urinary output
- Increasing proteinuria
- Severe frontal or occipital headache
- Drowsiness or confusion
- Visual disturbances such as blurring of vision or flashing lights
- Nausea and vomiting
- Epigastric pain which may be reported as indigestion

These are all due to increasing vasospasm and oedema.

Delivery

A decision on when to deliver the baby will depend partly on how effective the treatment is considered to be, which will be based on the interpretation of the observations. The timing can be a fine line drawn between maternal condition and fetal maturity. The mode of delivery similarly depends on the risks to mother and baby. Whether delivery is by induction of labour or caesarean section will depend on the urgency and suitability, including cervical ripeness, of the individual case.

ECLAMPSIA

If preeclampsia is of sudden onset or if the woman has not attended for antenatal care, about one in 1500 women will develop the generalised tonic-clonic convulsions and coma of eclampsia. The incidence of eclampsia is 45% in the antenatal period, 15% during labour and 40% within the first few hours after delivery. In the United Kingdom Douglas & Redman (1994) found that only 62% of cases of eclampsia were preceded by preeclampsia with hypertension and proteinuria. Arterial vasospasm, with blood vessel rupture and haemorrhage which trigger abnormal electrical discharges, is a possible cause of the convulsions.

Eclampsia constitutes an obstetric emergency and immediate care is necessary to prevent death. The complications of eclampsia are multisystem. There may be cerebral haemorrhage, acute renal failure, liver necrosis, heart failure, respiratory failure, temporary blindness, injuries to the tongue, fractures, fetal hypoxia and stillbirth. The most common causes of maternal death are intracranial bleeding and acute renal failure.

Emergency treatment

- Clear and maintain the mother's airway
- Administer oxygen
- Prevent injury during the convulsion

Anticonvulsive therapy

- Intravenous diazepam 10 mg as a bolus injection followed by continuous administration of 40 mg in 500 ml of 5% dextrose.
- In severe hypertension a slow intravenous injection of hydralazine hydrochloride (Apresoline) 20 mg followed by an intravenous infusion of 20–40 mg regulated as needed to control the blood pressure.
- Lytic cocktail, which is a combination of pethidine, promethazine and chlorpromazine in 5% dextrose, is no longer recommended.
- Magnesium sulphate is widely used in America to control the convulsive state. Chamberlain (1992) and Neilson (1995) suggest it could be used more often in the UK. Duley & Henderson-Smart (1997a,b) have reviewed the use of magnesium sulphate versus diazepam and phenytoin. They suggest that there is overwhelming evidence in favour of magnesium sulphate rather than diazepam, phenytoin or lytic cocktail for the treatment of eclampsia.

Other aspects of treatment

Blood is taken for crossmatching and haemoglobin in case severe bleeding occurs at delivery. If the fetus is still in utero, delivery should be completed as soon as the mother's condition is under control. An epidural anaesthetic may help control the blood pressure in labour and delivery.

HELLP syndrome

In a few women severe preeclampsia may affect the liver and be complicated by haemolytic anaemia, elevated liver enzymes and low platelet count (the HELLP syndrome). Immediate delivery will resolve the abnormal blood picture but there may be a need to give platelets or packed red cells to lessen the risk of haemorrhage.

Health implications

The long-term prognosis is that the blood pressure returns to normal within weeks. It is believed that there is no long-term link between hypertension in pregnancy and later onset of chronic hypertension. Proteinuria may persist for longer than the hypertension and may indicate underlying renal disease. Some women who develop preeclampsia may become hypertensive later but this is probably an association rather than a direct cause.

ESSENTIAL HYPERTENSION

Essential hypertension exists when blood pressure is raised without apparent cause. It occurs in families and often affects younger people so that it is often present during pregnancy. If a woman's blood pressure is 140/90 mmHg or more in early pregnancy with no renal or cardiac complications and no proteinuria or oedema, she is diagnosed as having essential hypertension. If the blood pressure can be contained at this level the outlook for the pregnancy is quite good. Blood pressure often falls in the middle trimester but rises again towards term.

Management

The woman is booked for care by a consultant obstetrician and for a hospital delivery. She is advised to take extra rest throughout pregnancy and to avoid too much weight gain. Fetal well-being is monitored closely. Pregnancy is not allowed to go beyond term and induction may be necessary if the blood pressure rises or the fetus shows signs of intrauterine growth retardation. In serious cases caesarean section may be necessary.

Summary of main points

- There is a changing pattern of heart disease with more women surviving congenital heart disease and an increase in coronary artery disease. In parts of the world rheumatic heart disease is still the most common problem and may affect recent immigrants. In some women the combined changes in the cardiovascular system in pregnancy may exceed the ability of the heart to function and congestive cardiac failure with pulmonary oedema may occur.
- The main effect of rheumatic heart disease is to cause valvular lesions. Mitral stenosis needs an increase in left atrial pressure to push blood into the left ventricle and will require a greater effort in pregnancy. The left atrium may fail and pulmonary oedema may develop.
- Atrial or ventricular septal defect and patent ductus arteriosus are the most likely uncorrected defects seen in pregnancy. All these allow communication between right and left sides of the heart and main arteries. The woman's well-being depends on the amount of blood flowing in the correct direction.
- The woman may already be aware of her heart disease and may have sought preconception advice. Occasionally the midwife may suspect a problem during history taking. The New York Heart Association classification has little predictive value of the effect of pregnancy on the disease process. If care of the woman is to be successful, social and psychological aspects need to be considered from first appointment to final post-natal visit. Major maternal complications must be avoided.
- Measures to prevent the onset of heart failure include bed rest and dietary salt restriction. Diuretics may be given but the reduction in plasma volume may be associated with poor fetal growth. Digoxin may be used to improve the contractility of the heart and prevent the development of ventricular tachycardia. Fetal growth retardation and preterm labour are common, probably because of compromised uteroplacental circulation.
- If possible, the labour should be spontaneous in onset with a vaginal delivery. The use of intravenous fluids will lead to an increase in circulating blood volume which may result in pulmonary oedema. If it is necessary to induce labour, prostaglandin pessaries are advocated. Some advise antibiotic prophylaxis because of the risk of bacterial endocarditis.

- Women are at greater risk from the effects of aortocaval compression and the lithotomy position could result in sudden heart failure. Epidural anaesthesia reduces pain and stress, decreases cardiac output, causes peripheral vasodilation and decreases venous return, reducing the risk of pulmonary oedema.
- The 2nd stage should be kept short and without exertion. The Valsalva manoeuvre should be avoided as it may provoke heart failure. Elective forceps delivery and avoiding the supine position may be advocated. Ergometrine should be avoided as it causes the sudden return of up to 500 ml of blood to the circulation but syntocinon may be used in order to prevent haemorrhage.
- Management of cardiac failure includes alleviating anxiety and the woman is nursed in a supported sitting position. Venesection may reduce venous congestion and relieve pressure on the right side of the heart. Morphine used as pain relief in labour may cause neonatal respiratory depression. A diuretic will relieve oedema, a bronchodilator will relieve dyspnoea and digoxin will correct cardiac dysrhythmias. Oxygen and prophylactic antibiotics may be given. Anticoagulants may be given to avoid the risk of developing thromboemboli.
- Hypertension which develops for the first time in the 2nd half of pregnancy and is caused by the pregnancy is common. Other hypertensive conditions occurring in pregnancy are essential hypertension, phaeochromocytoma and renal disease.
- Pregnancy-induced hypertension occurs mainly after the 28th week and disappears following delivery. Preeclampsia is more severe and is also associated with proteinuria. It may lead on to eclampsia. Pregnancy-induced hypertension is a multisystem disorder which may result in maternal and fetal morbidity and mortality. It is possible to classify PIH into mild, moderate and severe. More than one in 10 women develop pregnancy-induced hypertension.
- Preeclampsia is mainly a disease of primigravidae but may occur in a multiparous woman in a first pregnancy by a new partner. There is evidence that in a prolonged sexual relationship women develop an immune response to sperm and are immunologically protected in later pregnancies. Hypertensive women may have preeclampsia superimposed on the existing condition.
- In preeclampsia there is inadequate invasion of the spiral arterioles by trophoblastic cells so that a decreased uteroplacental perfusion occurs. The damaged endothelium of the spiral arteries undergoes acute atherosclerosis and the lumen is narrowed, causing a rise in blood pressure. Associated with vasoconstriction is a reduced plasma volume and haemoconcentration and usually oedema develops. There are two common features of preeclampsia – vasoconstriction and disseminated intravascular coagulation – leading to changes in the kidney, liver and placental bed.
- The aim of care is to prolong the pregnancy until the fetus is mature enough to survive. Low-dose aspirin inhibits thromboxane production but the multicentre CLASP trial did not show sufficient effect to be of use prophylactically in the prevention of preeclampsia. Antihypertensive drugs help to protect the woman's circulation against the risk of cerebrovascular accident but have no effect on the disease or on fetal growth.
- Calcium channel blockers such as nifedipine have been used in trials to try to achieve vasodilation. There is a significant rise in intracellular free calcium in preeclampsia with urinary calcium excretion falling in direct proportion to the severity of the condition. Diuretics are contraindicated in preeclampsia because there is already a low plasma volume.
- Maternal observations include urinalysis for protein, fluid balance, the presence of oedema, blood pressure and abdominal examination for pain and tenderness. Plasma urate concentrations are the only useful biochemical indicator of deterioration and severe disease is present if platelet counts begin to fall. Fetal observations include heart rate and rhythm, activity charts and serial ultrasonic assessments of growth. Doppler measurements of blood velocity in the placental bed and umbilical arteries are useful.
- A decision on when to deliver the baby will depend partly on how effective the treatment is considered to be, which will be based on the interpretation of the observations. The timing can be a fine line drawn between maternal condition and fetal maturity. The mode of delivery similarly depends on the risks to mother and baby.
- Not all cases of eclampsia are preceded by preeclampsia. Eclampsia constitutes an obstetric emergency and immediate care is necessary to prevent death. Complications may include cerebral haemorrhage, acute renal failure, liver necrosis, heart failure, respiratory failure, temporary blindness, injuries to the tongue, fractures, fetal hypoxia and stillbirth. Emergency treatment includes maintaining the mother's airway, administering oxygen and preventing injury.
- Further treatment involves anticonvulsive therapy. There is overwhelming evidence in favour of magnesium sulphate rather than diazepam, phenytoin or lytic cocktail for the treatment of eclampsia. Blood is taken for crossmatching and haemoglobin in case of severe bleeding at delivery and the fetus is delivered as soon as the mother's condition is controlled.
- In a few women severe preeclampsia may affect the liver and be complicated by the HELLP syndrome. Immediate delivery will resolve the abnormal blood picture but there may be a need to give platelets or packed red cells to lessen the risk of haemorrhage.
- The long-term prognosis is that the blood pressure returns to normal within weeks. It is believed that there is no long-term link between hypertension in pregnancy and later onset of chronic hypertension. Some women who develop preeclampsia may become hypertensive later but this is probably an association rather than a direct cause.
- Essential hypertension occurs in families and often affects younger people so that it is often present during pregnancy. If a woman's blood pressure is 140/90 mmHg or more in early pregnancy with no renal or cardiac complications and no proteinuria or oedema, she is diagnosed as having essential hypertension.
- The woman is booked for care by a consultant obstetrician and for a hospital delivery. She is advised to take extra rest throughout pregnancy and to avoid too much weight gain. Fetal well-being is monitored closely. Pregnancy is not allowed to go beyond term and induction may be necessary if the blood pressure rises or the fetus shows signs of intrauterine growth retardation.

References

Arias F. 1993 Practical Guide to High Risk Pregnancy and Delivery, 2nd edn. Mosby Year Book, Chicago.

Bewley C. 1997 Medical conditions complicating pregnancy. In Sweet BR with Tiran D (eds) Mayes Midwifery, 12th edn. Baillière Tindall, London, pp 548–569.

Blackburn ST, Loper DL. 1992 Maternal, Fetal and Neonatal Physiology, A Clinical Perspective. WB Saunders, Philadelphia.

Broughton Pipkin F. 1995 The hypertensive disorders of pregnancy. British Medical Journal 311, 609–612

Chamberlain G. 1991 Medical problems in pregnancy – 1. British Medical Journal 302, 1262–1264.

Chamberlain G. 1992 Raised blood pressure in pregnancy. In Chamberlain G (ed) ABC of Antenatal Care. BMJ Books, London, pp 51–55.

CLASP 1994 Collaborative Low-dose Aspirin Study in Pregnancy, collaborative group. Lancet 343(8898), 619–629.

Conde-Agudelo A, Lede R, Belizan J. 1994 Evaluation of methods used in the prediction of hypertensive disorders of pregnancy. Obstetrical and Gynaecological Survey 49(3), 210–222.

Department of Health 1996 Report on Confidential Enquiries into Maternal Deaths in the United Kingdom, 1991 to 1993. HMSO, London.

de Swiet M. 1989 Cardiovascular problems in pregnancy. In Turnbull A, Chamberlain G (eds) Obstetrics. Churchill Livingstone, London.

de Swiet M. 1991 The cardiovascular system. In Hytten F, Chamberlain G (eds) Clinical Physiology in Obstetrics, 2nd edn. Blackwell Scientific, Oxford, pp 3–38.

Douglas KA, Redman CWG. 1994 Eclampsia in the United Kingdom. British Medical Journal 309(6966), 1395–1400.

Duley L, Henderson-Smart D. 1997a Magnesium sulphate versus diazepam for eclampsia. In Neilson JP, Crowther CA, Hodnett ED, Hofmeyr GJ, Keirse MJNC (eds) Pregnancy and Childbirth module of the Cochrane Database of Systematic Reviews, The Cochrane Library. Update Software, Oxford.

Duley L, Henderson-Smart D. 1997b Magnesium sulphate versus phenytoin for eclampsia. In Neilson JP, Crowther CA, Hodnett ED, Hofmeyr GJ, Keirse MJNC (eds) Pregnancy and Childbirth module of The Cochrane Database of Systematic Reviews, The Cochrane Library. Update Software, Oxford.

Hearnshaw A. 1996 The trouble with terminology. APEC Newsletter no. 11, Spring, p17.

Kelly S. 1996 Disorders caused by pregnancy. In Bennett VR, Brown LK (eds) Myles Textbook for Midwives, 12th edn. Churchill Livingstone, Edinburgh, pp 306–319.

Lloyd C, Lewis V. 1996 Diseases associated with pregnancy. In Bennett VR, Brown LK (eds) Myles Textbook for Midwives, 12th edn, Churchill Livingstone, Edinburgh.

Lopez-Jaramillo P, Navarez M, Felix C, Lopez A. 1990 Dietary calcium supplementation and prevention of pregnancy induced hypertension. Lancet 335, 293.

Neilson JP. 1995 Magnesium sulphate: the drug of choice in eclampsia. British Medical Journal 311, 702–703.

Robillard PY, Hulsey TC, Perianin J. 1994 Association of pregnancy induced hypertension with duration of sexual cohabitation before conception. Lancet 344(8928), 973–975.

Wallenburg HCS. 1989 Detecting hypertensive disorders of pregnancy. In Chalmers I, Enkin M, Keirse MJNC (eds) Effective Care in Pregnancy and Childbirth. Oxford University Press, Oxford.

Weinstein L. 1982 Syndrome of hemolysis, elevated liver enzymes and low platelet count: a severe consequence of hypertension in pregnancy. American Journal of Obstetrics and Gynecology 142, 159–167.

Recommended reading

Broughton Pipkin F. 1995 The hypertensive disorders of pregnancy. British Medical Journal 311, 609–612

CLASP 1994 Collaborative Low-dose Aspirin Study in Pregnancy, collaborative group, Lancet 343(8898), 619–629.

Conde-Agudelo A, Lede R, Belizan J. 1994 Evaluation of methods used in the prediction of hypertensive disorders of pregnancy. Obstetrical and Gynaecological Survey 49(3), 210–222.

Douglas KA, Redman CWG. 1994 Eclampsia in the United Kingdom. British Medical Journal 309(6966), 1395–1400.

Neilson JP. 1995 Magnesium sulphate: the drug of choice in eclampsia. British Medical Journal 311, 702–703.

Weinstein L. 1982 Syndrome of hemolysis, elevated liver enzymes and low platelet count: a severe consequence of hypertension in pregnancy. American Journal of Obstetrics and Gynecology 142, 159–167.

Chapter **33**

Anaemia and clotting disorders

In this chapter

INTRODUCTION

Lloyd & Lewis (1996) define anaemia clearly as 'a reduction in the oxygen-carrying capacity of the blood which may be due to a reduced number of red blood cells, a low concentration of haemoglobin (Hb) or a combination of both'. The effects of anaemia involve both mother and fetus. The mother may develop symptoms such as dyspnoea, fainting, fatigue, tachycardia and palpitations. She may have reduced resistance to infection and her life may be threatened by antepartum or postpartum haemorrhage.

The fetus may suffer intrauterine hypoxia and growth retardation although it is difficult to separate the effects of anaemia from other factors such as social class, smoking and maternal age. Godfrey et al (1991) found that large placental weight with a reduction in fetal weight was associated with iron deficiency anaemia. Interesting work on the fetal origins of adult disease has been carried out by Barker et al (1990) which correlated this change in placental: fetal weight ratio with a risk of hypertension in later life. For those interested in the wider aspects of early predisposition to adult disease, Barker (1993) has edited a book.

RECOGNITION OF ANAEMIA

In 1972, the World Health Organization (WHO 1979) set criteria for diagnosis of anaemia in pregnancy as an Hb of less than (<)11 g/dl but because of increased understanding of the physiological changes in pregnancy, many doctors now only investigate women with an Hb of <10.0 or 10.5 g/dl, depending on local policy (Bewley 1997). The American Center for Disease Control suggest that a first and 3rd trimester Hb of <11 g/dl or haematocrit of <33% or a 2nd trimester Hb of

10.5 g/dl or haematocrit of <32% should be the threshold levels for the establishment of anaemia. Most cases of anaemia in pregnancy will be due to iron deficiency but Schwartz & Thurnau (1995) identify the following anaemias associated with pregnancy:

- iron deficiency anaemia (IDA);
- folic acid deficiency anaemia;
- sickle cell anaemias and the thalassaemias (hereditary haemoglobinopathies);
- anaemia due to blood loss.

IRON DEFICIENCY ANAEMIA

Incidence

Iron is present in all living cells and is essential for the bioavailability of oxygen. Iron deficiency is a common pathology of pregnancy but may be asymptomatic and difficult to diagnose as the physiological changes seen in pregnancy make it difficult to use normal criteria such as haemoglobin level except as an indicator of a potential problem. As mentioned above, local criteria for the indicators for IDA vary slightly. Schwartz & Thurnau (1995) state that IDA is the most common nutrient deficiency in the world, affecting about 15% of the world's population. Most anaemic people are found in the developing countries of the world and this may be due to nutritional deficiencies or to infections such as malaria, dysentery and parasite infestation.

Causes

In the developed world iron deficiency in women is usually due to one of the following conditions.

- Reduced intake or absorption of iron or protein
- Blood loss from heavy menses
- Iron deprivation from previous pregnancies
- Multiple pregnancy
- Chronic urinary tract infection

In a multicultural society such as Britain, the effects of nutrition and infection on iron status should be considered as well as the likelihood of the inherited haemoglobinopathies when caring for recent immigrants.

Investigations

Identification of IDA involves screening blood counts, history taking and investigations. Screening all pregnant women for Hb concentration on a regular basis will indicate the presence of anaemia but will not identify the cause. A history taken at booking may indicate women at risk of developing IDA and iron therapy may be used as a preventive measure. Women identified as having a low Hb should be questioned about nutritional habits, gastrointestinal upset and excessive menstrual bleeding and the presence of a multiple pregnancy should be excluded. Any of these may have precipitated iron deficiency.

IDA is a microcytic anaemia with a fall in mean corpuscular volume occurring before other changes. A fall in Hb is a late sign and iron stores have already been depleted. Serum ferritin estimations will show changes before the Hb falls and would be of great value in screening but the cost is prohibitive. (For normal pregnancy values, see Chapter 16.) A urine sample should be obtained to exclude urinary tract infection.

Management

Once IDA has been confirmed, it is usual to give an oral iron preparation. Absorption seems to be maximised if the iron is taken 30 min before meals but is reduced by up to 50% if the iron is taken with meals. The daily dose of iron needed to treat IDA is 100–200 mg in divided doses. Ferric salts are poorly absorbed but there is little difference in the absorption of the different ferrous salts. Typical preparations are ferrous sulphate, dried 200 mg tablets which contain 60 mg iron, and ferrous gluconate 300 mg tablets which contain 35 mg iron.

Iron can be given by intramuscular injection or intravenous infusion if necessary (Lloyd & Lewis 1996). **Intramuscular iron** is given in the form of iron sorbitol 50 mg/ml. The dose is 1.5 mg per kg body weight and it can be given daily or weekly. Deep intramuscular injection should be used to avoid staining the skin and fat necrosis. Oral iron therapy should be discontinued whilst the injections are being given to avoid toxic symptoms such as headache, nausea and vomiting.

Intravenous iron is given as a total dose slow infusion in normal saline in the form of iron dextran 50 mg/ml. The dose depends on body weight and the degree of iron deficiency. Anaphylactic shock is a major side effect so close observations of blood pressure, pulse, respiration and general condition should be made during the infusion and local policy for the management of severe allergic reaction followed if necessary. A test dose may be given 24 h before the total infusion. Joint pain may also occur.

Rarely, if late in pregnancy or if the iron deficiency is severe, **blood transfusion** may be given but care must be taken to avoid circulatory overload. The Hb level should increase by about 0.2 g/dl per day and a definite rise should be obtained in 1–2 weeks. It may take up to 2 months to become normal depending on the severity of the anaemia. If no response is seen in 4 weeks and the woman is able to tolerate the iron preparation and is complying with the treatment, there may be a problem with absorption or a severe cause of the anaemia. Further investigations are needed.

FOLIC ACID DEFICIENCY ANAEMIA

Incidence

Folic acid is necessary for cell proliferation and deficiency is likely to occur in pregnancy unless the intake of folic acid is increased. It can lead to megaloblastic anaemia which is seen when the deficiency is serious. There is a very small possibility that the megaloblastic anaemia is caused by vitamin B_{12} deficiency. Iron deficiency may conceal a mild megaloblastic anaemia. The deficiency is most likely to occur in late pregnancy or in the puerperium. Folic acid deficiency may cause pallor, lassitude and gastrointestinal symptoms such as anorexia, nausea and vomiting, glossitis and gingivitis and diarrhoea. Mental depression may also occur.

Investigations

Diagnosis of folic acid deficiency is made by examination of peripheral blood. The red cells are macrocytic but fewer in number so that the overall Hb level is low. Plasma folate and red cell folate can be estimated (Mahomed & Hytten 1989). There may be a low platelet and white cell count also. Serum folic acid is lower than 4 μg/ml. Diagnosis of true megaloblastic anaemia is by bone marrow aspiration. Prior to the onset of megaloblastic cell production, folate status can be ascertained and treated whilst the condition is subclinical.

Management

This is usually straightforward with the anaemia responding to folic acid supplementation of 5–15 mg folic acid daily. Prevention by administration of prophylactic folic acid 300–500 μg daily can be given to the following women:

- those with malabsorption syndrome;
- those with haemoglobinopathies (see below);
- those on anticonvulsant therapy;
- those with a multiple pregnancy.

Folate deficiency must be discussed in relation to its role in the causation of neural tube defects, as it is possibly a preventable condition.

Box 33.1 Neural tube defects in the fetus and folate deficiency

Neural tube defects (NTD) include conditions such as anencephaly and spina bifida with or without a meningocoele. Most of these defects are caused by failure of caudal neuropore closure towards the end of the 4th week of development (Moore 1989). α-fetoprotein (AFP) is a fetal protein that can be found in small amounts in the maternal serum in normal pregnancies. Any open defects of the fetus will lead to the leaking of AFP into the amniotic fluid with higher levels than usual entering maternal serum. Higher levels of AFP occur if the gestational age is overassessed or if more than one fetus is present.

Whyte (1996) records that about 1000 cases of NTD are detected through screening each year. Although most are aborted or stillborn, over 100 babies survive, mostly with severe disability. Whilst there is a fall in the absolute annual numbers due to better diet and screening, it is possible to prevent most such tragedies. Detection of open NTDs by the measurement of α-fetoprotein in maternal serum with confirmation by ultrasound scan has led to the termination of many affected pregnancies. However, many find this method of prevention unsatisfactory and would prefer to prevent their occurrence. The cause may involve both genetic and environmental triggers. A dietary factor in the causation of NTD has been suspected for a long time. Wald (1991) records that folic acid, a member of the B vitamin group, was implicated as early as 1964. Two studies in the 1980s suggested that folic acid supplementation might reduce the risk of recurrence of NTDs.

To rule out the bias of small group studies, a randomised double-blind prevention trial was conducted across 33 centres

Box 33.1 (cont'd) Neural tube defects in the fetus and folate deficiency

in seven countries. The aim was to see if supplementation with folic acid or a mixture of seven other vitamins around the time of conception could prevent NTDs. 1817 women at risk because they had already had one affected pregnancy were allocated to one of four groups:

1. folic acid supplementation;
2. other vitamins also likely to prevent the occurrence of a first NTD;
3. both treatments;
4. neither treatment.

The findings were that folic acid supplements prevented three-quarters of the cases of NTD recurrence. In the conclusion, the authors made the point that it was unlikely that the effect would be restricted to recurrences and that folic acid would probably prevent first-time occurrences of NTD. Despite this study, there seems to have been little publicity and most of the general public are not aware of the findings. Although the government is about to launch a publicity campaign, previous experience suggests it will be difficult to change people's eating habits and the most vulnerable section of society will still be at risk. Some doctors and health workers, including Nicholas Wald (mentioned above), believe that supplementing flour, including bread which is already fortified with other B vitamins, with folic acid would be a more successful venture.

HAEMOGLOBINOPATHIES

The incidence of single gene defects varies throughout the world but the most widespread are disorders of the red cell. The World Health Organization estimates that by the year 2000 7% of the world's population may be carriers for one of the disorders (Weatherall 1991). Two of the commonest diseases are the recessively inherited thalassaemias and sickle cell disease. Evidence suggests that these are common because inheriting one abnormal gene and one normal gene for haemoglobin, i.e. being a heterozygote, is protective against the organism *Plasmodium falciparum*, the cause of a severe form of malaria. Unfortunately inheriting two genes for the same Hb, i.e. being a homozygote, is often lethal with ill health leading to death in late childhood or early adulthood. It is possible to inherit genes for two abnormal haemoglobins and the resulting effect can be as severe as being homozygous for one disorder.

The globin chains

The gene for the α-globin chain family is located on chromosome 16 and for the β-globin chain family on chromosome 11. The α-globin chain is 141 amino acids long and the β-globin chain is 146 amino acids long. All haemoglobin variants have a tetramic structure with four protein chains in association with four haem molecules. The four protein chains in normal haemoglobin take up a particular shape which allows for maximum uptake, delivery and release into the tissues of oxygen.

Abnormal genes produce abnormal proteins that cannot carry out their function efficiently and the result is ill health with

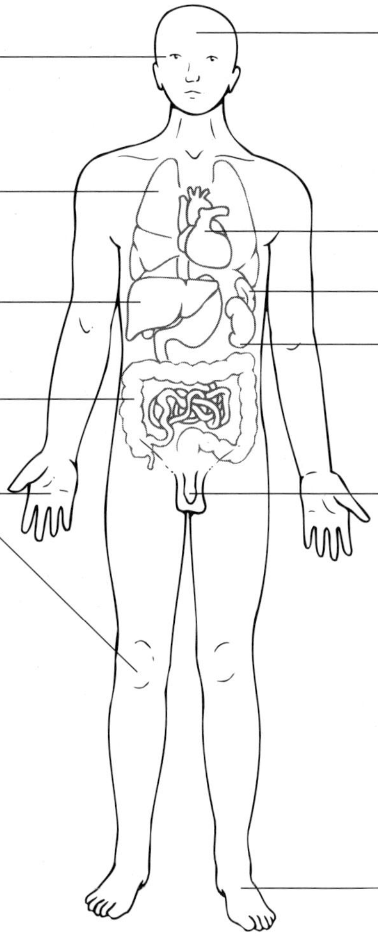

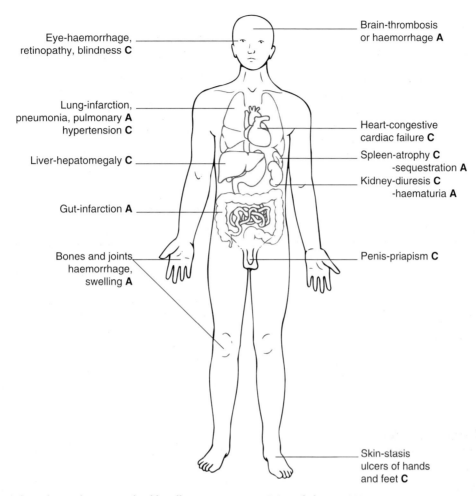

Figure 33.1 *Major clinical manifestations of sickle cell anaemia. Acute (A) and chronic (C).*

anaemia, hypoxia, tissue damage and haemolysis (Fig. 33.1). Hundreds of millions of people carry one of the many abnormal haemoglobin genes and are said to have the trait and more than 200 000 seriously affected homozygotes are born annually throughout the world, of which about half will have thalassaemia and half sickle cell disease.

There are three forms of inherited haemoglobinopathies:

1 structural Hb variants, where there is a fault in either the α-globin chain or the β-globin chain;
2 the thalassaemias, where there is reduced production of either α-globin chain or β-globin chain;
3 failure to switch from the production of HbF to HbA which is clinically insignificant.

Sickle cell disease

Sickle cell disease is the commonest and best known of the structural haemoglobin variants and over 400 have been described, of which 95% are due to a single amino acid substitute in either the α-globin or the β-globin chain. These haemoglobins were originally called after letters of the alphabet but there are so many of them that other tactics have been used to name them. There is thus an Hb Bart's, an Hb Constant Springs and an Hb Aida. Some structurally abnormal haemoglobin genes produce chains that are too long, such as Hb Constant Springs found in a suburb of Kingston, Jamaica, and some chains that are too short.

Table 33.1 *Common combinations of haemoglobin in Sickle cell disease (Bewley 1997)*

HbSS	Homozygous sickle cell disease (sickle cell anaemia)
HbSC	Heterozygous sickle cell disease (sickle cell C disease)
HbCC	Homozygous CC disease (not a sickling disorder)
HbS β/thal	Sickle-β thalassaemia
HbAs	Sickle cell trait

The most common form of sickle cell disease occurs when a child inherits two genes for the abnormal haemoglobin variant HbS. The abnormal β-globin chain has a base substitution which leads to the presence of the amino acid valine instead of glutamic acid at point 6 of the β-globin chain. The result is a haemoglobin molecule that is less soluble. When oxygen is low the molecules form long, linear stacks that distort the red cells into a sickle shape.

Incidence

The incidence of gene carriage varies from country to country and is about one in four in parts of Africa and one in 10 of the black population of the USA and UK (Weatherall 1991). Estimates of the annual birth rate of children with HbS/HbS for various countries are:

- Africa – 100 000;
- USA – 1500;
- Caribbean – 700;
- UK – 150 (one in 100 babies born to parents of Afro-Caribbean descent).

Pathophysiology

Deoxygenation is the most common cause of sickling but decreased plasma volume, hypothermia, infection and acidosis are other conditions that will precipitate it. This will occur with minor degrees of oxygen shortage in people with sickle cell disease but has to be severe to cause sickling in people with sickle cell trait. Normally sickle cell trait is asymptomatic and there is no anaemia, even with the added stress of pregnancy.

The sickled red cells are stiff and cannot pass through the capillaries so that vascular occlusion occurs anywhere in the body but especially in the kidney and brain. In pregnancy the placental bed may be affected. Pain is severe and death of tissues occurs within affected organs. Sickled cells are haemolysed in the spleen, resulting in anaemia. Sickling is not permanent and most of the red cells will regain their normal shape after reoxygenation and rehydration. The extent and clinical manifestations of sickling will depend on the percentage of haemoglobin that is HbS. This is why it is rare for a heterozygous person to suffer much sickling (McCance & Huether 1994).

Sickle cell crises

Extensive sickling can precipitate four types of crisis.

- **Thrombotic crisis**, where tangled red cells occlude small blood vessels. Thrombosis and infarction of the tissue may occur unless the process is reversed.
- **Aplastic crisis** consists of severe anaemia because of reduced erythropoiesis. Red cell survival in sickle cell disease may be as short as 10–20 days because of increased haemolysis. If the ability to respond to this by increased erythropoiesis is lost, an aplastic crisis will develop rapidly.
- **Sequestration crisis** where large amounts of blood become pooled in the liver and spleen. This is mainly seen in the young child.
- **Hyperhaemolytic crisis** is rare and may be associated with some drugs or infections. Another inherited problem of glucose-6-phosphate dehydrogenase deficiency (see below) may be present in people with hyperhaemolytic crisis.

Treatment

There is a need to provide supportive care so that anaemia and crises can be avoided. Avoidance whenever possible of infection, dehydration, acidosis and exposure to cold will help. Immediate correction of dehydration and acidosis with intravenous therapy is necessary. Blood transfusion to raise the level of normal haemoglobin can be considered. Oral folic acid and iron can be given.

Care in pregnancy

Women with sickle cell disease may not be very fertile but those who become pregnant may already have damaged tissues. Crises are more likely in pregnancy. All women are screened for Hb type in pregnancy. The author knew an Irish midwife who carried the sickle cell trait so race alone cannot be used as an indicator without a knowledge of historical population movements, a point made clear by Jones (1996).

Anyone with sickle cell disease needs specialised care from both haematologist and obstetrician with back-up from laboratory and sickle cell centre (Lloyd & Lewis 1996). Treatment may include a blood transfusion every 6 weeks or it may be necessary to carry out an exchange transfusion. During labour it is essential to avoid dehydration and ketosis and adequate pain relief is necessary. Prophylactic antibiotics are given and oxygen should be available.

Fetal testing

It is possible to test fetal blood for abnormal haemoglobin genes from 7 weeks onwards by **cordocentesis**. Chorionic villus sampling may also be used for DNA analysis. Genetic counselling may be needed whether or not termination of an affected pregnancy is decided on. Cord blood may be taken at birth for screening purposes. Testing the blood for sickling will not be effective until 4 months when HbF has receded enough. If the child is found to have sickle cell disease, some give prophylactic antibiotics to minimise the risk of death during a crisis.

Thalassaemia

Incidence

This disease is caused by the reduced rate of synthesis of either α-globin or β-globin chains. The heterozygote condition with the presence of one normal haemoglobin gene is not very harmful and usually results in chronic anaemia. The homozygous condition is serious and life threatening and if untreated, leads to death in childhood. Thalassaemia is a multivariant disorder with more than 60 variants of the genes. These may be due to chromosomal abnormalities, such as deletions along the gene, or to mistakes in the sequencing bases along the gene. This makes detection and counselling difficult.

Weatherall (1991) studied the population of Thailand to demonstrate aspects of thalassaemia. Its total population is about 50 million and about 500 000 children suffer severe ill health due to the interactions of different thalassaemias. Another haemoglobin variant, HbE, is carried by up to 50% of the population in parts of the country and people who inherit HbE and β-thalassaemia, a common genotype in Thailand, can be quite ill.

The thalassaemias also cause severe health problems with α-thalassaemia being a problem in parts of China, Cambodia and Vietnam and β-thalassaemia in Mediterranean countries of Italy,

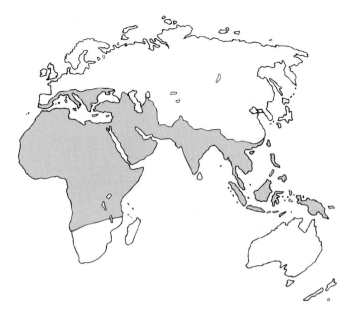

Figure 33.2 *The world distribution of thalassaemia. (Reproduced with permission from Weatherall 1991.)*

Greece, Cyprus and Sardinia (Fig. 33.2). About 7% of the population of the Greek mainland carry the gene for β-thalassaemia and about 250 homozygous babies are born annually. In Cyprus and Sardinia the carrier state reaches 15–20% and about one in 100 homozygous babies are born annually. Each new wave of immigration may lead to increased incidence of inherited disorders and the boat people from Vietnam are the latest thalassaemia sufferers to reach the UK. Weatherall (1991) makes the point that people who carry the gene for β-thalassaemia come from many different countries and that the provision of a comprehensive prenatal diagnosis programme may be expensive.

Pathophysiology

The thalassaemias can be categorised as:

1. **α+ thalassaemia**, where there is low production of α-globin chains due to one defective gene;
2. **α° thalassaemia**, where neither gene is producing an α-globin chain. Tetramers of β-chains and γ-chains are produced: β4, which is HbH, and γ4, which is Hb Bart's, are formed but the absence of α-globin chains means that oxygen cannot be released and the condition is incompatible with life;
3. **β+ thalassaemia**, where there is low production of β-globin chains, due to one defective gene;
4. **β° thalassaemia**, where neither gene is producing β-globin chains, there is production of HbF and α-globin chain excess which precipitate inside red cell precursors. These cells are destroyed by the immune system and this leads to ineffective erythropoiesis.

Clinical signs and symptoms

β-thalassaemia is much more common than α-thalassaemia and in the carrier state leads to mild microcytic hypochromic anaemia and hyperplasia of bone marrow. Haemolysis of immature erythrocytes may cause a slight raise in serum iron but there are usually no symptoms. Homozygous people are quite ill with severe anaemia and death from cardiac failure is common in untreated people. Blood transfusions can increase the lifespan by up to 20 years but there is an increasing problem of iron metabolism with iron overload. Enlargement of the liver and spleen occur and bronzing of the skin due to iron deposition is present.

People who inherit the α-thalassaemia trait are usually symptom free with a milder anaemia than seen in β-thalassaemia trait. However, homozygous α-thalassaemia leads to intrauterine congestive cardiac failure and hydrops fetalis with intrauterine death.

Treatment

People who carry one copy of the gene seldom need treatment and the treatment for homozygous β-thalassaemia is only partially successful. It involves:

- blood transfusions to top up the haemoglobin and haematocrit levels;
- iron chelation therapy with an agent such as desferrioxamine to allow the excess iron to be excreted from the body;
- splenectomy to reduce the amount of haemolysis.

Care in pregnancy

Anyone with thalassaemia trait is likely to develop anaemia that is similar to iron deficiency with microcytic cells but iron deficiency is not usually a problem as the reduced number of red cells and mild haemolysis ensure iron stores are available. Iron therapy is inappropriate unless deficiency is proven. Folic acid supplements are given. Without treatment, people with homozygous β-thalassaemia would die in childhood but treatment increases the likelihood of women with homozygous β-thalassaemia becoming pregnant. Such women need specialised care shared between the haematologist and obstetrician, preferably in a specialised centre (Lloyd & Lewis 1996). Treatment may include repeated blood transfusions and folic acid supplementation.

Fetal testing

Prenatal diagnosis and genetic counselling are important measures that should be available to couples susceptible to having an affected child. It is possible to test fetal blood for abnormal haemoglobin genes from 7 weeks onwards by cordocentesis. Chorionic villus sampling may also be used for DNA analysis. Genetic counselling may be needed whether or not termination of an affected pregnancy is decided on. The severity of the effect on the child's health is more complicated than in sickle cell anaemia and will depend on the nature of the abnormal genes inherited from each parent.

Glucose-6-phosphate dehydrogenase (G6PD) deficiency

G6PD deficiency is a rare X-linked enzyme deficiency. It affects people of African, Asian and Mediterranean origin. Certain drugs precipitate haemolytic crises, including antimalarial preparations, sulphonamides and some antibiotics such as nitrofurantoin, nalidixic acid and chloramphenicol. A gene frequency of 11% has been found in the American black male population (McCance & Huether 1994). The gene is also present in the Sephardic Jewish population. Neonates may have prolonged jaundice if they carry this gene.

THROMBOEMBOLISM AND PREGNANCY

Thrombosis in the childbearing woman is serious because of the association with deep vein thrombosis and with pulmonary embolism which remains the most common cause of maternal death, especially during the puerperium (DoH 1996). Thromboembolic diseases are much more likely to occur in the puerperium than in the antenatal period or in labour. The normal physiological changes in the cardiovascular system and the blood that take place in pregnancy lead to vascular stasis. Thrombosis can be divided clinically into:

- superficial thrombophlebitis;
- deep vein thrombosis (DVT).

Superficial thrombophlebitis

The superficial veins of the legs are affected and the effect can easily be recognised. The vein is tender and may be reddened and hard. It is usually a varicose vein that is affected and there is no risk of pulmonary embolism unless there is a concomitant deep vein thrombosis. Women who are at risk tend to be older, overweight and of high parity. This condition is treated by applying a supportive bandage. Some advise the application of a soothing agent such as glycerine and ichthyol (Ball 1996). The woman should elevate her legs when resting but there is no need to restrict movement and anticoagulant therapy is not necessary.

Deep vein thrombosis

The deep veins of the calf, thigh or pelvis are usually affected. If there is no accompanying inflammation (**phlebitis**) and the **thrombus** (blood clot) does not obstruct the blood vessel, there may be no clinical signs. If the clot is friable and pieces become detached from the vessel wall they will travel round the circulation, through the heart and into the pulmonary circulation, leading to a pulmonary embolism.

Pregnancy factors that predispose women to thromboembolism

- Caesarean section
- Age over 30 years
- High parity
- Obesity
- The use of oestrogens to suppress lactation
- Smoking
- Immobility, as when women are kept on bed rest
- Trauma to the legs
- Reduced plasma volume, as in dehydration or as seen in preeclampsia.

One of the more adverse set of conditions is seen in women with moderate to severe preeclampsia who have been confined to bed antenatally, are taken for delivery by caesarean section and kept sedated for a period of time in the puerperium.

Prevention

Exercise encourages the return of blood to the heart and helps to prevent stasis. Women should be discouraged from sitting with one leg resting across the other. During labour and delivery, care must be taken not to damage or bruise the woman's legs or apply too much pressure from equipment such as stirrups used to maintain the lithotomy position.

Some women at risk of thrombosis may be given prophylactic treatment with low-dose heparin. This is the preferred anticoagulant because oral warfarin crosses the placenta and may cause fetal abnormality if given in the first trimester and spontaneous fetal intracranial or neonatal haemorrhage if given late in pregnancy. Also, the effects of heparin are more readily reversed by giving protamine sulphate solution 10 mg/ml in a dose that will depend on the amount of heparin given and the time since its administration (Ball 1996). The effects of warfarin can be reversed by the administration of vitamin K.

Diagnosis

DVT is most common in the first few days after delivery. The woman may complain of pain or discomfort in the leg which is increased when the foot is dorsiflexed (Homan's sign). The affected leg may be swollen and measure 2–3 cm more than the unaffected leg. There may be a slight rise in systemic temperature. Diagnosis on clinical signs alone is difficult and there may be up to 50% error in diagnosing DVT of the lower extremity. Therefore ultrasound examination by listening for the Doppler effect and venography by injecting a radiopaque dye prior to X-ray may be used to study blood flow and confirm the clinical picture. Although venography is the most accurate method it can be painful and lead to local chemical phlebitis so is not a preferred treatment. In 80% of pregnant patients the thrombosis starts in the iliac and femoral veins and can be diagnosed by non-invasive methods such as Doppler ultrasound (Arias 1993). However, this method is not very accurate for diagnosing calf thrombosis.

Treatment

Anticoagulant therapy is commenced and movement is restricted until the clotting time improves. Intravenous heparin will be commenced and may be followed by oral warfarin, especially if the woman has delivered her baby. The danger of haemorrhage and haematoma formation should be kept in mind and the effects of warfarin can be monitored by serial estimation of blood prothrombin time. A woman with DVT is confined to bed until the swelling has reduced and the anticoagulant therapy has taken effect.

Pulmonary embolism

If a woman develops chest pain, dyspnoea and **haemoptysis** (bloodstained sputum) she must be immediately referred to a doctor and seen as soon as possible. More serious signs that constitute an emergency are sudden collapse, cyanosis and hypotension. The woman must be seen by a doctor at once. If these last symptoms occur the woman may develop respiratory failure and cardiac arrest within seconds. Oxygen and intravenous heparin can be administered and morphine or diamorphine can be given to relieve the pain and distress. An intravenous infusion of streptokinase may be given if the response to the usual anticoagulant therapy is poor. Tragically, some women will die suddenly despite all efforts. Rarely surgery may be needed to remove the embolus (**pulmonary embolectomy**).

CONSUMPTIVE COAGULOPATHIES

Disseminated intravascular coagulation (DIC)

Local activation of the clotting system carries a risk of DIC. In particular, this may complicate abrupt separation of the placenta where there is massive release of thromboplastin into the circulation. This causes intravascular formation of fibrin (microthrombi) with consumption of clotting factors and platelets, leading to severe bleeding. Fibrinolysis is stimulated by DIC and this results in the formation of **fibrin degradation products** (FDPs). These interfere with the formation of firm fibrin clots and a vicious circle is established, increasing the blood loss.

FDPs are also thought to interfere with myometrial contraction. Microthrombi may block the microcirculation, leading to cyanosis of the extremities, failure of organs such as the kidney and liver and cerebrovascular accidents (Rankin 1996). Other causes include prolonged fetal death in utero and amniotic fluid embolism. Septicaemia may also cause DIC. A low-grade DIC is thought to occur in preeclampsia.

Diagnosis

One of the most important aspects of diagnosis is observation of the nature of blood obtained from the woman, either as loss from the body such as in a nose bleed or during labour or a specimen taken for testing. Oozing from a venepuncture or intravenous needle site may occur.

Treatment

The replacement of blood cells and clotting factors is a priority, usually with the transfusion of fresh frozen plasma and platelet concentrates. Banked red cells may be given later. Whole blood is not usually given as it is easier to reestablish equilibrium if the factors are given separately.

Idiopathic thrombocytopenia

This rare disorder is characterised by an autoimmune destruction of the woman's platelets. Such women are usually asymptomatic but may report that they bruise easily and bleed excessively. Petechiae may develop on the skin, an example being when the blood pressure cuff is tightened. If maternal platelets fall very low there may be bleeding from the gastrointestinal and urinary tracts. Intracranial haemorrhage may be a complication. Unfortunately, treatment may also cause problems with splenectomy, corticosteroid therapy and immunosuppressant therapy, all having serious side effects in pregnancy. Fetal thrombocytopenia may be due to transplacental passage of antiplatelet antibodies. For a more detailed examination of this rare problem, see Arias (1993).

Summary of main points

- Most cases of anaemia in pregnancy will be due to iron deficiency but folic acid deficiency, sickle cell anaemias and the thalassaemias and anaemia due to blood loss may result in a low Hb. In the developed world iron deficiency in women is usually due to reduced intake or absorption of iron or protein, blood loss from heavy menses, iron deprivation from previous pregnancies, multiple pregnancy or chronic urinary tract infection.
- Identification of IDA involves screening blood counts, history taking and investigations. In iron deficiency iron can be given by oral preparation, intramuscular or intravenous infusion. In late pregnancy or if the iron deficiency is severe, blood transfusion may be given. If no response is seen in 4 weeks there may be a problem with absorption or other severe cause of anaemia.
- Folic acid deficiency or vitamin B_{12} deficiency in pregnancy can lead to megaloblastic anaemia. Folic acid deficiency responds to folic acid supplementation of 5–15 mg folic acid daily. Folic acid can be given to women with malabsorption syndrome or haemoglobinopathies, those on anticonvulsant therapy and with multiple pregnancy. Folic acid supplements from conception may prevent neural tube defect recurrence.
- By far the most widespread of single gene defects are red cell disorders such as the commonest ones – the recessively inherited thalassaemias and sickle cell disease. A heterozygote is protected against the organism *Plasmodium falciparum*, the cause of severe malaria. Being a homozygote is lethal in late childhood or early adulthood. The most common form of sickle cell disease occurs when a child inherits two genes for the abnormal haemoglobin variant HbS.
- When oxygen is low the red cells are distorted into a sickle shape and cannot pass through the capillaries so that vascular occlusion occurs, especially in the kidney and brain. Normally sickle cell trait is asymptomatic and there is no anaemia, even with the added stress of pregnancy. Most of the red cells will regain their normal shape after reoxygenation and rehydration.
- Extensive sickling can precipitate four types of crisis: thrombotic, aplastic, sequestration and hyperhaemolytic. In a crisis immediate correction of dehydration and acidosis with intravenous therapy is necessary followed by blood transfusion to raise the level of normal haemoglobin. Oral folic acid and iron can be given. In pregnancy treatment may include an exchange transfusion.
- Fetal blood can be tested for abnormal haemoglobin genes from 7 weeks onwards by cordocentesis. Chorionic villus sampling may also be used for DNA analysis. Cord blood may be taken at birth for screening purposes. Testing the blood for sickling will not be effective until 4 months.

- β-thalassaemia is much more common than α-thalassaemia and in the carrier state leads to mild microcytic hypochromic anaemia and hyperplasia of bone marrow. Homozygous people have severe anaemia and death from cardiac failure is common in untreated people. Blood transfusions can increase the lifespan by up to 20 years but there is an increasing iron overload. Enlargement of the liver and spleen and bronzing of the skin due to iron occur.
- Pregnant women with homozygous β-thalassaemia need specialised care shared between the haematologist and obstetrician. Treatment may include repeated blood transfusions and folic acid supplementation. Prenatal diagnosis and genetic counselling should be available to couples susceptible to having an affected child.
- G6PD deficiency is a rare X-linked enzyme deficiency. It affects people of African, Asian and Mediterranean origin. Certain drugs precipitate haemolytic crises. Neonates may have prolonged jaundice if they carry this gene.
- Thromboembolic diseases are more likely to occur in the puerperium than in the antenatal period or in labour. Thrombosis can be divided clinically into superficial thrombophlebitis and deep vein thrombosis. In superficial vein thrombosis the leg veins are tender and may be reddened and hard. Women at risk tend to be older, overweight and of high parity. This condition is treated by applying a supportive bandage.
- In deep vein thrombosis the deep veins of the calf, thigh or pelvis are usually affected. If there is no accompanying inflammation and the thrombus does not obstruct the blood vessel there may be no clinical signs. If the clot is friable and pieces become detached from the vessel wall, they will travel round the circulation, leading to a pulmonary embolism. Some women at risk of thrombosis may be given prophylactic treatment with low-dose heparin. Anticoagulant therapy is commenced and movement is restricted until clotting time improves.
- If a woman develops a pulmonary embolism, oxygen can be given and intravenous heparin administered. Morphine or diamorphine will relieve pain and distress. An intravenous infusion of streptokinase may be given and surgery may be needed to remove the embolus. Massive release of thromboplastin into the circulation leads to intravascular formation of microthrombi with consumption of clotting factors and platelets and severe bleeding leading to organ failure. Fibrinolysis is stimulated by DIC. The replacement of blood cells and clotting factors is a priority.
- Idiopathic thrombocytopenia is an autoimmune disease with destruction of platelets. It is usually asymptomatic but there may be easy bruising and excessive bleeding from the gastrointestinal and urinary tracts. Intracranial haemorrhage may be a complication. Treatments such as splenectomy, corticosteroids or immunosuppressant therapy have serious side effects in pregnancy.

References

Arias F. 1993 Practical Guide to High Risk Pregnancy and Delivery, 2nd edn. Mosby Year Book, Chicago.

Ball JA. 1996 Complications of the puerperium. In Bennett VR, Brown LK (eds) Myles Textbook for Midwives, 12th edn. Churchill Livingstone, Edinburgh.

Barker DJP (ed) 1993 Fetal and Infant Origins of Adult Disease. BMJ Books, London.

Barker DJP, Bull AR, Osmond C, Simmons SJ. 1990 Fetal and placental size and risk of hypertension in adult life. British Medical Journal 301, 259–262.

Bewley C. 1997 Medical conditions complicating pregnancy. In Sweet BR with Tiran D (eds) Mayes Midwifery, 12th edn. Baillière Tindall, London, pp 548–569.

Department of Health. 1996 Report on Confidential Enquiries into Maternal Deaths in the United Kingdom, 1991 to 1993. HMSO, London.

Godfrey KM, Redman CWG, Barker DJP, Osmond C. 1991 The effect of maternal anaemia and iron deficiency on the ratio of fetal weight to placental weight. British Journal of Obstetrics and Gynaecology 98, 886–891.

Jones S. 1996 In the Blood: God, Genes and Destiny. HarperCollins, London.

Lloyd C, Lewis V. 1996 Diseases associated with pregnancy. In Bennett VR, Brown IK (eds) Myles Textbook for Midwives, 12th edn. Churchill Livingstone, Edinburgh, pp 333–364.

Mahomed K, Hytten F. 1989 Iron and folate supplementation in pregnancy. In Chalmers I, Enkin M, Keirse MJNC (eds) Effective Care in Pregnancy and Childbirth, Vol 1. Oxford University Press, Oxford, pp 310–317.

McCance KL, Huether SE. 1994 Pathophysiology, The Biologic Basis for Disease in Adults and Children, 2nd edn. Mosby Year Book, Chicago.

Moore KL. 1989 Before We are Born, 3rd edn. WB Saunders, Philadelphia.

Rankin S. 1996 Disorders of pregnancy. In Bennett VR, Brown LK (eds) Myles Textbook for Midwives, 12th edn. Churchill Livingstone, Edinburgh, pp 320–334.

Schwartz WJ III, Thurnau GR. 1995 Iron deficiency anaemia in pregnancy. Clinical Obstetrics and Gynaecology 38(3), 443–454.

Wald N. 1991 Prevention of neural tube defects: results of the Medical Research Council Vitamin Study. Lancet 338 (8760), 131–137.

Weatherall DJ. 1991 The New Genetics and Clinical Practice, 3rd edn. Oxford Medical Publications, Oxford.

Whyte A. 1996 Fortifying the pregnancy message. MIDIRS Midwifery Digest 6(1), 38–40.

World Health Organization 1979 The Prevalence of Nutritional Anaemia in Developing Countries. WHO, Geneva.

Recommended reading

Barker DJP, Bull AR, Osmond C, Simmons SJ. 1990 Fetal and placental size and risk of hypertension in adult life. British Medical Journal 301, 259–262.

Department of Health 1996 Report on Confidential Enquiries into Maternal Deaths in the United Kingdom 1991 to 1993, HMSO, London.

Godfrey KM, Redman CWG, Barker DJP, Osmond C. 1991 The effect of maternal anaemia and iron deficiency on the ratio of fetal weight to placental weight. British Journal of Obstetrics and Gynaecology 98, 886–891.

Jones S. 1996 In the Blood: God, Genes and Destiny. HarperCollins, London.

Mahomed K, Hytten F. 1989 Iron and folate supplementation in pregnancy. In Chalmers I, Enkin M, Keirse MJNC (eds) Effective Care in Pregnancy and Childbirth, Vol 1. Oxford University Press, Oxford, pp 310–317.

Schwartz WJ III, Thurnau GR. 1995 Iron deficiency anaemia in pregnancy. Clinical Obstetrics and Gynaecology 38(3), 443–454.

Chapter 34

Respiratory, renal, gastrointestinal and neurological problems

In this chapter

RESPIRATORY PROBLEMS

Asthma

Blackburn & Loper (1992) define asthma as 'an obstructive disease characterised by increased airway resistance, decreased expiratory flow rates and hyperinflation with premature airway closure'. McCance & Huether (1994) add that asthma is an inflammatory disease with hyperresponsiveness of the airways characterised by constriction of the smooth muscle in the bronchioles, hypersecretion of mucus and mucosal oedema. The work of breathing is increased and excessive negative intrapleural pressures can increase the demands on the right ventricle. There will be a rise in pulmonary arterial pressure and a decrease in arterial systolic pressure and pulse pressure. The lung changes seen in asthma are reversible and occur in response to a variety of stimuli.

Aetiology

The mechanism of disease causation is complex, involving biochemical, autonomic nervous system, immunologic response, infectious, endocrine and psychological factors, and differs from person to person. Most attacks of bronchospasm are of short duration with freedom from symptoms between episodes. However, airway inflammation is present even when the person is symptom free.

There is a familial incidence in asthma and it affects about 5% of the population. Environmental factors such as dust, pollens, moulds, animal dandruff and foods interact with inherited factors to cause bronchospasm. Asthma is described as **extrinsic** (**atopic**) if triggered by allergens, the most common type, and **intrinsic** (**nonatopic**) if it is not. About half of sufferers develop asthma in childhood and another third before age 40. Complete remission is quite common in children but less so in adults in whom symptomatic episodes tend to occur more frequently.

Pathophysiology

In extrinsic asthma bronchoconstriction occurs within minutes of exposure to the allergen and usually resolves in a short time although there may be a secondary episode, called the late reaction, 6 h after the first reaction. Kumar & Busse (1995) highlight the pivotal role played by the mast cells in asthma. Exposure to the allergen causes IgE antigen to bind to receptors on the surface of the mast cells. These degranulate and release inflammatory substances such as histamine, bradykinin, prostaglandins and thromboxane A_2 and chemotactic factors for eosinophils, neutrophils, T lymphocytes and platelets. In extrinsic asthma, eosinophils produce a protein that stops epithelial cell cilia from beating, disrupts mucosal integrity and causes damage and sloughing of epithelial cells.

Intrinsic asthma has no known allergen and usually occurs in people aged over 35. It tends to be quite severe. The factors that precipitate attacks are known but the mechanisms by which they produce their effects are not clear. Factors involved in the triggering of intrinsic asthma seem to indicate abnormality in the autonomic neural regulation of airway function (Leatherman & Ingram 1992) and include:

- respiratory tract infections;
- some drugs such as aspirin and β-adrenergic antagonists;
- environmental irritants;
- cold dry air;
- exercise;
- emotional stress.

Parasympathetic dominance will result in bronchospasm and this may occur because of a decrease in the number or function of β-adrenergic receptors and an increase in α-adrenergic response.

Asthma in pregnancy

There is a varied response to pregnancy, with some asthmatic women improving, some having a deterioration and some experiencing no change in lung function. It is difficult to predict the course of events so that close monitoring and ensuring compliance with treatment are essential to ensure mother and fetus remain well. Asthma is increasing and is a common medical disorder found in pregnancy, complicating about 1% of all pregnancies. Uncontrolled asthma may result in maternal or fetal morbidity and mortality.

Treatment

Asthma requires long-term administration of drugs such as bronchodilators and antiinflammatory agents. Thomson (1996) writes that it is necessary to consider the effect of these drugs on early fetal development. The use of drugs has to be considered from the risk–benefit point of view, balancing bronchodilation and the risk of hypoxia against the possible risk of teratogenicity.

Management of asthma in pregnancy includes encouraging the patient to recognise the early symptoms of an attack so that hypoxia can be avoided. Blackburn & Loper (1992) state that up to 15% of asthmatic women require hospitalisation during their pregnancy for status asthmaticus or recurrent asthmatic episodes. Women must also be made aware of the necessity for compliance with the prescribed treatment and of avoiding over-the-counter drugs.

Tuberculosis

The prevalence of pulmonary tuberculosis (TB) in Great Britain is between 0.5% and 1% although its incidence is higher in certain sections of the population such as some Asians. The disease is caused by the bacillus *Mycobacterium tuberculosis*. Mycobacteria are soil-living organisms that are pathogenic to some animals. The organism probably first infected cattle and birds and then made a species leap to humans about 6000 years ago. Improvements in urban conditions during the 19th century led to a decrease in the incidence.

Incidence

The mycobacterium infects far more people than it causes to be ill and infected people have a 10% lifetime risk of developing the full disease. Although it is a slow-growing bacterium with a waxy outer coat that protects it from immune system attack, the body's response to the organism is to wall off the microbe by forming fibrinous tubercles (Brock & Madigan 1991).

The bacillus can lie dormant for years, surviving inside macrophages, but lowered resistance causes it to become active and the host to become sick. TB exploits the vulnerable, with poverty, overcrowding, institutionalisation, presence of other disease and immune suppression leading to an increase in active disease. It is highly contagious. In 1993 a girl in a Californian school infected 400 other students.

Some statistics (Karlen 1995)

- Around the world between 1985 and 1991 there was a 12% increase in cases in the USA, a 30% increase in cases in Europe and a 300% increase in cases in parts of Africa where HIV is prevalent.
- 1.7 billion (thousand million) people, about a third of all humans are thought to be infected.
- Ten million people have active tuberculosis.
- Three million people die every year from TB, which is 9000 people a day.

Inborn resistance

There may be a genetic link to resistance to TB. Ashkenazi Jewish people carry a mutated gene for a recessive inherited disorder where having two copies of the gene causes a central nervous system degeneration disorder called Tay–Sachs disease which leads to death in early childhood. Evidence suggests that having one mutated gene only (the carrier state) is protective against TB. In a further example, there is a gene that makes some people produce too much gastric hormone pepsinogen I which predisposes to gastric ulceration because of excess acidity of gastric juices. However, this may also protect against TB.

Signs and symptoms

The signs of pulmonary tuberculosis range from general malaise, with the person lacking energy, to non-specific symptoms such as anorexia, weight loss, low-grade fever and night sweats, and pulmonary specific symptoms such as productive cough with purulent sputum and **haemoptysis**. Although pregnancy increases the demands on the respiratory system, debilitation rather than dyspnoea may be the principal problem. There is a possibility of transplacental infection of the fetus though this is rare. The poor state of health of the woman may affect fetal growth adversely.

Management in pregnant women

A chest physician should be involved in the woman's care and if there are clinical signs of TB or the woman has been in contact with active TB, a chest X-ray will be performed using a lead apron to protect the fetus. Sputum specimens and pleural effusions may be cultured to confirm the presence of the bacillus. Positive sputum may necessitate the admission of the woman to an isolation unit and her family should be investigated for positive signs. Rest and drug therapy form the basis for treatment. Lloyd & Lewis (1996) write that early commencement of treatment can result in negative sputum by the time the baby is born although, as in any patient, drug treatment is prolonged. They outline the use of drugs in pregnancy as follows.

- **Isoniazid** 5 mg/kg/day is given during the first trimester although fetal abnormalities have been seen in animals. The drug interferes with the absorption of pyridoxine so that supplementation is necessary. It is found in significant amounts in breast milk.
- **Ethambutol hydrochloride** 15–20 mg/kg/day can be used in the first trimester of pregnancy as there is no apparent effect on the fetus.
- **Rifampicin** 6–12 mg/kg/day is added after the first trimester. Increased incidence of neural tube defects has been reported.

The baby

It is not always necessary to separate mother and baby; this will depend on the presence of active disease. However, without vaccination there is a 50% chance that the baby will catch the disease. Therefore, following delivery, the baby can be vaccinated with an isoniazid-resistant BCG whilst being protected by prophylactic use of isoniazid syrup 25 mg/kg/day. The vaccine will take effect in about 3–6 weeks and will be shown by a positive Mantoux test. Women who still have an active infection should not breastfeed and those who breastfeed whilst continuing their medication may need their treatment reviewed.

Emergence of multiple drug-resistant (MDR) tuberculosis

With the discovery of antibiotics in the 1940s, tuberculosis became curable and there was a further reduction of cases. The lowest point in the USA, for instance, was seen in 1984 and TB was thought to be conquered. Funding for medical research was withdrawn. However, by 1985 the disease was once more on the increase and in New York there is now an epidemic of MDR-TB. By 1994 many strains of *Mycobacterium* could resist up to seven different antibiotics (Karlen 1995). The disease has become more lethal, treatment has become more prolonged, taking up to 24 months, and the cost of treatment has therefore escalated.

The bacillus can be passed from high-risk to low-risk populations in crowded subways and buildings that recirculate air; for instance, in 1995 a business man working in the London Docklands found he had contracted TB. Several factors have been responsible for the resurgence. First, there has been an increase worldwide in immunosuppressed people with the spread of the human immunodeficiency virus. Second, there is inadequate health-care provision for the poor and socially marginalised population. Some people have no access to health care and others are refused care. Of those receiving treatment, many discontinued their antibiotics before it was safe to do so. This and self-discharge from hospital caused the development of MDR strains. People often difficult to treat include drug addicts, alcoholics and the mentally ill.

Vaccination

A vaccine for TB was discovered in the 1930s and has been used in many countries but not in the USA. This is the Bacillus Calmette-Guerin or BCG which is a live attenuated strain of bacillus developed from cattle TB. It is given to stimulate an increased immune response in humans. BCG is given by injection into the skin. In babies care must be taken not to inject under the skin as this may lead to abscess formation.

The vaccine is effective in the prevention of tuberculosis in children but of variable value when given to adults. It can reduce the incidence of pulmonary tuberculosis by up to 80% and minimises the risk of complications. The effectiveness of BCG programmes remains controversial. In the USA it is thought that vaccination creates difficulties in interpreting the results of any future tuberculin test performed to establish whether a person is infected with the bacillus. In the UK BCG vaccination is carried out in children aged 10–14 years if they demonstrate a negative tuberculin test. Some areas where the rate of incidence is less than 1% have discontinued the routine use of the vaccine. Parish (1991) believes this is a financial rather than medical decision.

Both children and adults who have contact with someone suffering from active pulmonary tuberculosis should be tuberculin tested and given BCG if the test is negative. Babies in contact with active TB should be vaccinated without having a tuberculin test as their immune systems may be too immature to show a response. Parish (1991) suggests that college students, trainee teachers and student nurses should be tested and vaccinated if necessary. In the UK it has been routine to test all immigrants from countries with a high incidence of TB and to give BCG vaccination to those with a negative result and to vaccinate all babies born to recent immigrants.

Contraindications to BCG

Harmful effects of BCG are rare. However, ulcers and abscess formation may occur at the site of the vaccination, sometimes with swollen lymph glands and inflammation of the underlying bone. Healing of such an ulcer may be slow and result in a keloid scar. Very rarely, **lupus vulgaris** (TB of the skin) may occur. BCG vaccine should not be given to people who have leukaemia, cancer or acute illness (including TB) or to patients taking corticosteroids or immune suppressant drugs. People with an immune system deficiency disorder such as HIV/AIDS should never be given the vaccine.

RENAL DISORDERS

Acute renal disease

Acute pyelonephritis

Arias (1993) states that the two most common presentations of kidney abnormalities in pregnancy are the acute onset of signs and symptoms of renal disease in patients with no history of kidney problems before pregnancy and the occurrence of pregnancy in a patient with known renal disease.

Pregnant women are more susceptible to infections in the renal tract than other women. There is an incidence of unsuspected asymptomatic bacteriuria in between 4% and 10% of pregnant women which, if not diagnosed and treated, results in about 25% of them developing pyelonephritis. Ascending infection caused by perineal bacteria is the most usual route and the most common causative organisms are Gram-negative bacilli such as *Escherichia coli*, *Klebsiella pneumoniae* and *Proteus mirabilis* with *E. coli* present in at least 80% of cases. Some strains of *E. coli* have fimbriae that bind to specific receptors on the surface of epithelial cells, increasing their selection of the urinary tract and their virulence. Women most at risk of urinary tract infections have been found to carry the Lewis antigen blood group on their red cells (Arias 1993).

Screening pregnant women for asymptomatic bacteriuria

Because testing urine is a simple procedure and is so effective at preventing pyelonephritis, every woman has a midstream specimen of urine taken and sent to the pathology laboratory for culture. If the culture of a specific bacterium exceeds 10^5 organisms per ml of urine (100 000 organisms/ml), asymptomatic bacteriuria is diagnosed. An antibiotic regime should be successful in treating the condition, depending on the sensitivity results.

Clinical implications

The fetus is at risk of:

- intrauterine growth retardation, even with asymptomatic bacteriuria alone;
- preterm labour;
- the possibility of congenital abnormality.

The woman is at risk of:

- endotoxic shock;
- chronic renal infection;
- renal failure.

Signs and symptoms

Acute pyelonephritis still occurs in 1–2% of pregnancies, usually in the 2nd and 3rd trimesters. It begins with the onset of malaise, fatigue, chills and back pain located in the upper lumbar region, accompanied by muscle guarding. The pain follows the path of the ureters and may radiate round to the suprapubic area. Some women also complain of nausea, vomiting and uterine contractions. Affected women may have a pyrexia as high as 40°C with a corresponding increase in pulse rate. There may be vomiting accompanied by dehydration and also frequency of micturition with scalding on voiding. The urine appears cloudy and even bloodstained and on urinalysis red blood cells, leucocytes and casts may be present as well as bacteria.

Management

It is essential to treat pyelonephritis immediately to avoid the serious side effects of the infection. It is necessary for the woman to be admitted to hospital and the following treatment should be instigated.

- Intravenous fluids may be required to correct any dehydration.
- A midstream specimen of urine should be sent to the laboratory for culturing and sensitivity tests. A blood specimen may be requested if the woman is obviously very ill.
- Antibiotic therapy should be commenced, intravenously if the woman is nauseated. Oral medication may be commenced after 48 h. *E. coli* is becoming increasingly resistant to ampicillin and a combination of antibiotics may be prescribed until the sensitivity reports are returned.
- Other drugs that may be given include buscopan 20 mg to relieve pain caused by muscle spasm and an antiemetic to counteract nausea (Rankin 1996).
- Renal function should be assessed both during the acute illness and as a follow-up.
- Maternal observations of temperature, pulse and blood pressure should be recorded at least 4 hourly. Tachycardia and hypotension may indicate the development of endotoxic shock.
- Fetal observations are as important as maternal and the onset of labour should be recognised.

Most women will respond to the combination of rehydration and antibiotics. In cases of reinfection or persistent problems, there may be an abnormality of the renal tract and such women should be referred to the appropriate consultant.

Acute renal failure

Diagnosis

The onset of acute renal failure (ARF) is said to have occurred if the urine output falls below 400 ml in 24 h or to less than 20 ml/h. There is a reduction in GFR and a rise in blood urea and creatinine. Arias (1993) gives the incidence as one in 10 000 pregnancies in developed countries and one in 2000–5000 in developing countries. Septic abortion may lead to ARF and probably accounts for the differences in incidence. ARF usually

Box 34.1 Association of ARF with pregnancy conditions

Severe preeclampsia	60%
Haemorrhage, especially from the placental site	30%
Kidney disease:	5%
acute pyelonephritis	
severe nephrotic syndrome	
Blood disorders:	5%
shock	
coagulopathy	

results from a severe deficit in cortical renal blood flow, resulting in ischaemia.

If cortical hypoperfusion is allowed to persist the result may be **acute tubular necrosis** (ATN) or **cortical necrosis**. Renal cortical necrosis is a severe form of ARF that is most likely to result from large, sudden blood loss or vascular collapse, such as in severe preeclampsia. There is sudden onset of oliguria or anuria and permanent loss of nephrons. The prognosis for recovery is poor and most women will require long-term dialysis and renal transplant.

Management

The aims of clinical management are to reestablish urinary output and treat the underlying condition. Blood samples should be sent to the laboratory for estimation of urea, electrolytes and plasma proteins. Haematocrit and blood osmolality findings will indicate the degree of dehydration. Blood culture and liver function tests will help to diagnose the cause. Urine samples will be tested for culture and sensitivity of organisms, protein estimation, specific gravity and osmolality.

Delivery

Delivery will benefit the mother and the fetus as once the 25% of renal output necessary for placental circulation is available for the kidney, there may be an immediate response with increased urinary output. Also, if preeclampsia has been the precipitating cause, delivery should lead to a fall in blood pressure and cessation of the pathological effect on the kidneys.

Reestablishing urine flow

Steps to reestablish urine flow are undertaken, depending on the underlying pathology. These may include:

- intravascular volume expansion with packed red cells, fresh frozen plasma or crystalloid solutions;
- dialysis if there is cardiovascular overload, hyperkalaemia, electrolyte imbalances, metabolic acidosis or uraemia;
- restricted fluid intake to the volume of fluid lost in the previous 24 h plus 500 ml to replace insensible fluid loss. If the woman is pyrexial an extra 200 ml may be added.

Diuretics and diet

Women who develop ATN may benefit from careful use of diuretics such as frusemide, depending on the ability of the tubules to respond to the drug. There is discussion on whether the diuretic administration prevents or ameliorates mild ATN. If there is no response after increasing doses, the patient is considered to have serious ATN. Intravenous mannitol may be used as it is both a plasma expander and a diuretic. The woman may need a high-calorie, low-protein, low-sodium and potassium diet until renal function improves.

Prognosis

Women with ATN but no cortical necrosis usually recover completely without long-term damage and return to normal kidney function.

Nephrotic syndrome

Nephrotic syndrome consists of proteinuria greater than 3 g/day, a serum albumin of less than 3 g/dl, oedema and hypercholesterolaemia (Arias 1993). It occurs in one in 1500 pregnancies.

Causes

The development of nephrotic syndrome in pregnancy is usually associated with:

- preeclampsia and eclampsia;
- diabetic nephropathy;
- chronic and acute renal diseases;
- lupus nephritis.

Diagnosis

If hypertension is present the underlying cause is most likely to be preeclampsia. The presence of red cells or red cell casts is indicative of acute glomerulonephritis. The diagnosis of lupus nephritis is difficult to make in pregnancy and the disease is often confused with preeclampsia. The size of proteins being lost from the kidney may indicate the type of damage to the glomerular membrane. The majority of cases are caused by preeclampsia.

Management

Diet is important. The woman may need a high-protein, low-sodium and potassium and low-cholesterol diet to try and prevent the onset of oedema. There is a tendency to develop renal vein thrombosis and anticoagulation with heparin may be advised. Glucocorticoids may be used if lupus erythematosus is the cause. Some may prescribe prophylactic antibiotics because of an increased risk of infection. Diuretics are only used if salt restriction does not prevent oedema developing. The fetus is at risk of intrauterine growth retardation, preterm delivery and antepartum fetal distress and should be monitored accordingly.

Acute glomerulonephritis

Acute glomerulonephritis is rare in pregnancy but should be considered if a woman presents with proteinuria but no hypertension and has a urinary sediment containing red cell casts.

Chronic renal disease

Lloyd & Lewis (1996) report that the chances of a woman becoming pregnant are reduced as renal function declines. Pregnancy is rare when the kidneys are functioning with less than 50% efficiency. The pathology of chronic renal disease is multiple and includes the following:

- glomerulonephritis;
- chronic pyelonephritis;
- renal calculi;
- polycystic kidney disease;
- nephrotic syndrome.

Arias (1993) suggests that the following three questions are important when caring for a woman with chronic renal disease.

1. What are the fetal and maternal prognoses?
2. What are the possible complications and risks?
3. What are the basic principles of the patient's management?

Fetal and maternal prognoses

Perhaps the most important consideration is what effect the pregnancy will have on the progress of the disease. Katz et al (1980) analysed data from 121 pregnancies in 89 women with renal disease. Renal function declined in 16% and there was increased proteinuria in 47%. The prognosis was worst in those with glomerulonephritis. The authors concluded that in patients with normal or mildly impaired renal function, pregnancy does not accelerate renal damage. Katz et al also reported that fetal outcome was good in women with chronic renal disease as long as there was no superimposed preeclampsia and renal function was not severely affected. There was a survival rate of 94% although 24% of the babies were growth retarded and 20% were delivered before term.

Prognostic indicators

Hypertension is the most reliable indicator of the likely outcome. If the diastolic blood pressure is 100 mmHg or more before the onset of pregnancy serious complications are likely to develop.

The next important factor is the **degree of renal impairment** as measured by creatinine clearance. The better the clearance, the better the prognosis.

The presence or absence of **proteinuria** is also important when trying to predict the risks of poor outcome for mother or baby. A patient who has a significant amount of proteinuria registered or an albumin- detecting reagent strip on ward testing or 3 g or more in a 24 h specimen of urine tested by the pathology laboratory at the beginning of pregnancy will tend to develop increasing proteinuria, culminating in the onset of nephrotic syndrome.

As noted, the pathology of kidney function is important. Women with glomerulonephritis have serious maternal and fetal complications.

Complications and risks

The complications of chronic renal disease mentioned below are developed elsewhere in the book.

- Hypertension is the most common and serious complication for pregnant women with chronic renal disease. Maternal mortality may occur because of cerebral haemorrhage, abruptio placentae or acute renal failure.
- Fetal growth retardation, with a significant reduction in the weight, length and head circumference, may occur.
- Preterm birth may occur, because of a medical need to intervene in the pregnancy or because of the spontaneous onset of labour due to poor placental function.
- Fetal distress occurs both antenatally and in labour in pregnancies complicated by intrauterine growth retardation.
- Fetal mortality may occur because of poor placental blood flow, abruptio placentae or fetal hypoxia.

Management

General measures that women can take when they become pregnant include stopping working and reducing their physical activity. Periods of bed rest in the lateral supine position have been found to be useful. Modifying the diet to increase the amount of protein and reduce the amount of sodium is necessary, especially in those women who are retaining sodium and water and have developed oedema. Antihypertensive treatment should be commenced and maintained throughout pregnancy if necessary. Diuretics may be added to the regime as necessary.

Kidney function should be monitored. It is useful to have a full renal creatinine clearance test early in pregnancy followed by serum creatinine measurements every 4–6 weeks. Women should test their urine for albumin each morning and report any significant change. Those with chronic pyelonephritis should be commenced on antibiotic therapy which is continued until after delivery. Pregnant women having renal dialysis or developing a need for dialysis should not pose too many problems. Both haemodialysis and peritoneal dialysis have been used successfully until the baby becomes viable. Fetal growth should be monitored by serial ultrasound from 16 weeks and any deviation from the expected growth curve should be considered carefully. The time and mode of delivery will depend on the findings of maternal and fetal condition.

Renal transplant recipients

If kidney function is adequate and there is no hypertension, women with renal transplants tolerate pregnancy well. Most women are prescribed azathioprine as an immunosuppressor and prednisone to prevent rejection of the transplanted kidney. There have been no reports of an increase in congenital malformations due to the taking of these drugs. Cyclosporine is a more potent immunosuppressing agent and it is recommended that this should be replaced by azathioprine for the duration of the pregnancy. The more common complications are preterm labour and delivery and preeclampsia. Vaginal delivery is recommended. Lloyd & Lewis (1996) quote a list of indicators of likely success from Davison (1987).

- Good health for 2 years following transplant
- Stature compatible with good obstetric outcome
- No proteinuria
- No significant hypertension
- No evidence of graft rejection
- No evidence of distension of the renal pelvis or calyces
- Plasma creatinine of 180 µmol/l or less
- Limited drug therapy

It is important that any pregnancy in a woman with chronic renal disease, on dialysis or following a renal transplant should be planned. Contraceptive and preconception advice is essential.

GASTROINTESTINAL PROBLEMS

Vomiting in pregnancy

Slight nausea and vomiting are common in pregnancy and may affect up to 70% of women in the first trimester. This so-called minor disorder is discussed fully in Chapter 30. Causes and management of moderate to severe vomiting will be discussed below.

Causes of vomiting

Although vomiting is commonly associated with pregnancy, it is important to remember that the pregnant woman is as likely to suffer from diseases not associated with pregnancy as the non-pregnant population. Other causes of vomiting such as gastric ulceration or infection must be considered and ruled out before accepting that moderate to severe vomiting is due to the pregnancy alone.

Vomiting is a reflex which occurs because of stimulation of two centres in the brain discovered by Borison & Wang in 1953 (Rang & Dale 1991). These are the **vomiting centre** (VC) in the medulla and the **chemoreceptor trigger zone** (CTZ) on the floor of the 4th ventricle close to the vagal nuclei.

The VC controls the movements of the smooth muscle in the stomach wall and the related skeletal muscle of the respiratory and abdominal muscles. The CTZ lies outside the blood–brain barrier and responds to circulating chemical stimuli from ingested drugs and endogenous toxins produced in uraemia and radiation sickness. This centre also produces motion sickness. Stimuli arising in the CTZ are passed to the VC which then activates the relevant respiratory and gastrointestinal muscles which result in the action of vomiting. Vomiting can be triggered by:

- stimulation of the sensory nerve endings in the stomach and duodenum;
- stimulation of the vagal sensory endings in the pharynx;
- drugs or endogenous toxins produced as a result of radiation damage, infection or disease;
- disturbance of the vestibular apparatus as in motion sickness;
- some stimuli to the heart and viscera such as distension, damage or infection of the uterus, renal pelvis or bladder and injury to the testicles;
- a rise in intracranial pressure;
- nauseating smells, sights or thoughts;
- endocrine factors such as increased concentration of oestrogen;
- migraine;
- a fall in blood pressure and reduced circulation to the brain.

Neurotransmitter involvement in the vomiting reflex

Substances produced locally in the brain are also involved in the vomiting reflex (Rang & Dale 1991). These include acetylcholine, noradrenaline, dopamine, serotonin (5-HT), histamine and endorphins. 5-HT appears to act both in the gut and on the CTZ and seems to be the cause of vomiting in cancer chemotherapy. Drugs which antagonise acetylcholine and histamine are useful antiemetics and a 5-HT antagonist called ondansetron is specific for the nausea caused by chemotherapeutic agents.

Aetiology

Lindsay (1997) explores the lack of clarity in the aetiology of vomiting in pregnancy and summarises the theoretical causes as follows:

- high levels of pregnancy hormones such as HCG or oestrogen;
- physiological changes in the gastrointestinal tract in pregnancy resulting in decreased motility and increased gastric reflux;
- metabolic changes including carbohydrate deficiency and alteration in lipid pathways;
- genetic incompatibility between mother and fetus;
- position of the right corpus luteum resulting in high concentrations of steroid hormones in the hepatic portal system;
- psychological factors.

Profet's (1992) theory of prevention of toxic substance ingestion during embryogenesis is explained in Chapter 30. Vomiting may also occur in the following conditions (Kelly 1996):

- acute polyhydramnios;
- preeclampsia;
- acute liver failure;
- gastroenteritis;
- renal tract infections;
- appendicitis;
- acute intestinal obstruction;
- torsion of an ovarian cyst;
- cerebral tumour.

Hyperemesis gravidarum

This severe condition resulting in vomiting in pregnancy may lead to maternal death, if not treated actively. It usually begins in the first trimester and is continuous, severe and often associated with excessive salivation. Kelly (1996) gives the incidence of hyperemesis as one in 500 pregnancies. The condition is associated with excessive placental tissue so that it is more common in multiple pregnancies and hydatidiform mole. These conditions should be suspected if the uterus appears large for dates. Tyack (1991) discusses hyperthyroidism as a cause of hyperemesis gravidarum and mentions the study by Valentine et al (1980) who found that the use of antithyroid therapy abolished vomiting in those cases where hyperthyroidism and hyperemesis gravidarum were present together.

Signs and symptoms

The woman complains of continuous nausea and vomiting throughout the day. Signs of dehydration such as loss of skin elasticity, sunken eyes and mouth dryness are present. There is marked oliguria and the urine is dark with high specific gravity and may contain ketones, bile, protein and sugar. Electrolyte disturbances include hyponatraemia and hypochloraemia as sodium and chloride ions are lost in the vomitus. The woman's breath smells offensive, she loses weight and her condition will deteriorate rapidly without treatment. The pulse will be rapid and the blood pressure reduced. Anaemia may occur because of the disruption in vitamin B_{12}, folic acid and vitamin C absorption.

Complications include liver and renal damage, resulting in jaundice, and vitamin B deficiency, resulting in neuropathy such as polyneuritis. Rarely, Wernicke's encephalopathy may occur, signalled by confusion leading to coma because of hypothalamic lesions caused by haemorrhage. Hyperthermia may occur due to disturbance of temperature control. The condition responds well to treatment with thiamine. Fetal growth may be impaired but there is no link to any other fetal condition.

Care

The woman is usually admitted to hospital so that investigations, treatments and investigations can be made as necessary. The cause of vomiting should be identified, antiemetics should be given and fluids and electrolytes replaced by intravenous infusion of a solution such as Hartmann's. Vitamins B_{12} and C, folic acid and iron will be needed to correct anaemia if present. Promethazine 25 mg, given intramuscularly, is the antiemetic of choice.

Observations of pulse, blood pressure and temperature enable the woman's condition to be monitored. All fluids taken in and put out by the woman should be recorded, including the vomitus. There is usually a rapid response to treatment and oral fluids may be recommenced when vomiting has ceased for 24 h. Solid food should then be introduced gradually. On the rare occasion when deterioration in the woman's condition continues, termination of pregnancy is needed to save the mother's life.

Appendicitis

The appendix is gradually displaced upwards by the growing uterus so that the typical signs of appendicitis may not be present. In early pregnancy appendicitis may be difficult to differentiate from threatened abortion. However, there will be no bleeding. Later in pregnancy the pain may be mistaken for urinary tract infection, abruptio placentae or the onset of labour. Careful consideration of the patient's symptoms should allow a differential diagnosis to be made. The appendix must be removed to save life. There is a risk of spontaneous abortion or preterm onset of labour.

Peptic ulceration

Blackburn & Loper (1992) write that peptic ulceration is uncommon in childbearing years as oestrogen may protect the gastric lining against ulcer formation. If peptic ulceration is present up to 80% of women experience an improvement although almost all will have a recurrence of their symptoms by 2 years following the pregnancy. The improvement may be due to the reduction of gastric acidity present in pregnancy.

Pregnancy in women with a stoma

An ileostomy or colostomy for urinary or alimentary diversion should not affect the course of pregnancy. About 75% of women with stomas will have a normal vaginal delivery. Problems that may need careful management include:

- changes in shape and position of the stoma as the uterus enlarges;
- leaking from the stoma as the opening changes shape;
- hormonal changes that alter skin secretions, leading to reduced adhesiveness of the appliance;
- reduced absorption of nutrients, for example vitamin B_{12} and folic acid. This may lead to anaemia;
- increased risk of gastrointestinal obstruction; the consequent abdominal pain is difficult to distinguish from appendicitis (Stables 1995).

NEUROLOGICAL DISORDERS

Epilepsy

Epilepsy is a general term for a group of conditions that cause **seizures**. The word epilepsy means to be seized by an outside force. A seizure can be described as 'a sudden, explosive, disorderly discharge of cerebral neurones' (McCance & Huether 1994). There is a brief alteration in brain function that can involve motor, sensory, autonomic or psychic clinical features accompanied by an alteration in the level of consciousness. The term convulsion refers to the clonic-tonic movements associated with some seizures.

Disorders associated with seizures

Pathological processes lead to seizures although some people may have a lower seizure threshold than others. Epilepsy may result from:

- metabolic disorders;
- congenital malformation;
- genetic predisposition;
- birth injury;
- postnatal trauma;
- motor syndromes;
- infection;
- brain tumour;
- vascular disease.

In people with any of the above disorders, seizures may be provoked by hypoglycaemia, lack of sleep, tiredness, raised temperature, emotional or physical stress, drinking large amounts of water, constipation, drugs, hyperventilation, blinking lights, loud noises, some music and being startled. Women may have seizures linked to the menstrual cycle.

Classification of seizures

A simplified version of an international classification is given by McCance & Huether (1994).

Generalised seizures involve neurones bilaterally, often without a focal onset and usually originating from a subcortical or even deeper brain focus. Consciousness is always impaired or lost. The term corresponds to **grand mal** and **petit mal** epilepsy.

Partial seizures (focal) involve neurones unilaterally, often have a local onset and usually originate from cortical brain tissue. **Temporal lobe epilepsy** and **Jacksonian epilepsy** come under this heading. Consciousness is maintained as long as the seizure is limited to one cerebral hemisphere. There may be involvement of the neurones in the other hemisphere, which is called **secondary generalisation**, and consciousness will then be lost.

In **status epilepticus**, a second or more seizures follows the first before consciousness is fully regained and the person is said to be in the **postictal state** (a state following a seizure) when the next seizure begins. Status epilepticus is most often caused by sudden discontinuation of antiseizure drugs or in people whose epilepsy is uncontrolled or inadequately controlled. Cerebral hypoxia means that this state is a medical emergency and failure to treat adequately may result in dementia, mental retardation and death. The individual is also at risk of aspiration.

Pathophysiology of seizures

Neuronal cells that act as a focus for seizures are activated easily and their firing becomes more frequent and increases in amplitude. The discharge of electricity may rapidly spread throughout the brain to involve the cortex, basal ganglia, thalamus and brainstem, leading to a tonic phase with generalised muscle contraction and increased muscle tone. This is followed by a clonic phase as inhibitory neurones begin to interrupt the seizure discharge, leading to an intermittent contract – relax pattern of muscle action. The clonic bursts gradually become more infrequent and the seizure ends. Immediately prior to the onset of a seizure there may be an **aura** which may involve a visual disturbance or sensing a peculiar smell. A **prodroma** is similar but occurs hours or days before the seizure.

Treatment of epilepsy

The underlying cause of the seizures is established by taking a health history and by physical examination. If there is a correctable cause, treatment is offered. If this is not possible antiseizure treatment is begun. Sodium valproate (Epilim) or phenytoin sodium (Epanutin) have been the drugs of choice. Phenobarbitone or benzodiazepines are sometimes used.

Epilepsy in pregnancy

Epilepsy affects one in 200 of the general population and pregnant women. It has caused maternal death. Pregnancy may affect the incidence of seizures with the possibility of both an increase and a decrease in seizures but there is often no change for most epileptic women. The more severe the disorder, the greater the effect on pregnancy. Pregnant epileptics have a successful outcome to their pregnancy in 90% of cases (Brodie 1990). Preconception advice is important so that the drug regime can be altered prior to conception.

Some of the drugs used to control epilepsy are teratogenic and there is an increased risk of orofacial clefts and heart defects (Lloyd & Lewis 1996) which may be related to folate antagonism. Phenytoin appears to have less risk than other drugs in the causation of defects. Folic acid supplements (5 mg daily) should be given. Carbamazepine is now considered to be the best drug to use in pregnancy as it is not a folic acid antagonist. There is an increased risk of congenital malformations even without treatment (Chamberlain 1992) but about 90% of fetuses will be unaffected. Other problems associated with anticonvulsant drugs are anaemia, because of the folate antagonism, and vitamin D deficiency. Seizures occurring during pregnancy may cause fetal hypoxia or placental abruption. Status epilepticus may cause the death of up to one-third of fetuses

The neonate

Anticonvulsants cross the placenta and decrease the production of vitamin K. This may lead to haemorrhagic disease of the newborn. Vitamin K should be administered to mothers from 36 weeks gestation (Brodie 1990) and to all infants of epileptic mothers. Some babies may be affected by the anticonvulsant drug and remain sleepy and difficult to feed. All the drugs are excreted in breast milk but as long as the dosage is not high, there is no contraindication to breastfeeding (Bewley 1997).

Summary of main points

- Asthma is characterised by increased airway resistance, decreased expiratory flow rates and hyperinflation with premature airway closure. There is a familial incidence in asthma and it affects about 5% of the population. Environmental factors such as dust, pollens, moulds, animal dandruff and foods interact with inherited factors to cause bronchospasm.
- There is a varied response to pregnancy with some asthmatic women improving, some having a deterioration and some experiencing no change in lung function. Asthma complicates about 1% of all pregnancies and, if uncontrolled, may result in maternal or fetal morbidity and mortality. The advantages of bronchodilators and antiinflammatory agents have to be balanced against the risk of fetal hypoxia and teratogenicity.
- The prevalence of pulmonary tuberculosis in Great Britain is between 0.5% and 1% although its incidence is higher in certain sections of the population such as some Asians. TB exploits the vulnerable, with poverty, overcrowding, institutionalisation, presence of other disease and immune suppression leading to an increase in active disease.
- There may be genetic links to resistance to TB. There is evidence suggesting that being a carrier of Tay–Sachs disease protects against TB. The genetic predisposition to produce too much of the gastric hormone pepsinogen I leads to gastric ulceration but may also protect against TB.
- The signs of pulmonary tuberculosis include general malaise, anorexia, weight loss, low-grade fever and night sweats, and pulmonary-specific symptoms such as productive cough with purulent sputum and haemoptysis. There is a rare possibility of transplacental infection of the fetus. Positive sputum may necessitate admission of the pregnant woman to an isolation unit and her family should be investigated for positive signs.
- Rest and drug therapy form the basis for treatment. Increased incidence of neural tube defects has been reported. It is not always necessary to separate mother and baby; this will depend on the presence of active disease but without vaccination there is a 50% chance that the baby will catch the disease. Following delivery the baby can be vaccinated with an isoniazid-resistant BCG whilst being protected by prophylactic use of isoniazid syrup 25 mg/kg/day.
- There is a worldwide developing epidemic of multiple drug-resistant TB – MDR-TB. Many strains of the mycobacterium may resist up to seven different antibiotics. Vaccination is effective in the prevention of tuberculosis in children but of variable value in adults. In the UK BCG vaccination is carried out in children aged 10–14 years if they demonstrate a negative tuberculin test. All immigrants from countries with a high incidence of TB are routinely given BCG vaccination if they have a negative result. People with an immune system deficiency disorder such as HIV/AIDS should never be vaccinated.
- A major problem in pregnancy is unsuspected asymptomatic bacteriuria. If the condition is not diagnosed and treated, about 25% of the women will develop pyelonephritis. If the culture of a specific bacterium exceeds 10^5 organisms per ml of urine, asymptomatic bacteriuria is diagnosed. An antibiotic regime should be successful in treating the condition.

- Acute pyelonephritis occurs in 1–2% of pregnancies, usually in the 2nd and 3rd trimesters of pregnancy. Pyelonephritis is treated immediately to avoid serious side effects. It is necessary for the woman to be admitted to hospital. Most women will respond to the combination of rehydration and antibiotics.
- In acute renal failure there is a reduction in GFR and a rise in blood urea and creatinine. Renal cortical necrosis is most likely to result from large, sudden blood loss or vascular collapse with sudden onset of oliguria and permanent loss of nephrons. The prognosis is poor and most women require long-term dialysis and renal transplant. The aims of clinical management are to reestablish urinary output and treat the underlying condition.
- Delivery will benefit the mother and the fetus as once the 25% of renal output necessary for placental circulation is available for the kidney, there may be an immediate response with increased urinary output. Steps to reestablish urine flow are undertaken depending on the underlying pathology.
- Diet is important in the management of nephrotic syndrome. The woman may need a high-protein, low-sodium diet. Acute glomerulonephritis is rare in pregnancy but should be considered if a woman presents with proteinuria but no hypertension and has a urinary sediment containing red cell casts.
- The chances of a woman becoming pregnant are reduced as renal function declines. The pathology of chronic renal disease is multiple and includes glomerulonephritis, chronic pyelonephritis, renal calculi, polycystic kidney disease and nephrotic syndrome. Perhaps the most important consideration is what effect the pregnancy will have on the progress of the disease.
- Hypertension is the most common and serious complication for pregnant women with chronic renal disease. Maternal mortality may occur because of cerebral haemorrhage, abruptio placentae or acute renal failure. Fetal mortality may occur because of poor placental blood flow, abruption placentae or fetal hypoxia. Fetal growth retardation may occur, as may preterm birth, with fetal distress likely both antenatally and in labour.
- When women with renal disease become pregnant they should reduce their physical activity. Periods of bed rest in the lateral supine position may be useful. Modifying the diet to increase the amount of protein and reduce the amount of sodium is necessary. Antihypertensive treatment should be commenced and maintained throughout pregnancy if necessary. Diuretics may be added to the regime. Kidney function should be monitored by creatinine clearance tests.
- Women with chronic pyelonephritis should be commenced on appropriate antibiotic therapy which is continued until after delivery. Both haemodialysis and peritoneal dialysis have been used successfully until the baby becomes viable. Fetal growth should be monitored and any deviation from the expected growth curve considered carefully. The time and mode of delivery will depend on the findings of maternal and fetal condition.
- If kidney function is adequate and there is no hypertension, women with renal transplants tolerate pregnancy well. The more common complications are preterm labour and delivery and preeclampsia. Vaginal delivery is recommended.
- Slight nausea and vomiting are common in pregnancy and may affect up to 70% of women in the first trimester. Other causes of vomiting must be considered and ruled out before accepting that vomiting is due to the pregnancy alone.
- Hyperemesis gravidarum may lead to maternal death if not treated actively. The condition is associated with excessive placental tissue and is more common in multiple pregnancies and hydatidiform mole. The woman is admitted to hospital so that investigations can be made. Antiemetics should be given and fluids and electrolytes replaced by intravenous infusion. Deterioration may rarely necessitate termination of pregnancy to save the woman's life.
- In early pregnancy appendicitis may be difficult to differentiate from threatened abortion. Later in pregnancy the pain may be mistaken for urinary tract infection, abruptio placentae or the onset of labour. Careful consideration of the patient's symptoms should allow a differential diagnosis to be made. The appendix must be removed to save life.
- If peptic ulceration is present up to 80% of women experience an improvement although almost all will have a recurrence of their symptoms by 2 years following the pregnancy. The improvement may be due to the reduction of gastric acidity present in pregnancy. An ileostomy or colostomy for urinary or alimentary diversion should not affect the course of pregnancy. About 75% of women with stomas will have a normal vaginal delivery.
- Epilepsy is a general term for a group of conditions that cause seizures. The term convulsion refers to the clonic-tonic movements associated with some seizures. Pathological processes lead to seizures although some people may have a lower seizure threshold than others. Seizures may be provoked by many triggers.
- In status epilepticus a second or more seizures follows the first before consciousness is fully regained and the person is said to be in the postictal state when the next seizure begins. Inadequately treated cerebral hypoxia may result in dementia, mental retardation and death. The individual is also at risk of aspiration.
- Immediately prior to the onset of a seizure there may be an aura and earlier there may have been a prodroma. The underlying cause of the seizures is established by taking a health history and by physical examination. If there is a correctable cause treatment is offered. If this is not possible, antiseizure treatment is begun.
- Epilepsy affects one in 200 pregnant women. There may be an increase or decrease in seizures but there is often no change for most epileptic women. Preconception advice is important so that the drug regime can be altered prior to conception. Some of the drugs used to control epilepsy are teratogenic. This may be related to folate antagonism. Folic acid supplements should be given.
- Seizures occurring during pregnancy may cause fetal hypoxia or placental abruption. Anticonvulsants cross the placenta and decrease the production of vitamin K, which may lead to haemorrhagic disease of the newborn. Vitamin K should be administered to mothers from 36 weeks gestation and to all infants of epileptic mothers.

References

Arias F. 1993 Practical Guide to High Risk Pregnancy and Delivery, 2nd edn. Mosby Year Book, Chicago.

Bewley C. 1997 Medical conditions complicating pregnancy. In Sweet BR with Tiran D (eds) Mayes Midwifery, 12th edn. Baillière Tindall, London, pp 548–569.

Blackburn ST, Loper DL. 1992 Maternal, Fetal and Neonatal Physiology, A Clinical Perspective. WB Saunders, Philadelphia.

Borison HL, Wang SC. 1953 Physiology and pharmacology of vomiting. Pharmacology Review 5, 193–230.

Brock TD, Madigan MT. 1991 Biology of Micro-organisms, 6th edn. Prentice-Hall International, New Jersey.

Brodie MJ. 1990 Management of epilepsy during pregnancy and lactation. Lancet 336 (8712), 426–427.

Chamberlain G. 1992 ABC of Antenatal Care. BMJ Books, London.

Davison JM. 1987 Pregnancy in renal allograft recipients: prognosis and management. Clinical Obstetrics and Gynaecology 1(4), 1027–1045.

Karlen A. 1995 Plagues Progress, A Social history of Man and Disease. Victor Gollancz, London.

Katz AI, Davison JN, Hayslett JP et al. 1980 Pregnancy in women with renal disease. Kidney International 18, 192–206.

Kelly S. 1996 Disorders caused by pregnancy. In Bennett VR, Brown LK (eds) Myles Textbook for Midwives, 12th edn. Churchill Livingstone, Edinburgh,

pp 306–319.
Kumar A, Busse WW. 1995 Airway inflammation in asthma. Scientific American 38–47.
Leatherman JW, Ingram RJ. 1992 Respiratory medicine: II asthma. In Rubenstein E, Federman D (eds), Scientific American Medicine, New York, Scientific American Inc. Cited in McCance KL, Huether SE. 1994 Pathophysiology, the Biologic Basis for Disease in Adults and Children, Mosby, St Louis, Missouri: p 1166.
Lindsay P. 1997 Vomiting. In Sweet BS with Tiran D (eds) Mayes Midwifery, 12th edn. Baillière Tindall, London, pp. 507–510.
Lloyd C, Lewis V. 1996 Diseases associated with pregnancy. In Bennett VR, Brown LK. (eds) Myles Textbook for Midwives, 12th edn. Churchill Livingstone, Edinburgh, pp 333–364.
McCance KL, Huether SE. 1994 Pathophysiology. The Biologic Basis for Disease in Adults and Children, 2nd edn. Mosby Year Book, Chicago.
Parish P. 1991 Medical Treatments: the Risks and Benefits. Penguin, Harmondsworth.
Profet M. 1992 Pregnancy sickness as adaptation: a deterrent to maternal ingestion of toxins. In Barkow JH et al (eds) The Adapted Mind. Oxford University Press, New York, pp 327–365.
Rang HP, Dale MM. 1991 Pharmacology. Churchill Livingstone, Edinburgh.
Rankin S. 1996 Disorders of pregnancy. In Bennett VR, Brown LK (eds) Myles Textbook for Midwives, 12th edn. Churchill Livingstone, Edinburgh, pp 320–334.
Stables D. 1995 Mother and child nursing: stomas and pregnancy. In Heath HBM (ed) Potter and Perry's Foundations in Nursing Theory and Practice. Mosby, London, p 477.
Thomson V. 1996 Psychological and physiological changes of pregnancy. In Bennett VR, Brown LK (eds) Myles Textbook for Midwives, 12th edn. Churchill Livingstone, Edinburgh.
Tyack AJ. 1991 Vomiting in pregnancy. Current Opinion in Obstetrics and Gynaecology 1, 93–96.
Valentine BV, Jones C, Tyack AJ. 1980 Hyperemesis gravidarum due to thyrotoxicosis. Postgraduate Medical Journal 56, 746–747.

Recommended reading

Brodie MJ. 1990 Management of epilepsy during pregnancy and lactation. Lancet 336(8712), 426–427.
Katz AI, Davison JN, Hayslett JP et al. 1980 Pregnancy in women with renal disease. Kidney International 18, 192–206.
Tyack AJ. 1991 Vomiting in pregnancy. Current Opinion in Obstetrics and Gynaecology 1, 93–96.
Valentine BV, Jones C, Tyack AJ. 1980 Hyperemesis gravidarum due to thyrotoxicosis. Postgraduate Medical Journal 56, 746–747.

Chapter 35

Metabolic disorders in pregnancy – diabetes mellitus and thyroid disorders

In this chapter

DIABETES MELLITUS

Diabetes mellitus is a group of disorders characterised by **impaired carbohydrate utilisation** caused by an absolute or relative deficiency of insulin production by the endocrine pancreas. Before reading on, it may be advisable to revise the topics concerning the metabolism of nutrients. The role of insulin and the digestion and absorption of glucose across cell membranes and its use by cells have been described in the chapters on the gastrointestinal tract (21) and nutrition (23).

Pathophysiology

The inability of the tissues to receive enough glucose results in inhibition of **glycolytic enzymes** and activation of the enzymes involved in **gluconeogenesis** (Bewley 1997). This results in more glucose being present in the bloodstream which cannot be utilised. Excessive glucose passes into the renal filtrate which cannot be reabsorbed and **glycosuria** occurs. Glucose is osmotically active and pulls water after it, resulting in **polyuria** and dehydration. Thirst increases to try and maintain body fluids at an adequate level.

The body tries to mobilise energy sources from fats and proteins. Amino acids are broken down during gluconeogenesis. Urea, which is produced as a by product of amino acid metabolism, is excreted in the urine. The release of fatty acids always results in **ketogenesis** but in the diabetic person, ketones will be produced in excess and again excreted in the urine. The ketones in the blood cause **metabolic acidosis**, resulting in a lowering of the pH. The buffer systems attempt to correct this and become exhausted. Other metabolic processes are also disturbed and all systems of the body are affected. If untreated, acidosis will lead to shock, coma and death.

Signs and symptoms

Diabetes is a syndrome which includes chronic hyperglycaemia and other disturbances of carbohydrate, fat and protein metabolism (McCance & Huether 1994). These authors describe the historical diagnosis of diabetes with weight loss, excessive urination (polyuria), thirst (**polydipsia**) and hunger (**polyphagia**).

Types of diabetes mellitus

The World Health Organization (WHO 1985) identified four major classes of diabetes mellitus.

Type 1 or Insulin-dependent diabetes mellitus (IDDM)

Onset is usually in juveniles and there is an almost total lack of insulin production. Hyperglycaemia, polyuria and ketosis are present at onset and insulin treatment is necessary.

Type II or non-insulin dependent diabetes mellitus (NIDDM)

Women with this type of diabetes will have an abnormal glucose tolerance test (GTT) but rarely have symptoms. There seems to be a resistance to insulin in the tissues and the onset is usually in later life and in obese people. There is a form of NIDDM called **mature-onset diabetes of the young (MODY)** which is caused by an autosomal dominant gene and has an age of onset under 25 years.

Malnutrition-related diabetes mellitus (MRDM)

This type of diabetes is found in developing countries in young people with severe protein malnutrition and emaciation (McCance & Huether 1994). It is unlikely that they would be fertile and the condition is unlikely to be seen in the developed countries. There is severe hyperglycaemia without ketosis.

Other types of diabetes mellitus

Diabetes also occurs secondary to other conditions such as pancreatic disease, hormonal disorders or the effect of drugs and chemical agents.

Related conditions

Impaired glucose tolerance (IGT)

This condition used to be known as **latent diabetes**. The GTT is normal except in situations where a woman is stressed and then she may develop diabetes. When this occurs in pregnancy it is called **gestational diabetes** although Jarrett (1993) concludes that gestational diabetes is no more than a special case of impaired glucose tolerance temporarily associated with pregnancy. About 15% of such women will develop NIDDM in later life. If obesity is present the incidence of later onset of diabetes rises to 70%. Jarrett agrees with this but states that any fetomaternal morbidity is more likely to be due to maternal age or obesity rather than to a diabetic state.

Aetiology

Type I or juvenile-onset diabetes (IDDM)

IDDM accounts for about 10% of diabetes in the developed countries. There are differences between populations both within and between countries. For instance, it is thought to be more prevalent amongst white members of a population and the incidence around the world is highest in Finland and lowest in Japan. There is a seasonal variation in the onset of IDDM with more new cases in the Northern hemisphere being reported in the autumn and winter.

There is a long period of subclinical diabetes as the β cells are progressively destroyed. Islet cell antibodies have been found years before the onset of clinical signs. There is considerable evidence that α cell function is impaired, leading to an excess of glucagon. This would exacerbate the hyperglycaemia. Autoantibodies have been found in the majority of people with juvenile-onset diabetes.

Type I diabetes mellitus can be subdivided into two distinct types.

1. IDDM type IA is thought to be due to a genetic–environmental interaction which results in destruction of the β cells in the pancreas. There is a link with a **human leucocyte antigen** (found on the surface of white cells) – HLA-DR4. The predisposing gene is carried on chromosome 6. Diagnosis is rare before 9 months and peaks at 12 years of age. About 12% of newly diagnosed diabetics of this type have a first-degree relative with the disease.
2. IDDM type IB is probably an autoimmune disorder with a link to carriage of HLA-DR3. It tends to occur later in life, between the ages of 30 and 50.

Type II or mature-onset diabetes (NIDDM)

Type II diabetes mellitus is four times as common as IDDM. Once again, incidence varies with ethnicity and environment, suggesting a genetic–environment interaction (McCance & Huether 1994). It is not usually until after the age of 40 that NIDDM affects people and many of them are obese. Obesity is a factor in three-quarters of individuals who develop NIDDM although a subtype of NIDDM, MODY, affects younger individuals who are usually of light to normal weight.

There are no specific pancreatic changes seen. **Amyloid deposits**, associated with islet cell destruction, are seen in about 25% and usually correlate with the age of the person and the degree of severity. The cause of the decrease in weight and number of islet cells is not yet clear. The ratio of α to β cells is normal and there is no reduction of insulin in the blood. The most important risk factor is obesity, often secondary to an excessive calorie intake. In obese people insulin has a decreased ability to influence cellular uptake of glucose. There are multiple explanations for this phenomenon but the most popular is increased insulin resistance because of decreased cellular insulin receptors.

Clinical diagnosis

Once suspected, a GTT will confirm the presence of diabetes. A drink containing 75 g of glucose is given in the morning after the patient has fasted. Venous blood samples are taken at intervals. Normally blood glucose rises but returns to normal within 2 h. The following abnormalities occur in the diabetic:

- a fasting plasma glucose of over 7 mmol/l;
- a blood glucose level over 10 mmol/l after 2 h;
- if the 2-h blood glucose level is between 7 and 10 mmol/l, glucose tolerance is impaired.

Pathological effects

Seventy years ago a young diabetic was likely to die within 2

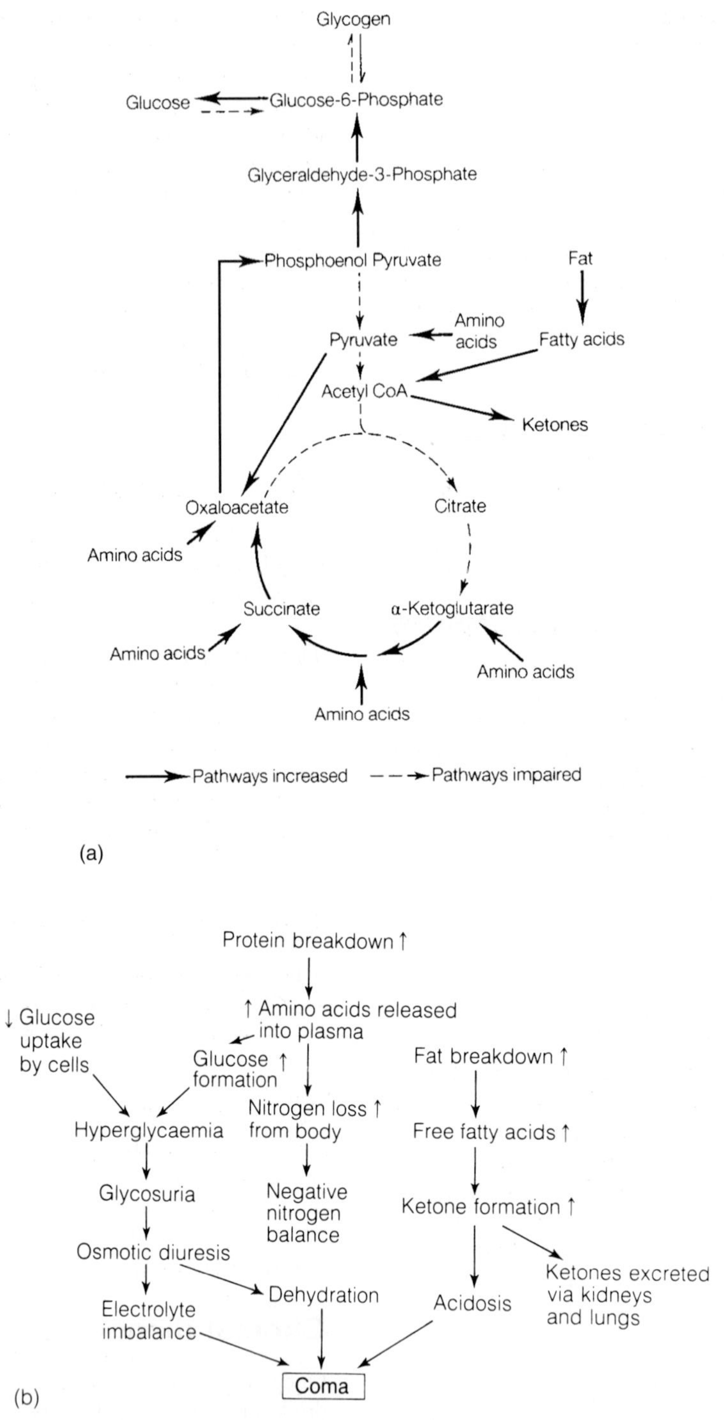

Figure 35.1 *Diabetes mellitus: (a) metabolic changes, (b) physiological effects (from Hinchliff SM, Montague SE, 1990, with permission).*

years of the onset of illness. The identification of insulin by Banting and Best and its development as a therapy led to survival but consequently, the acute and long-term effects became apparent. Deaths from cardiovascular disease and renal disease are much more common than in the general population. A brief review of these complications is given below. A good overview of diabetes mellitus can be found in McCance & Huether (1994). Acute complications include **hypoglycaemia** and **diabetic ketoacidosis**.

Hypoglycaemia

The term hypoglycaemia refers to a lowered plasma glucose level. It occurs at some time in 90% of IDDM and is also known as **insulin shock** or **insulin reaction**. The aim for a diabetic patient is to prevent hypoglycaemia by diet and insulin administration.

Symptoms

Symptoms vary between individuals but tend to be consistent for an individual. They result from cellular starvation. If neurones cannot obtain enough carbohydrate to maintain normal function, tachycardia, palpitations, tremors, pallor and anxiety occur. Other symptoms include headaches, dizziness, irritability, confusion, visual disturbances, hunger, convulsions and coma.

Management

Emergency treatment is to provide glucose. If the person is conscious ingestion of a fast-acting carbohydrate can be encouraged. If the individual has lapsed into coma intravenous glucose is necessary.

Diabetic ketoacidosis

Ketoacidosis is a serious condition which may lead to death. It develops when there is insufficient insulin and an increase in hormones antagonising the effect of insulin, such as catecholamines, glucagon, cortisol and growth hormone. Liver glucose production increases and peripheral glucose usage decreases. Fat mobilisation increases and ketogenesis occurs. In a known diabetic the most likely precipitating causes are infection, trauma, surgery or myocardial infarction. Interruption of insulin administration can also lead to ketoacidosis. Health education should enable people to avoid the precipitating causes.

Symptoms

The symptoms of ketoacidosis are often non-specific. Coma is rare. Polyuria, polydipsia and dehydration will occur because of **osmotic diuresis**. Sodium, magnesium and phosphorus deficits may occur but the most severe electrolyte disturbance is deficiency in potassium. Hyperventilation (Kussmaul respirations) may occur to attempt to compensate for the acidosis. Other symptoms may include postural dizziness, anorexia, nausea and abdominal pain. Both glucose and ketones will be present in urine. There may be a smell of acetone on the breath.

Management

Treatment of diabetic ketoacidosis is to decrease blood glucose levels by continual administration of low-dose insulin. Fluids and electrolytes are replaced as needed, depending on laboratory findings.

Chronic complications

Diabetic neuropathy with sensory deficits and microvascular disease with thickening of capillary basement membrane occur. The latter appears to be directly linked to the duration of the disease and blood glucose levels. Retinal ischaemia causes blood vessel changes (**retinopathy**) leading to loss of sight. The kidney is also commonly affected (**nephropathy**), resulting in endstage renal disease.

Macrovascular disease with atherosclerosis occurs, leading to coronary artery disease and stroke. This is unrelated to the severity of diabetes and appears in people who only have impaired glucose tolerance. Deposition of lipids in the atherosclerotic lesions may occur. The atherosclerosis appears at a younger age and progresses more rapidly in diabetic people. Peripheral vascular disease leading to gangrene and amputation due to atherosclerosis is often seen.

Infection is more likely to occur because pathogens use the increased tissue glucose to multiply and the function of phagocytic white cells is impaired. If neuropathy is present, breaks in the skin may go unnoticed and vascular disease may reduce the blood supply to tissues, impairing the body's ability to heal.

Effects in pregnancy

The incidence of carbohydrate metabolism abnormalities in pregnancy varies between 1% and 3%. Most of these women will have a genetic or metabolic predisposition to diabetes which leads to a failure to compensate for the diabetogenic effect of pregnancy, i.e. they develop carbohydrate intolerance (Arias 1993). Chamberlain (1992) states that four-fifths of women with diabetes will be known to their doctor prior to becoming pregnant. Diabetes becomes more difficult to control in pregnancy although immediately after delivery women return to their prepregnancy needs. Most women with carbohydrate intolerance show no signs or symptoms but there is a significant increase in fetal and maternal morbidity.

Maternal problems (Garner 1995)

Preeclampsia will develop in about 13% and infection is more common, with a high incidence of urinary tract and vaginal infections, chorioamnionitis and postpartum infection.

Fetal problems

- First-trimester abortions
- Congenital abnormalities
- Macrosomia
- Polyhydramnios
- Traumatic delivery
- Stillbirth
- Neonatal asphyxia
- In the newborn, respiratory distress syndrome
- Hyperviscosity syndrome

Congenital abnormalities, intrapartum and neonatal problems

Congenital abnormalities are more common, especially in poorly controlled diabetes. The embryonic and fetal abnormalities occur because development takes place in a metabolically abnormal environment. Glucose and ketones are two of the teratogenic agents responsible for a range of defects in poorly controlled diabetes (Sadler et al 1989). The first 6 weeks following conception are the most important; spontaneous abortion or congenital anomalies of the nervous, cardiovascular, renal and skeletal systems may occur (Buchanan & Kitzmiller 1994).

Buchanan & Kitzmiller differentiate between **embryopathy** or congenital abnormality and **fetopathy**, which results from fetal overnutrition and hyperinsulinaemia in the 2nd and 3rd trimesters. Poor diabetic control in the 2nd and 3rd trimesters may result in **macrosomia**, i.e. large-for-gestational-age babies with birth weights over the 90th centile. However, this is not a simple relationship between blood glucose levels and fetal size. Both protein (Metzger 1991) and triglyceride (Knopp et al 1985) metabolism have been implicated in excessive fetal growth.

Effect of pregnancy on the diabetes

The additional metabolic requirements of the fetus place large demands on the mechanisms that maintain adequate nutrient supply to the cells during both the absorptive and post-absorptive phases of metabolism. Maternal metabolism changes to allow more efficient storage of nutrients while minimising catabolism of the woman's own protein stores (Buchanan & Kitzmiller 1994).

As we have seen in Chapter 23, there is progressive insulin resistance in pregnancy which disappears immediately after delivery of the baby with its placenta. Normally the β cells increase the amount of insulin they release in the presence of insulin resistance. Insulin needs increase progressively during pregnancy, maintaining carbohydrate tolerance. Glucose metabolism in diabetic pregnant women is likely to become unstable and more insulin will be needed to achieve metabolic control.

Diabetic nephropathy

Diabetic nephropathy is present in 5% of pregnant women with IDDM and significant proteinuria in the first trimester is associated with poor outcome. In more than half of such pregnancies, delivery is before 37 weeks and by caesarean section (Garner 1995). Oedema, anaemia and hypertension further complicate the pregnancy. There is difficulty in choosing an appropriate drug for controlling hypertension. Although in the non-pregnant patient protein-restricted diet would be commenced, this is generally avoided in pregnancy because of the nutritional needs of the fetus. Even though the outcome may be satisfactory in that the woman has a live, healthy infant, long-term morbidity and mortality may affect her ability to raise her child.

Diabetic retinopathy

Diabetic retinopathy may worsen in pregnancy and there is also evidence that improved glycaemic control may add to this problem. Ophthalmologic examination and evaluation should be carried out at regular intervals and the Valsalva manoeuvre avoided in labour to prevent possible haemorrhage. Women who have proliferative retinopathy with **neovascularisation** (new growth of blood vessels) have a greater risk of loss of vision during pregnancy. New growth of blood vessels can be prevented or treated by laser photocoagulation before or during the pregnancy.

Type I diabetes mellitus

IDDM complicates less than 0.5% of pregnancies but as Garner (1995) writes, it is an enormous challenge to those caring for such women. Prior to the availability of insulin, fetal and neonatal mortality was 60% but vast improvements in care and outcomes have been made and the fetal/neonatal loss can be as low as 2%.

Care in pregnancy

Preconception advice

There is an urgent need to discuss pregnancy with the woman with confirmed diabetes mellitus prior to conception. Arias (1993) suggests the following important aspects of care:

- adequate blood glucose control;
- self-monitoring;
- fetal surveillance.

Achieving **adequate blood glucose control** prior to conception helps to reduce the number of early abortions, congenital abnormalities, fetal macrosomia, polyhydramnios and stillbirth. Research and experience have shown that diabetic women whose blood sugar is well controlled around conception and during pregnancy have abnormal pregnancy outcomes approaching the incidence of the non-diabetic population (Arias 1993). Ideally plasma glucose levels should be below 5.0 mmol/l in the fasting state and less than 7.8 mmol/l after a meal (Garner 1995).

The importance of **self-monitoring** needs to be discussed and the point made that good control can only be achieved by this means. Women must be told of the gastrointestinal disturbances likely to occur in the first trimester of pregnancy. Information should be provided about the manner in which glucose metabolism is changed by the presence of the fetus. Instant reporting of problems to the doctor will allow rapid adjustments to therapy to be made.

The necessity for **fetal surveillance** should be emphasised and likely fetal problems discussed. The risks of fetal abnormality and the methods of diagnosis and possible outcomes should be discussed prior to pregnancy so that the woman and her partner can take decisions based on an understanding of the problems. The effect of the pregnancy on the woman's lifestyle needs to be highlighted. The time and cost of care, the implications for maintaining a job, especially if it is a demanding one, and the need for medical leave should all be considered.

The role of Haemoglobin A_1 (HbA_1) concentration

Glycosylated haemoglobin (HbA_1) is a type of adult haemoglobin where glucose is attached to part of the β-chain. As this takes time to occur, HbA_1 levels indicate the blood glucose levels that were present about 2 months before the reading. They are increased in diabetes, especially if blood glucose control is not adequate. Pregnancy should be deferred until HbA_1 is less than 8% of the total (0.08 SI units). Following conception some advocate monthly HbA_1 readings but this may not be any better at predicting neonatal birth weight or neonatal hypoglycaemia than mean glucose concentration estimations (Garner 1995).

Management during pregnancy

It is important that health professionals collaborate with the diabetic woman in her care during pregnancy. The involvement of the diabetic team, the obstetrician and the midwife is essential. The woman should be booked for care and delivery in a consultant unit with attached neonatal care unit and is usually seen at least every 2 weeks.

Diabetic control

The management of diabetes before and during pregnancy in order to maximise normal fetal development requires control of blood sugar and prevention of ketosis. If control is too extreme so that there is hypoglycaemia this may endanger the mother and may cause fetal intrauterine growth retardation (Buchanan & Kitzmiller 1994). The woman's diet and insulin dosage should be monitored with blood glucose levels. Because of the altered renal threshold for glucose, urinary glucose levels are of no help. The adjustment of insulin dosage during the antenatal period is usually managed better at home so that the normal food and energy usage of the woman are adhered to rather than by admission to the unusual surroundings of a hospital.

Insulin

The need for insulin increases during pregnancy because of the increased energy requirements and the diabetogenic hormones produced by the placenta (Bewley 1997, Garner 1995). Better control can be obtained by altering the regimen to twice-daily soluble and intermediate insulin. This avoids the tendency to hypoglycaemia which occurs in pregnancy. Garner (1995) writes that only 1% of diabetic pregnancies are now complicated by ketoacidosis. It is mainly associated with hyperemesis gravidarum and infections and there may be minimal hyperglycaemia. If ketoacidosis does occur there may be a fetal loss of 20%.

Diet

Brenchley (1994) considers that dietary advice during pregnancy should aim 'to achieve good diabetes control together with ensuring optimum nutrition for both mother and baby'. A calorie intake of 35 kcal/kg body weight is recommended (Garner 1995). An ideal dietary composition would be 55% carbohydrate, 20% protein and 25% fats with polyunsaturated fats no more than 10%. This could be divided between three meals and three snacks. Ethnic differences in dietary habits should be understood and discussed with the woman. Obese women may be asked to eat fewer calories as long as they do not lose weight or develop ketonuria.

The newly diagnosed diabetic

Some women develop diabetes during pregnancy and will need the information education provided above about diet, insulin dosage, blood glucose monitoring and the recognition and management of hypoglycaemia, as well as more general aspects such as the effects of exercise and prevention of infection.

Monitoring the fetus

Ongoing fetal well-being should be monitored closely using the methods discussed in Chapter 13. Although fetal macrosomia is the main problem, the babies of women with renal disease or superimposed preeclampsia may suffer from intrauterine growth retardation.

Delivery

It is usual to deliver the woman with uncomplicated diabetes and no obstetric problems vaginally at 38 weeks. Women with unstable diabetes, complications or obstetric problems may be delivered earlier by caesarean section to avoid the possibility of intrauterine death. Following induced or spontaneous onset of labour, 5% dextrose is infused at a rate of 1 l every 8 h. Insulin is given according to hourly blood glucose results on a sliding scale to maintain blood glucose levels of 4.5–5.5 mmol/l. Immediately following delivery insulin requirements usually revert back to prepregnancy levels.

Care in the puerperium

Insulin requirements fall and restabilisation is necessary. It is important to avoid infection.

Breastfeeding is possible but it is necessary to remember that lactating women have a higher energy turnover and this means diet and insulin dosage need to be monitored carefully.

Family planning methods must be discussed. The oral contraceptive pill can be taken but may mimic pregnancy, increasing the need for insulin. The intrauterine contraceptive device may lead to infection and is not recommended for most diabetic women. A barrier method may be used by women wishing to add to their family.

The problems and care of the baby of a diabetic mother are discussed in Chapter 52.

Gestational diabetes (GDM)

Berkowitz et al (1992) define gestational diabetes as 'the onset or recognition of glucose intolerance during pregnancy'. They also write that gestational diabetes is associated with an increased risk of perinatal morbidity and mortality. There are usually no symptoms and diagnosis depends on abnormal blood glucose results, usually following a GTT (see above). Avery & Rossi (1994) write that GDM may be detected by screening or by clinical diagnosis.

GDM occurs in 2% of all pregnancies usually in the third trimester. Following delivery glucose metabolism may return to normal, stay impaired or diabetes mellitus may develop. McCance & Huether (1994) state that 60% of these women will develop diabetes mellitus within 15 years of the pregnancy. Gestational diabetes is likely to recur in subsequent pregnancies and such patients should be retested in each pregnancy (Philipson & Super 1989). Oats (1995) provides a useful review of diabetes in pregnancy concluding that at least 50% of women who develop GDM are at risk of developing NIDDM and that the prevention of obesity, consumption of high fibre diet and, in some cases, hypoglycaemic drugs may prevent this progression.

The Third International Workshop/Conference on GDM recommended screening of all pregnant women at 24–28 weeks gestation. However, there is still much controversy about the benefits of screening, summarised by Jarrett (1993) who states that screening for a condition where there is no agreement on definition or even treatment cannot be cost effective. Most obstetricians use clinical findings from history taking or from the present pregnancy to select out women for whom they order tests to diagnose the presence of GDM. Arias (1993) lists these as:

- a history of diabetes in close relatives;
- chronic hypertension;

- recurrent urogenital infections;
- age over 30 years;
- poor reproductive history (three or more spontaneous abortions);
- a previous baby weighing more than 4000 g;
- a previous unexplained perinatal death;
- a previous baby with unexplained congenital malformations;
- history of GDM in a previous pregnancy;
- an obese woman;
- glycosuria on two occasions at antenatal visit;
- the presence of polyhydramnios.

Population differences in incidence

Studies have been conducted into variations in the incidence of gestational diabetes between different ethnic groups (Berkowitz et al 1992, Dornhurst et al 1992, Shelley-Jones et al 1993). Berkowitz et al (1992) carried out their research in America and found that there was an excess risk of developing gestational diabetes in women from India and the Middle East, Oriental women and first-generation Hispanic women. They also found an increased risk in women of lower socioeconomic class, older women, obese women and those with infertility.

In Britain the study by Dornhurst et al (1992) found a high prevalence of gestational diabetes in women from ethnic minority groups, in older women, in increasing parity and in obesity. In particular, compared to white women, they found an 11-fold increase in gestational diabetes in women from the Indian subcontinent but only a threefold increase in black women.

Shelley-Jones et al (1993), working in Australia, examined variations in racial differences to ascertain why Asian-born (Oriental) women have such a high incidence of gestational diabetes. They compared in depth the physiology of 15 women with normal glucose tolerance, 16 Caucasian women with GDM and 19 Asian-born women with GDM, measuring body size, lipid metabolism and serum insulin response to an oral glucose load. Compared to the control group, the following findings were reported.

- **Obesity** The most significant finding was that Caucasian women, unlike the Asian women, were obese compared to the control group of women.
- **Insulin response** Both groups of women with GDM had a similar abnormal response to the glucose load.
- **Serum triglycerides** Fasting serum triglycerides were increased in all women with GDM. Asian women had significantly lower serum cholesterol levels than the Caucasian women, with or without GDM.

The authors concluded that it is difficult to know whether the differences in obesity and serum cholesterol 'reflect a dietary difference or a major difference in lipid metabolism'.

These research findings from around the world have been included to demonstrate how difficult it is to separate the relative importance of genetic or environmental factors in the causation of any of the types of diabetes mellitus.

Complications

There is an increased incidence of complications for both mother and fetus in GDM (Avery & Rossi 1994). Macrosomia, which is usually taken to mean a birth weight of 4000 g or more, is twice as frequent. This leads to a greater incidence of difficult births, including increased use of forceps delivery and caesarean section. Shoulder dystocia is a problem and may result in injury to the mother or baby.

Postnatally, women should be counselled about the possibility of developing NIDDM later in life and about ways to minimise the risk. They should be reminded of the need to maintain normal body weight, to exercise regularly, to have annual blood glucose tests and to ensure that they receive early care if they become pregnant again (Avery & Rossi 1994).

Management

Once GDM is diagnosed, treatment should begin aimed at controlling blood glucose, additional fetal surveillance and decreasing the incidence of macrosomia with its attendant problems. Modification of diet is the main target and is similar to that described above in the care of women with IDDM, with the carbohydrate content taken in complex starchy forms and fat to be less than 30% of total calories. Dietary control is usually sufficient in GDM but occasionally insulin injections will be necessary. The need for insulin should disappear after delivery.

Thompson et al (1990) carried out a randomised controlled research programme into the use of prophylactic insulin in the management of gestational diabetes. They explored the use of diet alone against the use of diet + insulin in 108 women with GDM who were randomly assigned to the two groups. They found that insulin therapy had no apparent detrimental effect on pregnancy and there was no incidence of hypoglycaemia. The best results were seen in the obese patients where larger reductions in birth weights were seen. However, there has been no suggestion that routine use of insulin should supersede its use in carefully selected women.

The baby of a diabetic mother

If there has been poor control of the diabetes mellitus the baby may be large, weighing over the 90th centile, and plethoric (Fig. 35.2). With the good control usually achieved in current practice, babies are more likely to be of a weight appropriate for gestational age (Bewley 1997). However, the baby may be physiologically immature and have problems similar to those of a preterm baby, including respiratory distress syndrome (Chapter 51). Congenital defects are also related to the control of the diabetes around the time of conception. Birth injuries may occur if the baby is large (Chapter 53).

Hypoglycaemia may also be a problem because the islets of Langerhans have hypertrophied during prenatal life and produce more insulin in response to high maternal blood glucose levels. Once delivered, the baby no longer has access to this high glucose source. Careful monitoring of neonatal blood glucose and early feeding should help to prevent severe side effects. Other problems encountered in this group of babies are skin infections, polycythaemia with hyperbilirubinaemia, weight loss and bleeding from the thick umbilical cord. The baby tends to be lethargic at first but development then proceeds normally.

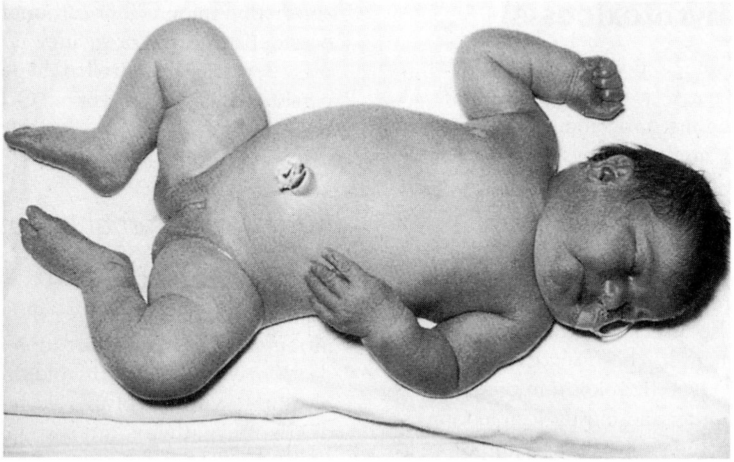

Figure 35.2 *A large-for-gestational-age baby from a diabetic mother (from Kelnar C, Harvey D, Simpson C, 1995, with permission).*

ABNORMALITIES OF THYROID FUNCTION

Overactivity and underactivity of the thyroid gland can produce serious illness with metabolic disturbances.

Hypothyroid disturbances may result from a defect in the thyroid gland or in the hormonal control pathway of TRH or TSH release. A deficiency in dietary iodine may also cause the problem. In adults hypothyroidism is called **myxoedema** and symptoms include a low BMR, feeling cold, constipation, thick, dry skin, puffy eyes, oedema, lethargy and mental sluggishness.

When the cause is lack of iodine the thyroid gland hypertrophies, producing an endemic goitre (this has been called Derbyshire neck because of its link with inland environments). The thyroid gland is stimulated by increasing amounts of TSH but unusable colloid is produced. In infants hypothyroidism is called **cretinism**. This disorder is discussed in Chapter 52.

The most common **hyperthyroid** disturbance is called **Graves' disease** which is considered to be an autoimmune disorder (Fig. 35.3). Thyroid-stimulating immunoglobulins or TSIs (antibodies) attach to and activate TSH receptors on the follicular cells, causing increased production of thyroid hormones. Signs include raised BMR, excessive perspiration, weight loss despite good calorific intake, a rapid irregular heart beat and nervousness. Protrusion of the eyeballs (**exophthalmos**) may occur if the tissue behind the eye becomes oedematous and then fibrous. Treatment may be either by surgical removal of the thyroid gland or ingestion of radioisotope-tagged iodine to destroy the most active thyroid cells.

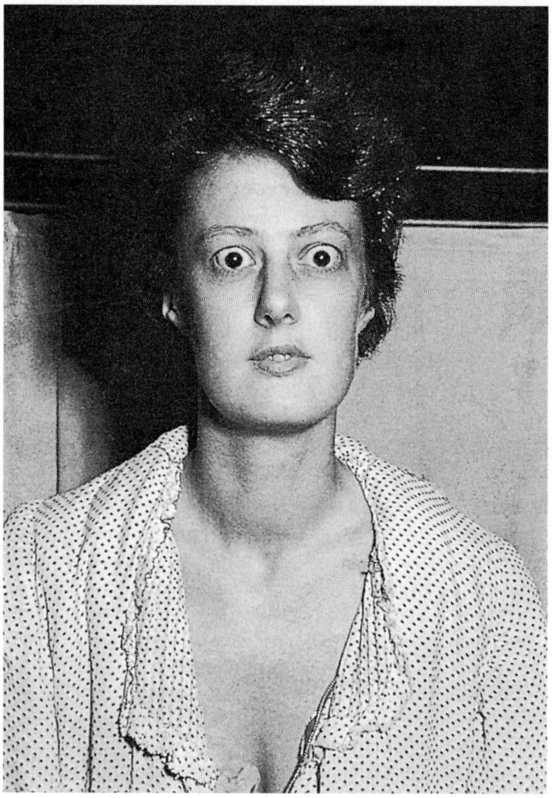

Figure 35.3 *A person with Graves' disease (from Hinchliff SM, Montague SE, 1990, with permission).*

Hypothyroidism

Hypothyroidism is more common than hyperthyroidism in pregnant women. Ramsay (1991) refers to an American study by Niswander & Gordon (1972) giving the statistics as nine per 1000 white women and three per 1000 black women. Untreated hypothyroidism is usually associated with infertility because TRH stimulation induces hyperprolactinaemia which prevents ovulation.

The hypothyroidism occasionally found in pregnancy is secondary to immune disorders or destruction of thyroid tissue, either surgically or with radioactive iodine. As long as the fetus is not exposed to iodine deficiency or teratogenic drugs, fetal development should be normal. Complications of increased fetal loss and prolonged pregnancy may occur. Diagnosis is suggested by excessive weight gain, cold intolerance, a slow pulse and a puffy face and confirmed by measurement of T_3 and T_4 levels. Treatment is by thyroxine medication.

Hyperthyroidism (thyrotoxicosis)

Hyperthyroidism occurs in about 2.2 per 1000 pregnant white women and 1.7 per 1000 black women (Ramsay 1991). Hypertension may occur for the first time about 12 weeks into the pregnancy. Because of the similar findings in normal pregnancy and hyperthyroidism, it may be difficult to diagnose the condition if it arises for the first time in pregnancy. However, failure to gain weight despite a good appetite, a rapid sleeping pulse and lid lag should raise the possibility. T_4 assays higher than the normal elevation of pregnancy will be present.

Severe hyperthyroidism is also associated with infertility but conception may occur if treatment has been successful or if the disease is mild (Bewley 1997). Hyperthyroidism in pregnancy is usually due to autoimmune disorder and mostly seen in Graves' disease, discussed above. If the hyperthyroidism is mild improvements to the woman's condition often accompany pregnancy. This is due to increase in TBG which can offset the increased production of thyroid hormones. Women with Graves' disease may also experience improvement during pregnancy due to the alterations in the immune system. Relapse is common within several weeks of delivery.

Management

Pregnant women with hyperthyroidism must take a diet with a higher calorific content than normal to compensate for the higher metabolic rate. Fluid loss may occur if the hyperthyroidism is accompanied by diarrhoea. Antithyroid drugs are used to control the disease but their effects must be monitored carefully so that the remission is not exacerbated with excessive levels of drug treatment. The antithyroid drugs commonly used are methyl thiouracil or carbimazole but treatment may need to be stopped during pregnancy. Care must be taken as the fetus may develop uncontrolled hyperthyroidism with a heart rate persistently above 160 bpm. Occasionally, it may be necessary to perform a **subtotal thyroidectomy** during the 2nd trimester if the disease is difficult to control or the woman has a large goitre.

Effect of maternal treatments on the fetus

Fetal hypothyroidism

If hyperthyroidism is poorly controlled during pregnancy, intrauterine growth retardation, preterm labour and perinatal death may occur. Antithyroid drugs may cross the placenta and block the synthesis of thyroid hormones by the fetus. The incidence of hypothyroidism is about one in 100 fetuses exposed to the drugs. Thyroid hormone supplements given to the mother to try to prevent fetal hypothyroidism will not succeed as the thyroid hormones and TSH do not cross the placenta.

Fetal hyperthyroidism

Thyroid-stimulating immunoglobulins (TSIs) may cross the placenta and lead to fetal hyperthyroidism. In pregnancies where there is placental transfer of long-acting thyroid stimulator (LATS) from mother to fetus, hyperthyroidism will result. Intrauterine treatment of the fetus is a growing area of research. Antithyroid drugs readily cross the placenta and can be used to treat fetal hyperthyroidism. If the mother then becomes hypothyroid she can be given thyroxine which does not cross the placenta. In some women who have thyrotoxicosis, placental transfer of LATS from mother to fetus will result in **neonatal hyperthyroidism**. The baby's thyroid function will return to normal within 3 weeks.

Summary of main points

- Diabetes mellitus is characterised by impaired carbohydrate utilisation caused by an absolute or relative deficiency of insulin production. Tissues cannot receive enough glucose, resulting in inhibition of glycolytic enzymes and activation of the enzymes involved in gluconeogenesis. There is hyperglycaemia and excess glucose passes into the renal filtrate, causing glycosuria, resulting in polyuria and dehydration with increased thirst.
- The body tries to mobilise energy sources from fats and proteins and ketone bodies released from fatty acids result in metabolic acidosis and a lowering of the pH. Other metabolic processes are also disturbed, affecting all body systems. If untreated, acidosis will lead to shock, coma and death.
- The development of diabetes in pregnancy is called gestational diabetes and occurs in 2% of all pregnancies, especially in the 3rd trimester. Following delivery, glucose metabolism may return to normal or stay impaired or diabetes mellitus may develop. Gestational diabetes is likely to recur in subsequent pregnancies.
- Insulin-dependent diabetes mellitus (IDDM) accounts for about 10% of diabetes in the developed countries. There are differences between populations both within and between countries and there is a seasonal variation in the onset of IDDM, with more new cases in the Northern hemisphere being reported in the autumn and winter. Autoantibodies have been found in the majority of people with juvenile-onset diabetes.
- Type II diabetes mellitus is four times as common as IDDM, occurring after the age of 40. In obese people insulin has a lowered ability to influence cellular uptake of glucose, possibly due to increased insulin resistance because of decreased cellular insulin receptors.
- Acute complications of diabetes mellitus include hypoglycaemia and diabetic ketoacidosis. Symptoms of hypoglycaemia include tachycardia, palpitations, tremors and pallor. Mental symptoms include anxiety, headaches, dizziness, irritability, confusion, visual disturbances, hunger, convulsions and coma. Emergency treatment is to provide glucose.
- Ketoacidosis may lead to death when there is insufficient insulin. Fat mobilisation increases and ketogenesis occurs. Treatment is to decrease blood glucose levels by continual administration of low-dose insulin. Fluids and electrolytes are replaced as needed. Chronic complications include diabetic neuropathy with sensory deficits.
- Most women who develop abnormalities of carbohydrate metabolism in pregnancy will have a genetic or metabolic predisposition to diabetes. Diabetes becomes more difficult to control in pregnancy although immediately after delivery women return to their prepregnancy needs.
- There is a significant increase in fetal and maternal morbidity and congenital abnormalities are more common, especially in poorly controlled diabetes. Glucose and ketones are teratogenic agents responsible for a range of defects. Poor diabetic control in the 2nd and 3rd trimesters may result in macrosomia. Both protein and triglyceride metabolism have been implicated in excessive fetal growth.

- Diabetic nephropathy is present in 5% of pregnant women with IDDM and significant proteinuria in the first trimester is associated with poor outcome. Diabetic retinopathy may worsen in pregnancy. Women who have proliferative retinopathy have a greater risk of loss of vision during pregnancy.
- Pregnancy should be discussed with the woman with confirmed diabetes mellitus prior to conception to achieve adequate blood glucose control and early fetal surveillance. Adequate blood glucose control prior to conception helps to reduce the number of early abortions and congenital abnormalities. Pregnancy should be deferred until HbA_1 is less than 8% of the total.
- The management of diabetes before and during pregnancy should aim to maximise normal fetal development which requires control of blood sugar and prevention of ketosis. The need for insulin increases and better control can be obtained by altering the regimen to twice-daily soluble and intermediate insulin.
- Dietary advice during pregnancy aims to achieve good diabetes control with optimum nutrition for both mother and baby. Ethnic differences in dietary habits should be understood and discussed with the woman. Obese women may be asked to eat fewer calories as long as they do not lose weight or develop ketonuria.
- Although fetal macrosomia is the main problem, babies of women with renal disease or superimposed preeclampsia may suffer from intrauterine growth retardation. Women with uncomplicated diabetes and no obstetric problems are usually delivered vaginally at 38 weeks. Women with unstable diabetes, complications or obstetric problems may be delivered earlier by caesarean section to avoid a risk of intrauterine death.
- In the puerperium insulin requirements fall and restabilisation is necessary. Breastfeeding is possible but lactating women have a higher energy turnover and this means diet and insulin dosage need to be monitored carefully. Family planning advisers should take the pathophysiology of diabetes mellitus into consideration.
- Gestational diabetes is associated with an increased risk of perinatal morbidity and mortality. There are usually no symptoms and diagnosis depends on abnormal blood glucose results, usually following a GTT. There is an excess risk of developing gestational diabetes in women from India and the Middle East, Oriental women and first-generation Hispanic women, in women of lower socioeconomic class, in older women, in obese women and those with infertility.
- There is an increased incidence of complications for both mother and fetus in GDM. Macrosomia is twice as frequent, leading to a greater incidence of difficult birth, including increased use of forceps delivery and caesarean section. Postnatally, women should be counselled about the risk of developing NIDDM later in life. Modification of diet is usually sufficient but occasionally insulin injections will be necessary.
- The baby may be physiologically immature and have problems similar to those of a preterm baby, including respiratory distress syndrome. Congenital defects are also related to the control of the diabetes around the time of conception. Birth injuries may occur if the baby is excessively large.
- Hypoglycaemia may also be a problem because the islets of Langerhans have hypertrophied during prenatal life and produce more insulin in response to high maternal blood glucose levels. Other problems include skin infections, polycythaemia with hyperbilirubinaemia, weight loss and bleeding from the thick umbilical cord.
- Untreated hypothyroidism is usually associated with infertility because TRH stimulation induces hyperprolactinaemia, which prevents ovulation. As long as the fetus is not exposed to iodine deficiency or teratogenic drugs, fetal development should be normal.
- Because of the similar findings in normal pregnancy and hyperthyroidism, it may be difficult to diagnose the condition if it arises for the first time in pregnancy. However, failure to gain weight despite a good appetite, a rapid sleeping pulse and lid lag should raise the possibility. Hyperthyroidism in pregnancy is usually due to autoimmune disorders, mainly Graves' disease.
- Pregnant women with hyperthyroidism must take a diet with a higher calorific content to compensate for the higher metabolic rate. The antithyroid drugs methyl thiouracil or carbimazole can readily cross the placenta and can be used to treat fetal hyperthyroidism. In some women who have thyrotoxicosis, placental transfer of long-acting thyroid stimulator from mother to fetus will result in neonatal hyperthyroidism which should return to normal within 3 weeks.

References

Arias F. 1993 Practical Guide to High Risk Pregnancy and Delivery, 2nd edn. Mosby Year Book, Chicago.

Avery MD, Rossi MA. 1994 Gestational diabetes. Journal of Nurse-Midwifery 39(2)(suppl) S9–S13.

Berkowitz GS, Lapinski RH, Wein R, Lee D. 1992 Race/ethnicity and other risk factors for gestational diabetes. American Journal of Epidemiology 135(9), 965–973.

Bewley C. 1997 Medical conditions complicating pregnancy. In Sweet BR with Tiran D (eds) Mayes Midwifery, 12th edn. Baillière Tindall, London, pp 548–569.

Brenchley S. 1994 Diabetes and pregnancy: current dietary advice. Professional Care of Mother and Child. 4(5): 128–130.

Buchanan TA, Kitzmiller JL. 1994 Metabolic interactions of diabetes and pregnancy. Annual Review of Medicine 45, 245–260.

Chamberlain G. 1992 ABC of Antenatal Care. BMJ Books, London, pp 38–40.

Dornhurst A, Paterson CE, Nicholls JSD, Wadsworth J, Chiu DC, Elkeles RS. 1992 High prevalence of gestational diabetes in women from ethnic minority groups. Diabetic Medicine 9, 820–825.

Garner P. 1995 Type I diabetes mellitus and pregnancy. Lancet 346, 157–161.

Hinchliff SM, Montague SE. 1990 Physiology for Nursing Practice. Baillière Tindall, London.

Jarrett RJ. 1993 Gestational diabetes: a non-entity? British Medical Journal 306, 37–38.

Kelnar C, Harvey D, Simpson C. 1995 The Sick Newborn Baby. Baillière Tindall, London.

Knopp RH, Bergelin RO, Wahl PW, Walden CE. 1985 Relationship of infant birth size to maternal lipoproteins, apoproteins, fuels, hormones, clinical chemistries and body weight at 36 weeks gestation. Diabetes 34(suppl 2), 71–77.

McCance KL, Huether SE. 1994 Pathophysiology, The Biologic Basis for Disease in Adults and Children, 2nd edn. Mosby Year Book, Chicago.

Metzger BE. 1991 Biphasic effects of maternal metabolism on fetal growth. Quintessential expression of fuel-mediated metabolism. Diabetes 40(suppl 2), 99–105.

Oats JN. 1995 Diabetes. Baillière's Clinical Obstetrics and Gynaecology 9(3), 481–495.

Philipson EH, Super DM. 1989 Gestational diabetes mellitus: does it recur in subsequent pregnancy? American Journal of Obstetrics and Gynecology 160(6), 1324–1331.

Ramsay ID. 1991 The thyroid gland. In Hytten F, Chamberlain G (eds) Clinical Physiology in Obstetrics. Blackwell Scientific, Oxford.

Sadler TW, Hunter ES III, Wynn RE, Phillips LS. 1989 Evidence for multifactorial origin of diabetes-induced embryopathies. Diabetes 38, 70–74.

Shelley-Jones DC, Wein P, Nolan C, Beischer NA. 1993 Why do Asian-born women have a higher incidence of gestational diabetes? An analysis of racial differences in body habitus, lipid metabolism and the serum insulin response to an oral glucose load. Australian and New Zealand Journal of Obstetrics and Gynaecology 33(2), 114–118.

Thompson DJ, Porter KB, Gunnells DJ, Wagner PC, Spinnato JA. 1990 Prophylactic insulin in the management of gestational diabetes. Obstetrics and Gynaecology 75(2), 960–964.

World Health Organization Study Group. 1985 Diabetes Mellitus Report of a Study Group. Technical report series 727. WHO, Geneva.

Recommended reading

Avery MD, Rossi MA. 1994 Gestational diabetes. Journal of Nurse-Midwifery 39(2)(suppl) S9–S13.

Buchanan TA, Kitzmiller JL. 1994 Metabolic interactions of diabetes and pregnancy. Annual Review of Medicine 45, 245–260.

Dornhurst A, Paterson CE, Nicholls JSD, Wadsworth J, Chiu DC, Elkeles RS. 1992 High prevalence of gestational diabetes in women from ethnic minority groups. Diabetic Medicine 9, 820–825.

Garner P. 1995 Type I diabetes mellitus and pregnancy. Lancet 346, 157–161.

Metzger BE. 1991 Biphasic effects of maternal metabolism on fetal growth. Quintessential expression of fuel-mediated metabolism. Diabetes 40(suppl 2), 99–105.

Shelley-Jones DC, Wein P, Nolan C, Beischer NA. 1993 Why do Asian-born women have a higher incidence of gestational diabetes? An analysis of racial differences in body habitus, lipid metabolism and the serum insulin response to an oral glucose load. Australian and New Zealand Journal of Obstetrics and Gynaecology 33(2), 114–118.

Section

3A

LABOUR – NORMAL

Section contents

Perhaps the most exciting aspect of childbearing is the birth. Midwives in the United Kingdom are privileged to be the major care-giver during this short but intensely meaningful time in the life of the woman and her family. Section 3A is about normal labour. There is no denial of the importance of social and psychological aspects of this major life event but these chapters concentrate on the management of labour that arises from a deep knowledge of physiology. In chapter 36 the onset and maintenance of labour are discussed. Although some researchers query the separation of labour into stages (discussed in the text), it is the author's opinion that such a division provides a basis for understanding the process. Therefore there is a chapter dedicated to each of the three stages of labour. Chapter 37 examines the physiology and management of the first stage of labour whilst chapter 38 concentrates specifically on pain pathways and pain relief in labour. Chapters 39 and 40 discuss the second and third stages of labour respectively.

Chapter

36 The onset of labour

In this chapter

INTRODUCTION

The two main issues about providing care for women in labour are how to meet the social, psychological and spiritual needs and to provide physiological safety for the woman and her baby. A major problem for anyone courageous enough to research the field of human behaviour, especially in physiological terms, is to place such behaviour in the context of cultural influences.

There are many textbooks devoted to the social meaning of pregnancy and labour and those by Sheila Kitzinger and Ann Oakley are worth reading for anyone considering how the management of childbearing is influenced by major changes and beliefs of society. The purpose of this chapter is to examine the physiological concepts associated with normal uncomplicated labour so that the reader can make caring decisions on the management of labour based on current concepts and theories.

Much of the core content of this chapter is derived from Blackburn & Loper (1992). Other references will be included in the text.

TIMING OF THE ONSET OF LABOUR

In humans the timing of the onset of labour is less precise than in many other species. The mean day of onset of labour in humans is probably about 39.6 weeks with a range of 3 weeks on either side of the mean. The timing may be related to fetal brain activity via ACTH and the pituitary adrenal axis. Progesterone is then metabolised to oestrogen which gradually increases the sensitivity of the uterus to prostaglandins and oxytocin produced by both the fetoplacental unit and maternal tissues. Many research projects into the onset of labour in cattle, sheep and humans have found that when there is an abnormality of the fetal hypothalamus and pituitary area of the brain, extreme prolongation of pregnancy may occur (Steer 1991).

The aetiology of labour is complex and at present not understood and therefore there are numerous hypotheses and theories. Because of this, there follows an outline only of key areas of discussion. If the sequence of events leading to the onset of labour was fully understood it might be easier to prevent the onset of preterm labour and the devastating fetal loss and morbidity resulting from extreme immaturity. There is good evidence for a central role for prostaglandins in the initiation of labour but the composition and biosynthesis of prostaglandins by the various tissues remains unclear (see below).

The role of the fetal endocrine system

There is evidence to support the concept that the fetus is largely responsible for triggering the onset of labour. However, there is still uncertainty about the role of the fetal hypothalamo-pituitary-adrenal axis in the initiation of labour in humans. It has become apparent that the extrapolation of experimental findings from one species to another is not reliable. In sheep, parturition is initiated by a surge of cortisol secreted by the fetal adrenal cortex. This acts on placental enzymes to convert progesterone to oestrogen. The rapid change in steroid balance stimulates the release of prostaglandins from both the placenta and the myometrium. There is increased sensitivity of the myometrium to oxytocin and uterine contractions powerful enough to expel the fetus are produced.

The adrenal cortex

Steer (1991) has summarised the research findings in humans and suggests it is unlikely that increased production of cortisol plays a major part as labour begins in the congenital absence of the fetal adrenals. Cortisol levels measured in the umbilical cord blood after delivery are difficult to assess as they may increase because of the stress of labour rather than being responsible for initiating labour. Scalp blood cortisol measurements made in early labour showed no difference in spontaneous or induced labour although there was a rise in fetal plasma cortisol as labour progressed. There is no dramatic rise in total cortisol level in fetal circulation prior to the onset of labour.

The administration of corticosteroids such as betamethasone to women in late pregnancy causes a fall in maternal circulating oestrogen levels but there is little effect on the placental progesterone synthesis or the duration of pregnancy. In the human placenta, although glucocorticoids do not induce the fall in progesterone and rise in oestrogen leading to labour, they are involved in the maturation of the fetus, in particular the fetal lung, allowing survival of a fetus born 6 weeks early. In the sheep cortisol produces both organ maturity and the onset of labour and a lamb born even 1 or 2 weeks early may be too immature to survive.

One hormone that may be implicated in fetal control of the onset of labour is dehydroepiandrosterone sulphate (DHAS) which is the major precursor of placental oestradiol and oestrone synthesis. The human fetal adrenal gland is relatively large at birth with a fetal zone occupying 80% of the cortex and being responsible for the size. The fetal function of the adrenal cortex is different from that of the adult and the fetal zone atrophies after birth. It has been found that HCG is a major stimulator of the fetal zone during pregnancy and ACTH can also stimulate the production of DHAS.

The fetal posterior pituitary gland

Higher concentrations of the posterior pituitary hormones vasopressin and oxytocin have been found in the umbilical circulation than in the maternal circulation. Although the source of this fetal oxytocin is not clear, the levels are higher in fetal arterial blood than venous blood, which suggests fetal origin. It is possible that as much as 1–3 mU/min of oxytocin is transferred from fetus to mother which is enough to promote uterine activity at term. An argument against the fetal role is that labour almost always follows fetal death in utero, depending on the gestational age of the fetus. Possibly the release of prostaglandins is more important and the mechanism of release differs when the fetus is dead, being provoked by the massive fall in progesterone level that accompanies fetal death.

The role of the placenta

Progesterone

It is now over 30 years since Csapo put forward a hypothesis that labour is initiated by the withdrawal of the progesterone block on myometrial activity. It has been difficult to prove or disprove this hypothesis (Steer 1991). All attempts to use progesterone to prolong labour, postpone preterm labour or prevent early abortion have been unsuccessful. Measurement of progesterone levels in the peripheral blood has not shown any withdrawal of progesterone at the end of pregnancy. However, this may not be significant if the progesterone acts locally and it may be an alteration in the binding of progesterone that is important rather than the level.

Oestrogens

Placental production of oestrogens rises as pregnancy progresses and DHAS of both maternal and fetal origin contributes to the placental production of oestrogens, most importantly of oestradiol. However, women do go into labour without the rise in the oestradiol concentration and there is no dramatic rise in oestradiol levels just before the onset of labour. It is probable that oestradiol facilitates rather than causes the onset of labour. As yet, there is no clear evidence that changing concentrations of oestrogens and progesterone alter at the onset of labour. However, these changes in balance between the two steroid hormones facilitate increasing myometrial activity.

Fetal membranes

Steroid hormones

The fetal membranes are known to have a relatively high concentration of progesterone. Both the chorion laeve and the amnion contain enzymes that can reduce the level of progesterone and also they both contain a protein which increases towards the end of pregnancy and that can bind progesterone. These two mechanisms would produce a local progesterone withdrawal effect. However, the membranes are avascular and any substance produced by them must travel by diffusion.

Prostaglandins

The amnion and chorion are both involved in the production of prostaglandins. Karim (1966) first suggested that prostaglandins played a role in the initiation of labour. It is still not clear whether prostaglandins initiate labour or maintain it. Earlier studies' findings have been unusable because of prostaglandin production by tissue trauma during sample collection. Measuring prostaglandins is extremely difficult as storage or temperature can affect the findings. Drugs such as aspirin act as prostaglandin inhibitors, preventing the first step in the metabolism of arachidonic acid. The fetal membranes contain significant amounts of arachidonic acid and research indicates that the membranes are significantly involved in the synthesis of prostaglandins but once again, there seems to be no significant change at the onset of labour.

Maternal influences

The decidua

The decidua is also implicated in the production of prostaglandins. Evidence suggests that it is a major source of prostaglandins during labour (McNabb 1997). Gustavii (1977) proposed that the decidual cells have lysosomes which contain phospholipase A_2, an enzyme necessary for the synthesis of prostaglandins. The evidence cited by Gustavii for the role of the decidua in controlling the onset of labour is presented in Steer (1991). These lysosomes are fragile and degenerate under the influence of oestrogen in late pregnancy when progesterone levels fall and oestrogen levels rise. Steer (1991) finds this hypothesis useful in the explanation of the onset of labour at term.

Work carried out by Keirse and his colleagues in the 1970s showed that the primary prostaglandins present were PGE_2 and $PGF_{2\alpha}$. The precursor of these two is an essential fatty acid called arachidonic acid derived from glycerophospholipids and their production involves several stages of conversion by enzymes. Both are known to stimulate myometrial contractions (McNabb 1997). Production rates of the two prostaglandins in decidual cells may be 30 times greater in labour than at elective caesarean section.

The endocrine system

The ovaries are not necessary for the initiation of labour and it seems that maternal oxytocin from the pituitary gland also plays

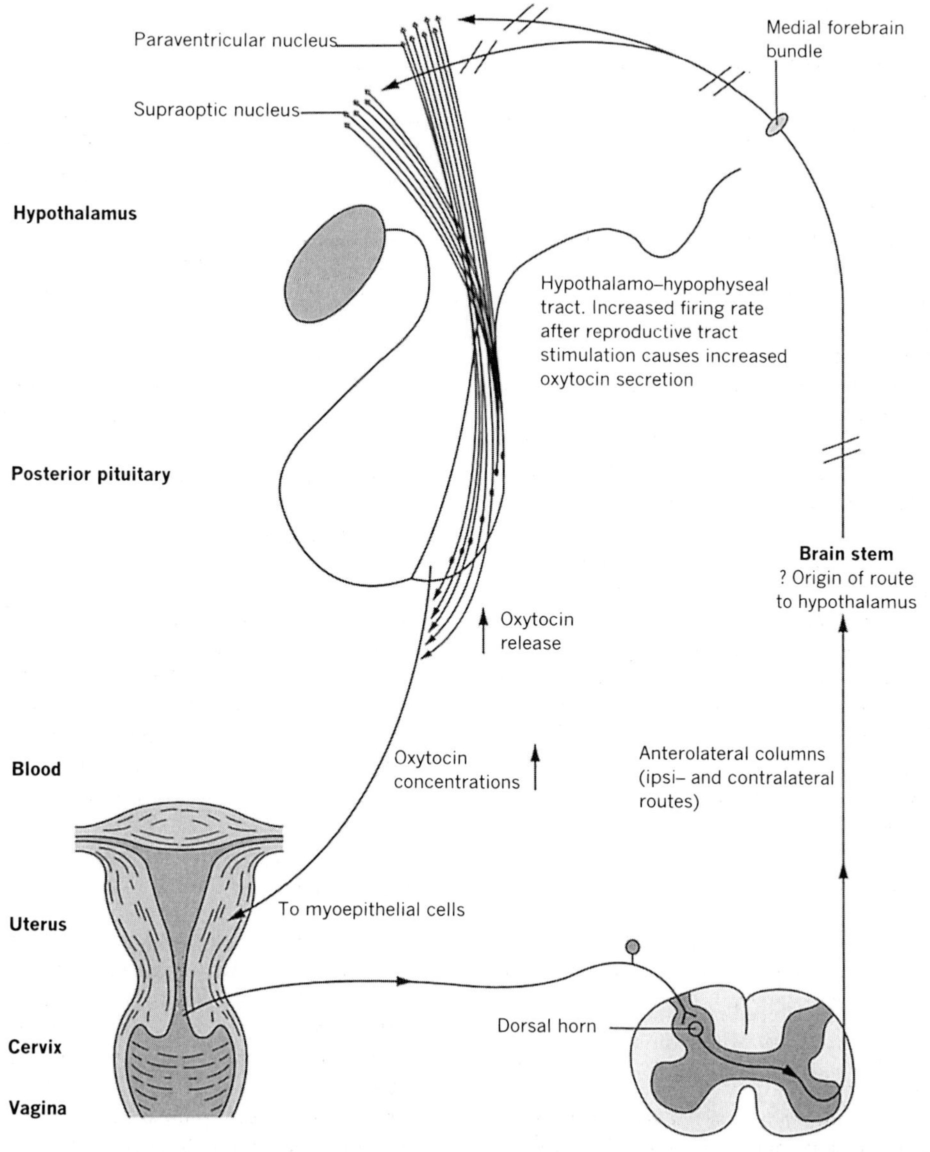

Figure 36.1 *The neuroendocrine reflex (Ferguson reflex) underlying oxytocin synthesis and secretion. (Reproduced with permission from Johnson and Everitt, 1995.)*

little part. The maternal adrenal glands do not seem to be involved.

Neurohormonal control

The **Ferguson reflex** is a neurohormonal reflex (Fig. 36.1) arising from the genital tract that may be involved in the release of both oxytocin and prostaglandin in labour. The release of oxytocin could lead to increasing prostaglandin production as it does in some animal species. If this were so, administration of epidural analgesia should block the spinal part of the reflex and oxytocin release, resulting in prolongation of the first stage of labour. There is no evidence that this happens so that prostaglandin release in human labour probably does not involve oxytocin release.

Control of cervical changes in labour

It is absolutely necessary that uterine contractions are coordinated with cervical dilatation. The increasing pressure placed on the cervix by the presenting part during active labour is said to aid dilatation of the cervix by the mechanism of Ferguson's reflex described above. Uterine contractions alone cannot bring about cervical softening and dilatation. Changes in the collagen content of the cervix must occur and evidence suggests that it is the hormone oestradiol that brings about the change. Prostaglandins also play a part in the ripening of the cervix and are often administered prior to the induction of labour if the cervix is unfavourable.

DEFINITIONS OF LABOUR

The previous section considered the role of the myometrium, decidua, fetus, placenta and membranes in the initiation of labour and the maintenance of contractions resulting in progress. This progress must be achieved without compromising maternal or fetal safety. Cassidy (1996) defines concepts associated with labour as follows.

- Labour – the process by which the fetus, placenta and membranes are expelled through the birth canal.
- Normal labour is spontaneous in onset at term, with the fetus presenting by the vertex, and is completed in 18 h with no complications arising.
- There are three stages of labour:
  Stage 1 – is the stage of dilatation of the cervix and begins with the onset of regular rhythmic contractions and is complete when the cervix is fully dilated
  Stage 2 – is the stage of expulsion of the fetus and begins when the cervix is fully dilated. It ends with complete expulsion of the fetus
  Stage 3 – is the stage of expulsion of the placenta and membranes and the control of bleeding. It begins following expulsion of the fetus and ends when the placenta and membranes are expelled.

The causes of onset of labour have been discussed above and the timing is important as it allows decisions to be made about the progress and ongoing management of labour, yet it is difficult to establish with accuracy. Gibb (1988) discusses the concept of **prelabour**, meaning the changes that occur in the last few weeks of pregnancy. It is often difficult to decide when the transition from the painless uterine contractions of prelabour develop into true labour. The length of labour is variable and is affected by parity, birth interval, psychological state, presentation and position, pelvic shape and size and the type of uterine contractions.

MATERNAL ADAPTATIONS IN LABOUR

The physiological changes in labour are examined separately from the process of labour so that sufficient depth can be achieved.

Cardiovascular system

There are profound changes in the cardiovascular system due to the effect of uterine contractions. The woman's emotional response to labour may affect the cardiovascular system, especially in primigravidae. The first stage of labour is associated with a progressive rise in cardiac output as each contraction adds 300–500 ml blood to the circulating blood volume. These changes are limited by epidural analgesia or supine position and by alleviation of pain and anxiety. Epidural analgesia appears to prevent the progressive increases in cardiac output whilst supine positioning lowers the cardiac output and decreases stroke volume but causes a compensatory increase in heart rate.

Pain, anxiety and apprehension may add to this effect, causing an increase in systolic and diastolic blood pressure and heart rate by increasing sympathetic tone. Blood pressure begins to rise 5 s before the contraction begins and returns to its baseline after the contraction has ended. During the first stage of labour there may be a blood pressure rise of 35 mmHg systolic and it may rise even higher in the 2nd stage. The diastolic pressure can rise 25 mmHg in the first stage of labour and up to 55 mmHg in the 2nd stage. There is only a small change in peripheral vascular resistance in labour so the increase is probably due to the transient rise in cardiac output during the contraction.

Following the delivery of the fetus, placenta and membranes, there may be cardiovascular instability because of dramatic haematological changes. The changes occur because of blood loss at delivery and compensatory mechanisms. Within 10 min of the delivery cardiac parameters fall to prelabour levels and may then take up to 4 weeks to return to prepregnancy levels.

Haematological system

There are changes in the haematological system and haemostasis to ensure that blood loss is kept to a minimum and tolerated. Haemoglobin levels tend to increase slightly in labour because of haemoconcentration. This is related to an increase in erythropoiesis due to stress, muscular activity and dehydration. WBC count increases during labour and immediately post-partum and may reach levels of $25–30 \times 10^9/l$. This is mainly due to an increase in neutrophils and is a probable response to stress.

The hypercoagulable state present in pregnancy is further magnified in labour. There is a transitory increase in the activity of the coagulation system during and immediately after placental separation so that clot formation in the torn blood vessels is maximised and blood loss from haemorrhage minimised. The placenta and decidua are rich in thromboplastin and release of this factor during separation activates coagulation via the extrinsic system.

There is also a decrease in fibrinolytic activity, enhancing clot formation at the placental site. The placental site is rapidly covered by a fibrin mesh which utilises about 5–10% of the circulating fibrinogen. Levels of fibrin/fibrinogen degradation products (FDPs) rise after delivery, increasing the risk of coagulation disorders in the immediate postpartum period.

Respiratory system

Maternal acidosis

There is an increase in the work of the uterine and other muscles during labour and therefore a greater need for oxygen. Alterations in ventilation and acid/base status occur. If the contractions are too frequent there will be a decrease in the oxygenation of the myometrium and a metabolic acidosis. In the presence of strong, frequent uterine contractions, ischaemia and consequent tissue hypoxia will occur with an increase in PCO_2 because of the change to anaerobic metabolism leading to a fall in pH (maternal acidosis). The ischaemia will increase the pain experienced during contractions.

In the 2nd stage of labour maternal PCO_2 may rise during pushing and also the use of voluntary muscles during bearing down. Fetal PCO_2 will rise if the mother is acidotic because the build-up of maternal PCO_2 will prevent placental transfer to the mother of fetal PCO_2. This will lead to significant fetal acidosis and distress.

Maternal alkalosis

In some women there is a tendency to hyperventilation leading to respiratory alkalosis. This appears to be mainly caused by pain. Anxiety, drugs, breath holding and antenatal breathing exercises will also add to the likelihood of hyperventilation.

The end result will be a fall in PCO_2 and a level of 25 mmHg can commonly occur. Blackburn & Loper (1992) report that levels as low as 17 mmHg have been seen in women during painful contractions. The woman may complain of tingling of the fingers and toes and dizziness due to overbreathing. She should be encouraged to change her respiratory rate, to lower it if necessary, to breathe when breath holding is inappropriate and to deep breathe if oxygen is needed, such as between contractions.

Renal system

There is an increase in maternal and fetal renin and angiotensin during labour and delivery which may be important in reducing uteroplacental blood flow following delivery. The changes in pregnancy outlined in Section 2 of the book affect fluid and electrolyte status so that administration of intravenous fluids and their electrolytic content must be carefully monitored to avoid water intoxication. Also, it is important to remember that oxytocin has an antidiuretic effect so that oxytocin infusion during labour reduces water excretion.

Gastrointestinal system

Gastric emptying

Gastric motility is decreased and gastric emptying is mildly delayed during labour, with or without epidural analgesia. Factors dramatically increasing this delayed gastric emptying include:

- fear and pain;
- the administration of opioid drugs;
- food intake during labour containing high levels of fibre and fat.

There is also a rise in gastric acidity, thus increasing the risk of aspiration pneumonitis, commonly known as **Mendelson's syndrome**, should a woman require general anaesthesia. Nutrition and hydration in labour and the prevention of acid aspiration are discussed in the section on clinical implications below.

Metabolism

Prior to labour women generally have a degree of respiratory alkalosis and metabolic acidosis and a reduced ability to utilise glucose in order to provide glucose for the fetus. Provision of glucose (gluconeogenesis) from the metabolism of body fat (lipolysis) occurs, causing an increase in plasma ketones throughout pregnancy. Labour has an effect on maternal metabolism and plasma electrolytes and these changes may affect the fetus.

The vigorous contractions of the uterus throughout labour require energy and glucose is the main substrate for this. Most women have little reserve for aerobic metabolism and glucose stores are quickly used up, especially with the modern tendency to restrict oral intake in labour. Swift (1991) suggests that a woman in labour has a calorific need for 700–1100 calories/h. Compensatory lipolysis occurs to meet the body's energy requirements, resulting in the production of ketones which, in excess, may depress fetal pH and interfere with myometrial activity (Liu & Fairweather 1985). Anaerobic metabolism causes the accumulation of lactate (see Krebs' cycle, Chapter 23) and this produces a small drop in maternal plasma pH to about 7.34, a reduction in base excess to –5 mEq/l and a fall in PCO_2.

CLINICAL IMPLICATIONS

Recognition of the onset of labour

Women themselves usually recognise that labour has begun, especially if they have received antenatal education about what to expect. The woman may notice a **show**, although this may occur following a vaginal examination in the antenatal clinic. **Contractions** which are regular, rhythmic and increase in **length, strength** and **frequency** occur but the woman may only be aware of backache with hardening of her uterus. When the presenting part of the fetus is not well applied to the cervix, the membranes may rupture and the woman has a sudden gush of fluid. This must be reported to the midwife immediately as there is a small risk of cord prolapse. Sometimes a steady trickle of amniotic fluid may be difficult to distinguish from urine and it is possible to pass a speculum into the vagina and test the fluid with a **nitrazine swab** which changes from orange to dark blue if amniotic fluid is present.

Initial examination

Although this is a book on physiology, it is important to realise that the social and psychological background and approach to care may interfere with the process of labour. This interaction between the mind and body will be discussed in full elsewhere in the book (Chapter 57). For now, it is necessary to remember that the approach taken at this initial meeting of the woman and her midwife (if they have not met during the antenatal period) may influence not only her perception of labour but also her physical progress towards delivery. Whilst it is desirable to provide a meaningful experience for the woman, it is of paramount importance that the physical safety of mother and fetus is ensured. This is the aspect of care that follows below.

The history

When a woman telephones her midwife, the decision needs to be made either to visit if there is to be a home confinement or admit her to hospital. If there are no complications and the woman is in early labour it will be beneficial for her to remain in her own surroundings for the time being. The history of the woman's health, any previous pregnancies and this pregnancy up to the onset of labour should be carefully scrutinised for any indications that complications may occur. True labour can be distinguished by the midwife from what is termed **spurious** or **false labour** by the nature of the contractions, which should show the pattern of increase in length, strength and frequency, and the state of the cervix, which will dilate progressively.

General examination

The general condition of the woman is important and her appearance may indicate aspects of her well-being to the midwife. Her general stance and gait may indicate pain or even imminent delivery The midwife should look for any abnormality in skin colour such as flushing, pallor or cyanosis which may indicate underlying problems. Her behaviour may indicate how well she is coping with contractions and whether she is anxious or afraid. Observations of temperature, pulse rate and blood pressure, signs of oedema and urinalysis are recorded.

Abnormal findings may indicate a problem with the woman's general health or be associated with an abnormality of labour. If the temperature and pulse rate are elevated, it is necessary to find the cause. Infection may be present and care must be taken to avoid passing this on to other women and their babies. A rise in blood pressure should be reported to the obstetrician. The presence of slight oedema of the feet and ankles may be normal, depending on the time of day, but pretibial oedema or puffiness of the fingers or face, especially if there is a raised blood pressure, may indicate the presence of pregnancy-induced hypertension (PIH). Urine is tested for protein, which may indicate that the woman has had a show or that her membranes have ruptured, both easily confirmed, but may also indicate PIH or urinary tract infection. Glucose and ketones are also tested for and are considered in the light of the woman's medical past history, when she last ate and how her labour is progressing.

Assessing progress in labour

When as much detail as possible has been ascertained about the progress of labour the woman is examined to confirm details given verbally and to establish a baseline on which to judge further progress. An abdominal examination is made and this may be followed by a vaginal examination. Progress can be considered as a function of descent of the presenting part through the pelvis and dilatation of the cervix. The presence of one in the absence of the other suggests lack of progress and is a cause for concern. These factors will be discussed in the next chapter.

Summary of main points

- In humans the timing of the onset of labour is less precise than in many other species and may be related to fetal brain activity via ACTH and the pituitary-adrenal axis. Progesterone is metabolised to oestrogen which gradually increases the sensitivity of the uterus to prostaglandins and oxytocin produced by both the fetoplacental unit and maternal tissues.
- If the sequence of events leading to the onset of labour were fully understood, it might be easier to prevent the onset of preterm labour and the devastating fetal loss and morbidity. Prostaglandins may play a central role in the initiation of labour but their composition and biosynthesis by various tissues remain unclear.
- There is still uncertainty about the role of the fetal hypothalamo-pituitary-adrenal axis in the initiation of labour in humans. It is unlikely that increased production of cortisol plays a major part because labour begins in the congenital absence of the fetal adrenals and there is no dramatic rise in total cortisol level in fetal circulation prior to the onset of labour
- The administration of corticosteroids such as betamethasone to women in late pregnancy causes a fall in maternal circulating oestrogen levels but there is little effect on placental progesterone synthesis or the duration of pregnancy.
- Dehydroepiandrosterone sulphate (DHAS), the major precursor of placental oestradiol and oestrone synthesis, may be implicated in fetal control of the onset of labour. Higher concentrations of the posterior pituitary hormones vasopressin and oxytocin have been found in the umbilical circulation than in the maternal circulation. The source of this fetal oxytocin is not clear but the levels are higher in fetal arterial blood than venous blood, which suggests a fetal origin.
- One argument against the fetal role is that labour almost always follows fetal death in utero, depending on the gestational age of the fetus. Possibly the release of prostaglandins is more important, being provoked by the massive fall in progesterone level that accompanies fetal death.
- The hypothesis that labour is initiated by the withdrawal of the progesterone block on myometrial activity is difficult to prove. Measurement of progesterone levels in the peripheral blood has not shown any withdrawal of progesterone at the end of pregnancy.
- Placental production of oestrogens rises as pregnancy progresses but women go into labour without a rise in oestradiol concentration and there is no dramatic rise just before the onset of labour. There is no clear evidence that concentrations of oestrogens and progesterone

alter at the onset of labour but changes in balance between them facilitate increasing myometrial activity.

- The fetal membranes have a relatively high concentration of progesterone. Both the chorion and amnion contain enzymes that can reduce the level of progesterone and both contain a protein which increases towards the end of pregnancy that can bind progesterone. There is still debate about whether prostaglandins initiate labour or maintain it.
- Maternal ovaries are not necessary for the initiation of labour and maternal oxytocin from the pituitary gland also plays little part. The maternal adrenal glands do not seem to be involved.
- Uterine contractions are coordinated with cervical dilatation. The increasing pressure placed on the cervix by the presenting part during active labour is said to aid dilatation of the cervix by the mechanism of Ferguson's reflex, which may be involved in the release of both oxytocin and prostaglandin in labour. Prostaglandin release in labour seems not to involve oxytocin release.
- Uterine contractions alone cannot bring about cervical softening and dilatation. Changes in the collagen content of the cervix must occur and evidence suggests that it is the hormone oestradiol that brings about the change. Prostaglandins also play a part in the ripening of the cervix.
- Normal labour is spontaneous in onset at term with the fetus presenting by the vertex and is completed in 18 h with no complications arising. The length of labour is affected by parity, birth interval, psychological state, presentation and position, pelvic shape and size and the type of uterine contractions.
- There are profound changes in the cardiovascular system due to the effect of uterine contractions. The woman's emotional response to labour may affect the cardiovascular system, especially in primigravidae. Pain, anxiety, apprehension and uterine contractions may cause an increase in systolic and diastolic blood pressure and heart rate. Within 10 min of the delivery, cardiac parameters fall to prelabour levels and may take up to 4 weeks to return to prepregnancy levels.
- Haemoglobin levels tend to increase slightly in labour because of haemoconcentration. WBC count increases during labour and immediately postpartum. There is a transitory increase in the activity of the coagulation system during and immediately after placental separation so that blood loss is minimised. Levels of FDPs rise after delivery, increasing the risk of coagulation disorders in the immediate postpartum period.
- There is an increase in the work of the uterine and other muscles during labour. If the contractions are too frequent there will be decreased myometrial oxygenation and metabolic acidosis. Fetal PCO_2 will rise if the mother is acidotic because the build-up of maternal PCO_2 will prevent placental trans-fer of fetal PCO_2 to the mother, leading to fetal acidosis and distress. In some women hyperventilation leads to respiratory alkalosis, resulting in a fall in PCO_2.
- During labour and delivery there is an increase in maternal and fetal renin and angiotensin which may be important in reducing uteroplacental blood flow following delivery. Oxytocin has an antidiuretic effect so that oxytocin infusion during labour reduces water excretion.
- Gastric motility is decreased and gastric emptying is delayed during labour. This delay increases in fear, pain, the administration of opioid drugs and food intake containing fat. The rise in gastric acidity increases the risk of Mendelson's syndrome if a general anaesthetic is required.
- Uterine contractions require energy and glucose is the main substrate. Most women have little reserve and glucose stores are quickly used up, especially with restricted oral intake. Compensatory lipolysis occurs resulting in the production of ketones which may depress fetal pH and interfere with myometrial activity.
- True labour can be recognised by the nature of the contractions and progressive dilatation of the cervix. Observations of temperature, pulse rate, blood pressure, signs of oedema and urinalysis are recorded. Abnormal findings may indicate a problem with the woman's general health or be associated with an abnormality of labour.

References

Blackburn ST, Loper DL. 1992 Maternal, Fetal and Neonatal Physiology, A Clinical Perspective. WB Saunders, Philadelphia.
Cassidy P. 1996 The first stage of labour: physiology and early care. In Bennett VR, Brown LK (eds) Myles Textbook for Midwives, 12th edn. Churchill Livingstone, Edinburgh, pp 149–167.
Gibb D. 1988 A Practical Guide to Labour Management. Blackwell Scientific, Oxford.
Gustavii B. 1977 Human decidual and uterine contractility. In The Fetus and Birth, Ciba Foundation Symposium, vol 47. Elsevier/Excerpta Medica/North Holland, Amsterdam, p 348.
Johnson and Everitt. 1995 Essential Reproduction. Blackwell Scientific, Oxford.
Karim SMM. 1966 Identification of prostaglandins in human amniotic fluid. Journal of Obstetrics and Gynaecology of the British Commonwealth 73, 903.
Liu DTY, Fairweather DVI. 1985 Labour Ward Manual. Butterworths, London.
McNabb M. 1997 Hormone interactions in labour. In Sweet BR with Tiran D (eds) Mayes Midwifery, 12th edn. Baillière Tindall, London, pp 343–354.
Steer PJ. 1991 The genital system. In Hytten F, Chamberlain G (eds) Clinical Physiology in Obstetrics, 2nd edn. Blackwell Scientific Oxford, pp 245–302.
Swift L. 1991 Labour and fasting. Nursing Times 87 (48), 64–65.

Recommended reading

Karim SMM. 1966 Identification of prostaglandins in human amniotic fluid. Journal of Obstetrics and Gynaecology of the British Commonwealth 73, 903.
McNabb M. 1997 Hormone interactions in labour. In Sweet BR with Tiran D (eds) Mayes Midwifery, 12th edn. Baillière Tindall, London, pp 343–354.
Swift L. 1991 Labour and fasting. Nursing Times 87 (48), 64–65.

Chapter 37 The first stage of labour

In this chapter

INTRODUCTION

It is essential to understand the physiology of any system or process so that observations and care are based on understanding. One problem of caring for women in labour is to define the acceptable parameters for progress and maternal and fetal responses so that the experience is viewed as satisfactory by women whilst safety is assured. In the past these parameters have been arbitrarily decided by empirical methods but research is increasingly utilised. Practitioners have a duty to women to ensure that they read widely, develop a discerning mind and base their practice on the best of this research.

PHYSIOLOGY

Uterine activity

In early labour contractions may be 15–20 min apart and are fairly weak, lasting for about 30 s. They may not be identified as labour by the mother for a while. In established labour the uterus contracts every 3–4 min and in advanced labour each contraction may last 50–60 s and is powerful. Contractions can be measured in mmHg by the pressure they exert on the amniotic fluid. This is called the **intrauterine hydrostatic pressure**. The resting pressure exerted by the muscular myometrium is about 5 mmHg. In pregnancy, the intensity of uterine contractions may reach 30 mmHg and up to 60–80 mmHg in labour.

Several concepts are described in relation to uterine activity in labour. The spread of each contraction across the uterine muscle is thought to begin in the fundus near the cornua, spreading outwards and downwards, remaining most intense in the fundus and being weakest in the LUS, a phenomenon known as **fundal dominance**. The spread of myometrial electrical activity to its maximum takes about 1 min and the same time is taken for the wave of contraction to pass off (Liu & Fairweather 1985). This allows progressive dilatation of the cervix and as the upper segment thickens and shortens, the fetus is propelled down the birth canal. During contractions, the upper and lower poles of the uterus act in harmony, with contraction and retraction of the upper pole and dilatation of the lower pole to allow fetal expulsion. This is known as **polarity**.

Uterine muscle in labour has the unique property of contraction and retraction (Fig. 37.1). Following each contraction, the muscle fibres do not completely relax but retain some of the shortening of contraction. This is called **retraction** and leads to the progressive shortening and thickening of the UUS and the diminishing of the uterine cavity. A ridge forms between the UUS and LUS, known as a **retraction ring**. The name **Bandl's ring** is usually applied only to the exaggerated pathological retraction ring that develops in obstructed labour and becomes visible above the symphysis pubis.

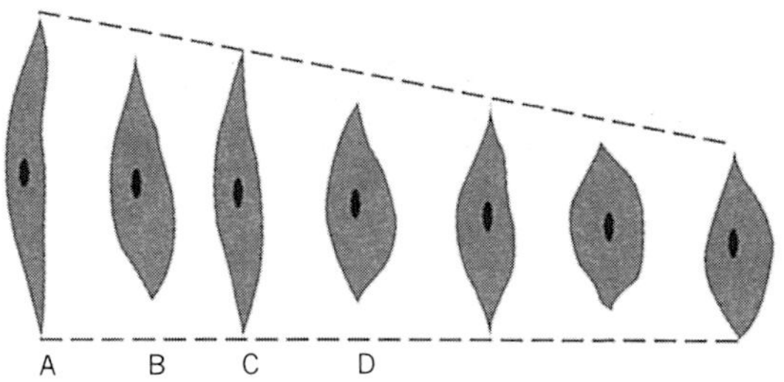

Figure 37.1 *Retraction of the uterine muscle fibres. (a) Relaxed. (b) Contracted. (c) Relaxed but retracted. (d) Contracted but shorter and thicker than those in (b) (from Sweet B, 1997, with permission).*

Effacement or taking up of the cervix into the LUS is often complete in primigravidae before the onset of labour. In multigravidae a perceptible cervical canal remains until labour is well established, a finding midwives refer to as a 'multip's os' when effacement and dilatation occur simultaneously. During labour there is **dilatation** of the external os (Fig. 37.2) until it is large enough for the widest diameter of the presenting part to pass through. In a fetus at term presenting by the vertex, the diameter of the cervix would have to reach 10 cm but in a preterm infant with a smaller head, this would be less. As the cervix begins to dilate, the operculum or mucus plug formed in pregnancy is lost and the woman will notice a bloodstained mucoid discharge around the time of the commencement of labour. This is termed the show. The blood originates from ruptured capillaries where the chorion has become detached from the dilating cervix.

Mechanical factors

Besides uterine action, there are mechanical forces that aid dilatation of the cervix. As the lower uterine segment is stretched the chorion is detached from it. In normal labour the increased intrauterine pressure during contractions forces a well-flexed head snugly against the cervix, trapping a small amount of amniotic fluid in front of the head separate from the rest of the fluid surrounding the body of the fetus. This small sac of fluid is known as the **forewaters** and the rest of the fluid as the **hindwaters**. The forewaters bulge through the cervix to a depth of 6–12 mm, becoming more tense during contractions (Fig. 37.2). This separation of the forewaters from the larger volume of the hindwaters keeps the membranes intact during the first stage of labour, providing a barrier against ascending infection.

When the membranes remain intact the pressure of each contraction is exerted on the fluid and as fluid is not compressible, pressure is equalised throughout the uterus. This is known as **general fluid pressure**. If the membranes are ruptured and amniotic fluid is reduced, contraction pressure is applied directly to the fetus. The placenta is compressed between the uterine wall and the fetus, which further reduces the oxygen supply to the fetus. Therefore, there are two good reasons for maintaining intact membranes: to reduce the risk of

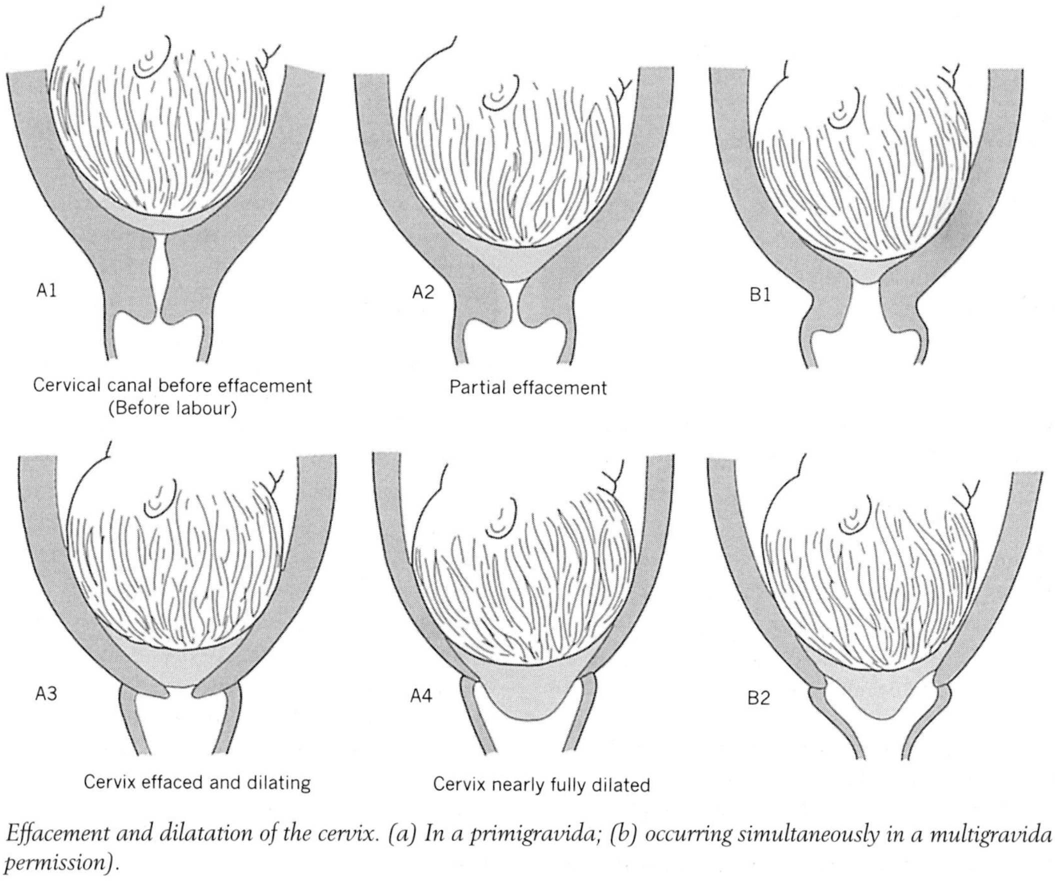

Figure 37.2 *Effacement and dilatation of the cervix. (a) In a primigravida; (b) occurring simultaneously in a multigravida (from Sweet B, 1997, with permission).*

infection and to maintain a good oxygen supply to the fetus. The physiological moment for the membranes to rupture is when the cervix is fully dilated and no longer able to support the forewaters and the force of the uterine contractions reaches maximum. Henderson (1990) points out that routine amniotomy during the first stage of labour is never justified.

During each contraction, the force of the fundal contraction is transmitted to the upper pole of the fetus and down the long axis of the fetal spine, causing increasing flexion of the head and ensuring that the smallest possible circumference, which is the circular vertex, is applied to the circular cervical os. This is known as **fetal axis pressure**. It becomes much more significant after the membranes have ruptured and during the 2nd stage of labour.

Phases

Arias (1993) writes that 'The present understanding of labour is based on the work of Emanuel A Friedman'. Friedman developed the graphic representation of labour by plotting cervical dilatation and descent of the presenting part against time. In normal labour, the rate of dilatation of the cervix follows a sigmoid-shaped curve. There are three distinct parts.

1 An initial part where there is little progress in cervical dilatation, which Friedman called the **latent phase**.
2 A part of the curve where there is rapid progress in dilatation, called the **active phase**.
3 A part of the curve where dilatation slows, called the **deceleration phase**.

The latent phase, which lasts until cervical dilatation is about 3 to 4 cm, can take 6–8 h in a primigravida. Rapid dilatation of the cervix in the active phase takes place at about 1 cm per hour in a primigravida and 1.5 cm per hour in a multigravida. Plotting the rate of cervical dilatation is commonly carried out in labour (a **cervicograph**) and an average duration is indicated in Figure 37.3.

Individualised care

Morrin (1997) highlights the nature of the dual biological and social event that the childbearing woman experiences. She suggests that the midwife should:

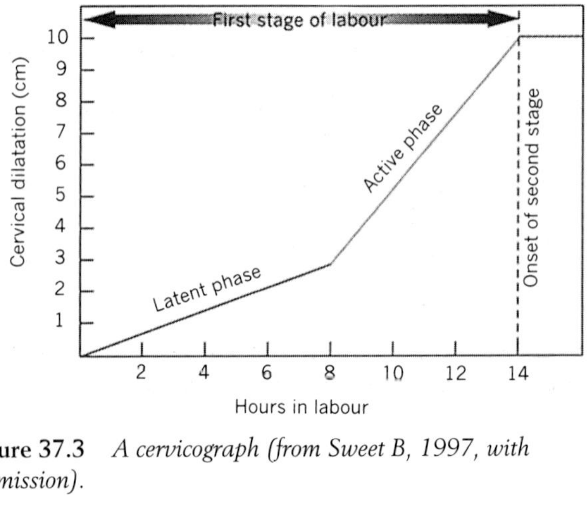

Figure 37.3 *A cervicograph (from Sweet B, 1997, with permission).*

- assess the needs and expectations of the labouring woman;
- plan care for each woman to meet specific needs and expectations;
- carry out the plan;
- evaluate the effect of the care and modify it if necessary.

The physiological aspects of care in labour include assessing progress, positioning of the woman, nutrition and hydration and monitoring the condition of mother and fetus.

ASSESSING PROGRESS

When as much detail as possible has been ascertained about the progress of labour prior to admission, the woman is examined to confirm details given verbally and to establish a baseline on which to judge further progress. An abdominal examination is made and this may be followed by a vaginal examination. Progress can be considered as a function of descent of the presenting part through the pelvis and dilatation of the cervix. The presence of one in the absence of the other suggests lack of progress and is a cause for concern.

Abdominal examination in labour

Most of the abdominal examination points considered by Thomson (1996) in the context of antenatal care apply equally well to labour. These are to assess fetal size and well-being, to diagnose the location of fetal parts in particular lie, presentation, position and engagement and to detect any deviation from normal. Abdominal examination should always be carried out prior to performing a vaginal examination and repeated abdominal examinations can be used to assess descent of the presenting part.

Inspection

The size and shape of the uterus can be of value in ensuring that there is a normal longitudinal lie. In the rare instance of a transverse lie, the uterus may appear to be low and broad. If there is a saucer-shaped depression below the umbilicus the fetus may be lying in an occipitoposterior position. Fetal movements may be seen and can help in the diagnosis of position.

Palpation

The following terms are used to describe fetal palpation:

Lie – The relationship of the long axis of the fetus to the long axis of the uterus
Presentation – That part of the fetus lying in the lower part of the uterus
Attitude – The relationship of the fetal head and limbs to its body
Denominator – The part of the presentation lying over the internal os
Position – The relationship of the denominator to 6 points on the maternal pelvic brim
Engagement of the fetal head – the widest transverse diameter has passed through the pelvic brim.

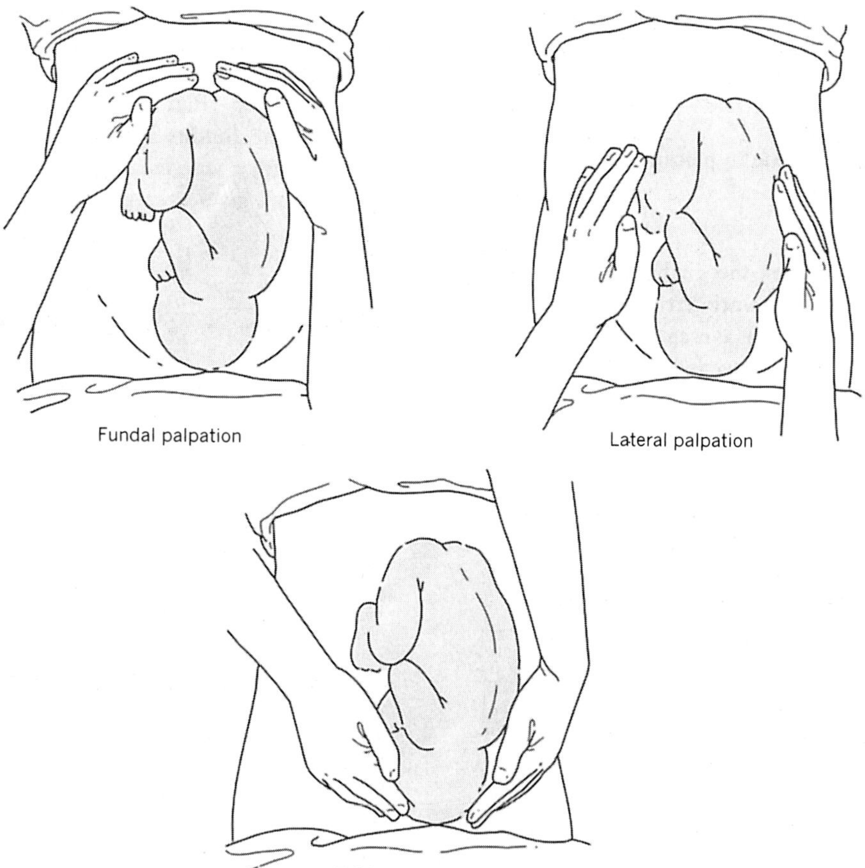

Figure 37.4 *Types of palpation per abdomen (from Sweet B, 1997, with permission).*

Fundal palpation (Fig. 37.4) (taking into account the overall size of the uterus) allows a judgement of the gestational age to be made (Fig. 37.5). It is also necessary to determine the lie of the fetus (Fig. 37.6). Lateral palpation is used to locate the fetal back to determine position. The length, strength and frequency of contractions should be noted by palpation rather than by the reaction of the woman.

Pelvic palpation using both hands can identify the presenting part (Fig. 37.7) and the amount of flexion (Fig. 37.8) and engagement of the head can be assessed by estimating the amount of head still present above the pelvic brim. If the head is engaged, less than half of it will be felt above the pelvic brim and the head will not be mobile. It may not be possible to palpate the occiput if the head is deeply engaged (Fig. 37.9). Engagement is a good sign and indicates that the bony pelvis is adequate for the passage of the fetus and a vaginal delivery should follow. Descent of the head can be measured abdominally and described in fifths of the head that can be felt above the pelvic brim.

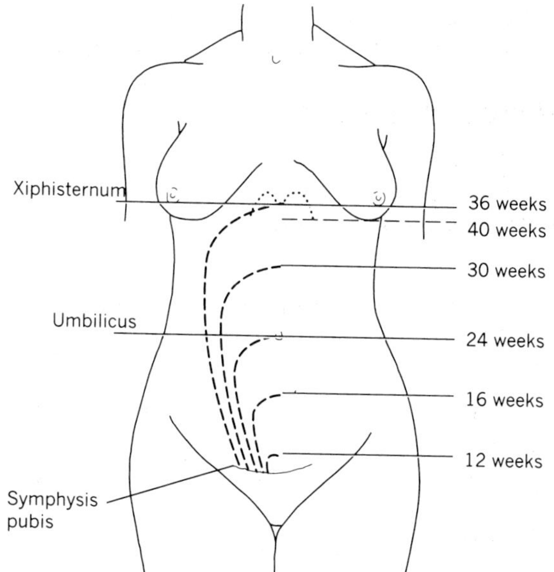

Figure 37.5 *The height of the fundus at different stages of pregnancy (from Sweet B, 1997, with permission).*

Auscultation

Listening to the fetal heart is an important part of any abdominal examination as it enables the practitioner to make an assessment of fetal well-being. The point of maximum intensity is located by considering the position of the fetus (Fig. 37.10).

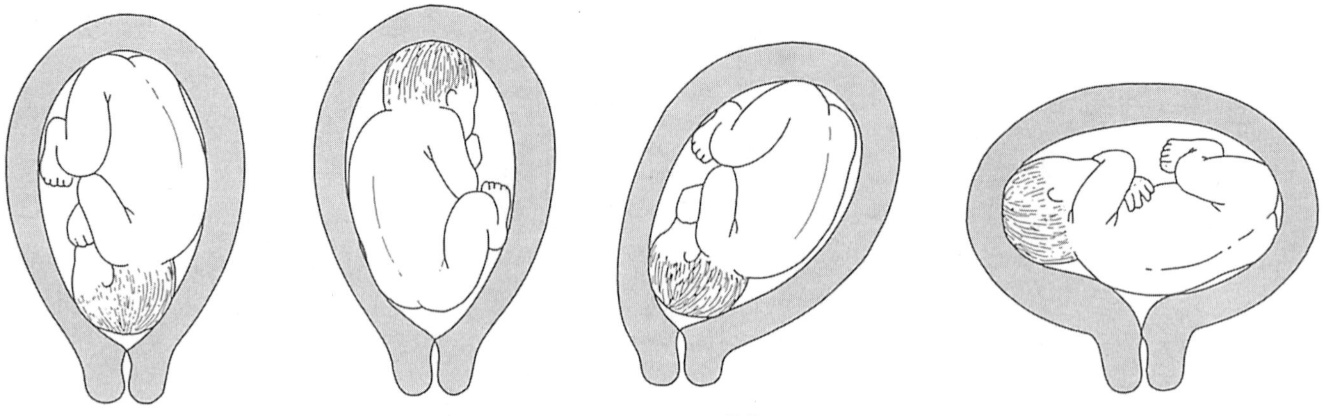

Figure 37.6 *The lie of the fetus (from Sweet B, 1997, with permission).*

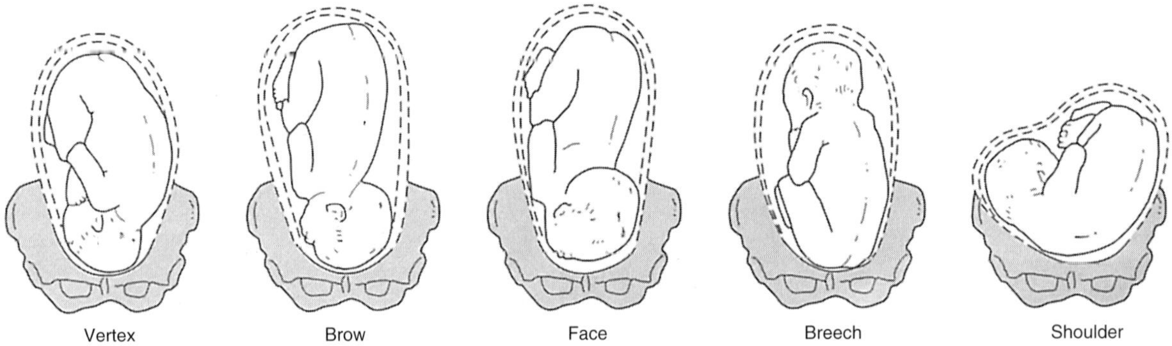

Figure 37.7 *The presentation of the fetus (from Sweet B, 1997, with permission).*

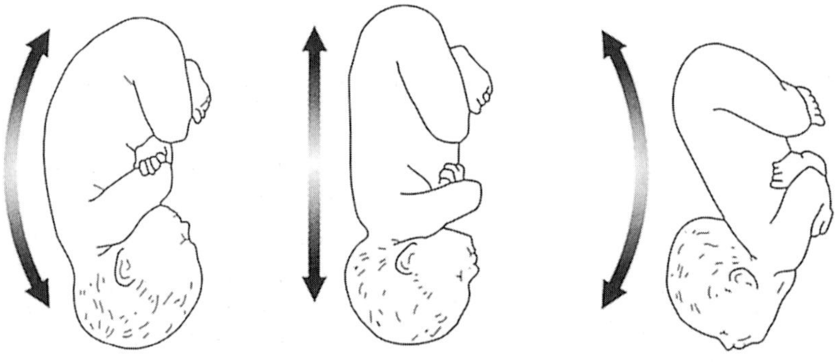

Figure 37.8 *The attitude of the fetus (from Sweet B, 1997, with permission).*

As labour progresses and descent takes place, the point of maximum intensity will change. Moving the stethoscope around will ensure the best possible clarity of the fetal heartbeat and its regularity, strength and frequency can be assessed. Continuous monitoring of the fetal heart may be necessary so that abnormalities can be diagnosed.

Vaginal examination in labour (VE)

Cassidy (1996) gives the following indications for vaginal examination in labour.

- To make a positive diagnosis of labour
- To make a positive identification of presentation
- To determine whether the head is engaged if there is doubt
- To ascertain whether the forewaters have ruptured or to rupture them artificially
- To exclude cord prolapse if the forewaters rupture and the presenting part is high
- To assess progress or delay in labour
- To apply a fetal scalp electrode
- To confirm full dilatation of the cervix
- In multiple pregnancy, after the birth of the first baby, to

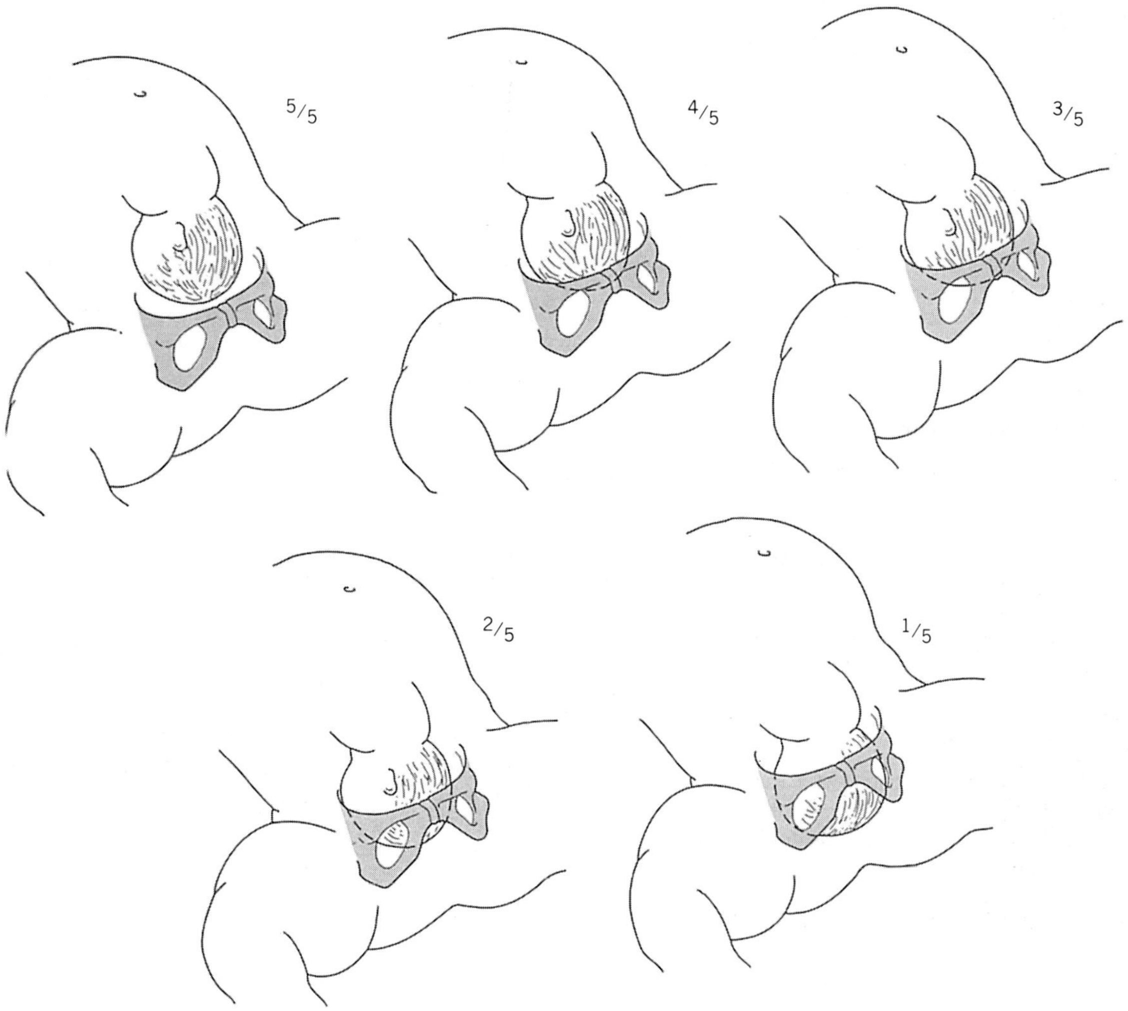

Figure 37.9 *Examination per abdomen to determine the descent of the fetal head in fifths (from Sweet B, 1997, with permission).*

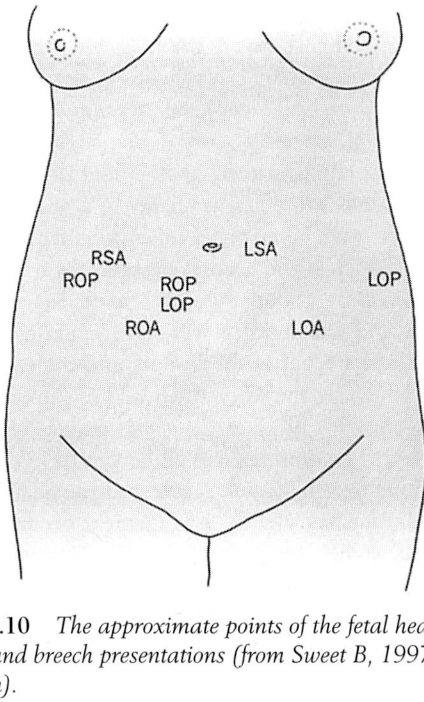

Figure 37.10 *The approximate points of the fetal heart sounds in vertex and breech presentations (from Sweet B, 1997, with permission).*

confirm the lie and presentation of the 2nd fetus and to puncture the 2nd amniotic sac.

There is a way in which such a list, whilst comprehensive, does not do justice to the value of a well-performed, carefully timed vaginal examination and Cassidy makes two points about this. First it is the combination of abdominal and vaginal findings that provides a clear picture of the progress in labour and second, continuous careful observation of the mother will enable the avoidance of unnecessary vaginal examinations.

In any clinical examination, it is sensible to use the same order of findings each time. This ensures that there is less chance of missing an important feature. It is also important to continue with the examination until satisfied in all aspects as it is essential to keep the number of vaginal examinations to a minimum to reduce the risk of infection. Morton Thompson's book *The Cry and the Covenant* should be essential reading for anyone caring for women in labour and full aseptic technique should be used at all times.

The concept of a 'quick VE' is dangerous for more than one reason. Adequate care to prevent infection is unlikely to be taken and important features of the examination are likely to be missed. When the author was a student midwife a senior colleague pulled on a glove and did a 'quickie' to confirm full cervical dilatation in a woman who seemed to be making no progress in the 2nd stage of labour. The cervix was confirmed as fully dilated and no other findings were sought! Twenty minutes later, following a drop in the fetal heart, yet another VE was performed by the obstetric registrar and a brow presentation necessitating an emergency caesarean section was discovered.

Findings

The following order is suggested for the performance and recording of a vaginal examination.

External genitalia

Prior to inserting fingers into the vagina, the external genitalia should be inspected as some findings may influence the course and management of labour. The labia should be examined for any varicosities or warts and the presence of oedema noted. The perineum should be inspected for scarring which could indicate a previous tear or episiotomy and, in some cultures, female circumcision. Signs of vaginal discharge or bleeding and, if the membranes have ruptured, the colour and quantity of any amniotic fluid should be recorded. Any offensive odour should be reported as this is likely to indicate the presence of infection.

Condition of the vagina

The normal vagina in labour should feel warm and moist. It is very rare but not impossible that the implications of a prolonged labour with obstruction would be seen. Women who have been cared for in pregnancy and have sought care early in their labour should never present with a hot and dry vagina but occasionally someone may have tried to conceal their pregnancy and labour and only ask for help when unable to deliver themselves. A cystocoele and/or rectocoele may be present in a multiparous woman. A loaded rectum can be easily felt through the posterior vaginal wall.

State of the cervix

The cervix is palpated for length and consistency to diagnose the length of the cervical canal and the degree of effacement. The position of the cervix relative to the fetal presenting part is noted – is it in the normal central position or, as is occasionally found in early labour, very posterior? A long closed cervix indicates that labour has not begun. The cervix in labour should feel soft and elastic and will usually be applied closely to the presenting part.

Dilatation of the cervical os

The two examining fingers are opened gently in the cervical os to judge the dilatation in centimetres. If this is done too forcibly, the os may be stretched sideways like a mouth so the cervix should be palpated in every direction. In particular, this will ensure that no lip of cervix remains if the VE is to confirm full cervical dilatation. Intact membranes can be felt through the dilating os. They feel a little like clingfilm and become tense during a contraction. If the membranes are absent the slightly rougher fetal scalp can be felt.

Level or station of the presenting part

The level of the presenting part is judged in relation to the ischial spines so that descent of the fetus through the pelvis can be monitored. The distance above or below the ischial spines is calculated in centimetres (Fig. 37.11). If there is a caput succedaneum care must be taken to establish the level of the bony skull above the swelling.

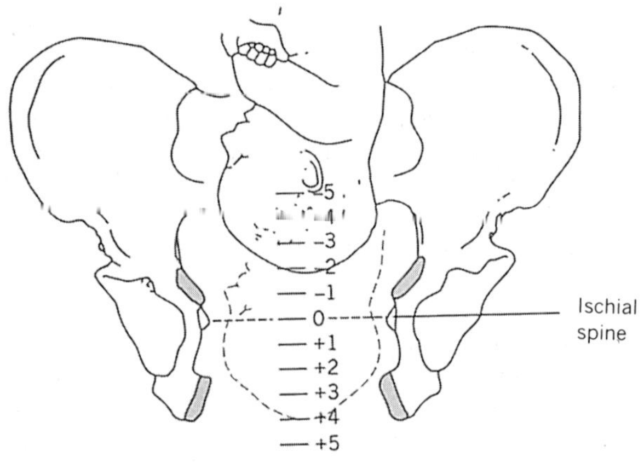

Figure 37.11 *The stations of the head. Descent in relation to the maternal ischial spines is expressed in centimetres (from Sweet B, 1997, with permission).*

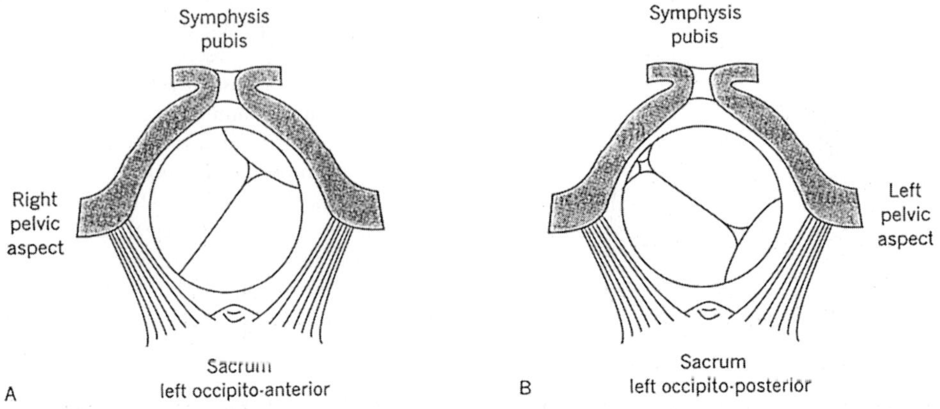

Figure 37.12 *Identifying the position of the fetus. (a) Left occipitoanterior: the sagittal suture is in the right oblique diameter of the pelvis. (b) Left occipitoposterior: the sagittal suture is in the left oblique diameter of the pelvis (from Sweet B, 1997, with permission).*

The presentation

In 96% of cases this will be vertex and easily confirmed. Only rarely will it be difficult to confirm presentation on VE and this usually indicates a very abnormal labour or, even more rarely, a fetal abnormality such as an encephalocoele which may have slipped through the vaginal os and feel too soft to be a head.

Position

Landmarks such as sutures and fontanelles on the fetal skull can be felt to diagnose or confirm the position of the presenting part (Fig. 37.12). The most commonly identified landmark is the sagittal suture as it is found in a vertex presentation (Fig. 37.13). It is identifiable by moulding that occurs with the leading anterior parietal bone overriding the posterior parietal bone and is usually in one or other of the oblique diameters. The posterior fontanelle can be identified because of its small size and the three sutures that leave it. The anterior fontanelle is larger, diamond shaped and has four sutures leaving it.

Moulding of the fetal skull

This is described in Chapter 24 and the most important aspect is to make a judgement on whether the amount of moulding is normal or excessive, suggesting disproportion between the fetal skull and the bony pelvis.

Pelvic capacity

An estimation of pelvic size has probably been made antenatally but the practitioner responsible for the safe conduct of the delivery should make their own estimation of the pelvic outlet by assessing the ischial spines and the angle of the subpubic arch. Prominent ischial spines often accompany a pubic arch that is less than 90° and the features suggest an android pelvis.

Fetal heart rate

An assessment of the fetal heart should always be made after the vaginal examination is completed, especially if the membranes are ruptured, to ensure that the examination has had no adverse effect on the fetus. This aspect was brought home to the author whilst conducting a vaginal examination where the fetal heart rate was being recorded by continuous external monitor. The position was occipitoposterior and the anterior fontanelle was immediately under the examining fingers. As the fontanelle was being gently palpated the fetal heart became erratic. When the fingers were removed it settled down into its normal pattern. The author believed that the fetus was aware of her presence.

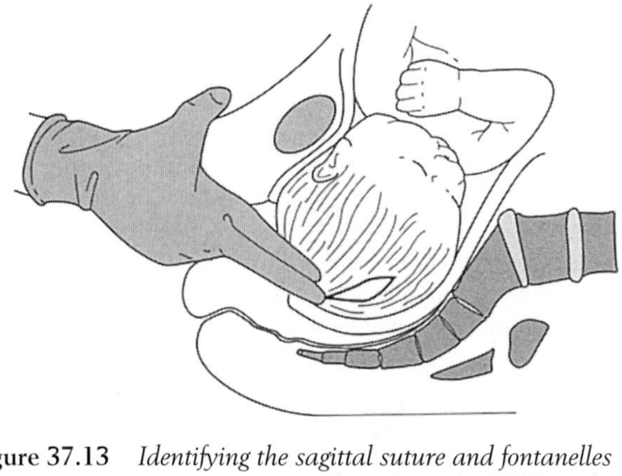

Figure 37.13 *Identifying the sagittal suture and fontanelles during examination per vaginam (from Sweet B, 1997, with permission).*

MATERNAL POSITION

Banks (1992) summarised the effect of women being mobile or adopting the upright position in the first stage of labour (Fig. 37.14). As well as adding to the discussion on placental perfusion, she quotes Flynn et al (1978) who suggested that there is better alignment between the descending presenting part and the pelvic brim so that engagement of the presenting part is facilitated and, in occipitoposterior presentation, rotation of the occiput to the anterior may be helped.

Also, the forces of gravity may lead to better application of the presenting part to the cervix which will promote Ferguson's reflex. Balaskas (1983) suggested that the strength and length of uterine contractions are increased, leading to a more rapid dilatation of the cervix. Less pain and backache are perceived by women adopting an upright posture and they often request delivery in an upright position for a subsequent labour.

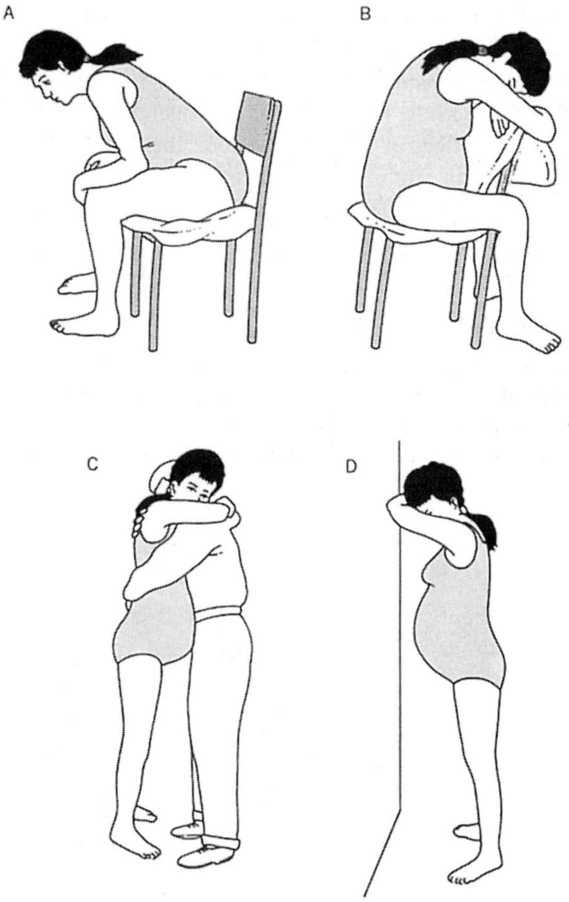

Figure 37.14 *Resting positions in labour. (a) In chair. (b) Astride chair. (c) Supported by partner. (d) Leaning. (Illustrations courtesy of Jim Morrin, 1993.)*

IMMERSION IN WATER

Immersion of the body in warm water has been in use for decades and is acceptable to many women. Although its main use is for relaxation and pain relief, it may also shorten the labour and decrease the need for augmentation. The warmth of the water relaxes the muscles and enhances a state of mental relaxation. There may be a decrease in the release of the stress hormones such as catecholamines resulting in better uterine perfusion and more efficient contractions (Schorn et al 1993). The woman feels weightless, can support her body in whatever position she prefers and is helped to cope with the discomfort of contractions. However, there may be problems such as unrealistic expectations, restricted choice of analgesia, restriction of mobility, inhibition of effective contractions, increase in perineal trauma, postpartum haemorrhage and uterine infections. Zimmerman et al (1993) state that emergency interventions may be delayed if there is difficulty in emptying the water bath quickly or getting the mother out of the water.

NUTRITION AND HYDRATION

Nutrition

The process of labour uses large amounts of energy. If insufficient carbohydrate is available, body fat will be utilised with the release of ketones and the development of ketoacidosis. Prior to admission it is advisable for the woman to take carbohydrate foods such as toast, cereal and plain biscuits. The main problem with food intake in normal labour is the possible need for a general anaesthetic. Coupled with delayed stomach emptying and the relative inefficiency of the cardiac sphincter brought about by the influence of progesterone is a risk of inhalation of acid gastric reflux, resulting in **inhalational pneumonitis** (Mendelson's syndrome).

Fasting in labour has been a feature of management since the relationship between anaesthesia and Mendelson's syndrome was established more than 40 years ago (Smith & Bogod 1995). However, Johnson et al (1991) suggested that withholding food does not necessarily ensure an empty stomach or reduce the acidity of stomach contents. Broach & Newton (1988a,b) trace the practice of withholding food and fluids in America to the use of general anaesthesia in normal births. They suggest that unless there is a reason why an epidural analgesia cannot be administered, there is no need to prevent women from eating and drinking sensible amounts in labour, a view supported by Elkington (1991).

There are a variety of opinions and policies in different hospitals (Michel et al 1991). In some units women are not allowed anything to eat after labour is established whilst in other units women may be allowed a low-residue, low-fat diet. Smith & Bogod (1995) state that whilst death due to aspiration pneumonitis is rare, there is little evidence that fasting in labour is harmful and that fasting in labour is effective in reducing the risk with little cost.

On the subject of oral nutrition in labour, Grant (1990) recommended that women who eat in the first stage of **normal** labour should take light meals such as clear soup, jelly, ice cream, tea, toast and marmalade, jam, boiled egg, fruit juices, cooked fruit or light cereals. Also, Grant suggests, a sensible protocol would be:

- where there is no risk of general anaesthetic or instrumental delivery, women should be allowed to eat a light diet and drink as required;
- when narcotic analgesia has been given oral food should be withheld and sips of water given.

Hydration

In a paper about fluid balance in labour, Millns (1991) examines four situations which may lead to the administration of intravenous fluids in labour. He advocates that any administration of fluid in labour should be given intravenously. The four situations are:

- during the administration of epidural analgesia;
- for the administration of oxytocic drugs;
- to correct ketonuria which has arisen because of metabolism of fat stores;
- to correct dehydration.

Nordstrom et al (1995) examined the effects of maternal glucose administration in labour. They compared continuous infusion of 5% dextrose with 0.9% saline solution. Whilst they found a significant rise in maternal and neonatal plasma glucose levels and maternal insulin levels during the administration of 5% dextrose, they found no evidence of fetal hyperinsulinism in healthy term fetuses. No differences in either maternal or fetal lactate levels were found and both regimes seemed to present no risk of increased fetal lactate levels or fetal hypoglycaemia. However, Stratton et al (1995) carried out similar research in women who required oxytocin and found significantly lowered serum sodium levels in both mothers and babies where the oxytocin had been infused in 5% dextrose, suggesting that non-electrolyte solutions administered in labour may lead to hyponatraemia.

MONITORING THE MATERNAL CONDITION

- Maternal temperature should be recorded 4 hourly and the pulse hourly unless there is an indication for more frequent recording.
- In the early part of labour blood pressure can be taken every 2 h and then hourly as labour progresses.
- Fluid intake and output should be measured and recorded and the woman should be encouraged to pass urine every 2 h.
- The urine is tested for protein, glucose and ketones. Small amounts of protein in the absence of known hypertensive or renal disease may indicate contamination by show or amniotic fluid. A small amount of ketosis is expected in normal labour and can be considered part of the physiological adaptation. Large amounts of ketones indicate exhaustion of the energy stores and may lead to uterine inertia if not corrected.
- The psychological response to labour and to pain should be assessed as any stress may interfere with the course of labour.

MONITORING THE FETAL CONDITION

Blood vessels in the myometrium which supply the fetus with oxygen and nutrients are compressed during each uterine contraction. Delivery of nutrients and oxygen is impeded when the strength of a contraction exceeds 40 mmHg. Therefore increased myometrial tone or rapidly occurring contractions may cause fetal hypoxia and distress. When the membranes remain intact the pressure of each contraction is exerted on the fluid and, as fluid is not compressible, pressure is equalised throughout the uterus and this is known as general fluid pressure.

If the membranes are ruptured and the amniotic fluid is reduced the pressure of contractions is applied directly to the fetus and the placenta is compressed between the uterine wall and the fetus, which further reduces the oxygen supply to the fetus. However Johnson et al (1991) conclude that although there is a theoretical improvement in oxygenation by the avoidance of vena caval compression, no research supports a clinical advantage to the fetus from any position taken in labour. The fetus is subjected to compression and hypoxic stress during uterine contractions and, if healthy, tolerates these conditions without a change in heart rate.

Fetal distress results in alterations in heart rate, development of acidosis, passage of meconium, presence of excessive moulding and excessive movements. Information about fetal well-being is mainly obtained by recording fetal heart rate and rhythm, either intermittently or continuously. Amniotic fluid can be inspected for the presence of meconium and the pH of fetal blood can be taken if necessary.

Heart rate

Intermittent monitoring

Intermittent monitoring of the fetal heart can be undertaken using Pinard's fetal stethoscope or a Doppler ultrasound apparatus such as Sonicaid. The **rate** is best counted over a full minute to allow for variations and should be between 120 and 160 beats per minute. If a Doppler apparatus is used the heart rate can be monitored throughout a contraction and the rate should normally be maintained. If there is bradycardia, hypoxia may be a problem. The **rhythm** of the fetal heart, as for any heart, is coupled and should remain steady. Any irregularity needs prompt action to establish the cause.

Continuous recording

Continuous recording of the fetal heart (**cardiography**) is usually combined with continuous monitoring of maternal uterine activity (**tocography**) by using a cardiotocograph apparatus (CTG). This allows recording of a graphic response of the fetal heart rhythm and rate to uterine activity (Fig. 37.15). CTG can be used for periods of 20 min (periodic CTG) or continuously for the whole of labour. Some women prefer to avoid

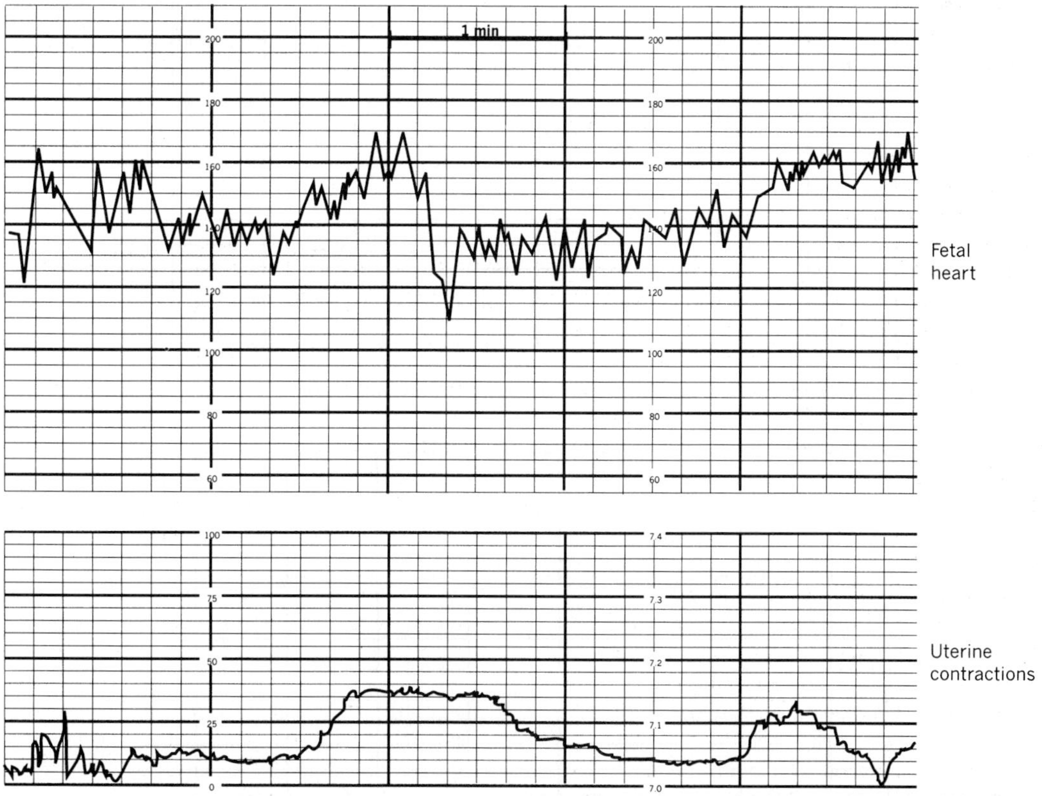

Figure 37.15 *Normal cardiotocograph: the fetal heart rate is normal and reactive. (Courtesy of J.A. Jordan, Birmingham Maternity Hospital.)*

continuous monitoring and, as there is no research to support the value of CTG in normal labour, this request can and should be respected. The woman should discuss antenatally her feelings concerning an urgent need to monitor the fetus arising in the course of her labour. A compromise is often reached with periodic monitoring being accepted.

External cardiotocography involves strapping an ultrasound transducer to the abdominal wall over the point of maximum fetal heart intensity and the contraction monitor to the fundus of the uterus. The reading can be affected by maternal or fetal movement, the thickness of the abdominal wall and uterine contractions but is non-invasive. Internal cardiography can be used by the application of an electrode to the fetal scalp and the membranes must be ruptured and the cervix at least 2–3 cm dilated. Wiring attaches the electrode to the CTG.

Telemetry

If available, internal cardiography can be recorded by a portable battery-operated transmitter used to pick up the signal from the fetal heart and the mother can be ambulant (telemetry). However, no recording of uterine activity can be made and the woman is requested to press a button at the onset of each contraction which will mark the strip chart accordingly.

Findings

The cardiotocograph provides information about:

- baseline fetal heart rate;
- baseline variability;
- fetal heart response to uterine contractions.

Each of the above will be discussed and graphs will be used to demonstrate the points and to begin to develop the skills of reading and interpreting recordings.

Baseline fetal heart rate

This is the fetal heart rate between contractions. If the heart rate is more than 160 bpm it is termed **baseline tachycardia** (Fig. 37.16) while a baseline of less than 120 bpm is called **baseline bradycardia** (Fig. 37.17). With no other alteration, these two features may indicate hypoxia but tachycardia may be a response to maternal ketosis and some fetuses have a normal baseline of 110–120 bpm. Continuous compression of the cord will cause a prolonged severe bradycardia.

Baseline variability

It is a normal function of hearts to have minute variations in the length of each beat. This is caused by electrical activity varying as a response to the environment and will produce a jagged rather than a smooth line on the graph, called baseline variability (Fig. 37.18). The baseline rate should vary by at least five beats over a period of 1 min. Loss of this (Fig. 37.19) may indicate fetal hypoxia but has also been noted for a short period

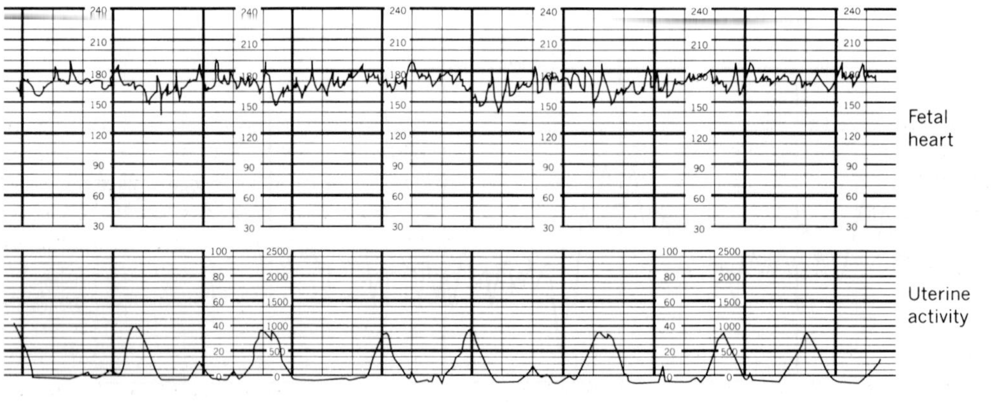

Figure 37.16 *Uncomplicated baseline tachycardia. (Courtesy of Sonicaid, Abingdon, Oxon.)*

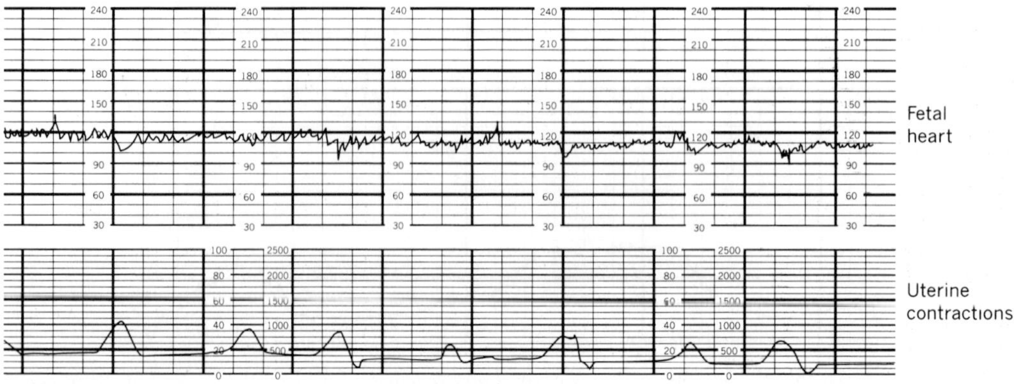

Figure 37.17 *Normal baseline bradycardia. (Courtesy of Sonicaid, Abingdon, Oxon.)*

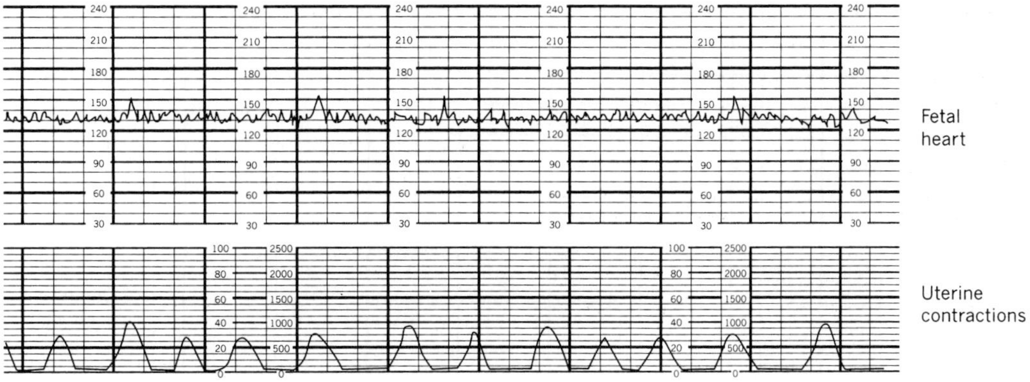

Figure 37.18 *ECG trace showing variability in fetal heart rate. (Courtesy of Sonicaid, Abingdon, Oxon.)*

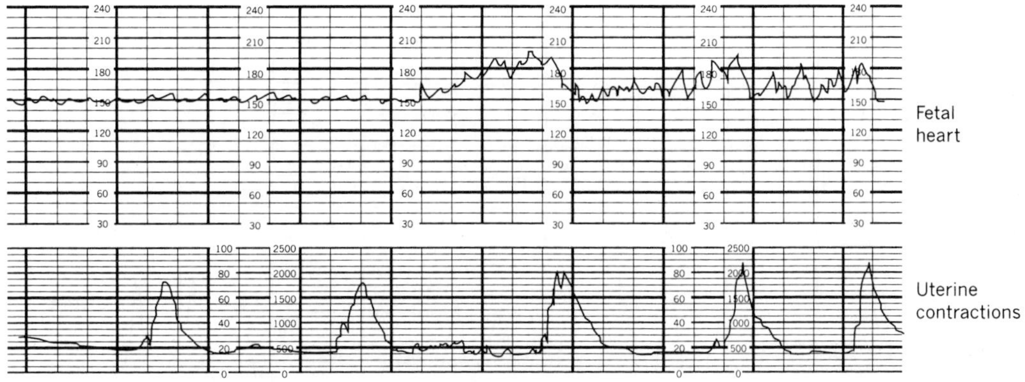

Figure 37.19 *Physiological reduction of baseline variability in fetal heart rate (left). Normal baseline variability (right). (Courtesy of Sonicaid, Abingdon, Oxon.)*

following the administration of pethidine to the woman, which depresses the cardiac centre in the fetal brain. Gibb (1988) found that periods of 'fetal sleep' will cause a loss of baseline variability lasting for about 29–30 min.

Response of the fetal heart to uterine contractions

It is normal for the fetal heart rate to remain steady or to accelerate during contractions (Fig. 37.20). The relationship of decelerations to the occurrence of uterine contractions must be considered closely to assess their significance. **Early decelerations** (Fig. 37.21) begin at or after the onset of a contraction, reach their lowest point at the peak of the contraction and return to the baseline rate by the time the contraction has finished. They are commonly associated with compression of the fetal head but may be an early sign of hypoxia.

A **late deceleration** (Fig. 37.22) begins during or after a contraction, reaches its lowest point after the peak of the contraction and has not recovered by the time the contraction

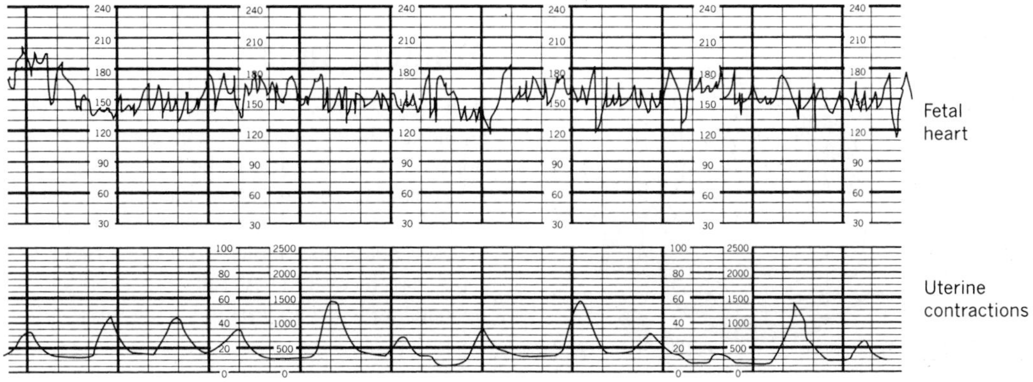

Figure 37.20 *Fetal heart rate accelerations. (Courtesy of Sonicaid, Abingdon, Oxon.)*

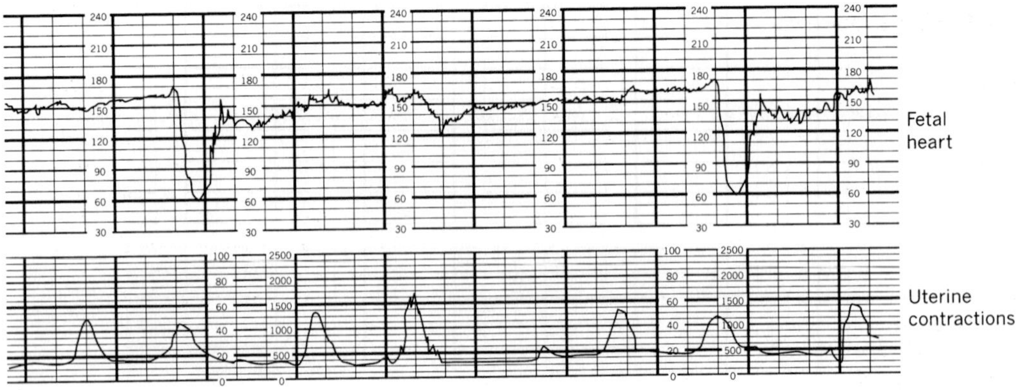

Figure 37.21 *Early fetal heart rate decelerations. (Courtesy of Sonicaid, Abingdon, Oxon.)*

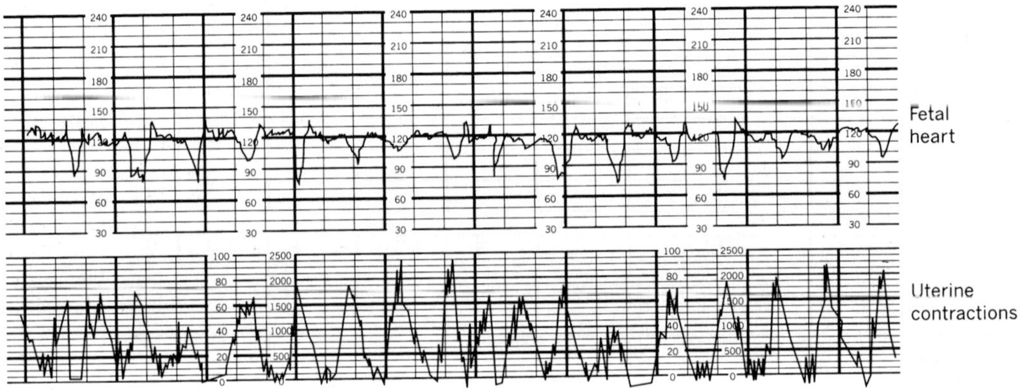

Figure 37.22 *Late fetal heart rate decelerations. (Courtesy of Sonicaid, Abingdon, Oxon.)*

ends. In severe deceleration the heart rate may not have returned to normal by the onset of the next contraction. The **time lag** between the peak of the contraction and the low point of the deceleration is more significant than the actual fall in rate. This always indicates fetal hypoxia and should be treated as an emergency. It is sensible to perform a vaginal examination to assess dilatation of the cervix and exclude cord prolapse prior to informing the obstetrician.

Fetal blood sampling

Hypoxia will lead to respiratory acidosis and a lowering of blood pH. The normal pH of fetal blood should be 7.35 or above. In the first stage of labour a pH of 7.25 calls for urgent action and in the 2nd stage a level of 7.2 can be accepted if delivery is imminent. Blood is taken by passing an amnioscope through the cervix and using a small blade to puncture the scalp skin (Fig. 37.23). A heparinised capillary tube is used to collect 0.5 ml blood for immediate analysis. The blood must not be allowed to clot or come into contact with atmospheric oxygen. Iron filings will be in the tube so that the blood can be gently agitated by moving a magnet backwards and forwards along the outside of the tube. The ends of the tube are sealed with wax to prevent spillage and exclude air whilst the tube is transported to the blood gas analyser.

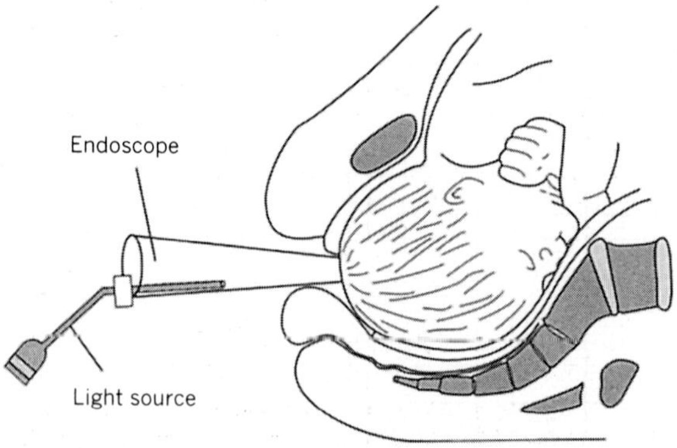

Figure 37.23 *Fetal blood sampling.*

Amniotic fluid

If the membranes have ruptured there is a continuous escape of amniotic fluids available for inspection. The fluid should normally remain clear but the fetus may pass meconium if there is hypoxia. Fresh meconium stains the amniotic fluid green and it is likely that the fetus is hypoxic at that time but a muddy yellow colour may indicate previous hypoxia from which the fetus has recovered. A full discussion on fetal distress and neonatal asphyxia appears in Chapter 46.

Summary of main points

- In early labour contractions may be 15–20 min apart and are fairly weak, lasting for about 30 s. In established labour the uterus contracts every 3–4 min and in advanced labour each contraction may last 50–60 s and is powerful. Contractions can be measured in mmHg by the pressure they exert on the amniotic fluid.
- Fundal dominance allows progressive dilatation of the cervix and as the upper segment thickens and shortens, the fetus is propelled down the birth canal. Polarity during contractions allows the upper and lower poles of the uterus to act in harmony, with contraction and retraction of the upper pole and dilatation of the lower pole. Uterine muscle also has the unique property of contraction and retraction, leading to the progressive shortening and thickening of the UUS and the diminishing of the uterine cavity. A retraction ring forms between the UUS and LUS. There is dilatation of the external os until it is large enough for the widest diameter of the presenting part to pass through.
- When the membranes remain intact there is general fluid pressure. If the membranes are ruptured the placenta is compressed between the uterine wall and the fetus, reducing fetal oxygen supply.
- During each contraction fetal axis pressure causes increasing flexion of the head. This is more significant during the 2nd stage of labour. If the woman adopts an upright posture engagement of the presenting part is facilitated. Gravity may lead to better application of the presenting part to the cervix, promoting Ferguson's reflex and a rapid cervical dilatation. In normal labour the rate of cervical dilatation follows a sigmoid-shaped curve with three distinct parts: the latent phase, the active phase and the deceleration phase.
- Immersion of the body in warm water has been in use for decades and is acceptable to many women. Although its main use is for relaxation and pain relief, it may also shorten the labour and decrease the need for augmentation.
- The process of labour uses large amounts of energy. If insufficient carbohydrate is available, body fat will be utilised with the release of ketones and the development of ketoacidosis. Prior to admission a woman should take carbohydrate foods such as toast, cereal and plain biscuits.
- The main problem with food intake in labour is the possible need for a general anaesthetic. Coupled with the delayed stomach emptying and the relative inefficiency of the cardiac sphincter is a risk of inhalation of acid gastric reflux, resulting in Mendelson's syndrome. Withholding of food does not ensure an empty stomach or reduce the acidity of stomach contents. In some units women are not allowed anything to eat after labour is established whilst in others women may be allowed a low-residue, low-fat diet.
- Research indicates that maternal glucose administration in labour may cause a significant rise in maternal and neonatal plasma glucose levels and maternal insulin levels during the administration of 5% dextrose. There is no evidence of fetal hyperinsulinism in healthy term fetuses and no differences in either maternal or fetal lactate levels.
- In women who require oxytocin, significantly lowered serum sodium levels may occur in both mothers and babies where the oxytocin has been infused in 5% dextrose, suggesting that non-electrolyte solutions administered in labour may lead to hyponatraemia.
- Blood vessels in the myometrium which supply the fetus with oxygen and nutrients are compressed during each uterine contraction with impeded delivery of nutrients and oxygen when the strength of a contraction exceeds 40 mmHg. Fetal hypoxia and distress may occur, especially if the membranes are ruptured. No research supports a clinical advantage to the fetus from any position taken in labour.
- Distress in the fetus results in alterations in heart rate, development of acidosis, passage of meconium, presence of excessive moulding and excessive movements. Information about fetal well-being is mainly obtained by recording fetal heart rate and rhythm, inspection of amniotic fluid for meconium and the pH of fetal blood.
- Cardiotocography allows recording of the response of the fetal heart rhythm and rate to uterine activity. There is no research to support the value of CTG in normal labour. In the first stage of labour a pH of 7.25 calls for urgent action and in the 2nd stage a level of 7.2 can be accepted if delivery is imminent.
- If the membranes have ruptured there is a continuous escape of amniotic fluid available for inspection. The fluid normally remains clear but the fetus may pass meconium if there is hypoxia. Fresh meconium stains the amniotic fluid green and it is likely that the fetus is hypoxic at that time but a muddy yellow colour may indicate previous hypoxia from which the fetus has recovered.

References

Arias F. 1993 Practical Guide to High Risk Pregnancy and Delivery, 2nd edn. Mosby Year Book, Chicago.

Balaskas J. 1983 Active Birth. Unwin, London.

Banks E. 1992 Labouring in comfort. Nursing Times 88 (31), 40–41.

Broach J, Newton N. 1988a Food and beverages in labor. Part 1: cross cultural and historical practices, Birth 15 (2), 81–85.

Broach J, Newton N. 1988b Food and beverages in labour. Part II: the effects of cessation of oral intake during labor. Birth 15 (2), 88–92.

Cassidy P. 1996 The first stage of labour: physiology and early care. In Bennett VR, Brown LK (eds) Myles Textbook for Midwives, 12th edn. Churchill Livingstone, Edinburgh, pp 149–167.

Elkington KW. 1991 At the water's edge: where obstetrics and anaesthesia meet. Obstetrics and Gynaecology 77 (2), 304–308.

Flynn AM, Kelly J, Lynch PF. 1978 Ambulation in labour. British Medical Journal 2 (6137), 591–593.

Gibb D. 1988 A Practical Guide to Labour Management. Blackwell Scientific, Oxford.

Grant J. 1990 Nutrition and hydration in labour. In Alexander J, Levy V, Roch C (eds) Intrapartum Care: A Research-based Approach. Macmillan, Basingstoke, pp 58–69.

Henderson C. 1990 Artificial rupture of the membranes. In Alexander J, Levy V, Roch S (eds) Intrapartum Care: A Research-based Approach. Macmillan, Basingstoke

Johnson N, Johnson VA, Gupta JK. 1991 Maternal positions during labour. Obstetrical and Gynaecological Survey 46 (7), 428–434.

Liu DTY, Fairweather DVI. 1985 Labour Ward Manual. Butterworths, London.

Michel S, Reilly CS, Caunt JA. 1991 Policies for oral intake during labour. A survey of maternity units in England and Wales. Anaesthesia 46, 1071–1073.

Millns JP. 1991 Fluid balance in labour. Current Opinion in Obstetrics and Gynaecology 1 (1), 35–40.

Morrin NA. 1997 Midwifery care in the first stage of labour. In Sweet BR with Tiran D (eds) Mayes Midwifery, 12th edn. Baillière Tindall London, pp 355–384.

Nordstrom L, Arulkumaran S, Chua S et al. 1995 Continuous maternal glucose infusion during labour: effects on maternal and fetal glucose and lactate levels. American Journal of Perinatology 12 (5), 357–362.

Schorn MN, McCallister JL, Blanco JD. 1993 Water immersion and the effect on labor. Journal of Nurse-Midwifery 38 (6), 338–342.

Smith ID, Bogod DG. 1995 Feeding in labour. Contemporary Reviews in Obstetrics and Gynaecology 7 (3), 151–155.

Stratton JF, Stronge J, Boylan PC. 1995 Hyponatraemia and non-electrolyte solutions in labouring primigravidae. European Journal of Obstetrics and Gynaecology and Reproductive Biology 59 (2), 149–151.

Sweet B. 1997 Mayes' Midwifery. Baillière Tindall, London.

Thomson V. 1996 Antenatal care. In Bennett VR, Brown LK (eds) Myles Textbook for Midwives, 12th edn. Churchill Livingstone Edinburgh, pp 123–148.

Zimmerman R, Huch A, Huch R. 1993 Water birth – is it safe? Journal of Perinatal Medicine 21 (1), 5–11.

Recommended reading

Alexander J, Levy V, Roch C. (eds) 1990 Intrapartum Care: A Research-based Approach. Macmillan, Basingstoke.

Balaskas J. 1983 Active Birth. Unwin, London.

Elkington KW. 1991 At the water's edge: where obstetrics and anaesthesia meet. Obstetrics and Gynaecology 77 (2), 304–308.

Flynn AM, Kelly J, Lynch PF. 1978 Ambulation in labour. British Medical Journal 2 (6137), 591–593.

Johnson N, Johnson VA, Gupta JK. 1991 Maternal positions during labour. Obstetrical and Gynaecological Survey 46 (7), 428–434.

Michel S, Reilly CS, Caunt JA. 1991 Policies for oral intake during labour. A survey of maternity units in England and Wales. Anaesthesia 46, 1071–1073.

Millns JP. 1991 Fluid balance in labour. Current Opinion in Obstetrics and Gynaecology 1 (1), 35–40.

Nordstrom L, Arulkumaran S, Chua S et al. 1995 Continuous maternal glucose infusion during labour: effects on maternal and fetal glucose and lactate levels. American Journal of Perinatology 12 (5), 357–362.

Stratton JF, Stronge J, Boylan PC. 1995 Hyponatraemia and non-electrolyte solutions in labouring primigravidae. European Journal of Obstetrics and Gynaecology and Reproductive Biology 59 (2), 149–151.

Zimmerman R, Huch A, Huch R. 1993 Water birth – is it safe? Journal of Perinatal Medicine 21 (1), 5–11.

Chapter 38 Pain relief in labour

In this chapter

INTRODUCTION

The experience of pain can be discussed on three levels: pain transmission and perception, pain reception and pain modulation. Pain is a complex process and is experienced differently depending on the physiological process, the context and the previous experience of an individual. Pain can be modulated at different points in the physiological pathway and by education aimed at achieving an understanding of the accompanying events and the meanings attached to them by individuals and by their culture.

PAIN PERCEPTION

The nature of pain depends not just on physiological parameters such as the part of the body affected and the extent of the injury but also on the psychological reaction to the pain (Allan et al 1996). McCaffery (1980) reminded us of the cognitive and emotional inputs into pain perception, stating that pain is what the patient says it is and exists when he says it does. Telfer (1997) wrote that pain 'is a complex, personal, subjective, multifactorial phenomenon which is influenced by psychological, biological, sociocultural and economic factors'. In similar fashion, Carlson (1991) reminds us that pain is not purely physical. It can be modified by placebo drugs, emotions and other stimuli such as acupuncture. The translation of pain messages into unpleasant feelings ensures that an individual avoids repeating the experience if possible. These are important factors in the management of pain.

Whereas the physiological threshold for pain sensation appears to be similar in all people (Sternbach & Tursky 1965, cited by Telfer 1997), the cognitive and emotive factors alter the individual's reaction to pain and the meaning attached to the experience. The anticipation of pain increases anxiety levels and the perceived intensity of pain. Hayward (1975) demonstrated that knowledge of events reduces anxiety and pain and this applies to pain in labour. Interesting work has been done by Walding (1991) on the **locus of control theory** which suggests that pain is perceived as less threatening and with less intensity if women believe they are in control of events. Placing the woman at the centre of her care should therefore make labour less painful and traumatic, even if problems such as occipitoposterior position occur.

Pain may also increase the level of catecholamines released into the blood. This in turn has the usual result of increased heart and respiration rate with decreased blood flow to the internal organs such as the uterus. The uterus in labour needs a good oxygen and nutrient delivery to enable efficient contractions and thus anxiety and fear increase pain, reduce uterine blood supply and may prolong labour (Heywood & Ho 1990).

PAIN RECEPTION

> The principle of pain reception is that several million bare sensory nerve endings weave their way through all the tissues and organs of the body (except the brain) and respond to noxious stimuli. (Marieb 1992).

A chemical released from damaged tissue seems to act as a universal pain stimulus. This is **bradykinin**, which in turn releases inflammatory chemicals such as histamine and prostaglandin. Bradykinin is thought to bind to receptor endings, resulting in an action potential. However, pain perception is much more than the simple sensation relayed by neurones.

Classification of pain

Pain can be classified as somatic or visceral. Somatic pain arising from skin, muscles or joints can be deep or superficial. **Superficial somatic pain** tends to be brief, highly localisable and sharp or pricking in character. This pain is transmitted along large myelinated fibres – the A-δ fibres. **Deep somatic pain** is more likely to be described as burning or aching; it is more diffuse and longer lasting and always indicates tissue destruction. Impulses travel along small unmyelinated fibres called C fibres. A third type of fibre, the myelinated A-β fibre, relays light touch.

Pain pathways

Visceral pain originates in the organs of the body cavities; it is described as burning, gnawing or aching. Visceral sensory neurones (afferents) accompany autonomic sympathetic and parasympathetic fibres and send information about chemical changes; distension or irritation of the viscera. Both somatic and visceral pain stimuli pass along the dendrites of the first-order neurones to their cell bodies in the **dorsal root ganglia**. Their axons leave the dorsal root ganglia to enter the spinal cord and synapse with second-order neurones in the dorsal horns of the spinal cord. The pain impulse causes the release of the pain neurotransmitter, **substance P**, from the presynaptic membrane into the synaptic cleft.

Anatomy of the dorsal horn

The cells in the spinal cord are arranged in **laminae** (layers) in a dorsal-ventral direction running the full length of the spinal cord (Fig. 38.1). The dorsal horn contains six laminae numbered from the tip of the horn inwards. The ventral horn contains another three laminae and another column of cells, lamina 10, is clustered around the central canal. Laminae 1 and 2 are visible to the naked eye as a clear zone and are together called the **substantia gelatinosa**.

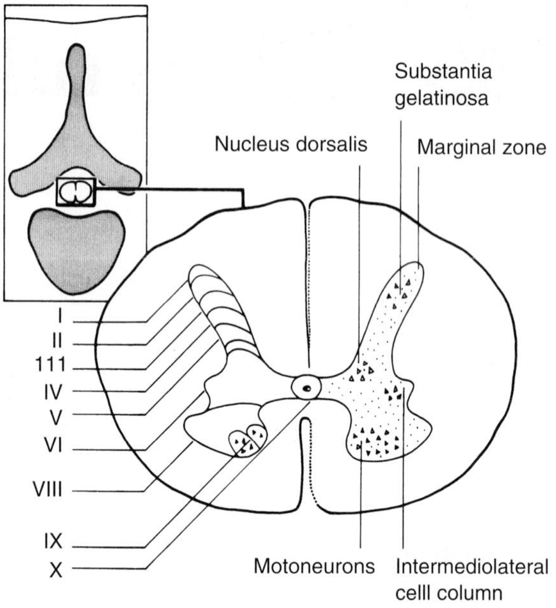

Figure 38.1 *Laminae (I–X) and named cell groups at mid-thoracic level (from Hinchliff SM, Montague SE, Watson R, 1996, with permission).*

Ascending pathways

Sensory fibres return to the dorsal horns in an orderly fashion (Fig. 38.2). The rule is that the thicker the fibre, the deeper it penetrates. The unmyelinated C fibres do not penetrate past lamina 2 and the small myelinated A-δ fibres mainly terminate in laminae 1 and 2 although a few make it to lamina 5. The large myelinated fibres from the skin end mainly in laminae 4, 5 and 6. The specialised large muscle stretch afferents reach level 6 (Melzack & Wall 1988).

The axons of most of the second-order neurones cross the cord and enter the anterolateral spinothalamic tracts to ascend to the thalamus (Fitzgerald 1992). There they synapse with third-order neurones to pass the pain message to the sensory cortex for interpretation. The second-order fibres may make abundant synapses in the brainstem, hypothalamus and limbic system before reaching the thalamus. This will add a state of arousal and emotion to the perception of pain.

PAIN MODULATION

Control systems descending from the brain

Nerve fibres descending in the white matter penetrate into the grey matter and innervate the nearest cells. The dorsolateral column is therefore able to send axons to the most dorsal laminae. In particular, fibres from the raphe, the locus coelureus in the reticular formation and the hypothalamus, as well as the pyramidal tract from the cortex, innervate dorsal laminae 3–6. Descending fibres synapse in the dorsal horns and further modify the final ascending message by releasing endogenous opiates such as endorphins and enkephalins, discovered by Hughes et al (1975), into the synaptic cleft. Endogenous opiates

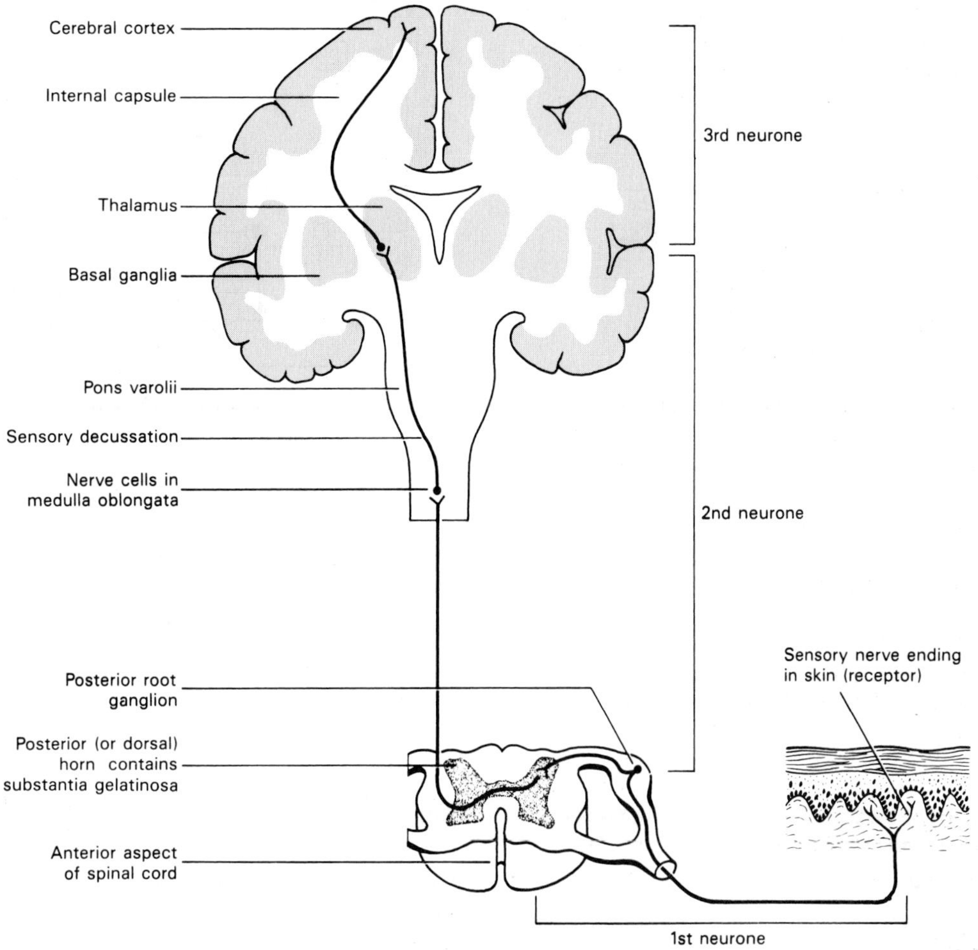

Figure 38.2 *The sensory pathway showing the structures involved in the appreciation of pain. (Reproduced with permission from Bevis 1984.)*

have been shown to inhibit prostaglandin production. Prostaglandin is thought to be a key chemical necessary for pain perception.

The gate control theory of pain

In order to understand the theory of Melzack & Wall (1988), it is necessary to keep in mind:

- the ascending and descending tracts in the spinal cord;
- the relative conduction speeds of sensory nerve fibres returning to the spinal cord;
- the anatomy of the dorsal horns of the spinal cord.

Any theory of pain must explain several facts about pain perception (Melzack & Wall 1988).

- The high variability between injury and pain
- The production of pain by innocuous stimuli
- The perception of pain in areas seemingly removed from the area of damage
- The persistence of pain in the absence of injury or after healing
- The change in the location and nature of pain over time
- The multidimensional nature of pain
- The lack of treatment for some types of pain such as arthritic pain and migraines

Melzack & Wall (1988) have updated their gate control theory of pain first proposed in 1965 (Fig. 38.3). Although they emphasise that there is still work to be done to complete their understanding, most people would agree that the gate control theory offers satisfactory explanations for some of the above unusual phenomena.

The essence of the gate control theory

Gating of the spinothalamic tract response to C fibre activity can be achieved by stimulating large myelinated mechanoreceptor afferents by rub or tickle. These impulses inhibit the ascending pain impulse. Inputs from the large myelinated fibres conveying touch and smaller A-δ and C fibres conveying pain interact at the level of the spinal cord. The large-diameter sensory nerve impulses come into the spinal cord more rapidly. This normally inhibits the slower, smaller fibre pain impulses presynaptically. This inhibition constitutes the **gate** that is normally closed against small-diameter fibre impulses unless the stimulation is so great that it overcomes the gate (Fig. 38.3).

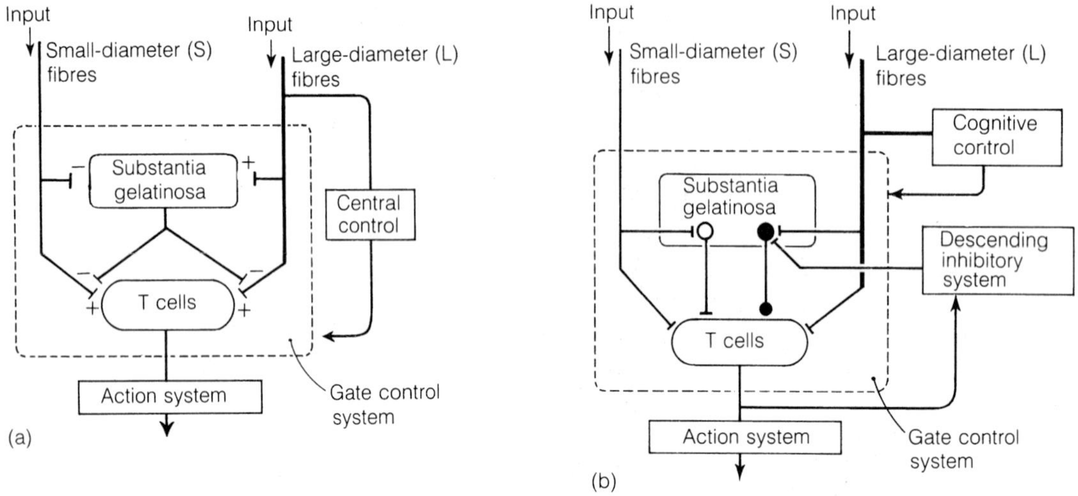

Figure 38.3 *The gate control theory of pain. (a) Original formulation of the theory. Large diameter (L) and small diameter (S) peripheral nerve fibres input to the substantia gelatinosa (SG) and to the first central transmission (T) cells of the spinal cord. The inhibitory effect exerted by the SG on the T cells is increased by activity of the S fibres (pain fibres). The central control mechanisms are represented as running from the L fibre system and feeding back to the gate control, (b) Updated model. On the basis of subsequent evidence, Melzack and Wall formulated the gate control theory to include excitatory (white circle) links from the SG to the T cells, as well as descending inhibitory control from the brain-stem. All synaptic connections are excitatory except the inhibitory link from SG to T. The round knob at this inhibitory synapse implies that its action may be presynaptic, postsynaptic, or both. (Reproduced with permission from Melzack & Wall 1988.)*

Other modifications of the ascending pain impulse takes place in the substantia gelatinosa.

- Interneurones in the substantia gelatinosa can regulate and amplify the impulse conducted to the brain via the ascending pathways.
- Descending fibres synapse in the same area of the spinal cord and further modify the final ascending message by releasing endogenous opiates such as endorphins and enkephalins into the synaptic cleft (see above).
- Virtually all the brain plays a part in pain perception; the thalamus, reticular system, limbic system and cortex add their effects to the physical, emotional and cognitive experience of pain.

Knowledge of the multidimensional nature of pain perception allows the management of pain to be approached in an equally multidimensional manner. Techniques to inhibit the gate include stimulation of the large nerve fibres so that the pain impulses from the smaller fibres are blocked. Methods include heat, massage and pressure. Transcutaneous electrical nerve stimulation (TENS) works by applying a stimulating electrode to the skin at the level of the noxious C fibre activity and delivering an electrical current sufficient to cause a buzzing sensation (Fitzgerald 1992). Descending fibre impulses can also inhibit transmission of pain by release of natural opiates and concentration techniques may work in this way (Blackburn & Loper 1992).

Visceral sensory neurones

Although the ANS is considered to be a motor system, there are sensory neurones, mainly visceral pain afferents, in autonomic nerves. These visceral pain afferents travel along the same pathways as somatic pain fibres. Pain perception is referred to the somatic area of the specific dermatome of the body surface. For example, the pain of a heart attack is felt in the chest and along the medial aspect of the left arm.

PAIN PATHWAYS IN LABOUR

Both visceral and somatic pain are perceived in labour. Visceral pain is caused by the uterine contractions, the dilatation of the cervix and, later, by the stretching of the vagina and pelvic floor. The body of the uterus is served by autonomic nerves originating in T-11 and T-12 and L-1 vertebrae (Fig. 38.4). Sensation from the body of the uterus is perceived as pain in response to stretch, infection and contraction and possibly ischaemia.

The cervix is innervated by the sacral plexus from S-2, S-3 and S-4 vertebral nerves (Fig. 38.4) which pass through the transcervical nerve plexi. Pain sensation from the cervix is in response to rapid dilatation. Somatic pain is caused by the pressure of the fetus as it distends the birth canal, vulva and perineum. Sensations from the pelvic floor are relayed from the pudendal nerve to the sacral plexus. Pain during the first stage of labour may be referred as nerve impulses from the uterus and cervix stimulate spinal cord neurones that innervate the abdominal wall. Pain may be felt between the umbilicus and the symphysis pubis and around the iliac crests to the buttocks. It may radiate down the thighs and into the lumbar and sacral regions of the back.

THE EFFECT OF PAIN

Besides the physical, emotional and cognitive factors affecting pain quality and perception, abnormalities of labour may cause

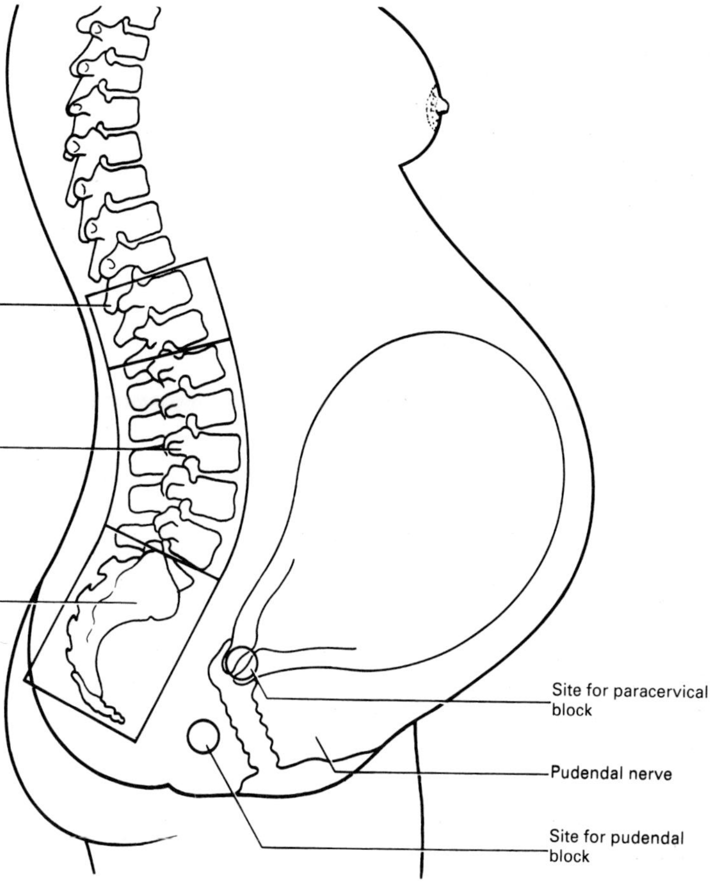

Figure 38.4 *Pain pathways in labour, showing the sites at which pain may be intercepted by local anaesthetic technique. (Reproduced with permission from Bevis 1984.)*

an increase in the pain perceived. Pain may be increased in labours complicated by prolongation, occipitoposterior position and borderline cephalopelvic disproportion.

Pain is a form of stress and may cause increased levels of catecholamine secretion which will cause the following signs:

- increased cardiac output;
- increased heart rate;
- a rise in blood pressure;
- hyperventilation;
- maternal alkalosis;
- decreased cerebral and uterine blood flow due to vasoconstriction;
- decreased uterine contractions;
- delayed stomach emptying leading to nausea and vomiting;
- delayed bladder emptying.

MANAGEMENT OF PAIN

Understanding of pain pathways and perception allows a reasonable range of interventions. Care may include pharmacological and non-pharmacological methods of pain relief. Carers can offer:

- non-pharmacological support;
- transcutaneous electrical nerve stimulation (TENS);
- systemic analgesia;
- tranquillisers;
- inhalational analgesia;
- regional and local (epidural) analgesia;
- alternative methods.

Non-pharmacological support

Antenatal preparation

Pain management ideally begins during the antenatal period. Women should be given the opportunity to discuss their anxieties and fears and obtain information about pain relief at a level they are able to understand. Every person's needs are different but all women should participate in the planning of care in labour, including the choice of pain relief. There should be no feeling of finality in the choice made; women need to feel reassured that they can change their minds during the course of labour, depending on their actual experience of pain. Some women may wish to attend preparation classes.

During labour

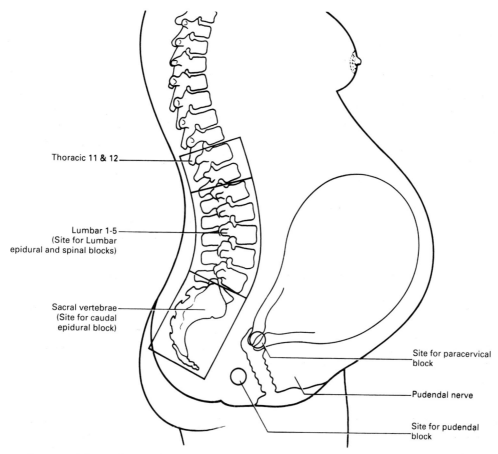

The **environment** is important. The room should be furnished comfortably but in such a way that any emergency treatment needed can be carried out swiftly and efficiently (Bevis 1996). Wallpaper, curtains and screens can be useful in creating a restful atmosphere. There is a move towards informal furnishings such as beanbags, reclining chairs and rocking chairs in many units. Music and television can provide pleasure and distraction for some women in early labour.

A **companion** of the woman's choice should be able to stay with her throughout labour. This may not be her partner as some men find the situation uncomfortable. Women may choose to give birth supported by a female relative or friend. If possible, a midwife known to the woman prior to labour should be available and should form a supportive relationship with the woman and her chosen companion.

Freedom to move about as and when she wants can give the woman control of her situation and shorten the process of birth. The perception of active participation in the birth is very important. The woman should be helped to find the position in which she is most comfortable, making full use of the range of furniture and equipment provided. Thus she may walk about, lie down, sit astride a chair or kneel as she wishes.

Relaxation techniques should be encouraged if the woman has learned them antenatally. It is also possible to teach women simple breathing techniques during the course of labour.

Communication of information about progress and encouragement to keep going will also reduce anxiety and add to the feeling of being in control. The woman and her companion should participate in any decision making such as the need for pain relief. Communication also includes physical contact but care should be taken to ascertain what the woman is comfortable with. Hand holding, back rubbing, massage and cuddling may be appreciated by some women while others prefer to be left alone.

Bathing may be soothing for some women both as a direct reliever of pain and indirectly through feeling refreshed. Clean clothing should be available if necessary. Mouth cleansing such as teeth cleaning or sucking ice can be most refreshing.

Transcutaneous electrical nerve stimulation (TENS)

This non-pharmacological method of pain relief depends on the physiology of the gate (Melzack & Wall 1988, Wall 1985). It stimulates the release of endogenous opiates (Simkin 1989). Electrodes are placed over the areas of the woman's back which overlie the thoracic and lumbar nerve endings and over the sacral nerves, as shown in Figure 38.5.

Accurate placing is important for maximising the pain relief. The equipment is operated by the woman herself and she should have been able to practise with it in the antenatal period. Pressing a button causes a small electrical current to pass through the electrodes. The current may be pulsed, that is, intermittent and low frequency, or it may be continuous and high frequency. Low-frequency TENS stimulates the release of endogenous opiates whilst high-frequency TENS closes the pain gate (Bevis 1996). TENS is most effective when commenced early in labour but will not provide adequate analgesia for some women if used on its own. It is probably best in the shorter multigravid labours although many primigravidae find it useful. The TENS equipment may interfere with some electronic fetal monitors and may need to be switched off to obtain an accurate reading.

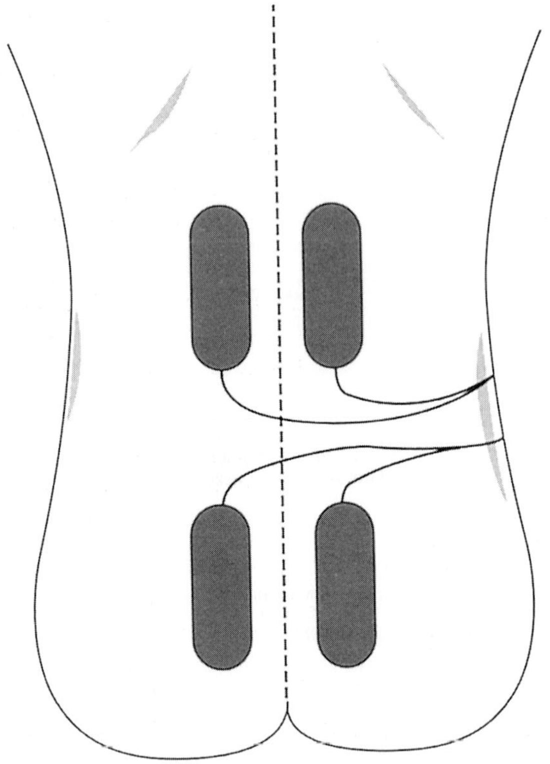

Figure 38.5 *Positions of TENS electrodes for pain relief in labour (from Sweet B, 1997, with permission).*

TENS was approved by the UKCC for use by midwives provided that:

- they had received adequate and appropriate instruction, that is, determined by local policy;
- safety standards conform to those laid down by the Department of Health Medical Devices Directorate or equivalent body in Scotland, Wales and Northern Ireland.

Systemic analgesia

An analgesic is a substance that reduces sensibility to pain without loss of consciousness and sense of touch. In labour the substance should not compromise the safety of mother or fetus and it is advisable that there should be a specific antagonist (Telfer 1997). A strong analgesic drug is called a **narcotic** and these include opioid drugs. The most commonly used is **pethidine**, a synthetic drug which has powerful analgesic, sedative and antispasmodic effects. The effect of intramuscular injection of pethidine is rapid and lasts up to 4 h. The dose is from 50 to 200 mg depending on the route of administration, the mother's weight, the progress of labour and the degree of pain. Pethidine may be given by intramuscular or intravenous injection or by self-administered infusion of 25 mg as needed. There is a built-in time limitation so that the woman does not take an overdose. Side effects include nausea, loss of self-control, a fall in blood pressure and perspiration. It crosses the placental membrane to affect the fetus and changes in fetal heart rate pattern, with a loss of baseline variability, may be seen within 40 min of administration. As it also depresses the fetal respiratory centre, it is preferably not given if delivery is expected within 2–3 h. Given within 1 h of delivery or more than 6 h before delivery, its effect on the neonate's respiration is minimal.

However, Barrett (1983) found that changes in sleep and arousal patterns, attention, motor competence and sucking and feeding patterns followed the administration of analgesics, especially pethidine. Babies were less alert, more likely to cry when disturbed and more difficult to settle. They were more difficult to attach to the nipple and sucked less efficiently. The antidote is naloxone hydrochloride (Narcan) and the neonatal dose is 0.01 mg/kg.

Meptazinol is an analgesic which has little effect on cardiovascular and respiratory function. The dose is 100–150 mg administered intramuscularly. There is little difference in the analgesic properties of pethidine and meptazinol but the latter may cause vomiting in the woman.

Tranquillisers which also have antiemetic properties may be given with the narcotic. The most commonly used are promazine (Sparine) 25–50 mg and promethazine (Phenergan) 25–50 mg.

Inhalational analgesia

Anaesthetics are used to make a patient unaware of and unresponsive to painful stimulation (Rang & Dale 1991). They are given systemically and have their effect on the central nervous system. In order to be a useful anaesthetic, a drug must induce anaesthesia rapidly, be easily adjustable and reversible. The use of the inhaled gaseous agent **nitrous oxide** (laughing gas) was suggested by Humphrey Davy in 1800. Like ether, it was first used in dental extractions.

James Simpson used the agent **chloroform** to relieve the pain of childbirth, which was opposed at first by the clergy. The administration of chloroform to Queen Victoria during the birth of her 7th child silenced the opposition. Inhalation anaesthetics include a wide variety of substances with no common chemical structure, such as halothane, nitrous oxide and xenon, and the mechanism for their action is not clear despite much research.

The inhalation of a low dose of an anaesthetic agent will provide analgesia. **Entonox gas**, which contains a mixture of equal parts of oxygen and nitrous oxide (laughing gas), is approved for use by midwives. Entonox may be available by cylinder or by piped supply (Fig. 38.6). There are four types of apparatus approved for use by midwives on their own responsibility:

- Entonox;
- PneuPac;
- SOS Nitronox, midwifery model;
- Peacemaker.

Entonox is colourless and odourless and the nitrous oxide is heavier than oxygen. If stored at a temperature below –7°C, the gases may separate. Therefore, cylinders should always be stored at 10°C and on their side until needed, when the cylinder should be inverted several times to mix the contents. Entonox does not flow from the cylinder and must be obtained via the facemask by inspiratory efforts. The analgesic begins to take effect after about 20 s, with maximum effect after 50 s. The mother is instructed to begin to breathe the gas as soon as the uterus begins to contract and before the sensation of pain is felt. Entonox can be used in conjunction with narcotic drugs. It is excreted rapidly via the lungs as the mother exhales and therefore toxic levels do not build up to affect the fetus. Entonox does cross the placental barrier in both directions following a concentration gradient.

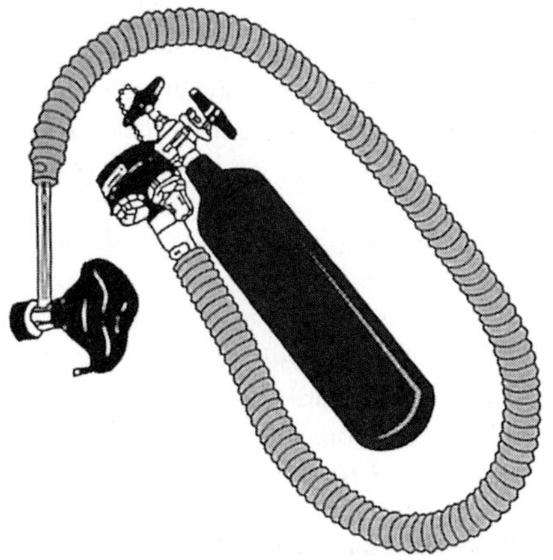

Figure 38.6 *The Entonox inhaler (from Sweet B, 1997, with permission).*

Stages of anaesthesia

When inhalational anaesthetics are given on their own, well-defined stages are passed through as the blood concentration increases.

- **Stage I – analgesia**. The person is conscious but drowsy and response to painful stimuli is reduced.
- **Stage II – excitement**. The subject loses consciousness and does not respond to non-painful stimuli but will respond in a reflex manner to painful stimuli. Cough and gag reflexes are also present. Irregular breathing may occur and this is a dangerous state that modern procedures are designed to eliminate.
- **Stage III – surgical anaesthesia**. Spontaneous movement ceases and respiration becomes regular. If the anaesthesia is light some reflexes are still present and muscle tone is still good. As the anaesthesia deepens muscles become flaccid and reflexes disappear. Respirations become progressively more shallow.
- **Stage IV – medullary paralysis**. Respiration and vasomotor control disappear and death would occur in a few minutes.

Obstetric use of inhalational anaesthetics

An important characteristic of an inhalational anaesthetic is the rapidity with which the arterial blood concentration changes as the amount of drug inhaled changes. These drugs are generally used as anaesthetics in obstetrics in two ways: either as pain relief or as part of a combination of drugs to induce general anaesthesia during a caesarean section. Commonly, anaesthesia is induced by an intravenous drug and then the state is maintained with an inhalational agent such as nitrous oxide or halothane. Muscle paralysis is obtained by the administration of a drug such as tubocurarine. Inhalation agents are time and dose dependent and may affect the fetus directly by being transported across the placenta or indirectly by altering uteroplacental blood flow.

Various factors, including the higher metabolic requirements and the presence of the fetus, make the pregnant woman more vulnerable to hypoxia should it occur during intubation. There is a rapid fall in PO_2 and hypoxia and respiratory acidosis may quickly follow. Supine hypotensive syndrome may exaggerate the effect by reducing venous return and cardiac output so that the uteroplacental blood flow is poor; a left lateral tilt on the operating table will reduce the incidence of this problem. However, with safe techniques, light to moderate anaesthesia and adequate oxygen administration, women with normal health should not have problems.

Epidural analgesia

Epidural analgesia involves the introduction of a local anaesthetic into the epidural space surrounding the spinal cord. A catheter is inserted so that further doses of local anaesthetic can be administered if needed. Epidural analgesia provides adequate pain relief in about 80% of women although the success rate may depend on the experience of the anaesthetist. The choice of epidural analgesia may be declining for women experiencing normal labour although it is becoming more common as a method for caesarean section.

Anatomy of the epidural space

The epidural space is a small space about 4 mm wide situated around the dura mater and contains blood vessels and fatty tissue (Figs 38.7 and 38.8). The spinal nerves pass through it. Engorgement of the veins reduces the size of the space during pregnancy and uterine contractions, which cause even more engorgement of the veins, reduce it even more. The aim is to surround specific fibres of the spinal nerves in order to remove the sensation of pain. The procedure is similar to a lumbar puncture but the meninges are not penetrated. Most commonly, the lumbar route is used and the alternative of caudal anaesthesia is not popular in Britain. The anaesthetic is introduced between lumbar vertebrae 3 and 4 or 2 and 3 (Fig. 38.9).

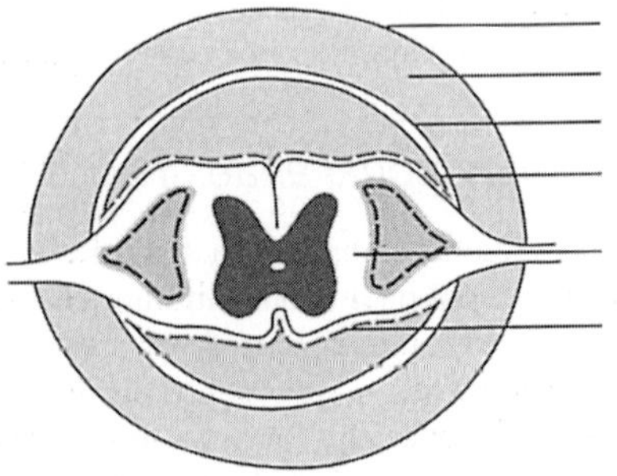

Figure 38.7 *The epidural space.*

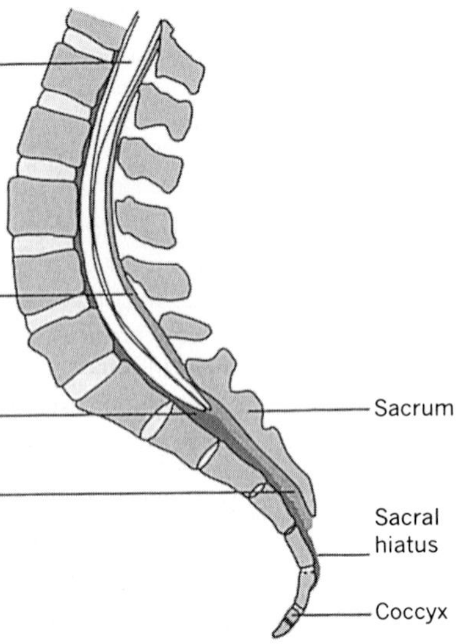

Figure 38.8 *The epidural space and sacral hiatus (from Sweet B, 1997, with permission).*

Preparation of the woman

The procedure and its risks are explained to the woman, who must give consent. Baseline readings of temperature, pulse, blood pressure and fetal heart are recorded. The woman is encouraged to empty her bladder. An intravenous infusion of a crystalloid solution such as Hartmann's is commenced to reduce the risk of hypotension. Resuscitation equipment and drugs should be available. The woman may be positioned on her left side or sitting up and she is asked to flex her back by drawing up her knees. This helps to separate the vertebrae and give better access to the epidural space.

Procedure

Using an aseptic technique, the skin is cleaned and sterile towels are placed around the area of skin to be breached. A small amount of local anaesthetic is injected and a special epidural needle (**Tuohy needle**), which is a blunt needle with stilette, is inserted. The needle is advanced carefully until the resistance of the ligamentum flavum is reached, just before the epidural space. The stilette is removed and a syringe containing air or normal saline is attached to the needle. Further advancement of the needle brings it into the epidural space, which is recognised by a sudden loss of resistance when the plunger of the syringe is depressed. Any leakage of cerebrospinal fluid would indicate that a dural tap has occurred.

If no blood or CSF is seen, the catheter is introduced through the epidural needle until its tip is in the epidural space. A test dose of 3–4 ml of local anaesthetic, usually bupivacaine (Marcain) 0.25%, is given. A bacterial filter is attached to the end of the catheter which is taped securely in place. Observations of maternal blood pressure and pulse are recorded, usually every 5 min for 30 min and then every 30 min.

Indications (Telfer 1997)

- Pain relief

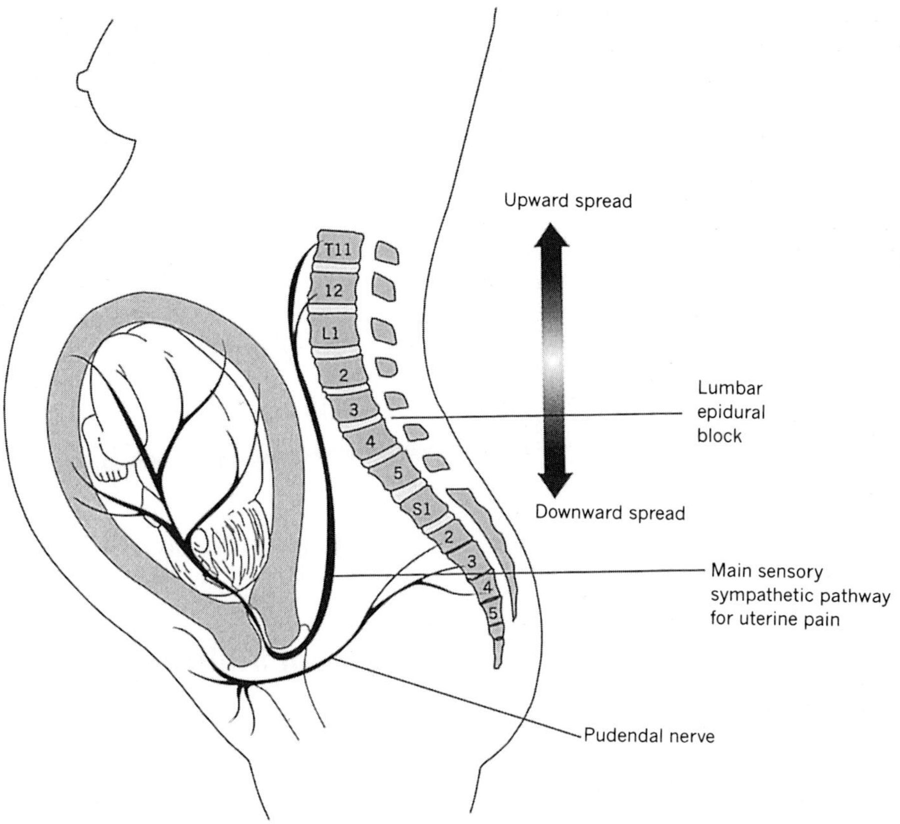

Figure 38.9 *Nerve supply in relation to epidural anaesthesia during labour (from Sweet B, 1997, with permission).*

- Hypertensive conditions, to prevent the rise of blood pressure (it may even cause a small fall in BP)
- Preterm labour, to avoid the use of narcotic drugs
- Prolonged labour, to allow rest and prevent exhaustion
- Malpresentations such as breech, to prevent premature pushing and in case manipulations are needed in the 2nd stage of labour
- Occipitoposterior malposition, to reduce pain and early pushing. However, there may be delay or no rotation of the head due to the reduced tone of the pelvic floor. 0.5% is given and if there are no adverse signs after 5 min, the remainder of the initial dose is completed
- Multiple pregnancy, to prevent the administration of narcotic drugs and in case manipulations are needed in the 2nd stage of labour
- Cardiac and respiratory disease
- Operative deliveries such as caesarean section
- Possible difficulties with intubation during administration of a general anaesthetic.

Contraindications (Telfer 1997)

- Maternal reluctance
- Sepsis near the site of the injection
- Systemic sepsis
- Haemorrhagic disease or clotting disorder
- Spinal deformity
- Neurological disease
- Hypovolaemia or hypotension
- Chronic back trouble

Complications (Bevis 1996)

Hypotension may occur because the local anaesthetic blocks the transmission of both motor and sensory nerves and affects the sympathetic nervous system. This causes vasodilation and a fall in blood pressure may occur unless blood volume is increased by infusion (a **preload**) prior to the epidural block.

Dural tap may occur if the dura mater is punctured. It should be recognised by a few drops of CSF leaking through the Tuohy needle. If more CSF leaks the woman may develop a severe headache which often lasts a week. Lying flat will relieve the headache but also removes her ability to care for her baby. A blood patch of 10–20 ml of blood introduced into the epidural space may provide a cure.

Total spinal block is a rare complication and occurs if the anaesthetist fails to recognise a dural puncture and proceeds to inject the local anaesthetic. There is a profound motor and sensory block and a dramatic fall in blood pressure. The woman collapses and may have a cardiac arrest. Resuscitation and ventilatory support are needed immediately. Prevention of maternal hypoxia and restoration of normal blood pressure may allow the baby to be delivered safely as soon as feasible.

A bloody tap occurs if the anaesthetist punctures an epidural vein. Blood will be seen in the epidural cannula. Resiting is necessary to avoid an intravenous injection of local anaesthetic.

A patchy block with a better effect on one side of the body may occur, usually the right side. A top-up by the anaesthetist with the woman lying on the affected side may work but for a few women, it may be impossible to provide total analgesia.

Other drugs

Opiates have been injected into the epidural space, including diamorphine, morphine, pethidine and fentanyl. They do not produce a block so that there is little risk of hypotension but they may reduce the amount of pain perceived, especially post-operatively. A dilute combination of opiate with local anaesthetic may give a longer, more effective analgesia with less motor blockade. The local anaesthetic blocks the A-δ fibres whilst the opiates remove pain transmitted by the smaller C fibres. This allows careful mobilisation of the woman and she can be more active in the 2nd stage of labour (Telfer 1997). The drugs commonly used are bupivacaine and fentanyl and they may be given by epidural infusion rather than by bolus injection. Wild & Coyne (1992) report side effects including pruritus, urinary retention, postural hypotension, nausea, vomiting and respiratory depression.

Spinal anaesthesia

Spinal anaesthesia is different from epidural anaesthesia in that the local anaesthetic solution is injected into the subarachnoid space directly into the cerebrospinal fluid rather than into the epidural space. It is quick, easy to perform and usually effective. It induces a total motor and sensory block below the anaesthetised area but there is more risk of profound hypotension occurring. It is useful for performing short procedures such as forceps delivery or manual removal of the placenta. It can be used for performing a caesarean section but care must be taken that its effects do not wear off before the end of the surgery. Spinal anaesthesia may be combined with epidural anaesthesia to prevent the above risk (Bevis 1996).

Pudendal block

This is the infiltration of a local anaesthetic agent via a transvaginal route into an area around the pudendal nerve (Fig. 38.10), carried out by an obstetrician. It originates from S2–4 and passes across the ischial spine. A special needle called a pudendal block needle, which has a guide, is used. Ten ml of lignocaine 1% is introduced just below each ischial spine. Analgesia of the lower vagina and perineum results and is suitable for use in forceps or breech deliveries. Perineal repair may be carried out using the same analgesia although perineal infiltration would be more usual.

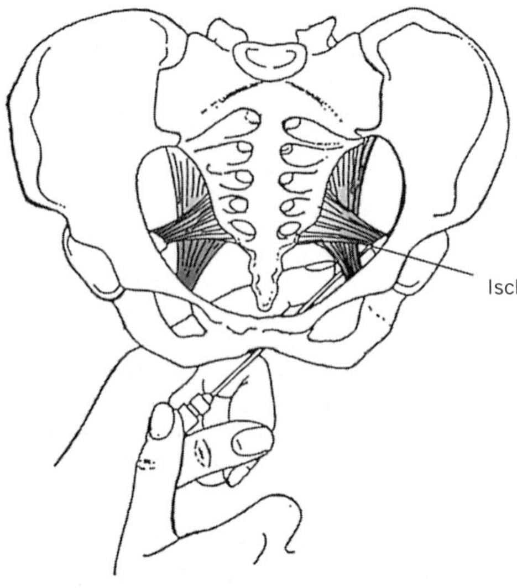

Figure 38.10 *Pudendal nerve block (from Sweet B, 1997, with permission).*

Perineal infiltration

This is the use of a local anaesthetic to infiltrate the perineum for either performance of an episiotomy or suturing. Ten ml of plain lignocaine 0.5% solution is distributed by fan-like injections. Precautions are taken to avoid the inadvertent intravascular injection of the drug.

Complementary pain relief methods

Some women wish to avoid using pharmacological methods of pain relief or the invasive technique of epidural analgesia. Some midwives are keen to learn complementary techniques so that they can offer a wider range of help to the women they care for but they should ensure that they are trained and that the therapy has no hidden dangers for the mother. Some women choose to be accompanied in labour by their complementary therapist. Many complementary therapies are now accepted by health professionals (Tiran 1997).

Some methods that have been found to benefit women in labour are massage, acupuncture (Budd 1992), hypnosis (Jenkins & Pritchard 1993), aromatherapy with oils placed in a warm bath (Burns & Blamey 1994), reflexology (Feder et al 1993) and biofeedback. Other allied therapies involve immersion in warm water, nipple stimulation to increase oxytocin production and listening to soothing music.

Summary of main points

- The chemicals bradykinin, prostaglandin and histamine are involved in the local production of inflammation and pain. The physiological threshold for pain sensation may be similar in all people but cognitive and emotive factors alter the individual's reaction to and experience of pain. The anticipation of pain increases anxiety levels and the perceived intensity of pain.
- Somatic pain may be deep or superficial. Superficial pain tends to be brief, highly localisable and sharp or pricking in character. Deep somatic pain is described as burning or aching, is more diffuse and longer lasting. Visceral pain originates from the organs of the body cavities and is often described as burning, gnawing or aching. The brain plays a large part in the modulation of pain.

- Melzack & Wall (1988) updated their gate control theory of pain. Inputs from large myelinated fibres conveying touch and fibres conveying pain interact at the level of the spinal cord. The large-diameter sensory nerve impulses come into the spinal cord more rapidly, which inhibits the slower pain impulses presynaptically. This constitutes the gate against small-diameter fibre impulses.
- Although the ANS is considered to be a motor system, there are sensory neurones, mainly visceral pain afferents, in autonomic nerves. These visceral pain afferents travel along the same pathways as somatic pain fibres. Pain perception is referred to the somatic area of the specific dermatome of the body surface. Both visceral and somatic pain are perceived in labour.
- Besides the physical, emotional and cognitive factors affecting pain perception, abnormalities of labour may cause an increase in the pain perceived. Pain may be increased in labours complicated by prolongation, occipitoposterior position and borderline cephalopelvic disproportion.
- Pain may cause raised levels of catecholamine secretion, leading to increased cardiac output and heart rate, a rise in blood pressure, hyperventilation with maternal alkalosis, decreased cerebral and uterine blood flow due to vasoconstriction, decreased uterine contractions and delayed stomach and bladder emptying.
- Understanding of pain pathways and perception leads to both pharmacological and non-pharmacological methods of pain relief. The environment of the woman in labour is important and a companion of the woman's choice should be able to stay with her throughout labour. The perception of active participation in the birth is very important. Communication of information about progress and encouragement will reduce anxiety and add to the feeling of being in control.
- Transcutaneous electrical nerve stimulation (TENS) depends on the physiology of the gate in the spinal cord. It works by interrupting the transmission of pain and also stimulates the release of endogenous opiates.
- In labour the most commonly used analgesic is pethidine. Meptazinol is an analgesic which has little effect on cardiovascular and respiratory function. There is little difference in the analgesic properties of pethidine and meptazinol but the latter may cause vomiting in the woman. Tranquillisers, which also have antiemetic properties, may be given with the narcotic.
- Anaesthetics are generally used in obstetrics either as pain relief or as part of a combination of drugs to induce general anaesthesia during a caesarean section. The inhalation of a low dose of an anaesthetic agent will provide analgesia. Entonox gas, which contains a mixture of equal parts of oxygen and nitrous oxide, is approved for use by midwives.
- Various factors, including the higher metabolic requirements and the presence of the fetus, make the pregnant woman more vulnerable to hypoxia should it occur during intubation. However, with safe techniques, light to moderate anaesthesia and adequate oxygen administration women with normal health should not have problems.
- Epidural analgesia provides adequate pain relief in about 80% of women who are given the technique. Indications for epidural analgesia include pain relief, hypertensive conditions, preterm, prolonged labour, malpresentations and malpositions, multiple pregnancy, cardiac and respiratory disease, operative deliveries and possible difficulties with intubation during general anaesthetic.
- Contraindications for epidural analgesia include maternal reluctance, sepsis near the site of the injection, systemic sepsis, haemorrhagic disease or clotting disorder, spinal deformity, neurological disease, hypovolaemia or hypotension or chronic back trouble. Complications of insertion include hypotension, dural tap, total spinal block and a bloody tap.
- A dilute combination of opiate with local anaesthetic may give a longer, more effective analgesia with less motor blockade. This allows careful mobilisation of the woman and she can be more active in the 2nd stage of labour.
- Pudendal block results in analgesia of the lower vagina and perineum and is suitable for use in forceps or breech deliveries. Perineal infiltration is used for either performance of an episiotomy or suturing. Precautions are taken to avoid the inadvertent intravascular injection of the drug.
- Some women do not wish to use pharmacological methods of pain relief or epidural analgesia. Midwives keen to use alternative techniques should ensure that they are trained and that the therapy has no hidden dangers for the mother. Methods used in labour include massage, acupuncture, hypnosis, aromatherapy, reflexology and biofeedback.

References

Allan D, Nie V, Hunter M. 1996 Control and co-ordination. In Hinchliff SM, Montague SE, Watson R (eds) Physiology for Nursing Practice, 2nd edn. Baillière Tindall, London.

Barrett JHW 1982 Prenatal influences on adaptation in the newborn. In Stratton P (ed) Psychobiology of the Human Newborn, John Wiley and Sons Ltd, New York, pp 267–295.

Bevis R. 1996 Pain relief and comfort in labour. In Bennett VR, Brown LK (eds) Myles Textbook for Midwives, 12th edn. Churchill Livingstone, Edinburgh, pp 184–198.

Blackburn ST, Loper DL. 1992 Maternal, Fetal and Neonatal Physiology, A Clinical Perspective. WB Saunders, Philadelphia.

Budd IS. 1992 Traditional Chinese medicine in obstetrics. Midwives' Chronicle, 105, 140–143.

Burns E, Blamey C. 1994 Using aromatherapy in childbirth. Nursing Times 9(9), 54–60.

Carlson NR 1991 Physiology of Behaviour. Allyn and Bacon, Boston, Massachusetts.

Feder E, Liisberg GB, Lenstrup C et al. 1993 Zone therapy in relation to birth. In Midwives: Hear the Beat of the Future. Proceedings of the 23rd International Congress of Midwives. International Confederation of Midwives, London, pp 651–656.

Fitzgerald MJT 1992 Neuroanatomy: Basic and Clinical, Bailliere Tindall, London.

Hayward J 1975 Information, a Prescription Against Pain, Royal College of Nursing, London.

Heywood AM, Ho E. 1990 Pain relief in labour. In Alexander J, Levy V, Roch S (eds) Intrapartum Care: A Research-based Approach. Macmillan, Basingstoke.

Hinchliff SM, Montague SE, Watson R. 1996 Physiology for Nursing Practice. Baillière Tindall, London.

Hughes J, Smith TW, Kosterlitz HW, Fothergill LA, Morgan BA, Morris HR. 1975 Identification of two related pentapeptides from the brain with opiate agonist activity. Nature 258, 577.

Jenkins MW, Pritchard M. 1993 Practical applications and theoretical considerations of hypnosis in normal labour. British Journal of Obstetrics and Gynaecology 100, 221–226.

Marieb EN. 1992 Human Anatomy and Physiology, 2nd edn. Benjamin/Cummings Publishing, California.

McCaffery M. 1980 Understanding your patient's pain. Nursing 80(10), 26–31.

Melzack R, Wall P. 1988 The Challenge of Pain. Penguin, Harmondsworth.

Rang HP, Dale MM. 1991 Pharmacology. Churchill Livingstone, Edinburgh.

Simkin P. 1989 Non-pharmacological methods of pain relief during labour. In Chalmers I, Enkin M, Kierse MJNC (eds) Effective Care in Pregnancy and Childbirth, Vol. 2. Oxford University Press, Oxford, pp 893–912.

Sternbach RA, Tursky B. 1965 Ethnic differences among housewives in psychophysical and skin potential responses to electric shock. Psychophysiology 1, 241.

Sweet B. 1997 Mayes' Midwifery. Baillière Tindall, London.

Telfer FM. 1997 Relief of pain in labour. In Sweet BR with Tiran D (eds) Mayes Midwifery, 12th edn. Baillière Tindall, London, pp 418–433.

Tiran D. 1997 Complementary therapies and childbearing. In Sweet BS with Tiran D (eds) Mayes Midwifery, 12th edn. Baillière Tindall, London, pp 268–284.

Walding MF. 1991 Pain, anxiety and powerlessness. Journal of Advanced Nursing 16, 338–397.
Wall PD. 1985 The discovery of transcutaneous nerve stimulation. Physiotherapy 7(8), 348–350.
Wild L, Coyne C. 1992 The basics and beyond: epidural analgesia. American Journal of Nursing, 26–30.

Recommended reading

Burns E, Blamey C. 1994 Using aromatherapy in childbirth. Nursing Times 9 (9), 54–60.
Budd IS. 1992 Traditional Chinese medicine in obstetrics. Midwives' Chronicle 105, 140–143.
Jenkins MW, Pritchard M. 1993 Practical applications and theoretical considerations of hypnosis in normal labour. British Journal of Obstetrics and Gynaecology 100, 221–226.
Melzack R, Wall P. 1988 The Challenge of Pain. Penguin, Harmondsworth.
Simkin P. 1989 Non-pharmacological methods of pain relief during labour. In Chalmers I, Enkin M, Kierse MJNC (eds) Effective Care in Pregnancy and Childbirth, Vol. 2. Oxford University Press, Oxford, pp 893–912.
Walding MF. 1991 Pain, anxiety and powerlessness. Journal of Advanced Nursing 16, 338–397.
Wall PD. 1985 The discovery of transcutaneous nerve stimulation. Physiotherapy 7(8), 348–350.
Wild L, Coyne C. 1992 The basics and beyond: epidural analgesia. American Journal of Nursing, 26–30.

Chapter

39 The second stage of labour

In this chapter

INTRODUCTION

Sleep (1996) comments that the duration of the 2nd stage is difficult to predict and in multigravidae may last for as little as 5 min whereas in primigravidae the process may take up to 2 h. However we analyse, divide and measure the 2nd stage of labour much physical effort is usually provided by the mother over a comparatively short period. The physiological changes are a continuation of the forces present in the first stage of labour but there is now no impediment to descent of the fetus through the birth canal.

The 2nd stage of labour begins when the cervix is fully dilated (Fig. 39.1) and ends when the fetus is fully expelled from the birth canal. This definition has been used by both midwives and their medical colleagues to manage the delivery of the baby according to a time regime. There have been challenges to the concept that the exact timing of the 2nd stage is possible and progress rather than an estimated time limit is probably more useful as an indicator of normality.

PHYSIOLOGY

Contractions

There is often a brief lull in uterine activity at the end of the first stage (the **latent phase**) before the contractions take on their expulsive nature. The character of the contractions changes from that of the first stage (Morrin 1997). They become longer and stronger but may be less frequent so that the woman and her baby can recover between each expulsive effort. There is continued contraction and retraction of the UUS. The fetus descends the birth canal and fetal axis pressure increases flexion and reduces the size of the presenting part.

The secondary powers

As pressure is exerted on the rectum and pelvic floor, a reflex occurs which the woman feels as a compelling urge to push (the **active phase**). Normal bearing down efforts made by women if left to their own devices occur for about 5–6 s several times during the contraction. Compaction of the fetus occurs during the contraction and pressure on the fetal head may evoke vagal stimuli, causing a transient fall in fetal heart rate with a rapid recovery. Reduction in oxygen supply due to compression of the placenta will add to this effect. Recent studies suggest that spontaneous pushing will prolong the 2nd stage but cause fewer fetal heart rate changes, higher arterial pH and less damage to the birth canal.

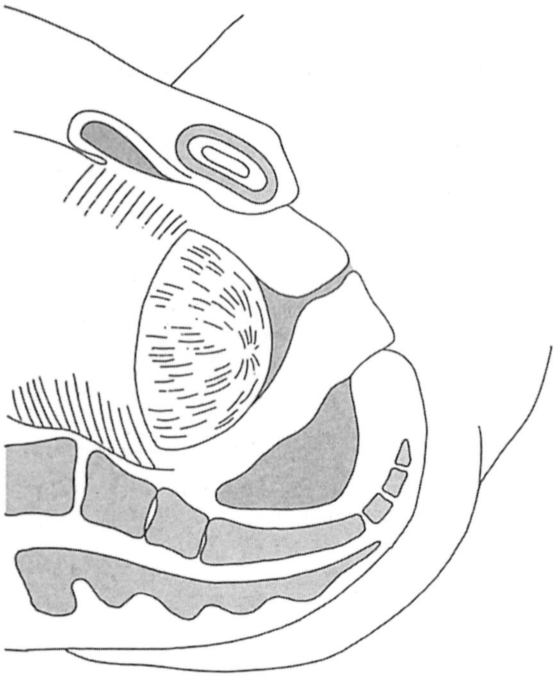

Figure 39.1 *The os uteri is fully dilated and the head enters the vagina (from Sweet B, 1997, with permission).*

Descent of the fetus

As the fetus descends it displaces the soft tissues contained in the pelvis. Anteriorly the bladder is pushed up into the abdominal cavity which results in stretching and thinning of the urethra. Posteriorly the rectum becomes flattened in the sacral curve and any faecal matter will be expelled. The levator ani muscles of the pelvic floor thin out and are displaced laterally. The perineal body is stretched and thinned.

The fetal head now becomes visible at the vulva and advances with each contraction to recede slightly between contractions until crowning of the head occurs (the **perineal phase**). The head is born first and the shoulders and body of the baby emerge with the next contraction, accompanied by a gush of amniotic fluid. The 2nd stage culminates as soon as the baby is completely born.

Onset

There is often no clear demarcation between the end of the first stage and the beginning of the 2nd. Several signs can be taken as indicative that the 2nd stage has begun but the midwife ought to have no difficulty in making the diagnosis. Sleep (1996) outlines the **presumptive signs** of the onset of the 2nd stage and differential diagnoses (Table 39.1). The appearance of several of the signs together may indicate that the 2nd stage has begun but if no progress can be seen after a few contractions, it is sometimes necessary to confirm the absence of cervix by vaginal examination.

Duration

Sleep (1996) comments that the duration of the 2nd stage is difficult to predict and in multigravidae may last for as little as 5 min whereas in primigravidae the process may take up to 2 h. Sleep et al (1989) concluded that there was no good evidence to impose a time limit for this stage of labour and it is more relevant to base decisions on evidence of progress with adequate uterine contractions and continuing good condition of mother and baby. Two phases of the 2nd stage can be described, as in the first stage: the **latent** and **active** phases.

The latent phase begins at full dilatation of the cervix but the presenting part may not yet be visible at the pelvic outlet and the woman may not have an urge to bear down. As the fetal head descends due to the force of uterine contractions and stretches the tissues of the vagina and pelvic floor, it will become visible at the vaginal orifice. Once the fetal head is visible pressure on the rectum will normally provide the reflex stimulus for maternal expulsive pushing and the active phase begins. Women are often encouraged to take a big breath and push as long and as hard as they can (the Valsalva manoeuvre). This manoeuvre causes the blood pressure to drop and rise again and women using the technique have shown alterations in heart rate and brain wave patterns. Inch (1989) implicates forced pushing as the cause of burst capillaries in the face and eyes and, rarely, cerebrovascular accidents (strokes) may occur.

Table 39.1 *The presumptive signs of the 2nd stage of labour*

Presumptive sign	*Differential diagnosis*
Expulsive uterine contractions	There may be an urge to push before full cervical dilatation if the rectum is full, the head is in the occipitoposterior posterior position or the woman is highly parous
Rupture of the forewaters	This may occur at any time in labour
Dilatation and gaping of the anus	Deep engagement of the presenting part and premature maternal pushing may cause this
Appearance of the presenting part	Excessive moulding and caput succedaneum formation may protrude through the cervix prior to full dilatation, as may a breech presentation
Show	This must be distinguished from bleeding due to premature separation of the placenta
Congestion of the vulva	Pushing before full dilatation of the cervix may produce this

MECHANISMS OF LABOUR

The fetus is in effect a cylinder which has to negotiate the curved birth canal formed of the bony pelvis and soft tissues of the flattened and distended perineal body. There are two problems with being human and giving birth. One is the curve of the birth canal, generated by the upright posture and walking on two legs (bipedalism), and the other is the large size of the baby's head due to the size of the human brain. Even so, the brain is only one-quarter of the size it will grow to in the adult. Moulding of the skull in order to reduce the presenting diameters is described elsewhere and this section will concern itself with the passive movements that the fetus makes in response to the forces exerted on it by the birth canal.

Collectively, these movements are called the mechanism of labour and the fetus is turned slightly to take advantage of the widest part of each plane of the pelvis. The reader will remember that the plane of the inlet is widest in the transverse diameter whilst the outlet is widest in the anteroposterior diameter. Knowledge of mechanisms enables the midwife to facilitate birth with the least trauma to mother and fetus. Therefore it is important to take a fetal doll and pelvis and practise these mechanisms until they can be visualised in relation to the unseen movements during the birth of the baby. It is helpful to silently run through these when observing deliveries. It may be life saving to understand what is occurring inside the woman's body so that external manoeuvres can be used to complete delivery.

Different mechanisms occur depending on the presentation and position of the fetus and there are principles common to all.

- Descent of the fetus takes place.
- The part of the fetus that leads and meets the resistance of the pelvic floor will rotate forwards to lie anteriorly under the symphysis pubis.
- Whatever part of the fetus emerges will pivot around the pubic bone.

Mechanism of a normal labour

There is a classic way of recalling the situation of a fetus at the commencement of the 2nd stage. The terms are described in Chapter 37. The following is for a normal labour.

- The **lie** is longitudinal.
- The **presentation** is cephalic.
- The **position** is right or left occipitoanterior.
- The **attitude** is one of good flexion.
- The **denominator** is the occiput.
- The **presenting part** is the posterior part of the anterior parietal bone.

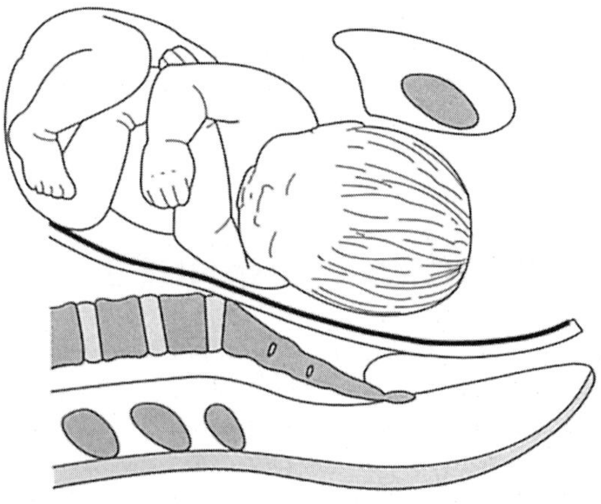

Figure 39.2 *Descent of a well-flexed head into the pelvis. The sagittal suture is in the transverse diameter of the pelvis (from Sweet B, 1997, with permission).*

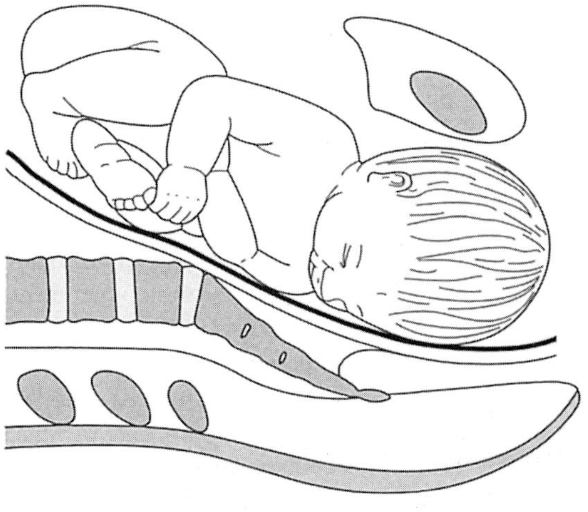

Figure 39.3 *Internal rotation occurs. The sagittal suture is in the oblique diameter of the pelvis (from Sweet B, 1997, with permission).*

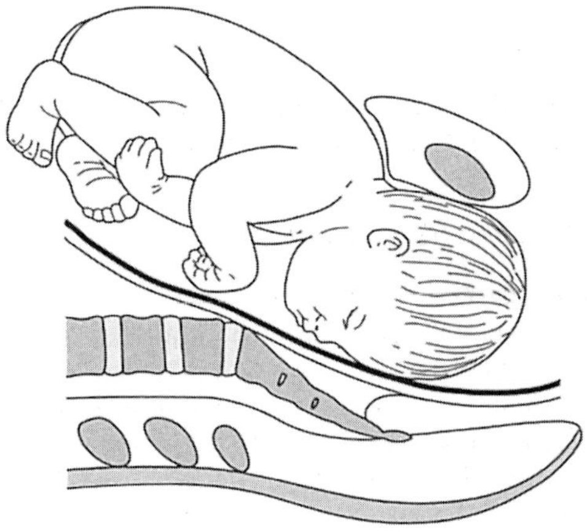

Figure 39.4 *Internal rotation complete – further descent occurs. The sagittal suture is now in the anteroposterior diameter of the pelvis (from Sweet B, 1997, with permission).*

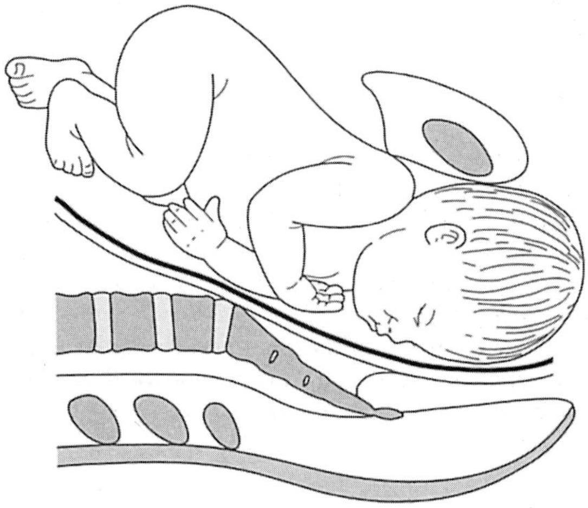

Figure 39.5 *The head descended to the vulval outlet (from Sweet B, 1997, with permission).*

The movements

Descent

Descent of the fetal head into the pelvis may have occurred in the antenatal period so that the woman, especially a primigravida, begins labour with the head engaged. This usually indicates that vaginal delivery is likely. There is continued descent during the first stage of labour and this is speeded by maternal effort during the 2nd stage.

Flexion

Flexion of the fetal head on the trunk is increased during labour because the skull is attached to the fetal spine nearer to the occiput than the sinciput. Pressure transmitted from the uterine fundus down the fetal spine will force the occiput lower than the sinciput, increasing flexion and resulting in the conversion of the suboccipitofrontal diameter of 10 cm to the favourable suboccipitobregmatic diameter of 9.5 cm.

Internal rotation of the head

As the leading part is driven onto the pelvic floor, the resistance of the muscular diaphragm and its gutter shape, sloping downwards anteriorly, cause the occiput to rotate forwards in the pelvis by one-eighth of a circle to lie under the symphysis pubis. The anteroposterior diameter of the head now lies in the anteroposterior diameter of the pelvis. This causes a slight twist on the neck of the fetus so that the head is no longer aligned with the shoulders.

Extension of the head

The occiput escapes from beneath the subpubic arch and the smallest possible diameters, which are the suboccipitobregmatic diameter of 9.5 cm and the biparietal diameter of 9.5 cm, distend the vaginal orifice. The head is now born by extension as it pivots on the suboccipital region around the pubic bone. The sinciput, face and chin sweep the perineum. The widest diameter to distend the vagina is the suboccipitofrontal as the sinciput is born.

Restitution

Restitution is a movement made by the head following delivery which brings it into correct alignment with the shoulders. This will be one-eighth of a circle towards the side of the occiput.

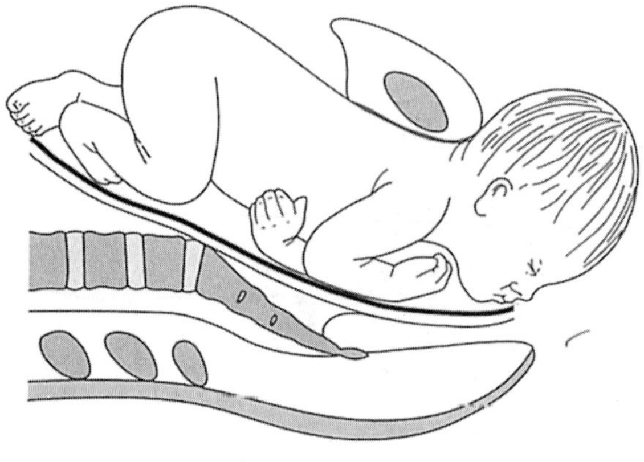

Figure 39.6 *The head is crowned (from Sweet B, 1997, with permission).*

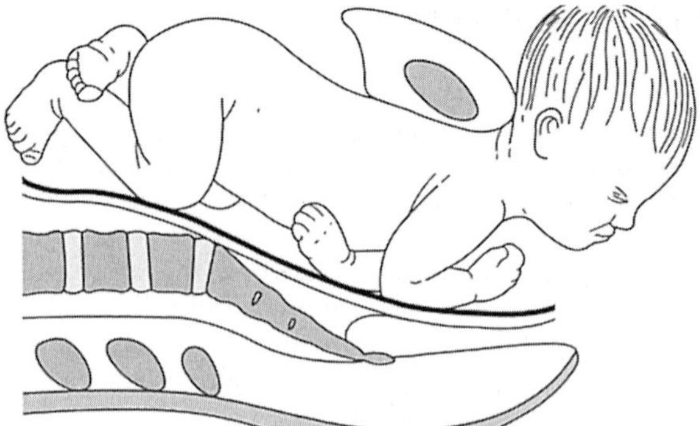

Figure 39.7 *The face is delivered (from Sweet B, 1997, with permission).*

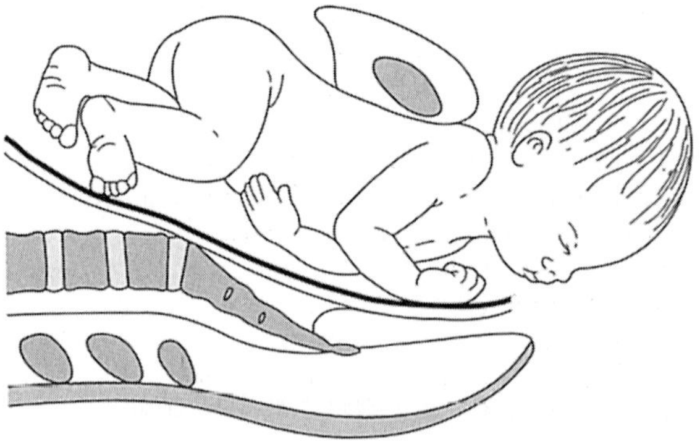

Figure 39.8 *Restitution has taken place and internal rotation of the shoulders occurs (from Sweet B, 1997, with permission).*

Internal rotation of the shoulders

The anterior shoulder is the first to reach the pelvic floor and this now rotates forwards to lie under the symphysis pubis. This movement is accompanied by external rotation of the head by one-eighth of a circle more in the direction of restitution. The occiput now lies laterally turned towards the woman's thigh.

Lateral flexion

The anterior shoulder is usually born first and slips under the pubic arch and the posterior shoulder passes over the perineum. The remainder of the body is born by lateral flexion as the spine bends laterally on its way through the curved birth canal.

PHYSIOLOGICAL CHANGES

Edwards (1995) outlines the physiological principles which underlie the management of the 2nd stage.

- Fetal hormone secretion aimed at adaptation to independent life
- The condition of mother and baby
- The bearing down reflex
- Thinning of the perineum
- Position of the mother

MANAGEMENT

The question must be asked about stages and phases of labour as to whether they are physiological entities or human imagination. Before describing the physiology and management of the 2nd stage, the concepts need to be examined.

The second stage of labour – two or three phases

Crawford (1983) believed that the division of labour into three stages and subdividing the stages into phases was contrary to the actual events of labour and that basing the management of labour on these concepts may lead to distress and hazard for mother and fetus. Whilst he discussed the division of the first stage of labour into the latent and active phases, he stated that the 'distinction between the first and second stages leads to the greatest trouble in clinical practice'. He believed that the difficulty occurs because there is a lack of clear definition as to when the 2nd stage begins. Some women wish to bear down before the cervix is fully dilated and sometimes a woman will not bear down until the presenting part is distending the perineum. If the woman has had epidural analgesia, she may not have an urge to bear down at all.

Aderhold & Roberts (1991) examined the concept of phases in the 2nd stage with an in depth study of four nulliparous women. They describe the above concept of two phases to the 2nd stage as follows:

> The early phase from complete dilation until the presenting part becomes visible which lasts 10 to 30 minutes and generally occurs with mild or no urge to bear down. Then the period of active bearing down … follows as the fetal scalp becomes visible, and proceeds until the birth of the baby. Pushing becomes more pronounced and there is a sudden change in the woman's demeanour.

They remind readers that some authorities have gone further and described three phases of the 2nd stage: the latent phase or lull, the descent or active phase and the perineal phase. In their small study of four nulliparous women, they found evidence to support the three phases.

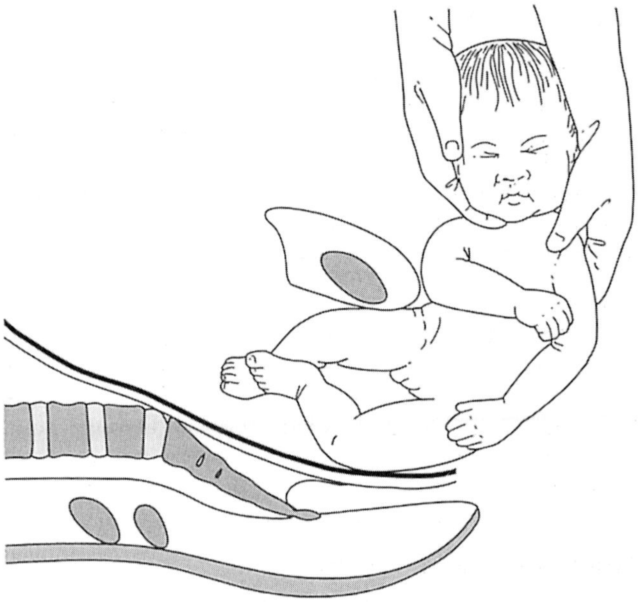

Figure 39.10 *The posterior shoulder is delivered and then the trunk by lateral flexion (from Sweet B, 1997, with permission).*

These researchers suggest that if further research verifies the phases of the 2nd stage, midwives and other obstetric care providers will be able to use this deeper understanding to inform their management. In particular, they agree with Crawford that forced expulsive efforts before the woman is ready could impose hypoxic stress on the fetus and maternal exhaustion could occur.

The length of the second stage

Normal bearing down efforts made by women if left to their own devices occur for about 5–6 s several times during the contraction (Caldeyro-Barcia 1979). Saunders et al (1992) investigated both neonatal and maternal morbidity in relation to the length of the 2nd stage. They found no relation between the length of the 2nd stage and the frequency of low Apgar scores

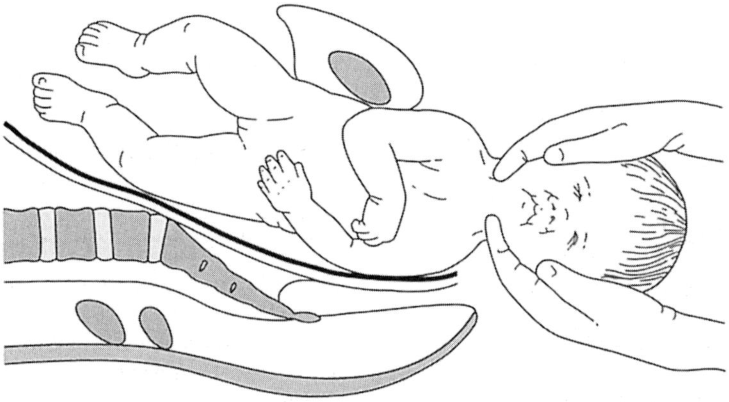

Figure 39.9 *Gentle downward traction is applied to deliver the anterior shoulder (from Sweet B, 1997, with permission).*

or of admissions to a SCBU. They concluded that current management allowing spontaneous pushing, even in 2nd stages lasting up to 3 h, did not carry any undue fetal risk. Recent studies suggest that spontaneous pushing will prolong the 2nd stage but cause fewer fetal heart rate changes, higher arterial pH and less damage to the birth canal.

If the three factors discussed above are considered together and applied to clinical practice, it appears that the best way to manage the 2nd stage is to allow the woman to push as and when she wishes as long as maternal and fetal condition remain good and progress is occurring. However, Chamberlain & Drife (1995) stated that whilst there may be indications to change practice, further research must be carried out, especially following up the infants into childhood.

Chamberlain & Drife (1995) summarised the previous decade of thinking thus:

> ... ideas about the length of the second stage of labour have swung from a regimented time table to a go-as-you-please regime according to the attitudes of the mother, the midwife and possibly the fetus.

They add that the division between the first and second stages cannot be timed and go on to outline a possible history of why clinicians have been so keen to establish full dilatation of the cervix, concluding it is because that is the point at which vaginal delivery can be accomplished by the use of obstetrical forceps. They finally state that no rules can be laid down about the length of the 2nd stage but that research should be continued into the effects on the fetus and long-term effects on the child.

The definition at the beginning of this chapter stated that the 2nd stage begins with full cervical dilatation but how can this exact moment be recognised? The author remembers a woman in preterm labour at 32 weeks who was receiving drugs to attempt to stop the labour. She was examined by the obstetric registrar at 09.00 hours one morning. In the absence of recognisable contractions, the cervix was found to be fully dilated. There was no fetal distress and no urge to bear down and the baby was delivered safely. Nobody could tell when the 2nd stage of labour had begun.

Medical control

Crawford stated that clinicians believe they know when the 2nd stage of labour begins and that they have an 'entrenched opinion' about how long it should last. The problem is that the woman is then asked to bear down once full cervical dilatation is established, regardless of whether she feels she wants to, creating a situation with developing maternal exhaustion, metabolic acidosis and ending in an instrumental delivery. This may result in birth trauma to the woman or her baby. He believed that the woman should not be urged to bear down until she wished to or until the presenting part was distending the perineum and that if there was no maternal or fetal distress there was no need for instrumental delivery. These views were supported by Westcott (1984), who summarised Crawford's views in an article looking at the wider issue of medical control of labour intended to be read by pregnant women.

In an attempt to clarify definitions, she suggested that the first part of the 2nd stage begins at full cervical dilatation and ends when the mother voluntarily bears down. She found that there were two distinguishable parts and that the 2nd part was more likely to lead to fetal acidosis and birth asphyxia than the first. In her last paragraph, she suggests that the first part of the 2nd stage should 'really be considered as the end of the first stage of labour'. Once again, the distinction between the end of the first stage and beginning of the 2nd is ill defined.

Midwifery thinking

Thomson (1988) reviewed the management of women in the 2nd stage of normal labour. She described with feeling and accuracy the control exerted over the labouring woman including position, forced expulsive efforts and the concentration on the vulva. She concluded that the available literature on managing the 2nd stage 'suggested an inter-relationship between three factors:

1 the position of the woman;
2 the means by which the woman exerts pressure to assist the uterus to expel the baby;
3 the length of the second stage of labour.'

These three factors will be used as a plan for discussing the physiological management of labour.

POSITION OF THE WOMAN

In most other cultures in the world and in Europe until the 18th century, women used a variety of positions during the 2nd stage of labour. Russell (1982) commented that whatever the position used for delivery, women have tended to deliver with abducted thighs in an upright position. In most cases women adopt upright positions so that the 3rd lumbar vertebra is above the 5th (Thomson 1988). Upright positions include standing, kneeling, sitting on birthing chairs and squatting. The lying down dorsal position may have originated in France because of Louis XIV's wish to witness the delivery of his mistress's baby but has been perpetuated for the ease of the medical profession. In Britain the left lateral position may have originated as the 'London position' advocated by Smellie in 1752 (Thomson 1988).

Although the recumbent position has been the most common position for delivery until the last two decades, it is known that it leads to supine hypotension which may adversely affect fetal oxygenation (Watson 1994). If the mother lies on her back there will be a significant reduction in maternal cardiac output and circulation of oxygenated blood through the placental tissue due to compression of the inferior vena cava and descending aorta (Banks 1992). This does not happen if the woman lies on her side or if the uterus is tilted to the left. The upright posture has at least four beneficial effects on the progress of the 2nd stage.

1 It allows gravity to play its part in the descent of the fetus.
2 It increases the pelvic outlet diameters by up to 1 cm in the transverse diameter and 2 cm in the anteroposterior diameter in the squatting position, producing a 28% increase in the area of outlet over women delivered in the supine position (Russell 1969).

3 It increases the efficiency of uterine contractions.
4 It reduces the incidence of fetal distress and neonatal asphyxia.

Morrin (1997) summarises findings on some of the alternative positions.

Squatting

Squatting is probably the most common position for childbirth in the developing world. The mother may need the support of two people or she may support herself with her back to a wall or firm surface. The flexion and abduction of the thighs brought about by squatting have a number of advantages.

- The thighs support the abdominal muscles and the weight of the uterus.
- Gravity can tilt the uterus forwards so that the longitudinal axis of the birth canal is straightened.
- Expulsive efforts are maximised.
- Pelvic diameters are increased.

Birthing chairs

Electronically controlled birthing chairs appeared to be an alternative for supporting women in the squatting position, giving the midwife good vision and access to the fetus. However, there have been problems associated with their use. There appears to be a higher mean blood loss and an increase in postpartum haemorrhage in multigravidae. This finding may be due to the increased accuracy in measuring blood loss or there may be more actual blood loss from perineal trauma caused by obstructed venous return because of pressure on the buttocks and perineum. This pressure may also be responsible for the increase in perineal oedema and haemorrhoids in women delivered in the upright position in birthing chairs.

Hands and knees/all-fours positions

This position appears to give relief to women suffering from backache. It allows an excellent view of the fetus and perineum and it aids rotation and descent and causes less perineal trauma. There may be an increase in vulval trauma.

MATERNAL EFFORT

We may then accept that the 2nd stage of labour begins with full dilatation of the cervix but the presenting part may not yet be visible at the pelvic outlet and the woman may not have an urge to bear down. As the fetal head descends due to the force of uterine contractions and stretches the tissues of the vagina and pelvic floor, it will become visible at the vaginal orifice. Once the fetal head is visible, pressure on the rectum will normally provide the reflex stimulus for maternal expulsive pushing and the active phase begins.

Watson (1994) wrote that it is 'customary practice for birth attendants to give women formal instructions during the second stage of labour'. The rationale for this has been to reduce the length of the 2nd stage and prevent too much stress for the fetus.

Effect on pelvic soft tissues

There are two ways of interpreting early pushing in the 2nd stage of labour: pushing in the early part of each contraction, as discussed above, and pushing in the latent phase. A paper by Beynon (1957) explains the effect that forceful pushing from the commencement of each contraction has on the soft tissues of the pelvic floor. Beynon theorised that in the early part of a contraction the vaginal muscles are drawn taut to prevent the bladder supports and transverse cervical ligaments being pushed down in front of the baby's head. Early expulsive effort may lead to incontinence and prolapsed uterus later in life. Sleep (1996) writes that active pushing during the latent phase of the 2nd stage may strain the uterine supports and the vaginal and perineal muscle before these tissues have a chance to stretch gradually.

Perineal lacerations

During the 2nd stage of labour, perineal lacerations may occur. In order to control the extent of these lacerations, an **episiotomy** may be performed. Depending on the depth of tissue involved in the tear, perineal lacerations can be classified as follows.

- A **first-degree tear** involves just the skin of the fourchette.
- A **2nd-degree tear** involves the skin of the fourchette, the perineum and perineal body. The muscles of the perineal body involved are the superficial muscles – the bulbocavernosus and transverse perinei – and the deep muscle – the pubococcygeus.
- A **3rd-degree tear** involves all the above tissues and the anal sphincter.
- Sweet (1997) includes a **4th-degree tear** which includes the anal sphincter and extends into the rectal mucosa.

An episiotomy includes the same structures as a 2nd-degree tear.

Other tissues may be lacerated during delivery. **Labial** lacerations are not usually severe enough to require suturing but can be very painful, especially during micturition. **Vaginal** and **cervical** lacerations may bleed severely and need immediate pressure to control bleeding followed by suturing.

The episiotomy

An episiotomy is a deliberate incision through the structures involved in a 2nd degree tear. The rationale for the incision is to enlarge the vulval outlet immediately before delivery. A midwife in the United Kingdom is allowed to infiltrate the perineum with local anaesthetic and to perform an episiotomy if thought necessary. Sweet (1997) records the historical use of the episiotomy. Studies by Sleep (1984) and Begley (1986, 1987) led to a reduction from a high of 50% in the 1970s and early 1980s to a more sensible and considered 20–30%. Sleep (1984a, b) demonstrated that the usual reason given for performing an episiotomy, to prevent perineal trauma, has no validity. There was no reduction in trauma to the pelvic floor nor did women suffer less pain or swelling; indeed, many women feel more pain following an episiotomy. The perineal wound, whether tear or episiotomy, healed in a similar manner.

Indications for performing an episiotomy

During the antenatal period women should be given a chance to discuss the possible needs for the midwife to make an episiotomy to avoid confrontation situations in an emergency. It is unlikely that a woman will refuse if she is able to make an informed choice based on knowledge acquired calmly. Her wishes should be recorded on her birth plan.

The indications can be divided into fetal and maternal and include the following (Sweet 1997).

- To expedite delivery if the fetal head is on the perineum and there is evidence of fetal distress.
- If the fetus is preterm or is presenting by the breech, to reduce the risk of intracranial trauma.
- To minimise the effort of delivery when a woman is hypertensive or has cardiac disease or shows signs of distress.
- To prevent trauma when women have had previous surgery to the pelvic floor.
- If there is serious delay in the 2nd stage thought to be due to the nature of the perineal tissues (often called a **rigid perineum**).

The incision

There are two types of incision: the **mediolateral** and the **midline**. The mediolateral is most commonly used because it avoids damage to Bartholin's gland and is unlikely to extend in the midline to involve the anal sphincter (Fig. 39.11).

The perineum is infiltrated along the line of the intended episiotomy using 10 ml of lignocaine solution 0.5% or 5 ml of lignocaine 1%. The practitioner should check carefully to avoid giving the injection intravenously because of the risk of causing bradycardia or collapse. The anaesthetic takes effect in about 4 min and the incision can then be made using episiotomy scissors. The incision is best made during a contraction when the perineum is thinned out and should be at least 4 cm long. During the administration of the local anaesthetic and the making of the episiotomy the fetal head should be protected by inserting two fingers between it and the perineum (Figs 39.12 and 39.13).

Suturing the perineum

Midwives are allowed to suture the perineum if they have been taught the procedure and pronounced proficient. This includes being able to recognise situations where it is not appropriate for the midwife to suture; for instance, if a 3rd-degree tear has unfortunately been sustained. The advantage to the woman is that the suturing is carried out immediately and she doesn't have to wait until a doctor is available. The midwife should comply with the local policies for the use of suture materials, hopefully based on up-to-date research. Aseptic technique is universal. The most important point is to explore the depth of the wound and ensure that the first suture is placed above its apex to prevent the development of a vaginal haematoma. The perineum is then sutured in layers from the inside tissues outwards. Absorbable sutures are preferred for the skin.

THE FETUS

It is traditional to view the 2nd stage of labour as the most dangerous stage for the fetus with an increased risk of asphyxia and trauma. This has led to attempts to deliver the baby as quickly as possible. Although the Valsalva manoeuvre will significantly shorten the 2nd stage of labour, studies have indicated that sustained breath holding leads to abnormalities in the fetal heart (Caldeyro-Barcia 1979) and adversely affects fetal condition and neonatal outcome (Barnett & Humenick 1982, Bassell et al 1980, Paine & Tinker 1992). Compaction of the fetus occurs during the contraction and pressure on the fetal head may evoke vagal stimuli, causing a transient fall in fetal heart rate with a rapid recovery.

Reduction in oxygen supply due to compression of the placenta will add to this effect. This may cause prolongation of

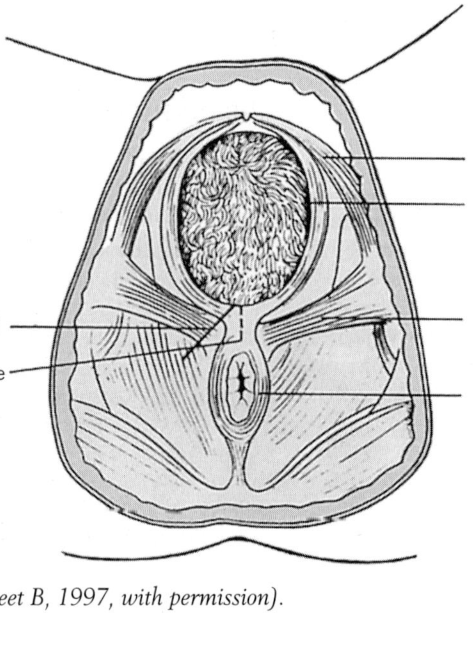

Figure 39.11 *Episiotomy (from Sweet B, 1997, with permission).*

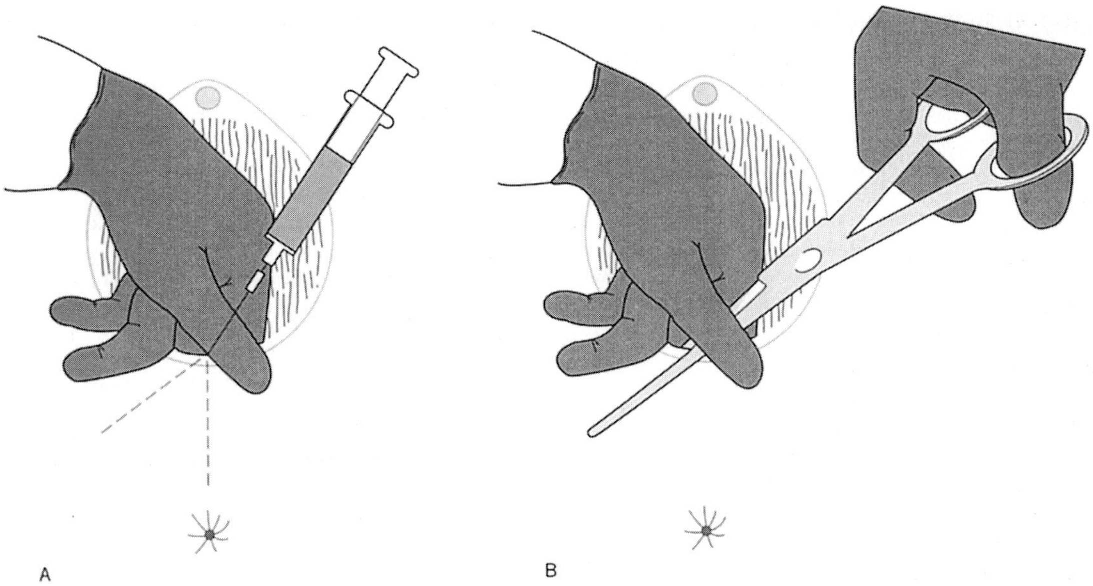

Figure 39.12 *(a) Infiltration of the perineum. (b) Making a mediolateral incision (from Sweet B, 1997, with permission).*

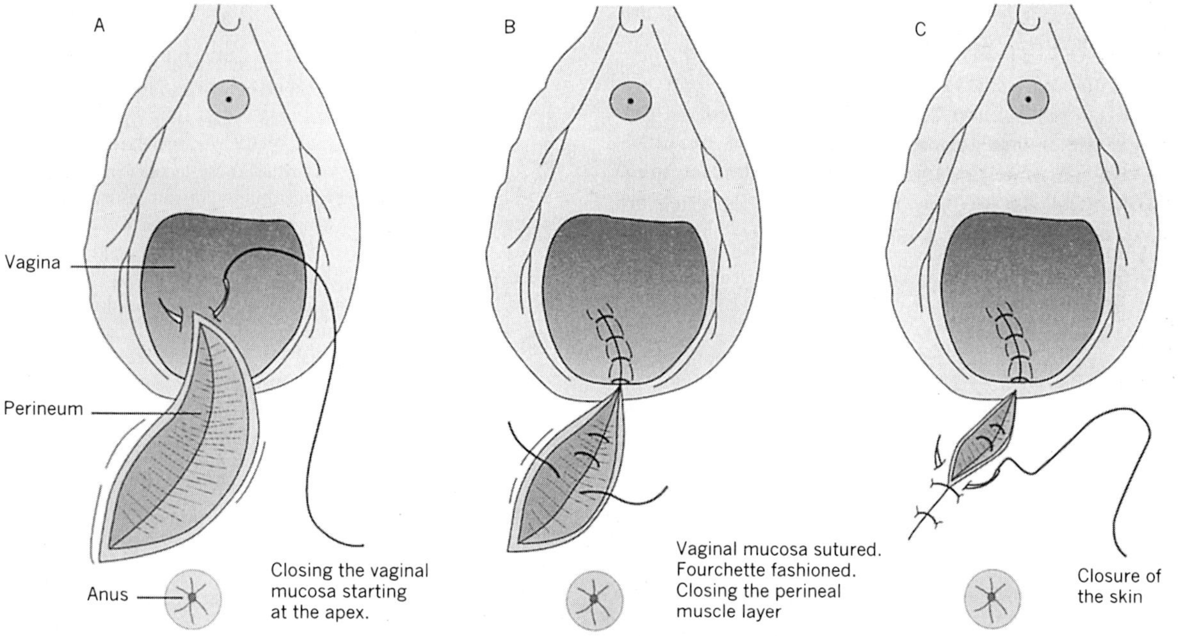

Figure 39.13 *Suturing the perineum. (a) Closing the vaginal mucosa, starting at the apex. (b) Vaginal mucosa sutured, fourchette fashioned, closing the perineal muscle layer. (c) Closure of the skin (from Sweet B, 1997, with permission).*

the normal fall in fetal heart rate seen after contractions in the 2nd stage. Also, if the mother lies on her back there will be a significant reduction in cardiac output and circulation of oxygenated blood through the placental tissue due to compression of the inferior vena cava and descending aorta (Banks 1992). This does not happen if the woman lies on her side or of the uterus is tilted to the left.

Piquard et al (1988) examined the validity of fetal heart rate monitoring in the 2nd stage of labour and whether a time limit should be placed on the 2nd stage to safeguard the fetus. They cited evidence that umbilical artery pH decreased significantly if the 2nd stage exceeded 45 min. In 1989 Piquard et al analysed fetal distress in relation to the concept of two biological parts to the 2nd stage of labour. They agreed with clinicians that the 2nd stage is a time of risk for the fetus with distress related not only to hypoxia but also to mechanical stress.

Summary of main points

- There is often a brief lull in uterine activity at the end of the first stage of labour before the contractions take on their expulsive nature, becoming longer and stronger but less frequent so that the woman and her baby can recover between each expulsive effort. The fetus descends the birth canal and increasing flexion reduces the size of the presenting part.
- As pressure is exerted on the rectum and pelvic floor, the woman feels a compelling urge to push. Compaction of the fetus occurs during the contraction and pressure on the fetal head, coupled with a reduced oxygen supply, may evoke vagal stimuli, causing a transient fall in fetal heart rate with a rapid recovery.
- There is often no clear demarcation between the end of the first stage and the beginning of the 2nd. Several signs can be taken as indicative that the 2nd stage has begun but the midwife ought to have no difficulty in making the diagnosis. If no progress can be seen, the absence of the cervix can be confirmed by vaginal examination.
- Different mechanisms of labour occur depending on the presentation and position of the fetus and there are principles common to all: descent of the fetus, the part of the fetus that leads and meets the resistance of the pelvic floor will rotate forwards to lie anteriorly under the symphysis pubis, and the part of the fetus that emerges will pivot around the pubic bone.
- The 2nd stage of labour is said to begin with full dilatation of the cervix and ends when the fetus is fully expelled from the birth canal. There have been challenges to the concept that the exact timing of the 2nd stage is possible and it is probable that progress rather than an estimated time limit is more useful as an indicator of normality.
- The duration of the 2nd stage in multigravidae may last for as little as 5 min whereas in primigravidae the process may take up to 2 h. Two phases of the 2nd stage of labour can be described: latent and active. The latent phase begins at full dilatation of the cervix but the woman may not have an urge to bear down. Pressure on the rectum normally provides the stimulus for maternal expulsive pushing and the active phase begins. Some authorities describe three phases: the latent phase or lull, the descent or active phase, and the perineal phase.
- The division of labour into three stages and subdividing the stages into phases may be contrary to the actual events of labour and basing the management of labour on these concepts may lead to distress and hazard for mother and fetus. If the woman is asked to bear down once full cervical dilatation is established, she may develop maternal exhaustion, metabolic acidosis and end with an instrumental delivery and birth trauma to herself or her baby.
- In most other cultures in the world women use a variety of positions during the 2nd stage of labour. In most cases women adopt upright positions so that the 3rd lumbar vertebra is above the 5th lumbar vertebra.
- The upright posture allows gravity to aid descent of the fetus, increases uterine contraction efficiency and reduces the incidence of fetal distress and neonatal asphyxia. The squatting position increases the diameters of the pelvic outlet by up to 1 cm in the transverse diameter and 2 cm in the anteroposterior.
- Squatting is probably the most common position for childbirth in the developing world. It has a number of advantages: the thighs support the abdominal muscles and the weight of the uterus, gravity can tilt the uterus forwards so that the longitudinal axis of the birth canal is straightened, expulsive efforts are maximised and pelvic diameters are increased. The hands and knees position appears to relieve backache, aids rotation and descent and causes less perineal trauma.
- Women are often encouraged to take a big breath at the start of each contraction and bear down as long and as hard as they can. This Valsalva manoeuvre causes the blood pressure to drop and rise again and women using the technique have shown alterations in heart rate and brain wave patterns. Forced pushing may cause burst capillaries in the face and eyes and, rarely, cerebrovascular accidents have occurred. Early expulsive effort may lead to incontinence and prolapsed uterus later in life. Although the Valsalva manoeuvre will significantly shorten the 2nd stage of labour, studies have indicated that it may lead to fetal heart abnormalities and adversely affects fetal condition and neonatal outcome.
- Compaction of the fetus occurs during the contraction and pressure on the fetal head may evoke vagal stimuli, causing a transient fall in fetal heart rate with a rapid recovery. Reduction in oxygen supply due to compression of the placenta will add to this effect. This may cause a prolonged fall in fetal heart rate after contractions in the 2nd stage of labour.
- During the 2nd stage of labour perineal lacerations may occur. In order to control the extent of these lacerations, an episiotomy may be performed. Labial lacerations are not usually severe enough to require suturing but can be painful during micturition. Vaginal and cervical lacerations may bleed severely and need immediate pressure to control bleeding followed by suturing.
- The rationale for the incision of an episiotomy is to enlarge the vulval outlet immediately before delivery. Indications for episiotomy may be fetal or maternal but it should rarely be performed just to prevent a tear occurring. During the antenatal period women should be given a chance to discuss the possible needs for an episiotomy to avoid confrontation situations in an emergency. It is unlikely that women will refuse if they can make an informed choice based on knowledge.
- Midwives may suture the perineum if they have been taught the procedure and pronounced proficient. It is most important to explore the depth of the wound and ensure that the first suture is placed above its apex to prevent the development of a vaginal haematoma. The perineum is then sutured in layers from the inside tissues outwards. Absorbable sutures are preferred for the skin.

References

Aderhold KJ, Roberts JE. 1991 Phases of second stage labor: four descriptive case studies. Journal of Nurse-Midwifery 36(5), 267–275.

Banks E. 1992 Labouring in comfort. Nursing Times 88(31), 40–41.

Barnett MM, Humenick SS, 1982 Infant outcome in relation to second stage labor pushing method, Birth, 9(4) 221–228.

Bassell GM, Humayun SG, Marx GF. 1980 Maternal bearing-down efforts – another fetal risk? Obstetrics and Gynaecology 5(1), 39–47.

Begley CM. 1986 Episiotomy: use or abuse? Nursing Review 4, 4–7.

Begley CM. 1987 Episiotomy – a change in midwives' practice. Irish Nursing Forum and Health Service 5(6), 12–14.

Beynon C. 1957 The normal second stage of labour. Journal of Obstetrics and Gynaecology of the British Commonwealth 64(6), 815–820.

Caldeyro-Barcia R. 1979 The influence of maternal bearing-down efforts during second stage on fetal well-being. Birth Family Journal 6(1), 17–21.

Chamberlain G, Drife J. 1995 What is a prolonged second stage of labour? Contemporary Review of Obstetrics and Gynaecology 7, 69–70.

Crawford JS. 1983 The stages and phases of labour: an outworn nomenclature that invites hazard. Lancet 321, 271–272.

Edwards NP. 1995 Birthing Your baby: The Second Stage. Association for Improvements in the Maternity Services (AIMS), London.

Inch S, 1989 Birthrights, Hutchinson, London.

Morrin NA, Midwifery care in the second stage of labour. In Sweet BR with

Tiran D (eds) 1997 Mayes Midwifery. Baillière Tindall, London: 385–402.
Paine LL, Tinker DD. 1992 The effect of maternal bearing-down efforts on arterial umbilical cord pH and length of the second stage of labor. Journal of Nurse-Midwifery 37(1), 61–63.
Piquard F, Hsiung R, Schaefer A, Habery P, Dellenbach P. 1988 The validity of fetal heart rate monitoring during the second stage of labor. Obstetrics and Gynaecology 72(5), 746–751.
Piquard F, Schaefer A, Hsiung R, Dellenbach P, Habery P. 1989 Are there two biological parts in the second stage of labor? Acta Obstetrica et Gynaecologica Scandinavica 68, 713–718.
Russell JGB, 1969 Moulding of the pelvic outlet. Journal of Obstetrics and Gynaecology of the British Commonwealth, 76: 817–820.
Russell JGB 1982 The rationale of primitive delivery positions. British Journal of Obstetrics and Gynaecology, 89 (September): 712–715.
Saunders NStG, Paterson CM, Wadsworth J. 1992 Neonatal and maternal morbidity in relation to the length of the second stage of labour. British Journal of Obstetrics and Gynaecology 99, 381–385.
Sleep J. 1984a Episiotomy in normal delivery, 1. Nursing Times 80(47), 29–30.
Sleep J. 1984b Episiotomy in normal delivery, 2. The management of the perineum. Nursing Times 80(48), 51–54.
Sleep J, 1996 Physiology and management of the second stage of labour. In Bennett VR & Brown LK (eds) 1996, Myles Textbook for Midwives, Churchill Livingstone Edinburgh 199–215.
Sleep J, Roberts J, Chalmers I, 1989 Care during the second stage of labour. In Chalmers I, Enkin M Keirse M (eds), Effective Care in Pregnancy and Childbirth, Oxford University press, Oxford.
Sweet BR. 1997 The pelvic floor and its injuries. In Sweet BR with Tiran D (eds) Mayes Midwifery, 12th edn. Baillière Tindall, London, pp 444–454.
Thomson AM. 1988 Management of the woman in normal second stage of labour: a review. Midwifery 4, 77–85.
Watson V. 1994 Maternal position in the second stage of labour. Modern Midwife 4(7), 21–24.
Westcott VP. 1984 The revolution starts here. Mother and Baby, April 19–23.

Recommended reading

Bassell GM, Humayun SG, Marx GF. 1980 Maternal bearing-down efforts – another fetal risk? Obstetrics and Gynaecology 5(1), 39–47.
Chamberlain G, Drife J. 1995 What is a prolonged second stage of labour? Contemporary Review of Obstetrics and Gynaecology 7, 69–70.
Cottrell BH, Shannahan MD. 1986 Effect of the birth chair on duration of second stage labour and maternal outcome. Nursing Research 35, 364–367.
Crawford JS. 1983 The stages and phases of labour: an outworn nomenclature that invites hazard. Lancet 321, 271–272.
Piquard F, Schaefer A, Hsiung R, Dellenbach P, Habery P. 1989 Are there two biological parts in the second stage of labor? Acta Obstetrica et Gynaecologica Scandinavica 68, 713–718.
Saunders NStG, Paterson CM, Wadsworth J. 1992 Neonatal and maternal morbidity in relation to the length of the second stage of labour. British Journal of Obstetrics and Gynaecology 99, 381–385.
Turner MJ, Romney ML, Webb JB, Gordon H. 1986 The birthing chair – an obstetric hazard? Journal of Obstetrics and Gynaecology, 6: 232–235.
van Dongen PWJ, deGroot ANJA 1995 History of ergot alkaloids from ergotism to ergometrine. European Journal of Obstetrics and Gynaecology and Reproductive Biology, 60: 107–116.
Watson V. 1994 Maternal position in the second stage of labour. Modern Midwife 4(7), 21–24.
Westcott VP. 1984. The revolution starts here. Mother and Baby, April 19–23.

Chapter 40 The third stage of labour

In this chapter

INTRODUCTION

The 3rd stage of labour begins with the completion of delivery of the fetus and ends with the control of bleeding. During this period vigilance is required as there are emergencies which may arise to threaten the health and life of the mother. An understanding of the normal physiology allows choice between physiological management or active management of the 3rd stage and minimises the risk of complications by preventive treatment or rapid emergency treatment if necessary.

PHYSIOLOGY

The 3rd stage of labour begins immediately following the birth of the baby. During the 3rd stage separation and expulsion of the placenta and membranes occur and bleeding from the placental site is minimised. This stage is most hazardous for the mother because of the risk of haemorrhage and other complications to be discussed in Chapter 45. The physiological 3rd stage normally lasts from 5 to 15 min but may take up to an hour. The uterus is steadily emptied accompanied by accelerated myometrial contraction and retraction.

Separation of the placenta

Separation of the placenta usually begins with the contraction that delivers the baby's body (Fig. 40.1). The placental site begins to diminish in size and the placenta is compressed so that blood in the intervillous spaces is forced back into the spongy layer of the decidua. Retraction of the oblique muscle fibres constricts the blood vessels supplying the placenta so that the blood cannot drain into the maternal vascular tree. The uterine vessels become tense and congested and burst so that a small amount of blood collects between the spongy layer of the decidua and the maternal surface of the placenta, stripping it from its attachment.

The non-elastic placenta is detached from the uterine wall. Separation normally begins from the centre of the placenta so that no blood escapes and a retroplacental clot forms. This probably provides a 3rd means of separation of the placenta as the developing blood clot increases pressure and helps to strip the adherent lateral borders. The weight of the placenta strips the membranes off the uterine wall and the placenta descends fetal side first, enclosing the blood clot in a complete bag of membranes into the vagina and out of the body. This method was described by Schultze and generations of midwifery students have referred to this method of separation as 'shiny Schultze', referring to the glistening appearance of the fetal surface of the placenta.

There is an alternative mechanism of placental separation which begins unevenly at one of the lateral borders. Blood escapes from behind the placenta so that there is no formation of a retroplacental clot. The placenta folds in on itself with the maternal surface outwards and descends edge-on to appear maternal surface first. It is accompanied by a fluid blood loss which the inexperienced may perceive as the onset of a postpartum haemorrhage. This process takes longer and there is more risk of incomplete expulsion of the membranes, often referred to as **ragged membranes**. This process was first described by Matthews & Duncan and has been called 'dirty Duncan' as an *aide-memoire*.

Control of bleeding

Once separation is complete the uterus contracts strongly (Fig. 40.2) and the placenta and membranes fall into the lower uterine segment and then into the vagina. It is important to remember that at least 500 ml of blood/min flows through the placental site. This flow must be stopped in seconds to prevent serious haemorrhage. Four factors are involved in the process.

1 to see whether or not the placenta and membranes have been completely delivered;
2 to detect abnormalities which might provide information about any intrauterine problems. This may be of help in planning neonatal care.

- Gloves should be worn to prevent the transmission of bloodborne diseases such as hepatitis or HIV. The placenta should be held up by the cord to inspect the membranes for completeness. There should be a single hole through which the fetus was delivered.
- The amnion is stripped back from the chorion to the cord insertion to ensure that both membranes are present.
- The maternal surface of the placenta should be examined to make sure all the lobes are present. Any infarctions should be noted.
- The umbilical cord should be measured. The number of cord vessels should be ascertained. The absence of one of the umbilical arteries is sometimes associated with renal agenesis.
- The placenta is weighed and should be about one-sixth of the fetal weight if the baby was born at term.
- Blood loss is measured and added to the estimated loss present in the bed linen and pads. A blood loss of more than 500 ml is considered to be a postpartum haemorrhage and should be reported to the obstetric team.
- Cord blood should be obtained as routine practice or as requested.

The midwife should remain with the woman for at least 1 h following completion of the delivery, whether this is in the maternity unit or the mother's home. The uterus should now be palpated gently to ensure that it remains well contracted. Her temperature, pulse and blood pressure are taken and recorded. The mother's lochia is inspected and she is encouraged to pass urine. An all-over wash, clean clothing and refreshment will be appreciated. Immediate care of the baby and the role of parenting will be discussed in other chapters.

Summary of main points

- In the 3rd stage of labour separation and expulsion of the placenta and membranes occur and bleeding from the placental site is minimised. It begins immediately following the birth of the baby and normally lasts from 5 to 15 min but may take up to an hour.
- The placental site begins to diminish in size and the placenta is compressed so that blood in the intervillous spaces is forced back into the spongy layer of the decidua. Retraction of the oblique muscle fibres constricts the blood vessels supplying the placenta, preventing blood from draining into the maternal vascular tree. The uterine vessels become tense and congested and burst so that a small amount of blood collects between the spongy layer of the decidua and the maternal surface of the placenta, detaching it from the uterine wall.
- Separation normally begins from the centre of the placenta so that no blood escapes and a retroplacental clot forms. This probably provides a 3rd means of separation of the placenta as the developing blood clot increases pressure and helps to strip the adherent lateral borders and the membranes.
- There is an alternative mechanism of placental separation which begins at one of the lateral borders. Blood escapes from behind the placenta so that there is no formation of a retroplacental clot. The placenta folds in on itself with the maternal surface outwards and descends edge-on to appear maternal surface first accompanied by blood.
- Once separation is complete, the uterus contracts strongly and the placenta and membranes fall into the lower uterine segment and then into the vagina to be delivered. Three factors are involved in haemostasis: the action of the living ligatures, the walls of the uterus applying pressure to the placental site and a transitory increase in the activity of the coagulation system.
- Discussion of the management of the 3rd stage of labour centres on the benefits of actively managing the third stage of labour by using oxytocic drugs followed by controlled cord traction versus physiological management with the placenta and membranes being expelled by maternal effort.
- Syntometrine is the drug of choice in active management. Many women requested that oxytocic drugs should be omitted in the 3rd stage unless thought necessary in an emergency. This led to a series of trials to ascertain the safety of physiological management of the 3rd stage.
- Active management may be associated with unpleasant side effects such as nausea and vomiting and though some believe that active management should be the management of choice in maternity units where it is still standard practice, there is a need to examine the implications for deliveries in other settings.
- The placenta and membranes should be examined as soon after delivery as possible to see whether or not the placenta and membranes have been completely delivered and to detect abnormalities which might provide information about any intrauterine problems. Gloves should be worn to prevent the transmission of bloodborne diseases such as hepatitis or HIV.
- The midwife should remain with the woman for at least 1 h following completion of the delivery. The uterus should remain well contracted. Her temperature, pulse and blood pressure are taken and recorded. The mother's lochia is inspected and she is encouraged to pass urine. An all-over wash, clean clothing and refreshment will be appreciated.

References

Begley CM. 1990 A comparison of active and physiological management of the third stage of labour. Midwifery 6, 3–17.
Elbourne D. 1996 Care in the third stage of labour. In Robinson S, Thomson AM (eds) Midwives, Research and Childbirth, Vol 4. Chapman and Hall, London, pp 192–207.
Elbourne D, Harding J. 1991 Routine management for the third stage of labour: evidence from two random controlled trials. Journal of Obstetrics and Gynaecology 11 (suppl 1), S23–S27.
Gilbert L, Porter W, Brown VA. 1987 Postpartum haemorrhage – a continuing problem. British Journal of Obstetrics and Gynaecology 94, 67–71.
Harding JE, Elbourne D, Prendiville WJ. 1989 Views of mothers and midwives participating in the Bristol randomised controlled trial of active management of the third stage of labor. Birth 16(1), 1–6.
Inch S. 1985 Management of the third stage of labour – another cascade of intervention? Midwifery 1, 114–122.
Morrin NA 1997 Midwifery care in the third stage of labour. In Sweet BR with Tiran D (eds) Mayes Midwifery. Baillière Tindall, London 403–417.
Prendiville WJ, Harding JE, Elbourne D, Stirrat GM. 1988 The Bristol third stage trial: active versus physiological management of the third stage of labour. British Medical Journal 297.

Prendiville WJ, Elbourne DR, McDonald S. 1996 Active versus expectant management of the third stage of labour. In Neilson JP, Crowther CA, Hodnett ED, Hofmeyr GJ, Keirse MJNC (eds) Pregnancy and Childbirth module of The Cochrane Database of Systematic Reviews, The Cochrane Library. Update Software, Oxford.
Sweet B. 1997 Mayes' Midwifery. Baillière Tindall, London.
Thilaganathan B, Cutner A, Latimer J, Beard R. 1993 Management of the third stage of labour in women at low risk of postpartum haemorrhage. European Journal of Obstetrics and Gynaecology and Reproductive Biology 48, 19–22.
Van Dongen PWJ, de Groot ANJA. 1995 History of ergot alkaloids from ergotism to ergometrine. European Journal of Obstetrics and Gynaecology and Reproductive Biology 60, 109–116.
Yuen PM, Chan NST, Yim SF, Chang AMZ. 1995 A randomised double blind comparison of syntometrine and syntocinon in the management of the third stage of labour. British Journal of Obstetrics and Gynaecology 102, 277–380.

Recommended reading

Begley CM. 1990 A comparison of active and physiological management of the third stage of labour. Midwifery 6, 3–17.
Elbourne D, Harding J. 1991 Routine management for the third stage of labour: evidence from two random controlled trials. Journal of Obstetrics and Gynaecology 11 (suppl 1), S23–S27.
Inch S. 1985 Management of the third stage of labour – another cascade of intervention? Midwifery 1, 114–122.
Prendiville WJ, Elbourne D, McDonald S. 1996 Active versus expectant management of the third stage of labour in Neilson JP, Crowther CA, Hodnett ED, Hofmeyr GJ, Keirse MJNC (eds). Pregnancy and Childbirth module of The Cochrane Database of Systematic Reviews, The Cochrane Library. Update Software, Oxford.
Thilaganathan B, Cutner A, Latimer J, Beard R. 1993 Management of the third stage of labour in women at low risk of postpartum haemorrhage. European Journal of Obstetrics and Gynaecology and Reproductive Biology 48, 19–22.
Yuen PM, Chan NST, Yim SF, Chang AMZ. 1995 A randomised double blind comparison of syntometrine and syntocinon in the management of the third stage of labour. British Journal of Obstetrics and Gynaecology 102, 277–380.

Section
3B

LABOUR PROBLEMS

Section contents

Although the majority of labours progress normally, problems may be present at the onset or develop rapidly within labour that are life threatening to both mother and fetus. The knowledge and experience required to recognise these problems and to summon help from the obstetric and paediatric team is vital to the midwife. This section is concerned with abnormal labour. Traditionally these problems can be grouped as the effects of the 'powers, passenger and passages' on the progress of labour. Chapter 41 examines the 'powers' and presents the different problems of abnormal uterine action in detail. The following two chapters discuss problems with the passenger, taking this literally to mean the fetus. Although technically the placenta and membranes are part of the passenger, problems arising from these are discussed in chapter 45. Chapter 42 is concerned with the fetus that presents by the breech and chapter 43 discusses all other abnormal positions and presentations. Except in extreme cases it is artificial to discuss problems with 'the passages' as these almost always are related to the size of the particular passenger. Chapter 44 is mainly concerned with cephalo-pelvic disproportion. Chapter 46 is about perinatal asphyxia and sits at the junction of labour and neonatal care. Finally chapter 47 discusses operative procedures such as delivery by forceps, vacuum extraction or Caesarean section.

Chapter 41

Abnormalities of uterine action and onset of labour

In this chapter

INTRODUCTION

The length of labour is variable and is affected by the type of uterine contractions, parity, birth interval, psychological state, presentation and position, pelvic shape and size. Each of these factors will be considered in turn over the next few chapters although in practice there may be interaction between them. This chapter on abnormal uterine action will include active management of labour. The association between the pattern of contractions and the progress of labour is highly variable and the outcome difficult to predict. Abnormal uterine action may be inefficient, resulting in prolongation of labour, or overefficient, resulting in precipitate labour.

Normal labour begins spontaneously at term, i.e. after 37 completed weeks and before 42 completed weeks of pregnancy. The contractions increase in length, strength and frequency, resulting in progressive descent of the fetus and dilatation of the cervical os until the fetus, placenta and membranes are expelled from the uterus and bleeding is controlled. Normal labour is also characterised by harmonious interaction between the two poles of the uterus: the upper uterine segment contracts and retracts and the lower uterine segment thins out and the cervix dilates. A retraction ring forms between the two.

ABNORMALITIES OF UTERINE ACTION

Prolonged labour

The first stage of labour can be described as having latent, active and deceleration phases. The latent phase lasts until cervical dilatation is about 3–4 cm and can take 6–8 h in a primigravida. In the active phase rapid dilatation of the cervix occurs at about 1 cm per hour in a primigravida and 1.5 cm per hour in a multigravida. Defining the term prolonged labour is problematic and related to a chosen length mainly because of a belief that the longer labour lasts, the more danger there is for mother and fetus. It is important to remember that although prolonged labour is common in primigravidae, it occurs less often in multigravidae and may be due to obstruction of labour. Rupture of the uterus may follow careless use of oxytocic drugs in a multigravid labour.

Over the last 40 years, there has been a trend to reduce the accepted length of labour in a primigravida from 24 to 12 h. If the length of the latent phase of the first stage of labour in a primigravida is accepted as 6 h, resulting in a dilatation of 4 cm and average progress of dilatation is 1 cm per hour up to 10 cm in the active and deceleration phases, it is easy to see how 12 h has become the accepted norm. Labour may be prolonged in the latent, active or deceleration phases.

Timing of the onset of labour

A further difficulty is how to define the onset of labour. As discussed in Chapter 36, the timing is important as it allows decisions to be made about the progress and ongoing management of labour yet it is difficult to establish with accuracy. Gibb (1988) discusses the concept of **prelabour**, meaning the changes that occur in the last few weeks of pregnancy. It is often difficult to decide when the transition from the painless uterine contractions of prelabour develop into true labour.

Latent or active phase?

There is lack of agreement about whether to count the onset of labour from the onset of the latent phase or the active phase of the first stage (O'Brien 1997). The most frequently used marker for the commencement of labour is the time of admission. This is an arbitrary point in time rather than a biologically correct starting point (Enkin et al 1995). Vaginal examination of women at the time of admission demonstrates that the decision to present for admission varies depending on the advice the woman has been given on recognising the onset of labour and her anxieties and expectations.

Dangers of prolonged labour to the mother and fetus

Maternal risks

The physical effort, pain and anxiety of a prolonged labour result in dehydration, ketosis and tiredness. If this were to be allowed to continue maternal distress could occur. The temperature, pulse and blood pressure rise, dehydration, oliguria and ketosis develop and the woman may vomit.

If the membranes are ruptured, intrauterine infection is a risk and if undetected cephalopelvic disproportion is present, the uterus may rupture. Other risks include general anaesthesia, operative interventions and postpartum haemorrhage.

Fetal risks

- Intrapartum hypoxia may cause acidosis, fetal distress, neonatal asphyxia and meconium aspiration, possibly leading to perinatal death.
- Cerebral trauma may occur due to severe hypoxia or excessive moulding.
- Prolonged rupture of the membranes may result in neonatal pneumonia.

Inefficient uterine action

Uterine contractions are inefficient if they do not result in dilatation of the cervix. Inefficient uterine action was the commonest cause of abnormal labour in primigravidae (O'Driscoll et al 1993) and of delay in 65% of 9018 nulliparous women with prolonged labour. The remaining cases were caused by persistent occipitoposterior position (24%) and cephalopelvic disproportion (11%) (Malone et al 1996). There is slow progress and the length of labour is prolonged. Inefficiency may arise because the contractions are too weak (**hypotonic uterine action**) or because there is loss of co-ordination between the upper and lower uterine segments (**incoordinate uterine action**).

Hypotonic uterine action

The uterine contractions are weak and short. There is slow or absent dilatation of the cervix and the woman does not find the contractions too painful or distressing. The fetus remains in good condition. If hypotonic contractions occur from the commencement of labour, they are said to be **primary**. The cause of primary hypotonic uterine action is unknown but it is more commonly seen in primigravidae. If hypotonic contractions begin after a period of normal uterine action they are said to be **secondary** and there may be abnormalities of labour such as cephalopelvic disproportion (CPD), malposition of the occiput, a malpresentation, maternal dehydration or ketosis. The commencement of epidural analgesia sometimes causes hypotonic uterine action (O'Brien 1997).

Incoordinate uterine action

There is loss of polarity and an increase in resting tone of the uterus. The contractions are frequent and painful with backache and pain between contractions. The woman feels the contraction before and after it is palpable abdominally. The cervix dilates slowly or not at all. Placental blood flow is decreased, leading to fetal distress. This type of uterine action is associated with malpositions of the occiput.

Active management of labour

Active management of labour (AML) was introduced by O'Driscoll et al (1986) in the 1960s for the management of labour in primigravidae. There must be accurate diagnosis of the onset of labour with painful uterine contractions and one of the following: complete effacement of the cervix, a show or spontaneous rupture of the membranes (Henderson 1996). Amniotomy is carried out shortly after admission with augmentation of labour with syntocinon if there is inadequate progress after 2 h. All women are given adequate emotional support and ongoing peer review to assess the efficiency and effectiveness of the protocol is essential (Gerhardstein et al 1995, O'Brien 1997).

Acceleration of labour

A modified version of AML is used to manage prolonged labour when progress is slow but otherwise normal. This is acceleration or augmentation of labour. Once delay has been diagnosed and abnormalities of presentation or CPD ruled out the membranes are ruptured and an intravenous infusion of an oxytocic drug commenced to stimulate labour contractions. Any abnormality of fluid and electrolyte balance is corrected and both mother

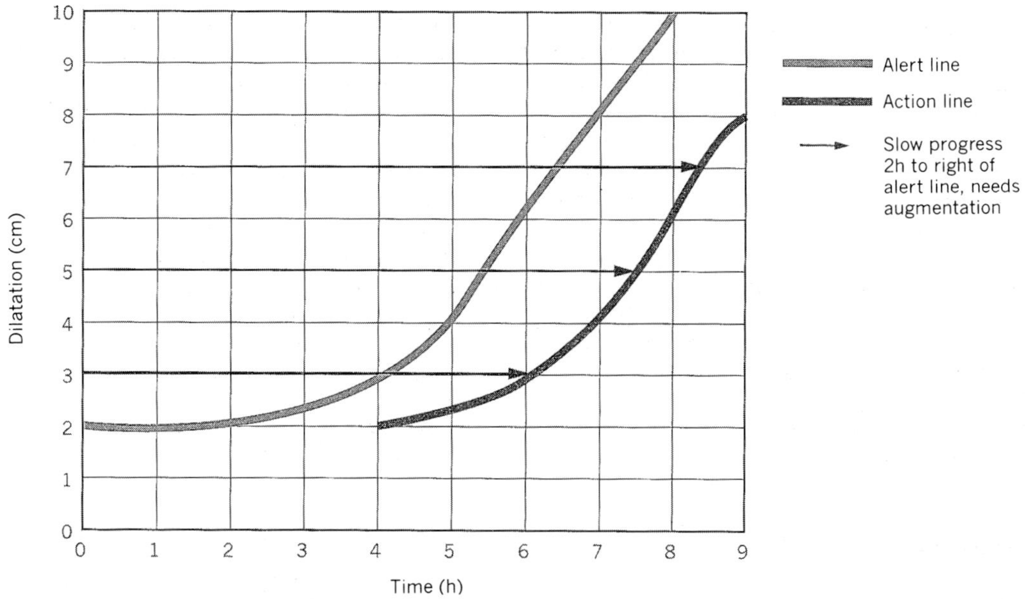

Figure 41.1 *Normogram/partogram of cervimetric progress commencing at 2 cm dilatation. 'Alert' line outlines normal progress. 'Action' line indicates when augmentation should be instituted. (After Studd (1973).)*

and fetus monitored carefully. Adequate pain relief should be provided. Findings regarding the progress of labour should be recorded graphically on a partogram (Fig. 41.1) so that deviations from normal can be immediately recognised. There should be good psychological support of the woman.

Reduction of caesarean section births

Gerhardstein et al (1995) discussed the effect of AML on the reduction of caesarean section births (CS) in the USA where the rate of CS has risen dramatically. Their study found that women whose labours had been managed actively had a lower rate of caesarean birth than the control group of women who laboured spontaneously. Similarly Henderson (1996) wrote that CS rates have escalated in all Western countries, reaching 20% of all deliveries in some units in the UK and 25% in the USA. Concern over the increased maternal morbidity and financial cost has led to attempts to reduce the CS rate to that of 5–7% of all births achieved by O'Driscoll and his colleagues in Dublin. Henderson analysed how the Dublin figures had been maintained at this low level despite the noted increase in other countries.

Other factors that could account for the low use of CS in Dublin included 'an avoidance of innovations seen in most obstetric units in the 1970s and 1980s'. These innovations include induction of labour and electronic fetal monitoring. Henderson quotes Barrett et al (1990) who concluded that 30% of CS performed for fetal distress were unnecessary.

AML is a package and it is necessary to examine the individual parts of the package. Henderson concluded 'that research has failed to demonstrate that the two widely used elements of the O'Driscoll protocol, artificial rupture of the membranes and the infusion of oxytocin, reduce the rate of Caesarean section'.

Amniotomy

The benefits of intact membranes throughout labour include reduced risk of intrauterine infection and of fetal hypoxia because of less placental compression and less reduction of size of the placental site. Artificial rupture of the membranes has been practised for several decades. The membranes are usually ruptured to accelerate labour. Amniotomy may also be done to examine the amniotic fluid for the presence of meconium.

A metaanalysis of early amniotomy in women with spontaneous onset of labour, carried out by Fraser et al (1997), concluded that amniotomy was associated with a reduction in the length of labour by 60–120 min. They also found a reduction in the proportion of women reporting the most severe level of pain at some point in labour in those who were given amniotomy. However, a survey by the National Childbirth Trust (1989) reported that women who had been given an amniotomy found labour harder to cope with.

Fraser et al (1997) found an upward trend in the number of CS and evidence of an increase in fetal heart rate monitoring abnormalities in women following amniotomy and suggest that amniotomy should be reserved for use in labours which are progressively slowing. In similar fashion, O'Brien (1997) believes there should be a clear indication of the need for amniotomy before it is carried out.

Oxytocic infusion

O'Brien (1997) reports that the use of oxytocin can be as high as that quoted by O'Driscoll et al (1993) – 45%. As described above, the benefits are correction of inefficient uterine action, a shorter labour, a reduced rate of CS with a corresponding increase in vaginal delivery. Byrne et al (1993) found no evidence that an oxytocic infusion generated excessive intrauterine pressure. However, women experience more painful contractions and are restricted in their ability to move about.

The division of the first stage of labour into latent, active and deceleration phases is important to the use and efficacy of oxytocin. Olah et al (1993) found that cervical muscle fibres constrict in response to oxytocin in the latent phase, leading to a poor response, high intrauterine pressures and the possibility of fetal distress although O'Driscoll et al (1993) found no evidence of this.

Expectations of childbirth have developed and the medicalisation of a normal physiological process has been criticised in the last decade (Walkinshaw 1994). There is much variation in practice between units and until recently, maternal satisfaction with delivery has not been considered in research protocols. Enkin et al (1995) summarised the evidence and did not think there was any benefit to women and their babies of liberal use of oxytocic infusions. They concluded that although the use of an oxytocic infusion had its place in the management of women enduring a prolonged labour, other measures such as ambulation and allowing intake of appropriate nutrition should be considered before labelling a labour as abnormal and using medical intervention.

Prolonged second stage of labour

A discussion on the acceptable length of the 2nd stage of labour is presented in Chapter 39. Delayed progress may be due to:

- inefficient uterine action (primary powers);
- inefficient maternal effort (secondary powers);
- a full bladder or rectum, a rigid perineum;
- a contracted pelvic outlet;
- a large baby;
- a fetal abnormality such as hydrocephaly or abdominal enlargement;
- persistent occipitoposterior position;
- deep transverse arrest of the head;
- a malpresentation.

Management

The condition of mother and fetus should be carefully assessed and as long as progress is being made, although slowly, more time may be given. Adopting an upright position may enlarge the pelvic outlet and direct the presenting part against the posterior vaginal wall, utilising Ferguson's reflex with the release of oxytocin. If maternal or fetal condition becomes worrying or there is obviously no progress, an assisted vaginal delivery or, more rarely, a CS may be needed.

Overefficient uterine action

Precipitate labour

A precipitate labour is when the uterine contractions are frequent and intense. Delivery occurs within an hour. This condition is much commoner in the multigravid woman and is usually caused because of a lack of resistance of the maternal soft tissues. There may have been minimal pain in the first stage of labour and the woman becomes aware of imminent delivery when the head is about to be born. The author remembers 'Mrs Murphy' who delivered her 5th baby in the day room whilst watching television. When the excitement had died down and mother and baby were safe, the author asked the other women for their perceptions of the event. One woman reported that Mrs Murphy had just said 'Oo-er, the baby's coming' and delivered!

Dangers of precipitate labour

The woman may have lacerations to the cervix and perineum. Postpartum haemorrhage may follow. The baby may be hypoxic and may sustain intracranial injuries because of rapid descent through the birth canal. If the birth takes place in an inappropriate place the baby may fall to the ground and be injured. Any woman with a history of a previous precipitate delivery should be admitted to hospital before term.

Tonic contraction of the uterus

This rare event, where the tone of the uterus is continuously high and there is no relaxation of the uterine muscle, is accompanied by intense pain. The fetus becomes distressed as the placental circulation is grossly restricted. Intrauterine death may occur. Causes may be obstructed labour or misuse of oxytocic drugs such as syntocinon and prostaglandins. This is an emergency and immediate treatment may save the baby's life and prevent uterine rupture.

- If an oxytocic infusion is in progress, turn it off.
- Turn the mother onto her left side to enhance uteroplacental blood flow.
- Administer oxygen.
- Inform the obstetrician who will carry out a CS.

Cervical dystocia

Cervical dystocia, where the cervix dilates slowly if at all, may be congenital or acquired. Congenital problems may be fibrosis, stenosis or poor cervical development. Acquired cervical dystocia may be due to fibrosis and scarring of the cervix following surgery, cautery or irradiation. In the past when there was failure to recognise the condition, prolonged pressure would result in ischaemia and there would be annular detachment of the cervix.

If the anterior part of the cervix is trapped between the pelvic brim and the fetal head, venous return is restricted and the anterior lip may become swollen and oedematous and feel as thick as a finger during vaginal examination. The first stage of labour will be prolonged and occasionally the cervix may be seen blue and glistening between the fetal head and the symphysis pubis (Williams 1996). The most likely cause is the woman bearing down before full cervical dilatation and it is commonly the result of a persistent occipitoposterior position. If the woman lies on her side and is encouraged to use inhalational analgesia, she will be helped to avoid pushing. Elevating the foot of her bed may also help. Epidural analgesia may occasionally be needed. It is sometimes possible to push an anterior lip of cervix up behind the fetal head but care must be taken not to tear the cervix.

PROBLEMS IN THE TIMING OF THE ONSET OF LABOUR

Preterm onset of labour

Preterm labour is one that begins before the end of the 37th week of pregnancy. A baby born from such a labour is a preterm baby irrespective of birth weight. Not all preterm babies are of low birth weight (LBW), weighing less than 2000 g, but many babies are both preterm and of low birth weight. Babies weighing less than 1500 g are very low birth weight (VLBW) while those weighing less than 1000 g are named extremely low birth weight (ELBW). Preterm babies have different problems and needs from LBW babies with growth retardation and the care of the babies will be discussed in Section 4A.

To quote Lindsay (1997), 'The incidence of preterm delivery as a proportion of all births ranges from 6 to 10% in developed countries and has changed little over the past 20 years'. Maternal mortality and morbidity are rarely affected by preterm onset of labour (Arias 1993) although women may suffer feelings of inadequacy as a result of perceiving themselves to have failed. However, preterm birth is responsible for almost all neonatal deaths not due to congenital malformations and for much morbidity. As gestational age increases, so does the rate of preterm delivery. Less than a quarter of such births occur before 32 weeks.

Aetiology

Preterm births may follow a spontaneous onset of labour or be elective because of a problem for the woman or the fetus. The following conditions may lead to an elective induction of preterm delivery.

- Severe preeclampsia
- Maternal disease such as renal disease, diabetes mellitus and maternal infection
- Severe intrauterine growth retardation
- Rhesus isoimmunisation
- Premature rupture of the membranes
- Prolapsed cord
- Placental abruption

In about 40% of cases onset of labour occurs spontaneously with no known cause. Lindsay (1997) summarises the risk factors which have been associated with preterm labour (Table 41.1). Whilst they are not directly causative, they may indicate which women have an increased risk of preterm delivery. Although the above list is comprehensive, it is difficult to predict which woman will begin labour before term. A further problem is that even if the onset of preterm labour could be predicted, it is difficult to prevent the progress to delivery.

As the risk factors are so varied, attempts at reducing some of the physical or social factors have had limited success. Risk-scoring systems have been developed using the above factors but have been found to be poor predictors, especially in primigravid women. Home monitoring of uterine activity has had no effect on the rate of preterm birth. Cervical effacement can be assessed but not only is it not a good predictor of preterm birth but it may introduce infection.

Fetal fibrinectin

High levels of fetal fibronectin, a component of the extracellular matrix secreted by the anchoring trophoblastic villi, have been found in cervical and vaginal secretions prior to the onset of preterm labour (Lockwood et al 1991). Separation of maternal and fetal tissue at the choriodecidual junction leads to a leakage of fibronectin and a test has been developed. The test is accurate in up to 80% of cases and can be carried out every 2 weeks after the 24th week of pregnancy. Both blood and amniotic fluid contain fibronectin, limiting the use of the test (Lindsay 1997).

Preterm rupture of the membranes

Spontaneous preterm prelabour rupture of the membranes is associated with cervical incompetence and genital tract infection. Labour may begin soon after the event but if delayed, bacteria may ascend the genital tract to colonise the uterus and fetus. The woman must be admitted to a hospital with a neonatal intensive care unit. No vaginal examination is performed in the absence of signs of labour but a speculum examination is carried out to visualise the cervix. A cervical swab is taken for culture and sensitivity testing.

Table 41.1 *A summary of the risk factors given by Lindsay (1997)*

Biological/medical factors	*Reproductive history*	*Current pregnancy*	*Socioeconomic and psychological (Peacock et al 1995)*
Age less than 15 or more than 35	History of previous preterm birth	Failure to gain weight adequately	Poverty and social deprivation
Low body weight (less than 50 kg at conception)	Bleeding in previous pregnancy	Bleeding in this pregnancy	Psychological distress
History of hypertension, renal disease or diabetes mellitus	Uterine abnormality	Retained intrauterine contraceptive device	Late antenatal booking and poor attendance for care
Cigarette, alcohol or drug use	Abdominal surgery		
Short interpregnancy interval		Infections, e.g. pyelonephritis	
		Genital tract infection e.g. bacterial vaginosis (Hillier et al 1995), *Chlamydia*, group B haemolytic streptococcus	
		Fetal problems: multiple pregnancy, fetal malformation, rhesus disease, fetal death, polyhydramnios	

The use of drugs

Corticosteroids

The risk of hyaline membrane disease for the neonate is high and the steroid dexamethasone is given to the mother to accelerate surfactant production in the lungs. Crowley (1997) has provided an extremely well-detailed review of the use of corticosteroids prior to preterm delivery, analysing 18 trials and 3700 babies between 1976 and 1994. Her findings were that antenatal administration of corticosteroids to women expected to deliver preterm reduced mortality, respiratory distress syndrome and intraventricular haemorrhage in preterm infants. Crowley concluded that 'Every effort should be made to treat women with corticosteroids prior to preterm delivery'. A typical regime is two doses of 12 mg given by intramuscular injection 12 h apart. The effects of the drug take 24 h to develop and it is effective for up to 7 days.

Antibiotics

Chorioamnionitis is the cause of preterm labour in up to 30% of cases. Intraamniotic infection may exist without a rise in temperature, rise in white cell count, uterine tenderness or fetal tachycardia and the cause is poorly understood (Arias 1993). Preterm labour possibly follows infection because of an increased production of prostaglandin by the decidua and the amnion. In preterm prelabour rupture of the membranes with clear evidence of infection or vaginal colonisation with pathogenic bacteria, antibiotic therapy is commenced. Prophylactic use of antibiotics has resulted in reduction of the risk of preterm delivery occurring within 1 week and the prevention of infection in the mother or baby (Enkin et al 1995).

Tocolytic drugs

If preterm labour is diagnosed and the membranes are intact, β-adrenergic drugs such as ritodrine hydrochloride, salbutamol and terbutaline, which relax smooth muscle, may be administered by intravenous infusion. No effect on perinatal mortality has been found but the delay of onset of labour by 48 h gives time for the corticosteroids to be effective (British National Formulary 1996).

These drugs affect all smooth muscle and the woman may suffer side effects of tachycardia, cardiac dysrhythmias, palpitations and peripheral vasodilation resulting in hypotension and flushing may occur (Rang & Dale 1991). Nausea and muscle tremors can be a problem. Pulmonary oedema may occur because of increased permeability of the alveolar – capillary barrier (Watson & Morgan 1989). There may be stimulation of the renin-aldosterone system with increased secretion of antidiuretic hormone, leading to fluid retention. No attempt should be made to stop labour if the fetus is more than 34 weeks gestation or estimated to be more than 2500 g (Pearce 1985).

Prostaglandin synthesis inhibitors such as indomethacin may also be used which block production of the enzyme endoperoxide synthase responsible for the conversion of arachidonic acid to prostaglandin. Maternal side effects are nausea, vomiting, diarrhoea, dizziness and headaches. Fetal effects may be premature closing of the ductus arteriosus, right heart failure and death in utero. Major et al (1994) found an increased incidence of necrotising enterocolitis in neonates following exposure to indomethacin in utero. Indomethacin may be the best current tocolytic agent but it is not the first choice because of the side effects on the fetus (Arias 1993).

Calcium channel blockers such as nifedipine inhibit muscle contraction (Marieb 1992). Because of the side effects of the drugs, careful observations of mother and fetus must be made, including blood glucose monitoring (RCOG 1994). If cervical dilatation progresses to 4 cm or if the membranes rupture delivery is probably inevitable (Lindsay 1997).

Labour and delivery

All tocolytic drugs are stopped and careful monitoring of the condition of the woman and her fetus carried out. Analgesic drugs such as pethidine and morphine should be avoided if possible and the preferred methods of pain relief are epidural anaesthesia or Entonox, neither of which affects the fetus adversely. An obstetrician and paediatrician should be present at the delivery and an elective episiotomy performed to reduce pressure on the fetal head and minimise cerebral trauma. Forceps may offer better protection. Some obstetricians prefer to deliver VLBW babies, especially if presenting by the breech, by CS. The cord should be clamped at least 10 cm away from its insertion into the abdominal wall to facilitate care in the neonatal unit. Vitamin K 0.5–1 mg is usually given to lessen the risk of haemorrhage.

Prolonged pregnancy

A pregnancy is considered to be postterm if the gestational age is accurate and it is prolonged beyond 42 completed weeks (294 days). The risk of prolonged pregnancy is higher in primigravidae, being about 20% higher than in women who have given birth previously. Fetal maturity can be estimated by calculation if the first day of the last menstrual period is known and the woman has a regular cycle.

Abdominal examination is not an accurate way of measuring gestational age. An early ultrasound scan will provide good assessment of fetal age and serial scans later in pregnancy can monitor continuing fetal growth. If the woman has not been seen until late in pregnancy it is possible to find ossification centres by X-ray but this is not reliable as ossification may vary by up to 5 weeks between fetuses in late pregnancy. Static maternal weight, abnormal fetal heart rate patterns and reduced fetal movements may indicate a deterioration in fetal condition.

Risk factors

Postterm pregnancy is associated with a higher incidence of perinatal death and congenital malformation. After term, there may be progressive placental insufficiency and perinatal asphyxia is more common. The volume of amniotic fluid may diminish so that oxygen supply may be interrupted during contractions due to compression of the placenta. Meconium staining of the liquor is common, with the risk of meconium aspiration syndrome. Babies born after 42 weeks are more likely to weigh more than 4000 g and the increased size of the fetus may result in shoulder dystocia, accompanied by the typical trauma of brachial and facial palsy and fractured clavicle.

Management

Conservative management of pregnancy is becoming more common if there are no complications. It is possible to monitor the well-being of the fetus by cardiotocography, ultrasound measurement of amniotic fluid volume and biophysical profile but there is no evidence that their use improves the outcome for the fetus. Unrestricted breast stimulation and coitus after 39 weeks may decrease the incidence of postterm pregnancy and digital separation of the membranes from the lower pole of the uterus (**sweeping the membranes**) may also help. Induction of labour after 41 weeks has been shown to lessen the incidence of perinatal death but there is no support for the use of induction in postterm pregnancies before 41 weeks (Enkin et al 1995).

Induction of labour

The term induction refers to the initiation of labour by artificial means. Induction is carried out for medical or obstetric reasons, when it is thought that the health of the mother or fetus would be compromised by the continuation of pregnancy (Table 41.2).

Contraindications

These include placenta praevia, cephalopelvic disproportion, oblique or transverse lie, severe fetal compromise and lack of maternal consent.

Method

Induction should be timed when the presence of favourable factors indicates readiness. The success of induction depends on the state of the cervix (Enkin et al 1995) which can be assessed by the Bishop's scoring system (Table 41.3). The prognosis for induction is good with a score of 6 or more.

Cervical ripening

Prostaglandins

There are few oxytocin receptors in the cervix, making oxytocin inefficient as a ripening agent. There is a high failure of induction leading to long labours and an increase in the need for CS if the cervix is unfavourable at the commencement of induction. The introduction of vaginal administration of prostaglandins (PGE_2) or a smaller dose by the endocervical route for cervical ripening has increased the likelihood of a successful induction of labour leading to spontaneous vaginal delivery within 12–24 h (Enkin et al 1995). However, uterine hypertonus occurs more often among women in whom prostaglandin ripening of the cervix has been used than in those women who received placebo or no prostaglandins. Abnormalities of fetal heart rate are also more likely to occur but neither trend appears to result in an increase in operative delivery (Enkin et al 1995).

Table 41.2 *Some indications for induction of labour*

Maternal indications	*Fetal indications*	*Joint indications*
Prolonged pregnancy	Placental insufficiency	Preeclampsia
Following spontaneous rupture of membranes	Rhesus isoimmunisation with haemolysis	Placental abruption
Medical conditions such as diabetes mellitus	Intrauterine death	Previous precipitate labour
Poor obstetric history such as a previous stillbirth	Severe congenital abnormalities	An unstable lie
Maternal request for social/psychological reasons		

Table 41.3 *Modified Bishop's scoring system*

Assessment features	0	1	2	3
Dilatation of the cervix (cm)	0	1–2	3–4	5–6
Consistency of the cervix	Firm	Medium	Soft	–
Length of cervical canal (cm)	> 2	1–2	0.5–1	< 0.5
Position of cervix	Posterior	Mid	Anterior	–
Station of presenting part related to ischial spines	–3	–2	–3	+1, +2

Sweeping the membranes

As mentioned above, stripping the membranes from the lower uterine segment possibly produces increased amounts of prostaglandin. In a randomised controlled trial of 142 nulliparous and multiparous women, membrane stripping was found to be a safe and possible effective way of avoiding induction by promoting spontaneous onset of labour at term (Berghella et al 1996). However, the authors agree with Enkin et al (1995) that a larger trial is necessary to judge the effectiveness of this procedure.

Amniotomy with or without oxytocin

Rupturing the membranes is a point of no return in obstetric management of labour. Once performed, the risk of intrauterine infection increases with the time interval before delivery. Amniotomy may be used on its own, followed by commencement of an oxytocic infusion in contractions do not commence after a few hours, or with the simultaneous commencement of an oxytocic infusion. Syntocinon infusion must be carefully regulated to avoid the complications of hyperstimulation of uterine action and water retention. Amniotic fluid embolism is a rare complication which follows hyperstimulation of uterine action.

Moldin & Sundell (1996) carried out a randomised controlled trial of amniotomy versus amniotomy with oxytocin infusion with 196 participants. All the women had a favourable Bishop's score and were at term with an indication for induction. Group A had the combined induction regime whilst group B had amniotomy alone. The addition of an oxytocic drug led to a shorter induction – delivery interval due to a shorter latent phase of labour but no difference in the active phase or the 2nd stage of labour. Of the group B women who had amniotomy alone, 32% eventually received oxytocin although the length of time of oxytocin administration was nearly five times less than in group A where oxytocin had been commenced soon after the amniotomy. The authors concluded that the minor differences between the groups justified an individual management policy with attention paid to both the indication for induction of labour and the woman's choice.

Summary of main points

- The length of labour is affected by the type of uterine contractions, parity, birth interval, psychological state, presentation and position, pelvic shape and size. Each of these factors must be considered although there may be interaction between them.
- Normal labour begins spontaneously at term. The contractions increase in length, strength and frequency resulting in progressive descent of the fetus and dilatation of the cervical os until the fetus, placenta and membranes are expelled from the uterus and bleeding is controlled.
- The first stage of labour can be described as having latent, active and deceleration phases. The term prolonged labour is used because of a belief that the longer labour lasts, the more danger there is for mother and fetus. Labour may be prolonged in the latent, active or deceleration phases.
- The timing of the onset of labour is important as it allows decisions to be made about the progress and ongoing management of labour yet it is difficult to establish with accuracy. It may be difficult to decide when the painless uterine contractions of prelabour develop into true labour.
- There is lack of agreement about whether to count the onset of labour from the onset of the latent or the active phase of the first stage. The most frequently used marker for the commencement of labour is the time of admission.
- The dangers of prolonged labour to the mother are the physical effort, pain and anxiety, dehydration, ketosis and tiredness. If this is allowed to continue, maternal distress could lead to maternal morbidity and mortality. For the baby, risks include intrapartum acidosis, fetal distress, neonatal asphyxia and meconium aspiration, perinatal death, cerebral trauma and ascending neonatal infections.
- Uterine contractions are inefficient if they do not result in dilatation of the cervix. Inefficient uterine action because of hypotonic uterine action or incoordinate uterine action is the commonest cause of abnormal labour in primigravidae. Progress is slow and the length of labour is prolonged.
- Active management of labour (AML) was introduced for the management of labour in primigravidae. Amniotomy is carried out shortly after admission with augmentation of labour with syntocinon if there is inadequate progress after 2 h. A modified version is used to manage prolonged labour when progress is slow but otherwise normal – acceleration or augmentation of labour. Studies have shown a reduction of CS births in women whose labours had been managed actively.
- The benefits of intact membranes throughout labour include reduced risk of intrauterine infection and of fetal hypoxia because of less placental compression and less reduction of size of the placental site. There may be an upward trend in the number of CS and an increase in fetal heart rate monitoring abnormalities in women following amniotomy and it is possible that amniotomy should be reserved for use in labours which are progressively slowing.
- Oxytocin administration will correct inefficient uterine action, shorten labour and reduce the rate of CS. However, women experience more painful contractions and are restricted in their ability to move about. Other measures such as ambulation and allowing appropriate nutrition should be considered before labelling a labour as abnormal and using medical intervention.
- Delayed progress in the 2nd stage may be due to inefficient uterine action or inefficient maternal effort, a full bladder or rectum, a rigid perineum, cephalopelvic disproportion or obstructed labour. Adopting an upright position may enlarge the pelvic outlet and direct the presenting part against the posterior vaginal wall, bringing about increased uterine action. If maternal or fetal condition deteriorates or there is no progress, an assisted vaginal delivery or CS may be needed.
- In precipitate labour, uterine contractions occur frequently and are intense, delivery occurring within an hour. It is commoner in multigravid women and is usually caused by lack of resistance of the maternal soft tissues. The woman may have lacerations to the cervix and perineum and postpartum haemorrhage may follow. The baby may be hypoxic and sustain intracranial injuries. Women with a history of precipitate delivery should be admitted to hospital before term.
- Tonic uterine action is usually accompanied by intense pain. The fetus becomes distressed as the placental circulation is grossly restricted and intrauterine death may occur. Causes may be obstructed labour or misuse of oxytocic drugs such as syntocinon and prostaglandins. Immediate treatment may save the baby's life and prevent uterine rupture.
- Cervical dystocia, where the cervix dilates slowly if at all, may be congenital or acquired. Congenital problems may be fibrosis, stenosis or poor cervical development. Acquired cervical dystocia may be due to fibrosis and scarring of the cervix following surgery, cautery or irradiation.
- If the anterior part of the cervix is trapped between the pelvic brim and the fetal head, venous return is restricted and the anterior lip may become swollen and oedematous, prolonging the first stage of labour. Bearing down before full cervical dilatation should be avoided and elevating the foot of the bed may help. Epidural analgesia may occasionally be needed.
- Preterm labour is responsible for almost all neonatal deaths not due to congenital malformations and for much morbidity. Preterm births may be spontaneous or elective because of a problem for the woman or the fetus. Risk factors are varied and attempts at reducing some of the physical or social factors have had limited success. Risk-scoring systems have been developed but are poor predictors, especially in primigravidae.
- Spontaneous preterm prelabour rupture of the membranes is associated with cervical incompetence and genital tract infection. Chorioamnionitis is the cause of preterm labour in up to 30% of cases. Labour may begin soon after the event but if delayed, bacteria may ascend the genital tract to colonise the uterus and fetus. Prophylactic use of antibiotics may prevent infection.
- If preterm labour is diagnosed and the membranes are intact, tocolytic drugs may be administered by intravenous infusion. The delay of onset of labour by 48 h gives time for the corticosteroids to be effective in maturation of the fetal lungs. If delivery is inevitable, tocolytic drugs are discontinued. Analgesic drugs such as pethidine and morphine should be avoided if possible.
- During the delivery an elective episiotomy is performed to minimise cerebral trauma. Forceps may offer better protection. Some obstetricians prefer to deliver VLBW babies, especially if presenting by the breech, by CS. The cord should be clamped at least 10 cm away from the abdominal wall to facilitate care. Vitamin K 0.5–1 mg is usually given.
- A pregnancy is prolonged if it persists beyond 42 completed weeks. Meconium staining of the liquor is common with the risk of meconium aspiration syndrome. The baby may be large and shoulder dystocia, nerve palsies and bone fractures are more common.

Induction of labour after 41 weeks has been shown to lessen the incidence of perinatal death.

- Induction of labour is carried out for medical or obstetric reasons. Contraindications include placenta praevia, cephalopelvic disproportion, oblique or transverse lie, severe fetal compromise and lack of maternal consent. The success of induction depends on the state of the cervix, which can be assessed by the Bishop's scoring system.
- The introduction of vaginal or endocervical administration of prostaglandins (PGE_2) for cervical ripening has increased the likelihood of a successful induction of labour. Stripping the membranes from the lower uterine segment possibly produces increased amounts of prostaglandin and may be a safe way of avoiding induction by promoting spontaneous onset of labour at term.
- Rupturing the membranes increases the risk of intrauterine infection. Amniotomy may be used on its own, followed by commencement of an oxytocic infusion if contractions do not commence after a few hours, or with the simultaneous commencement of an oxytocic infusion. Amniotic fluid embolism is a rare complication which follows hyperstimulation of uterine action.

References

Arias F. 1993 Practical Guide to High Risk Pregnancy and Delivery, 2nd edn. Mosby Year Book, Chicago.

Barrett JFR, Jarvis GJ, McDonald NH. 1990 Inconsistencies in clinical decisions in obstetrics. Lancet 336, 549–551.

Berghella V, Rogers RA, Lescale K. 1996 Obstetrics and Gynaecology 87(6), 927–931.

British National Formulary. 1996 British Medical Association and the Royal Pharmaceutical Society of Great Britain, London.

Byrne BM, Keane D, Boylan P, Stronge JM. 1993 Intra-uterine pressure and the active management of labour. Journal of Obstetrics and Gynaecology 13, 433–436.

Crowley P. 1997 Corticosteroids prior to preterm delivery. In Neilson JP, Crowther CA, Hodnett ED, Hofmeyr GJ, Keirse MJNC (eds) Pregnancy and Childbirth module of the Cochrane Database of Systematic Reviews, The Cochrane Library. Update Software, Oxford.

Enkin M, Keirse MJNC, Renfrew M, Neilson J. 1995 A Guide to Effective Care in Pregnancy and Childbirth, 2nd edn. Oxford Medical Publications, Oxford.

Fraser WD, Krauss I, Brisson-Carrol G, Thornton J, Breadt G. 1997 Amniotomy to shorten spontaneous labour. In Neilson JP, Crowther CA, Hodnett ED, Hofmeyr GJ, Keirse MJNC (eds) Pregnancy and Childbirth module of the Cochrane Database of Systematic Reviews, The Cochrane Library. Update Software, Oxford.

Gerhardstein LP, Allswede MT, Sloan CT, Lorenz RP. 1995 Reduction in cesarean birth with active management of labor and intermediate-dose oxytocin. Journal of Reproductive Medicine 40(1), 4–8.

Gibb D. 1988 A Practical Guide to Labour Management. Blackwell Scientific, Oxford.

Henderson J. 1996 Active management of labour and caesarean section rates. British Journal of Midwifery 4(3), 132–149.

Hillier SL, Nugent RP, Eschenbach DA. 1995 Association between a bacterial vaginosis and preterm delivery of a low birth-weight infant. New England Journal of Medicine 333(26), 1736–1742.

Lindsay P 1997 Preterm Labour. In Sweet BR with Tiran D (eds) Mayes Midwifery. Baillière Tindall: 603–609.

Lockwood C, Senyei A, Dishe M et al. 1991 Fetal fibronectin in cervical and vaginal secretions as a predictor of preterm delivery. New England Journal of Medicine 325(10), 669–674.

Major C, Lewis D, Harding J, Porto M, Garite T. 1994 Tocolysis with indomethacin increases the incidence of necrotising enterocolitis in the low weight neonate. American Journal of Obstetrics and Gynecology 170(1), 102–106.

Malone FD, Geary M, Chelmow D et al. 1996 Prolonged labor in nulliparas: lessons from the active management of labor. Obstetrics and Gynaecology 88(2), 211–215.

Marieb E. 1992 Human Anatomy and Physiology. Benjamin/Cummings Publishing, California,

Moldin PG, Sundell G. 1996 Induction of labour: a randomised clinical trial of amniotomy versus amniotomy with oxytocin infusion. British Journal of Obstetrics and Gynaecology 103(4), 306–312.

National Childbirth Trust. 1989 Rupture of the Membranes in Labour: Women's Views. National Childbirth Trust, London.

O'Brien W. 1997 Prolonged labour and disordered uterine action. In Sweet BR with Tiran D (eds). Mayes Midwifery, 12th edn. Baillière Tindall, London.

O'Driscoll K, Meagher D, Boylan P. 1986 Active Management of Labour, 2nd edn. Mosby, London.

O'Driscoll K, Meagher D, Boylan P. 1993 Active Management of Labour, 3rd edn. Mosby, London.

Olah KSJ, Gee A, Brown JS. 1993 Cervical contractions: the response of the cervix to oxytocic stimulation in the latent phase of labour. British Journal of Obstetrics and Gynaecology 100, 535–640.

Peacock JL, Bland JM, Anderson HR. 1995 Preterm delivery: effects of socio-economic factors, psychological stress, smoking, alcohol and caffeine. British Medical Journal 311(7004), 532–536.

Pearie MJ. 1985 The Management of Preterm Labour. In Studd T (ed) The Management of Labour. Blackwell Scientific, Oxford.

Rang HP, Dale M. 1991 Pharmacology, 2nd edn. Churchill Livingstone, Edinburgh.

Royal College of Obstetricians and Gynaecologists. 1994 Guidelines No. 1 – For the Use of Ritodrine. RCOG, London.

Walkinshaw SA. 1994 Is routine active intervention in spontaneous labour beneficial? Contemporary Review of Obstetrics and Gynaecology 6, 13–17.

Watson N, Morgan B. 1989 Pulmonary oedema and salbutamol in preterm labour. British Journal of Obstetrics and Gynaecology 96(12), 1445–1448.

Williams J. 1996 Prolonged pregnancy and disorders of uterine action. In Bennett VR, Brown LK (eds) Myles Textbook for Midwives, 12th edn. Churchill Livingstone, Edinburgh, pp 386–403.

Recommended reading

Gerhardstein LP, Allswede MT, Sloan CT, Lorenz RP. 1995 Reduction in cesarean birth with active management of labor and intermediate-dose oxytocin. Journal of Reproductive Medicine 40(1), 4–8.

Hillier SL, Nugent RP, Eschenbach DA. 1995 Association between a bacterial vaginosis and preterm delivery of a low birth-weight infant. New England Journal of Medicine 333(26), 1736–1742.

Malone FD, Geary M, Chelmow D et al. 1996 Prolonged labor in nulliparas: lessons from the active management of labor. Obstetrics and Gynaecology 88(2), 211–215.

O'Driscoll K, Meagher D, Boylan P. 1993 Active Management of Labour, 3rd edn. Mosby, London.

Walkinshaw SA. 1994 Is routine active intervention in spontaneous labour beneficial? Contemporary Review of Obstetrics and Gynaecology 6, 13–17.

Chapter

42 Breech presentation

In this chapter

INTRODUCTION

Any presentation of the fetus other than a vertex is called a **malpresentation**. These include breech, face, brow and shoulder presentations which have in common an ill-fitting presenting part which may be associated with early rupture of the membranes. There is also the likelihood of poor uterine action leading to prolongation of labour. Each malpresentation leads to a different mechanism for descent and there may be difficulties in delivery. An understanding of the movements made by the fetus in response to the maternal pelvis will help to prevent injury to a woman or her baby. The risk of morbidity and mortality for the fetus is increased and malpresentations may result in operative delivery. Breech presentation is discussed in this chapter and the other malpresentations in Chapter 43.

BREECH PRESENTATION

Breech presentation is where the lie is longitudinal but the fetal buttocks lie in the lower segment of the uterus. It is found in 3–4% of all deliveries (Arias 1993, Sweet 1997). One in four fetuses will present by the breech at some stage in pregnancy but as pregnancy progresses spontaneous version to a vertex presentation is likely to occur, especially in multigravidae. Westgren et al (1985) found that this occurred in 57% of pregnancies after 32 weeks and 25% after 36 weeks.

Types of breech presentation

Depending on the relationship of the lower limb to the fetal trunk, four types of breech presentation can be described (Fig. 42.1). This can influence the diagnosis of breech antenatally and the complications likely to occur at delivery.

1 **Complete or flexed breech** The thighs and knees are flexed and the feet close to the buttocks. This type is commonest in multigravidae.
2 **Extended or frank breech** The fetal thighs are flexed and the legs extended at the knees. The legs lie alongside the trunk with the feet near the head. This is the most common of the four types of breech presentation and is seen most commonly in primigravidae near to term. The firm uterine and abdominal muscles prevent fetal movement so that the fetus is unable to flex its knees and there is little likelihood of a turn to cephalic presentation.
3 **Footling presentation** One or both hips and knees are extended and the feet present below the buttocks. This rare complication is more common in preterm labour.
4 **Knee presentation** One or both hips are extended and the knees flexed. The knee(s) present below the buttocks. This is the least common of the four presentations.

As in vertex presentations, the baby presenting by the breech can take up different positions (Figure 42.2).

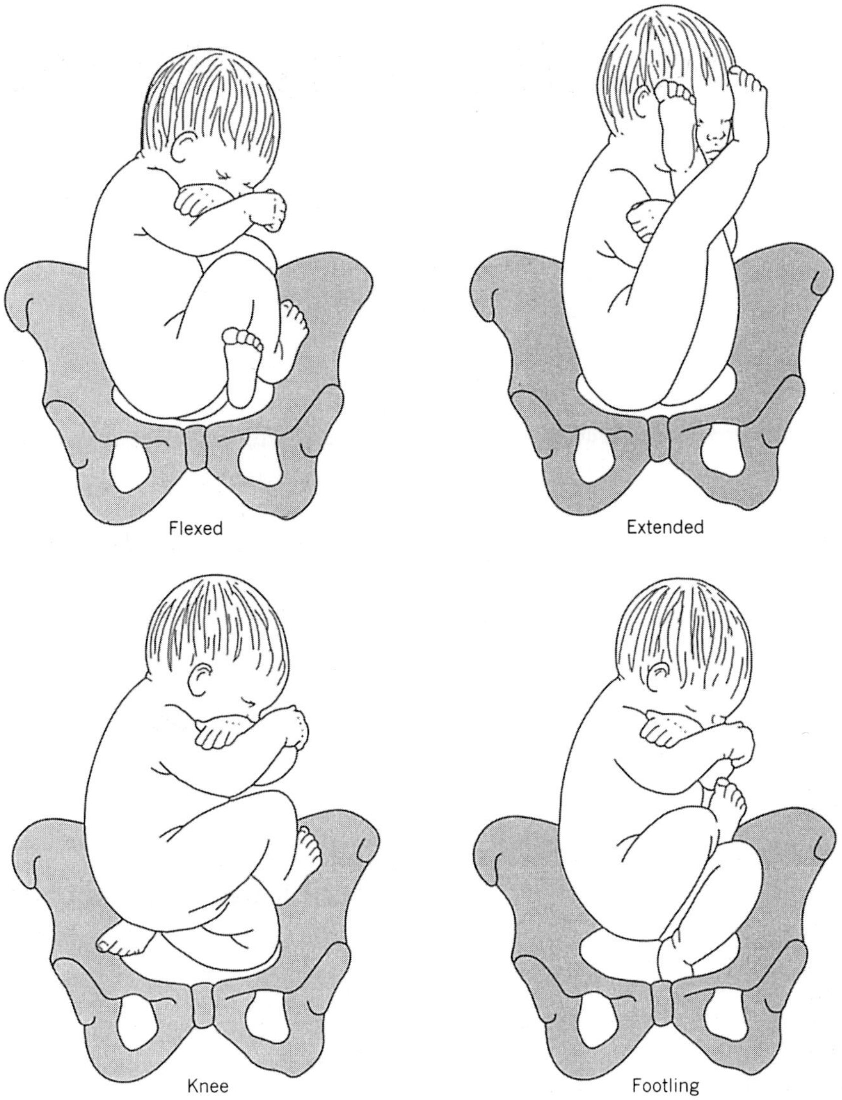

Figure 42.1 *Types of breech presentations (from Sweet B, 1997, with permission).*

Aetiology

Many of the causes of persistent breech presentation are associated with conditions which either restrict or allow excessive movement of the fetus. Others involve the health of the fetus (Table 42.1).

Diagnosis

On discussion

A past history of a previous breech presentation could suggest a uterine anomaly and an increased risk of repeated breech. If the woman complains of discomfort under the ribs it may be due to the presence in the fundus of the hard fetal head. She may also be aware of fetal kicking movements below the umbilicus.

On abdominal examination

- **Inspection**: usually reveals nothing unusual.
- **Palpation**: the presenting part feels firm but not hard or smooth. The head may be felt in the fundus, hard, round and ballottable.
- **Auscultation**: fetal heart sounds may be heard above the umbilicus.

On vaginal examination

A vaginal examination will exclude a deeply engaged head in either pregnancy or labour. It is sometimes difficult to

> Although abdominal examination is the main diagnostic tool it may not be so useful in the primigravid woman with an extended breech. The breech may be deep in the pelvis and simulate an engaged head. Also, the feet lie alongside the head which makes identification by palpation difficult and prevents movement of the head on the neck elicited by ballottment. Also, if the breech is engaged, the fetal heart may be heard in the expected position for a vertex presentation.

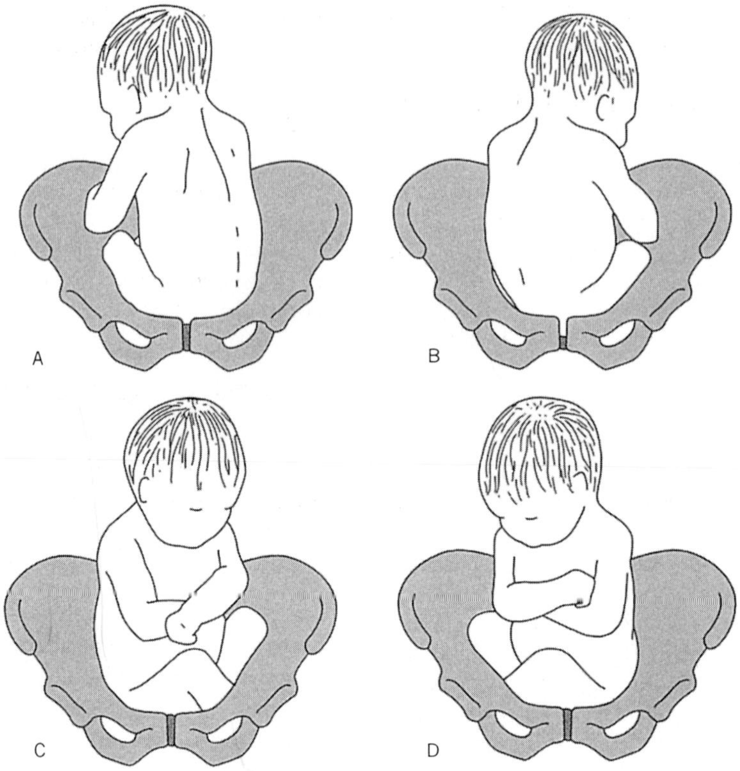

Figure 42.2 *Breech positions. (a) Left sacroanterior. (b) Right sacroanterior. (c) Right sacroposterior. (d) Left sacroposterior (from Sweet B, 1997, with permission).*

Table 42.1 *Possible causes of breech presentation*

Restricted space	*Excessive intrauterine space*	*Fetal causes*
Primigravidae with firm uterine and abdominal muscles	Grand multiparity because of lax uterine and abdominal muscles	Fetal abnormalities
Uterine malformations such as bicornuate uterus	Polyhydramnios	Fetal death in utero
Uterine fibroids		Decreased fetal activity
Contracted pelvis preventing engagement of the presenting part		Impaired fetal growth
Multiple pregnancy		Short umbilical cord
Placenta praevia		
Oligohydramnios		

differentiate the shoulders, which lie at the level of the pelvic brim, from the breech.

Ultrasound scan

Diagnosis in a suspected breech presentation can be made by ultrasound or occasionally by radiography. The fetus should be examined for anomalies at the same time.

Associated risk factors

The increased risk of morbidity and mortality in breech deliveries may be four times that of cephalic presentation but is partly dependent on associated factors. These include prematurity, congenital abnormalities, placenta praevia and placental abruption (Arias 1993). Prolapse of the umbilical cord may lead to anoxia and fetal death, as may entrapment of the fetal head behind an incompletely dilated cervix. The woman is also placed at risk because of the possibility of delivery by CS.

Congenital abnormality

Congenital abnormality occurs more frequently with a breech presentation than with a vertex. The risk of congenital abnormality may be as high as 15% in babies of less than 1500 g (Arias 1993). The most common major abnormality is a defect of the neural tube such as meningomyelocoele, hydrocephaly or anencephaly. Anomalies of the internal organs such as the gastrointestinal, respiratory, cardiovascular and urinary systems are also found. Congenital dislocation of the hip is the most common problem, occurring in three times as many girls as boys.

Risks at delivery

The fetus is at risk from:

- **intrauterine and extrauterine asphyxia**, because of the delay in delivery of the head after the birth of the thorax and arms. Placental separation may occur before the birth is complete and cord compression is inevitable. The hypoxia may stimulate breathing leading to the inhalation of blood, liquor and mucus;

- **intracranial haemorrhage**, which used to be thought to be due to rapid compression and decompression of the brain as the head descended through the pelvis, resulting in a torn tentorium cerebelli. However, it is now thought that the main cause is anoxia and congestion of the cerebral vessels;
- **skeletal fractures and dislocations**, damage to muscles and nerves and rupture of abdominal organs due to difficulties arising during delivery or to faulty delivery technique;
- **genital oedema** and bruising because of the formation of a caput succedaneum.

Long-term problems may possibly include growth hormone deficiency. Albertsson-Wikland et al (1990), cited in Sweet (1997), believe this may be due to brain damage in the hypothalamic-pituitary region but as yet this association has not been confirmed.

MANAGEMENT

Any woman found to have a breech presentation after 32 weeks should be seen by an obstetrician. With her full involvement, a decision needs to be made about the safest option for delivery. An attempt will probably be made to move the fetus to a cephalic presentation to reduce the risks mentioned above.

Cephalic version

Promotion of spontaneous cephalic version

Hofmeyr (1997a) has reviewed the postural techniques 'used by doctors, midwives and birth attendants to promote cephalic version'. He reported Elkins' (1982) study where women were encouraged to maintain a knee-chest position for 15 min every 2 h for 5 days. In 71 women where breech presentation was confirmed by ultrasound after 37 weeks of gestation, 65 proceeded to normal cephalic delivery.

The studies considered by Hofmeyr were:

- Chenia & Crowther (1987), who modified Elkins' procedure asking women to adopt the posture three times a day for 7 days with a full bladder;
- Bung et al (1997), who used a different technique – the 'Indian' version – where women are encouraged to lie down once or twice a day in a supine head-down position with the pelvis supported on a wedge-shaped cushion;
- Hartadottir et al (1992), who carried out a randomised controlled trial in women with a diagnosed breech presentation after 34 weeks. One group were taught how to take up the knee-chest position for 15 min twice a day. The results were compared to a control group of normally managed women.

Because all the trials mentioned above involved women taking up a relaxed position where the pelvis was elevated above the level of the shoulders, Hofmeyr (1997a) combined the findings from the three studies. He concluded that the studies showed a non-significant trend towards a reduction in breech presentation with no measurable effects on the number of CSs carried out or babies born with an Apgar of less than 7 at 1 min. He advised that larger trials are needed to assess the clinical value of postural management of breech presentation.

Moxibustion

Sweet (1997) discusses the findings that 80% of breech presentations after 34 weeks can be corrected by the use of a Chinese acupuncture technique called moxibustion where 'the herb *Artemis vulgaris* (mugwort) is applied to the B67 acupuncture point at the base of the little toenails twice a day for 5 days' (Budd 1992).

External cephalic version

During external cephalic version (ECV) the fetus is manipulated through the abdominal wall to turn it from a breech to a cephalic presentation (Fig. 42.3). This manual manoeuvre has always been controversial, especially if carried out before 36 weeks. There are risks of bleeding from the placental site, cord entanglement, causing fetal distress, converting the lie and presentation to an undeliverable one and initiating preterm labour. To reduce these risks to a minimum, the following contraindications are described.

- A history of infertility
- Elderly primigravidae
- Hypertension
- A rhesus-negative mother
- Cephalopelvic disproportion
- A uterine scar
- Placenta praevia or placental abruption
- Multiple pregnancy
- Congenital malformations
- Intrauterine fetal death

Hofmeyr also reviewed the role of external cephalic version in three separate ways.

1. External cephalic version before term (Hofmeyr 1997b)
2. External cephalic version at term (Hofmeyr 1997c)
3. Routine tocolysis for external cephalic version at term (Hofmeyr 1997d)

The research into the efficacy of preterm ECV demonstrated no significant effect on the incidence of breech presentation, CS, perinatal mortality and Apgar scores below 7 at 1 min. Hofmeyr (1997b) concluded there was no place for ECV before term although its use in spontaneous or induced preterm labour needs evaluating.

Hofmeyr (1997c) found 'compelling evidence that ECV attempt at term materially reduces the chance of non-cephalic birth and CS' and 'In individual cases the risk of ECV needs to be weighed against the current and future risks of continued breech presentation to mother and fetus'.

Tocolysis involves the use of drugs that the uterine musculature, such as salbutamol and ritodrine, prior to carrying out ECV. Hofmeyr (1997d) found no significant support for the routine use of tocolytic agents prior to ECV.

The advantages of delaying ECV until term include (Sweet 1997):

- allowing more time for spontaneous version to occur;

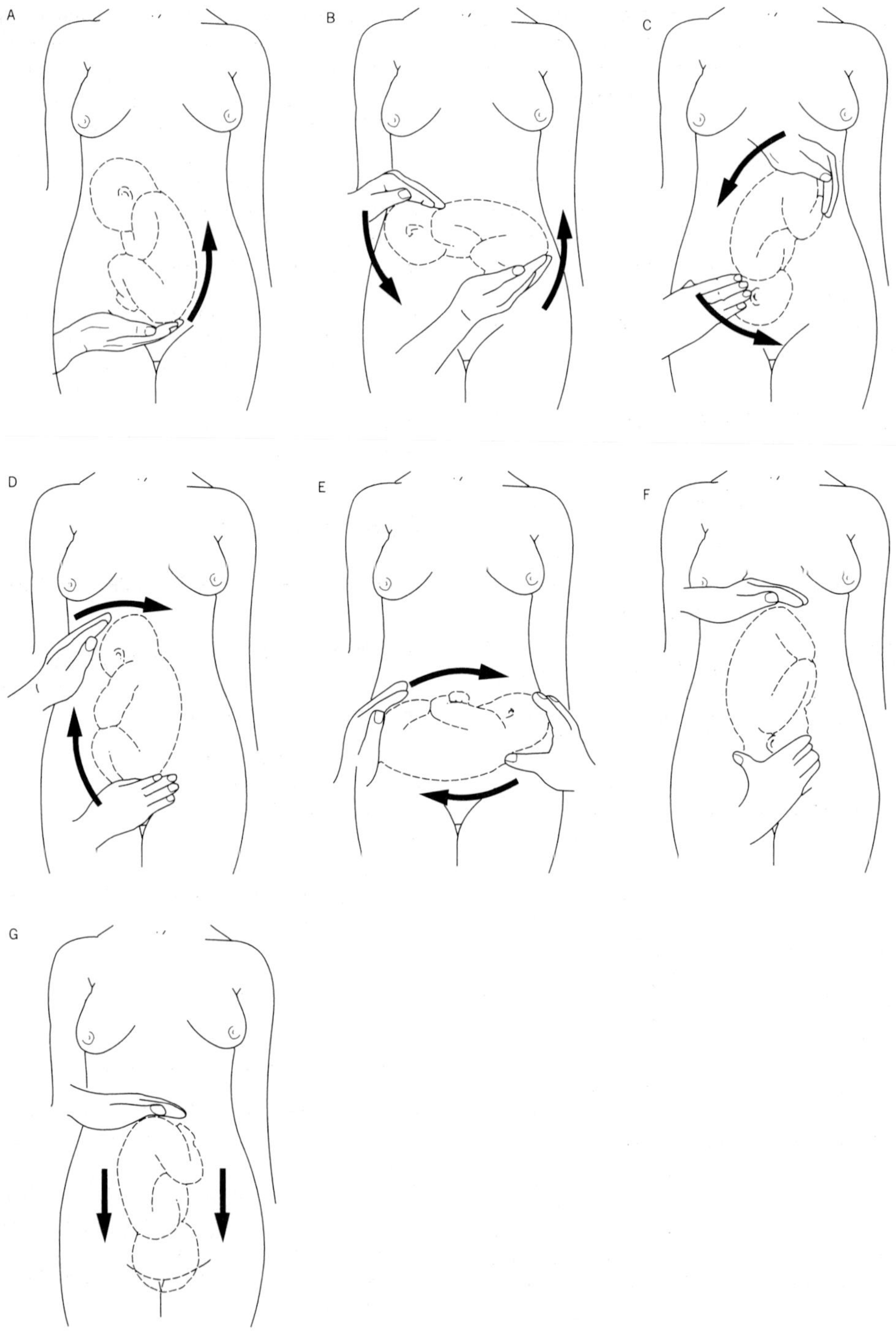

Figure 42.3 *External cephalic version. (a) Palpation and mobilisation of the breech. (b) Manual forward rotation using both hands, one to push the breech and the other to guide the vertex. (c) Completion of forward roll. (d) Backward flip using both hands. (e) Quarter turn accomplished. Continue to push breech upwards and vertex downward. (f) Completion of external version. (g) Gently push the breech downwards to direct vertex into pelvis. (Reproduced with permission from* Clay et al 1993.*)*

- fewer reversions to breech presentation;
- a reduction in fetal mortality;
- other pregnancy complications may become apparent;
- if complications occur the fetus is mature enough to be delivered;
- reducing the incidence of breech deliveries;
- reducing the incidence of CS.

Disadvantages are that the membranes may rupture and labour commence before version is attempted.

The procedure for ECV

The woman is asked to empty her bladder and she then lies flat on a couch or bed. A cardiotocography reading of the fetal heart may be obtained prior to the procedure. A tocolytic drug may be used. Talcum powder is sprinkled over the abdomen. The obstetrician disimpacts the breech from the pelvis and then, applying pressure to both poles of the fetus, rotates it into a cephalic presentation. It is safer to achieve this by making the fetus turn a forward somersault or 'follow its nose', as the author's tutor used to say. A backward somersault may sometimes achieve the version more easily but there is a risk of extension of the neck, resulting in a brow presentation. On completion of the manoeuvre the fetal heart should be recorded for 30 min to ensure there is no fetal distress. Uterine contractions, signs of rupture of the membranes and any vaginal bleeding are watched for and reported immediately.

The role of planned caesarean section at term

Over the last 20 years it has been accepted that CS should be the mode of delivery for fetuses presenting by the breech (Hannah & Hannah 1996) but few studies have been carried out to evaluate this use of planned CS. Hofmeyr (1997e) reviewed two studies on elective CS at term for frank breeches (Collea et al 1980) and non-frank breeches (Gimovsky et al 1983). He found the studies to be too small to make clear statements about the role of CS in these cases. However, in the combined results of the studies, there was a trend to reduce short-term perinatal morbidity but an increase in maternal morbidity. Hofmeyr suggests the need for larger studies to clarify the issues involved in planned CS policies for breech presentation at term.

Hannah & Hannah (1996) suggest that the results of Hofmeyr's metaanalysis do not support policies of planned CS. They undertook a systematic review comparing the outcomes of planned CS and planned vaginal birth and found significantly lower perinatal mortality and neonatal morbidity with the planned CS over the planned vaginal deliveries. The question of which method of delivery is safest for mother and baby is still unanswered and Hannah & Hannah (1996) suggest more research is needed.

In a study of long-term outcomes of children with breech presentation at term, Danelian et al (1996) reviewed data on preschool children and found that planned delivery by CS was not associated with better long-term outcomes. A handicap rate of 19.4% in 1387 children whose records were available was present in both CS and vaginal delivery groups, suggesting that planned vaginal delivery is as safe as elective CS when long-term outcome is considered. A further problem is that as more breech babies are delivered by CS, practitioners lose their skills, thus endangering the fetus. What appears to be more certain is the role of elective CS in the delivery of the preterm breech. A trend towards increased risk of neonatal death has been found when the baby weighs less than 1750 g (Kiely 1991) and 1600 g (Gilady et al 1996.) Babies with birth weights over 3000 g are also at risk.

VAGINAL DELIVERY

In the event of a persistent breech presentation vaginal delivery may be attempted after consideration of the following factors (Sweet 1997).

- **Maternal age and par**
  parity have increased
  1991).
- **Period of gestation** –
- The **history of the** p
  obstetric or medical
- **Past obstetric histor**
- **Size and shape of t**
  fetus.
- The **condition of t**

If women are selecte
dimensions in relation to the ...
adverse factors, they should be able to deliv...
vaginam. It is essential to understand the mechanism of a breech delivery so that management of the delivery can be completed without trauma.

Management

The mechanism of a breech delivery

There are six possible positions for a breech delivery. These are right or left sacroanterior, right or left sacroposterior, right or left sacrolateral. The mechanism of the left sacroanterior position will be described in full.

- The **lie** is longitudinal.
- The **presentation** is breech.
- The **denominator** is the sacrum.
- The **attitude** is one of complete flexion.
- The **presenting part** is the anterior (left) buttock.
- The **bitrochanteric diameter**, 10 cm, enters the pelvis in the left oblique diameter of the pelvic brim.

The movements

It is necessary to consider the birth of the fetus in three parts: the buttocks, the shoulders and the head.

1. **Compaction and flexion** Descent takes place with increasing compaction due to increased flexion of the limbs on the trunk.
2. **Internal rotation of the buttocks** The anterior buttock reaches the pelvic floor and rotates forwards in the pelvis one-eighth of a circle to lie under the symphysis pubis. The bitrochanteric diameter now lies in the anteroposterior diameter of the pelvis.
3. **Lateral flexion of the trunk** The anterior buttock escapes under the symphysis pubis, the posterior buttock sweeps the perineum and the buttocks are born by a movement of lateral flexion (Fig. 42.4).
4. **Restitution** The anterior buttock turns slightly to the mother's right side.
5. **Internal rotation of the shoulders** With the birth of the buttocks, the bisacromial diameter (11 cm) of the shoulders enters the pelvis in the same diameter as the buttocks, the left oblique. The anterior (left) shoulder reaches the pelvic floor and rotates forwards one-eighth of a circle to lie behind the symphysis pubis.
6. **Birth of the shoulders** The anterior shoulder and arm

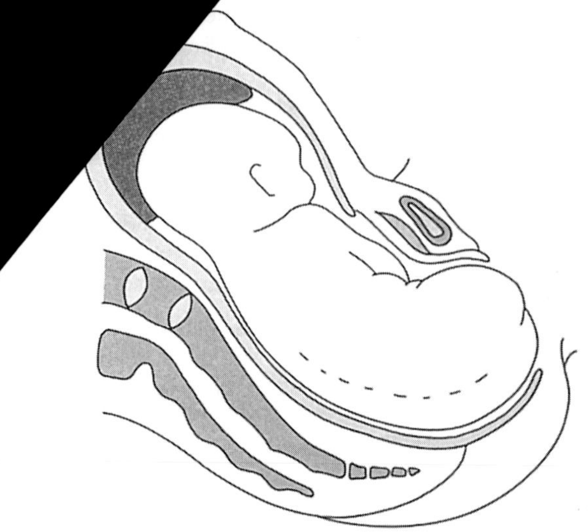

Figure 42.4 *Lateral flexion and birth of the buttocks (from Sweet B, 1997, with permission).*

escape under the symphysis pubis and the posterior shoulder and arm pass over the perineum.

7 **Internal rotation and delivery of the head** The flexed head engages with the suboccipitobregmatic diameter of 9.5 cm or the suboccipitofrontal diameter of 10 cm lying in the right oblique or transverse diameter of the pelvic brim. Internal rotation of the head carries the occiput behind the symphysis pubis. The face lies in the hollow of the sacrum. Internal rotation of the head is accompanied by external rotation of the trunk. The chin, face, vertex and occiput are born over the perineum by a movement of flexion.

First stage

The first stage does not differ from normal labour. However, the risks of the delivery mean that the birth should take place in a consultant unit with an anaesthetist and paediatrician available. Labour is normally induced at term and some obstetricians prefer to induce labour at 38 weeks when the fetus will be smaller. If the breech is flexed and not engaged, there may be early rupture of the membranes with the risk of prolapse of the umbilical cord. If the legs are extended the breech is likely to be engaged and the risk of cord prolapse is minimal.

The woman may be ambulant if the breech is engaged and continuous monitoring of the fetus should be undertaken.

Epidural analgesia can be useful as pain relief and because it prevents the desire to push too early, when the buttocks slip through the incompletely dilated cervical os with a risk of entrapment of the head. However, Chadha et al (1992) found that the contractions in both first and 2nd stages of labour decrease in intensity following the commencement of epidural analgesia. This appeared to increase the frequency of breech extraction (see below) or CS and its use is not advocated by all. Epidural analgesia top-ups can be managed to ensure that the woman is able to bear down when requested.

Second stage

The woman must be encouraged not to push until the cervix is confirmed as fully dilated by vaginal examination. The delivery will be conducted by an experienced obstetrician who usually prefers the woman's legs to be placed in lithotomy position for the actual delivery. All midwives should be familiar with the manoeuvres necessary to deliver the baby in case of an emergency. Simulated practice is essential. An anaesthetist and paediatrician should be present at the delivery in case of a sudden need for intervention.

Breech delivery may be spontaneous with little help needed, usually in a multigravida or with a preterm baby, or assisted where the manoeuvres are performed to assist the birth of the baby. Breech extraction may occasionally be necessary where the fetus is extracted from the birth canal by manipulation rather than assisting the normal mechanism. This is dangerous and not often used in developed countries.

Assisted breech delivery

The buttocks

The woman's bladder is emptied prior to commencement. The perineum is infiltrated with local anaesthetic and an episiotomy is performed when the posterior buttock distends the perineum. No handling is necessary until the baby is born as far as the umbilicus. If the legs have not slipped out they should be carefully delivered. Unless the cord is under obvious tension there is no need to pull down a loop.

The shoulders

With the next contraction, the shoulder blades appear. If the arms are flexed across the chest they should be slipped out and the shoulders are born.

The head

There are two alternative methods for delivering the head: the Burns-Marshall manoeuvre (Fig. 42.5) and the Mauriceau-Smellie-Veit manoeuvre (Fig. 42.6).

Burns-Marshall

The baby is allowed to hang by his own weight to encourage descent and flexion of the head, taking care not to let the baby's head deliver suddenly. Once the nape of the neck and hairline can be seen, the baby's ankles are grasped and with slight traction the trunk is carried in a wide arc up over the mother's abdomen. The other hand should support the perineum to prevent sudden delivery of the head. Once the mouth is clear the baby can breathe and time should be taken to complete the delivery of the cranium.

Mauriceau-Smellie-Veit

This method, also described as jaw flexion-shoulder traction, allows good control of the head and is easier if the practitioner is small. It can also be used to deliver the head if there is extension and delay.

The practitioner straddles the baby across one arm, usually the left in a right-handed person, and inserts three fingers of the other hand into the mother's vagina. The head can now be

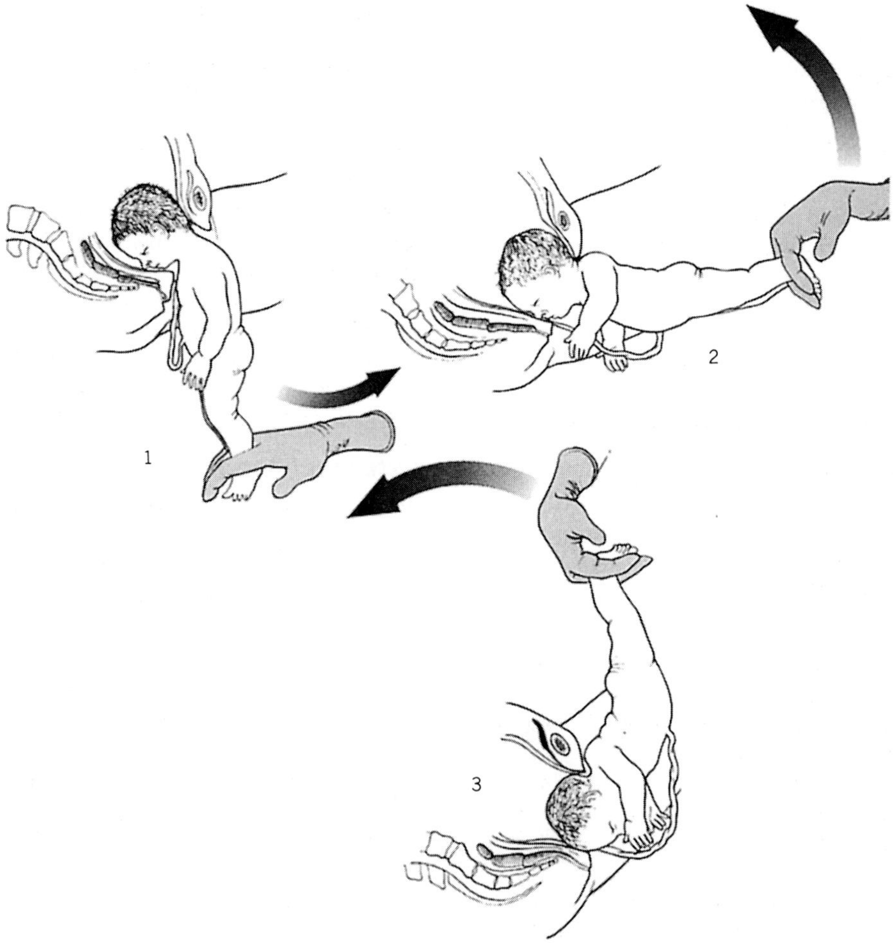

Figure 42.5 *The Burns-Marshall manoeuvre (from Sweet B, 1997, with permission).*

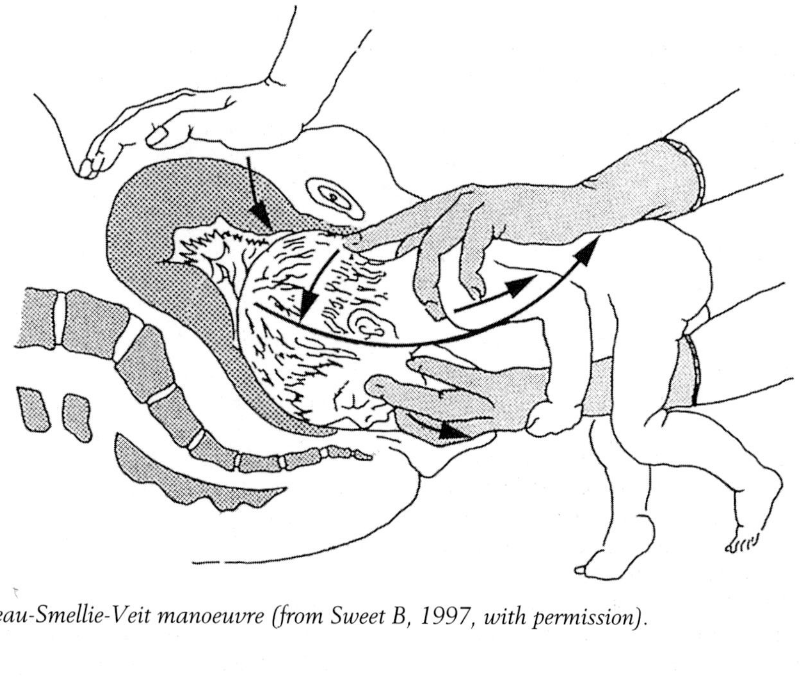

Figure 42.6 *The Mauriceau-Smellie-Veit manoeuvre (from Sweet B, 1997, with permission).*

flexed if necessary. The middle finger is placed in the baby's mouth and the other two fingers are placed on his cheek bones. An assistant can apply suprapubic pressure if necessary. The outer two fingers are now hooked over the baby's shoulders and the middle finger presses on the occiput to maintain flexion. The baby's head is carefully delivered following the curve of the birth canal.

Sweet (1997) advises a midwife conducting a breech delivery to remember a golden rule: '**Flexion before traction**'.

Extended legs

If the legs are extended they may splint the body and prevent lateral flexion of the trunk. Gentle traction is applied with a finger in each of the baby's groins until it is possible to see the back of the knees. Popliteal pressure is applied to abduct and flex the knees.

Extended arms

If the baby's arms cannot be found crossed over the chest they may be extended alongside the head, making the total diameter of the presenting part too large to descend into the pelvis. This often happens when the breech is pulled on to deliver the legs and trunk. The arms must be brought down before the head can be delivered and this is done by Lövset's manoeuvre (Fig. 42.7). The success of the manoeuvre arises from the relative positions of the two shoulders. The posterior shoulder is below the sacral promontory whilst the anterior shoulder is above the symphysis pubis.

The obstetrician grasps the baby's thighs with his thumbs placed over the sacrum. The baby is pulled gently downwards while the back is kept uppermost. The baby is rotated through 180° to bring the posterior shoulder to the anterior position but beneath the symphysis pubis. Friction of the arm against the pelvic walls will bring the arm down and it can be released. The manoeuvre is repeated in the opposite direction and the second arm released.

Extended head

If the hairline does not become visible after a few seconds of allowing the baby to hang by its weight, the head is probably extended. Forceps are usually used to deliver the head but the Mauriceau-Smellie-Veit manoeuvre may be used if the midwife has to conduct the delivery.

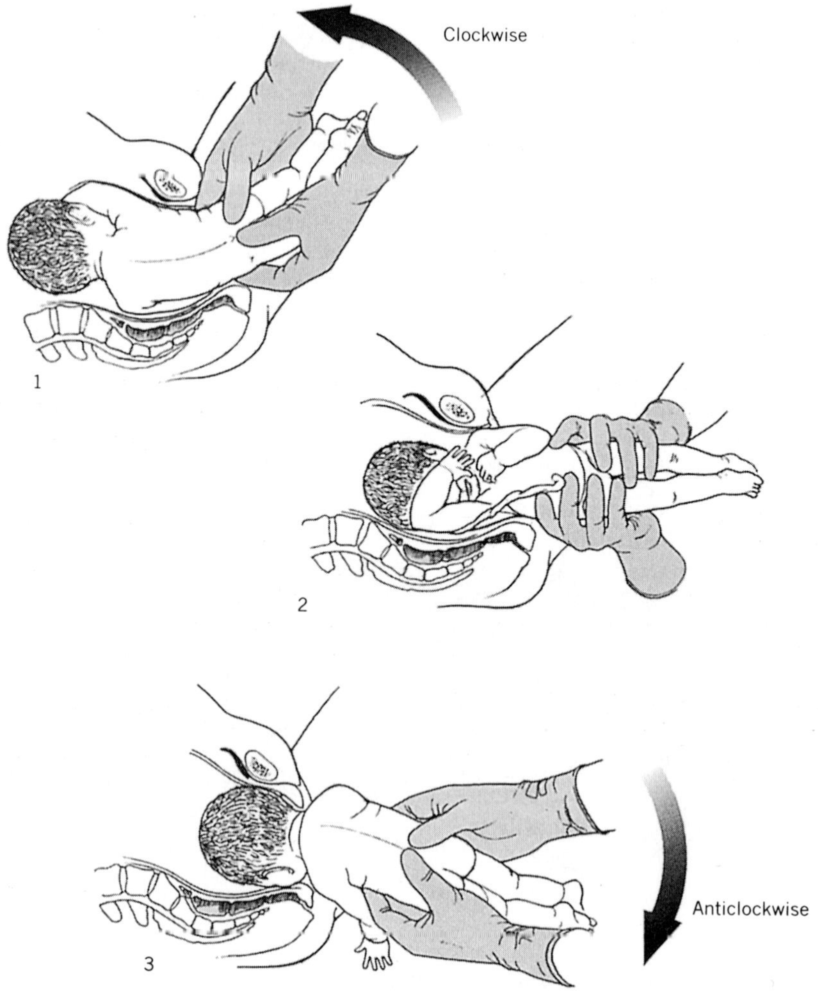

Figure 42.7 *Birth of the arms using Lövset's manoeuvre (from Sweet B, 1997, with permission).*

Entrapment of the fetal head

This dangerous situation arises when the fetal body slips through an incompletely dilated cervix and the head is trapped behind the cervix. In the immediate absence of medical aid it may be possible to make an airway for the baby by placing fingers or a Simm's speculum in the vagina, thus holding maternal tissues away from the baby's mouth and nose.

The obstetrician will try to release the baby's head from the cervix and one method that may help is McRobert's manoeuvre (Sweet 1997), which is also useful in the delivery of a fetus with shoulder dystocia. The woman lies on her back, lifts her knees up to her chest and raises her buttocks off the bed. Arias (1993) stated that 'There is no adequate description in the literature of the incidence, methods of management and outcome of infants when the fetal head is entrapped during a breech delivery'. He suggested incisions into the cervix as the quickest way of freeing the head, although these are known to extend into the lower segment and cause cervical incompetence. He also suggested trying an injection of diazoxide or other drugs to relax the cervix. However, mortality and morbidity rates for the neonate are high.

Undiagnosed cephalopelvic disproportion

In an unbooked woman or where there has been failure to diagnose a degree of hydrocephaly, this dire emergency may arise as the delivery proceeds. If the breech is delivered up to the head, it is usually difficult to perform a CS. Symphysiotomy may save the baby's life.

Posterior rotation of the occiput

This rare complication is usually due to mismanagement so that the back of the baby is turned towards the mother's buttocks. To deliver the head, the chin and face are allowed to escape under the symphysis pubis as far as the root of the nose, then the baby is lifted towards the mother's abdomen to allow the occiput to sweep the perineum.

Summary of main points

- One in four fetuses will present by the breech at some stage in pregnancy but spontaneous version to a vertex presentation is likely to occur, especially in multigravidae. Depending on the relationship of the lower limb to the fetal trunk, breech presentation may be complete or flexed, extended or frank, footling or knee presentation.
- Many of the causes of persistent breech presentation are associated with conditions which either restrict or allow excessive movement of the fetus. Others involve the health of the fetus, for example an open neural tube defect.
- There is an increased risk of morbidity and mortality in breech deliveries. Associated factors include prematurity, congenital abnormalities, placenta praevia and placental abruption, prolapse of the umbilical cord and entrapment of the fetal head behind an incompletely dilated cervix. The woman is also placed at risk during CS.
- At delivery, the fetus is at risk from asphyxia, intracranial haemorrhage, skeletal fractures and dislocations, damage to muscles and nerves and rupture of abdominal organs, genital oedema and bruising. Long-term problems are thought to include growth hormone deficiency.
- Any woman found to have a breech presentation after 32 weeks should be seen by an obstetrician. A decision needs to be made with her about the safest option for delivery. External cephalic version may be attempted. Postural techniques used to promote cephalic version may reduce the numbers of term breech presentations but not the number of CSs carried out or babies born with an Apgar of less than 7 at 1 min.
- Risks of external cephalic version include bleeding from the placental site, cord entanglement, fetal distress, converting the lie and presentation to an undeliverable one and initiating preterm labour. There are no findings supporting the use of tocolytic drugs prior to carrying out ECV.
- The advantages of delaying ECV until term include allowing more time for spontaneous version to occur, fewer reversions to breech presentation and a reduction in fetal mortality. Other pregnancy complications which would exclude ECV may become apparent. Disadvantages are that the membranes may rupture and labour commence before version is attempted.
- Over the last 20 years it has been accepted that CS should be the mode of delivery for fetuses presenting by the breech. However, the combined results of studies demonstrated reduction in perinatal morbidity but an increase in maternal morbidity. There is a definite advantage in elective CS for the delivery of the preterm breech.
- Carefully selected women with pelves of adequate dimensions in relation to the fetus and with no other adverse factors should be able to deliver a baby presenting by the breech safely per vaginam. The risks of the delivery mean that the birth should take place in a consultant unit. Labour is normally induced at term and some obstetricians prefer to induce labour at 38 weeks when the fetus will be smaller. If the breech is flexed and not engaged, there may be early rupture of the membranes with the risk of prolapse of the umbilical cord.
- Epidural analgesia can be useful as pain relief because it prevents the desire to push before full cervical dilatation. In the 2nd stage full cervical dilatation is confirmed by vaginal examination. The delivery will be conducted by an experienced practitioner. All midwives should be familiar with the manoeuvres necessary to deliver the baby in case of an emergency.
- An anaesthetist and paediatrician should be present at the delivery in case of a sudden need for intervention. There are two alternative methods for delivering the head: the Burns-Marshall manoeuvre and the Mauriceau-Smellie-Veit manoeuvre. Dangerous but rare complications such as entrapment of the fetal head, late diagnosis of cephalopelvic disproportion and posterior rotation of the occiput may lead to fetal death.

References

Albertsson-Wikland K, Niklasson A, Karlberg OP. 1990 Birth data for patients who develop GHD: preliminary analysis of a national register. Acta Paediatrica Scandinavica 370 (Suppl), 115–120.

Arias F. 1993 Practical Guide to High Risk Pregnancy and Delivery, 2nd edn. Mosby Year Book, Chicago.

Budd S. 1992 Traditional Chinese medicine in obstetrics. Midwives' Chronicle 105 (1253), 140–143.

Bung P, Huch R, Huch A. 1997 Is Indian version a successful method of lowering the frequency of breech presentations? Geburtshilfe Frauenheilkd 47, 202–205.

Chadha YC, Mahmood TA, Dick MJ, Smith NC, Campbell DM, Templeton A. 1992 Breech delivery and epidural analgesia. British Journal of Obstetrics and Gynaecology 99, 96–100.

Chenia F, Crowther CA. 1987 Does advice to assume a knee-chest position reduce the incidence of breech presentation at delivery? A randomised clinical trial. Birth 14, 75–78.

Collea JV, Chein C, Quilligan EJ. 1980 The randomised management of term frank breech presentation: a study of 208 cases. American Journal of Obstetrics and Gynecology 137, 235–244.

Danelian PJ, Wang J, Hall MH. 1996 Long-term outcome of term breech presentation by method of delivery. British Medical Journal 312 (7044), 1451–1453.

Elkins VH. 1982 Materials and methods used in synthesizing evidence to evaluate the effects of care during pregnancy and childbirth. In Enkins M, Chalmers I (eds) Effectiveness and Satisfaction in Antenatal Care. Spastics International Medical Publishers, London, p 216.

Gilady Y, Battino S, Reich D et al. 1996 Elective Caesarean Section in the Delivery of the Preterm Breech. Israel Journal of Medical Sciences 32(2), 116–120.

Gimovsky ML, Wallace RL, Schifrin BS, Paul RH. 1983 Randomised management of the non-frank breech presentation at term: a preliminary report. American Journal of Obstetrics and Gynecology 146, 34–40.

Hannah M, Hannah W. 1996 CS or vaginal birth for breech presentation at term? British Medical Journal 312 (7044), 1433–1434.

Hartadottir H, Thornton JG. 1992 A randomised trial of the knee-chest position to encourage spontaneous version of breech pregnancies. Proceedings of the 26th British Congress of Obstetrics and Gynaecology, Manchester, UK, p 356.

Hofmeyr GJ. 1997a Cephalic version by postural management. In Neilson LJ, Crowther CA, Hodnett ED, Hofmeyr GJ, Keirse MJNC (eds) Pregnancy and Childbirth module of the Cochrane Database of Systematic Reviews, The Cochrane Library. Update Software, Oxford.

Hofmeyr GJ. 1997b External cephalic version before term. In Neilson LJ, Crowther CA, Hodnett ED, Hofmeyr GJ, Keirse MJNC (eds) Pregnancy and Childbirth module of the Cochrane Database of Systematic Reviews, The Cochrane Library. Update Software, Oxford.

Hofmeyr GJ. 1997c External cephalic version at term. In Neilson LJ, Crowther C A, Hodnett ED, Hofmeyr GJ, Keirse MJNC (eds) Pregnancy and Childbirth module of the Cochrane Database of Systematic Reviews, The Cochrane Library. Update Software, Oxford.

Hofmeyr GJ. 1997d Routine tocolysis for external cephalic version at term. In Neilson LJ, Crowther CA, Hodnett ED, Hofmeyr GJ, Keirse MJNC (eds) Pregnancy and Childbirth module of the Cochrane Database of Systematic Reviews. The Cochrane Library. Update Software, Oxford.

Hofmeyr GJ. 1997e Planned elective CS for breech presentation. In Neilson LJ, Crowther CA, Hodnett ED, Hofmeyr GJ, Keirse MJNC (eds) Pregnancy and Childbirth module of the Cochrane Database of Systematic Reviews, The Cochrane Library. Update Software, Oxford.

Kiely JL. 1991 Mode of delivery and neonatal death in 17587 infants presenting by the breech. British Journal of Obstetrics and Gynaecology 98 (9), 898–904.

Roumen FJ, Luyben AG. 1991 Safety of term vaginal breech delivery. European Journal of Obstetrics, Gynaecology and Reproductive Biology 40 (3), 171–177.

Sweet BR. 1997 Malpresentations. In Sweet BR with Tiran D (eds) Mayes Midwifery, 12th edn. Baillière Tindall, London, pp 631–657.

Westgren M, Edvall H, Nordstrom E, Svalenius E. 1985 Spontaneous cephalic version of breech presentation in the last trimester. British Journal of Obstetrics and Gynaecology 92, 19–22.

Recommended reading

Chenia F, Crowther CA. 1987 Does advice to assume a knee-chest position reduce the incidence of breech presentation at delivery? A randomised clinical trial. Birth 14, 75–78.

Collea JV, Chein C, Quilligan EJ. 1980 The randomised management of term frank breech presentation: a study of 208 cases. American Journal of Obstetrics and Gynecology 137, 235–244.

Hannah M, Hannah W. 1996 CS or vaginal birth for breech presentation at term. British Medical Journal 312 (7044), 1433–1434.

Hofmeyr GJ. 1997b External cephalic version before term. In Neilson LJ, Crowther CA, Hodnett ED, Hofmeyr GJ, Keirse MJNC (eds) Pregnancy and Childbirth module of the Cochrane Database of Systematic Reviews, The Cochrane Library. Update Software, Oxford.

Hofmeyr GJ. 1997c External cephalic version at term. In Neilson LJ, Crowther CA, Hodnett ED, Hofmeyr GJ, Keirse MJNC (eds) Pregnancy and Childbirth module of the Cochrane Database of Systematic Reviews, The Cochrane Library. Update Software, Oxford.

Hofmeyr GJ. 1997e Planned elective CS for breech presentation. In Neilson LJ, Crowther CA, Hodnett ED, Hofmeyr GJ, Keirse MJNC (eds) Pregnancy and Childbirth module of the Cochrane Database of Systematic Reviews, The Cochrane Library. Update Software, Oxford.

Kiely JL. 1991 Mode of delivery and neonatal death in 17587 infants presenting by the breech. British Journal of Obstetrics and Gynaecology 98 (9), 898–904.

Roumen FJ, Luyben AG. 1991 Safety of term vaginal breech delivery. European Journal of Obstetrics, Gynaecology and Reproductive Biology 40 (3), 171–177.

Chapter 43

Malposition and cephalic malpresentations

In this chapter

INTRODUCTION

If the vertex is the denominator in a cephalic presentation the term malpresentation is not used. The correct word to use for occipitoposterior position of the vertex is **malposition**. True cephalic malpresentations are face and brow. Shoulder presentation resulting from oblique or transverse lie is a rare but dangerous event. Each of these situations may affect the length and outcome of the labour and require vigilance to prevent maternal and fetal morbidity and, rarely, mortality. The more common occipitoposterior position will be discussed first as it may lead to secondary brow or face presentation.

OCCIPITOPOSTERIOR POSITION OF THE VERTEX

In occipitoposterior position of the vertex, the occiput occupies one or other of the posterior quadrants of the mother's pelvis and the sinciput points towards the opposite anterior quadrant (Fig. 43.1). Malposition is common and affects about 10% of all labours. Although the outcome of such labours is generally normal with rotation of the occiput to the anterior and normal vertex delivery, there may be prolonged labour and mechanical difficulties associated with the delivery (Sweet 1997).

Causes

There is no single satisfactory cause for occipitoposterior position. However, if the forepelvis is small, as found in android and anthropoid pelves, the head may take up a posterior position. Sweet (1997) mentions other possible causes of a pendulous abdomen, a flat sacrum or an anterior placenta.

Attitude

Instead of the normal well-flexed attitude with the limbs and head flexed on the trunk and the rounded back pointing towards the mother's soft abdominal wall, the fetal spine faces

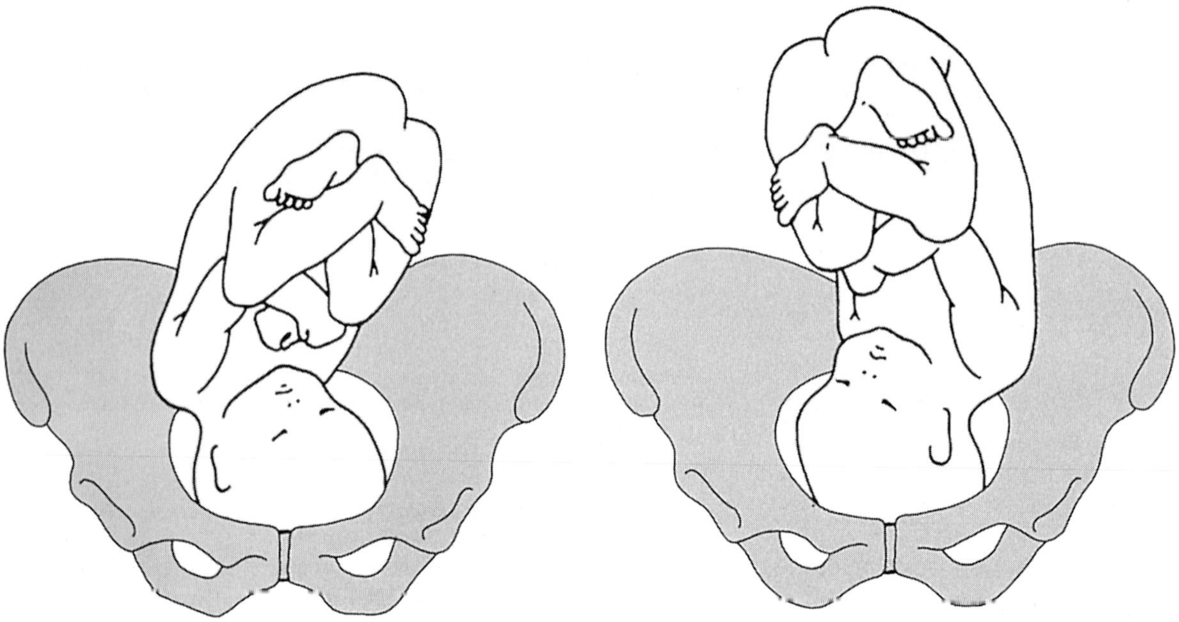

Figure 43.1 *Right and left occipitoposterior positions (from Sweet B, 1997, with permission).*

the forward curve of the maternal lumbar spine and good flexion is not possible. The fetal spine is straightened, the head is held in a deflexed position known as the **military position** and the anterior fontanelle is found directly over the internal os. The term bregmatic presentation is sometimes used (Sweet 1997). This position of the head brings larger diameters into relationship with the pelvic brim and engagement of the head may not occur.

Risks (Williams 1996)

- Obstructed labour if either deep transverse arrest or brow presentation result.
- Maternal perineal trauma such as a 3rd-degree tear and bruising.
- Cord prolapse if there is early spontaneous rupture of the membranes.
- Neonatal cerebral haemorrhage due to upward moulding of the fetal skull. The falx cerebri may be pulled away from the tentorium cerebelli, resulting in a tear of the great vein of Galen. Chronic hypoxia, if present, results in venous distension which increases the likelihood of haemorrhage.

Diagnosis in pregnancy

Occipitoposterior position is the commonest cause of a non-engaged head in late pregnancy in primigravidae. The woman may complain that the baby has too many hands and feet and that she is having to pass urine more frequently in the absence of infection (El Halta 1996). Abdominal examination will point to the diagnosis.

- **On inspection** – the abdomen appears flattened. There may be a saucer-shaped depression below the umbilicus between the fetal head and limbs (Fig. 43.2).
- **On palpation** – the fetal head is high and deflexed. It may feel large if the occiput is more lateral but small if the occiput is quite posterior and the bitemporal diameter is palpated. Fetal limbs may be felt on both sides of the midline of the uterus and the fetal back may be felt out in the flank (Fig. 43.3).

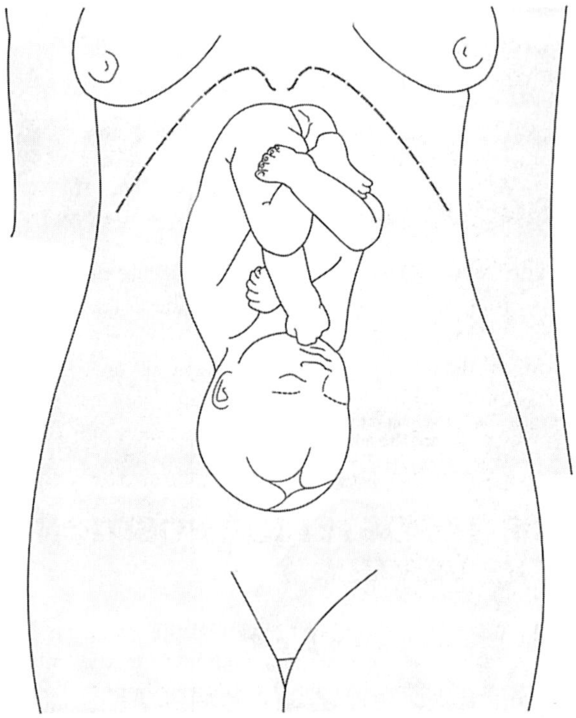

Figure 43.2 *In occipitoposterior positions the anterior shoulder is well out from the midline and fetal limbs are readily palpable. This may cause a mistaken diagnosis of multiple pregnancy. (Reproduced with permission from Beischer & Mackay 1986 Obstetrics and the Newborn. Baillière Tindall, London.)*

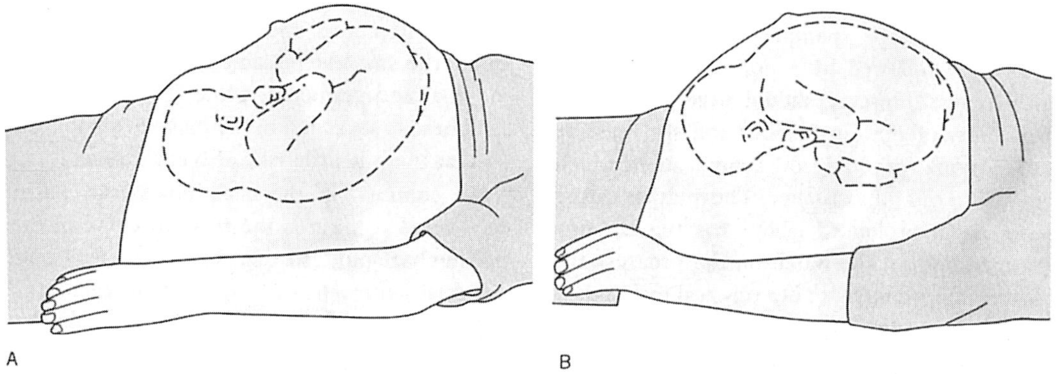

Figure 43.3 *(a) Abdominal contour with occipitoposterior position, showing depression at umbilicus. (b) Rounded abdominal contour with occipitoanterior position (from Sweet B, 1997, with permission).*

- **On auscultation** – the fetal heart may be heard at or just above the umbilicus or out in one flank.

Diagnosis in labour

Abdominal examination, as described above, will indicate the presence of an occipitoposterior position although the head may have flexed and engaged.

On **vaginal examination**, palpation of the anterior fontanelle is likely. If the head is reasonably well flexed the anterior fontanelle will be felt anteriorly and it may be possible to feel the posterior fontanelle. When the head is deflexed the anterior fontanelle is almost central and easy to feel by its shape and size (Fig. 43.4).

First stage

The course of labour partly depends on the degree of descent and flexion that takes place (Fig. 43.5). This in turn is influenced by the strength of uterine contractions. If the head flexes, it is likely that labour will proceed normally. The engaging diameter is the suboccipitofrontal of 10 cm. When the occiput reaches the pelvic floor it rotates three-eighths of a circle and the baby is born with the occiput anterior.

If the head remains deflexed, problems may arise. The engaging diameter is the occipitofrontal which measures 11.5 cm. The head may be non-engaged at the commencement of labour and early rupture of the membranes may happen. Because the presenting part is high and not well applied to the cervix, there is a risk of cord prolapse.

Labour is prolonged because of poor stimulation of the cervix and dilatation is slow and uneven. Contractions may be excessive but uncoordinated and painful and the woman experiences severe backache. Encouraging the mother to take up a knee-chest position for 45 min may help rotation of the vertex to an anterior position (El Halta 1996). Augmentation of labour may be necessary (see Chapter 41). Care must be taken to prevent maternal loss of confidence, ketosis and dehydration and fetal distress. There may be difficulty in micturition with retention of urine and the woman needs encouragement to empty her bladder frequently. Catheterisation may be necessary.

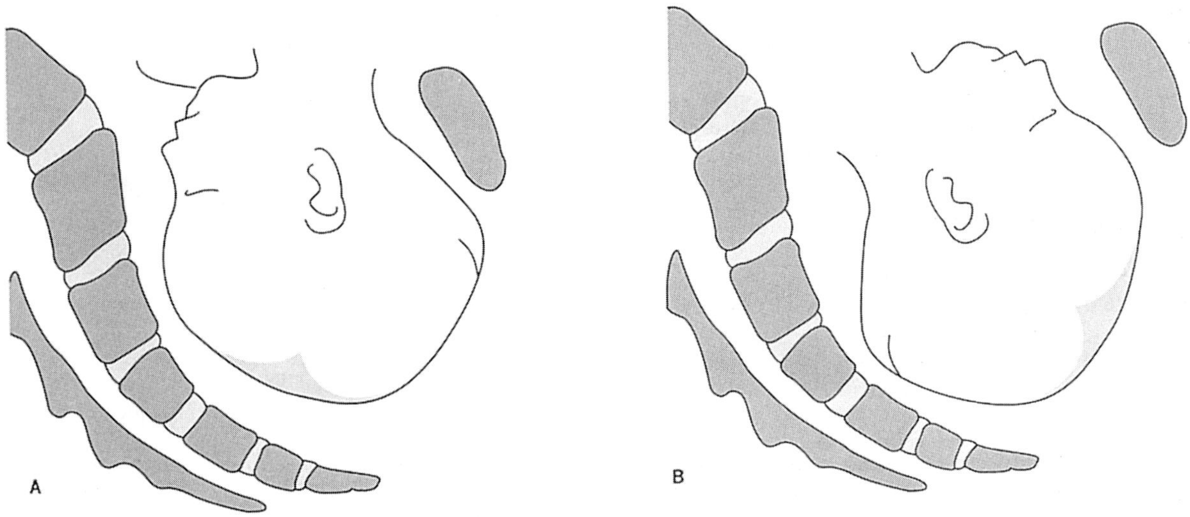

Figure 43.4 *Position of the anterior and posterior fontanelles. (a) Occipitoanterior. (b) Occipitoposterior (from Sweet B, 1997, with permission).*

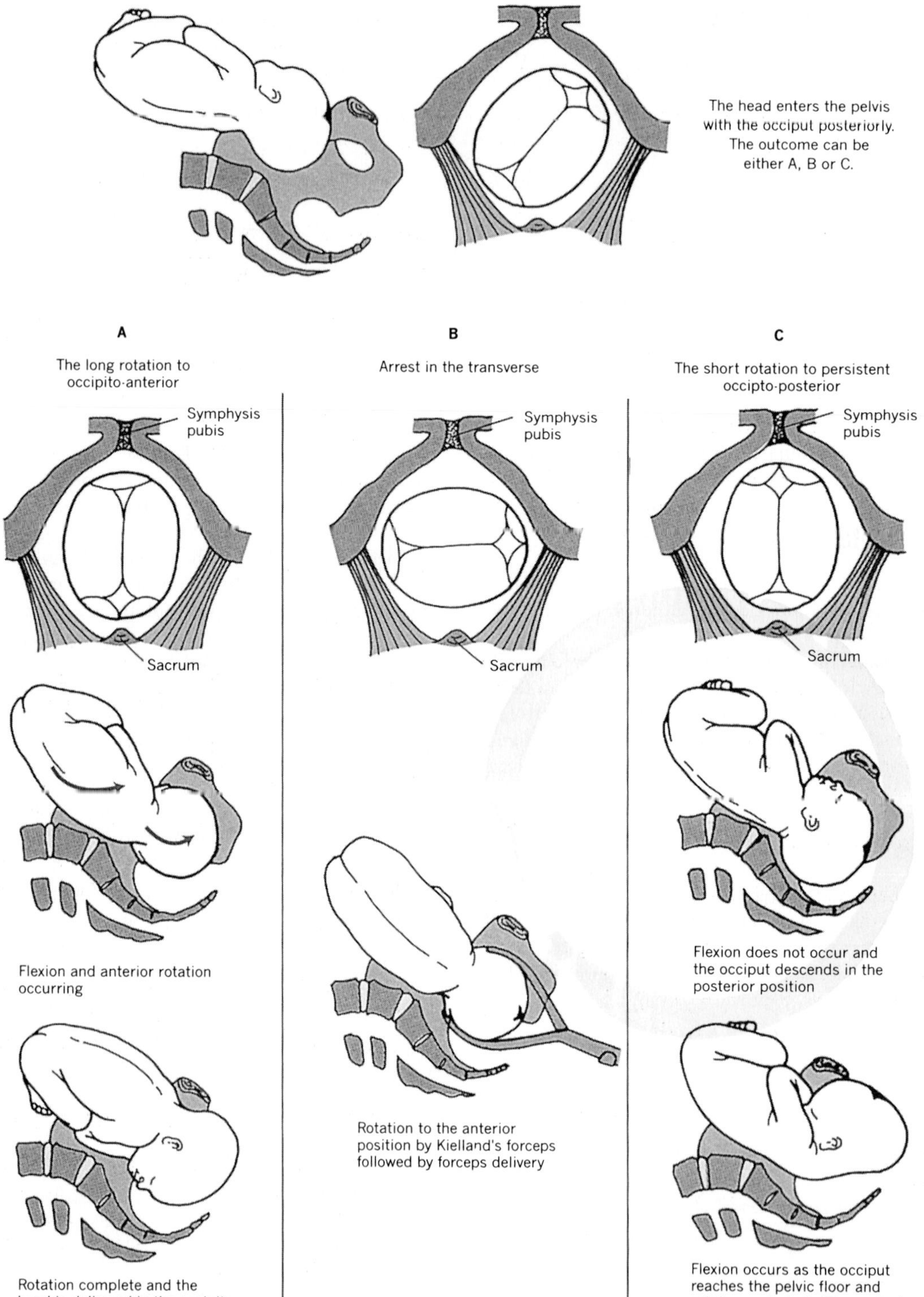
The head enters the pelvis with the occiput posteriorly. The outcome can be either A, B or C.
A
The long rotation to occipito-anterior
Symphysis pubis
Sacrum
Flexion and anterior rotation occurring
Rotation complete and the head is delivered in the occipito-anterior position
B
Arrest in the transverse
Symphysis pubis
Sacrum
Rotation to the anterior position by Kielland's forceps followed by forceps delivery
C
The short rotation to persistent occipto-posterior
Symphysis pubis
Sacrum
Flexion does not occur and the occiput descends in the posterior position
Flexion occurs as the occiput reaches the pelvic floor and rotates posteriorly. The occiput delivers followed by the brow and face under the symphysis pubis

Figure 43.5 *Outcome of an occipitoposterior position. The head enters the pelvis with the occiput posteriorly. The outcome can be A, B or C (from Sweet B, 1997, with permission).*

The role of maternal position

Sutton (1996) discusses the benefits of upright and leaning forward postures in order to encourage the fetal head to engage in the optimal occipitoanterior position. Avoidance of a reclining position with knees higher than hips will reduce the incidence of occipitoposterior position of the fetal head at the commencement of labour. Taking up an all-fours posture may reduce the pressure of the fetus on the maternal spine and help to alleviate backache. It may also aid rotation of the fetus to an occipitoanterior position (Johnson et al 1991).

Sweet (1997) summarises the research on ambulation and position in labour. Freedom to move around in the first stage and the maintenance of an upright position such as sitting astride a chair and leaning on its back have been shown to be beneficial to women with an occipitoposterior presentation. Descent of the fetal head is encouraged and good uterine contractions should follow. Progress is more likely to be normal culminating in long internal rotation of the occiput (see below). In the 2nd stage the squatting position increases the anteroposterior position of the outlet and may aid rotation and delivery.

Relieving backache

To relieve the backache, many women find the kneeling position beneficial. This will also aid rotation of the head to an occipitoanterior position. In the 2nd stage perineal trauma is reduced (Grant 1987). Massaging the woman's back in the lumbosacral region may also help to relieve the backache and a warm bath has been found to be helpful. Epidural analgesia is the most effective method of relieving the pain.

A difficult problem for the woman in the late first stage is feeling a strong urge to push before full cervical dilatation. Pushing presses the fetal head against the anterior lip of the cervix and oedema may occur, thus lengthening the transitional stage of labour. Brayshaw & Wright (1994) suggest that a kneeling position with the head resting on the forearms may lessen the pressure on the anterior lip of cervix.

Second stage

The possible outcomes of an occipitoposterior position are:

1. long internal rotation of the occiput and delivery as an occipitoanterior;
2. deep transverse arrest of the head;
3. short internal rotation of the sinciput and delivery as 'face to pubes';
4. partial extension of the head to a brow presentation;
5. full extension of the head to a mentoposterior face presentation.

Mechanism of long internal rotation of a right occipitoanterior position

- The **lie** is longitudinal.
- The **attitude** of the head is deflexed.
- The **presentation** is vertex.
- The **position** is right occipitoposterior.
- The **denominator** is the occiput.
- The **presenting part** is the middle to anterior area of the left parietal bone.

The movements

Descent and flexion

There is continued descent with flexion during the first stage and the presenting diameter of occipitofrontal (11.5 cm) is converted to suboccipitofrontal (10 cm).

Internal rotation of the head

The occiput reaches the pelvic floor first and rotates forwards along the right side of the pelvis three-eighths of a circle to lie under the symphysis pubis. The anteroposterior diameter of the head now lies in the anteroposterior diameter of the pelvis. The shoulders follow and rotate two-eighths of a circle. The occiput escapes from beneath the subpubic arch.

Extension of the head

The head is now born by extension as it pivots on the suboccipital region around the pubic bone. The sinciput, face and chin sweep the perineum.

Restitution

Restitution is a movement made by the head following delivery which brings it into correct alignment with the shoulders. This will be one-eighth of a circle towards the side of the occiput.

Internal rotation of the shoulders

The anterior shoulder is the first to reach the pelvic floor and rotates forwards to lie under the symphysis pubis. This movement is accompanied by external rotation of the head one-eighth of a circle more in the direction of restitution. The occiput now lies laterally turned towards the woman's thigh.

Lateral flexion

The anterior shoulder is usually born first and slips under the pubic arch and the posterior shoulder passes over the perineum. The remainder of the body is born by lateral flexion.

This outcome is the most common, occurring in about 65% of births.

Deep transverse arrest of the head

If the head remains deflexed, deep transverse arrest may occur. The fetal head has begun long internal rotation but there is insufficient flexion to complete the process. The occipitofrontal diameter is caught above the ischial spines in the bispinous diameter. Labour is obstructed. A straight sacrum or narrow outlet, as found in the android pelvis, may lead to this, as may weak contractions.

Diagnosis and management

Diagnosis is made by finding the sagittal suture in the transverse diameter of the pelvis with a fontanelle at each end of the suture. Caput succedaneum may obscure the landmarks. It will be necessary to rotate the head to an occipitoanterior position either manually or with Kielland's forceps prior to delivery by forceps. An alternative way of rotating and delivering the fetal head is by vacuum extraction.

The use of the vacuum extractor is preferable to the forceps as it reduces the incidence of maternal injuries (Enkin et al 1995). Johanson & Menon (1997) found that although vacuum extraction was related to increased incidence of neonatal cephalhaematoma and retinal haemorrhages, there was less incidence of maternal trauma and CS. In the light of their review, they recommended the use of vacuum extraction.

Short internal rotation of the sinciput and delivery as 'face to pubes'

In about 5% of labours the occiput fails to rotate spontaneously to an anterior position (Arias 1993). This is known as persistent occipitoposterior position or POP. The head remains deflexed and the sinciput reaches the pelvic floor first and rotates forwards. The occiput comes to lie in the hollow of the sacrum and the head of the baby is born facing the pubic bone. Incidentally, this is the normal birth position of the great apes such as chimpanzees.

Diagnosis

- There may be delay in the 2nd stage of labour.
- There is gaping of the vagina and dilatation of the anus due to the presence of the large occiput.
- Confirmation is by finding the anterior fontanelle directly behind the symphysis pubis. This may be masked by caput succedaneum and feeling for the pinna of the ear will aid confirmation. In a POP the pinna will point towards the sacrum.

Management of the spontaneous delivery

The 2nd stage is likely to be prolonged and even when the woman wishes to push, there may be incomplete cervical dilatation (Kuo et al 1996). The squatting position may assist rotation and descent of the presenting part (Romond & Baker 1985). Once the perineal phase of delivery is reached, to maintain the smallest possible diameters distending the perineum, the sinciput is allowed to emerge under the symphysis pubis as far as the root of the nose. Flexion is maintained and the occiput is allowed to sweep the perineum. The rest of the face is brought down from under the symphysis pubis. There is a high risk of perineal trauma, especially a 'buttonhole' tear in the centre of the perineum. An episiotomy is usually required.

FACE PRESENTATION

The incidence of face presentation at term is about one in 500. In this presentation, the head and spine are fully extended and the limbs fully flexed. The fetal occiput lies against its shoulder blades and the face is directly above the internal os (Fig. 43.6).

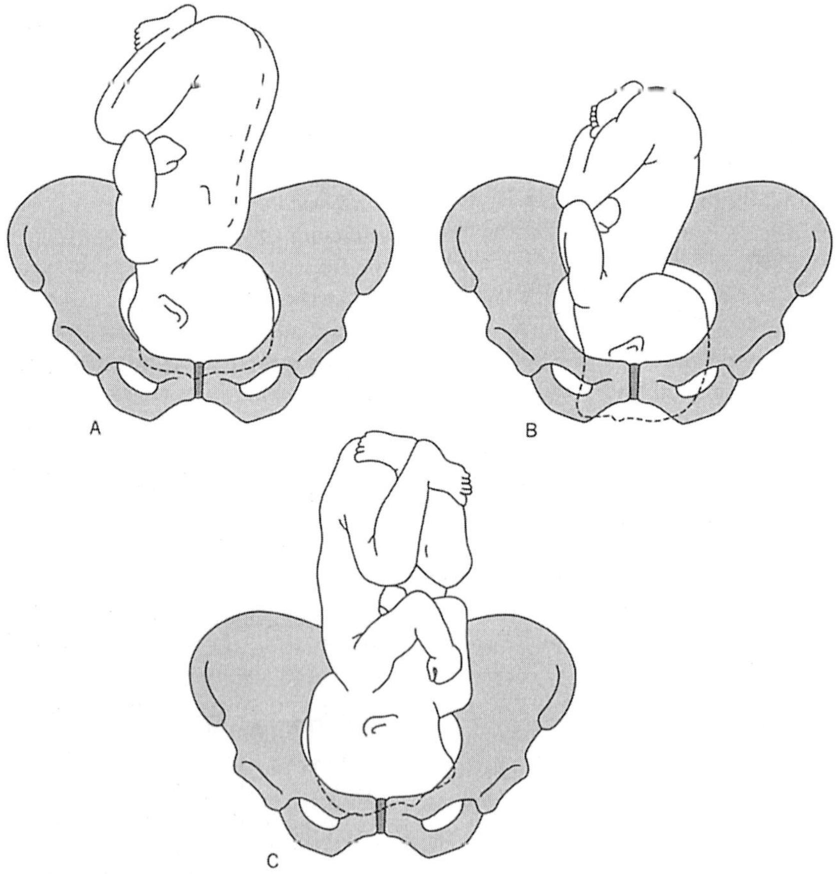

Figure 43.6 *Face presentations. (a) Right mentoposterior. (b) Right mentolateral. (c) Left mentoanterior (from Sweet B, 1997, with permission).*

Causes

Face presentation may be described as primary when it is present before the onset of labour. The fetus is often abnormal and anencephaly is common whilst a rarer cause is due to fetal goitre which prevents the head from flexing. A secondary face presentation is one that develops as labour proceeds. In a deflexed occipitoposterior position, the biparietal diameter of the fetal head may be unable to pass through the sacrocotyloid diameter of the pelvic brim. The bitemporal diameter descends more quickly and the head extends first to a brow presentation and ultimately to a face presentation. Other causes of face presentation include a flat pelvis and lax uterine muscle tone, prematurity, polyhydramnios or multiple pregnancy.

Risks (Williams 1996)

- Obstructed labour if either deep transverse arrest or brow presentation result.
- Maternal perineal trauma such as a 3rd-degree tear and bruising.
- Cord prolapse if there is early spontaneous rupture of the membranes.
- Facial bruising as the caput forms over the face.
- Cerebral haemorrhage due to excessive moulding of the cranium.

Diagnosis

Per abdomen

Face presentation is rarely found in pregnancy as the majority of cases develop in labour (Williams 1996). It may be difficult to diagnose face presentation. A deep groove may be palpated between the fetal head and back. The chest wall may be pressed up against the anterior wall of the uterus and heart sounds are heard clearly on the side where limbs are palpated. However, in mentoposterior positions where the chest faces posteriorly, heart sounds may be difficult to hear. In women who have a late ultrasound, a face presentation is sometimes found.

Per vaginam

In labour, the possibility of a face presentation should be suspected if the head remains high. On vaginal examination, feeling orbital ridges and a mouth with gum margins will confirm the diagnosis. The fetus may help, as the author has encountered, by sucking the examining finger! The mouth feels very different from the soft and clinging anal orifice which would be found if the presentation was breech. Also, the examining finger may have meconium coating it if the breech was presenting. It is important to determine whether the fetus is presenting in a mentoposterior or mentoanterior position. Unless a posterior face rotates to anterior, there will be an obstructed labour. The position of the chin is the important diagnostic tool.

Progress and outcomes of labour

As in many labours where there is an irregular high presenting part there may be early spontaneous rupture of the membranes with the risk of cord prolapse and contractions may be inefficient leading to a prolonged labour. The face bones cannot mould and large diameters must enter the pelvis.

Mentoanterior position

If contractions are good, descent and rotation of the head occur and labour progresses to a spontaneous delivery.

Mechanism of a left mentoanterior position

There are six possible positions: right mentoanterior, mentolateral and mentoposterior, and left mentoanterior, mentolateral and mentoposterior.

- The **lie** is longitudinal.
- The **attitude** of the head and back is one of extension.
- The **presentation** is face.
- The **position** is left mentoanterior.
- The **denominator** is the mentum.
- The **presenting part** is the left malar bone.

The movements

Descent

There is continued descent with increasing extension. The mentum is the leading part.

Internal rotation of the head

The mentum reaches the pelvic floor first and rotates forwards one-eighth of a circle to lie under the symphysis pubis. The chin escapes from beneath the subpubic arch (Fig. 43.7).

Flexion of the head

The head is now born by flexion. The sinciput, vertex and occiput sweep the perineum.

Restitution

Restitution occurs as the chin turns one-eighth of a circle towards the woman's left side.

Internal rotation of the shoulders

The anterior shoulder is the first to reach the pelvic floor and rotates forwards to lie under the symphysis pubis. This movement is accompanied by external rotation of the head one-eighth of a circle more in the direction of restitution.

Lateral flexion

The anterior shoulder is usually born first and slips under the pubic arch and the posterior shoulder passes over the perineum. The remainder of the body is born by lateral flexion.

Mentoposterior positions

If the head is completely extended and the mentum reaches the pelvic floor first, it rotates forwards into a mentoanterior position and delivery is possible. If the head is incompletely extended there is a persistent mentoposterior position and the sinciput reaches the pelvic floor first. The chin comes to lie in the hollow of the pelvis and there can be no further progress as in order to move further, the head and chest of the fetus

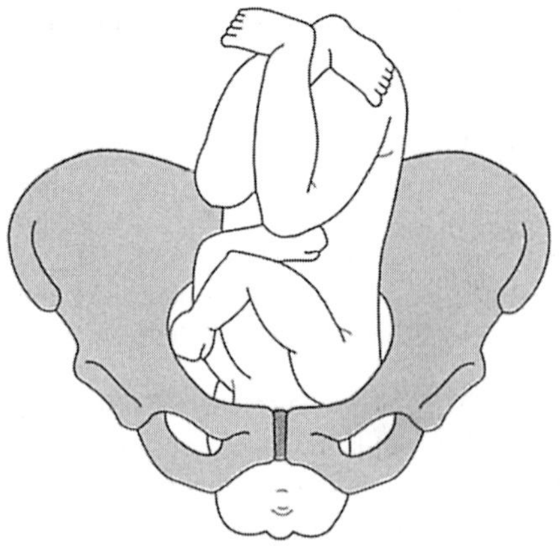

Figure 43.7 *The face at the outlet, the chin passing under the pubic arch (from Sweet B, 1997, with permission).*

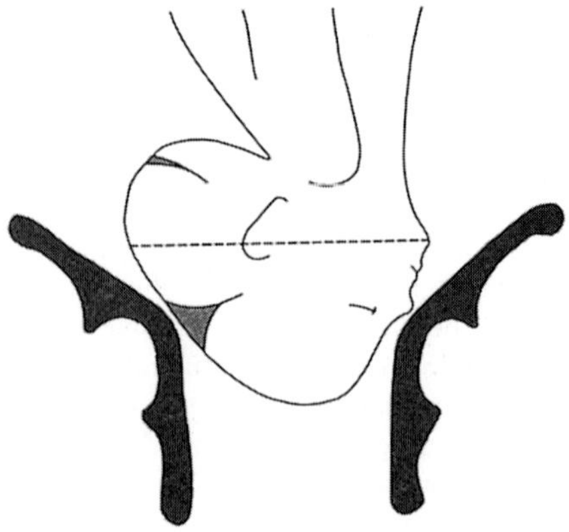

Figure 43.8 *Brow presentation (from Sweet B, 1997, with permission).*

would have to be in the pelvic cavity together. In order to be born, the presenting fetal part must pivot round the subpubic arch either by flexion or extension. If the chin is posterior, this cannot happen as the fully extended head cannot extend further and labour is obstructed.

Management of labour

The first stage of labour is managed according to the risks. During vaginal examination, note should be taken of the descent of the mentum. If the head remains high or there is a suspicion of cephalopelvic disproportion, a CS may be necessary.

In the 2nd stage, when the face appears at the vulva, the sinciput must be held back to permit extension. This allows the mentum to escape under the pubic arch before the occiput sweeps the perineum. This allows the smallest possible diameter, which is the submentovertical of 11.5 cm to distend the vaginal orifice rather than the large mentovertical diameter of 13.5 cm. An elective episiotomy must be made because of the large diameters distending the vaginal orifice. If there is delay in descent or if the fetus remains in a persistent mentoposterior position, a forceps delivery, with rotation if necessary, may be successful. Otherwise a CS will be needed.

BROW PRESENTATION

Brow presentation occurs in about one in 2000 deliveries. Except for anencephaly, the causes are the same as those resulting in face presentation. The head is midway between flexion and extension and the largest diameter of the head, the mentovertical which is 13.5 cm, cannot enter the widest possible diameter of the pelvic brim which is the transverse of 13 cm (Fig. 43.8). Unless the brow presentation extends fully to a face presentation and the mentum becomes anterior, labour is obstructed.

Diagnosis

Per abdomen

The head is very high and the presenting diameter is very wide. A groove may be felt between the occiput and the back.

Per vaginam

The presenting part may be so high it cannot be reached. If the brow is within reach, the orbital ridges are felt at one side and the anterior fontanelle on the other with the frontal suture running between them. Diagnosis can be confirmed by X-ray or ultrasound.

Management

If the brow presentation is diagnosed early in labour and both maternal and fetal conditions are satisfactory, time may be allowed to see if the head will flex to a vertex or extend to a face presentation. If the brow presentation persists, a CS will be necessary.

SHOULDER PRESENTATION

Shoulder presentation in labour is the result of an uncorrected abnormal lie in pregnancy. Instead of the normal longitudinal lie, the fetus lies across the uterus either obliquely or transversely. The lie may be unstable. Shoulder presentation leads to obstructed labour and must be prevented.

Causes

The commonest cause is seen in the grand multiparous woman, i.e. laxity of the uterine and abdominal muscles. More than 80% of cases occur in women with three or more previous pregnancies (Arias 1993). Other causes include anything which prevents the fetus from adopting a longitudinal lie or the fetal head from engaging. These include placenta praevia, multiple pregnancy, polyhydramnios, a uterine abnormality, a large uterine fibroid or a contracted pelvis. When the fetus dies in utero it may slump into an abnormal lie.

Diagnosis

Per abdomen

A transverse lie is easy to diagnose in pregnancy because of the

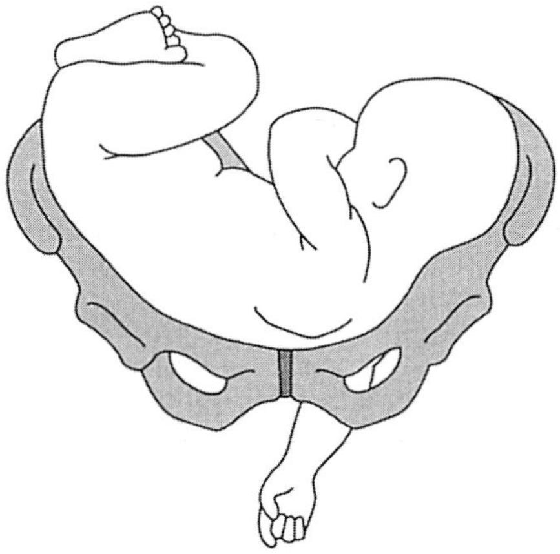

Figure 43.9 *Shoulder presentation with prolapse of one arm (from Sweet B, 1997, with permission).*

abnormal shape of the uterus. The uterus is broader and the fundal height lower than normal and there may be a discernible bulge at either side of the uterus. On palpation, the fetal head will be felt on one side of the uterus and the breech on the other. The fetal back may be anterior (dorsoanterior) or posterior (dorsoposterior). There is no presenting part entering the pelvis (Fig. 43.9). In an oblique lie the shape of the uterus may be indicative and one or other pole of the fetus is found in one or other iliac fossa. Ultrasound is useful both to confirm the diagnosis and detect the cause.

Per vaginam

A vaginal examination should not be done if a transverse lie is suspected on abdominal examination in case there is a placenta praevia. Rarely, a woman will be admitted already in labour with the shoulder impacted at the brim of the pelvis. It may be mistaken for a breech presentation. The fetal cord and arm may prolapse into the vagina. On vaginal examination the shoulder is recognised by feeling the fetal ribs and the hand, which must be differentiated from a foot by the length of the digits and the presence of a heel. CS is the safest method of delivery even if the fetus is dead.

Management

A full examination is made to exclude causes such as placenta praevia and if no major pregnancy abnormality is found, the obstetrician may attempt to correct the lie to a longitudinal lie and cephalic presentation. However, reversion to the original lie is common and some doctors do not perform repeated ECV before the onset of labour, planned or otherwise. As pregnancy progresses some lies will stabilise as longitudinal. Sweet quotes Phelan et al (1986) who found that after 37 weeks of pregnancy a transverse lie persisted in only 17% of cases.

Phelan et al recommended that the woman should be admitted to hospital at 37–38 weeks, when the fetus is mature, for ECV and induction of labour. There is a risk of labour commencing spontaneously with early rupture of the membranes and cord prolapse. The lie can be maintained as longitudinal by gentle pressure on the uterus. When the contractions are established and the fetal head enters the pelvis the membranes can be ruptured. If complications arise or if the woman has a poor obstetric history, a CS is performed.

If after the birth of a first twin, the 2nd fetus takes up a transverse or oblique lie, it must be turned by ECV, the 2nd set of membranes ruptured and the delivery completed.

COMPOUND PRESENTATION

This is a presentation where a hand or foot lies alongside the head. It is a rare complication and Arias (1993) gives the incidence as 0.1% of all deliveries. Cord prolapse may occur in up to 20% of cases. It is more likely to happen if the fetus is small and the pelvis large or there is any condition that prevents the descent of the head such as contracted pelvis, prematurity or multiple pregnancy. Usually the limb will recede as the head advances and the delivery proceeds normally. It is rarely necessary to attempt to move the limb.

Summary of main points

- There is no single cause for occipitoposterior position of the vertex but if the forepelvis is small, as found in android and anthropoid pelves, the head may take up a posterior position. Other causes include a pendulous abdomen, a flat sacrum or an anterior placenta. Risks include obstructed labour, maternal perineal trauma, cord prolapse and neonatal cerebral haemorrhage.
- Antenatally occipitoposterior position is the commonest cause of a non-engaged head in late pregnancy in primigravidae. It may be detected by a combination of maternal complaints and abdominal examination. In labour during a vaginal examination, palpation of the anterior fontanelle is likely.
- The course of labour partly depends on the degree of descent and flexion that takes place, which is influenced by the strength of uterine contractions. If the head flexes, it is likely that labour will proceed normally. If the head remains deflexed, problems may arise. Early rupture of the membranes may happen and there is a risk of cord prolapse.
- Labour may be prolonged because of poor cervical stimulation and slow dilatation. Contractions may be excessive, uncoordinated and painful with severe backache. There may be difficulty in micturition with retention of urine and the woman needs encouragement to empty her bladder frequently. Catheterisation may be necessary.
- Upright and leaning forward positions encourage the fetal head to engage in the occipitoanterior position. Taking up an all-fours posture may help to reduce backache and aid rotation of the fetus to an occipitoanterior position. Encouraging the mother to take up a knee-chest position for 45 min may help anterior rotation of the vertex.
- In the late first stage of labour the woman may have an urge to push before full cervical dilatation. Oedema of the anterior lip of cervix may occur, lengthening the transitional stage of labour. The adoption of the kneeling position with the head resting on the forearms may lessen the pressure on the anterior lip of cervix.
- The possible outcomes of an occipitoposterior position are long internal rotation of the occiput and delivery as an occipitoanterior, deep transverse arrest of the head, short internal rotation of the

sinciput and delivery as 'face to pubes', partial extension of the head to a brow presentation or full extension of the head to a mentoposterior face presentation.

- If there is deep transverse arrest of the head, it must be rotated to an occipitoanterior position either manually or with Kielland's forceps prior to delivery by forceps or by vacuum extraction. The use of the vacuum extractor is preferable to the forceps as it reduces the incidence of maternal injuries and of CS.
- If there is persistent occipitoposterior position the 2nd stage of labour may be prolonged and the woman may commence pushing before complete cervical dilatation. The squatting position may assist rotation and descent of the presenting part. At delivery the sinciput is allowed to emerge under the symphysis pubis as far as the root of the nose. Flexion is maintained and the occiput is allowed to sweep the perineum. The rest of the face is brought down from under the symphysis pubis. An episiotomy is usually required.
- Face presentation may be primary, when it is present before the onset of labour, or secondary, which develops as labour proceeds. In pregnancy face presentation is rarely found as the majority of cases develop in labour. Risks include obstructed labour, maternal perineal trauma, cord prolapse, facial bruising and cerebral haemorrhage.
- The irregular high presenting part may result in early spontaneous rupture of the membranes with the risk of cord prolapse and contractions may be inefficient, leading to a prolonged labour. The face bones cannot mould and large diameters must enter the pelvis.
- In labour it is important to determine whether the fetus is presenting in a mentoposterior or mentoanterior position. The position of the chin is the important diagnostic tool. In a mentoanterior position with good contractions, descent and rotation of the head occur and labour progresses to a spontaneous delivery. In a mentoposterior position the usual outcome is that the fully extended head cannot extend further and labour is obstructed.
- In brow presentation the mentovertical diameter is too large to enter the transverse, widest possible diameter of the pelvic brim. Unless the head extends fully to a face presentation and the mentum becomes anterior, labour is obstructed. If brow presentation is diagnosed early in labour and maternal and fetal conditions are satisfactory, time may be allowed to see if the head will flex to a vertex or extend to a face presentation. If brow presentation persists, CS is necessary.
- Shoulder presentation in labour is the result of an uncorrected abnormal lie in pregnancy. The fetus lies across the uterus either obliquely or transversely. Shoulder presentation leads to obstructed labour and must be prevented. The commonest cause is laxity of the uterine and abdominal muscles, most often in multiparous women. Other causes include factors which prevent the fetus from adopting a longitudinal lie or the fetal head from engaging.
- Per abdomen, the uterus is broader and the fundal height lower than normal and there may be a discernible bulge at either side of the uterus. On palpation, the fetal head will be felt on one side of the uterus and the breech on the other with no presenting part above the pelvic brim. In an oblique lie, the shape of the uterus may be indicative and one or other pole of the fetus is found in one or other iliac fossa. Ultrasound is useful both to confirm the diagnosis and detect the cause.
- A full examination is made to exclude causes such as placenta praevia. If no major pregnancy abnormality is found, the obstetrician may attempt to correct the lie to a longitudinal lie and cephalic presentation. The woman should be admitted to hospital at 37–38 weeks, when the fetus is mature, for ECV and induction of labour to avoid risk of early rupture of the membranes and cord prolapse. When the contractions are established and the fetal head enters the pelvis, the membranes can be ruptured. If any difficulty arises a CS is performed.
- In compound presentation a hand or foot lies alongside the head. It is more likely to happen if the fetus is small and the pelvis large or there is any condition that prevents the descent of the head. Usually the limb will recede as the head advances and the delivery proceeds normally. It is rarely necessary to attempt to move the limb.

References

Arias F. 1993 Practical Guide to High Risk Pregnancy and Delivery, 2nd edn. Mosby Year Book, Chicago.

Brayshaw E, Wright P. 1994 Teaching Physical Skills for the Childbearing Year. Books for Midwives Press, Hale.

El Halta V. 1996 Posterior labor – a pain in the back! Its prevention and cure. Clarion 11(1), 12–13.

Enkin M, Keirse MJNC, Renfrew M, Neilson J. 1995 A Guide to Effective Care in Pregnancy and Childbirth, 2nd edn. Oxford University Press, Oxford.

Grant A. 1987 Reassessing the second stage. Journal of the Association of Chartered Physiotherapists in Obstetrics and Gynaecology 60, 26–29.

Johanson RB, Menon V. 1997 Vacuum extraction versus forceps delivery. In Neilson JP, Crowther CA, Hodnett ED, Hofmeyr GJ, Keirse MJNC (eds) Pregnancy and Childbirth module of The Cochrane Database of Systematic Reviews, The Cochrane Library. Update Software, Oxford.

Johnson N, Johnson VA, Gupta JK. 1991 Maternal positions during labor. Obstetrical and Gynecological Survey 46(7), 428–434.

Kuo Y-C, Chen C-P, Wong K-G. 1996 Factors influencing the prolonged second stage and the effects on perinatal and maternal outcomes. Journal of Obstetrics and Gynaecology Research 22(3), 253–257.

Phelan JP, Boucher M, Mueller E, McCart D, Horenstein J, Clark SL. 1986 The non-labouring transverse lie: a management dilemma. Journal of Reproductive Medicine 31, 184–186.

Romond JL, Baker IT. 1985 Squatting in childbirth: a new look at an old tradition. Journal of Obstetric, Gynaecological and Neonatal Nursing 14, 712–715.

Sutton J. 1996 A midwife's observations of how the birth process is influenced by the relationship of the maternal pelvis and the foetal head. Journal of the Association of Chartered Physiotherapists in Women's Health 79, 31–33.

Sweet BR. 1997 Malpresentations. In Sweet BR with Tiran DL (eds) Mayes Midwifery, 12th edn. Baillière Tindall, London, pp 631–657.

Williams J. 1996 Malposition of the occiput and malpresentations. In Bennett VR, Brown LK (eds) Myles Textbook for Midwives, 12th edn. Churchill Livingstone, Edinburgh, pp 404–431.

Recommended reading

El Halta V. 1996 Posterior labor – a pain in the back! Its prevention and cure. Clarion 11(1), 12–13.

Johnson N, Johnson VA, Gupta JK. 1991 Maternal positions during labor. Obstetrical and Gynecological Survey 46(7), 428–434.

Kuo Y-C, Chen C-P, Wong K-G. 1996 Factors influencing the prolonged second stage and the effects on perinatal and maternal outcomes. Journal of Obstetrics and Gynaecology Research 22(3), 253–257.

Romond JL, Baker IT. 1985 Squatting in childbirth: a new look at an old tradition. Journal of Obstetric, Gynaecological and Neonatal Nursing 14, 712–715.

Sutton J. 1996 A midwife's observations of how the birth process is influenced by the relationship of the maternal pelvis and the foetal head. Journal of the Association of Chartered Physiotherapists in Women's Health 79, 31–33.

Chapter 44

Cephalopelvic disproportion, obstructed labour and other obstetric emergencies

In this chapter

INTRODUCTION

Two evolutionary adaptations lead to problems of fit between the female pelvis and the fetal head. The birth canal and the pathway taken by the fetus are complex as the human pelvis is adapted to a bipedal posture (Aiello & Dean 1990). Compared to other primates such as the chimpanzee:

- the anteroposterior diameter is reduced at the brim, cavity and outlet;
- there is widening of the transverse diameters;
- the sacral promontory protrudes into the pelvic inlet;
- the sacrum makes an angle with the lumbar spine – the **lumbosacral angle**;
- there is inward protrusion of the ischial spines in order to support the strong pelvic floor;
- the sacrum is curved;
- the superior ramus is thinned and elongated with widening of the subpubic angle.

The fetal head is able to negotiate the pelvis successfully because of three features:

1. spheroid shape of the vertex;
2. mobility of the head on the neck, allowing flexion or extension;
3. moulding of the bones of the vault (Abitol 1993).

CEPHALOPELVIC DISPROPORTION

Any condition leading to a misfit between the fetal head and the maternal pelvis, with failure of descent of the head into the pelvis despite good contractions, results in cephalopelvic disproportion (CPD). The presenting diameters of the fetal head are larger than the diameters of the pelvis. The shape of the pelvis may be abnormal but as long as the diameters allow passage of the fetal head, delivery should follow and there should be no problem with the rest of the fetus. Cephalopelvic disproportion is an absolute cause of obstructed labour and there are tremendous dangers for mother and fetus.

Diagnosis

In a primigravida it is expected that the fetal head should engage in the last 2–3 weeks of pregnancy. If it does not, an attempt to make it engage is tried and, if unsuccessful, CPD should be suspected. The most common cause for non-engagement of the head is **occipitoposterior position**, with deflexed head and a presenting occipitofrontal diameter of 11.5 cm. However, in such cases the head flexes and descent occurs in labour. Other causes of a non-engaged head include pelvic tumours, placenta praevia and polyhydramnios.

A steep **angle of inclination** between the pelvic brim and the horizontal is found in some Afro-Caribbean women and may delay engagement until late in labour.

Maternal indications of possible CPD include:

- bone conditions such as rickets or osteomalacia, which may have resulted in alterations in the size and shape of the pelvis;
- spinal deformities such as scoliosis;
- pelvic trauma and fractures which may have altered the size and shape of the pelvis;
- previous obstetric conditions such as prolonged labour, difficult delivery or caesarean section;
- short stature of the woman. Mahmoud et al (1988) found that the height of the woman was a better predictor of CPD than the shoe size although 80% of women under 1.6 m still achieved vaginal delivery. Haig's (1993) work on the conflict between maternal and paternal genes for the control of fetal size is of interest (discussed in Chapter 13).

In the fetus, size in relation to the maternal pelvis is obviously the main consideration. In a multigravida with deliveries of normal-sized infants, CPD is less likely but in the event of a larger fetus there may be a problem. Abdominal palpation is an inaccurate method of judging fetal size although experienced practitioners may become quite adept. Estimation of fetal size is becoming easier as ultrasound technology advances.

Assessing the pelvis

A combination of careful history taking and clinical expertise backed up by technology should enable selection of women at risk (Brock 1997). Head fitting or pelvic assessment examinations may be carried out. However, Enkin et al (1995) write that there is 'reasonable correlation between clinical and radiological assessment of pelvic dimensions but neither are particularly accurate in predicting the outcome of labour and opinion varies about the value of pre-labour assessments'.

Head fitting

In head fitting, an attempt is made to provoke engagement of the non-engaged head. The woman is asked to empty her bladder and to lie flat on the examination couch. The symphysis pubis is located with the fingers of the right hand and the fetal head is held between the thumb and fingers of the left hand. The woman takes a deep breath and as she breathes out the head is pushed downwards and backwards into the brim of the pelvis. The fingers of the right hand palpate to assess whether the widest diameter of the head has entered the pelvic brim.

Pelvic assessment

Pelvic assessment of the shape and size of the pelvis is carried out by the obstetrician in the last few weeks of pregnancy, if the head cannot be made to engage. The tissues will be softer, allowing ease of examination, and the fetus is large enough to relate to the size of the pelvis. The aim is to assess the brim, cavity and outlet of the pelvis. An attempt is made to measure the diagonal conjugate which runs from the lower border of the symphysis pubis to the sacral promontory and so assess the anteroposterior diameter of the pelvic brim, also known as the **true** or **obstetric conjugate**, through which the fetus has to pass.

During a vaginal examination an attempt is made to reach the sacral promontory but in a good-sized pelvis this is unlikely as the diagonal conjugate measures 12–13 cm. If it is reached, 2 cm are subtracted to allow for the depth of the pubic bone and the obstetric conjugate is estimated. The size of the pelvic cavity is assessed by examination of the length and curve of the sacrum and by feeling the length of the sacrospinous ligament, which should accommodate two fingers.

Finally, the shape and size of the pelvic outlet can then be assessed. The ischial spines are located to see whether or not they are prominent, which may suggest a narrow transverse diameter of the outlet. The subpubic angle should be more than 90° and should accommodate the width of two fingers. One external measurement, the distance between the ischial tuberosities, should accommodate a large fist.

X-ray pelvimetry

An erect lateral X-ray pelvimetry provides information about the size and shape of the pelvis and the relationship of the fetal head to the pelvic brim. However, there has been criticism of its use because of an association between prenatal irradiation and childhood leukaemia. It may also be a poor predictor of CPD and the results do not appear to affect the management and therefore an X-ray pelvimetry should seldom if ever be necessary in pregnancy (Enkin et al 1995). Details that can be seen are:

- the shape of the pelvis;
- the shape of the sacrum;
- the inclination between the sacrum and pelvic brim;
- the anteroposterior diameters of the brim, cavity and outlet;
- the width of the sacrosciatic notch;
- the depth of the pelvic cavity.

Pelvimetry may be ordered for (Brock 1997):

- any primigravida with the fetal head not engaged at term in whom clinical assessment suggests pelvic contraction;

- a primigravida with a breech presentation if external cephalic version has failed or is contraindicated and vaginal delivery is being considered;
- any multipara with a history of difficult labour, such as failure to progress in labour, prolonged labour and operative delivery, although these women should be offered a pelvimetry in the postnatal period to avoid the risks of radiation to the fetus in any subsequent pregnancy. A previous CS for a reason other than CPD is not a contraindication for trial of labour (Flamm et al 1994).

Proud (1996) adds the following:

- women with a history of injury or disease of the pelvis and spine;
- women with a limp or deformity.

Brock (1997) mentions a small study by Moore et al (1992) examining the benefits of magnetic resonance imaging (MRI). More accurate measurements of the pelvic outlet without the danger of radiation may be achievable but more research is needed. Depending on the antenatal findings discussed above, there are three possibilities: disproportion is not present and vaginal delivery will be possible; there is CPD of such a degree that vaginal delivery will not be possible; and there is a degree of CPD which may be overcome in labour.

Trial of vaginal delivery

If there are no obstetric or medical complications, the woman can be admitted to hospital for a trial of labour. The aim is to allow time for the contractions of labour, aided by the abdominal and pelvic floor muscles, to cause sufficient flexion and moulding of the fetal head so that descent occurs (Abitol 1993). Engagement of the head is likely to be followed by vaginal delivery. Brock (1997) writes that all primigravidae with a non-engaged head are considered to be undergoing a trial of labour. An old but probably useful saying is that the fetal head is the best pelvimeter.

Selection of women for trial of vaginal delivery

- The presentation must be cephalic.
- There should be no major degree of CPD.
- The woman should be healthy with a good obstetric and medical history.
- There should be no pregnancy complications such as hypertension.

Management

There must be careful monitoring of mother and fetus and facilities to carry out an immediate CS if needed. All observations are plotted on a partogram and any changes in the conditions of mother, fetus or progress noted by the midwife must be reported to the obstetrician who is the decision maker. The obstetrician may wish to conduct all vaginal examinations. Ambulation and adoption of an upright position encourage flexion and descent of the head, maintenance of good uterine action and cervical dilatation.

Assessment of progress

Successful progression to a vaginal delivery should occur if the contractions are good, the fetal head flexes and the skull bones mould, the pelvic joints relax and maternal and fetal heart remain satisfactory. Progress is assessed by observation of descent of the head by abdominal palpation and vaginal examination and dilatation of the cervix by vaginal examination. Progress in dilatation should be 1 cm per hour.

If progress is slow due to inefficient uterine action and thought to be unrelated to CPD, active management of labour can be undertaken and oxytocic drugs can be used. However, it is important to remember that the injudicious use of oxytocic drugs in the presence of more than a minor degree of CPD may lead to rupture of the uterus (see below). If hyperstimulation occurs the syntocinon infusion should be stopped immediately and the obstetrician informed. A CS may be necessary if:

- the progress of labour remains slow following the commencement of the oxytocin infusion;
- the head fails to descend in the presence of efficient contractions;
- fetal distress arises.

OBSTRUCTED LABOUR

Obstructed labour occurs whenever there is an impassable barrier to the descent of the fetus through the birth canal in spite of efficient uterine action. There is a large increase in maternal and fetal morbidity and mortality if labour is allowed to proceed in the presence of unrecognised obstructed labour. The situation is more common in remote parts of the world such as villages in Africa or India where women do not have access to trained personnel but it can also occur in the developed world if a woman fails to disclose her pregnancy or to present herself for care in labour.

Causes

- Cephalopelvic disproportion is a cause of obstructed labour unresolvable except by CS (in remote parts of the world division of the symphysis pubis – **symphysiotomy** – or a fetal destructive operation may save the life of the mother).
- Malpositions and malpresentations of the head, such as brow, posterior face or deep transverse arrest of the head.
- Fetal abnormalities such as hydrocephalus.
- Maternal tumours.

Signs and symptoms

Early signs

- There is little progress in labour, with no descent of the head despite efficient uterine action.
- On vaginal examination, the presenting part is high.
- The cervix dilates slowly and may be felt like a curtain or empty sleeve (Brock 1997) hanging in front of the presenting part.
- The membranes have usually ruptured early and there is an ever-present risk of cord prolapse.

- In a primigravida there may be active phase arrest and the contractions stop for a while, finally restarting with increased strength. The woman may complain of severe and continuous pain.
- The multiparous woman may have tumultuous contractions proceeding rapidly to uterine rupture.

Late signs

- If nothing was done for the woman or, much more likely in the UK, if she presented herself for care late in labour, she may progress to having a raised temperature, rapid pulse and dehydration.
- On abdominal inspection, the uterus would appear to be moulded around the fetus because of tonic contraction and loss of liquor amnii.
- A Bandl's pathological retraction ring may be seen as a ridge of tissue running obliquely across the abdomen. This denotes an extremely thinned lower uterine segment and imminent rupture of the uterus.
- Fetoplacental blood supply and fetal oxygen supply will be cut off and the fetus will die.
- On examination the vagina feels hot and dry and the presenting part is high. There may be excessive moulding and a large caput succedaneum obscuring the presenting part in a cephalic presentation.
- Urinary output is reduced and a vesicovaginal fistula may occur due to sloughing of tissue due to prolonged pressure.

Management

A high standard of antenatal care and observations in early labour will allow early detection of likely difficulties and treatment before obstructed labour occurs. Brock (1997) gives the following examples: removal of an ovarian cyst, correction of an abnormal lie or performing a planned CS. If labour is advanced when the woman is first seen, an emergency CS is carried out regardless of whether the fetus is dead or alive. Rarely, especially in developing countries, if the fetus is dead and the cervix is fully dilated destructive operations such as **cleidotomy** (division of the clavicles) or **craniotomy** (perforation of the skull) may allow vaginal delivery but there is risk of perforation of the thin lower uterine segment (Gupta & Chitra 1994, cited in Brock 1997).

UTERINE RUPTURE

Rupture of the uterus is an obstetric emergency and the fetus and mother may die. Rupture of the uterus may involve a previous scar, spontaneous rupture of an intact uterus or traumatic rupture. Four cases of death due to ruptured uterus occurred in Britain between 1991 and 1993 (DOH 1996). One of these involved a previous scar, two were spontaneous ruptures and the fourth occurred during a failed vacuum extraction and forceps delivery. Although it appears that the incidence of uterine rupture has fallen in developed countries it may be rising in the developing countries due to vaginal delivery following a previous CS and to the use of oxytocic infusions (Grace et al 1993).

Types of uterine rupture

Scar rupture is usually due to a previous CS. A longitudinal scar in the uterus (classic incision) is more likely to rupture than a transverse scar in the lower segment. Rupture of the classic scar may occur in about 2% of cases and is more likely to occur in late pregnancy when the upper segment is stretched to its limit. Caesarean section at 38 weeks may help to reduce this rate. Rupture of a transverse lower segment scar is more likely to happen in labour as the lower segment is thinned and extended. Uterine rupture following a lower segment CS is less than 1%.

Traumatic rupture of the uterus may be caused by the use of obstetric instruments, such as by tearing of the cervix which extends into the lower segment. Intrauterine manipulations, such as internal podalic version where the foot of the fetus is grasped at delivery to convert a transverse lie, usually of the 2nd twin, to breech or correction of a shoulder presentation in labour, may lead to uterine rupture, as may the misuse of oxytocic drugs.

Spontaneous rupture of the uterus may follow strong spontaneous uterine action such as occurs in obstructed labour. The rupture is found most often in the lower segment. Abruptio placentae, where there is extravasation of blood into the uterine muscle (**Couvelaire uterus**), facilitates such a rupture.

Signs and symptoms

Complete rupture

Rupture of the uterus may be complete or **true**, involving the full thickness of the uterine wall and the pelvic peritoneum. This is usually an acute event associated with sudden intense pain, blood loss and collapse followed by maternal and fetal death. The uterine contractions cease and there is vaginal bleeding. The fetus may pass into the abdominal cavity and be palpable outside the uterus directly under the abdominal wall.

Incomplete rupture

Incomplete or **silent** rupture involves the myometrium but the peritoneum remains intact. It is more frequently associated with a previous lower segment CS. Because scar tissue tends to be avascular, there are fewer dramatic signs. The mother's condition deteriorates slowly. Abdominal pain or scar tenderness may be present and a rise in maternal heart rate may be an indicator of impending rupture (Rachagan et al 1991).

Management

If the mother is shocked she must be resuscitated and prepared for theatre. A blood transfusion will be necessary. The baby is delivered and the uterus repaired if possible. A hysterectomy may be necessary if the rupture is severe and bleeding difficult to control. Postoperative treatment should include observation of severe side effects of haemorrhage such as renal failure or, later, onset of Sheehan's syndrome. The psychological effect of the experience on the woman and her family should be anticipated and explanations and counselling made available.

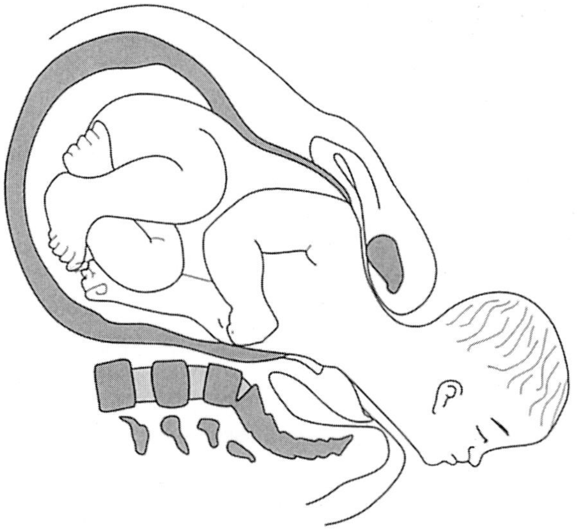

Figure 44.1 *Shoulder dystocia (from Sweet B, 1997, with permission).*

SHOULDER DYSTOCIA

Shoulder dystocia is another obstetric emergency which may end in fetal and occasionally maternal morbidity and mortality. There is difficulty in delivering the anterior shoulder and urgent manoeuvres are necessary (Fig. 44.1). There are two causes:

1 a large baby;
2 failure of the shoulders to rotate into the anteroposterior diameter following delivery of the head.

The incidence of shoulder dystocia is about 0.2% and the risk rises as pregnancy becomes prolonged and with increasing birth weight.

Recognition

The head fails to advance and the fetus looks to be burying its chin in the perineum. This happens because the anterior shoulder is wedged firmly behind the symphysis pubis. Difficulty in delivering the face and the chin are warning signs (Williams 1996a,b).

Risk factors

The following factors, most of them associated with a large fetus, should be taken into consideration so that the woman can be delivered in an appropriate setting.

- If the mother is over 35 there may be an associated increase in birth weight.
- A maternal weight of more than 90 kg is the most frequent associated factor.
- Maternal diabetes mellitus, whether insulin dependent or gestational, is associated with fetal macrosomia and difficulty in delivering the shoulders.
- Infants of increased birth weight in non-diabetic mothers have less incidence of shoulder dystocia, with a 10% risk rather than the 31% risk of the diabetic woman (Spellacy et al 1985).
- High maternal birth weight is associated with high birth weight of her own fetus.
- Women with a platypelloid pelvis, where the anteroposterior diameter is reduced, may develop shoulder dystocia with a normal-sized infant.

Management

Pulling on the head before rotation of the shoulders will only further impede delivery. If possible, the midwife should summon an obstetrician, paediatrician and anaesthetist. However, there is little time to save the life of the baby and the woman may be in her own home so the midwife must attempt to complete the delivery. It may be necessary to try more than one manoeuvre so it is necessary to keep calm and think clearly about what is happening inside the mother's pelvis. It is recommended that an episiotomy be performed. Even though the obstruction is bony, it will give room for the manoeuvres and prevent maternal trauma.

Manoeuvres (Brock 1997)

McRoberts' manoeuvre

This method was developed by McRoberts in Houston, Texas. The woman is helped to lie on her back with her knees drawn up to her chest (Fig. 44.2). Easy delivery of the shoulders should then be possible by minimising some of the problems of parturition discussed by Abitol (1993). Smeltzer (1986) suggests that the manoeuvre may help by:

- rotating the symphysis pubis superiorly by as much as 8 cm;
- elevating the anterior shoulder;
- pushing the posterior shoulder over the sacrum;
- flexing the fetal spine;
- straightening maternal lordosis;
- opening the pelvic inlet to its maximum possible diameter;
- bringing the inlet perpendicular to the maximum expulsive force;
- removing the weight-bearing forces from the sacrum;
- removing the sacral promontory as a point of obstruction.

This manoeuvre can be tried twice as a first resort when shoulder dystocia has been diagnosed.

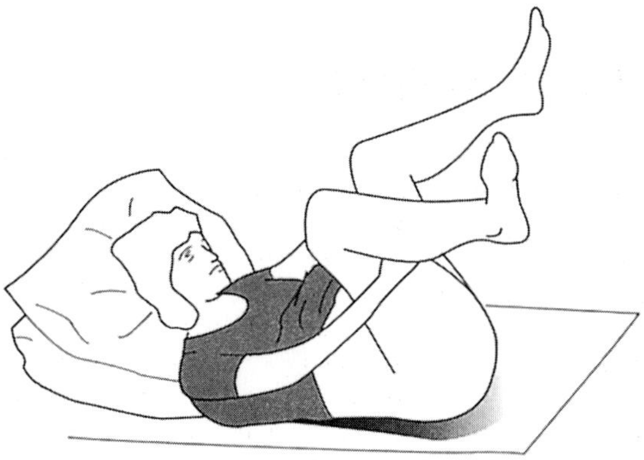

Figure 44.2 *McRoberts' position (from Sweet B, 1997, with permission).*

Woods' manoeuvre and Rubin's manoeuvre

If there is no success with McRoberts' manoeuvre, these two manoeuvres, which involve manual rotation of the shoulders into the anteroposterior diameter of the pelvic outlet, can be attempted. The woman is helped into the lithotomy position with her buttocks well over the edge of the delivery bed. An alternative position which removes pressure from the sacrum is the all-fours.

Woods' manoeuvre

One hand is placed on the fetal buttocks and firm gentle pressure applied. Two fingers of the other hand are inserted into the vagina and the clavicle of the posterior shoulder is located. This shoulder is rotated 180° in the direction of the fetal back. This rotation should disimpact the anterior shoulder and enable the posterior shoulder to enter the pelvic brim, thus facilitating delivery.

Rubin's manoeuvre

If both shoulders are adducted, the circumference of the baby's body is greatly reduced than if they are abducted (we use this position to squeeze through narrow spaces by bringing our shoulders forward to make ourselves smaller). A hand is inserted into the vagina as far as is necessary to locate a shoulder. Working from behind the fetal back, this shoulder is pushed towards the fetal front to take the bisacromial diameter into an oblique pelvic diameter (Fig. 44.3). This frees them from the symphysis pubis and they can be delivered.

Delivery of the posterior arm

A hand is inserted into the vagina along the sacral curve to locate the posterior arm or hand. The fetal arm is taken across its chest and delivered (Fig. 44.4). The anterior shoulder should then be easy to deliver but if still delayed, the Woods' or Rubin's manoeuvre can be used to rotate the delivered arm to the anterior position so that the anterior arm is freed from behind the symphysis pubis.

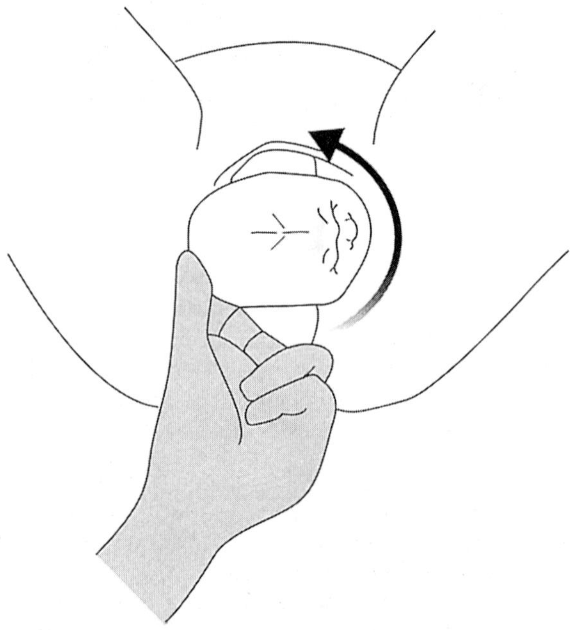

Figure 44.3 *Rubin's manoeuvre. The posterior shoulder is rotated anteriorly; the shoulders are adducted (from Sweet B, 1997, with permission).*

Other manoeuvres

Zavanelli manoeuvre

This manoeuvre of cephalic replacement does not result in vaginal delivery and has not been much used. The obstetrician returns the head to its prerestitution position and then flexes it and returns it to the vagina. Delivery is then by CS.

Cleidotomy

This is deliberate fracture of the clavicle but is difficult and rarely done. Spontaneous fracture may occur and facilitate delivery.

Outcome for mother and fetus

Maternal death is rare but can happen. Maternal morbidity is more common, with perineal, vaginal and cervical lacerations, uterine rupture, vaginal haematoma and haemorrhage possibly occurring. Postpartum haemorrhage should be anticipated and the genitalia carefully examined for lacerations.

For the baby, birth asphyxia is a complication of shoulder dystocia. Meconium aspiration may occur due to the asphyxia. Birth injury is also commonly reported with brachial plexus injury.

CORD PRESENTATION AND PROLAPSE

Lewis & Chamberlain (1990) state that one in 300 births is complicated by presentation of the umbilical cord when the cord lies in front of the presenting part. If a loop of cord lies alongside the fetal presenting part, this is called an **occult cord presentation**. If the membranes rupture, the cord is prolapsed. Murphy & Mackenzie (1995) found cord prolapse in 132 babies born in the John Radcliffe Hospital (Oxford) between January 1984 and December 1992. This gave a rate of one in 426 total births. There were six stillbirths and six neonatal deaths, giving an uncorrected perinatal mortality rate of 91 per 1000. Of 120 survivors, only one baby was known to have developed a major neurological handicap.

Causes

- A high presenting part: multiparous women, malposition of the occiput and malpresentations – brow, face, shoulder presentation (in 20%) – and breech presentation (in 5%), the high assimilation pelvis found in Afro-Caribbean women, cephalopelvic disproportion, placenta praevia, fibroids.
- Preterm labour because of the increased ratio of liquor amnii to fetus and the prevalence of malpresentations.
- Multiple births, especially following the birth of the first baby.

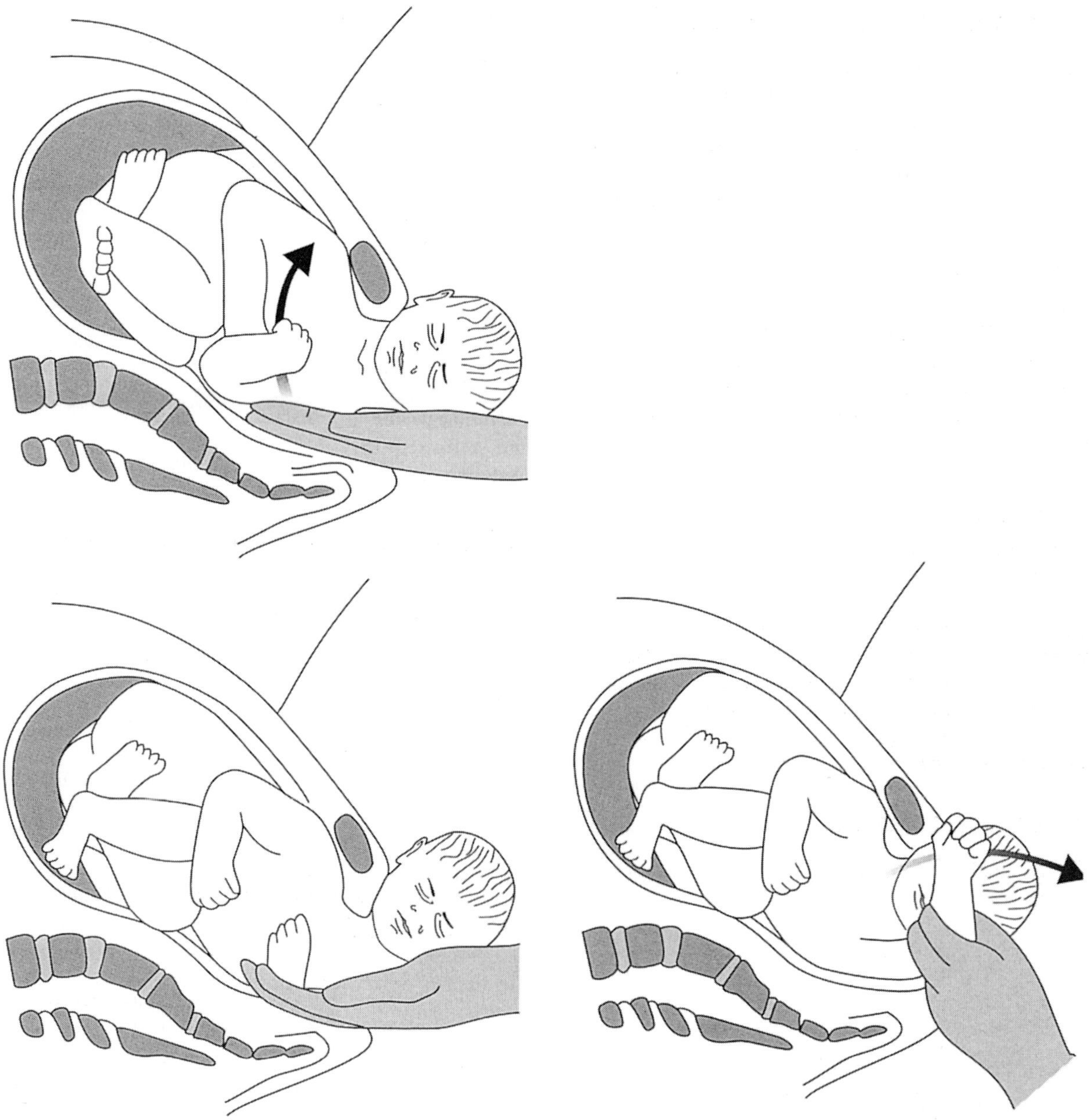

Figure 44.4 *Delivery of posterior arm (from Sweet B, 1997, with permission).*

- Polyhydramnios.
- An unusually long cord.
- Following obstetric manipulations such as external cephalic version.

Diagnosis

Cord presentation may be diagnosed in pregnancy by ultrasound scanning, especially in women with any of the risk factors mentioned above (Lange et al 1985). In early labour vaginal examination may occasionally find the rope-like cord between the presenting part and the membranes. It will be pulsating in time with the fetal heart rate. If cord presentation is suspected, it is essential to ensure that the membranes do not rupture. The mother is best placed in an exaggerated Simm's position with her pelvis, hips and buttocks elevated to take pressure off the cord and membranes. Medical assistance should be obtained immediately. If cord presentation persists, a CS will be needed. If the membranes have ruptured, the cord may prolapse through the cervix, into the vagina or even outside the vulva.

If the cord is prolapsed it may be compressed, especially if the presentation is cephalic because of the hardness of the fetal head, and the fetal oxygen supply cut off. If the cord is external to the vagina, cooling, drying and handling may precipitate spasm in the umbilical vessels. If the woman is in hospital the prognosis can be good, as Murphy & MacKenzie (1995) found. However, if the woman is at home fetal loss may be high.

Management

Factors to take into consideration are the stage in labour and whether or not the fetus is dead. If fetal death is confirmed, labour can be allowed to continue unless other conditions such as obstructed labour contraindicate vaginal delivery. If the fetus is thought to be alive the treatment is immediate delivery. In the first stage of labour a CS is arranged. Meanwhile, pressure must be kept off the cord by positioning the woman in a knee-chest or exaggerated Simm's position. The cord can be replaced gently back in the vagina and oxygen therapy may be of use if there is some fetoplacental circulation remaining.

In the early part of the 2nd stage of labour with no cephalopelvic disproportion or malpresentation, a forceps delivery is performed. If the woman is multiparous and in late 2nd stage an episiotomy may allow early delivery.

Summary of main points

- Any condition leading to a misfit between the fetal head and the maternal pelvis with failure of descent of the head into the pelvis despite good contractions results in cephalopelvic disproportion. Cephalopelvic disproportion is an absolute cause of obstructed labour and there are tremendous dangers for mother and fetus.
- In a primigravida the fetal head should engage in the last 2–3 weeks of pregnancy. The most common cause for non-engagement of the head is occipitoposterior position. A steep angle of inclination between the pelvic brim and the horizontal found in some Afro-Caribbean women may delay engagement until late in labour when engagement is followed by a normal vaginal delivery.
- Maternal indications of possible CPD include bone conditions, which may have resulted in alterations in the size and shape of the pelvis, spinal deformities, pelvic trauma and fractures, previous difficulties with delivery and short stature of the woman. The size of the fetus in relation to the maternal pelvis is the most obvious fetal consideration.
- A combination of careful history taking and clinical expertise backed up by technology should enable selection of women at risk. Head fitting or clinical or radiological pelvic assessment examinations may be carried out. An erect lateral X-ray pelvimetry provides information about the size and shape of the pelvis and the relationship of the fetal head to the pelvic brim. Magnetic resonance imaging may allow more accurate measurements of the pelvis.
- If there are no obstetric or medical complications, the woman can be admitted to hospital for a trial of labour. There must be facilities for an immediate CS to be carried out if needed. If progress is slow but unrelated to CPD, oxytocic drugs can be used. A CS may be necessary if the progress of labour remains slow following the commencement of the oxytocin infusion, the head fails to descend or fetal distress arises.
- Obstructed labour occurs whenever there is an impassable barrier to the descent of the fetus through the birth canal in spite of efficient uterine action. There is a large increase in maternal and fetal morbidity and mortality if labour is allowed to proceed. Causes of obstructed labour are CPD, malpositions and malpresentations of the head, such as brow, posterior face or deep transverse arrest of the head, fetal abnormalities such as hydrocephalus and maternal tumours.
- In a primigravida there may be active phase arrest and the contractions stop for a while, finally restarting with increased strength. The woman may complain of severe and continuous pain. The multiparous woman may have tumultuous contractions proceeding rapidly to uterine rupture.
- Rarely, the woman may progress to having a raised temperature, rapid pulse and dehydration. On abdominal inspection the uterus would appear to be moulded around the fetus and a Bandl's pathological retraction ring may be seen, denoting imminent rupture of the uterus. The fetus may die from anoxia. If labour is advanced when the woman is first seen, an emergency CS is carried out regardless of whether the fetus is dead or alive.
- Rupture of the uterus may involve a previous scar, spontaneous rupture of an intact uterus or traumatic rupture. Although it appears that the incidence of uterine rupture has fallen in developed countries it may be rising in the developing countries due to vaginal delivery following a previous CS and to the use of oxytocic infusions.
- Rupture of the uterus may be complete. This is usually an acute event associated with sudden intense pain, blood loss and collapse followed by maternal and fetal death. Incomplete or silent rupture is more frequently associated with a previous lower segment CS. Because scar tissue tends to be avascular there are fewer dramatic signs. Abdominal pain or scar tenderness may be present and a rise in maternal heart rate may be an indicator of impending rupture.
- If the mother is shocked she must be resuscitated and prepared for theatre. The baby is delivered and the uterus repaired if possible. A hysterectomy may be necessary if the rupture is severe and bleeding difficult to control.
- Shoulder dystocia is another obstetric emergency which may end in fetal and occasionally maternal morbidity and mortality. It may be due to a large baby and failure of the shoulders to rotate into the anteroposterior diameter following delivery of the head. An episiotomy will give room for the manoeuvres and help to prevent maternal trauma. Maternal morbidity is more common with risk of lacerations, uterine rupture and haemorrhage. The baby may suffer birth injuries.
- Causes of cord presentation and prolapse include high presenting part, breech presentation, cephalopelvic disproportion, placenta praevia, fibroids, preterm labour, multiple births, polyhydramnios, a long cord and external cephalic version. If cord presentation persists a CS will be needed. If the membranes rupture the cord may prolapse and become compressed, cutting off the fetal oxygen supply. If the cord is external, cooling, drying and handling may precipitate the umbilical vessel spasm.
- If fetal death is confirmed, labour can be allowed to continue unless other conditions such as obstructed labour contraindicate vaginal delivery. If the fetusis thought to be alive the treatment is immediate delivery. In the first stage of labour a CS is arranged. In the early part of the 2nd stage with no cephalopelvic disproportion or malpresentation, a forceps delivery is performed. If the woman is multiparous and in late 2nd stage, an episiotomy may allow early delivery.

References

Abitol MM. 1993 Adjustment of the fetal head and adult pelvis in modern humans. Journal of Human Evolution 8(3), 167–185.

Aiello L, Dean C. 1990 Human Evolutionary Anatomy. Academic Press, New York.

Brock MI. 1997 Cephalopelvic disproportion, obstructed labour and uterine rupture. In Sweet BR with Tiran D (eds) Mayes Midwifery, 12th edn. Baillière Tindall, London, pp 673–681.

Department of Health 1996 Report on Confidential Enquiries into Maternal Deaths in the United Kingdom 1991–1993. HMSO, London.

Enkin M, Keirse MJNC, Renfrew M, Neilson J. 1995 A Guide to Effective Care in Pregnancy and Childbirth, 2nd edn. Oxford Medical Publications, Oxford.

Flamm BL, Goings JR, Liu Y, Wolde-Tsadik G. 1994 Elective repeat Caesarean delivery versus trial of labour: a prospective multi-centre study. Obstetrics and Gynaecology 83(6), 927–932.

Grace D, Lavery G, Loughran PG. 1993 Acute uterine rupture and its sequelae. International Journal of Obstetric Anaesthesia 2, 41–44.

Gupta U, Chitra R. 1994 Destructive operations still have a place in developing countries. International Journal of Gynaecology and Obstetrics 44(1), 15–19.

Haig D. 1993 Genetic conflicts in human pregnancy. Quarterly Review of Biology 68(4), 495–519.

Lange IR, Manning FA, Morrison I, Chamberlain PF, Harman CR. 1985 Cord prolapse: is antenatal diagnosis possible? American Journal of Obstetrics and Gynecology 1512, 1083–1085.

Lewis T, Chamberlain G. 1990 Obstetrics by Ten Teachers. Hodder and Stoughton, Sevenoaks.

Mahmood TA, Campbell DM, Wilson AW. 1988 Maternal height, shoe size and outcome of labour in white primagravidas: a prospective study. British Medical Journal, 297: 515–517.

Moore NR, Dickenson DRM, Gillmer MD. 1992 Royal College of Radiologists annual meeting – abstract. Clinical Radiology 46, 414.

Murphy DJ, MacKenzie IZ. 1995 The mortality and morbidity associated with umbilical cord prolapse. British Journal of Obstetrics and Gynaecology 102(10), 826–830.

Proud J. 1996 Specialised antenatal investigations. In Bennett VR, Brown LK (eds) Myles Textbook for Midwives, 12th edn. Churchill Livingstone, Edinburgh, pp 660–674.

Rachagan SP, Raman S, Balasundram G, Balakrishnan S. 1991 Rupture of the uterus – a 21 year review. Australia and New Zealand Journal of Obstetrics and Gynaecology 31(1), 37–40.

Smeltzer JS. 1986 Prevention and management of shoulder dystocia. Clinical Obstetrics and Gynaecology 29(2), 299–308.

Spellacy WN, Miller S, Winegar A, Peterson PQ. 1985 Macrosomia, maternal characteristics and infant complications. Obstetrics and Gynaecology 66(2), 158–161.

Sweet B. 1997 Mayes' Midwifery. Baillière Tindall, London.

Williams J. 1996a Malposition of the occiput and malpresentations. In Bennett VR, Brown LK (eds) Myles Textbook for Midwives, 12th edn. Churchill Livingstone, Edinburgh, pp 404–431.

Williams J. 1996b Obstetric emergencies. In Bennett VR, Brown LK (eds) Myles Textbook for Midwives, 12th edn. Churchill Livingstone, Edinburgh, pp 432–440.

Recommended reading

Abitol MM. 1993 Adjustment of the fetal head and adult pelvis in modern humans. Journal of Human Evolution 8(3), 167–185.

Flamm BL, Goings JR, Liu Y, Wolde-Tsadik G. 1994 Elective repeat Caesarean delivery versus trial of labour: a prospective multi-centre study. Obstetrics and Gynaecology 83(6), 927–932.

Grace D, Lavery G, Loughran PG. 1993 Acute uterine rupture and its sequelae. International Journal of Obstetric Anaesthesia 2, 41–44.

Murphy DJ, MacKenzie IZ. 1995 The mortality and morbidity associated with umbilical cord prolapse. British Journal of Obstetrics and Gynaecology 102(10), 826–830.

Spellacy WN, Miller S, Winegar A, Peterson PQ. 1985 Macrosomia, maternal characteristics and infant complications. Obstetrics and Gynaecology 66(2), 158–161.

Chapter

45 Postpartum haemorrhage and other third-stage problems

In this chapter

INTRODUCTION

Once the baby has been born, delivery of the placenta and membranes may seem an anticlimax. However, the 3rd stage of labour is the most dangerous for the woman. The management of the 3rd stage should be aimed at minimising these possible serious complications while interfering as little as possible with the physiological process and the mother's enjoyment of her baby (Enkin et al 1995). A major role of the midwife is to explain the need for active interventions, such as giving an oxytocic drug or commencing an intravenous infusion, to the mothers prior to labour so that women are enabled to make informed choices should the need arise suddenly.

POSTPARTUM HAEMORRHAGE

Definition

Postpartum haemorrhage (PPH) is defined as excessive bleeding from the genital tract from the birth of the child to the end of the puerperium. If bleeding occurs in the first 24 h, it is called **primary PPH** and this complicates about 6% of labours. If the bleeding occurs after the first 24 h and before the end of the 6th week, it is called **secondary PPH**, a much less common occurrence complicating less than 1% of deliveries. Despite recommendations (DOH 1994), haemorrhage remains a major cause of maternal death, especially following a previous CS, and is associated with many deaths due to childbirth (Coulter-Smith et al 1996).

Postpartum haemorrhage is also classified according to the site of bleeding. Most commonly, the bleeding is from the placental site and there is poor tone of the uterine muscle. This is **atonic haemorrhage**. Bleeding may also be traumatic due to a laceration of the genital tract. In primary PPH, bleeding is said to be excessive if the amount exceeds 500 ml or is sufficient to cause a deterioration in the woman's condition.

Because of the diuresis and haemoconcentration that follow delivery, smaller amounts of blood loss are detrimental in secondary PPH.

Primary PPH is one of the most serious complications of labour that a midwife has to deal with until medical aid arrives. At term maternal blood is circulating to the placenta at about 500 ml per minute. Blood loss may be rapid and devastating if the bleeding is not controlled. PPH is still a significant cause of maternal mortality (DOH 1996). Measuring blood loss at delivery can be difficult. It is important to remember that blood soaks into sheets and towels and that it separates into clot and serum. Any clot placed in a jug and measured will only be 40% of the total loss so that it is easy to underestimate the total loss by up to 50%.

Primary postpartum haemorrhage

Causes

Failure of the uterine muscle fibres to contract and retract to compress the blood vessels is the immediate cause. Risk factors are:

- a history of previous postpartum haemorrhage;
- high parity – para three or more;
- overdistension of the uterus in multiple pregnancy, polyhydramnios and a large fetus;
- fibroids, which may interfere with efficient contraction and retraction;
- antepartum haemorrhage – bleeding into the muscle during placental abruption will reduce the fibres' ability to contract and retract and in placenta praevia there is little contractile ability in the lower uterine segment;
- prolonged labour with weak or uncoordinated contractions;
- atony, caused by drugs such as antihypertensives, general anaesthesia and tocolytics;
- retained placenta;
- anaemia, because even a small amount of blood loss may precipitate shock;
- inversion of the uterus;
- mismanagement of the 3rd stage of labour by fiddling with the uterus;
- coagulation defects – disseminated intravascular coagulation may complicate concealed placental abruption, amniotic fluid embolus, severe preeclampsia and eclampsia and intrauterine death;
- medical disorders of clotting.

Despite the long list of risk factors above, many cases of primary PPH occur in normal labours with no explanation.

Management – prophylaxis

In the antenatal period

Prevention is the best form of management and begins with the booking interview. If any of the risk factors described above are present, the woman should be delivered in hospital so that if bleeding does occur treatment is immediately available. As pregnancy progresses detection and treatment of anaemia is important and it would be advantageous to raise the Hb to at least 11 g/dl before delivery (Lindsay 1997).

In labour

Women at risk of PPH must be managed carefully to minimise the likelihood of bleeding. When labour commences an intravenous cannula is inserted and blood is taken for estimation of Hb and confirmation of blood group. Serum is saved to facilitate cross matching should it become necessary. Prolonged labour, with its problems of dehydration and exhaustion, is avoided and a syntocinon infusion commenced if needed. The woman's bladder should be kept empty by encouraging micturition or catheterisation as the full bladder may inhibit uterine muscle activity and add to the risk of atony.

Management of the 3rd stage should have been discussed with the woman antenatally. She should be informed that physiological management of the 3rd stage is considered unsafe and that it would be preferred if she would agree to active management with the use of an oxytocic drug. An intramuscular injection of syntometrine 1 ml containing syntocinon 5 units and ergometrine 500 μg is given with the birth of the anterior shoulder. An intravenous injection of ergometrine 500 μg may be required if bleeding should commence. The placenta is delivered by controlled cord traction.

Signs of PPH

It would be difficult to miss the visible bleeding and maternal collapse that can occur. The following signs may be present if blood loss is not visible; for instance, if clots were retained in an atonic uterus.

- Pallor
- A rising pulse rate and falling blood pressure
- Altered levels of consciousness
- Air hunger
- An enlarged boggy-feeling uterus

Management – treatment

It is important that a midwife is familiar with the sequence of actions needed to deal with a PPH and to minimise the effects of blood loss.

If bleeding begins **before the placenta is delivered**, the following actions should be taken.

1. Ensure that medical aid is available.
2. Massage the uterus to 'rub up' a contraction. Bleeding indicates that the placenta has begun to separate and it is no longer necessary to await events.
3. Give an oxytocic drug. Intramuscular syntometrine 1 ml will act to contract the uterus in 2.5 min and an intravenous injection of either syntometrine 1 ml or ergometrine 500 μg will act in 45 s. Note that the midwife should not give more than two injections of ergometrine 500 μg as the drug may cause severe peripheral vasodilation and a sudden rise in blood pressure.
4. Attempt to deliver the placenta before the uterus contracts.
5. If it is not possible to deliver the placenta pass a catheter into the bladder and ensure that it is completely empty and try once more.

6 In the event of inability to deliver the placenta, the doctor will need to carry out a manual removal of placenta under general anaesthesia.

Whilst awaiting help, do not elevate the foot of the bed as blood will pool in the uterus and prevent contraction. Instead, ensure that as much blood as possible is available to the vital centres by raising the woman's legs.

If bleeding begins **after delivery of the placenta**, massage the uterus to obtain a contraction and expel any blood clots remaining in the uterus. An injection of an oxytocic drug, either intramuscular syntometrine 1 ml or ergometrine 500 μg, should then stop bleeding by achieving a sustained contraction. Ensure that the urinary bladder is empty. If bleeding continues it is necessary to carry out bimanual compression of the uterus. Following delivery of the placenta and membranes, they should be examined for completeness. If the placenta appears incomplete exploration and evacuation of the uterus under general anaesthesia will be carried out by the doctor.

Bimanual compression of the uterus

Bimanual compression may be performed externally or internally. In **external** bimanual compression, one hand is dipped down as far as possible behind the uterus whilst the other is placed flat on the abdomen. The uterus is compressed between the two hands and pulled upwards in the abdomen. This ensures that the bleeding area of the placental site is compressed whilst the uterine veins are straightened out to allow free drainage, relieve congestion and decrease the bleeding (Lindsay 1997).

Internal bimanual compression is carried out if the mother is anaesthetised and still bleeding after manual removal of placenta. One hand is closed to form a fist and inserted into the anterior vaginal fornix. The other hand is placed on the abdominal wall behind the uterus and dips down to pull the uterus towards the symphysis pubis (Fig. 45.1). This applies compression to the placental site until the uterus is felt to contract.

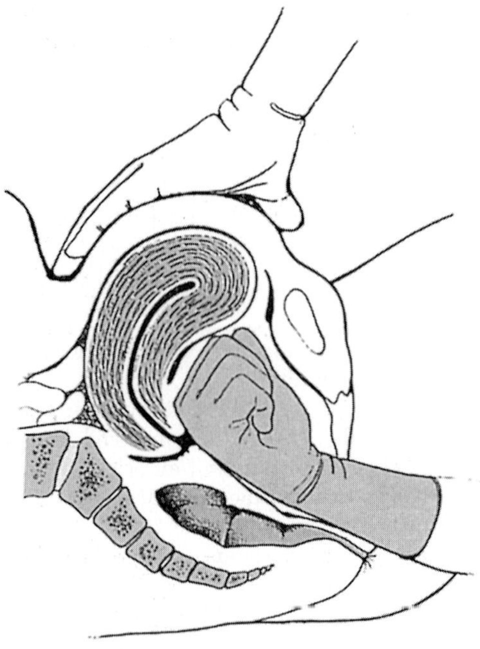

Figure 45.1 *Internal bimanual compression of the uterus (from Sweet B, 1997, with permission).*

Once bleeding is controlled an intravenous infusion containing oxytocin 20–40 units in 500 ml Hartmann's solution is commenced to maintain uterine contraction. Blood transfusion may also be required and it is important not to underestimate the amount of blood lost. As early as 1967 Brant found that estimates of blood loss became more inaccurate as the amount lost increased. If haemorrhage has been torrential an anaesthetist will manage fluid replacement. Dextran infusion should be avoided as not only can it interfere with cross-matching but it can prolong bleeding times (DOH 1994). Group O rhesus-negative blood must be available and, if necessary, should be passed through a warming coil.

If the uterus refuses to contract even though oxytocic drugs have been used, a deep intramuscular injection of the prostanoid carboprost, which is 15-methyl-$PGF_{2\alpha}$ (Rang & Dale 1991), can be given in a dose of 250 μg and repeated at intervals of 1.5 h. Carboprost is contraindicated in women with cardiac, renal, pulmonary and hepatic disease as well as in acute pelvic inflammation. It should be used with care in women who have asthma, hypertension, diabetes, epilepsy, hypotension or hypertension (BNF 1996). In continuing haemorrhage, often with DIC, aortic compression and internal iliac artery ligation may be needed and if all fails, a hysterectomy may be life saving.

Observations

Once blood loss is controlled, the total loss is estimated remembering how difficult this can be and that estimates are more inaccurate as blood loss increases. Fluid intake is recorded on a chart, as is the hourly output of urine from a self-retaining urinary catheter. Central venous pressure is monitored to ensure that the correct amount of fluid is replaced intravenously. Maternal pulse and blood pressure are recorded 1/4 hourly to ensure her condition remains satisfactory. The uterine fundus is palpated frequently to ensure it remains contracted and the lochia are observed.

If the problem involves failure of blood coagulation, a haematologist should be consulted. Fresh blood is usually the best treatment as it contains both platelets and coagulation factors but fresh frozen plasma, containing factors V and VIII and fibrinogen, can be used.

Traumatic PPH

If the blood loss is from a laceration of the genital tract bleeding should be stopped by direct pressure if possible and then sutured. Bleeding from a cervical or lower uterine tear should be suspected if the uterus is well contracted, no superficial bleeding can be seen and the blood loss is slow and steady. Tears of the upper part of the vagina, the cervix and lower uterine segment should be sutured under general or epidural anaesthesia. If the bleeding is from a tear in the uterus and is severe, a hysterectomy is occasionally necessary.

Secondary postpartum haemorrhage

Secondary PPH is a complication of the puerperium. It occurs after the first 24 h from delivery and is seen most often between days 4 and 14. It is usually due to a retained piece of placenta but other causes include the presence of blood clot or a fibroid in the uterine wall. Infection is also commonly associated with secondary PPH. There may have been warning signs of heavy, red, offensive lochia and subinvolution. If infection is present a low-grade pyrexia and tachycardia may ensue.

Management

If the uterus is palpable it is massaged to make it contract. Any clots are expelled and the bladder must be emptied. An injection of intravenous ergometrine 500 μg or intramuscular syntometrine 1 ml is given if bleeding is severe. If the woman is at home she should be transferred to hospital once her condition is under control. A blood transfusion is given and the uterus evacuated under general anaesthetic. If bleeding is slight it may be managed at home with antibiotics and oral ergometrine tablets.

Complications

Unless adequately treated, the woman is likely to develop **chronic iron deficiency anaemia**. Infection is more common and lactation may be poor. If shock develops acute renal tubular necrosis may present with anuria. Anterior pituitary necrosis leading to Sheehan's syndrome may occur if the haemorrhage was severe. All women who have suffered a postpartum haemorrhage should be advised to book into a hospital for any subsequent deliveries.

Haematoma formation

Postpartum haemorrhage may be concealed if progressive haematoma formation occurs in the perineum or lower vagina. A site of haematoma formation which is more difficult to diagnose is bleeding into the broad ligament. Up to 1 litre of blood may collect in the tissues, leading to increasing maternal pain due to pressure. The mother may collapse with signs of shock.

Management

The woman should be taken to theatre so that the haematoma can be drained and haemostasis achieved under a general anaesthetic. Replacement of the lost blood may be necessary. Infection is a risk and antibiotics are usually prescribed.

PROLONGED THIRD STAGE

Failure of the placenta to deliver spontaneously is an important cause of postpartum haemorrhage (Combs & Laros 1991). In their research these authors found that the incidence of postpartum haemorrhage remained constant up to 30 min and then rose progressively to reach a plateau at 75 min. If labour is managed actively the placenta and membranes should be delivered within 10 min.

If the delivery is delayed until 30 min the 3rd stage is considered to be prolonged. With physiological management of the 3rd stage, up to 1 h may be allowed before considering the procedure to be prolonged. The placenta may be separated but retained, trapped behind the reforming cervix, and bleeding is likely. Alternatively the placenta may be morbidly adherent to the uterine wall and if there is no separation, bleeding will not occur.

Causes

- Uterine inertia.
- Full bladder.
- Mismanagement of the third stage where 'fiddling' with the uterus causes irregular contractions and partial separation of the placenta.
- The formation of a constriction ring or spasm between the upper and lower uterine segments.
- A uterine abnormality such as bicornuate uterus.
- Morbid adherence of the placenta, more likely to occur in women who have had a previous CS or placenta praevia.

Types of adherent placenta

1 **Placenta accreta** where the decidua basalis is deficient and the chorionic villi have attached to the myometrium.
2 **Placenta increta** where the villi penetrate deeply into the myometrium.
3 **Placenta percreta** where the villi have penetrated to the serous external coat of the uterus.

Management

As long as the placenta remains in the uterus, haemorrhage is a threat. If, after emptying the bladder and attempting to remove the placenta, there is no success, manual removal of the placenta by the obstetrician is necessary (Fig. 45.2). The procedure may cause shock if conducted without adequate anaesthesia. If the placenta is only retained or if the area of

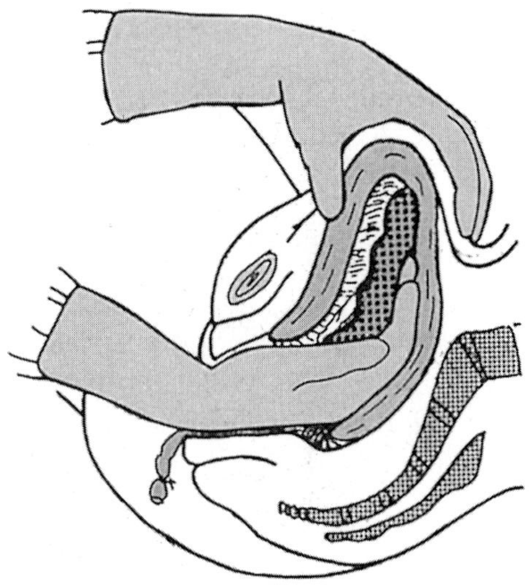

Figure 45.2 *Manual removal of the placenta (from Sweet B, 1997, with permission).*

adherence is only partial, manual removal of placenta may be successful.

The obstetrician has two choices in deeply adherent placentae. A hysterectomy can be performed or the placenta can be left in situ to be reabsorbed. The drug methotrexate has been used to hasten the absorption of the placental tissue but is not always successful (Lindsay 1997). An intravenous oxytocic injection is given after successful manual removal followed by an intravenous infusion of 20 units of syntocinon in 500 ml of solution. Antibiotic therapy is commenced as manual removal of placenta may have introduced organisms into the uterus.

ACUTE INVERSION OF THE UTERUS

In this rare condition, which occurs in about one in 100 000 deliveries, the uterus is partly or completely turned inside out (Fig. 45.3). In **partial inversion**, the inner surface of the fundus is drawn down into the uterine cavity but in **severe inversion** the inside of the fundus protrudes through the cervix into the vagina. If the uterus is fully turned inside out, it may appear outside the vulva. Profound neurogenic shock due to traction on the uterine supportive ligaments is likely to occur. There will be pain and possibly haemorrhage if there is partial placental separation.

Causes

- Mismanagement of the 3rd stage by applying fundal pressure or cord traction with the uterus relaxed.
- A short cord, where the fundus descends with the fetus.
- Manual removal of placenta if the operator withdraws the hand in the uterus whilst still applying fundal pressure.
- Spontaneous inversion, possibly due to straining which raises intrabdominal pressure, such as a sudden cough or sneeze.

Diagnosis and management

The woman will complain of pain and may collapse suddenly.

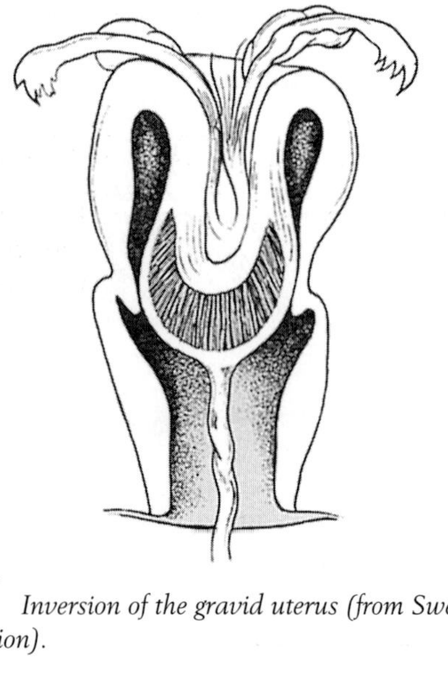

Figure 45.3 *Inversion of the gravid uterus (from Sweet B, 1997, with permission).*

On palpation of the uterus, it will be difficult to find the fundus of the uterus. A distinct hollow in the fundus may be felt. The woman may complain of a feeling that something is in her vagina.

The rapid replacement of the uterus will prevent the development of shock. Replacement is easier if it is carried out immediately, before uterine congestion and oedema develop. Pressure is applied first to the part of the lower segment nearest the cervix, gently proceeding upwards towards the fundus. If replacement is not possible the uterus should be replaced in the vagina and the foot of the bed elevated to reduce traction on the uterine ligaments, fallopian tubes and ovaries. An injection of morphine 15 mg will reduce pain. If the placenta is still attached to the uterine wall it should not be removed.

Methods of replacement

If there has been delay the woman is anaesthetised and the uterus replaced manually, as described above, by pressure in the fornices to replace the lower segment, which was last to invert, and then the fundus. If a retraction ring has developed between the upper and lower uterine segments, replacement may be difficult. Inhalation of amyl nitrite vapour or a deep general anaesthetic may be needed to relax the uterine muscle.

O'Sullivan's hydrostatic method is preferred by some obstetricians. Two to three litres of warm normal saline is infused via a douche nozzle into the vagina whilst the introitus is sealed around the forearm by the other hand (Lindsay 1997). The fluid container is held about a metre above the level of the uterus with the woman in lithotomy position. The pressure of the liquid distends the vagina and the uterus replaces itself quite quickly. Following replacement, an intravenous injection of ergometrine 500 μg will ensure it remains in its correct position. The placenta may now be removed if necessary.

AMNIOTIC FLUID EMBOLISM

This obstetric emergency occurs when amniotic fluid is forced from the uterine venous sinuses of the placental bed into the maternal circulation. It may occur not only in the 3rd stage but near to term, before labour begins, at any time during labour or immediately after delivery. The embolus travels around the systemic circulation, through the heart and into the pulmonary circulation to obstruct pulmonary arterioles or alveolar capillaries. The mortality rate is as high as 86% with 25% of the deaths occurring in the first hour (Williams 1996).

Risk factors

Amniotic embolism is more likely to occur in women where intraamniotic pressures are raised:

- hypertonic uterine action, spontaneous or induced by oxytocic drugs;
- older multiparous women with rapid labours;
- multiple pregnancy;
- polyhydramnios;
- uterine trauma such as CS, ruptured uterus, internal podalic version or manual removal of placenta.

Diagnosis

The diagnosis can only be made with certainty if amniotic fluid is detected in the maternal circulation and often this is postmortem when fetal desquamated skin and lanugo are also found in the lungs. There is usually sudden onset of **maternal respiratory distress** with cyanosis, chest pain, dyspnoea, blood-stained frothy sputum and collapse. **Cardiovascular collapse** soon follows with tachycardia and hypotension. Amniotic fluid is rich in thromboplastins and its release into the blood may cause **disseminated intravascular coagulation** (DIC) and coagulation failure (Davies & Harrison 1992).

Management

This is an obstetric emergency. The uterus must be emptied as rapidly as possible, by CS if necessary. Unfortunately, this rare complication often results in the death of the woman and her baby despite active treatment. Oxygen is given by facemask and cardiopulmonary resuscitation commenced if the woman collapses. Intravenous aminophylline may help relieve bronchospasm and hydrocortisone will relieve the inflammatory effect of amniotic fluid on lung tissue. An attempt is made to reverse the DIC and control haemorrhage, should they occur. If the woman survives there may be **renal failure** and dialysis may be necessary if the kidneys do not respond to diuretic drugs such as mannitol.

SHOCK IN OBSTETRICS

McCance & Huether (1994) define shock as 'a condition in which the cardiovascular system fails to perfuse the tissues adequately, resulting in widespread impairment of cellular metabolism'. Three functions of the cardiovascular system may be altered and result in shock. If the heart is thought of as a pump, these can be summarised as:

1 **heart function** – loss of the pump;
2 **blood volume** – nothing to pump;
3 **blood pressure** – no force in the pump.

Shock from any condition will inevitably cause progress to organ failure and death unless some compensatory mechanisms occur to reverse the situation or clinical treatments are successful.

If shock remains untreated, the body's compensatory mechanisms are overwhelmed and a downward spiral towards death will occur. The compensatory mechanisms function to maintain blood pressure and blood flow to vital organs such as the brain and the heart (Hinchliff et al 1996).

Recognition

Because the body has many systems, all involving cells at microscopic level, shock presents with many signs and symptoms. Tissue damage is diverse and subjective symptoms can be vague. A person may report nausea, weakness, feeling cold or hot, dizziness, confusion, fear and anxiety, thirst and shortage of breath with air hunger. Clinical measurements will find pulse and respiration rate increased, blood pressure and cardiac output decreased, diminished urinary output, cold, clammy skin, pallor and reduced core temperature.

Classification

There are various ways of classifying shock, for example by pathophysiological processes, by clinical manifestations or by cause (Campbell 1993). Classification by cause is the most useful as it will also indicate the likely pathophysiology

Table 45.1 *Types of shock and their immediate cause*

Type	*Cause*
Cardiogenic	Heart failure
Hypovolaemic	Reduced blood volume
Neurogenic	Neural alterations of smooth muscle tone resulting in vasodilation
Anaphylactic	Immune system pathology resulting in vasodilation
Septic	Resulting in cardiac depression and dilatation with vasodilation

Table 45.2 *Pathophysiological causes of shock in childbearing*

Cardiogenic shock	*Hypovolaemic shock*	*Neurogenic shock*	*Anaphylactic shock*	*Septic shock*
Pulmonary embolism	Haemorrhage associated with childbearing	Acute inversion of the uterus	Adverse drug reactions	Infection in septic abortion and puerperal infection
Severe anaemia	Ruptured ectopic pregnancy	Aspiration of acid gastric contents (Mendelson's syndrome)		
Cardiac disorders such as valvular or congenital problems	Ruptured uterus	Intrauterine manipulations without adequate anaesthesia		
Severe hypertension	Coagulopathy following amniotic fluid embolism Diabetic crisis			

underlying the shock and highlight the disorder that will need treating to reverse the shock (Tables 45.1 and 45.2). The three main cardiovascular functions that are impaired are obvious. All of the following types of shock may occur in childbearing women and will first be described in detail. Possible causes of obstetric shock will then be discussed. The danger is that the compensatory mechanisms may mask the signs of shock until maternal and fetal lives are at risk.

Cardiogenic shock

Heart failure is the cause of cardiogenic shock and most cases are due to myocardial infarction. Shock may also occur in congestive cardiac failure, myocardial ischaemia and drug toxicity. It is not very responsive to treatment and often leads to death.

The compensatory sequence of events is as follows.

- As cardiac output begins to decrease, renin produced by the kidneys stimulates aldosterone release so that sodium and water are retained.
- Hypothalamic responses cause catecholamine release from the adrenal glands, resulting in vasoconstriction to maintain blood pressure.
- Cardiac performance is enhanced but there is increased demand for oxygen and nutrients.
- Tissue perfusion begins to fall and nutrient and oxygen delivery to the cells decreases.
- Cellular metabolism is impaired and signs of shock appear.

Hypovolaemic shock

Hypovolaemic shock with inadequate blood volume is the most common form. Shock begins to develop when intravascular volume is decreased by 15%. The first sign is a thready pulse as intense vasoconstriction attempts to move blood from the periphery to supply the vital organs. A sharp decline in blood pressure is a late and serious sign (Marieb 1992). It may occur because of:

1. loss of whole blood in haemorrhage;
2. loss of plasma, as in burns;
3. loss of interstitial fluid;
4. diabetes mellitus;
5. excessive vomiting or diarrhoea.

The compensatory sequence of events is as follows.

- Adrenal release of catecholamines increases heart rate and systemic vascular resistance (SVR).
- Interstitial fluid moves into the vascular compartment.
- The liver and spleen disgorge stored red blood cells and plasma into the circulation.
- Renin produced by the kidneys stimulates aldosterone release and sodium and water are retained.
- Tissue perfusion begins to fall and nutrient and oxygen delivery to the cells decreases.
- Cellular metabolism is impaired and signs of shock appear.

Neurogenic shock

Another name for neurogenic shock is **vasogenic shock**, referring to the massive vasodilation that results because of a loss of balance between the sympathetic and parasympathetic stimulation of vascular smooth muscle. Although blood volume does not change, the vascular compartment is increased drastically, resulting in relative hypovolaemia with a decrease in SVR. Vascular resistance is normally maintained by the sympathetic stimulus and if this is interrupted or inhibited for any length of time, neurogenic shock will follow.

Causes include:

- trauma to the spinal cord;
- cerebral hypoxia;
- medullary hypoglycaemia;
- anaesthetics and other depressive drugs;
- pain and severe emotional distress.

The compensatory sequence of events is as follows.

- An increase in sympathetic activity will correct the bradycardia and very low SVR.
- Fainting ensures that the person is prevented from maintaining an upright posture so that blood pressure is equalised from head to toe and cerebral blood supply is maximised.

Anaphylactic shock

Anaphylactic shock results from a widespread hypersensitivity reaction. The pathophysiology is similar to that of neurogenic shock with widespread vasodilation and pooling of blood in the periphery. This type of shock is very serious because it involves multiple body systems. It begins as an allergic reaction with an immune and inflammatory response to a proteinous substance such as insect venom, pollens, shellfish, penicillin and foreign serum. The vascular component of this response includes vasodilation and increased vascular permeability so that the relative hypovolaemia brought about by peripheral pooling is exacerbated by tissue oedema. There is bronchoconstriction so that the ability to provide oxygen to the tissues is severely compromised.

The onset of anaphylactic shock is rapid and can progress to death in minutes unless emergency treatment is available. Ingesting peanuts causes anaphylactic shock in some people and the effects have been widely reported in the press and illustrate the condition well. The signs are anxiety, difficulty in breathing, gastrointestinal cramps, oedema and urticaria with severe itching and burning sensations in the skin (McCance & Huether 1994). A steep fall in blood pressure follows with confusion and coma.

Emergency management

There is little time for spontaneous compensatory mechanisms and the person may die unless medical intervention is possible.

- Adrenaline injection will reverse airway constriction and cause vasoconstriction.
- Intravenous volume expanders will reverse the relative hypovolaemia.
- Steroids will end the inflammatory process.

Septic shock

Septic shock is a very complex process and the explanations for its progress are still being developed. More than half the cases are caused by Gram-negative bacteria and the most common sources of infection in the non-pregnant population are the respiratory tract and the gastrointestinal tract. Infections of the genital tract are of prime importance in the childbearing woman.

Septic shock is triggered by bacteraemia and bacteria may be present in the blood for some time before shock develops. The elderly, critically ill or immune compromised are most likely to develop bacteraemic shock and one of the authors remembers a woman who became severely ill following insertion of an intrauterine contraceptive device. Uterine infection was followed by generalised infection and bacteraemia.

Four major body chemicals have been implicated in the development of bacteraemic shock (McCance & Huether 1994).

1 **Interleukins (Il)** Cytokines produced by the white blood cells which cause vasodilation and increase vascular permeability. They influence the hypothalamus to cause fever, initiate the complement cascade and stimulate the release of TNF.
2 **Tumour necrosis factor (TNF)** A cytokine produced by macrophages, natural killer cells and mast cells. It activates both clotting and complement cascades. In addition TNF causes vasodilation and increases vascular permeability.
3 **Platelet-activating factor (PAF)** Released from mononuclear phagocytes, platelets and some endothelial cells in response to the presence of an endotoxin. It is directly toxic to multiple organs and causes vasodilation and increased vascular permeability. PAF also mobilises white cells, activates platelets and stimulates the release of TNF.
4 **Myocardial depressant substance (MDS)** Secreted by white blood cells in response to an endotoxin. The heart responds to MDS by becoming depressed and dilated, leading to pump failure and hypotension.

As shock increases carbohydrate metabolism is altered with a serum increase in both insulin and glucagon. Serum glucose levels fluctuate and glucose usage by the tissues is enhanced. Glucose and glycogen stores become depleted. Depletion of glucose leads to heart failure and oxygen shortage and **multiple organ dysfunction syndrome** (MODS) may develop.

Multiple organ dysfunction syndrome

In multiple organ dysfunction syndrome (MODS) there is failure of two or more organ systems after severe illness or injury (Fig. 45.4). Sepsis and septic shock are the most common precipitating causes. Mortality is high and it is the most common cause of death following sepsis, trauma and burns. The following processes occur.

- Release of the stress hormones cortisol, adrenaline, noradrenaline and endorphins.
- Stimulation of the sympathetic nervous system.
- Vascular endothelial damage by endotoxins or inflammatory substances.
- Interstitial oedema.
- Disseminated intravascular coagulation with microvascular thrombi and capillary obstruction.

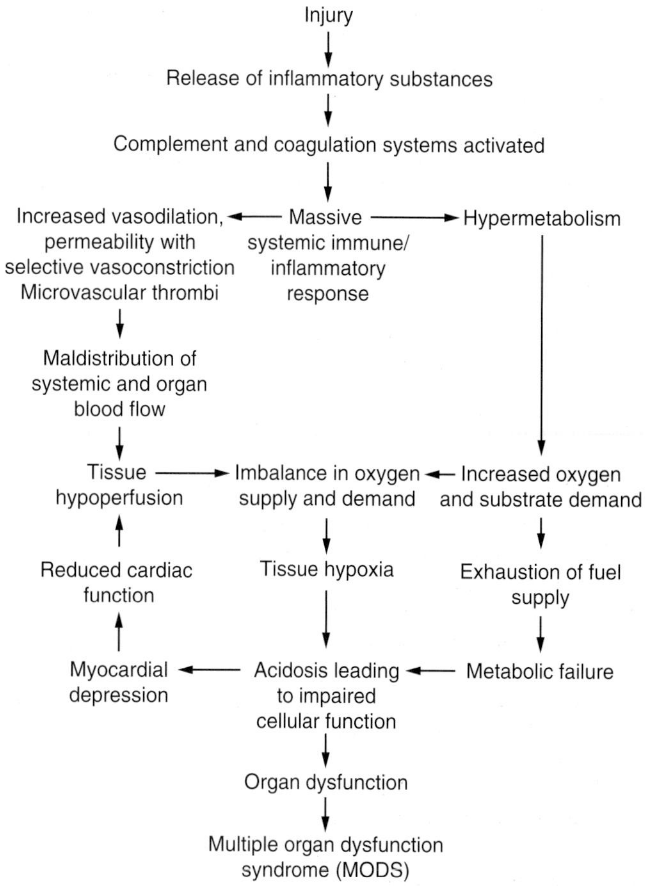

Figure 45.4 *The pathogenesis of multiple organ dysfunction. (Reproduced with permission from McCance & Huether 1994.)*

- Hyperdynamic circulation with increased venous return.
- Hypermetabolism with elevated carbohydrate, lipid and protein breakdown to provide energy, leading to weight loss.

Failure of the lungs develops first with adult respiratory distress syndrome (ARDS). If this occurs, there is a mortality of over 80% (Pearlman & Faro 1990). Renal and liver failure follow and there is gastrointestinal and immune system failure. Cardiovascular collapse with myocardial depression of function causes the death of the patient after about 3 weeks if treatment is unsuccessful. The normal supply of oxygen to the tissues is based on need and is met by alterations in blood flow distribution. This system fails and oxygen supply depends only on how much the circulation is able to deliver. This is known as **supply-dependent oxygen consumption**.

Outline of the management of MODS

The reader is referred to McCance & Huether (1994) for a fuller description of the management of MODS. Briefly, early recognition is extremely important followed by treatment of the precipitating cause, for example removing the source of infection. Restoration of tissue oxygenation and nutrition is very important. Individual organs such as the kidney may need supporting through the crisis.

Summary of main points

- In primary postpartum haemorrhage, the bleeding may be from the placental site but may occasionally be due to a laceration of the genital tract. Risk factors include previous PPH, high parity, overdistension of the uterus, fibroids, retained products of conception, inverted uterus, 3rd stage mismanagement and coagulation defects.
- If any of the risk factors are present the woman should be delivered in hospital. Physiological management of the 3rd stage is considered unsafe. An injection of intramuscular syntometrine 1 ml or intravenous ergometrine 500 µg is given with the birth of the anterior shoulder. The placenta is delivered by controlled cord traction.
- If bleeding commences before the placenta is delivered, the uterus is massaged to encourage contractions, an oxytocic drug is given and an attempt to deliver the placenta is made. A manual removal of placenta under general anaesthesia may be necessary. If bleeding begins after delivery of the placenta, the uterus is massaged to obtain a contraction and expel any blood clots remaining in the uterus. An injection of an oxytocic drug should sustain contractions to stop bleeding.
- If the placenta is incomplete, evacuation of the uterus under general anaesthesia will be carried out. Once bleeding is controlled an intravenous infusion containing oxytocin is commenced to maintain uterine contraction. Blood transfusion and fluid replacement may be required. Antibiotics will be prescribed following any operative intervention.
- If the blood loss is from a laceration of the genital tract, bleeding should be stopped by direct pressure if possible and then sutured. If severe bleeding is from a tear in the uterus, a hysterectomy is occasionally necessary.
- Secondary PPH is usually due to a retained piece of placenta. Other causes include the presence of blood clot, a fibroid or infection. If the uterus is palpable it is massaged until it contracts, clots are expelled and the bladder emptied. An intravenous injection of an oxytocic drug is given if bleeding is severe followed by evacuation of the uterus. Slight bleeding is managed at home with antibiotics and oral ergometrine. Inadequate treatment may lead to iron deficiency anaemia, acute renal tubular necrosis or anterior pituitary necrosis and Sheehan's syndrome.
- PPH may be concealed if progressive haematoma formation occurs in the perineum or lower vagina. The mother may collapse with shock. The haematoma is drained and haemostasis achieved under a general anaesthetic.
- Failure of the placenta to deliver spontaneously is an important cause of PPH. The placenta may be separated but retained, when bleeding is likely, or morbidly adherent to the uterine wall and bleeding will not occur. Manual removal may be necessary. In deeply adherent placentae a CS can be performed or the placenta can be left in situ to be reabsorbed.
- Causes of acute inversion of the uterus include mismanagement of the 3rd stage but spontaneous inversion does occur. Rapid replacement of the uterus will prevent shock. If replacement is not possible the uterus should be returned to the vagina and the foot of the bed elevated. An injection of morphine 15 mg will reduce pain. If still attached, the placenta should not be removed. If there has been delay the woman is anaesthetised and the uterus replaced manually followed by an intravenous injection of ergometrine 500 µg. O'Sullivan's hydrostatic method is preferred by some obstetricians.
- An amniotic fluid embolus travels into the pulmonary circulation to obstruct pulmonary arterioles or capillaries. It is more likely to occur where intraamniotic pressures are raised and in uterine trauma. Sudden onset of maternal respiratory distress is followed by cardiovascular collapse and possibly DIC. Oxygen is given and cardiopulmonary resuscitation commenced if needed. Mortality is high and renal failure may be a complication.
- Three functions of the cardiovascular system may be altered and result in shock. These are heart function, blood volume and blood pressure. Shock progresses to organ failure and death unless compensatory mechanisms or clinical treatments can reverse the pathology. Because the body has many systems, shock presents with many signs and symptoms including nausea, weakness, feeling cold or hot, dizziness, confusion, fear and anxiety, thirst and air hunger. There is diminished urinary output, cold, clammy skin, pallor and reduced core temperature.
- Classification of shock by cause is the most useful as it will also indicate the likely pathophysiology and highlight the underlying disorder that will need treating. Types of shock are cardiogenic, hypovolaemic, neurogenic, anaphylactic and septic.
- Cardiogenic shock due to heart failure is not very responsive to treatment and often leads to death. Hypovolaemic shock may occur because of loss of whole blood in haemorrhage, loss of plasma or interstitial fluid, diabetes mellitus, vomiting or diarrhoea. Neurogenic shock results from a loss of balance between the sympathetic and parasympathetic stimulation of vascular smooth muscle with vasodilation, resulting in relative hypovolaemia. Anaphylactic shock results from a widespread hypersensitivity reaction. Septic shock is caused by Gram-negative bacteria. Multiple organ dysfunction syndrome (MODS) may develop, with high mortality.

References

Brant H. 1967 Precise estimation of postpartum haemorrhage: difficulties and importance. British Medical Journal 1, 389–400.

British National Formulary 1996 British Medical Association and Royal Pharmaceutical Association of Great Britain, Number 32.

Campbell J. 1993 Making sense of shock. Nursing Times 89(5), 34–36.

Combs CA, Laros RK. 1991 Prolonged third stage of labor: morbidity and risk factors. Obstetrics and Gynaecology 77(6), 863–867.

Coulter-Smith SD, Holohan M, Darling MRN. 1996 Previous caesarean section: a risk factor for major obstetric haemorrhage. Journal of Obstetrics and Gynaecology 16(5), 349–352.

Davies M, Harrison J. 1992 Amniotic fluid embolism: maternal mortality revisited. British Journal of Hospital Medicine 14(10), 775–776.

Department of Health 1994 Report on Confidential Enquiries into Maternal Deaths in the United Kingdom 1988–1990. HMSO, London.

Department of Health 1996 Report on confidential enquiries into maternal deaths in the United Kingdom 1991 and 1993 HMSO, London.

Enkin M, Keirse MJNC, Renfrew M, Neilson J. 1995 A Guide to Effective Care in Pregnancy and Childbirth, 2nd edn. Oxford Medical Publications, Oxford.

Hinchliff SM, Montague SE, Watson R. 1996 Physiology for Nursing Practice, 2nd edn. Baillière Tindall, London.

Lindsay P. 1997 Complications of the third stage of labour. In Sweet BR with Tiran D (eds) Mayes Midwifery, 12th edn. Baillière Tindall, London, pp 703–718.

Marieb EN. 1992 Human Anatomy and Physiology. Benjamin/ Cummings Publishing, California

McCance KL, Huether SE. 1994 Pathphysiology: The Biologic Basis for Disease in Adults and Children, 2nd edn. Mosby, St Louis.

Pearlman M, Faro S. 1990 Obstetric septic shock: a pathophysiological basis for management. Clinics in Obstetrics and Gynaecology 33(3), 482–492.

Rang HP, Dale MM. 1991 Pharmacology, 2nd edn. Churchill Livingstone, Edinburgh.

Sweet B. 1997 Mayes' Midwifery. Baillière Tindall, London.

Williams J. 1996 Obstetric emergencies. In: Bennett VR, Brown LK (eds) Myles Textbook for Midwives, 12th edn. Churchill Livingstone, Edinburgh, pp 432–440.

Recommended reading

Campbell J. 1993 Making sense of shock. Nursing Times 89(5), 34–36.

Combs CA, Laros RK. 1991 Prolonged third stage of labor: morbidity and risk factors. Obstetrics and Gynaecology 77(6), 863–867.

Coulter-Smith SD, Holohan M, Darling MRN. 1996 Previous caesarean section: a risk factor for major obstetric haemorrhage. Journal of Obstetrics and Gynaecology 16(5), 349–352.

Davies M, Harrison J. 1992 Amniotic fluid embolism: maternal mortality revisited. British Journal of Hospital Medicine 14(10), 775–776.

Pearlman M, Faro S. 1990 Obstetric septic shock: a pathophysiological basis for management. Clinics in Obstetrics and Gynaecology 33(3), 482–492.

Chapter 46 Perinatal asphyxia

In this chapter

INTRODUCTION

Labour has been known to be dangerous for the fetus for centuries. Uterine contractions interfere with umbilical and uteroplacental blood flow and affect fetal gas exchange. The result is a normal tendency to mild metabolic acidosis in the active phase of the first stage and in the early 2nd stage of labour. At the end of the 2nd stage there may be transient respiratory acidosis (Arias 1993).

Definitions for this chapter (Anderson et al 1994)

- **Fetal distress** A general-purpose term to indicate the fetus is in jeopardy, sometimes but not always because of hypoxia.
- **Acidosis** An increased concentration of hydrogen ions in blood and at cellular level resulting from an accumulation of acid or loss of base with a blood pH of less than 7.4.
- **Hypoxia** A decreased concentration of oxygen in blood (**hypoxaemia**) and at cellular level.
- **Hypercapnia (hypercarbia)** An increased concentration of carbon dioxide in blood and at cellular level.
- **Asphyxia** A severe abnormality of gas exchange resulting in hypoxia, hypercapnia and acidosis. The term **fetal asphyxia** is preferred to that of **fetal distress**, which refers to a state of fetal danger which may or may not be caused by asphyxia.

FETAL GAS EXCHANGE AND pH REGULATION

The bicarbonate buffer system which regulates fetal acid/ base balance is not as efficient as in the neonate because of a decreased ability to eliminate carbon dioxide (CO_2). As CO_2 cannot be expelled by the fetus into the air it must be eliminated as molecular CO_2 via the placenta to be dealt with by the maternal respiratory system.

Respiratory acidosis

In the placenta there is a gradient between maternal and fetal circulations down which fetal CO_2 can diffuse. Fetal scalp blood PCO_2 is about 38–44 mmHg and maternal blood PCO_2 is 18–24 mmHg. In most cases interference with fetal gas exchange involves a problem of CO_2 elimination resulting in respiratory acidosis. An excessive rise in fetal PCO_2 causes fetal H^+ ions to be released from the unstable carbonic acid (H_2CO_3), which lowers fetal blood pH (**acidosis**). The buffering bicarbonate ions also released are insufficient to correct the acidosis. The full equation is:

$$CO_2 + H_2O \leftrightarrow H_2CO_3 \leftrightarrow H^+ + HCO_3^-$$

Metabolic acidosis

Decreased oxygen transfer to the fetus will also cause acidosis. Oxygen deficiency causes cells to switch to anaerobic respiration, with the release of lactic acid and H^+ ions into the blood. If hypoxia persists the excess H^+ ions cause CO_2 and water (H_2O) to be released from the buffer bicarbonate to add respiratory acidosis to the metabolic acidosis. Water is transferred across the placenta to the maternal circulation but there is a delay in removing the CO_2. Anaerobic respiration is inefficient and utilises more energy, resulting in a decrease in glucose.

INTRAUTERINE HYPOXIA

Oxygenation of the fetus depends on maternal oxygenation, perfusion of the placental site, the fetoplacental circulation and adequate fetal haemoglobin (Michie 1996). Disruption or impairment to the flow of oxygen from the air to the fetus will result in fetal hypoxia.

Possible causes

- Maternal oxygenation may be impaired by respiratory or cardiovascular disease.
- Perfusion of the placental site may be reduced in:
  - hypertension, because of vasoconstriction;
  - hypotension, due to blood loss;
  - aortocaval occlusion;
  - shock;
  - excessive uterine contractions.
- Prolapse, compression or a true knot in the umbilical cord may cause fetal hypoxia.
- Placental disease.
- There may be a reduction in fetal red cells caused by haemolysis.

Fetal response to hypoxia

The fetal response to hypoxia is an acceleration of heart rate to maintain oxygen supply to the brain and delivery of excess CO_2 to the placenta. As glycogen reserves become depleted, the increased supply of glucose demanded by the heart muscle because of the tachycardia cannot be met and the heart slows (**bradycardia**). The anal sphincter relaxes and fresh meconium is passed into the amniotic fluid. Hypoxia may stimulate the fetus to make gasping movements and meconium may be inhaled (Michie 1996).

Physiological control of the fetal heart

The cardiac regulatory centre is situated in the medulla oblongata. Baroreceptors found in the arch of the aorta and carotid sinus are responsive to changes in the blood pressure and chemoreceptors in the same blood vessels respond to changes in blood gas tensions (Marieb 1992). These receptors send messages to the cardiac regulatory centre which in turn sends messages via the sympathetic and parasympathetic nervous system to the heart. Sympathetic stimulation via the sinoatrial node will increase the heart rate whilst parasympathetic stimulation via the vagus nerve will decrease the heart rate. The continuous interaction between these two branches of the autonomic system cause small fluctuations in heart rate which leads to variability on heart rate tracings.

MONITORING THE FETUS IN LABOUR

The fetal response to labour may be monitored clinically by observing the amniotic fluid and the rate and rhythm of the fetal heart, either intermittently using a Pinard fetal stethoscope or Doppler ultrasound heart rate detector or by continuous use of Doppler ultrasound strapped to the mother's abdomen. Electronic monitoring is possible using electrodes attached to the fetal skull which produces a direct **fetal electrocardiogram** (Morrin 1997). Contraction length, strength and frequency can also be monitored externally by a transducer or internally by an intrauterine catheter pressure device.

Meconium

The presence of meconium in amniotic fluid is suggestive of intrapartum asphyxia in the fetus, but it is a non-specific finding that may be associated with problems other than asphyxia (Miller et al 1975). However, if the pregnancy is known to be high risk and the meconium is freshly passed, as indicated by it being dark green or black, thick and tenacious, the likelihood of asphyxia is high. Old or stale meconium giving rise to lightly stained yellowish or greenish amniotic fluid does not correlate well with fetal asphyxia (Arias 1993, Morrin 1997).

Classification of meconium-stained liquor

Meiss et al (1978) classified meconium into early light, early heavy and late meconium staining. Early staining was present during the active phase of labour and late was newly passed in the 2nd stage of labour. Early heavy staining and late staining were associated with a significant increase in meconium aspiration. Similarly, thick, fresh meconium at the onset of labour is associated with increased morbidity from meconium aspiration (McNiven et al 1994).

Prophylactic amnioinfusion for meconium-stained fluid

Thick, undiluted meconium reflects reduced amniotic fluid volume which is itself a risk factor (Enkin et al 1995). Morrin (1997) summarises the arguments for and against use of amniotomy to visualise the amniotic fluid for meconium staining. A randomised controlled trial which included nulliparous women found that routine amniotomy had little effect on the important outcomes of labour and is not to be recommended (UK Amniotomy Group 1994).

Spong et al (1994) concluded that amnioinfusion does dilute amniotic meconium but prophylactic amnioinfusion did not improve perinatal outcome and increased the risk of chorioamnionitis and endometritis. They suggested that the benefit of amnioinfusion resulted from the alleviation of variable fetal heart rate decelerations rather than meconium dilution. Hofmeyr (1997) reviewed the use of amnioinfusion for meconium-stained liquor and suggested that the benefits seen are more likely to be due to an improvement in oligohydramnios than dilution of meconium.

Fetal heart monitoring

Intermittent auscultation

Dover & Gauge (1995) wrote that the frequency of fetal heart monitoring used by the midwife is decided by the frequency and strength of the uterine contractions and the effects on the fetus. Other risk factors likely to affect fetal oxygenation were also taken into account. Intermittent auscultation is usually carried out hourly in early labour, every 15 min as contractions increase and between each contraction in the late first stage and 2nd stage of labour. The heart rate and rhythm should be listened to, commencing immediately after a contraction and counted over a full minute (Morrin 1997), to assess whether decelerations are present. The normal rate is between 110 and 150 bpm; the faster rate is found in preterm babies and the slower in term and postterm babies. The rhythm is regular with a coupled beat.

Electronic monitoring

Continuous electronic FHR monitoring was introduced in the 1970s and adopted by obstetricians enthusiastically as 'a significant improvement in intrapartum fetal assessment' (Arias 1993). The technique was introduced before evidence of its efficacy or safety had been sought. Electronic fetal monitoring (EFM) is used in the monitoring of labour in three out of four pregnancies in the USA. EFM can be used continuously or intermittently, for instance, for 15–30 min periodically.

Concerns have been raised about the safety and efficiency of continuous EFM (Arias 1993, Thacker 1987). Thacker et al (1997) compared EFM with intermittent auscultation during labour using the results of nine randomised controlled trials (RCTs). They reviewed studies including 58 855 pregnant women and their 58 324 infants. Data from each study were used to calculate a combined risk estimate for eight outcomes.

- 1-minute Apgar score below 7
- 1-minute Apgar score below 4
- Neonatal seizures
- Neonatal intensive care admissions (NICU)
- Stillbirths
- Neonatal deaths
- Caesarean delivery
- Operative vaginal delivery

When the value of EFM was compared with intermittent FHR monitoring, the results were as follows.

- No trial showed a significant decrease in babies with a 1-minute Apgar score of less than 7.
- Outside the USA, there was a significant decrease in the risk of 1-minute Apgar score of less than 4.
- Only one trial showed a significant decrease in the numbers of babies having neonatal seizures.
- Only one trial showed a significant decrease in perinatal mortality.
- Only one trial showed a significant decrease in the number of NICU admissions.
- There was a significant increase in the number of vaginal operative deliveries.
- There was a significant increase in the numbers of CS deliveries and risk of caesarean delivery was highest in low-risk pregnancies.

Implications for practice

The review found no measurable impact on morbidity or mortality, with the exception of reduced incidence of neonatal seizures although outside the USA studies there was a decrease in the 1-minute Apgar scores below 4. The increase of CS rates with added risk to the mother is a worrying factor. Expert panels in the USA and Canada have advised against routine EFM in low-risk pregnancies and have found weak evidence for its inclusion in high-risk pregnancies. Some believe the technology was introduced before it was well developed and that more research is needed. However, there seems to be no likelihood of a reduction in such monitoring at present (Thacker et al 1997). Arias (1993) believes this is because, despite the controversy, EFM.

- confirms fetal well-being;
- shows the possibility of the presence of fetal problems;
- determines the presence of severe problems.

Waveform analysis

Westgate et al (1993) carried out a prospective randomised clinical trial to compare conventional cardiotocography (CTG) with waveform analysis of changes in the ST waveform of the electrocardiogram. The subjects were 2434 high-risk labouring women in Plymouth, England. The criteria used for analysis were the incidence of operative intervention and neonatal outcome. They found that ST waveform analysis discriminated between cardiotocogram changes and reduced the incidence of operative deliveries and low 5-min Apgar scores. They conclude that more research into waveform analysis is warranted. Van Wijngaarden et al (1996), in similar fashion, used PR interval analysis and found they were able to reduce the number of fetuses undergoing scalp blood sampling.

Fetal heart patterns

The following terms are used to interpret CTG readings (Cassidy 1996).

Baseline fetal heart rate

There is a baseline rate per minute (bpm) of 110–160 which is the rate present between periods of acceleration and deceleration. A rate over 160 is called **baseline tachycardia** and below 120 is **baseline bradycardia**. Both tachycardia and bradycardia may be associated with fetal hypoxia. Tachycardia may be seen if the woman is ketotic. Some fetuses normally have a bpm of 110–120. A prolonged bradycardia occurs when there is continuous compression of the umbilical cord.

Baseline variability

Continuous adjustments in the autonomic nervous stimulation of the heart due to fetal response to the environment lead to minute variations in the length of each heart beat. The CTG tracing has a jagged appearance as the baseline rate is continuously adjusting rather than being a straight line because each beat is the same length. There should be variance in the baseline rate of at least five beats per minute. Loss of variance may be due to hypoxia. It is also seen after administration of pethidine because of depression of the cardiac regulatory centre in the fetal brain. Fetal sleep lasting 20–30 min may also cause a reduction in variability (Gibb 1988).

Response to uterine contractions

The fetal heart normally remains steady or **accelerates** during a contraction. Acceleration of 15 bpm above the baseline is associated with fetal activity and stimulation (Spencer 1993). The presence of two within a 20-min period is thought to be a sign of fetal health and the tracing is said to be **reactive** (Gibb 1988). **Decelerations**, dips of more than 15 bpm below baseline, are more worrying.

- An **early deceleration** mirrors the pattern of the contraction. It commences at or after the onset of a contraction, reaches its lowest point at the peak of the contraction and then returns to normal by the end of the contraction. It is associated with compression of the fetal head and vagal response but may also indicate early fetal hypoxia.
- A **late deceleration** begins during or just after a contraction, reaches its lowest point after the peak of the contraction and may not recover until the onset of the next contraction. This time lag between the peak of the contraction and the low point of the deceleration is more significant than the drop in heart rate. It indicates fetal hypoxia and inadequate fetal brain oxygenation (Aldrich et al 1995) and is suggestive of cord compression. Prolapse of the cord should be excluded by vaginal examination and the doctor informed.
- **Variable decelerations**, where the heart rate varies in timing, frequency and amplitude, are associated with cord compression where there is obstruction to venous flow and a corresponding rise in fetal blood pressure. This pattern can be considered benign but if the decelerations are below 60 bpm, 60 bpm below the baseline or last for longer than 1 min the fetus may be in danger (Morrin 1997).

Two other unusual and rare patterns (Morrin 1997) are **sinusoidal**, where there is a regular trace with a wave pattern of 3–6 per minute with an amplitude of 5–30 bpm. This is associated with rhesus isoimmunisation, fetal anaemia and asphyxia. The second is the **saltatory pattern** with excessive variability of more than 25 bpm. This may be associated with fetal acidosis but the cause is unclear.

Fetal blood sampling

Cardiotocography can suggest the presence of fetal hypoxia but acidosis can be confirmed only by fetal blood sampling. The normal pH of fetal blood is 7.35 and above. If this falls below 7.25 in the first stage of labour or below 7.2 in the 2nd stage, the fetus may be in danger and immediate delivery of the baby is required (Morrin 1997).

The membranes need to be ruptured and the cervix at least 3 cm dilated to carry out the procedure. An amnioscope is passed through the cervix to access the fetal scalp. The scalp is sprayed with ethyl chloride to produce a reactive hyperaemia and a thin layer of silicone gel applied to ensure blood collects in a droplet. The skin is punctured and 0.5 ml of blood is collected in a heparinised capillary tube for immediate analysis of blood gas tension, bicarbonate and pH.

MANAGEMENT OF CONFIRMED FETAL ASPHYXIA

Severe hypoxia may result in the baby being stillborn, asphyxiated at birth or suffering brain damage. If the condition of the fetus monitored by the above findings suggests a major problem, a doctor must be called to see the woman and her fetus. If labour is being augmented by administration of syntocinon, it is sensible to reduce the force of the uterine contractions by discontinuing the infusion. Administration of oxygen to the mother may be useful if the underlying cause of the fetal hypoxia is maternal disease. Delivery will probably be undertaken, either by CS in the first stage of labour or by operative delivery (forceps or ventouse extraction) in the 2nd stage. If delivery is imminent an episiotomy may be all that is required. A paediatrician should be called to the delivery room in all cases as the neonate may need resuscitation.

NEONATAL ASPHYXIA AND RESUSCITATION

Initiation of respirations at birth

From about 22 weeks surfactant is produced in the fetal lung. The amount present increases until birth and there is a surge of production at about 34 weeks gestation. Surfactant has two main functions: to reduce surface tension in the alveoli so that they can expand more easily and to help prevent the alveoli collapsing at the end of each expiration. Fetal breathing movements have been identified as early as 11 weeks gestation and these increase in strength and frequency until they are present for over 50% of the time. The rate varies between 30 and 70 breaths per minute.

Establishing respiration at birth

This topic is fully explored in Chapter 48.

- As the fetal chest is compressed by the birth canal, it is squeezed and lung and amniotic fluid are forced out of the alveoli into the upper respiratory tract. Passive recoil of the chest after delivery helps to draw air into the lungs.
- Hypoxia during the late stage of delivery occurs with the birth of the head and the beginning of placental separation. The oxygen content of the blood falls and the carbon dioxide content rises, stimulating chemoreceptors to send a message to the respiratory centre causing onset of breathing.
- The respiratory centre is also bombarded with stimuli from handling, the change in temperature in the nasopharynx and on the skin.
- Circulatory changes direct the blood away from the placental circulation to the pulmonary circulation and lungs for oxygenation.

- Effective oxygenation is achieved by respiratory exchange in the alveoli and by adequate circulation. Most neonates establish respirations within 1 min of birth.

Birth asphyxia

Failure to initiate or sustain respirations at birth is called birth asphyxia or **asphyxia neonatorum**.

Causes

- Obstruction of the airway by mucus, blood, meconium or amniotic fluid may occur, especially if intrauterine anoxia has been present. Because of stimulation of the respiratory centre the fetus may have gasped in utero, drawing the above substances into the trachea and bronchi.
- The airways may not be patent due to congenital anomalies such as choanal atresia, hypoplastic lungs or diaphragmatic hernia.
- Lung function may be compromised by abnormalities in the cardiovascular or central nervous system.
- Pain-relieving drugs such as pethidine and morphine and narcotic drugs such as diazepam, as well as general anaesthetics, if given in large doses, may depress the fetal respiratory centre.
- Intracranial haemorrhage may cause pressure on the cerebellum and medulla, affecting the cardiovascular and respiratory centres.
- Severe intrauterine infections following prolonged rupture of the membranes, leading to pneumonia, meningitis and septicaemia, may inhibit the efficient establishment of respiration.
- Immaturity of the neonate may lead to mechanical dysfunction because of poor lung development, lack of surfactant and a soft rib cage.

Recognition

Birth asphyxia may be classified as mild, moderate or severe, depending on scoring systems such as that devised by Virginia Apgar. Arias (1993) relates that several studies carried out in the 1980s, such as that of Sykes et al (1982), demonstrated that **Apgar scores** are poor predictors of hypoxia and acidosis. The Apgar score (Fig. 46.1) assesses the condition of the baby at birth and may be affected by all the above causes of neonatal asphyxia. It follows that babies may not always have shown pre-delivery signs of impending asphyxia, many of the causes arising suddenly after delivery. Respiratory depression by fetal hypoxia is only one factor that may cause a baby to fail to breathe at birth (Roberton 1986).

For each of the vital signs in Figure 46.1, the neonate may be given a score of 0, 1 or 2 depending on the descriptors. A 1-min Apgar score is recorded and suggested parameters are:

- 7–10 No asphyxia;
- 4–6 Mild to moderate asphyxia, response to treatment usually good;
- 3 or less Severe asphyxia, requires urgent resuscitation.

Case study

This case illustrates that there may be no way to predict asphyxia. When I was a junior sister I and a close friend had been caring for a multigravid woman in labour. Labour had commenced spontaneously, there had been no sign of fetal heart rate abnormalities and the delivery by my friend was normal.

I received the baby who seemed to be breathing spontaneously and, anticipating no problems, he was wrapped and given to his mother. Within 1 min he became extremely cyanosed and stopped breathing. I took him to the resuscitaire, gave oxygen by facemask and he recommenced breathing rapidly. This happened once more and I called the paediatric houseman. He examined the baby who was once more pink all over and breathing well. Put him in the cot was the guidance! Once more the baby collapsed. I then called the consultant who quickly diagnosed transposition of the great vessels of the heart. The baby, who is now a strapping 22-year-old, was transferred for immediate corrective surgery.

Management

A simple way to remember the steps in resuscitation is the **ABC method** (with D added).

A = airway – ensure patency
B = breathing – ensure that oxygen enters the lungs

Score	0	1	2
Sign Heart rate	Absent	Slow – below 100	Fast – above 100
Respiratory effort	Absent	Slow, irregular	Good, crying
Muscle tone	Limp	Some flexion of the extremities	Active
Reflex irritability	No response	Grimace	Crying, cough
Colour	Blue, pale	Body pink, extremities blue	Completely pink

Figure 46.1 *The Apgar scoring system based on points being awarded for five physiological signs*

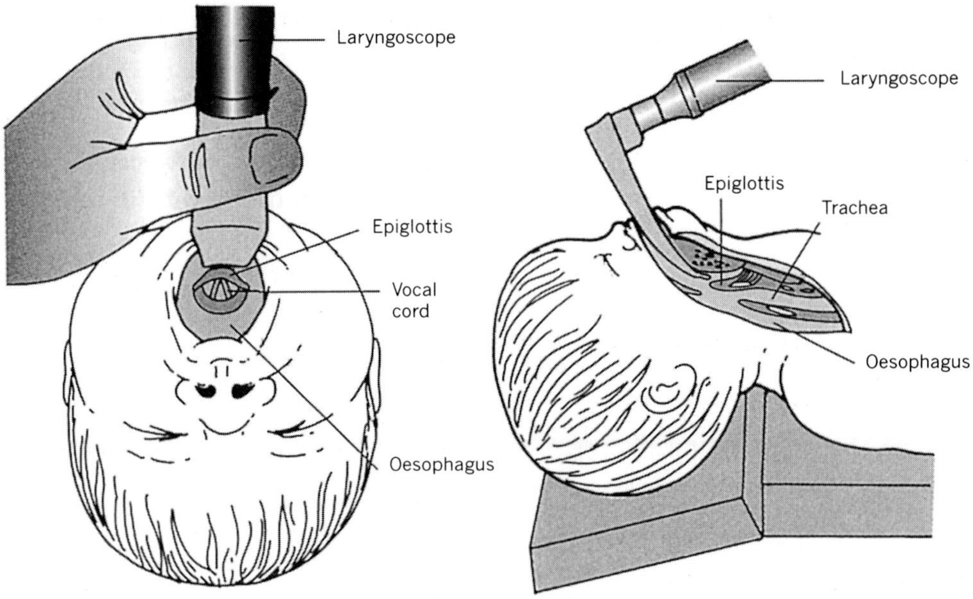

Figure 46.2 *Intubation of the neonate (from Sweet B, 1997, with permission).*

C = cardiac function – ensure there is an adequate heart beat and circulation
D = drugs – have available the resuscitation trolley with all its required components

Mild to moderate asphyxia

The upper airways should be cleared gently with suction. Intermittent positive pressure ventilation (IPPV) via a facemask should be given using a resuscitation bag such as the Ambu-bag attached to an oxygen supply. This should always include a means of limiting pressure to no more than 30 cm-H_2O to prevent pneumothorax from overinflation. The baby should become pink as oxygen supply is ensured and this should lead to an improvement in heart rate. When the baby breathes spontaneously oxygen should be maintained until the baby's condition is judged to be satisfactory.

If the baby's temperature is allowed to fall, the demands for oxygen and glucose will increase so the baby must be kept warm throughout the procedure. If the mother has received pethidine or morphine within the last 2–3 h naloxone hydrochloride (Narcan), which is a narcotic antagonist, should be given. The dose is 0.01 mg/kg and it can be given intramuscularly or into the umbilical vein.

Severe asphyxia

If the paediatrician is not present he or she should be called as an emergency. The midwife should commence IPPV with mask and bag. Endotracheal intubation will be necessary and all midwives should become proficient at this technique so that they can carry it out in the absence of a doctor (Fig. 46.2).

An appropriately sized laryngoscope is passed over the tongue to the posterior pharynx. It is then advanced carefully over the epiglottis until the glottis comes into view (Fig. 46.3). If the epiglottis cannot be seen gentle pressure on the cricoid cartilage may assist. Another technique is to advance the tip of the laryngoscope blade further and then slowly withdraw it. This

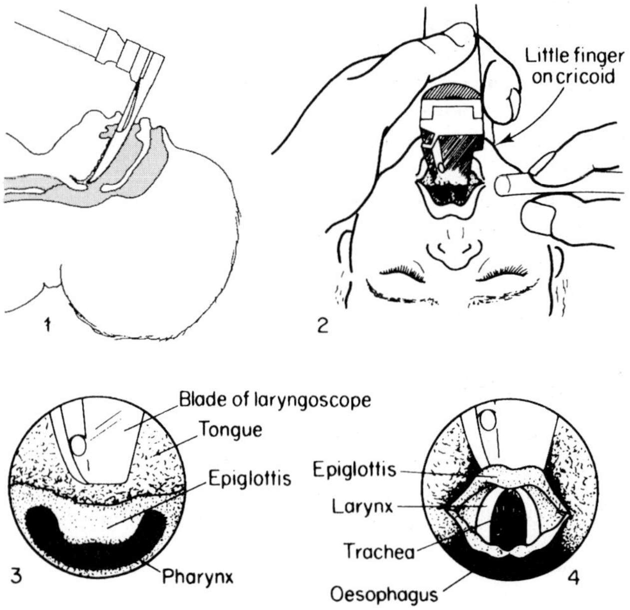

Figure 46.3 *How to intubate. 1. Lie the baby on its back if possible, with the head tilted slightly downwards. Extend the neck so that the chin points upwards. 2. Take the infant laryngoscope with a straight blade and insert the blade into the infant's mouth, gently lifting the tongue. 3. The epiglottis can be seen at the base of the tongue; it hangs down obscuring the entrance to the larynx. 4. Slide the laryngoscope to the base of the epiglottis and tilt the tip of the blade upward. At the same time, press gently on the cricoid cartilage with the little finger. The entrance to the larynx will then come into view. An endotracheal tube can then be guided carefully into the trachea (from Kelnar C, Harvey D, Simpson C, 1995, with permission).*

should allow the glottis to slip into view. Aspiration of mucus can be carried out directly if necessary.

A size 2.5 or 3.0 endotracheal tube is passed 1–2 cm through the glottis into the trachea and the laryngoscope removed. The trachea can be cleared by passing a fine catheter through the endotracheal tube which can then be attached to the oxygen supply connected to a water manometer. IPPV is commenced at 15 times per minute. The initial pressure should be 30 cmH_2O, reduced to 25 cmH_2O. This should be continued until the baby is pink, has a heart beat of over 100/min and is breathing spontaneously.

Cardiac massage using two fingers depressing the sternum 1–2 cm 120 times per minute should be commenced if the baby's heart rate is below 80 bpm or if the carotid or femoral pulses are weak or cannot be felt (Simpson 1997). The Apgar should be repeated at 5 min and until the baby's condition is satisfactory. A 5-min Apgar score has more prognostic value than a 1-min score.

For midwives practising in the community it is reassuring to remember that severe neonatal asphyxia rarely occurs unannounced and warning signs identified during fetal monitoring in labour should result in the woman being transferred to a maternity unit to safeguard the fetus. A resuscitation bag such as the Ambu-bag should usually be sufficient. When the delivery has been an emergency and no equipment is available, mouth-to-face (over mouth and nose) resuscitation has saved lives. Just the air in the cheeks should be blown into the baby's airways.

Drugs

Drugs that may be required and should always be available on the resuscitation trolley are as follows.

- Naloxone hydrochloride if a narcotic antagonist is needed.
- Adrenaline is a cardiac stimulant.
- Dextrose 10% is given if hypoglycaemia is confirmed
- Calcium is given slowly if there is hypocalcaemia.
- Vitamin K_1 is given to prevent haemorrhagic disease of the newborn.

Sodium bicarbonate to counteract acidosis is not now recommended as it has been associated with intraventricular haemorrhage in preterm babies.

Transfer to the neonatal unit

A baby who has suffered severe asphyxia should be transferred to the neonatal unit for further observation. Complications such as cerebral oedema, hypoglycaemia, hypothermia and electrolyte disturbance should be anticipated and prevented if possible and treated if they occur. Paediatric follow-up is important to detect long-term problems such as developmental delay or cerebral palsy.

Correction of acidosis

If only one of the two types of acidosis is present, the other system can be used to compensate. The lungs are central to the control of carbon dioxide level in respiratory acidosis whilst the kidneys control bicarbonate level in metabolic acidosis. Acidosis in neonates tends to be mixed and the buffering systems may fail. As stated above, the administration of sodium bicarbonate is controversial and should always follow blood gas analysis. The bicarbonate combines with hydrogen ions to form carbonic acid. This then dissociates into water and carbon dioxide:

$$H^+ + HCO_3^- \leftrightarrow H_2CO_3 \leftrightarrow CO_2 + H_2O$$

If the carbon dioxide can leave the body by the lungs, there is no problem but in respiratory difficulties it may accumulate in the body. It crosses cell membranes and the blood–brain barrier to cause intracellular acidosis, even if there seems to be a blood picture improvement in acidosis. This is because the bicarbonate buffer cannot cross cell membranes as readily as the carbon dioxide. The sodium content in sodium bicarbonate may cause an overloading of the baby's vascular system, resulting in cellular overhydration and damage.

Summary of main points

- The bicarbonate buffer system which regulates fetal acid/base balance is not as efficient in the neonate because of a decreased ability to eliminate carbon dioxide. It is common to find metabolic acidosis following respiratory acidosis to give a mixed picture in the fetus.
- Impairment of the distribution of oxygen to the fetus will result in fetal hypoxia with acceleration of heart rate to maintain oxygen supply to the brain and deliver excess CO_2 to the placenta. As glycogen reserves become depleted, the heart muscle slows. The anal sphincter relaxes and fresh meconium is passed into the amniotic fluid. Hypoxia may stimulate the fetus to make gasping movements and meconium may be inhaled.
- Messages from baroreceptors and chemoreceptors arrive at the cardiac regulatory centre which sends messages via the sympathetic and parasympathetic nervous system to the heart. Sympathetic stimulation will increase the heart rate whilst parasympathetic stimulation via the vagus nerve will decrease it.
- The presence of meconium in amniotic fluid is only suggestive of intrapartum asphyxia in the fetus but it is a non-specific finding that may be associated with other problems. Only if the meconium is fresh is asphyxia likely to occur.
- Thick, undiluted meconium reflects reduced amniotic fluid volume which is itself a risk factor. Amnioinfusion does dilute amniotic meconium but prophylactic amnioinfusion did not improve perinatal outcome and increased the risk of maternal infection. The benefits are more likely to be due to an improvement in oligohydramnios than dilution of meconium.
- Concerns have been raised about the efficiency of continuous electronic fetal monitoring. A review found no measurable impact on morbidity or mortality except reduced incidence of neonatal seizures. Expert panels in the USA and Canada advised against routine EFM in low-risk pregnancies and found weak evidence for its inclusion in high-risk pregnancies.
- Both tachycardia and bradycardia may be associated with fetal hypoxia. Tachycardia may be seen if the woman is ketotic. A prolonged bradycardia suggests continuous compression of the umbilical cord.
- There should be variance in the baseline rate of at least five beats per minute. Loss of variance may be due to hypoxia. It is also seen after the administration of pethidine because of depression of the cardiac regulatory centre in the fetal brain. Fetal sleep lasting 20–30 min may also cause a reduction in variability.

- Acceleration of 15 bpm above the baseline is associated with fetal activity and stimulation and the tracing is said to be reactive. Decelerations of more than 15 bpm below baseline are more worrying. Early decelerations are associated with compression of the fetal head and vagal response but may also indicate early fetal hypoxia. Late decelerations are suggestive of cord compression.
- Variable decelerations are associated with cord compression where there is obstruction to venous flow and a corresponding rise in fetal blood pressure. This pattern can be considered benign but if the decelerations are below 60 bpm, 60 bpm below the baseline or last for longer than 1 min the fetus may be in danger.
- Fetal acidosis can be confirmed by fetal blood sampling. Severe hypoxia may result in the baby being stillborn, asphyxiated at birth or suffering brain damage. Administration of oxygen to the mother may be useful if the underlying cause of the fetal hypoxia is maternal disease. Delivery will probably be undertaken as soon as possible.
- Surfactant reduces surface tension in the alveoli so that they can expand more easily and also helps prevent the alveoli collapsing at the end of each expiration. Fetal breathing movements have been identified as early as 11 weeks gestation.
- Passive recoil of the chest after delivery helps to draw air into the lungs. Mild hypoxia occurs with the birth of the head and the beginning of placental separation and chemoreceptor messages to the respiratory centre cause onset of breathing. The respiratory centre is also bombarded with other external stimuli.
- Birth asphyxia may be caused by obstructed airways or congenital anomalies of the respiratory, cardiovascular or central nervous systems. Pain-relieving drugs may depress the fetal respiratory centre. Intracranial haemorrhage may affect the cardiovascular and respiratory centres. Intrauterine infection or immaturity may inhibit the efficient establishment of respiration. The Apgar score assesses the condition of the baby at birth.
- In mild to moderate asphyxia the upper airways should be cleared gently with suction. Intermittent positive pressure ventilation via a facemask should be given. The baby becomes pink as oxygen supply is ensured and this leads to an improvement in heart rate. If the mother has received pethidine or morphine within the last 2–3 h naloxone hydrochloride (Narcan) 0.01 mg/kg, a narcotic antagonist, is given.
- If severe asphyxia is present the paediatrician should be called. Endotracheal intubation will be necessary and all midwives should become proficient at this technique. Cardiac massage should be commenced if the baby's heart rate is below 80 bpm or if the carotid or femoral pulses are weak or cannot be felt. The Apgar should be repeated at 5 min and until the baby's condition is satisfactory. A 5-min Apgar score has more prognostic value than a 1-min score.
- When the delivery has been an emergency and no equipment is available, mouth-to-face resuscitation has saved lives. Just the air in the cheeks should be blown into the baby's airways. Drugs that should always be available on the resuscitation trolley are naloxone hydrochloride, adrenaline, sodium bicarbonate, dextrose, calcium and vitamin K_1.
- A baby who has suffered severe asphyxia should be transferred to the neonatal unit for further observation. Complications such as cerebral oedema, hypoglycaemia, hypothermia and electrolyte disturbance should be anticipated, prevented if possible and treated if they occur.
- The administration of sodium bicarbonate to correct acidosis is controversial and should always follow blood gas analysis. The bicarbonate combines with hydrogen ions to form carbonic acid which dissociates into water and carbon dioxide. In babies with respiratory difficulties, carbon dioxide may accumulate in the body and cross cell membranes and the blood–brain barrier to cause intracellular acidosis. The sodium content in sodium bicarbonate may overload the baby's vascular system, resulting in cellular overhydration.

References

Aldrich CJ, d'Antona D, Spencer JA. 1995 Late fetal heart decelerations and changes in cerebral oxygenation during the first stage of labour. British Journal of Obstetrics and Gynaecology 102(1), 9–13.

Anderson KN, Anderson LE, Glanze WD. (eds) 1994 Mosby's Medical, Nursing and Allied Health Dictionary. Mosby, St Louis.

Arias F. 1993 Practical Guide to High Risk Pregnancy and Delivery, 2nd edn. Mosby Year Book, Chicago.

Cassidy P. 1996 Management of the first stage of labour, In Bennett VR, Brown LK (eds) Myles Textbook for Midwives, Churchill Livingstone, Edinburgh. 168–183.

Dover SL, Gauge SM. 1995 Fetal monitoring – Midwifery attitudes. Midwifery 11(1) 18–27.

Enkin M, Keirse MJNC, Renfrew M, Neilson J. 1995 A Guide to Effective Care in Pregnancy and Childbirth, 2nd edn. Oxford Medical Publications, Oxford.

Gibb DME. 1988 A Practical Guide to Labour Management. Blackwell Scientific, Oxford.

Hofmeyr GJ. 1997 Amnioinfusion for meconium-stained amniotic fluid. in Neilson JP, Crowther CA, Hodnett ED, Hofmeyr GJ, Keirse MJNC (eds) Pregnancy and Childbirth module of the Cochrane Database of Systematic Reviews, The Cochrane Library. Update Software, Oxford

Kelnar C, Harvey D, Simpson C. 1995 The Sick Newborn Baby. Baillière Tindall, London.

Marieb EN. 1992 Human Anatomy and Physiology, 2nd edn. Benjamin/Cummings Publishing, California.

McNiven P, Roch B, Wall J. 1994 Meconium-stained amniotic fluid. Modern Midwife 4(7), 17–20.

Meiss PJ, Hall M, Marshall JR et al. 1978 Meconium passage: a new classification for risk assessment during labor. American Journal of Obstetrics and Gynecology 131, 509.

Michie MM. 1996 Asphyxia and resuscitation. In Bennett VR, Brown LK (eds) Myles Textbook for Midwives, 12th edn. Churchill Livingstone, Edinburgh, pp 498–504.

Miller FC, Sacks DA, Yeh SY et al. 1975 Significance of meconium during labor. American Journal of Obstetrics and Gynecology 122, 573.

Morrin NA. 1997 Midwifery care in the first stage of labour. In Sweet BR with Tiran D (eds) Mayes Midwifery, 12th edn. Baillière Tindall, London, pp 355–384

Roberton NRC. 1986 Resuscitation of the newborn. In Roberton NRC (ed) Textbook of Neonatology. Churchill Livingstone, Edinburgh.

Spencer JA. 1993 Clinical overview of cardiotocography (review). British Journal of Obstetrics and Gynaecology 100 (suppl 9), 4–7.

Spong CY, Ogundipe OA, Ross MG. 1994 Prophylactic amnioinfusion for meconium-stained amniotic fluid. American Journal of Obstetrics and Gynecology 171, 931–935.

Sweet B. 1997 Mayes' Midwifery. Baillière Tindall, London.

Sykes GS, Johnson P, Ashworth F et al. 1982 Do Apgar scores indicate asphyxia? Lancet 1, 494.

Thacker SB. 1987 The efficacy of intrapartum electronic fetal monitoring. American Journal of Obstetrics and Gynecology 156, 24–30.

Thacker SB, Stroup DF, Peterson HB. 1997 Continuous electronic fetal heart monitoring during labor. In Neilson JP, Crowther CA, Hodnett ED, Hofmeyr GJ, Keirse MJNC. (eds) Pregnancy and Childbirth module of The Cochrane Database of Systematic Reviews, The Cochrane Library. Update Software, Oxford.

UK Amniotomy Group, 1994 Comparing routine versus delayed amniotomy in spontaneous first labour at term. A multicentre randomised trial. Online Journal of Current Clinical Trials, Document number 122, April 1.

Van Wijngaarden WJ, Sahota DS, James DK et al. 1996 Improved intrapartum surveillance with PR interval analysis of the fetal electrocardiogram: a randomised trial showing a reduction in fetal blood sampling. American Journal of Obstetrics and Gynecology 174, 1295–1299.

Westgate J, Harris M, Curnow JS, Greene KR. 1993 Plymouth randomised trial of cardiotocogram only versus ST waveform plus cardiotocogram for intrapartum monitoring in 2400 cases. American Journal of Obstetrics and Gynecology 169, 1151–1160.

Recommended reading

Aldrich CJ, d'Antona D, Spencer JA. 1995 Late fetal heart decelerations and changes in cerebral oxygenation during the first stage of labour. British Journal of Obstetrics and Gynaecology 102(1), 9–13.

Hofmeyr GJ. 1997 Amnioinfusion for meconium-stained amniotic fluid. In Neilson JP, Crowther CA, Hodnett ED, Hofmeyr GJ, Keirse MJNC (eds) Pregnancy and Childbirth module of the Cochrane Database of Systematic Reviews, The Cochrane Library. Update Software, Oxford.

McNiven P, Roch B, Wall J. 1994 Meconium-stained amniotic fluid. Modern Midwife 4(7), 17–20.

Spencer JA. 1993 Clinical overview of cardiotocography (review). British Journal of Obstetrics and Gynaecology 100 (suppl 9), 4–7.

Thacker SB, Stroup DF, Peterson HB. 1997 Continuous electronic fetal heart monitoring during labor. In Neilson JP, Crowther CA, Hodnett ED, Hofmeyr GJ, Keirse MJNC (eds) Pregnancy and Childbirth module of The Cochrane Database of Systematic Reviews, The Cochrane Library. Update Software, Oxford.

Van Wijngaarden WJ, Sahota DS, James DK et al. 1996 Improved intrapartum surveillance with PR interval analysis of the fetal electrocardiogram: a randomised trial showing a reduction in fetal blood sampling. American Journal of Obstetrics and Gynecology 174, 1295–1299.

Chapter 47 Operative delivery

In this chapter

INTRODUCTION

'Achievement of a safe vaginal delivery depends, in many cases, on the ability of the obstetrician to effect an operative delivery with forceps or vacuum' (Arias 1993). Operative vaginal delivery should be undertaken for three basic reasons American College of Obstetricians and Gynecologists (1991).

1 To shorten the 2nd stage of labour, if there is a problem with maternal or fetal condition
2 To manage a prolonged 2nd stage of labour
3 Presumed fetal jeopardy

Telfer (1997) adds a fourth indicator: to protect the baby's head as in preterm labour or breech delivery. It is equally important to choose when caesarean section is necessary for maternal or fetal safety and well-being.

FORCEPS DELIVERY

Obstetric forceps have been utilised in difficult deliveries since their invention by the Chamberlen family in the 17th century. Since then, there have been attempts to modify and improve their effectiveness and safety, leading to a variety of instruments available for use in different obstetric situations (Fig. 47.1). Obstetric forceps consist of two blades, each with a shank and handle (Telfer 1997). The blades are marked 'L' left and 'R' right (Bevis 1996). There may be a locking or traction device incorporated into the mechanism. Whatever the variation in shape, two considerations are important leading to the addition of pelvic and cephalic curves:

- the shape and size of the fetal head;
- the curve, shape and size of the bony pelvis.

The use of forceps

The shape and size of forceps depend on its use. Forceps may be applied in midcavity or at the pelvic outlet. They may be used to *rotate* the fetal head followed by **traction** in the direction of the curve of Carus to complete the delivery or to apply traction only.

For traction without rotation, non-rotational forceps such as those designed by Wrigley or Simpson are used for low-cavity delivery, mainly now for delivery of the aftercoming head of the

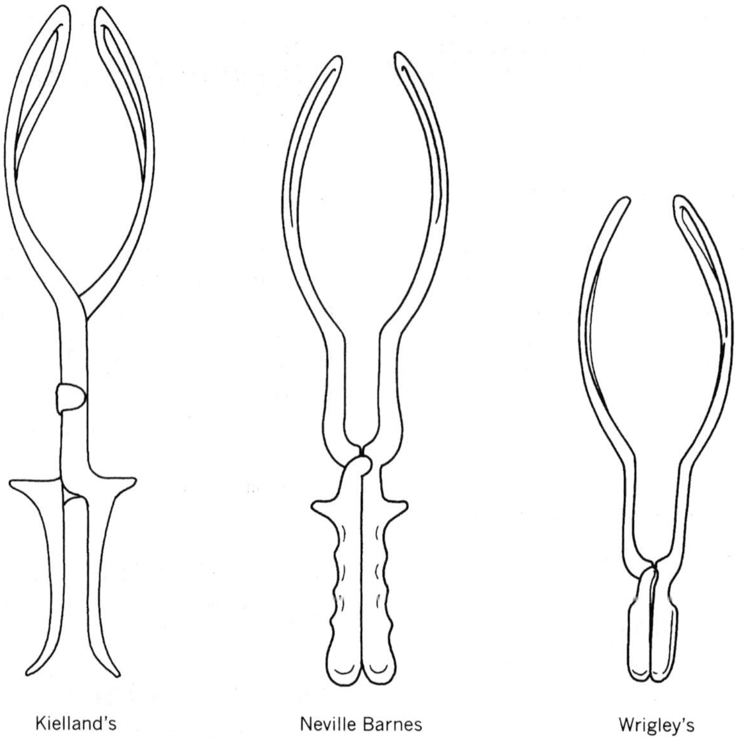

Figure 47.1 *Obstetric forceps (from Sweet B, 1997, with permission).*

breech. Neville Barnes or Haig Fergusson forceps, used for midcavity delivery, have a pelvic and cephalic curve although these are now used exclusively for low-cavity non-rotational delivery and the axis traction attachments are rarely used.

It is important to understand that mid and high-cavity forceps deliveries (when the fetal head is higher than +2) are no longer undertaken because of the possibility of trauma. Caesarean section is more likely to be the method of choice in these cases.

To correct malposition from occipitolateral or occipito-posterior to occipitoanterior prior to traction, rotational forceps such as Kielland's forceps are the only design commonly used. So that they can be rotated in the confines of the birth canal, these forceps have no pelvic curve. In malpositions there is often **asynclitism** (lateral tilting of the fetal head). Kielland's forceps have a sliding lock so that this can be corrected prior to rotation and traction. There is a gap between the handles when the blades are in place and there is a danger that too much pressure may be applied to the fetal head with the risk of cerebral trauma.

Applying the forceps

Positioning

The blades are inserted separately on either side of the fetal head so that they are located alongside the head and over the ears (Fig. 47.2). They should be situated symmetrically between the eye orbits and the ears, reaching from the parietal eminences to the malar area and cheeks (Vacca & Kierse 1989). They should come together and lock easily without the use of strength if they are applied correctly. Myerscough (1982) cited

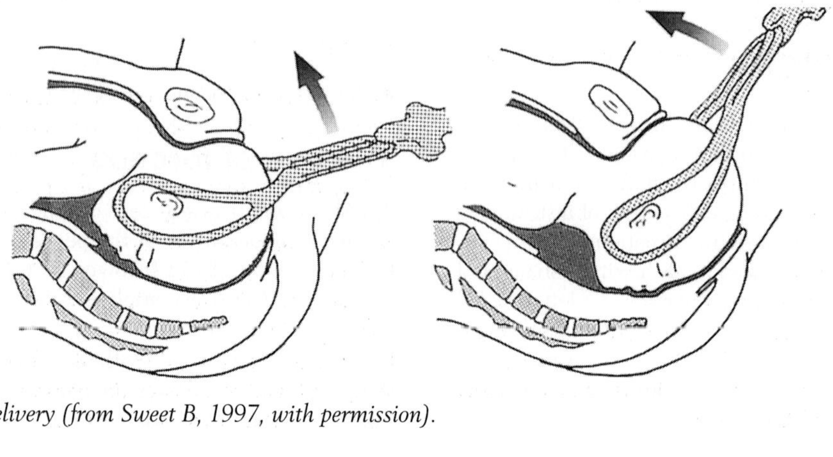

Figure 47.2 *Forceps delivery (from Sweet B, 1997, with permission).*

in Bevis (1996) described the line of application extending from the point of the chin to a point on the sagittal suture near the posterior fontanelle.

The skill of the operator

Enkin et al (1995) state that 'The operator is a major determinant of the success or failure of instrumental delivery. Unfavourable results are almost always caused by the user's unfamiliarity with either the instrument or the rules governing its use'. It is important that the skills of using any instrument are acquired under supervision because of the devasting consequences that could arise if the baby or mother is damaged during the operation.

Prerequisites

No obstruction to the descent of the fetus must be present.

- There must be full dilatation of the os uteri.
- The membranes must be ruptured.
- The bladder must be empty.
- There should be no cephalopelvic disproportion.
- The head must be engaged.

The mother should be safeguarded.

- Adequate anaesthesia must be available by epidural or pudendal block.
- A full explanation of the procedure should be given to the woman and her partner and consent obtained.
- There should be as much safety, comfort and dignity for the woman as possible although the lithotomy position is essential.
- An episiotomy is usually performed.
- The procedure is carried out aseptically with sterile instruments.

The baby should be safeguarded.

- There should be careful and accurate identification of the presentation and position of the fetal head.
- The forceps blades are applied correctly and their position checked before rotation and/or traction is commenced.
- A paediatrician should be present at the delivery.
- Neonatal resuscitation equipment should be available.
- Manual rotation of the head may be preferred by some obstetricians as it is thought to be less traumatic than instrumental rotation (Bevis 1996). Rotational forceps delivery may cause a significant deterioration in fetal acid/base balance (Baker & Johnson 1994).

Complications

Maternal

- There may be soft tissue damage to the lower uterine segment, cervix, vagina and perineum.
- Bleeding from tissue trauma may lead to postpartum haemorrhage and shock.
- Retention of urine may occur if there is bruising and oedema of the urethra and neck of the bladder.
- Perineal pain may be present once the anaesthesia has worn off.
- Dyspareunia may occur in the long term.
- Psychological effects may lead to avoidance of future pregnancy.

Fetal

- A cephalhaematoma may form due to friction between the fetal head and the blades or pelvic walls.
- Facial or scalp abrasions are common.
- Bruising of the scalp may lead to neonatal jaundice.
- Intracranial haemorrhage is a rare but serious problem which may lead to convulsions.
- These problems are more often seen with rotational forceps, as is failed forceps delivery resulting in emergency CS (Johanson et al 1992).

VACUUM EXTRACTION (VENTOUSE DELIVERY)

Use of the vacuum extractor

Delivery by the use of vacuum extraction has a history as long as that of forceps delivery. The modern version was developed by Malmström in the 1950s and has been modified by others (Vacca 1992). Originally the vacuum extractor consisted of a rounded metal cup in three sizes, 40, 50 and 60 mm in diameter (Bird 1969), and this type of cup is still in use. It is attached to a chain and handle and a suction pump to extract air and create a vacuum. The largest cup size which can be passed through the cervix is chosen.

Cups are now available made of silastic, silicone rubber and plastic. Johanson & Menon (1997a) have compared the use of soft versus rigid vacuum extractor cups. Soft cups deform to follow the contours of the baby's head during application but the application is poor if there is moderate to severe caput succedaneum. Also, there is limited ability to place the cup correctly if the head is deflexed and the success rate is lower than with metal cups. However, they are less likely to be associated with scalp trauma (Chenoy & Johanson 1992).

Applying the vacuum extractor

Positioning

The cup is attached by suction to the fetal scalp as near to the occiput as possible, taking care to avoid the anterior fontanelle (Fig. 47.3). A vacuum is created with a negative pressure of 0.2 kg/cm, drawing an artificial caput (**chignon**) into the cup (Telfer 1997). The cup is checked for position and to ensure that no maternal soft tissue, such as the cervix, has been included within the rim (Fig. 47.4). The vacuum pressure is increased to 0.8 kg/cm. This can either be done in stages or in one step. One to two minutes should be allowed for the chignon to develop. Traction is then applied following the curve of Carus along with and to enhance the natural forces of uterine contractions and maternal expulsive effort.

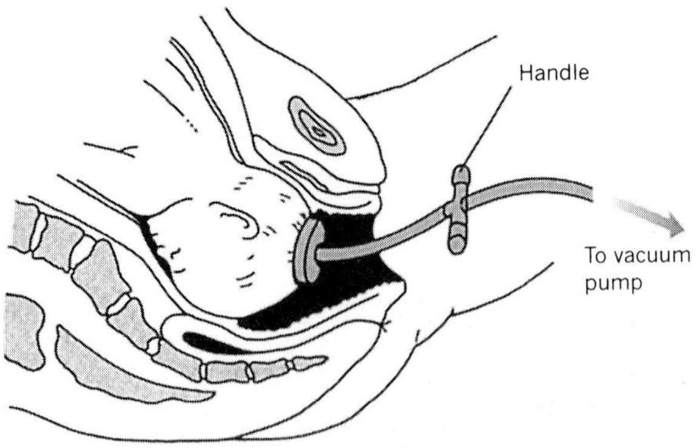

Figure 47.3 *Vacuum extraction (from Sweet B, 1997, with permission).*

The skill of the operator

Used skilfully, the advantages of the ventouse are that there is no increase to the presenting diameters and the instrument can be used to complete dilatation, to flex and rotate the head naturally and to assist the mother to deliver her infant. However, some operators may be too hasty or unskilled and apply traction before suction has been achieved, resulting in the cup coming away from the scalp. The technique is suitable for use by midwives working alone without obstetric colleagues in remote areas of the world.

Prerequisites

- These are as for forceps delivery with the exception that the os uteri may only need to be 7 cm or more dilated. This last is a controversial factor and there is a need for caution. The state of the cervix, whether it is thin or thick, soft or rigid and likely to recede under pressure, is as important as the dilatation of the os.
- The vacuum extractor is not suitable for application in babies under 36 weeks gestation or in those with suspected coagulability.
- It should not be used where contractions are weak or maternal effort is poor.

Complications

Maternal

There is minimal trauma to maternal tissues if the cup has been applied carefully.

Fetal

- Trauma to the fetal scalp is the most common complication although this is reported as minimal if soft cups are used (Chenoy & Johanson 1992).
- All babies will have a chignon which is a combination of oedema and bruising.
- Abrasions of the scalp may be caused by pulling the cup off during inexpert traction.
- Jaundice, which is usually mild and responds to phototherapy, may be due to the reabsorption of the red cells which have escaped the circulatory system during bruise formation (O'Grady 1988, cited by Telfer 1997).
- Neonatal retinal haemorrhages are more common following vacuum extraction than forceps delivery (Vacca 1992, Williams et al 1991) but there are no long-term problems.
- Vacuum extraction has been found to be associated with umbilical cord blood acid/base changes but these changes in pH and PCO^2 were not associated with increased perinatal morbidity or mortality or acidaemia at birth. These findings suggest that vacuum extraction can be used to deliver babies with fetal distress in the 2nd stage of labour.

COMPARISON OF FORCEPS AND VACUUM EXTRACTION

Although assisted vaginal delivery is performed worldwide, there is a large variation in its application, ranging from 1.5% of all deliveries in the Czech Republic to 15% in Australia and Canada (Stephenson 1992). Comparative studies have been undertaken of assisted vaginal delivery by obstetric forceps versus ventouse extraction (Chalmers & Chalmers 1989, Johanson et al 1992, Williams et al 1991).

Although some studies show that the ventouse is less likely to injure both mother and baby than forceps, it is possible to select papers that argue this point (Drife 1996). For instance, Williams et al (1991) found no significant differences in maternal and neonatal outcome. There were associations with mild neonatal hyperbilirubinaemia and neonatal retinal haemorrhages in babies delivered by vacuum extraction and with facial injury in those delivered by forceps. Johanson & Menon (1997b) have reviewed the studies. To quote Telfer citing in Vacca (1992), 'Use appears to be based on tradition and varies between countries and obstetricians'.

CAESAREAN SECTION

Births by caesarean section (CS), a surgical procedure in which the abdomen and uterus are incised to facilitate delivery (Anderson et al 1994), are recorded prior to the discovery of anaesthetic drugs, usually for delivery of the fetus when the mother had died. Caesarean section may be carried out as an emergency in response to adverse conditions developing in late pregnancy or in labour. Elective CS is a planned event where the timing is chosen to maximise safety for mother and fetus.

Current rates

Savage (1996) stated that the rates of CS worldwide have risen over the last 25 years. In the UK they have doubled and in the USA and Canada they have tripled. The WHO (1985) said that CS rates should not need to be more than 10–15% while Savage believes it should not need to be more than 6–8%. By 1993 the rate in the UK had reached the upper limit suggested by the WHO of 15%. Some 25–30% of births in the USA are for CS (Anderson et al 1994).

Indications

The majority of CS are performed for hypertensive disorders of

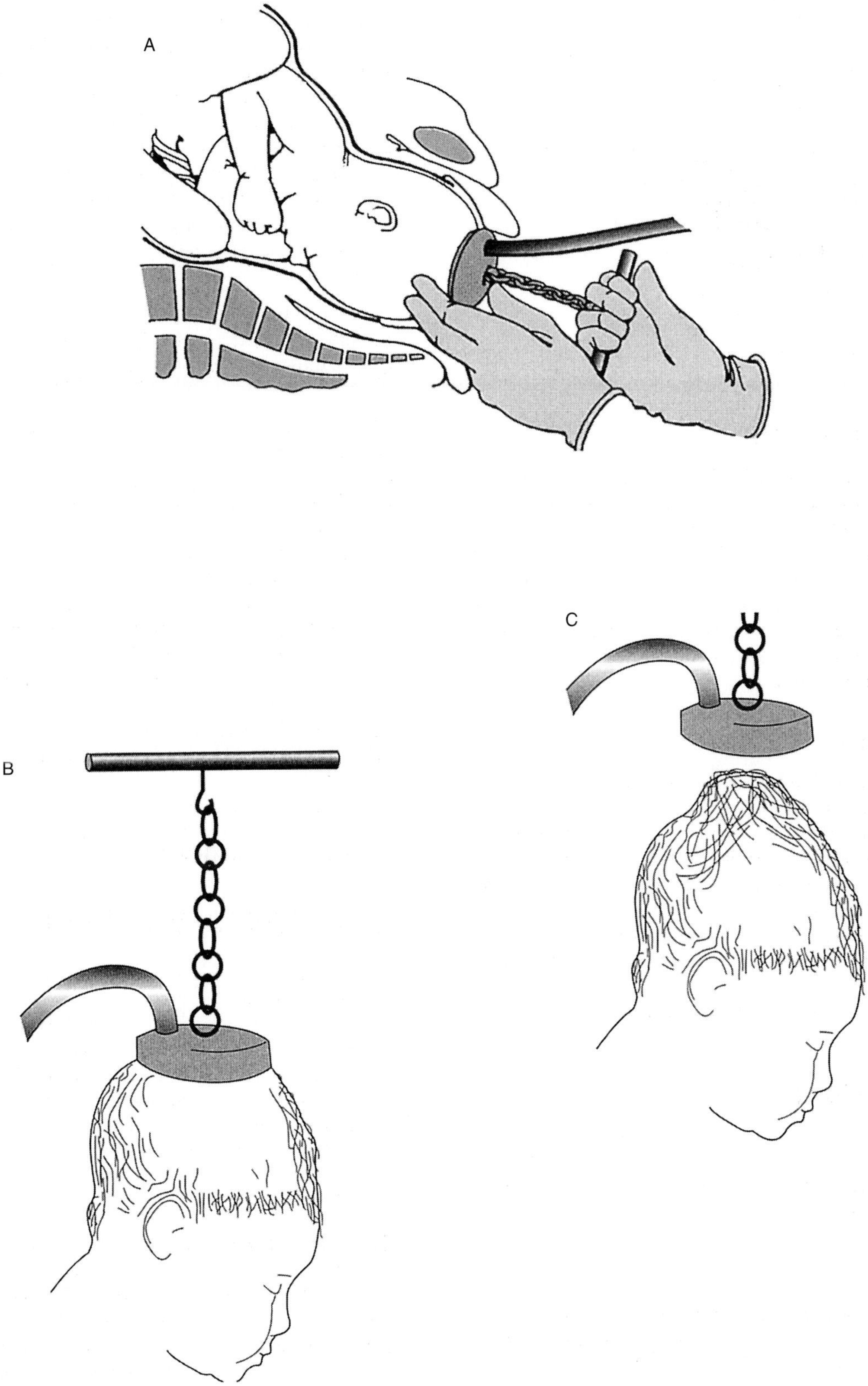

Figure 47.4 *(a) Outlet vacuum extraction using three-finger grip traction with a metal cup vacuum extractor (Bird's modification). (b) Correct midoccipital application of a rigid cup vacuum extractor. (c) Chignon produced by a rigid cup vacuum extractor. (Reproduced with permission from O'Grady 1988.)*

pregnancy, antepartum haemorrhage or fetal distress (DOH 1996). The major reasons for the increase in CS rate are for breech presentation, repeat CS or dystocia. The following list includes the likely reasons for carrying out a CS.

Maternal

- Severe pregnancy-induced hypertension
- Previous vaginal reconstructive surgery

Fetal

- Severe rhesus isoimmunisation
- Cord prolapse
- Multiple fetuses (three or more)
- Breech presentation
- Brow or shoulder presentations
- Intrauterine growth retardation
- Fetal distress in labour
- Fetal abnormality where damage may be increased by vaginal delivery
- Active genital herpes

Maternal with fetal

- Cephalopelvic disproportion
- Pelvic tumours
- High-risk obstetric history
- Antepartum haemorrhage
- Uterine rupture
- Failure to progress in labour
- Fetal macrosomia

Method

Any person called on to assist at a CS must be aware of the surgical techniques involved. Technically, there are two types of CS according to the incision in the uterus: the **lower segment** and the **classic**. There is no association with the type of abdominal wall incision although a lower uterine CS is most often performed through a transverse incision, also called the **Pfannenstiel** or **bikini-line incision** (Bevis 1996). The lower segment forms from about 32 weeks of pregnancy and is less muscular than the upper segment. A transverse incision into the lower segment heals more rapidly than a vertical incision into the upper uterine segment and there is less risk of rupture of the uterus in a subsequent pregnancy. For this reason, classic CS is rarely performed unless the fetus is to be delivered prior to the 32nd week of pregnancy or there is an anterior placenta praevia.

Anatomical layers to be incised and sutured

- Skin
- Fat
- Rectus sheath
- Muscle (rectus abdominis)
- Abdominal peritoneum
- Pelvic (visceral peritoneum or perimetrium)
- Uterine muscle (sutured in two layers)

As the uterus is incised, the membranes are ruptured with the escape of amniotic fluid. There is likely to be substantial bleeding because of the increased blood supply to the uterus. Immediate postoperative care is as for any surgery but the woman will wish to see her baby as soon as possible and to breastfeed if that is her intention. Because of the proximity of the bladder to the lower uterine segment, urine output must be observed as there may be difficulty in micturition at first. Any presence of haematuria must be reported. Postoperative analgesia, depending on the mode of anaesthesia for the surgery, may be:

- epidural top-up;
- epidural opiate;
- intramuscular analgesia.

Safety

Lilford (1990) warned that any increase in the proportions of elective CS would lead to increase in the CS rate and probably in maternal mortality. CS carried out for the safety of the fetus therefore puts the mother's life at risk (Hillan 1991). Even with the benefit of modern surgical techniques it is still less safe for the woman than a vaginal delivery. The major hazard is **pulmonary embolism** which is difficult to prevent (Savage 1996). Haemorrhage and infection, as well as thromboembolic disorders, may occur (Francome et al 1993). Long-term morbidity with infertility, voluntary or involuntary, may be a problem. The overall mortality rate due to CS is 0.33 per 1000 CS performed. Maternal deaths following CS were reported to be 48.8% of all direct deaths (DOH 1996). The immediate causes were found to be pulmonary embolism, hypertensive disease and haemorrhage.

Neonatal behaviour

There is a profound effect on neonatal behaviour attributable to at least the following four factors (Trevathen 1987).

1. Caesarean section is often carried out before term.
2. Maternal medication is greater than in vaginal births.
3. In elective CS the baby is not subjected to the stress of labour.
4. Hormonal influences vary depending on the time and mode of delivery.

Babies are less active if delivered by CS, they sleep more and cry less. The influence of drugs in labour on neonatal behaviour will be examined in more detail in Section 4A.

GENERAL ANAESTHESIA IN PREGNANCY AND CHILDBIRTH

Reversible anaesthesia, which is a state of unconsciousness and muscle relaxation, is brought about by pharmacological preparations. There is a great difference in obstetric anaesthesia from general surgery as two lives have to be cared for – the mother and the fetus. Telfer (1997) reminds us that obstetric anaesthesia is full of difficulties. A recent report (DOH 1996) states that there is a need for vigilance in the care of the pregnant woman undergoing general anaesthesia.

The altered physiology of the woman, which increases the danger, includes raised maternal intragastric pressure, acidity of gastric contents and delayed gastric emptying leading to the risk of acid aspiration syndrome. Aortocaval occlusion, the effect of drugs on the fetus, maternal hypoxia or hypotension, placental insufficiency and intrapartum fetal hypoxia also increase the risk of neonatal respiratory depression (Telfer 1997).

General anaesthetic agents

For a drug to be used as an anaesthetic agent, it must affect the central nervous system appropriately and be controllable so that anaesthesia can be induced rapidly, be adjusted during the operation to provide the correct level of consciousness and recovered from quickly (Rang & Dale 1991). Humphry Davy suggested the use of the gas nitrous oxide for relieving the pain of surgery in 1800. He tested its effects on himself and a few others, including the then Prime Minister. It was found to cause euphoria, analgesia and loss of consciousness but became famous as laughing gas until an American dentist, Horace Wells, had a tooth extracted under its influence.

Inhalational anaesthetics were used in surgery in 1846 when William Morton used ether to extract a tooth. He persuaded the chief surgeon at Massachusetts General Hospital to use it during a surgical procedure in October 1846 and it was successful. In 1847 James Simpson, professor of obstetrics in Glasgow, used the agent **chloroform** to relieve pain in childbirth but it became popular only after Queen Victoria gave birth to her 7th child under the influence of chloroform in 1853.

Modern drugs

Although many CS are now performed under epidural anaesthesia (see Chapter 36), general anaesthesia is still used. It is now common practice to preoxygenate pregnant women prior to induction of a general anaesthetic although this may lead to stress for the woman (Bevis 1996). The choice made by the woman is important (Pearson & Rees 1989). Holdcroft et al (1995) found that one-third of the women in their small study opted to be unconscious during CS. Induction agents used to initiate anaesthesia include barbiturates such as **thiopentone**, which causes loss of consciousness in 20 s if given intravenously (Rang & Dale 1991), or **propofol**, which appears to be a good alternative. Maternal unconsciousness follows rapidly with minimal side effects and fetal depression can be avoided.

Anaesthesia is then maintained by inhalational anaesthetic agents such as nitrous oxide combined with a volatile agent such as halothane (Fluothane) or enflurane (Ethrane). Halothane has limited usefulness as an obstetric anaesthetic agent as it causes relaxation of the uterine muscle (Rang & Dale 1991). These agents deepen the anaesthesia, improve uterine blood flow by reducing circulating catecholamines and improve fetal acid/base status (Capogna & Celluno 1993).

Problems

Failed intubation

Failed intubation is an obstetric emergency requiring prompt and calm action. Most maternal deaths attributed directly to anaesthesia have been reported to be due to a misplaced endotracheal tube. It is usual to have a failed intubation drill (Bevis 1996). The anaesthetist may choose to maintain an airway with a Guedel airway and facemask with an assistant maintaining cricoid pressure throughout the anaesthetic or **spinal anaesthesia** may be chosen.

Effect of anaesthetics on the nervous system

The mode of action of anaesthetic drugs is as yet unexplained. The brain has a large blood flow and the blood–brain barrier is freely permeable to anaesthetic agents (Rang & Dale 1991). Theories involve interaction with the lipid bilayer of the cell membrane or with hydrophobic binding sites on protein molecules. Anaesthetics inhibit the conduction of cellular action potentials and synaptic transmission.

It is probable that anaesthetics must act on two main parts of the brain: the **reticular formation** and the **hippocampus**. Loss of consciousness is probably due to the effect of the drug on the reticular formation of the brain. Anaesthetics also cause short-term amnesia and the hippocampus is likely to be the site for this action. Many other brain functions are affected such as motor control and reflex action. It is not helpful to look for one site of action as all neurones are affected.

Muscle relaxation is achieved by drugs which **depolarise** neuromuscular messages postsynaptically, such as suxamethonium (Scoline), or **non-polarising agents** which act postsynaptically such as pancuronium (Pavulon) (Rang & Dale 1991).

Acid aspiration syndrome (Mendelson's syndrome)

This life-threatening syndrome arises from the inhalation of acid gastric contents and was first described by Mendelson in 1946. The result of such aspiration is a chemical pneumonitis leading to adult respiratory distress syndrome (ARDS) with acute bronchospasm, dyspnoea, cyanosis, wheezing and tachycardia (Telfer 1997). The factors predisposing to this arise from the physiological effect of progesterone on the smooth muscle of the stomach which causes delayed emptying, decreased lower oesophageal tone, which leads to reflux, and the altered position of the stomach due to the enlarged uterus. There is also gastric hypersecretion in labour and there is still no consensus on nil-by-mouth policies. Water only is recommended in most units once a drug such as pethidine has been given, which is often associated with the change to active phase of labour with delivery likely to occur within 6–8 h.

Prevention

Prevention of this syndrome is essential. Prior to anaesthetic induction drugs such as **antacid preparations** like sodium citrate 30 ml and **H_2 antagonists** such as ranitidine 150 mg are recommended. Another drug is **metoclopramide**, which acts centrally in the nervous system but also locally in the gastrointestinal tract. It is an antiemetic and acts as a stimulant to gastric motility, accelerating emptying without stimulating gastric juice production. It increases tone in the lower oesophagus and prevents gastrooesophageal reflux (Rang & Dale 1991).

During induction of the general anaesthetic and intubation, **cricoid pressure** (Sellick's manoeuvre), part of what is referred to as **crash induction** along with the immediate passing of a cuffed endotracheal tube, is essential to prevent aspiration of acid stomach contents. The cricoid cartilage is compressed between the thumb and finger towards the cervical spine in order to occlude the oesophagus (Bevis 1985). Deaths have occurred due to inexperience of the practitioner and the DOH (1996) recommend that only an experienced anaesthetist should be involved in obstetric anaesthesia.

Aortocaval occlusion

The alternative name for aortocaval occlusion is **supine hypotensive syndrome**. Bevis (1996) believes this is misleading as the fall in blood pressure is a late sign and reduced placental perfusion will have occurred before the drop in maternal blood pressure. A reduction in venous return and a fall in cardiac output are produced by the weight of the gravid uterus pressing on and partly occluding the inferior vena cava. It will occur whenever the woman lies supine in late pregnancy. If fetal distress is present the interference with placental circulation will increase the severity of hypoxia.

Prevention

If the woman has to lie supine the sequence of events can be avoided by placing a folded blanket or a small rubber wedge under the mattress to tilt her body 15° to the left. Modern operating tables and delivery beds have this function built into their design. Enkin & Wilkinson (1997) reviewed the use of lateral tilt during CS but found the data to be poor. However, they stated that low Apgar scores were fewer and neonatal pH measurements and oxygen tensions appeared to be better if lateral tilt was used.

Summary of main points

- Obstetric forceps consist of two blades, each with a shank and handle. Forceps may be used to rotate the fetal head followed by traction in the direction of the curve of Carus to complete the delivery or to apply traction only. Prior to performing an obstetrics forceps delivery, no obstruction to the descent of the fetus must be present and the safety of both mother and baby must be assured.
- Maternal complications include soft tissue damage to the lower uterine segment, cervix, vagina and perineum, bleeding from tissue trauma, retention of urine, postdelivery perineal pain and dyspareunia in the long term. Neonatal complications are more often seen with rotational forceps and include cephalhaematoma, facial or scalp abrasions, neonatal jaundice, and intracranial haemorrhage which may lead to convulsions.
- The modern version of the vacuum extractor was developed by Malmström in the 1950s and has been modified by others. Cups are now available made of silastic, silicone rubber and plastic as well as the original metal. Soft cups deform to follow the contours of the baby's head during application and are less likely to be associated with scalp trauma.
- The instrument can be used to complete dilatation, to flex and rotate the head naturally and to assist the mother to deliver her infant. The technique is suitable for use by midwives working alone in remote areas of the world. The os uteri may only need to be 7 cm or more dilated but the state of cervical tissue is as important as the dilatation of the os.
- There is minimal trauma to maternal tissues. Trauma to the fetal scalp is the most common complication and may be accompanied by jaundice which is usually mild and responds to phototherapy. Neonatal retinal haemorrhages are more common following vacuum extraction than forceps delivery but there are no long-term problems.
- Worldwide CS rates have risen over the last 25 years, doubling in the UK and tripling in the USA and Canada, the majority being performed for hypertensive disorders of pregnancy, antepartum haemorrhage or fetal distress. Even with modern surgical techniques, it is still less safe for the woman than a vaginal delivery. During CS the altered physiology of the woman increases the danger of acid aspiration syndrome but the major hazard is pulmonary embolism. Maternal deaths following CS were reported as 48.8% of all direct deaths.
- Delivery by CS has a profound effect on neonatal behaviour. Babies are less active if delivered by CS, they sleep more and cry less. Aortocaval occlusion, drugs, maternal hypoxia or hypotension, placental insufficiency and intrapartum fetal hypoxia increase the risk of neonatal respiratory depression.
- Although many CS are now performed under epidural anaesthesia, general anaesthesia is still used. It is now common practice to preoxygenate pregnant women prior to induction of a general anaesthetic. Induction agents used to initiate anaesthesia include barbiturates and propofol. Anaesthesia is maintained by inhalational anaesthetic agents such as nitrous oxide combined with halothane.
- The blood–brain barrier is freely permeable to anaesthetic agents. It is probable that anaesthetics act on the reticular formation to cause loss of consciousness and the hippocampus to cause short-term amnesia. Muscle relaxation is achieved by drugs which depolarise neuromuscular messages postsynaptically or non-polarising agents which act postsynaptically.
- Acid aspiration syndrome arises from the inhalation of acid gastric contents, resulting in chemical pneumonitis and adult respiratory distress syndrome. There is still no consensus on nil-by-mouth policies but once a drug such as pethidine has been given, water only is recommended in most units. Prevention is essential and antacid preparations and H_2 antagonists are recommended. Most maternal deaths attributed directly to anaesthesia are due to a misplaced endotracheal tube. During induction of the general anaesthetic and intubation, cricoid pressure is essential to prevent aspiration of acid stomach contents.
- Aortocaval occlusion or supine hypotensive syndrome causes a reduction in venous return and a fall in cardiac output and is produced by the weight of the gravid uterus occluding the inferior vena cava. If fetal distress is present the interference with placental circulation will increase the severity of hypoxia. If the woman has to lie supine, the sequence of events can be avoided by placing a folded blanket or a small rubber wedge under the mattress to tilt her body 15° to the left.

References

American College of Obstetricians and Gynecologists, 1991 Operative vagina delivery, ACOG technical bulletin 152. ACOG, Washington DC.

Anderson KN, Anderson LE, Glanze WD. 1994 Mosby's Medical, Nursing and Allied Health Dictionary, 4th edn. Mosby, St Louis.

Arias F. 1993 Practical Guide to High Risk Pregnancy and Delivery, 2nd edn. Mosby Year Book Chicago.

Baker PN, Johnson IR. 1994 A study of rotational forceps delivery on fetal acid-base balance. Acta Obstetrica et Gynaecologica Scandinavica 73, 787–789.

Bevis R. 1985 Anaesthesia in Midwifery. Baillière Tindall, London.

Bevis R. 1996 Obstetric anaesthesia and operations. In Bennett VR, Brown LK (eds) Myles Textbook for Midwives, 12th edn. Churchill Livingstone, Edinburgh, pp 441–461.

Bird GC. 1969 Modification of Malmström's vacuum extractor. British Medical Journal 3, 526.

Capogna G, Celluno D. 1993 The effects of anaesthetic agents on the newborn. In Reynolds F (ed) Effects on the Baby of Maternal Analgesia and Anaesthesia. WB Saunders, London.

Chalmers JA, Chalmers I. 1989 The obstetric vacuum extractor is the instrument of first choice for operative vaginal delivery. British Journal of Obstetrics and Gynaecology 96, 505–509.

Chenoy R, Johanson RB. 1992 A randomised prospective study comparing delivery with metal and silicone rubber vacuum extractor cups. British Journal of Obstetrics and Gynaecology 99, 360–364.

Department of Health 1996 Report on Confidential Enquiries into Maternal Deaths in the United Kingdom 1991–1993. HMSO, London.

Drife J. 1996 Choice and instrumental delivery. British Journal of Obstetrics and Gynaecology 103, 608–611.

Enkin M, Wilkinson C. 1997 Lateral tilt during Caesarean section. In Neilson JP, Crowther CA, Hodnett ED, Hofmeyr GJ, Keirse MJNC (eds) Pregnancy and Childbirth module of The Cochrane Database of Systematic Reviews, The Cochrane Library. Update Software, Oxford.

Enkin M, Keirse MJNC, Renfrew M, Neilson JP. 1995 A Guide to Effective Care in Pregnancy and Childbirth, 2nd edn. Oxford Medical Publications, Oxford.

Francome C, Savage W, Churchill H, Lewison H. 1993 Caesarean Birth in Britain, Middlesex University Press, National Childbirth Trust, London.

Hillan E. 1991 Caesarean section: maternal risks. Nursing Standard (50), 26–29.

Holdcroft A, Parshall AM, Knowles MG et al. 1995 Factors associated with mothers selecting general anaesthesia for lower segment Caesarean section. Journal of Psychosomatic Obstetrics and Gynaecology 16(3), 167–170.

Johanson R, Menon V. 1997a Soft versus rigid vacuum extractor cups (protocol). In Neilson JP, Crowther CA, Hodnett ED, Hofmeyr GJ, Keirse MJNC (eds) Pregnancy and Childbirth module of The Cochrane Database of Systematic Reviews, The Cochrane Library. Update Software, Oxford.

Johanson R, Menon V. 1997b Vacuum extraction versus forceps delivery (protocol) In Neilson JP, Crowther CA, Hodnett ED, Hofmeyr GJ, Keirse MJNC (eds) Pregnancy and Childbirth module of The Cochrane Database of Systematic Reviews, The Cochrane Library. Update Software, Oxford.

Johanson R, Rice C, Doyle M et al. A randomised prospective study comparing the new vacuum extractor policy with forceps delivery. British Journal of Obstetrics and Gynaecology 100, 524–530.

Lilford R. 1990 Maternal mortality and Caesarean section. British Journal of Obstetrics and Gynaecology 97, 883–892.

Myerscough PR. 1982 Munro Kerr's Operative Obstetrics, 10th edn. Baillière Tindall, London.

O'Grady JP. 1988 Modern Instrumental Delivery. Williams and Wilkins, Baltimore.

Pearson J, Rees G. 1989 Technique of Caesarean section. In Chalmers I, Enkin M, Keirse MJNC (eds) Effective Care in Pregnancy and Childbirth, Vol 2. Oxford University Press, Oxford.

Rang HP, Dale MM. 1991 Pharmacology, Churchill Livingstone, Edinburgh.

Savage W. 1996 The caesarean section epidemic: a psychological problem? Journal of the Association of Chartered Physiotherapists in Women's Health 79, 13–16.

Stephenson PA. 1992 International Differences in the Use of Obstetrical Interventions. WHO, Copenhagen, 112.

Sweet B. 1997 Mayes' Midwifery. Baillière Tindall, London.

Telfer FM. 1997 Anaesthesia and operative procedures in obstetrics. In Sweet BR with Tiran D (eds) Mayes Midwifery, 12th edn. Baillière Tindall, London, pp 682–702.

Trevathen W. 1987 Human Birth: an Evolutionary Perspective, Aldine de Gruyter, New York.

Vacca A. 1992 Handbook of Vacuum Extraction Obstetric Practice. Edward Arnold, London.

Vacca A, Kierse MJNC. 1989 Instrumental vaginal delivery. In Chalmers I, Enkin M, Keirse MJNC (eds) Effective Care in Pregnancy and Childbirth, Vol 2. Oxford University Press, Oxford, pp 1217–1233.

Williams MC, Knuppel RA, O'Brien WF, Weiss A, Kanarek KS. 1991 A randomised comparison of assisted vaginal delivery by obstetric forceps and polyethylene vacuum cup. Obstetrics and Gynaecology 78, 789–794.

World Health Organization 1985 Appropriate technology for birth. Lancet ii, 436–437.

Recommended reading

Bevis R. 1996 Obstetric anaesthesia and operations. In Bennett VR, Brown LK (eds) Myles Textbook for Midwives, 12th edn. Churchill Livingstone, Edinburgh, pp 441–461.

Capogna G, Celluno D. 1993 The effects of anaesthetic agents on the newborn. In Reynolds F (ed) Effects on the Baby of Maternal Analgesia and Anaesthesia. WB Saunders, London.

Chenoy R, Johanson RB. 1992 A randomised prospective study comparing delivery with metal and silicone rubber vacuum extractor cups. British Journal of Obstetrics and Gynaecology 99, 360–364.

Drife J. 1996 Choice and instrumental delivery. British Journal of Obstetrics and Gynaecology 103, 608–611.

Johanson R, Menon V. 1997 Vacuum extraction versus forceps delivery (protocol). In Neilson JP, Crowther CA, Hodnett ED, Hofmeyr GJ, Keirse MJNC (eds) Pregnancy and Childbirth module of The Cochrane Database of Systematic Reviews, The Cochrane Library. Update Software, Oxford.

Lilford R. 1990 Maternal mortality and Caesarean section. British Journal of Obstetrics and Gynaecology 97, 883–892.

Savage W. 1996 The caesarean section epidemic: a psychological problem? Journal of the Association of Chartered Physiotherapists in Women's Health 79, 13–16.

World Health Organization 1985 Appropriate technology for birth. Lancet ii, 436–437.

Section

4A

PUERPERIUM – THE BABY

Section contents

Section 4 considers the mother and her baby in the puerperium. Section 4A consists of six chapters (48–53). Midwives may care for mothers and their babies for up to 28 days and it is imperative that they are able to recognise both normal appearance and behaviour and any deviations present. Chapters 48 and 49 provide a detailed account of the adaptation of the fetus to independent extrauterine life. The remaining chapters provide an introduction to some commonly encountered serious disorders. These chapters cannot take the place of a specifically written book on neonatal care and the reader is referred to one of the many excellent texts available and given in the chapter reference lists. Chapter 50 is about the care of the low birth weight infant, chapter 51 examines cardiovascular and respiratory problems, chapter 52 is concerned with neonatal jaundice and some metabolic disorders whilst chapter 53 discusses problems arising from infection or trauma.

Chapter

48 Adaptation to extrauterine life 1 – respiration and cardiovascular function

In this chapter

INTRODUCTION

During the following chapters about the neonate, a baby will be referred to using masculine pronouns. This is simply to distinguish him from his nearest carer, his mother.

Whilst he remains in utero, the fetus is dependent on his mother for many aspects of his survival. At the time of birth the fetus must rapidly adapt to life outside the uterus and every system of the baby's body must contribute to the maintenance of homeostasis. Of immediate importance are the anatomic and physiological changes which occur in the baby's respiratory and cardiovascular system. The initiating physiological principle appears to be the considerable but necessary rise in the partial pressure of CO_2 in the fetal blood when contact with the placenta is lost.

This mechanism stimulates the respiratory centre which in due course induces the baby's first gasp for breath commonly resulting in lung expansion. The inspired oxygen stimulates the subsequent haemodynamic alteration which involves the circulating blood volume, cardiac and respiratory functions. This chapter will discuss the above systems and include the renal system because of its contribution to maintaining the acid/base balance of the body.

THE APPEARANCE OF THE NORMAL BABY

Skin and hair

The normal baby at term weighs about 3500 g (just over 7 lb) and is 50 cm long (20 inches). His occipitofrontal head circumference averages 35 cm and his head is about 25% of his total body surface area (Michie 1996). The full-term infant may be plump with a rounded abdomen due to the deposition of subcutaneous fat. The high volume of total body water also contributes to this. The baby's nails should reach to the ends of his fingers and toes (Anderson 1992). The scalp is covered with varying amounts of fine silky hair. Some babies appear bald but some have luxuriant hair that may be straight or curly. Some

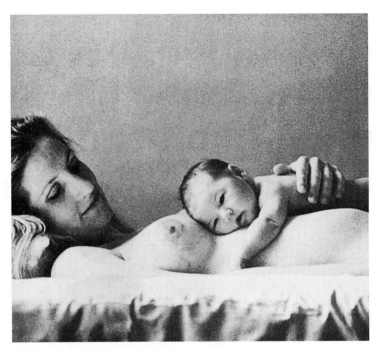

Figure 48.1 *Skin-to-skin contact in a warm labour ward. (Courtesy of Professor J Hedgecoe.)*

remnants of lanugo, the fine hair that completely covered his body in the middle weeks of pregnancy, may be left on his shoulders. The cartilage of his ears is well formed.

Depending on his race, as long as he is well oxygenated, the baby may have a pink skin or be lightly pigmented but pinkish. The mucous membranes of the mouth and lips and the nail beds should always appear pink. Pigmentation of the genitalia and nipples is deeper in babies with dark skins and a **linea nigra** may be present in the lower abdominal midline. Depending on his racial origin, a diffuse bluish-black skin colouration may be present, usually over the sacral area. This is known as the **Mongolian blue spot**. The creases of his palms and soles are well defined (Michie 1996).

Humans are unique amongst the primate species in having large sebaceous glands whose function is to produce sebum over the scalp, face and upper part of their backs (Morgan 1994). Although they have been very active in utero, the sebaceous glands of the baby have become inactive by birth and will stay dormant until puberty when their activity may lead to acne. At birth distended sebaceous glands called **milia** may be present over the nose and cheeks. The baby's skin will have remnants of the sebaceous gland excretion mixed with dead skin cells called **vernix caseosa** in places, usually the groins and axillae.

Morgan (1994) believes that during their evolutionary path humans spent large portions of their life in water on the edge of a large inland sea, an interesting idea that explains many human attributes such as hairlessness and the presence of a diving reflex, shared with aquatic mammals but which no land mammal has. She also places the human fetus in context with aquatic mammals and postulates a protective role for the vernix in protecting the lanugo, as in aquatic mammals, keeping it sleek and water repellent.

At about 5 months the fetus develops sweat glands (**eccrine glands**) on the palms of its hands and the soles of its feet. At the same time it develops scent glands (**apocrine glands**) all over its body, used by many mammals for sweat cooling. By 7 months the fetus loses its apocrine glands except for the armpits, pubic area, around the nipples and lips and the eccrine glands spread all over the body. In humans but no other primate, these are the glands used for sweat cooling when the body temperature rises above a critical physiological point (Morgan 1994). These sweat glands are inactive for the first few days of life (Michie 1996).

Eyes

The irises of the eyes of most babies are dark blue-grey. Although some dark-skinned babies may have brown eyes at birth, permanent colouring of the iris may take several years to develop. Oriental babies have an epicanthic fold which changes the shape of the soft tissue covering the orbital region. A newborn baby cannot generally shed tears which provide a natural lubricant and antiseptic for the eyes. This absence may contribute to a higher incidence of eye infections such as conjunctivitis. This clinical phenomenon may be further complicated by temporary blockage of the infant's lacrimal ducts which would normally remove accumulated conjunctival secretions.

Sexual characteristics

Both boys and girls have a small nodule of breast tissue about 1 cm in diameter around the nipple. This may be swollen as a consequence of the high plasma oestrogen acquired from the mother and, for a short time, milk may even be present in the baby's breasts. Traditionally this was called witch's milk. No attempt to remove this milk should be made as squeezing the tissue may lead to bruising and abscess formation.

In boys born at term the testes are descended into the scrotum. However, these may still be undescended in the preterm baby. The foreskin is still adherent to the glans penis. The deposition of fat in the genital area of girls ensures that the labia majora cover and conceal the labia minora. This feature is not present in preterm babies. If the labia are parted the urethral and vaginal orifices can be seen. A thick white vaginal discharge may be present as a response to maternal oestrogen. The linings of the uterus and vagina are quite mature and the baby may have a small pseudomenstruation. Once maternal oestrogen levels are reduced, the genital tract returns to an infantile state.

Posture

The baby usually lies in a flexed position and resists extension of his limbs. If his arms are extended they will reach out. If he is placed on his back he will turn his head to one side, usually the right side, and elevate his left shoulder. If he is placed in the prone position he will draw his knees under his abdomen and elevate his buttocks and turn his head to one side. The baby is usually quite active and should move his limbs freely, spontaneously and equally on both sides of his body.

PHYSIOLOGICAL CHARACTERISTICS OF THE NEWBORN BABY

The haematological system

Circulatory volume

A major transitional event for the fetus is his separation from the placenta circulation following his birth. The umbilical arteries taking deoxygenated blood from the fetus to the placenta for oxygenation constrict at birth but the umbilical vein remains dilated. Blood volume can vary from 75 to 125 ml/kg depending on the direction and amount of blood flow between fetus and placenta at the time of birth (Blackburn & Loper 1992). In the normal course of events where delivery results in the baby being held for 2 or 3 min at or below the level of the placenta, blood will flow from the placenta to the neonate by the force of gravity. In practice, the transfer of blood to the fetus also depends on the timing of the clamping of the umbilical cord (Fig. 48.2).

Yao & Lind (1969) found that if the baby was held at the level of the introitus until the cord was clamped or was held 40 cm below the level of the introitus for 30 s, he received a transfusion of blood from the placenta of approximately 80 ml. However, if the baby was held more than 50 cm above the introitus the transfusion of blood was negligible. There have been arguments for and against early or late clamping of the cord but little consensus (Blackburn & Loper 1992). In the normal neonate, late clamping of the cord may lead to increased total circulating blood volume but by 3 days of age there is little difference from babies where the cord has been clamped early as postbirth fluid shifts modify the baby's fluid volume.

Early clamping of the umbilical cord

In preterm infants, late cord clamping is associated with hyperbilirubinaemia due to the increased volume of RBCs and respiratory distress, possibly due to the accumulation of fluid in the vascular compartment and extravascular space in the lungs causing a decrease in lung compliance and functional residual capacity. However, a Horizon programme shown on BBC2 (March 1998) suggested that late clamping of the cord (after at least 30 s) may benefit preterm babies by ensuring an adequate transfer of oxygen-carrying red cells.

Other groups of infants who may be harmed by delayed cord clamping are those at risk of hydrops fetalis, those with rhesus isoimmunisation and babies at risk of polycythaemia such as of diabetic mothers or severely growth-retarded babies. The cord of the first baby in a multiple birth should be clamped early to prevent possible blood loss from unborn babies through a communicating placental circulation.

Changes in other haematologic parameters

The circulating blood volume in newborn infants at term averages 90 ml/kg of body weight. As in adults, each of the cellular components of the blood has a finite lifespan and must be continually replaced. In health, the collective process of **haematopoiesis** proceeds at a relatively fixed pace, consequently maintaining the necessary circulating concentrations of each cell type within remarkably narrow limits.

Despite this relative stability, the haematopoietic system is highly responsive, with a unique capacity to upregulate or downregulate production of any of the various cell types on

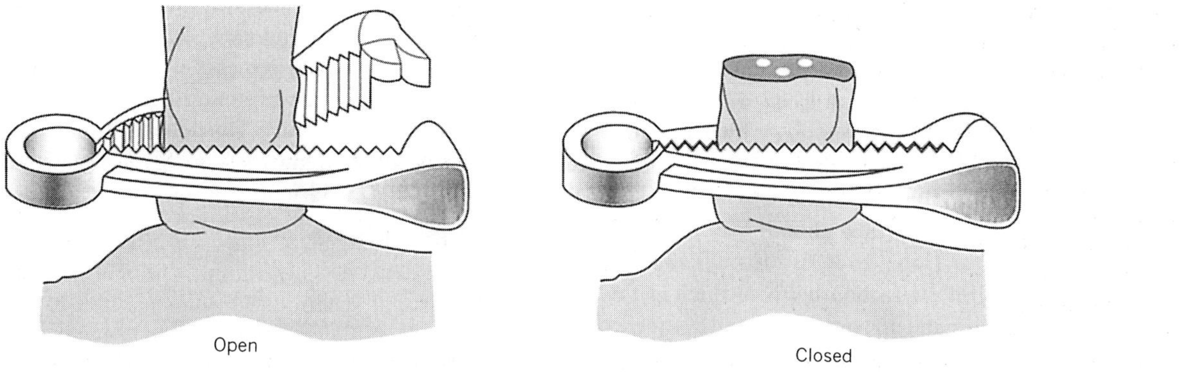

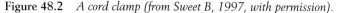

Figure 48.2 *A cord clamp (from Sweet B, 1997, with permission).*

demand. Not only does the blood volume found in neonates differ from that found in adults but changes continue to occur in the first week of life during the transitional period. Oxygen uptake and release has to adapt and the type and quantity of haemoglobin changes.

The processes regulating haematopoiesis are necessarily complex. This microanatomic and physiological intricacy seems essential not only for the maintenance of equilibrium between cellular production and utilisation, but also for the unique demands of various cellular metabolic activities. For instance, in adults mature, competent erythrocytes circulate for approximately 120 days, platelets for about 10 days and neutrophils for 6–8 h.

Erythrocytes (red blood cells)

The erythrocyte count at birth is about 5 million/ml. Although there is a relative increase in the RBC count in the first few hours/days of life due to plasma reduction and haemoconcentration, this is just a transitional phenomenon. Consequently, as the relatively rapid but fairly controlled destruction of the excess RBCs occurs, acceptable, physiological erythrocyte count is achieved by the end of the first 6 months of life (Rudolph 1996). Nucleated RBCs are seen during the first 24 h, possibly due to the stresses of delivery, but have generally disappeared by 4 days. After the first 24 h erythropoietin is not found in the blood until after 2–3 months. Its return coincides with the resumption of bone marrow activity and red cell production (Blackburn & Loper 1992).

Haemoglobin

The average haemoglobin levels are 16.5–17.5 g/dl. This may increase by a further 6 g/dl over the first 24 h due to the shift in fluid distribution leading to haemoconcentration. A decrease in plasma volume results in a net increase in RBCs. The haemoglobin concentration decreases back to cord blood values by the end of the first week. By the age of 3 months the haemoglobin level has fallen to 12 g/dl (Sweet 1997).

Bannister et al (1995) consider the erythrocytes to be more specialised in their composition than most other cells in the body. Their major constituent, haemoglobin, accounts for 95% of the total protein content of the individual cell. Haemoglobin has a molecular weight of 68 000 and consists of four subunits, each containing one iron atom linked to a porphyrin ring to form the haem structure which in turn attaches to a globin chain. Each molecule of haemoglobin contains two identical pairs of globin chains: a pair of α chains and a pair of β chains. At term birth, fetal haemoglobin averages 75% and haemoglobin A accounts for most of the remaining 25%. The rate of decline of fetal haemoglobin production after birth is considerable: at 4 months of age fetal haemoglobin will be less than 20%.

Cord blood Hb content varies with gestational age but contains the types of haemoglobin in the following proportions (Sweet 1997).

- Fetal haemoglobin (HbF): 50–85%
- Adult haemoglobin (HbA): 15–40%
- Haemoglobin A_2 (HbA_2): less than 2%

The function of haemoglobin is to combine reversibly with oxygen, permitting erythrocytes to deliver oxygen from the lungs to the tissues for use in cellular metabolic processes. According to Guyton (1994) this function is demonstrated by the **oxygen dissociation curve** where the oxygen saturation of the blood is plotted against oxygen tension or partial pressure of the whole blood. The oxygen dissociation curve in the neonate is generally placed firmly to the left, denoting the high affinity of fetal haemoglobin for oxygen, necessary to allow efficient extraction of oxygen from the maternal circulation. Although this high affinity for oxygen suits the intrauterine environmental conditions, it does not allow the release of equally large proportions of oxygen to the tissues after birth.

2,3-diphosphoglycerate (DPG)

Mature red blood cells lack mitochondria so that their metabolism of glucose is totally anaerobic. After birth the basis of the shift in the oxygen dissociation curve to the right is attributable to certain organic phosphates which can decrease the affinity of haemoglobin A for oxygen by competing for the same binding sites as oxygen. One of these organic phosphates, a unique substance called 2,3-diphosphoglycerate (2,3-DPG), is formed during anaerobic glycolysis and acts as an intermediate compound enhancing the release of oxygen from haemoglobin. 2,3-DPG is produced when the metabolic need for oxygen is increased.

Because HbF has a lower affinity for 2,3-DPG than HbA it is able to bind oxygen more tenaciously, accounting for the shift of the oxygen disassociation curve to the left in the fetus and neonate. The postnatal shift of the oxygen disassociation curve to the right is indirectly attributable to the decreasing production of HbF and its gradual replacement by HbA which lowers the affinity of the haemoglobin for oxygen. This enhances oxygen release to the tissues (Marieb 1997).

White blood cells

White blood cells are specialised in defending the body against undesirable cells, microorganisms and proteins. There is an initial increase in the number of white cells in the circulation at birth. This may be due to displacement of white cells from other sites provoked by the stress of birth. There is a reduction to normal levels by about 5 days. Two critical functions are the **phagocytic activities** brought about by the neutrophils and the monocytes and the **competent immune response** brought about by the lymphocytes and plasma cells. Monocytes engage in both functions as they are phagocytic but are also capable of processing antigens and producing lymphokines as an initiating event in the production of antibodies.

Differential cell counts in the newborn infant indicate that neutrophils account for approximately 50% and lymphocytes account for about 30% of the white blood cells present at birth. The proportion of lymphocytes then increases rapidly within the first few months to an average of 60%, a value which persists for the first 2 years of life. Monocytes are the most abundant cells in the first few weeks of life but gradually decline to the much lower adult value.

Haemostasis

Haemostasis is designed to stop haemorrhage without disturbing the natural systemic and pulmonary blood flow. This process depends on the critical interaction of the blood vessel walls, the platelets and a group of clot-promoting factors that make up the coagulation system. The neonate is at risk of spontaneous bleeding between the 3rd and 6th days of life due to a lack of vitamin K. By the end of the first week when milk feeding is established, the bacteria necessary for the manufacture of vitamin K are established in the gut (Sweet 1997).

Platelet counts at birth are little lower than normal but neonatal platelets sometimes have decreased ability to aggregate and form a clot. Platelet release of other substances enhancing the clotting cascade may also be reduced. There is a reduction in the amount of prothrombin because of a lack of vitamin K and factors VII, IX and X, which are also vitamin K dependent, are also reduced. Neonatal fibrinogen levels are similar to those of an adult (Blackburn & Loper 1992).

The cardiovascular system

The fetal circulation

At birth the fetal circulation (Fig. 48.3) changes to the configuration of the adult circulation (Fig. 48.4). The immediate part of the changes takes place within 60 s but the full transformation may take up to 6 weeks (Blackburn & Loper 1992). At the same time oxygenation of blood is changed from a placental source to a pulmonary source. The fetal circulation differs from that of the adult in having several modifications which bypass the lungs and transfer blood to and from the placenta for exchange of respiratory gases and oxygenation via the maternal circulation as well as for the exchange of nutrients and waste products.

The temporary structures are:

- Two sets of blood vessels to ferry blood between the fetus and his placenta:
  1 the ductus venosus
  2 two hypogastric arteries;
- Two right-to-left shunts to bypass the lungs:
  1 the ductus arteriosus;
  2 the foramen ovale.

Box 48.1 Vitamin K and haemorrhagic disease of the newborn

The reduction of the vitamin K clotting factors is a result of poor placental transfer of vitamin K to the fetus as well as the lack of intestinal flora. There is a further decline in these factors over the first few days following birth which is worse in breastfed babies as breast milk contains very low levels of the vitamin although it is higher in colostrum and hindmilk. Breastfed babies may eventually develop prolonged prothrombin deficiency. Haemorrhagic disease of the newborn occurs in 0.4–1.7% of all babies in the first week of life (Merenstein et al 1993).

The amount of vitamin K in cow's milk and formula is considered to be greater than in breast milk (Enkin et al 1995). Since the 1950s there has been a growth in the administration of prophylactic vitamin K to neonates to prevent the risk of spontaneous haemorrhage, in particular from the gastrointestinal tract, with haematemesis and the passage of melaena stools, as well as the umbilical cord. There is also a serious risk of intracranial haemorrhage in susceptible babies such as preterm or birth injured. However, many of the early studies were carried out when breastfeeding practices were restricted and neonates did not receive as much colostrum. At the same time supplementary feeds were given.

Golding et al (1990, 1992) suggested a link between the intramuscular administration of vitamin K and childhood cancer although this was not substantiated by Hull (1992) nor did the group set up by the American Academy of Pediatrics find a correlation between the introduction of vitamin K prophylaxis and any increase in the incidence of childhood leukaemia (Ekelund et al 1993, Merenstein et al 1993, von Kries et al 1996).

The British Paediatric Association recommended that oral vitamin K 0.5 mg is given with a repeat dose at 8 days. Most paediatricians recommend giving 0.5–1 mg vitamin K to all babies at birth as it is difficult to identify which babies might be at risk of haemorrhage (Blackburn & Loper 1992). Enkin et al (1995) recommend giving vitamin K to all breastfed babies until further research is carried out. However, by 1993 there were reports of late haemorrhagic disease in infants who had been given oral vitamin K. Preterm babies and others at risk of haemorrhage can be given intramuscular or intravenous vitamin K 0.5–1 mg. Babies with haemorrhagic disease should be given Konakion 1 mg intravenously. If bleeding has been severe a blood transfusion may be necessary.

Administration of vitamin K to mothers

Nishigushi et al (1996) examined three strategies for prevention of vitamin K deficiency in neonates.

1. Routine oral prophylaxis at birth
2. Additional vitamin K for breastfeeding mothers as well as routine oral prophylaxis
3. Screening and treatment of babies at greatest risk

Their findings were that giving babies two doses of oral vitamin K did not totally abolish the risk of haemorrhagic disease. However, in the group where the mothers took a 15 mg capsule of vitamin K daily for 2 weeks starting 2 weeks after delivery, no babies were found to be vitamin K deficient. Because of the lack of evidence of an association between intramuscular vitamin K and childhood leukaemia and the failure of oral vitamin K to prevent haemorrhagic disease, Zipursky (1996) suggests a return to prophylactic use of intramuscular vitamin K.

Arguments against the policy

The need for this treatment of all neonates has been questioned. Some studies cited by Blackburn & Loper (1992) suggest that the neonate is not vitamin K deficient and that concentrations of vitamin K-dependent factors do not always increase after the administration of vitamin K. In particular, the route of administration has come under scrutiny. Slattery (1996) suggests that the policy of routine administration of vitamin K is not evidence based. To assess the status of neonates against an adult norm may be inappropriate. In evolutionary terms, to suggest that a whole population suffers a dangerous disadvantage is suspect, yet this is what vitamin K prophylaxis does. Slattery suggests there is a need for a clinical trial to consider the administration of vitamin K to all neonates.

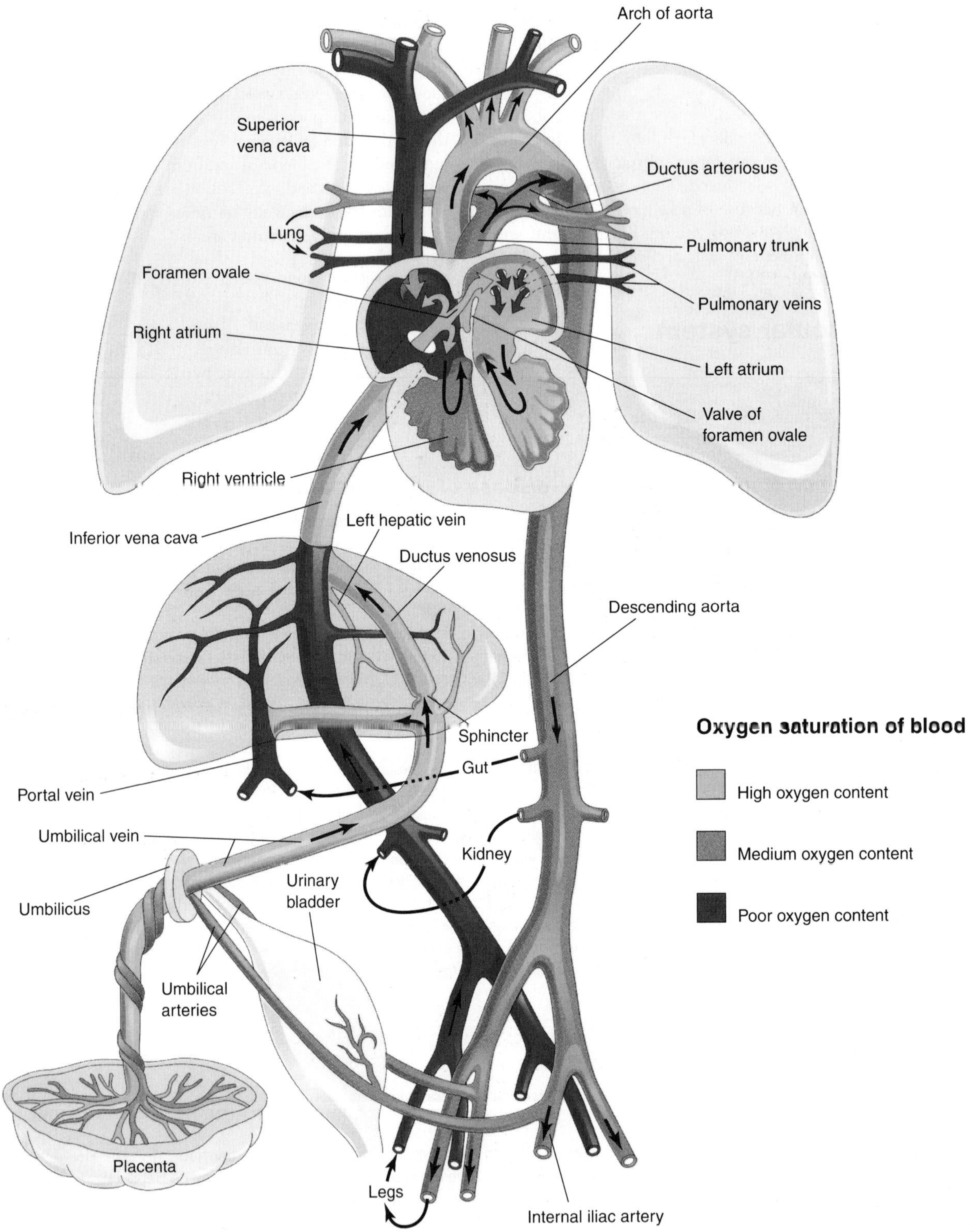

Figure 48.3 *Schematic illustration of the fetal circulation. The colours indicate the oxygen saturation of the blood and the arrows show the course of the blood from the placenta to the heart. The organs are not drawn to scale. Observe that three shunts permit most of the blood to bypass the liver and lungs: (1) ductus venosus, (2) foramen ovale, and (3) ductus arteriosus. The poorly oxygenated blood returns to the placenta for oxygen and nutrients through the umbilical arteries. (Reproduced with permission from Moore 1989.)*

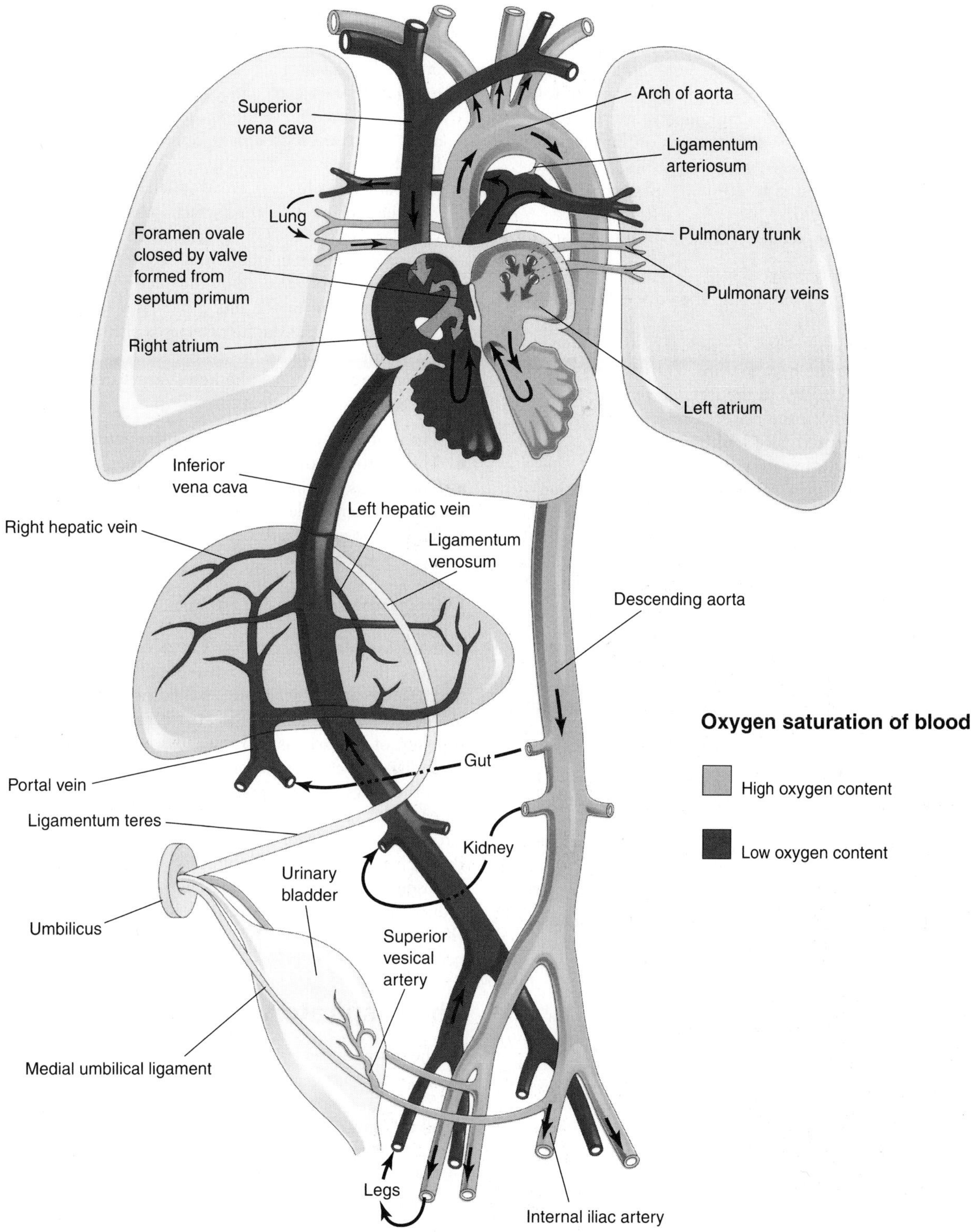

Figure 48.4 *Schematic illustration of the neonatal circulation. The adult derivatives of the fetal vessels and structures that become non-functional at birth are also shown. The arrows indicate the course of the blood in the infant. The organs are not drawn to scale. After birth, the three shunts that short-circuited the blood during fetal life cease to function and the pulmonary and systemic circulations become separated. (Reproduced with permission from Moore 1989.)*

The **ductus venosus** connects the umbilical vein to the inferior vena cava. The **hypogastric arteries** branch off from the internal iliac arteries and where they enter the umbilical cord, they become known as the umbilical arteries. The **ductus arteriosus** leads from the bifurcation of the pulmonary arteries to the descending aorta, entering it just after the exit of the subclavian and carotid arteries. The foramen ovale is a temporary opening between the right and left atria to divert blood away from the lungs (Bennett & Brown 1996).

The path taken by the fetal circulation, beginning at the placenta, is as follows.

- Oxygenated blood returns from the placenta via the umbilical vein.
- About half of this blood passes through the liver to join the inferior vena cava via the hepatic veins. The rest transfers via the ductus venosus directly to the inferior vena cava where the blood returning from the placenta mixes with the small amount of deoxygenated blood returning from the lower limbs, which reduces its oxygen content.
- As the inferior vena cava enters the heart, its position is aligned with the foramen ovale. The free edge of the atrial septum (the **crista dividens**) separates the flow of blood into two streams. Most of it passes straight through the foramen ovale, a right-to-left shunt, to enter the left atrium, the left ventricle and the aorta to supply oxygenated blood to the head, trunk and limbs.
- A small amount enters the right atrium and then into the right ventricle and about 10% of this goes on to the lungs for oxygenation of the lung tissue. The other 90% passes into the aorta via the 2nd right-to-left shunt, the ductus arteriosus, to mingle with the blood from the ductus venosus.
- Deoxygenated blood from the head and neck returns to the right atrium via the superior vena cava. This stream of blood crosses the stream coming from the inferior vena cava and enters the right ventricle, thus reducing the oxygen content of that blood even further.
- The two streams in the right atrium remain separate due to the shape of the atrium although there is some mixing of about 25% of the blood to allow oxygen and nutrients to be taken to the lungs.
- By the time the blood enters the internal iliac arteries it is effectively deoxygenated and returns to the placenta via the umbilical arteries for reoxygenation.
- A small amount of blood descends to supply oxygen to the lower limbs via the external iliac arteries and then returns to the heart via the inferior vena cava.

Changes at birth

These structures must change at birth if the fetus is to survive as an independent being. The change from fetal to neonatal circulation is linked directly to cardiovascular changes in the lungs. The following changes incorporate aspects of both the cardiovascular and respiratory systems.

- Once the baby is separated from the placental circulation there is collapse of the umbilical vein and arteries, the ductus venosus and the hypogastric arteries.
- This results in a reduction in flow to the right atrium, causing a lower pressure in the right atrium. Blood flow through the hypogastric arteries ceases, causing an increase in systemic vascular resistance (SVR), and the return of large quantities of blood from the lungs causes an increase in pressure in the left side of the heart. The equalising of pressures in the two atria closes the flap of the foramen ovale and the right-to-left atrial shunt of blood ceases, although it may remain patent for a few days.
- The baby takes his first breath, the lungs expand and there is vasodilation of the pulmonary vascular bed. Pulmonary vascular resistance (PVR) falls by 80% and there is a dramatic increase in pulmonary blood flow and a fall in the amount of blood shunted by the ductus arteriosus.
- Oxygen tension in the blood increases, causing constriction and closure of the ductus arteriosus although it may remain patent for a few hours.

Vestigial remnants of the fetal structures which are now obsolete remain as ligaments.

- The umbilical vein becomes the ligamentum teres.
- The ductus venosus becomes the ligamentum venosum.
- The ductus arteriosus becomes the ligamentum arteriosum.
- The foramen ovale becomes the fossa ovalis.
- The hypogastric arteries are known as the obliterated hypogastric arteries.

Persistent fetal circulation

If there are respiratory or cardiac disorders with hypoxia and acidosis, there may be persistent fetal circulation with patent ductus arteriosus or even a reversal in the cardiovascular changes in the heart and lungs (Sweet 1997). This exacerbates the problem of hypoxia as deoxygenated blood from the right side of the heart is able to mix with the oxygenated blood returning from the lungs to the left side of the heart. Throughout fetal life patency of the ductus arteriosus is maintained by high circulating levels of PGE_2 and local release of PGI_2. Prostaglandin synthetase inhibitors such as indomethacin may be used to close the ductus chemically. Indomethacin may reduce urinary output so that frusemide may also be given (Kelnar et al 1995). If this fails surgical ligation may be necessary.

The respiratory system

In the fetus at term, the acinar portion of the lung is well developed and more than 25% of true alveoli are present (Fig. 48.5). The pulmonary blood vessels are quite narrow and only a small amount of blood perfuses the lungs, just enough to meet the nutritional needs of the cells. The fetus obtains oxygen and excretes carbon dioxide via the placenta and maternal circulation. The lungs at term hold about 25 ml/kg of fluid (100 ml in total) which is expelled when the chest is compressed at vaginal delivery (Blackburn & Loper 1992). Any remaining fluid is absorbed by the lymphatic and pulmonary vascular systems. The fetus exercises the muscles of respiration by making fetal breathing movements.

Surfactant

As the fetus matures, from about 32 weeks gestation, increasing amounts of surfactant are produced by the type II pneumocytes

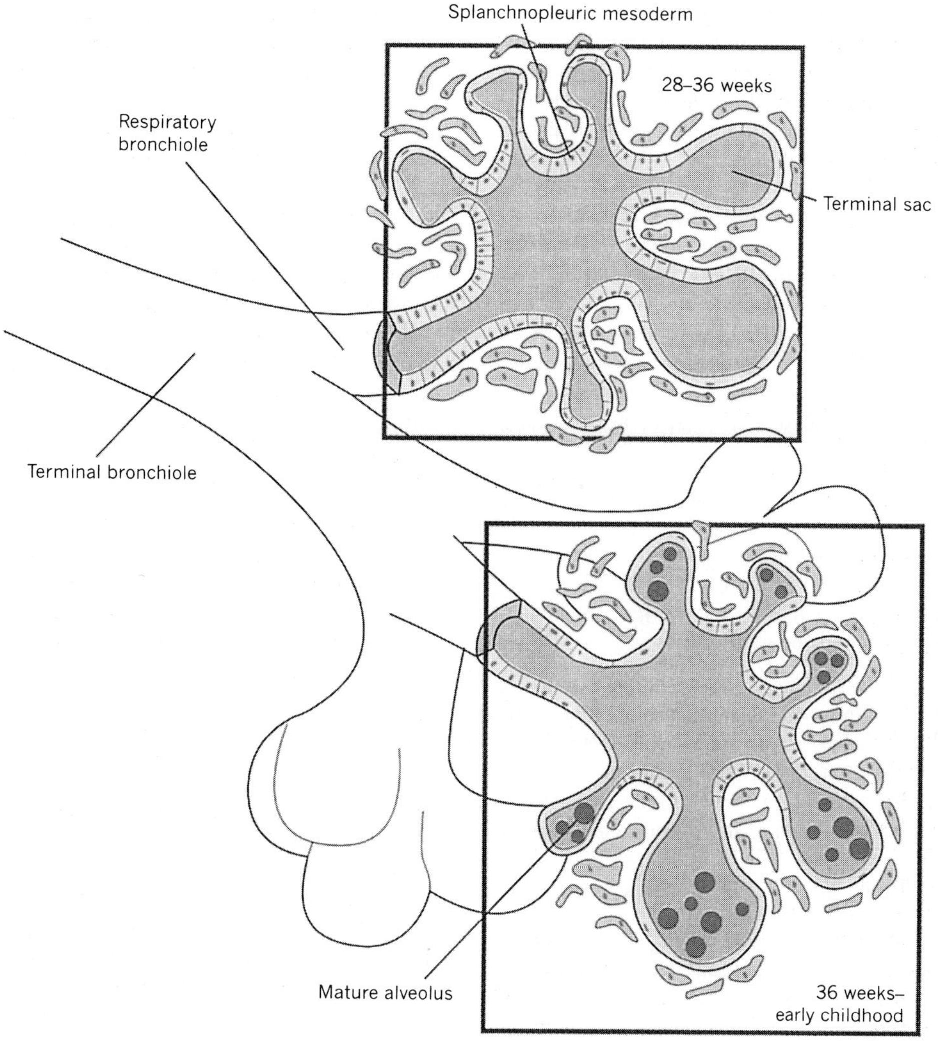

Figure 48.5 *Maturation of the lung tissue. Terminal sacs (primitive alveoli) begin to form between weeks 28 and 36 and begin to mature between 36 weeks and birth. Only 5–20% of all terminal sacs produced by the age of 8, however, are formed prior to birth. (Reproduced with permission from Larsen 1993.)*

of the alveoli. Surfactant is composed of a number of phospholipids and specialised protein molecules (McNabb 1997) (Fig. 48.6). At the same time the lining of the alveoli becomes thinner, increasing the surface area for gas exchange. The molecule platelet-activating factor (PAF) is thought to stimulate production of the phospholipids by triggering enzymes involved with their synthesis in the endoplasmic reticulum of the cells. By term, surfactant forms a monolayer lining to the alveoli which acts as an air–liquid interface, reducing surface tension of the terminal sacs (imagine blowing a soap bubble). This prevents the alveoli from collapsing at each expiration once breathing commences.

Onset of respirations

Most infants achieve sustained regular respiration within 60 s of birth and take their first breath as soon as their head is delivered (Michie 1996). The function of respiration is to meet the cellular need for oxygen and to remove carbon dioxide, the waste product of cellular metabolism. The respiratory centre in the medulla oblongata of the brain is responsible for matching

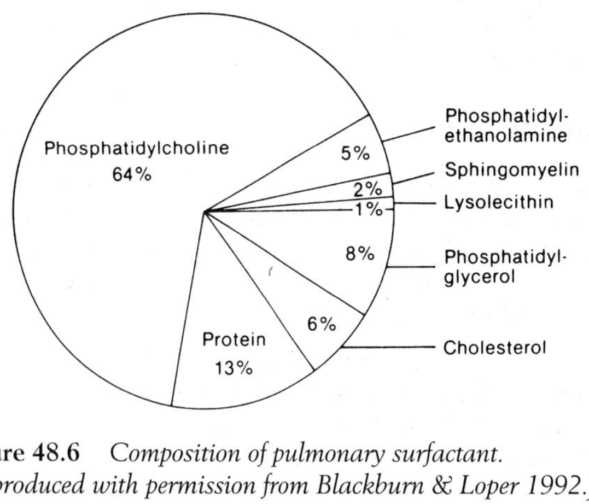

Figure 48.6 *Composition of pulmonary surfactant. (Reproduced with permission from Blackburn & Loper 1992.)*

respiratory effort to the cellular metabolic need. The medulla is influenced by chemoreceptors and stretch reflexes but the neonatal response to chemoreceptor stimulus is weak.

The emptying of the fluid from the lung plus the expansion of the pulmonary vascular bed and tissue creates a negative pressure of up to 100 cm H_2O (9.8 kPa) to assist the first breath (Michie 1996). The elastic recoil of the rib cage at delivery increases this capacity and the baby is stimulated to take an inspiration. The total amount of work performed by the lungs at the first breath is equal to the cry of a baby who is several days old (Blackburn & Loper 1992).

During descent through the birth canal, the fetus experiences a reduction in oxygen and an accumulation of carbon dioxide. These changes become more profound with the cessation of the placental circulation. Factors initiating the first breath and lung expansion include:

- the compression of the chest wall during delivery and its recoil after birth;
- chemoreceptor stimulation by the reduction in oxygen and increase in carbon dioxide in the blood;
- sensory stimuli on the skin such as touch, pressure and cold;
- stimulation of the senses by light and noise.

Initially the baby's respiratory rate is about 50 per minute, settling to about 40 per minute. Respirations are irregular with short periods of apnoea and are mainly abdominal. Respiratory effort must overcome the resistive forces of tissue, the viscosity of lung fluid and the surface tension forces. Once respirations have become established the control of respiratory effort is as in the adult.

Inflation of a normal lung in a newborn infant is completed within the first few breaths and most alveoli are expanded within the first hour, establishing a fairly constant lung volume of about 25 ml/kg body weight. The inflation of the lungs encourages the intraalveolar fluid to move into the interstitium, particularly the peribronchial and perivascular spaces. Its absorption into the vasculature and lymphatic drainage extends over a number of days. Any delays in the removal of this alveolar fluid will interfere with the efficiency of respiratory gas transfer and may cause cardiorespiratory distress.

The renal system

In late pregnancy

The kidney of the newborn baby differs from that of the older child and adult in both glomerular and tubular function. The number of nephrons is complete by 35 weeks but the nephrons are shorter and not as functionally mature, the cortex being more mature than the medulla (Sweet 1997). Bernstein (1982) suggests that by the end of the 36th week of gestation nephrogenesis ceases and at this point each normal kidney is likely to contain between 850 000 and 1000 000 nephrons. In premature infants, however, nephrogenesis does appear to continue for a variable period of time.

Postnatal development of the kidneys

At birth the kidneys must rapidly take over renal functions such as the control of fluid and electrolyte balance and excretion of metabolic wastes. Renal growth in early infancy depends on hypertrophy of existing units. Existing evidence suggests that in infancy kidney size correlates well with age and the usual parameters of somatic growth. The functional maturity of the infant's kidneys has been assessed by histological appearance of the glomeruli and by the size and disposition of the different types of nephrons. The rate of glomerular growth varies, with immature glomeruli being present for many months after birth. It is believed that superimposed diseases such as inflammatory changes and urinary tract obstructions may contribute to some persistence of the immature form of glomeruli.

Brenner & Rector (1991) hold that the anatomic development of the kidneys proceeds from the corticomedullary junction out towards the periphery in a centrifugal pattern. They believe that a process of budding from the ends of the collecting ducts ensures that new nephrons are added to the outermost part of the kidney. This phenomenon appears to ensure that the cortex contains the most recently formed nephrons.

Neonatal renal physiology

Activity of the systems influencing blood pressure control, such as the renin-angiotensin system, increase at birth, possibly due to stimulation by the excess catecholamines produced by the fetus as a response to the stress of labour and birth (Blackburn & Loper 1992). Both phenomena contribute to an adequate distribution of blood to vital organs.

The glomeruli

In normal circumstances of relatively rapid renal growth, the functional relationship between the glomeruli and the nephrons is achieved efficiently. The average glomerular size of 100 μm at birth increases to 300 μm but can be retarded or accelerated by certain pathological changes. For instance, cyanotic congenital heart disease is associated with striking glomerular enlargements.

Guignard (1982) argues that the clamping of the umbilical cord is a signal for a large increase in renal function. The most likely factors which contribute to this rapid maturation in renal function in newborn infants are of a haemodynamic and morphological nature. Thus, a decrease in renal vascular resistance and the increase in systemic blood pressure at birth contribute to a more effective filtration pressure and an increase in glomerular permeability and filtration area. The haemodynamic changes may be in part mediated by vasoactive substances such as prostaglandins.

The tubules

Postnatally, tubular length and, consequently, filtrate volume increase. The growth of the tubules appears to be relatively greater than the growth of the glomeruli and seems to contribute to the ongoing maintenance of the all-important **glomerulotubular balance** as glomerular filtrate increases after birth. Finally, tubular growth is an important factor in enhancing tubular capacity for transport and metabolic functions.

The bladder

The bladder of a newborn baby is **fusiform** (cigar shaped) rather than pyramidal as in the adult. It is situated almost entirely in the abdominal cavity until the pelvic cavity begins to increase as the child grows, when the bladder descends into the pelvis and the ureters lengthen. Distension of the bladder increases intraabdominal pressure and may exacerbate respiratory difficulties.

Renal function

The kidneys have a high rate of oxygen consumption, accounting for approximately 7% of the total oxygen used by the body. Indeed, a linear relationship can be demonstrated between changes in oxygen consumption and sodium changes; active transport of sodium reflects the most significant energy expenditure of the kidney other than that required for basic metabolic needs.

The renal blood flow is reduced in comparison with an older infant for the first few days after birth. The glomerular filtration rate (GFR) is also lower. These two parameters of renal function rapidly increase after birth and double by the end of the 2nd week. Removal of the placental circulation increases the systemic circulatory pressure and thus the blood flow to the kidneys. The tubular thresholds for reabsorption of solutes is lower in the neonate and infants are more likely to lose sodium, glucose and other solutes in their urine. Both term and preterm infants are able to excrete normal excess acid via the kidneys but have little reserve to cope with increased levels. The mechanism of water regulation is similar to that of the adult but the neonate's ability to dilute or concentrate urine is limited. The ability to excrete drugs is also limited.

Urine output

Urine is passed by reflex emptying of the bladder. Urine output varies depending on fluid and solute intake and events at the time of birth. Term infants normally excrete between 15 and 60 ml/kg of urine each day, increasing fourfold by the end of the first week as fluid intake increases. The initial passing of urine occurs within 24 h but may be delayed. About 25% of babies pass urine at or shortly after delivery when the event may pass unobserved or unrecorded. The urine is dilute, straw coloured and odourless. It is important to observe the force and direction of the stream of urine and in boys, whether the stream leaves the tip of the penis. The use of magnesium sulphate to control eclampsia may delay neonatal voiding of urine.

Body composition

Neonates have a higher total body and extracellular water content (ECF) and a lesser intracellular (ICF) water content than an adult. In relationship to an adult, a neonate's body has three times more interstitial volume. Quite soon after birth the ECF increases, possibly resulting from the withdrawal of maternal hormones, and infants may become slightly oedematous. The ECF content peaks at about 3 days and results in a diuresis as the fluid compartments are adjusted, possibly due to the decrease in atrial natriuretic peptide (ANP), important for the regulation of sodium, which occurs at the same time (Blackburn & Loper 1992). A loss of 5–10% of body weight is seen in the first week following birth, mainly because of this diuresis.

> Fluid therapy in the first few days must take account of these physiological differences to avoid fluid overload with a risk of congestive heart failure, necrotising enterocolitis and symptomatic patent ductus arteriosus (Blackburn & Loper 1992).

Summary of main points

- In utero the fetus is dependent on his mother for survival but at birth the fetus must adapt to independent life. Each physiological system must work to maintain homeostasis. Of immediate importance is the adaptation to obtaining oxygen from the surrounding air.
- The normal baby at term is plump with a rounded abdomen due to the deposition of subcutaneous fat. The scalp is covered with varying amounts of fine silky hair and some lanugo may be left on his shoulders. The cartilage of his ears is well formed. The creases of his palms and soles are well defined. Milia may be present over the nose and cheeks at birth. Vernix caseosa, usually found in the groins and axillae, will be absorbed within a few hours. The sweat glands all over his body will not be active for the first few days of life. A newborn baby cannot shed tears.
- Both boys and girls have a small nodule of breast tissue about 1 cm in diameter around the nipple. The breast tissue may be swollen in response to oestrogen from the mother and milk may even be present in the breasts. In boys the testes are descended into the scrotum by term and the foreskin is still adherent to the glans penis. In girls the labia majora cover the labia minora. A thick white vaginal discharge may be present as a response to maternal oestrogen.
- Blood volume at birth can vary from 75 to 125 ml/kg depending on the direction and amount of blood flow between fetus and placenta at birth. Late clamping of the cord may lead to increased total blood volume but by 3 days of age there is little difference from babies where the cord has been clamped early.
- The red blood cell count at birth is about 5 million/ml. There is an increase in the first few hours due to plasma reduction and haemoconcentration. The average haemoglobin is 16.5–17.5 g/dl. This may increase up to 6 g/dl over the first 24 h due to haemoconcentration. By the age of 3 months the haemoglobin level has fallen to 12 g/dl.
- Cord blood Hb content varies with gestational age but contains mainly HbF with some HbA. Mature red blood cells lack mitochondria so that their metabolism of glucose is totally anaerobic. 2,3-diphosphoglycerate binds to haemoglobin which lowers its affinity for oxygen.
- The neonate is at risk of spontaneous bleeding between the 3rd and 6th days of life due to a lack of vitamin K. There is a reduction in the amount of prothrombin and factors VII, IX and X. There is a further decline in these factors over the first few days following birth which is worse in breastfed babies who may develop prolonged prothrombin deficiency.
- Since the 1950s there has been a growth in the administration of prophylactic vitamin K to neonates to prevent the risk of spontaneous haemorrhage. A link between the intramuscular administration of vitamin K and childhood cancer has not been substantiated. The British Paediatric Association recommended that oral vitamin K 0.5 mg is given with a repeat dose at 8 days. By 1993 there were reports of late haemorrhagic disease in infants who had

been given oral vitamin K. The need for this treatment of all neonates has been questioned.

- The fetal circulation differs from that of the adult in having modifications which bypass the lungs and transfer blood to and from the placenta for exchange of respiratory gases and oxygenation. Two sets of blood vessels ferry blood between the fetus and his placenta: the ductus venosus and two hypogastric arteries. Two right-to-left shunts bypass the lungs: the ductus arteriosus and the foramen ovale. The changes at birth from fetal to neonatal circulation are linked to cardiovascular changes in the lungs.
- Respiratory or cardiac disorders with hypoxia and acidosis may lead to persistent fetal circulation with patent ductus arteriosus. Deoxygenated blood from the right side of the heart is able to mix with the oxygenated blood returning from the lungs. Prostaglandin synthetase inhibitors such as indomethacin may close the ductus chemically. If this fails surgical ligation may be necessary.
- From about 32 weeks gestation, increasing amounts of surfactant are produced by the type II pneumocytes lining the lung alveoli. The lining of the alveoli becomes thinner, increasing the surface area for gas exchange. By term, surfactant forms a monolayer lining to the alveoli providing an air–liquid interface and reducing surface tension of the terminal sacs. This prevents the alveoli from collapsing at the end of each expiration.
- Most infants achieve sustained regular respirations within 60 s of birth and take their first breath as soon as their head is delivered. The respiratory centre in the medulla oblongata of the brain is responsible for matching respiratory effort to cellular need. Initially the baby's respiratory rate is about 50 per minute, settling to about 40 per minute. Respirations are irregular with short periods of apnoea and are mainly abdominal.
- The number of nephrons is complete by 35 weeks but the nephrons are shorter and not as functionally mature, the cortex being more mature than the medulla. In premature infants nephrogenesis does appear to continue for a variable period of time. Renal growth in early infancy depends on hypertrophy of existing units. Superimposed diseases such as inflammatory changes and urinary tract obstructions may contribute to persistence of the immature form of glomeruli.
- The clamping of the umbilical cord may be a signal for an increase in renal function. The most likely factors which contribute to this are of a haemodynamic and morphological nature. The haemodynamic changes may be in part mediated by vasoactive substances such as prostaglandins. Postnatally tubular length and filtrate volume increase. Tubular growth is important in enhancing tubular capacity for transport and metabolic functions.
- Neonates have a higher total body and ECF and a lesser ICF water content than older people. Soon after birth the ECF increases and infants may become slightly oedematous. A diuresis results in a loss of 5–10% of body weight in the first week. The renal blood flow is reduced for the first few days after birth and GFR is also lower than at other ages. These rapidly increase after birth and double by the end of the 2nd week.
- The tubular thresholds for reabsorption of solutes are lower in the neonate and infants are more likely to lose sodium, glucose and other solutes in their urine. Infants are able to excrete normal excess acid via the kidneys but have little reserve to cope with increased levels. The neonate's ability to dilute or concentrate urine is limited.
- Term infants normally excrete between 15 and 60 ml/kg of urine each day, increasing fourfold by the end of the first week as fluid intake increases. Most infants pass urine within 12 h of birth. It is important to observe the force and direction of the stream of urine and, in boys, whether the stream leaves the tip of the penis.

References

Anderson M. 1992 The Anatomy and Physiology of Obstetrics. Wolfe Publishing, London.

Bannister L, Barry M, Collins P et al, 1995 Gray's Anatomy, Churchill Livingstone, Edinburgh.

Bennett VR, Brown LK. 1996 The fetus. In Bennett VR, Brown LK (eds) Myles Textbook for Midwives, 12th edn. Churchill Livingstone, Edinburgh, pp 51–64.

Bernstein J. 1992 The kidneys and the urinary tract. In Rudolph A (ed) Pediatrics. Appleton-Century-Crofts, New York.

Blackburn ST, Loper DL. 1992 Maternal, Fetal and Neonatal Physiology, A Clinical Perspective. WB Saunders, Philadelphia.

Brenner B, Rector F. 1991 The Kidney, Vol 1. WB Saunders, Philadelphia.

Ekelund H, Finnstrom O, Gunnarskog I, Kallen B, Larsson Y. 1993 Administration of vitamin K to newborn infants and childhood cancer. British Medical Journal 301, 89–91.

Enkin M, Keirse MJNC, Renfrew M, Neilson JP. 1995 A Guide to Effective Care in Pregnancy and Childbirth, 2nd edn. Oxford Medical Publications, Oxford.

Golding J, Paterson M, Kinlen LJ. 1990 Factors associated with childhood cancer in national cohort study. British Journal of Cancer 62, 304–308.

Golding J, Greenwood R, Birmingham K, Mott M. 1992 Childhood cancer, intramuscular vitamin K, and pethidine given in labour. British Medical Journal 305, 341–346.

Guignard J. 1982 Renal function in the newborn infant. In Fine R (ed) Pediatric Nephrology. WB Saunders, Philadelphia.

Guyton A. 1994 Textbook of Medical Physiology. WB Saunders, Philadelphia.

Hull D. 1992 Vitamin K and childhood cancer. The risk of haemorrhagic disease is certain; that of cancer is not. British Medical Journal 305, 326–327.

Kelnar CJH, Harvey D, Simpson C. 1995 The Sick Newborn Baby, 3rd edn. Baillière Tindall, London.

Larsen WJ 1993 Human Embryology. Churchill Livingstone, Edinburgh.

Marieb EN. 1992 Human Anatomy and Physiology, 2nd edn. Benjamin/Cummings Publishing, Company Inc, California.

McNabb M. 1997 The biological adaptations of the fetus to labour. In Sweet BR with Tiran D (eds) Mayes Midwifery, 12th edn. Baillière Tindall, London, pp 335–338.

Merenstein K, Hathaway WE, Miller RW, Paulson JA, Rowley DL. 1993 Controversies concerning vitamin K and the newborn. Pediatrics 91, 1001–1002.

Michie MM. 1996 The baby at birth. In Bennett VR, Brown LK (eds) Myles Textbook for Midwives, 12th edn. Churchill Livingstone, Edinburgh, pp 492–504.

Moore KL. 1989 Before We Are Born, 3rd edn. WB Saunders, Philadelphia.

Morgan E. 1994 The Descent of the Child. Souvenir Press, London.

Nishigushi T, Saga K, Sumimito K et al. 1996 Vitamin K prophylaxis to prevent neonatal vitamin K deficient intracranial haemorrhage in Shizuoka prefecture. British Journal of Obstetrics and Gynaecology 8(11), 1078–1084.

Rudolph A, Hoffman J, Rudolph C et al, 1996 Rudolph's Pediatrics. Prentice-Hall, New Jersey.

Slattery J. 1996 Treating all babies with vitamin K: an 'unnatural' policy? British Journal of Obstetrics and Gynaecology, 103(5) 400–401.

Sweet BR. 1997 Physiology and care of the Newborn. In Sweet BR with Tiran D (eds) Mayes Midwifery, 12th edn. Baillière Tindall, London, pp 783–800.

von Kries R, Gobel U, Hachmeister A et al, 1996 Vitamin K and childhood cancer: a population based case-control study in Lower Saxony, Germany. British Medical Journal 313(7051), 199–203.

Yao AC, Lind J. 1969 Distribution of blood between the infant and placenta at birth. Lancet 2, 505.

Zipursky A. 1996 Vitamin K at birth. British Medical Journal 313(1051), 179–180.

Recommended reading

Ekelund H, Finnstrom O, Gunnarskog I, Kallen B, Larsson Y. 1993 Administration of vitamin K to newborn infants and childhood cancer. British Medical Journal 301, 89–91.

Golding J, Greenwood R, Birmingham K, Mott M. 1992 Childhood cancer, intramuscular vitamin K, and pethidine given in labour. British Medical Journal 305, 341–346.

Hull D. 1992 Vitamin K and childhood cancer. The risk of haemorrhagic disease is certain; that of cancer is not. British Medical Journal 305, 326–327.

Kelnar CJH, Harvey D, Simpson C. 1995 The Sick Newborn Baby, 3rd edn. Baillière Tindall, London.

Merenstein K, Hathaway WE, Miller RW, Paulson JA, Rowley DL. 1993 Controversies concerning vitamin K and the newborn. Pediatrics 91, 1001–1002.

Morgan E. 1994 The Descent of the Child. Souvenir Press, London.

Rudolph A Hoffman J, Rudolph C et al, 1996 Rudolph's Pediatrics. Prentice-Hall, New Jersey.

Yao AC, Lind J. 1969 Distribution of blood between the infant and placenta at birth. Lancet 2, 505.

Chapter 49

Adaptation to extrauterine life 2 – nutritional and metabolic adjustments

In this chapter

INTRODUCTION

Whilst the fetus is in utero his nutritional, metabolic and excretory needs and protection against pathogenic organisms and toxins are met to a large extent by an efficient placental circulation. After birth the highly complex physiological systems of the intestinal tract and its accessory organs devoted to the above functions must begin to work independently.

THE GASTROINTESTINAL TRACT

Fetal development

The development of the gut is described in detail in Chapter 10. The primitive gut of the embryo forms at approximately 6 weeks of pregnancy as a hollow tube stretched between the primitive pharyngeal and cloacal membranes. Bannister et al (1995) and Larsen (1993) suggest that the primitive gut consists of three distinct parts – the foregut, midgut and hindgut – each corresponding to important vascular territories that become clearly defined in later stages of embryonic development. The components of the nervous system essential to the functioning of the digestive tract are thought to develop from the derivatives of the neural crest.

The neonate

There are functional, anatomical and physiological limitations in the gastrointestinal (GI) tract of the newborn baby (Blackburn & Loper 1992). Following birth, the GI tract must supply the infant's needs for energy, nutrients and fluids. Polin & Fox (1992) suggest that at birth the newborn infant manifests some anatomical and physiological limitations in relation to its gastrointestinal system which are partly influenced by the requirement of the fetus to swallow amniotic fluid. The swallowing actions of the small bolus of amniotic fluid may be an important contributing factor in the maintenance of gastrointestinal patency. There appears to be no evidence to suggest that the gastrointestinal system in utero serves any digestive or absorptive functions.

The stomach at birth

The stomach has a small capacity, holding only 15–30 ml at first, but increases rapidly within the first few weeks of life. Gastric emptying time is 2–3 h but can be influenced by the intake of nutrients; for example, carbohydrate increases emptying time and fats decrease it. The presence of mucus in the stomach during the first 24 h delays gastric emptying (Blackburn & Loper 1992). As the cardiac sphincter is weak, regurgitation of milk is common. Gastric acidity, which is equal to that of an adult at first, soon diminishes and there is little stomach acid produced by the 10th day, making the baby vulnerable to infection (Michie 1996).

Also, during the first 6 months the intestinal mucosal barrier remains immature so that antigens and other macromolecules can be transported across the epithelium into the systemic circulation. Colostrum is rich in antibodies, easily swallowed and helps the passage of meconium. Postnatal maturation of the gut is stimulated by increases in peptide hormones such as gastrin and motilin (Chapter 20) which follow the commencement of enteral feeding. Differences can be seen between babies who are breastfed and those given modified formula feeds. In particular, there is an insulin surge in formula-fed babies that lasts at least 9 months. Such insulin surges can be triggered by very small amounts of feeding but are absent in unfed babies (Aynsley-Green 1985).

The intestine of a neonate is long in relation to its size and there are large numbers of secretory glands and a large surface area for absorption of nutrients. Enteric intake stimulates the intestinal mucosa cells to divide and mature. Digestive enzymes are synthesised and released as required. Because there is a relative deficiency of the enzymes amylase and lipase, the human baby has difficulty in digesting carbohydrates and fats. The entry of food into the stomach produces a gastrocolic reflex with opening of the ileocaecal valve. As the contents of the ileum enter the colon, they appear to stimulate a forceful peristalsis which is in turn accompanied by a reflex emptying of the rectum (Michie 1996).

Meconium

Meconium is a material that collects in the intestines of the fetus from the 16th week and forms the first stools of the newborn. Its consistency is thick and sticky and it is greenish-black in colour. It is composed of secretions from the intestinal glands, amniotic fluid, debris from inside the uterus such as vernix, lanugo, bile salts, fatty acids, epithelial cells, mucus and blood cells (Anderson et al 1994). Initially meconium is sterile but within 24 h it begins to be colonised with bacteria. Most infants pass meconium within 24 h of birth. Failure to do so could be a sign of intestinal malfunction, obstruction or imperforate anus.

Once milk feeding is established, babies' stools begin to change as meconium is passed and digested milk enters the colon. By day 3–5 there is a transitional or 'changing' stool which is brownish-yellow in appearance. Following this, the normal yellowish stool of the neonate is established and the consistency and frequency of the stools depend on the type of feeding. Breastfed babies pass loose, bright yellow, inoffensive stools. The numbers passed vary from as many as 10 in 24 h in the early days to once every 2 or 3 days when feeding is established. Bottlefed babies pass paler, more formed stools with a recognisable smell less frequently and there is a tendency towards constipation.

THE LIVER

Fetal development

The fetal liver is formed in the first trimester of pregnancy. Subsequent hepatic growth continues linearly through the remainder of gestation. In fetal life the left hepatic lobe is approximately 10% larger than the right. Since this phenomenon is precisely opposite to the postnatal hepatic lobe relationship, it may be indicative of an altered blood supply. As with most developing tissues and embryonic organs, initial liver growth results largely from hepatocellular proliferation, i.e. cell hyperplasia, which peaks during the 2nd trimester of pregnancy. By the 3rd trimester mitosis begins to decrease as enlargement of the individual hepatocytes increasingly contributes to the eventual size of the whole organ (Bannister et al 1995).

The neonate

After birth liver growth continues until the end of the 2nd decade of life. This gradual growth and hepatic maturation is attributed to ongoing mitosis. Given that the liver of the neonate has less than 20% of the total hepatocytes of the mature adult liver, the ongoing mitosis is critical to the ultimate construction and physiological scope of the mature organ.

The liver is physiologically immature although it accounts for 5% of the neonate's weight. In the mature liver substances undergo oxidation and conjugation under enzymatic control to produce water-soluble byproducts. In the neonatal liver there is low production of some of the enzymes, for instance glucuronyl transferase which conjugates bilirubin. There is a high breakdown of superfluous red cells, releasing excess unconjugated bilirubin into the blood. This attaches itself to fatty tissue and there may be a transient jaundice on days 3–5. Feeding stimulates liver function and colonisation of the gut which allows vitamin K to be produced (Michie 1996).

METABOLISM

Whilst the fetus was in utero his metabolic processes were

geared towards anabolism and growth of tissue. He did not need to use energy to maintain his body temperature and functions which utilise energy such as respiration and digestion were carried out by the placenta. After birth an adequate supply of essential nutrients coupled with normal enzymatic and hormonal controls will ensure that most newborn infants sustain an anabolic state as they maintain independent homeostasis.

The fetus prepares for the transition to independence by laying down a fuel store of glycogen and lipids during the last few weeks of pregnancy so that the newborn infant has reserves of glycogen, fat and other nutrients. Once oxygen requirements have been met, the next immediate need for survival is an adequate supply of water. The relative excess of water confers no protection against dehydration since the obligatory daily turnover of water is equal to 15–20% of the total body water.

Following birth, heat production is by brown adipose tissue (BAT) and hepatic triiodothyronine synthesis is stimulated, resulting in a transition from a net anabolic to a catabolic state as glycogen and lipid reserves are mobilised to meet the required increase in metabolic rate (Blackburn & Loper 1992). The extent of these adaptations is strongly influenced by the state of maternal nutrition in the late stages of pregnancy as well as the maturity of the infant at birth.

Glucose metabolism

Garrow & James (1993) hold that glucose is the major substrate for carbohydrate metabolism in the newborn infant. At birth, the infant's plasma glucose concentration depends upon such factors as the timing of the last maternal meal, the duration of labour, the route of delivery and the type and quantity of intravenous fluid administered to the mother. After birth the neonate loses the maternal glucose source which he has relied on almost totally for energy production and growth. Falling insulin levels and slow production of insulin prevent glucose being taken up by the cells. This, coupled with an increase in serum glucagon levels, mobilises glucose from the cells from glycogen stores.

Hepatic glycogen stores decrease with 90% usage during the first 24 h after birth and 50–80% of muscle glycogen is also used up. Gluconeogenesis develops after birth, regulated by changes in the serum insulin:glucose ratio, catecholamine release, fatty acid oxidation and activation of liver gluconeogenic enzyme production. Concentrations of these liver enzymes continue to increase for the next 14 days. Once milk feeding begins, additional changes in hepatic function occur (Blackburn & Loper 1992).

Neonatal blood glucose levels fall to their lowest between 2 and 6 h after a normal delivery. They then become stable and rise, equilibrating at approximately 3.6 mmol/l as the baby adapts to his extrauterine environment (Dodds 1996). Most paediatricians believe that the lowest safe level for neonatal blood glucose is no less than 2 mmol/l (Koh & Vong 1996). In developed countries the method of feeding can influence neonatal blood glucose levels. Hawdon et al (1992) found the average neonatal blood glucose levels in 132 term, breastfed babies was 3.6 mmol/1 with a range of 1.5–5.3 mmol/1 but these levels were significantly lower than in bottlefed babies.

Fat metabolism

Lipolysis increases rapidly after birth and reaches a maximum within a few hours. This results in a rise in plasma free fatty acids which reach adult levels by 24 h after birth. During this time about two-thirds of the baby's energy is produced from oxidation of fat which is the major form of stored calories in the newborn. Fat is also the preferred energy source for the tissues which have high energy needs, such as the heart and adrenal cortex.

Mature human milk has a fat content of 3.5–4.5% contained within membrane-enclosed fat globules. The core of the globule comprises triglycerides whilst the membrane is constructed of phospholipids, cholesterol and proteins. This characteristic packaging of the triglycerides permits dispersion of the lipids in the aqueous environment of the milk and protects them from hydrolysis by milk lipase. Colostrum contains less fat content, averaging 2%, but phospholipids and cholesterol are found in higher concentrations. The major differences between human milk and formula milk are the absence of long chain unsaturated fatty acids in the formulae compared with high concentrations of long chain unsaturated fatty acids and cholesterol in mature human milk (see also Chapter 54).

The alternative substrates of fat stores and ketone bodies are used, stimulated by catecholamine release associated with cooling of the body after birth. Ketone bodies produced during fatty acid metabolism are important metabolites for the infant. Acetate is metabolised by the mitochondria and the resulting energy is released. Ketone bodies may be a major energy source for the developing brain (Polin & Fox 1992, Rudolph et al 1996).

Protein metabolism

Whereas in fetal life the basic building blocks are supplied by the placenta directly to the fetus, after birth the neonate has to digest milk proteins into amino acids and oligopeptides. This process requires proteolytic enzymes released into the stomach and the pancreas as well as the intestinal brush border. The relatively high concentration of free amino acids and peptides in human milk probably enhances the release of gastrin and cholecystokinin which in turn promote the release of the proteolytic enzymes. The newborn baby has little ability to synthesise protein because of relative immaturity of the liver enzyme systems. Serum amino acid levels are higher than normal later values in the first few weeks of life and there is significant urinary amino acid excretion.

Calcium, phosphorus and magnesium metabolism

If the neonate is compared with his mother, he is hypercalcaemic and hyperphosphataemic.

Calcium

Calcium is probably the most abundant mineral in the body. Polin & Fox (1992) postulate that at term most newborn infants would have accumulated between 20 and 30 g of calcium, 80% of which would have been accrued in the last trimester of pregnancy. Of this total body pool of calcium, 99% is located in the infant's developing skeletal frame. Serum calcium exists in three separate fractions which are present in dynamic equilibrium.

- Protein-bound calcium represents approximately 40% of the total serum concentration, with albumin serving as the primary binding protein.
- Calcium is also found bound to a number of other anions such as citrate, phosphate, bicarbonate and sulphate.
- Free, ionised calcium represents the physiologically active form of calcium.

Garrow & James (1993) postulate that the ultimate balance in plasma calcium is at least in part determined by ongoing exchange between the skeletal system, the intestine and the kidney. This significant movement of calcium is controlled by the calciotrophic enzymes, the parathyroid hormone 1,25-dihydroxycholecalciferol and calcitonin. Calcium metabolism is also influenced by growth hormones, corticosteroids and a variety of locally acting hormones such as the cytokines.

The neonate must move from intrauterine dependence on maternal calcium sources to independent metabolism. The normal range for blood calcium in a neonate is 1.8–2.2 mmol/l (Simpson 1997). During the first 2 days of life serum calcium levels fall and there is a physiological hypocalcaemia, increasing back to normal at between 5–10 days once intestinal absorption of calcium matures. Renal excretion of calcium is efficient and increases as the days pass (Pitkin 1985).

Aspects of calcium metabolism

- As serum calcium levels decrease, parathyroid hormone (PTH) levels increase. By 3–4 days the parathyroid glands are responding adequately to calcium levels.
- Calcitonin levels are normal at birth but this is followed by a surge in the next 24 h. After 36 h the calcitonin levels fall back to normal. This may act to protect the neonate from the effects of increased PTH and reabsorption of calcium from bone. Neither oral nor intravenous calcium administration seems to affect calcitonin levels.
- Term infants can metabolise vitamin D in the liver and kidneys although absorption of exogenous vitamin D may be limited because of immature fat absorption.

Phosphorus

As with calcium, approximately 80% of the phosphorus present in the neonate is accumulated by the fetus in the last trimester of pregnancy. As with calcium, body phosphorus is divided into three component parts.

- At least 85% of the infant's total phosphorus is contained in the skeletal system.
- The phosphorus contained in body fluids is divided between an organic fraction composed of a number of phospholipids and phosphoesters and
- Inorganic phosphate.

Although phosphorus levels decrease in the first 2 days after birth they still remain higher than in the adult. Renal excretion of phosphorus is delayed with a decreased glomerular filtration rate and increased tubular reabsorption rate. Also, increased energy release with conversion of adenosine triphosphate (ATP) to adenosine diphosphate (ADP) leads to increased phosphate release. If feeding is delayed this catabolic process is increased even further.

Magnesium

Magnesium is the 2nd most common intracellular cation in the body. According to Polin & Fox (1992), the newborn term infant contains about 20 mg of magnesium/100 g fat-free weight. The infant's total body magnesium is again divided between three compartments.

- The skeletal system contains about 60%.
- Muscle tissue holds about 29%.
- The remainder is distributed through soft tissue.

Plasma magnesium

Only 1% of the total body magnesium appears to be located in the extracellular space. In plasma about 60% of the magnesium exists as free ion whilst 20% is bound to various anions such as phosphate and oxalate. The remaining plasma magnesium is bound to serum proteins. This binding capacity is maintained within relatively tight limits and is thought to be essentially the same in neonates, children and adults. The normal range for plasma magnesium is 0.7–1.0 mmol/1. To date, no definitive hormones have been identified as essential to the fine tuning of plasma magnesium levels. However, the kidneys appear to be the primary organs for the regulation of serum magnesium concentrations.

THE NEONATAL NERVOUS SYSTEM

In a human adult the central nervous system is thought to consist of about 100 billion neurones. These are intricately connected with one another in a manner that makes possible consciousness, learning, thought, memory, vision and many other properties characteristic of the human nervous system. The achievement of precision of the adult neural pattern is in part dependent on some form of environmental stimulation (Fig. 49.1) as infants who spend most of their first year of life lying in their crib develop abnormally slowly (Shatz 1992).

Nervous system activity has been increasing steadily throughout gestation so that at term the baby is prepared to process incoming information from the environment and produce behaviour appropriate for his physical and physiological status. Transitional functions of the nervous system to be discussed are those suggested by Blackburn & Loper (1992): autonomic, sensory, motor and state regulation.

Autonomic functions

At birth the fetus must take over control of functions he has not needed during intrauterine life. Hunger, thirst and satiety centres in the hypothalamus must stimulate the baby to provide cues for the mother such as crying and sucking. A physiological steady state or homeostasis must be achieved by regulation of respiration, heart beat and his own temperature. He must adjust his metabolic needs to provide warmth.

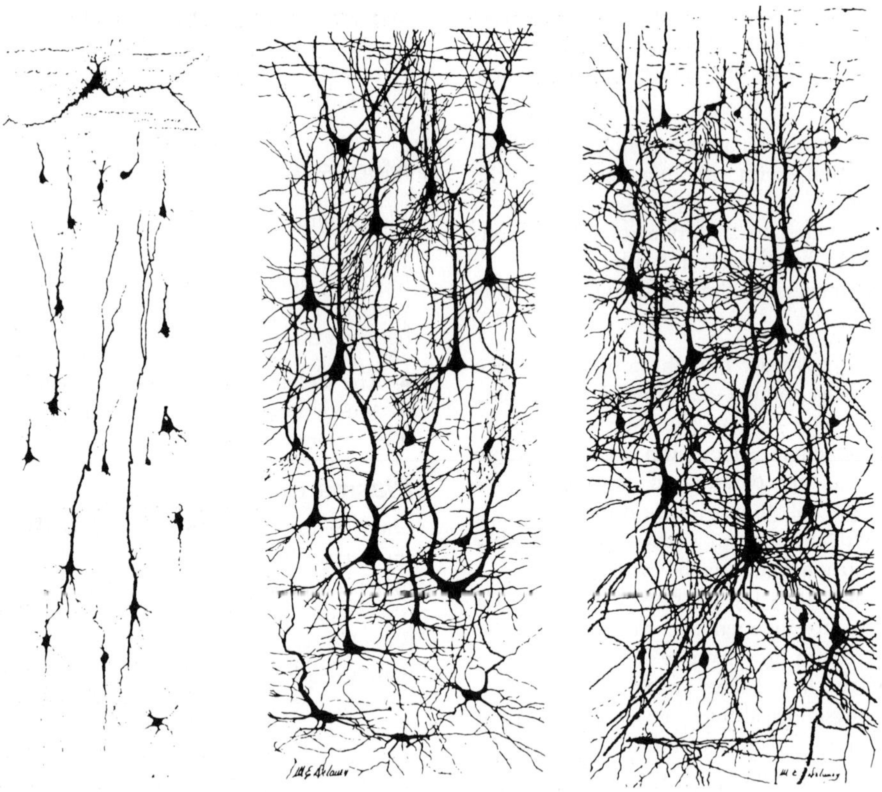

Figure 49.1 *Dendritic growth. (Reproduced with permission from Blackburn & Loper 1992.)*

Sensory functions

The neonate can detect odour, differentiate between tastes, see and observe preferential stimuli, hear and discriminate sounds; all sensory modalities that he uses to interact with his carers (see Chapter 57 for more detail).

Motor functions

Movements in neonates, as in adults, may be reflexive or volitional. **Volitional** movement is under the control of the motor cortex and at first glance it may appear that the baby makes few volitional movements. Most infants manifest gradual motor control as the myelination of the major central and peripheral nerve tracts progresses. It is possible that environmental stimulation results in new interneurone connections which may ultimately contribute to the fullness and complexity of the many integrated functions of the central nervous system.

Ongoing neural development

In the newborn baby the number of neurones is thought to be completed by birth but in the first year the brain enlarges to three times its size at birth. This is mainly due to the ongoing development of the neuroglia which form the supporting framework and protective structures for the conducting neurones. During infancy the brain and spinal cord are thought to enjoy a degree of plasticity contributing to the ongoing modifications of the developing nervous system in response to environmental stimuli. The baby learns through observation and perception (Greenfield 1997).

The term infant demonstrates a typical pattern of muscle tone that changes in a predictable way as he develops. At first there is strong but passive flexion but soon this passive muscle action disappears to be replaced by purposive movement with increasing control and accuracy. Control proceeds in a cephalocaudal direction and amongst the first to develop are head control, turning over, reaching and grasping.

Reflexes

Reflexes are automatic, 'built-in' motor behaviours which occur at spinal level (Blackburn & Loper 1992). They are critical for the baby's safety and care as he has no experience of the world and must use them to survive. They also provide carers with signs of his motor capabilities, responsiveness and needs. The absence of reflexes or their persistence may signify brain damage.

- The **Moro (startle) reflex** involves adduction and extension of the arms with the fingers fanned out, followed by abduction of the arms with flexed elbows in an 'embrace' position. There is a similar response by the legs. It is often accompanied by crying and should disappear by the 8th week of life (Michie 1996).
- The **palmar grasp reflex** involves a newborn baby closing his fingers tightly around any object placed in his palm. Trevathean (1987) mentions a series of photographs by Eibl-Eibesfeldt (1975) showing a preterm baby suspending herself

without help from a rope. Trevathen mentions that far from being useless, the Moro reflex and the grasp reflex, along with the walking and crawling movements, may have evolved to help the infant readjust itself when being carried.

- The **tonic neck (fencing) reflex** happens when the baby's head is turned to one side. He will extend the arm and leg on that side of the body and flex the arm and leg on the other side. This is a behaviour aimed at stabilising the baby and preventing him from rolling over.
- The **stepping reflex** is seen if the neonate is held upright with his feet touching a solid surface. Alternating stepping movements are made.
- **Rooting reflex** If the side of the mouth or cheek is gently stroked the baby will turn his head towards the source of the stimulus and open his mouth ready to suckle.
- **Sucking and swallowing reflexes** are well developed in the term neonate. Sucking and swallowing are coordinated with respirations including gag, cough and sneeze reflexes.
- **Traction response** If the baby is held by the wrists and pulled upright into a sitting position his head will lag at first, then right itself on his neck before falling forward.

State regulation

An excellent description of behavioural states is given by Prechtl & O'Brien (1982). The term refers to the recognisable combination of behaviours seen and repeated in the neonate over time. Behavioural states have been investigated by observational studies, electroencephalography and polygraphy where various physiological signals such as respiration rate are studied. Prechtl defines five states using the four parameters of eyes open, respirations regular, gross movements and vocalisation. Brazelton (1984) uses similar criteria to describe neonatal state. This is outlined in Michie (1996).

Sleep states

Deep sleep

The baby's eyes are closed, respirations are regular, no eye movements are present, response to stimuli is delayed. Jerky movements may be present.

Light sleep

Rapid eye movements (REM) occur, respirations are irregular, sucking movements may occur, response to stimuli is rapid and may result in an alteration of state, random movements are noticed.

Awake states

Drowsy state

The baby's eyes may be open or closed with some eyelid flutter, smiling may occur, smooth limb movements are seen, interspersed with startle responses, alteration of state occurs readily following stimulation.

Quiet alert state

Motor activity is minimal but the baby is alert to visual or auditory stimuli.

Active alert state

The baby is active and reactive to the environment. In this state he will mimic facial expressions.

Active crying state

The baby cries vigorously and may be difficult to console. There is considerable muscular activity. Babies cry for different needs such as hunger, thirst, pain, a need to change position or unsatisfactory room temperature. It is their only means of attracting attention to their needs. Although crying causes anxiety at first, mothers usually soon learn to recognise and respond to the different cries. Informing parents of the different behavioural states they will observe in their babies may lead to a better understanding and care, lessen anxiety and allow greater parental enjoyment.

THE IMMUNE SYSTEM

Lymphopoiesis is aimed at the production of competent cells capable of distinguishing between foreign and self antigens, facilitating the elimination of antigens detected to be foreign and maintaining a memory of previous exposure to foreign antigens. In order to accomplish these tasks, lymphoid tissue development proceeds along the two classic pathways culminating in the formation of competent B lymphocytes which are necessary for antibody-mediated immunity and T lymphocytes which are predominantly responsible for cell-mediated immunity.

The fetus and neonate are compromised because the immune responses are immature and also they lack experience of common organisms so that there is delayed response. In particular, the neonate is prone to gastrointestinal infections. Not only cell-mediated and humoral immunity are affected; the inflammatory response and complement cascade are also limited. This immaturity of the immune system may also predispose to allergy formation.

When the baby is born, he leaves a usually sterile intrauterine environment and enters an environment full of potentially pathogenic organisms. His skin, respiratory system and gastrointestinal tract must develop normal microbe commensal populations and respond appropriately to pathogens and allergens. The initial colonisation is via the mother's genital tract during birth, then her skin organisms and finally environmental organisms.

Organisms such as *Lactobacillus*, *E. coli* and protective anaerobes are provided by the mother's genital tract. Pathogens such as group B streptococcus and *Chlamydia trachomatis* may also be present. Newborn skin and mucous membranes are fragile and easily breached by pathogenic organisms. Colonisation occurs initially on the skin, umbilical stump and genitalia followed by mucous membranes of the eyes, nose and throat (Blackburn & Loper 1992).

The gut

The acidity of stomach secretions may afford some protection against ingested pathogens. Colonisation of meconium occurs within a few hours of birth and increases rapidly over the next few days. Breastfed babies develop a different pattern of bacterial colonisation than artificially fed babies. There is an acid environment in the gut in which protective organisms such as *Lactobacillus* can grow, thus preventing colonisation by pathogenic organisms (Chapter 54). The development of gut defence mechanisms is called **gut closure**, the development of the mucosal barrier and other defences to render the epithelium impermeable to organisms. Two specific immune responses concern IgA (humoral-mediated immunity) and maturation of T cells (cell-mediated immunity).

Specific immune responses

Humoral-mediated immunity

During fetal life there is transfer of IgG via the placenta from mother to fetus, affording some immunity. However, IgA does not cross the placenta and neonatal levels are low. Colonising IgA is provided in the colostrum. IgA is attached to human colostrum and milk and this protects the IgA molecule from the acidic contents and proteolytic enzymes in the baby's gastrointestinal tract. IgM is too large a molecule to cross the placental barrier. However, the neonate is capable of producing sufficient amounts of IgM in response to a challenge by organisms such as the TORCH organisms (Toxoplasmosis, Other viruses, Rubella, Cytomegalovirus and Herpes simplex).

Cell-mediated immunity

Numbers of T cells at birth are similar to levels in the adult but their function is decreased. Cytotoxic activity of T cells in the neonate is only 30–60% that of the adult. The newborn T cells are inexperienced and it appears to take about 5 weeks to achieve minimal protection.

THERMOREGULATION

Thermoregulation is the balance between heat production and heat loss.

Adult mechanisms

Humans are homeothermic animals, that is, they maintain a constant body temperature independent of their environment. Skin receptors in various parts of the body send messages to the hypothalamus to trigger autonomic nervous system responses and to the cerebral cortex to trigger behavioural responses. A rise in body temperature in humans is accompanied by an autonomically triggered peripheral vasodilation and sweating and a behavioural seeking for a cooler environment and wearing of appropriate clothing. If the body temperature falls there is usually a reflex peripheral vasoconstriction and shivering and the person seeks a warmer environment and puts on additional clothes (Michaelides 1997).

Neonatal mechanisms

Following birth the neonate passes from a thermoconstant intrauterine temperature of 37.7°C to a delivery room temperature between 21 and 25°C and can lose heat very rapidly because his skin is wet with amniotic fluid (Michie 1996). Heat may be

Table 49.1 *Sources of heat gain and heat loss in the neonate*

Heat gain	*Heat loss*
Metabolic processes such as oxidative metabolism of glucose, fats and proteins	Evaporation – water loss from the skin and respiratory tract, most common at birth. Heat is also lost in urine and faeces
Physical activity such as crying, restlessness and hyperactivity	Convection – heat lost into the air around the baby
Non-shivering thermogenesis generated through metabolism in brown adipose tissue	Radiation – heat radiated to nearby cold solid surfaces, most common after the first week of life
	Conduction – heat lost by direct contact with cold surfaces touching the baby

transferred down the internal gradient from body core to skin surface and then down the external gradient from body surface to the environment. The speed with which heat passes through the internal gradient depends upon capillary blood flow and the amount of subcutaneous fat present. The loss down the external gradient depends on the difference between the skin temperature and the external environment and involves the four processes of evaporation, convection, radiation and conduction (Blackburn & Loper 1992).

Neonatal thermoregulation is a problem because the baby is not able to utilise adult methods (Michaelides 1997). In the first few days of life infants can lose sweat only from their head region. The infant has a large surface area three times that of the adult from which to lose heat, relative to his small mass to produce heat, and his head makes up 25% of the area. The usual neonatal rectal temperature is 36.5–37°C and his skin temperature is 36–36.5°C.

Babies are unable to shiver and are limited in their ability to move about to generate heat from muscle action. They can decrease their surface area exposed to the environment by flexing their limbs and taking up the fetal position. After the first 24 h babies can increase their body heat production by 2.5 times as a response to cold. This heat comes from catecholamine stimulation of lipolysis of brown adipose tissue (BAT), a tissue found in other animal neonates and in hibernating animals.

Heat production and BAT

About 2–7% of the weight of a newborn is thought to consist of brown adipose tissue (BAT), mainly situated around the kidney, in the mediastinum, around the nape of the neck and scapulae, along the spinal column and around the large blood vessels in the neck (Fig. 49.2). BAT cells begin to proliferate at 26–30 weeks' gestation and continue developing until 4 weeks after birth.

The **adipocytes** (fat cells) of BAT differ from the normal adipocyte by the huge increase in metabolic processes and heat production of which they are capable. The cells contain many small fat vacuoles instead of one large fat accumulation. They also contain numerous mitochondria and the tissue is well supplied with blood capillaries, giving it the characteristically brown colour, and sympathetic nerve fibres. During cold stress,

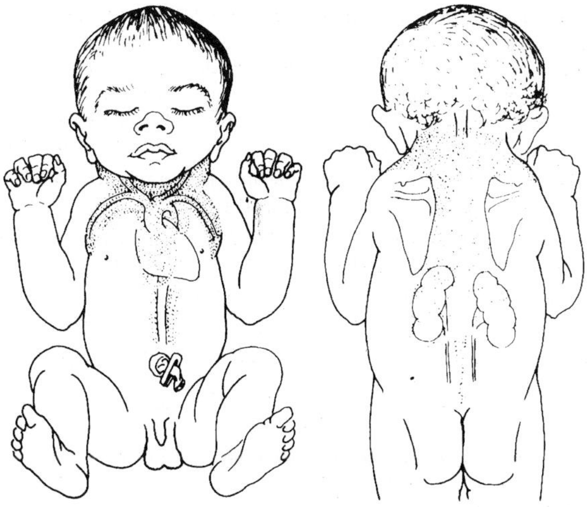

Figure 49.2 *The areas where brown fat is found. (Reproduced with permission from Wallis & Harvey 1979.)*

sympathetic nervous activity causes the adrenal glands to release catecholamines. Their local release of noradrenaline (norepinephrine) stimulates the anterior pituitary gland to release thyroid-stimulating hormone (TSH), causing the thyroid gland to increase its production of thyroxine (T_4). Adrenaline and thyroxine increase the metabolism of the brown fat cells and heat is produced but this requires extra oxygen and glucose.

Care of the neonate

It is important that parents as well as professionals caring for newborn babies are aware of the need to keep the head and nape of the neck warm and to adjust both the environmental temperature and the amount of clothing worn by the baby to maximise heat regulation. At delivery the infant should be dried and covered and given to his mother to hold if possible. The best source of heat is from the mother's body. Implications for the care of the small and sick neonate will be discussed in Chapter 50.

Summary of main points

- Whilst the fetus is in utero his nutritional needs, excretory needs, many metabolic needs and protection against pathogenic organisms and toxins are met by the placenta. After birth the complex physiological systems devoted to the above functions must begin to work independently.
- At birth the newborn infant manifests some anatomical and physiological limitations in relation to its gastrointestinal system, partly influenced by the phase of intrauterine life that requires the fetus to swallow amniotic fluid. The swallowing actions of the small bolus of amniotic fluid may be an important contributing factor in the maintenance of gastrointestinal patency.
- Following birth the GI tract supplies the infant's needs for energy, nutrients and fluids. Sucking and swallowing reflexes are present. The stomach has a small capacity but increases rapidly within the first few weeks of life. The cardiac sphincter is weak and regurgitation is common.
- The intestinal mucosal barrier remains immature so that antigens and other macromolecules can be transported across the epithelium into the systemic circulation. Colostrum is rich in antibodies, easily swallowed and helps the passage of meconium. Differences can be seen between babies who are breastfed and those given modified formula feeds. The relative deficiency of the enzymes amylase and lipase means that the human baby has difficulty in digesting carbohydrates and fats.
- A gastrocolic reflex ensures that feeding is often accompanied by reflex emptying of the bowel. Most infants pass meconium within 24 h of birth. Failure to do so could be a sign of intestinal obstruction. Once milk feeding is established the stools of the baby begin to change.
- The liver is physiologically immature and there is low production of some of the enzymes such as glucuronyl transferase. Feeding stimulates liver function and colonisation of the gut which allows vitamin K to be produced.
- The fetus prepares for the transition to independence by laying down a fuel store of glycogen and lipids during the last few weeks of pregnancy. After birth glycogen stores are broken down and the alternative substrates of fat stores and ketone bodies are used, stimulated by catecholamine release associated with cooling of the body.
- Neonatal blood glucose levels fall to their lowest between 2 and 6 h after birth. They then become stable and rise as the baby adapts to his extrauterine environment. Gluconeogenesis develops after birth. The method of feeding can influence neonatal blood glucose levels. Lipolysis increases rapidly after birth, reaching a maximum within a few hours. In the first 24 h about two-thirds of the baby's energy is produced from oxidation of fat.
- The newborn baby has little ability to synthesise protein because of relative immaturity of the liver enzyme systems. Serum amino acid levels are higher than normal later values in the first few weeks of life and there is significant urinary amino acid excretion.
- During the first 2 days of life serum calcium levels fall and there is a physiological hypocalcaemia, increasing back to normal at between 5 to 10 days once intestinal absorption of calcium matures. Renal excretion of calcium is efficient and increases as the days pass. Infants can metabolise vitamin D in the liver and kidneys although absorption of exogenous vitamin D may be limited because of immature fat absorption.
- Renal excretion of phosphorus is delayed with a decreased glomerular filtration rate and increased tubular reabsorption rate. Increased energy release with conversion of ATP to ADP leads to increased phosphate release.
- Only 1% of the total body magnesium appears to be located in the extracellular space. In plasma about 60% of the magnesium exists as free ion whilst 20% is bound to various anions. The remaining plasma magnesium is bound to serum proteins. The kidneys appear to be the primary organs for the regulation of serum magnesium concentrations.
- Nervous system activity increases steadily throughout gestation. At term the baby is prepared to process incoming information from the environment and produce behaviour appropriate for his status. The neonate can detect odour, differentiate between tastes, see and observe preferential stimuli and can hear and discriminate sounds to interact with his carers. During the first year the brain is plastic so that the connections can be modified by environmental stimuli as the baby learns through observation and perception.
- The term infant demonstrates a typical pattern of muscle tone that changes as he develops. At first there is strong but passive flexion but this soon disappears to be replaced by purposive movement. Reflexes are critical for the baby's safety and care as he has no experience of the world and must use them to survive. The absence of reflexes or their persistence may signify brain damage.

- The term behavioural state refers to the recognisable combination of behaviours repeated in the neonate over time. These include two sleep states – deep and light – and four awake states – drowsy, quiet alert, active alert and active crying. Helping parents to recognise these different behavioural states may lead to a better understanding and care, lessen anxiety and allow greater parental enjoyment.
- Lymphopoiesis is aimed at the production of competent cells capable of distinguishing between foreign and self antigens, facilitating the elimination of antigens detected to be foreign and maintaining a memory of previous exposure to foreign antigens. Lymphoid tissue development culminates in the formation of competent B and T lymphocytes.
- The fetus and neonate are immune compromised because the immune responses are immature and they lack experience of common organisms so that there is delayed response. This immaturity of the immune system may predispose to allergy formation. In particular, the neonate is prone to gastrointestinal infections.
- When the baby is born his skin, respiratory system and gastrointestinal tract must develop normal microbe commensal populations and respond appropriately to pathogens and allergens. The initial colonisation is via the mother's genital tract during birth, then her skin organisms and finally environmental organisms.
- Breastfed babies develop a different pattern of bacterial colonisation from artificially fed babies. The acid environment in the gut facilitates the growth of *Lactobacillus*, preventing colonisation by pathogenic organisms. Neonates must develop gut closure to render the epithelium impermeable to organisms. Two specific immune responses concern IgA and maturation of T cells.
- Thermoregulation in the neonate is a problem because the baby is not able to utilise adult methods. The infant has a large surface area from which to lose heat, relative to his small mass to produce heat. Babies are unable to shiver and are limited in their ability to move about to generate heat from muscle action. After the first 24 h babies can increase their body heat production by 2.5 times as a response to cold by lipolysis of brown adipose tissue.

References

Aynsley-Green A. 1985 Metabolic and endocrine interrelations in the human fetus and neonate. American Journal of Clinical Nutrition 41, 399.

Anderson KN, Anderson LE, Glanze WD. (eds) 1994 Mosby's Medical, Nursing and Allied Health Dictionary. Mosby, St Louis.

Bannister L, Berry M, Collins P et al. 1995 Gray's Anatomy. Churchill Livingstone, Edinburgh.

Blackburn ST, Loper DL. 1992 Maternal, Fetal and Neonatal Physiology, A Clinical Perspective. WB Saunders, Philadelphia.

Brazelton TB. 1984 Neonatal Behaviour Assessment Scale, 2nd edn. Spastics International Medical Publications, Blackwell Scientific, Oxford.

Dodds R. 1996 When policies collide: breastfeeding and hypoglycaemia. MIDIRS Midwifery Digest 6(4), 382–386.

Eibl-Eibesfeldt I. 1975 Ethology: The Biology of Behaviour. Holt, Rinehart and Winston, New York.

Garrow J, James W. 1993 Human Nutrition and Dietetics. Churchill Livingstone, Edinburgh.

Greenfield S. (ed) 1997 The Human Mind Explained. Cassell, London.

Hawdon JM, Platt MPW, Aynsley-Green A. 1992 Patterns of metabolic adaptation for preterm and term infants in the first neonatal week. Archives of Disease in Childhood Fetal and Neonatal Edition, 67(4), 357–365.

Koh T, Vong SK. 1996 Definition of neonatal hypoglycaemia: is there a change? Journal of Paediatrics and Child Health 344(4), 302–305.

Michie MM. 1996 The baby at birth. In Bennett VR, Brown LK (eds) Myles Textbook for Midwives, 12th edn. Churchill Livingstone, Edinburgh, pp 492–504.

Michaelides S. 1997 Thermoregulation and the neonate. In Sweet BR with Tiran D (eds) Mayes Midwifery, 12th edn. Baillière Tindall, London, pp 819–832.

Pitkin RM. 1985 Calcium metabolism in pregnancy and the perinatal period: a review. American Journal of Obstetrics and Gynecology 151, 99.

Polin R & Fox W. 1992 Fetal and Neonatal Physiology, WB Saunders, Philadelphia.

Prechtl HFR, O'Brien MJ. 1982 Behavioural states of the full-term newborn. The emergence of concept. In Stratton P (ed) Psychobiology of the Human Newborn. John Wiley, Chichester.

Rudolph A, Hoffman J, Rudulph et al 1996 Rudolph's Pediatrics. Prentice-Hall, New Jersey.

Shatz C. 1992 The developing brain. Scientific American 9, 35–41.

Simpson C. 1997 Metabolic and endocrine disorders of the newborn. In Sweet BR with Tiran D (eds) Mayes Midwifery, 12th edn. Baillière Tindall, London, pp 889–895.

Trevathen WR. 1987 Human Birth: An Evolutionary Perspective. Aldine de Gruyter, New York.

Wallis S, Harvey D. 1979 Intensive Care of the Newborn, 3. Disorders of the Newborn I. Nursing Times, 75 (31): 1319–1327.

Recommended reading

Aynsley-Green A. 1985 Metabolic and endocrine interrelations in the human fetus and neonate. American Journal of Clinical Nutrition 41, 399.

Dodds R. 1996 When policies collide: breastfeeding and hypoglycaemia. MIDIRS Midwifery Digest 6(4), 382–386.

Koh T, Vong SK. 1996 Definition of neonatal hypoglycaemia: is there a change? Journal of Paediatrics and Child Health 344(4), 302–305.

Polin R & Fox W. 1992 Fetal and Neonatal Physiology. WB Saunders, Philadelphia.

Shatz C. 1992 The developing brain. Scientific American 9, 35–41.

Chapter

50 The low birthweight baby – common problems and care

In this chapter

INTRODUCTION

This chapter provides an overview of common problems found in the neonate. General causes and diagnosis of congenital abnormalities have already been discussed in Chapter 13. It is not possible to give detail at the level required for those involved in neonatal intensive care units and there are many good textbooks on the market, some of which will be referred to in the text. The most relevant concepts of physiology and biological sciences applied to pathophysiological problems will be concentrated on. The application of those concepts to the necessary care will be briefly outlined.

LOW BIRTHWEIGHT BABIES

About 70% of perinatal mortality, that is, the total of stillbirths and neonatal deaths, occurs in the 7% of babies whose birth weight is low (Kelnar et al 1995). The concept of low birth weight is a complex one. The following parameters are applied regardless of the cause of a baby's low birth weight (Simpson 1997a, Thomson 1996).

- Low birth weight (LBW) is usually taken to include babies weighing 2500 g or less at birth.
- Very low birthweight (VLBW) babies are those weighing below 1500 g at birth.
- Extremely low birthweight (ELBW) babies weigh under 1000 g at birth (Simpson 1997a).

Causes of low birth weight

There are two main reasons why babies may be small at birth. They may have been born too early or they may not have grown well in utero (Fig. 50.1). The first category are the **preterm babies**. Preterm babies are those born before 37 completed weeks of pregnancy calculated from the first day of the last menstrual period, regardless of birth weight.

The second category is those babies who are **small for gestational age** (SFGA). This term refers to a baby who weighs less at birth than would be predicted for gestational age. It is usual to include babies born below the 10th centile. These two major groups of babies are likely to develop different problems and require different care. Some babies are born with both problems and are very much at risk. It is important to identify

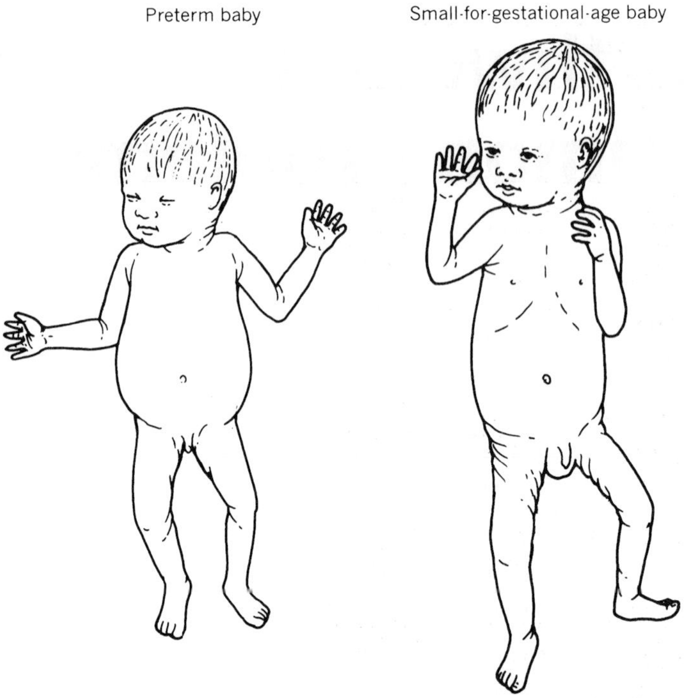

Figure 50.1 *Low birthweight babies (from Sweet B, 1997, with permission).*

the group to which a small baby belongs so that optimum care can be provided. Centile charts such as the one where birth weight is plotted against gestational age are quite useful for a rapid assessment (Fig. 50.2).

Assessment of gestational age

The obstetrician in most cases will have based the assessment during pregnancy on the length of gestation by taking into account the date of the beginning of the last menstrual period,

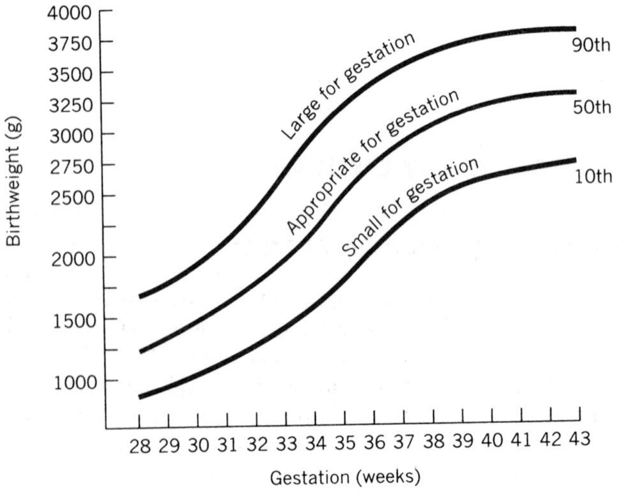

Figure 50.2 *A centile chart, showing weight and gestation (from Sweet B, 1997, with permission).*

the size and shape of the growing uterus and clinical tests such as the use of ultrasound and amniocentesis. The likely status of the baby is often known before delivery and the paediatric team are forewarned so that they can prepare for the necessary care.

As soon as is feasible after birth, small babies must be examined by a paediatrician so that their gestational age can be confirmed by the observation of physical characteristics and neurological development. Of the scoring systems devised to help assess gestational age, the Dubowitz scale (Dubowitz et al 1970) is most used in Britain (Fig. 50.3). However, as this scale awards points for neurological state as well as external criteria, it may not be suitable for use with sick and/or ventilated infants. The Parkin score (Parkin et al 1976), which relies totally on external criteria, although not quite as accurate, is quicker to use and may be more appropriate for some babies (Fig. 50.4) (Simpson 1997a).

THE PRETERM BABY

The problems of the preterm baby arise because of immaturity of the body systems (Fig. 50.5). They are not ready to adapt to extrauterine life in the ways discussed in the previous two chapters.

The main features include the following.

- A large head in proportion to their body, with a small face.
- Brain tissue is fragile and neurological damage more likely.
- In babies born before 24 weeks the eyelids may still be fused.
- Soft skull bones with widely spaced sutures and large fontanelles.
- Red, thin skin with absent subcutaneous fat and prominent surface veins.
- Lanugo may be present depending on the gestational age.
- A small narrow chest with little breast tissue.
- A large prominent abdomen with a low-set umbilicus.
- Thin limbs with soft nails not reaching to the ends of the digits.
- Small genitalia. In girls the labia majora do not cover the labia minora, in boys the testes have not descended into the scrotum.
- Muscle tone is poor and the limbs may be held extended.
- Reflexes, including sucking, may be absent or feeble.

Causes of preterm birth

Preterm deliveries may be spontaneous or medically controlled for maternal or fetal safety. In 40% of cases no known cause can be identified. Known causes often include factors arising from an interplay between maternal and fetal physical disorders and social class and it is difficult sometimes to separate these clearly. This is not surprising as many suboptimal health problems arise from the interplay of genes and environment (Chapters 7 and 15).

Fetal causes

- Multiple pregnancy
- Polyhydramnios
- Congenital abnormalities

External (superficial) Criteria

EXTERNAL SIGN	SCORE 0	1	2	3	4
OEDEMA	Obvious oedema hands and feet: pitting over tibia	No obvious oedema hands and feet: pitting over tibia	No oedema		
SKIN TEXTURE	Very thin, gelatinous	Thin and smooth	Smooth: medium thickness. Rash or superficial peeling	Slight thickening. Superficial cracking and peeling esp. hand and feet	Thick and parchment-like; superficial or deep cracking
SKIN COLOUR (Infant not crying)	Dark red	Uniformly pink	Pale pink: variable over body	Pale. Only pink over ears, lips, palms or soles	
SKIN OPACITY (trunk)	Numerous veins and venules clearly seen, especially over abdomen	Veins and tributaries seen	A few large vessels clearly seen over abdomen	A few large vessels seen indistinctly over abdomen	No blood vessels seen
LANUGO (over back)	No lanugo	Abundant; long and thick over whole back	Hair thinning especially over lower back	Small amount of lanugo and bald areas	At least half of back devoid of lanugo
PLANTAR CREASES	No skin creases	Faint red marks over anterior half of sole	Definite red marks over more than anterior half; indentations over less than anterior third	Indentations over more than anterior third	Definite deep indentations over more than anterior third
NIPPLE FORMATION	Nipple barely visible; no areola	Nipple well defined; areola smooth and flat diameter <0.75 cm.	Areola stippled, edge not raised; diameter <0.75 cm.	Areola stippled, edge raised diameter >0.75 cm.	
BREAST SIZE	No breast tissue palpable	Breast tissue on one or both sides <0.5 cm. diameter	Breast tissue both sides; one or both 0.5–1.0 cm.	Breast tissue both sides; one or both >1 cm.	
EAR FORM	Pinna flat and shapeless, little or no incurving edge	Incurving of part of edge of pinna	Partial incurving whole of upper pinna	Well-defined incurving whole of upper pinna	
EAR FIRMNESS	Pinna soft, easily folded, no recoil	Pinna soft, easily folded, slow recoil	Cartilage to edge of pinna, but soft in places, ready recoil	Pinna firm, cartilage to edge, instant recoil	
GENITALIA MALE	Neither testis in scrotum	At least one testis high in scrotum	At least one testis right down		
FEMALE (With hips half abducted)	Labia majora widely separated, labia minora protruding	Labia majora almost cover labia minora	Labia majora completely cover labia minora		

(Adapted from Farr et al., *Develop. Med. Child Neurol.* (1966) **8**, 507)

Figure 50.3 *(a) Dubowitz score. (Adapted from Dubowitz LMS, Dubowitz V, Goldberg C 1970.)*

Maternal causes

- Diseases associated with pregnancy such as preeclampsia or antepartum haemorrhage
- Rhesus incompatibility
- Serious disease in the mother such as renal disease
- Illnesses associated with pyrexia such as viral infections
- Smoking, alcohol and drug abuse, where the baby might also be SFGA
- Maternal short stature
- Cervical incompetence
- Maternal age and parity

Immediate management

The care of the preterm baby is aimed at supporting the many physiological functions that the baby cannot perform adequately and this should begin in labour. Preterm infants should be delivered in a maternity hospital with a suitable neonatal unit as transfer after birth may lead to exacerbation of problems or even death.

In labour

Corticosteroids should be administered to the mother in

Neurological Criteria

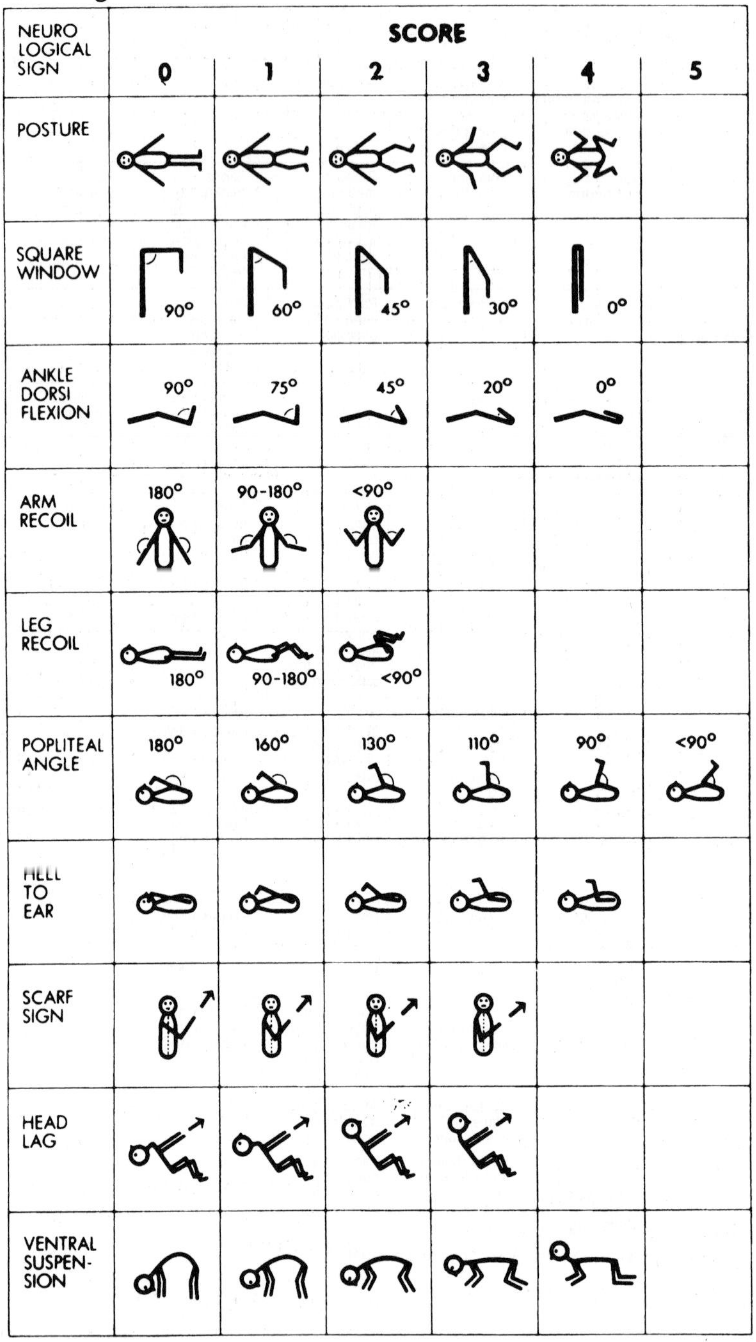

NEURO LOGICAL SIGN
SCORE
0
1
2
3
4
5
POSTURE
SQUARE WINDOW
90°
60°
45°
30°
0°
ANKLE DORSI FLEXION
90°
75°
45°
20°
0°
ARM RECOIL
180°
90-180°
<90°
LEG RECOIL
180°
90-180°
<90°
POPLITEAL ANGLE
180°
160°
130°
110°
90°
<90°
TO EAR
SCARF SIGN
HEAD LAG
VENTRAL SUSPEN-SION

Figure 50.3 *(b) Dubowitz score. (Adapted from Dubowitz LMS, Dubowitz V, Goldberg C 1970.)*

preterm labour. Crowley (1997), in a review of the literature, noted that the administration of 24 mg betamethasone or dexamethasone in divided doses or 2 g hydrocortisone has been found to reduce respiratory distress syndrome and intraventricular haemorrhage and no adverse effects have been seen.

The choice of mode of delivery needs careful consideration. Although there has been insufficient research to support a policy of elective CS for the delivery of all small babies (Grant 1997), there is some evidence that prophylactic CS delivery improves the outcome for very low birthweight babies, weighing between 1000 and 1600 g, presenting by the breech (Gilady et al 1996). If vaginal delivery is chosen an episiotomy is necessary and some obstetricians advocate forceps delivery to lessen the risk of intracranial haemorrhage. Care must be taken not to give the mother any drugs that will depress the fetal respiratory centre.

At birth

The equipment likely to be needed to resuscitate the baby should be prepared before the delivery is imminent and the

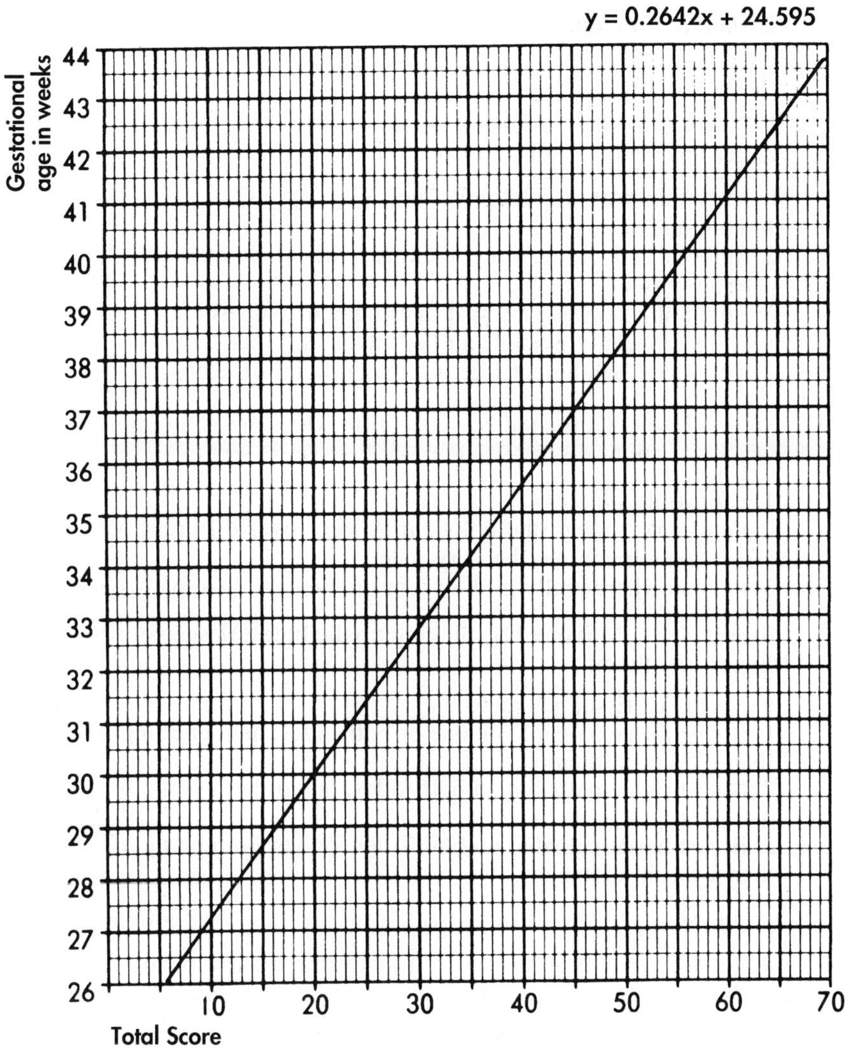

Figure 50.3 *(c) Dubowitz score. (Adapted from Dubowitz LMS, Dubowitz V, Goldberg C 1970.)*

paediatric team informed. An experienced paediatrician should be present at the delivery. The respiratory muscles of some babies may be weak and the respiratory centre immature. It may be difficult to establish adequate respirations. Some paediatricians prefer to intubate all low birthweight babies and there are studies to show that this policy may improve survival and well-being. Many babies that appear well at birth develop respiratory problems soon after.

The baby must be prevented from losing body heat at birth by having the room temperature at 24°C. The baby should be dried and warmly wrapped. If his respiratory and cardiovascular functions are satisfactory the parents will wish to hold him. If the mother wishes skin-to-skin contact, mother and baby will need to be covered with warmed blankets (Simpson 1997a). If the baby needs resuscitation the overhead radiant heater should be switched on.

Ongoing care of preterm babies

Potential problems

The preterm baby may present with a range of potential problems which will be discussed in detail under the relevant headings. These may include:

- respiratory problems such as apnoea, respiratory distress syndrome, bronchopulmonary dysplasia;
- metabolic problems such as jaundice, hypoglycaemia, hypocalcaemia, necrotising enterocolitis, intraventricular haemorrhage;
- persistent fetal circulation and anaemia.

The following aspects of care need attending to.

- The maintenance of temperature
- Respirations and cardiovascular function
- Nutrition and excretion
- Kidney function
- Prevention of infection
- The emotional relationship between mother and baby needs to be considered continuously.

Maintenance of temperature

The preterm baby needs all the calories it can assimilate to

2 Parkin, Hey and Clowes score

This is quicker to perform but may not be quite so accurate.

Skin texture. Tested by picking up a fold of abdominal skin between finger and thumb, and by inspection.

0 Very thin with a gelatinous feel.
1 Thin and smooth.
2 Smooth and of medium thickness, irritation rash and superficial peeling may be present.
3 Slight thickening and stiff feeling with superficial cracking and peeling especially evident on the hands and feet.
4 Thick and parchment-like with superficial or deep cracking.

Skin colour. Estimated by inspection when the baby is quiet.

0 Dark red.
1 Uniformly pink.
2 Pale pink, though the colour may vary over different parts of the body, some parts may be very pale.
3 Pale, nowhere really pink except on the ears, lips, palms and soles.

Breast size. Measured by picking up the breast tissue between finger and thumb.

0 No breast tissue palpable.
1 Breast tissue palpable on one or both sides, neither being more than 0.5 cm in diameter.
2 Breast tissue palpable on both sides, one or both being 0.5–1 cm in diameter.
3 Breast tissue palpable on both sides, one or both being more than 1 cm in diameter.

Ear firmness. Tested by palpation and folding of the upper pinna.

0 Pinna feels soft and is easily folded into bizarre positions without springing back into position spontaneously.
1 Pinna feels soft along the edge and is easily folded but returns slowly to the correct position spontaneously.
2 Cartilage can be felt to the edge of the pinna though it is thin in places and the pinna springs back readily after being folded.
3 Pinna firm with definite cartilage extending to the periphery and springs back immediately into position after being folded.

Score each external sign in turn. Add them up. Read off the baby's gestational age on the following chart:

Score	Gestational age	
	days	weeks
1	190	27
2	210	30
3	230	33
4	240	34.5
5	250	36
6	260	37
7	270	38.5
8	276	39.5
9	281	40
10	285	41
11	290	41.5
12	295	42

Figure 50.4 *Parkin, Hey and Clowes score. (Reproduced from Parkin et al 1976.)*

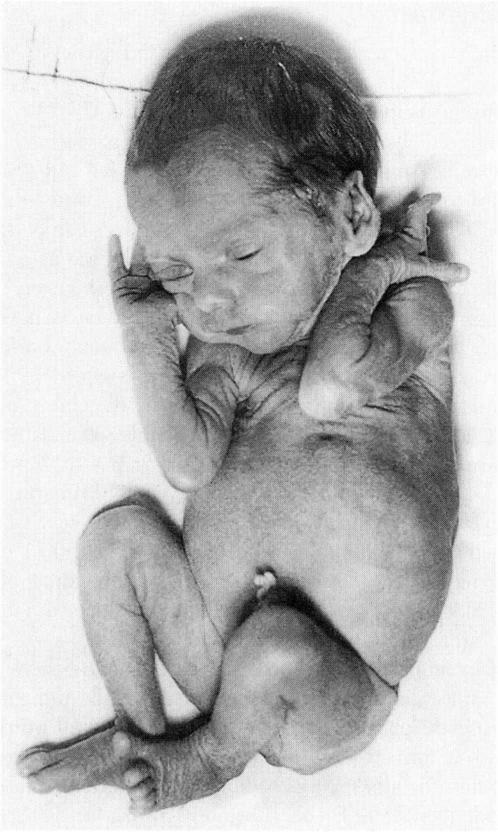

Figure 50.5 *A preterm baby born in 1954 at 28 weeks gestation and weighing 1.1 kg. He was discharged in good health after 11 weeks in hospital (from Kelnar C, Harvey D, Simpson C, 1995, with permission).*

supply its needs for growth and maturation. The use of glucose and oxygen to supply energy expended to maintain body warmth must be reduced to a minimum. This is achieved by providing an ideal environmental temperature for the baby, the **thermoneutral environment**, which is a very narrow range for a small naked baby (Kelnar et al 1995). SCBU room temperature is held between 26 and 28°C and the incubator temperature between 33 and 37°C to maintain an ideal body temperature for the baby of about 37°C. A skin probe is attached to the baby and the incubator temperature will be automatically adjusted as the skin temperature changes (Simpson 1997a). Infants born before 30 weeks of gestation have porous skin through which water passes and evaporates, causing an increase in heat loss. These babies should be nursed in a humid atmosphere for the first week or so. Heat loss by radiation can be prevented by using a heat shield.

Respiration

The respiration rate should be between 40 and 60/min and should be sufficient to keep the baby pink all over, including the extremities. Hourly observations will enable an accurate assessment of the baby's needs to be made. These should include (Thomson & Torley 1996):

- the chest shape: is it overinflated, concave, asymmetrical?
- the colour of the baby and any colour change;
- the rate and regularity of respiration;
- breath sounds on auscultation.

Oxygen therapy

Oxygen therapy may be necessary to relieve cyanosis if respiratory problems develop (see Chapter 51). The temperature, humidity, flow rate and concentration of inspired oxygen must be adequately controlled and monitored (Kelnar et al 1995). Oxygen may be given by enriched air in a headbox (Fig. 50.6) or by ventilation. The amount given should be adjusted to keep arterial oxygen tension in the normal range. Too high a concentration of oxygen can have adverse effects including the development of **retrolental fibroplasia** (retinopathy of prematurity) and pulmonary damage may follow long-term oxygen therapy. On the other hand, inadequate oxygenation may lead to hypoxic brain damage. Methods of monitoring oxygen administration include transcutaneous oxygen monitoring, arterial catheterisation, especially in the very ill baby, and oxygen saturation monitoring by an infrared probe attached to the foot or hand. Continuous monitoring is much better than intermittent sampling. Babies should be weaned off their assisted ventilatory support as early as possible. Signs to begin

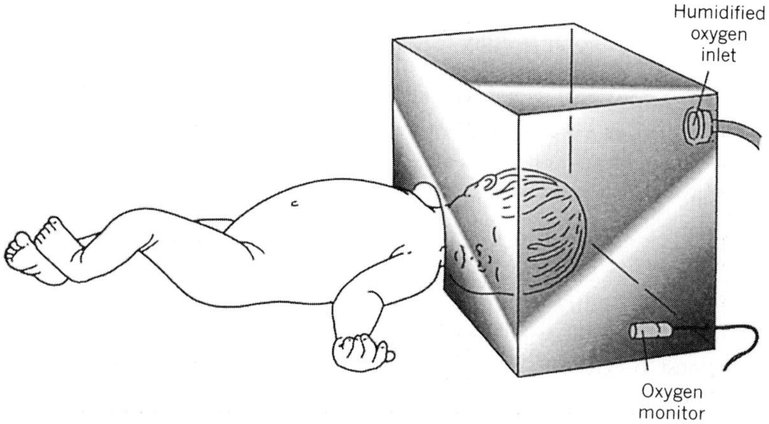

Figure 50.6 *Baby being nursed in a headbox (incubator not shown) (from Sweet B, 1997, with permission).*

this are falling oxygen requirements or attempts at spontaneous breathing.

Nutrition

The specific nutritional requirements of a newborn baby depend upon total body stores of fat, protein and glycogen. However, the infant's intestinal uptake and assimilation of nutrients, as well as elimination of the byproducts of digestion, cellular utilisation and energy expenditure also need to be taken into consideration when planning a nutritional programme. For practical reasons, a newborn infant's energy requirements may be divided into two major components: those required to support growth and those needed to support metabolic activities. In general, the energy requirements for metabolic activities take precedence over those needed for growth. If nutritional energy supply is insufficient for metabolic activities, the baby will fail to grow.

For the healthy term infant, most paediatricians and midwives are likely to recommend breastfeeding wherever circumstances make this feasible. Greer (1991) supports this policy by suggesting that it would be logical to establish an infant nutrition strategy that would mimic, for at least a short period of time, the fetal intrauterine nutritional needs and growth pattern.

In comparison with a healthy term infant born with adequate energy stores, the prematurely born infant is poorly equipped to make the physiological adaptation necessary to the maintenance of metabolic and nutritional homeostasis. Nutritional support for the low birthweight infant continues to be a challenge to midwives and clinicians. Ideally such appropriate nutritional support should commence within minutes of birth. However, the initial period of the infant's life tends to be complicated by a range of acute medical problems. Following the resolution of the identified clinical problems, the nutritional requirements for initiating and maintaining growth become a major concern for all who care for the infant.

Fats

Fats are the main dietary source of energy in the newborn infant, providing up to 50% of the total caloric needs (see also Chapter 54). Fats are thought to be essential for the development of the nervous system. Fats also play a critical role in the formation of all cell membranes. They can be stored in large quantities as major energy reserves in a growing and developing infant.

Proteins

Although dietary proteins supply less than 10% of the daily caloric needs, a daily intake of proteins is critical as it serves as a source of amino acids essential for growth in all newborn infants but particularly so in premature and low birthweight infants. Protein intake must supply the amino acids necessary to replace nitrogen lost in protein turnover which may be up to 10% of the total body protein per day. Greer (1991) suggests that although newborn infants have the ability to synthesise some amino acids, the essential amino acids which must be given are histidine, isoleucine, leucine, lysine, methionine, phenylalanine, threonine, tryptophan and valine. Low birthweight infants may require additional amino acids such as cystine and taurine.

Carbohydrates

According to Greer (1991), enterally fed growing newborn infants use carbohydrates as a major source of energy, glucose being the principal source. Thus the minimal 24-h glucose utilisation rate by the resting term infant is estimated to be 4 mg/kg/min. An intake of glucose less than that rate may result in gluconeogenesis from non-carbohydrate sources such as amino acids. Excess glucose, on the other hand, can be stored in the liver as glycogen and converted into glucose as and when required to support metabolic activities. However, in low birthweight infants glycogen stores are usually lower in the early neonatal period, accounting for the frequent episodes of hypoglycaemia these infants commonly experience.

The method of feeding chosen for a baby depends on his size, maturity and condition. Whenever possible, if a baby is well enough and shows inclination to suck, breast or bottle feeds should be offered with careful supervision. Immature babies may have poor sucking and swallowing ability so that enteral tube feeding, which may be nasojejunal (Fig. 50.7) or nasogastric, may be necessary. Intragastric feeding may be intermittent or continuous if overdistending the stomach with consequent regurgitation and inhalation is a risk.

Ill babies, such as those being ventilated, where there is a risk of milk aspiration or where the presence of milk in the stomach embarrasses respiration, may need total **parenteral nutrition**. It is usual to commence with intravenous water and dextrose with the addition of salts such as sodium, phosphate and calcium. If parenteral feeding is to be continued amino acids, lipids and vitamins are added. Trace elements are also given. When the baby's condition improves enteral feeding is slowly commenced and intravenous feeding slowly reduced and discontinued.

Requirements

A problem with nutrition is the extra nutritional requirements

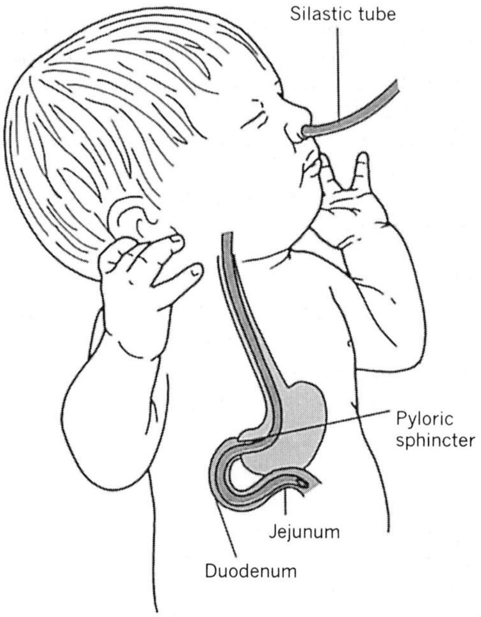

Figure 50.7 *Baby with nasojejunal tube in situ (from Sweet B, 1997, with permission).*

of the small or sick neonate. Whether enteral or parenteral feeding is chosen, the amount of fluid in which the nutrients are given must not exceed the kidneys' ability to cope with its excretion. Preterm babies grow more rapidly than term babies and need 600 kJ/kg/day. To achieve this level 180–200 ml/kg/day of breast milk or standard formula milk is necessary. This amount is excessive and the energy needs may be met by giving smaller amounts of low birthweight formula milk or adding calorific supplements to standard milk. Lucas et al (1992) reported that breast milk may be advantageous to central nervous system development and should be given whenever possible.

Nutritional supplements

As the baby grows, nutritional supplements are necessary. These include vitamins A and D from the age of 1 month to 2 years as preterm babies have poor stores of the fat-soluble vitamins. Vitamin C is also needed both for growth and healing and to aid absorption of iron. There is a delay in the production of red cells by the bone marrow and preterm babies become very anaemic, sometimes requiring blood transfusion. Iron supplements are recommended from 4 weeks until they are weaned.

As usual, treatment itself may lead to problems. Blood transfusion may suppress the manufacture of red blood cells and too much iron supplementation increases the risk of infection by inhibiting the antiinfective properties of lactoferrin and allowing *E. coli* to multiply. Very small babies may need folic acid supplementation. Calcium and phosphate supplementation are needed because of an increased rate of bone mineralisation.

Excretion

Urine

As with all babies the preterm baby should pass urine within 24 h of delivery and the amount should increase as fluid intake increases. All babies in the neonatal unit should have their urinary output measured and the urine tested for glucose and osmolality. Glycosuria may indicate a lower renal threshold for glucose and the amount of glucose administered will have to be reduced to avoid dehydration. The osmolality of the urine will indicate whether there is fluid retention or normal excretion so that the amount of fluid being administered can be adjusted. Failure of micturition occurs with hypotension, acute renal failure or urinary obstruction (Simpson 1997a).

Faeces

The passage of meconium may be delayed in small preterm babies, especially in those with respiratory distress syndrome. The presence of blood and mucus in the stools may indicate the serious disorder necrotising enterocolitis.

Pain

For many years clinicians took little account of the pain suffered by small babies. Many believed neonates felt little pain. However, multiple studies have now demonstrated that the nervous system is developed well enough to feel and react to painful stimuli. From an evolutionary point of view, this would seem to be an essential adaptation to extrauterine life!

Keeble & Twaddle (1995) discussed the benefits of developing an adequate tool for assessment of pain in the neonate. Response to pain stimuli may be **behavioural**, with crying, grimacing, startle or withdrawing limbs, **physiological**, with tachycardia, bradycardia, hypertension and increased oxygen requirements, or **metabolic**, with increased metabolic rate in response to decreased insulin secretion and increased corticosteroid release leading to hyperglycaemia. There may also be glycosuria, proteinuria, ketonuria and a raised urine pH (Simpson 1997b).

The relief of pain includes considering the environment, as discussed below, and development of expertise in the necessary techniques such as heel prick and intravenous line siting. Comfort interventions such as stroking, non-nutritive sucking, positioning and cuddling can be provided to reduce pain as well as the more clinical pharmacological methods. Anaesthesia should be used for invasive techniques and analgesia given postoperatively. Some narcotic drugs may depress respiration and their use in babies with respiratory problems is limited (Simpson 1997b).

Environmental neonatology

The preterm baby is adapted to an intrauterine environment and the effect of noise, light, handling and positioning may influence the well-being of the baby in the neonatal unit (Kelnar et al 1995). The preterm baby spends most of the time asleep and yet neonatal units are not necessarily the most restful places for their occupants. Noise and light levels can be high and care often necessitates much handling. These factors are associated with apnoea and bradycardia.

Noise

Noise level is measured in logarithmic units called **decibels** (dB). The human ear is very sensitive and can hear sound over a wide range from a pin dropping to a steam whistle shrieking, a range from 0.1 dB to 120 dB. In an adult there is a pain threshold of 130 dB. Severe hearing loss occurs with continuous exposure to sound over 90 dB. Some common noise levels are the background noise in a home (50 dB), a noisy restaurant (80 dB) and amplified rock music (over 90 dB) (Marieb 1992).

There is much ongoing research into the effects of noise on these babies, for instance the continuous noise levels inside the incubator. Kelnar et al (1995) quote the British safety standard that 'the mean noise inside an incubator should not exceed 60 decibels' and note that some incubator alarms can exceed 85 dB! Sudden loud noise can cause sleep disturbance, crying, tachycardia, hypoxaemia and raised intracranial pressure in the baby (Long et al 1980). Special care should be taken when closing portholes and cupboard doors and in moving incubators (Thomson 1996).

Light

In order to observe babies adequately, the level of light in NICUs has increased five- or 10-fold in the last two decades. With the use of phototherapy lamps, this increases the risk of the preterm baby developing retinopathy of prematurity (Kelnar et al 1995). The harmful effect of light can be reduced by establishing a day/night pattern of lighting and dimming lights when not in use. Mann et al (1986) found that when noise and light stimulus was reduced at night, babies slept on average 2 h in 24 more and increased their weight gain more rapidly than babies who did not undergo the day/night cycling. The practice of covering the eyes of neonates undergoing phototherapy is essential. Bright sunlight should be avoided.

Handling

A further problem is the need to carry out investigations and give care. Forward planning so that interventions are carried out together, leaving longer periods for the baby to rest, is helpful. Soothing and comforting interventions including baby massage and 'kangaroo care' have been assessed for their benefits and drawbacks by Lacy & Ohlsson (1993). Facilitated tucking (containment of the infant's arms and legs in a flexed position close to his trunk) has been utilised to deal with mild pain and to provide comfort by Corff et al (1995).

Positioning

Kelnar et al (1995) cite various studies on the effects of faulty positioning in preterm babies (Fig. 50.8); for instance, Bellefeuille-Reid & Jakubek (1989) on sensorimotor development and the effects of long periods of static nursing. Bottos & Stefani (1982) found that prolonged nursing in the prone position will result in externally rotated hips and everted feet, both of which may delay standing and walking. Fetters (1986) wrote that a lack of careful positioning to mimic the flexed position that the normal baby will take up during the last few weeks in utero and extension from about 40 weeks may result in developmental delay.

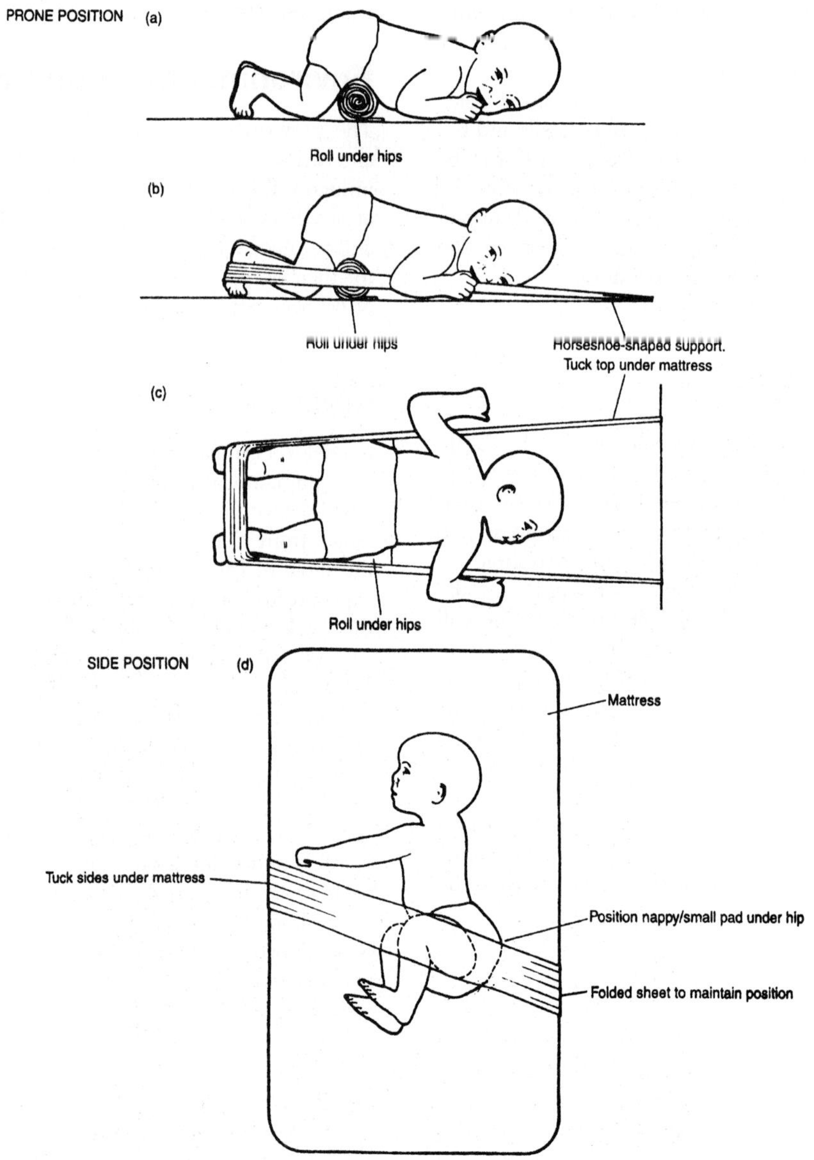

Figure 50.8 *Prone positioning and side lying (from Kelnar C, Harvey D, Simpson C, 1995, with permission).*

Preterm babies often develop flattened, elongated and asymmetrical head shapes. This can be avoided by frequent changes in the position of the baby's head. Periods of prone lying should be interspersed with side lying and articles such as folded nappies and rolled sheets can be used to maintain optimal positions for the hips and knees (Kelnar et al 1995).

Prevention of infection

The immaturity of the preterm baby's immune system makes it easy for infectious organisms to enter his body. The most important aspect of infection prevention is careful washing of hands and forearms both before and after attending to the baby. Liquid cleansing agents should be used and the hands and arms dried thoroughly. Gloves may need to be worn if body secretions are thought to be infected (Thomson 1996).

Each baby should have his own equipment which can be stored in the cupboards under the incubator or cot. There should be sufficient space between cots or incubators to prevent crossinfection. Disposable items are useful when available. Continuous vigilance with cleaning of equipment is essential. Staff or visitors with infections such as herpes simplex, upper respiratory tract infections, gastroenteritis or septic wounds should not enter a neonatal unit until their treatment is concluded.

THE SMALL-FOR-GESTATIONAL-AGE BABY

Babies who are small for gestational age (SFGA), sometimes referred to as 'light for dates', may be affected by **asymmetrical** growth retardation or **symmetrical** growth retardation (see Chapter 13). Most of these babies are born after the 37th week of gestation and are neurologically mature but lack subcutaneous fat (Fig. 50.9). The fetal brain undergoes a growth spurt in the last trimester of pregnancy and is vulnerable to lack of oxygen and nutrients. Other problems also arise from their lack of energy stores during birth. They are at risk of hypoxia

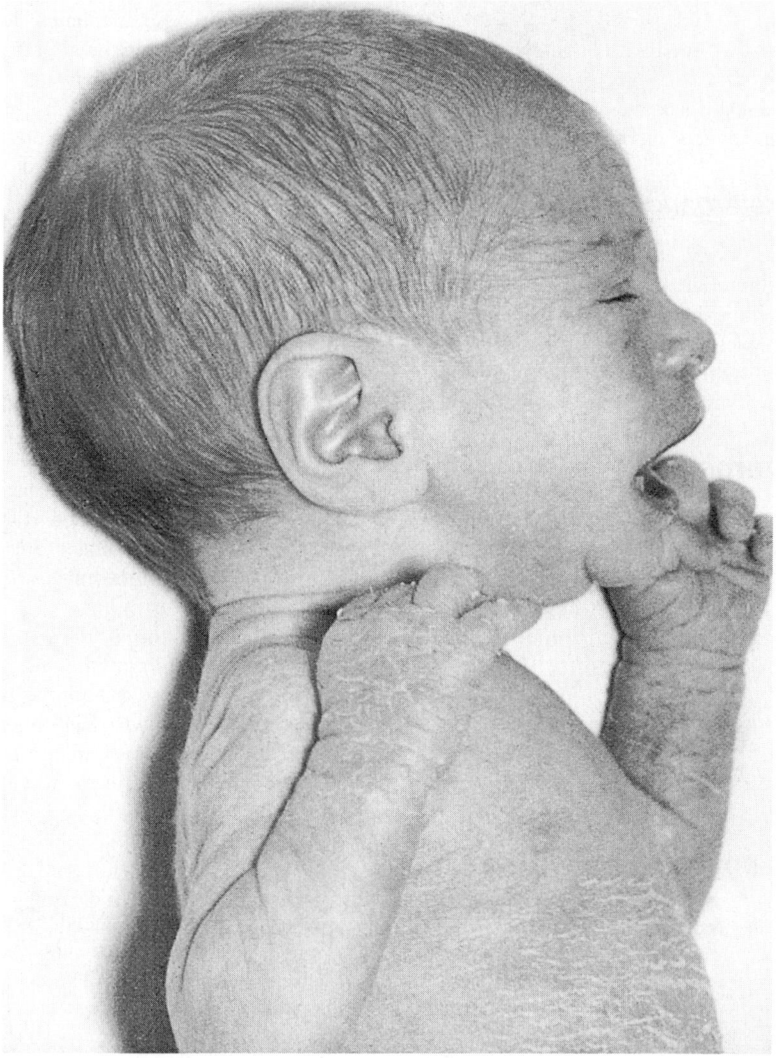

Figure 50.9 *The small-for-gestational-age (SFGA or dysmature) baby (from Kelnar C, Harvey D, Simpson C, 1995, with permission).*

during labour and hypoglycaemia after delivery. Recent research (e.g. Barker 1992) has indicated that SFGA babies may have long-term problems, such as hypertension and cardiovascular disease and mature-onset diabetes mellitus, as well as those in the neonatal period.

Asymmetrical growth retardation

Babies affected by asymmetrical growth retardation have grown normally in utero until the 3rd trimester. Conditions such as preeclampsia affect placental function and the fetus suffers from malnutrition, leading to the following features of appearance (Simpson 1997a).

- The birth weight is low but the head circumference and length of the baby are normal for gestational age.
- There is a lack of subcutaneous fat and the body and limbs appear wasted.
- The ribs are visible and the abdomen is flat or hollowed due to the small size of the liver.
- The skin is dry, loose and peeling and may be stained with meconium.
- The umbilical cord is thin and may also be stained with meconium.
- The face often looks old and wizened with large eyes and an anxious expression.
- Muscle tone is good and the baby is active.
- The baby appears very hungry and sucks his fist.

Symmetrical growth retardation

These babies have grown poorly throughout pregnancy. Common causes include intrauterine infections, chromosome abnormalities, malformations and maternal substance abuse. The head circumference of these babies is in proportion to their body size and weight. They suffer more morbidity and mortality than babies who have suffered from asymmetrical growth retardation.

Immediate management

SFGA infants should be delivered in a maternity hospital with a suitable neonatal unit where immediate care is available. Complications include perinatal asphyxia (see Chapter 46), meconium aspiration syndrome, hypothermia, hypoglycaemia, polycythaemia and pulmonary haemorrhage. Some of these problems will be discussed in the next chapter.

Labour and delivery

The baby in whom growth retardation has been noted in utero will have poor energy reserves of both fat and glycogen. It is essential to monitor the fetal condition by continuously observing fetal heart rate patterns and the presence of fresh meconium in the liquor. A clinician skilled in resuscitation should be present at the delivery. These babies lack subcutaneous fat and lose heat rapidly. They should be quickly dried and wrapped.

Ongoing care of SFGA babies

The SFGA baby has different problems from the preterm baby but the following aspects of care should still be attended to: the maintenance of temperature, respirations, cardiac function, nutrition, kidney function and excretion. Prevention of infection is a priority. The babies are usually active, vigorous and alert, feed well and many of them do not need admitting to a neonatal unit.

Transitional care

Transitional care wards have been developed in many maternity units, ideally situated near to the neonatal unit, to allow mothers to care for neonates with minor problems with supervision from experienced staff. Babies who are small but only have minor problems such as heat loss benefit from being cared for by their mothers in a transitional care unit. Mothers and babies are not separated and the mother is enabled to develop caring skills. It is no longer policy to keep babies in hospital until they weigh 2500 g and well babies may be transferred home as long as the surroundings are suitable.

The early care of these babies in the first 48 h is aimed at prevention of the complications, especially hypoglycaemia which is more likely if there has been asphyxia or hypothermia. Frequent recordings of blood glucose level are important and should take place 4 hourly for the first 48 h or until they are stable. There is also a risk of the rare condition transient neonatal diabetes mellitus in SFGA babies. The baby develops hyperglycaemia and glycosuria but will have no ketones in the urine, becoming dehydrated and failing to thrive (Stirling & Kelnar 1995). Breastfeeding reduces the risk of infection but low birthweight formula milks are energy dense and may be advantageous.

It is essential to offer follow-up care to ensure that these babies meet their growth and developmental milestones, especially those whose growth has been symmetrically retarded. Poor intrauterine growth has ongoing implications for health. Later in life these babies are prone to develop cardiovascular conditions and diabetes, as mentioned above.

Summary of main points

- About 70% of perinatal mortality occurs in the 7% of babies whose birth weight is low. Babies may be small at birth because they are preterm or small for gestational age. Some babies are born with both problems. As soon as is feasible after birth, the gestational age should be confirmed. Scoring systems for assessment of gestational age are the Dubowitz scale and the Parkin score.
- The care of the preterm baby is aimed at supporting the physiological functions that the baby cannot perform adequately. Preterm infants should be delivered in a maternity hospital with a suitable neonatal unit. Administration of corticosteroids reduces respiratory distress syndrome and intraventricular haemorrhage.
- Care must be taken not to give the labouring woman any drugs that will depress the fetal respiratory centre. An experienced paediatrician should be present at the delivery. The respiratory

muscles of some babies may be weak and the respiratory centre immature and it may be difficult to establish adequate respirations.

- The baby must be prevented from losing body heat at birth by having the room temperature at 24°C. The baby should be dried and warmly wrapped and if he is in good condition the parents will wish to hold him. Maintenance of body temperature is achieved by providing a thermoneutral environment.
- Respiration rate should be sufficient to keep the baby pink all over, including the extremities. Oxygen therapy may be necessary to relieve cyanosis if respiratory problems develop. The temperature, humidity, flow rate and concentration of inspired oxygen must be adequately controlled and monitored and the amount given should be adjusted to keep arterial oxygen tension in the normal range.
- The specific nutritional requirements of a newborn baby depend upon total body stores of fat, protein and glycogen. Intestinal uptake and assimilation of nutrients, elimination of the byproducts of digestion, cellular utilisation and energy expenditure are considered when planning a nutritional programme. A newborn infant's energy requirements may be divided into those required to support growth and those needed to support metabolic activities.
- The premature infant is poorly equipped for maintenance of metabolic and nutritional homeostasis. Following the resolution of other clinical problems, the requirements of nutrients for initiating and maintaining growth become major concerns.
- Fats are the main dietary source of energy in the newborn infant, providing up to 50% of the total caloric needs. Fats are thought to be essential for the development of the nervous system and play a critical role in the formation of all cell membranes. They can be stored in large quantities as major energy reserves in a growing and developing infant.
- Dietary proteins supply less than 10% of the daily caloric needs. However, protein intake must supply the amino acids necessary to replace nitrogen lost in protein turnover which may be up to 10% of the total body protein per day.
- Enterally fed babies use carbohydrates as a major source of energy. An intake of glucose less than the optimal rate may result in gluconeogenesis from non-carbohydrate sources such as amino acids. In low birthweight infants glycogen stores are usually lower in the early neonatal period, leading to frequent episodes of hypoglycaemia.
- The method of feeding chosen for a baby depends on his size, maturity and condition. If possible, breast or bottle feeds should be offered but immature babies may have poor sucking and swallowing ability and tube feeding may be necessary. Ill babies may need total parenteral nutrition. The amount of fluid in which the nutrients are given must not exceed the kidneys' ability to cope with its excretion.
- As the baby grows nutritional supplements are necessary. These include vitamins A and D from the age of 1 month to 2 years. Vitamin C is needed both for growth and healing and to aid absorption of iron. Iron supplements are recommended from 4 weeks until the baby is weaned.
- The preterm baby should pass urine within 24 h of delivery and the amount should increase as fluid intake increases. Babies in the neonatal unit should have their urinary output measured and the urine tested for glucose and osmolality. Glycosuria may indicate a lower renal threshold for glucose and reduction of the glucose administered will avoid dehydration. Urine osmolality allows decisions to be made about the amount of fluid being administered.
- The passage of meconium may be delayed in small preterm babies, especially in those with respiratory distress syndrome. The presence of blood and mucus in the stools may indicate the serious disorder necrotising enterocolitis.
- The nervous system is developed well enough to feel and react to painful stimuli. Response to pain stimuli may be behavioural, physiological or metabolic. Pain relief includes considering the environment and development of expertise in techniques such as heel prick. Comfort interventions such as stroking can reduce pain as well as pharmacological methods.
- The preterm baby is adapted to an intrauterine environment and the effect of noise, light, handling and positioning may influence the well-being of the baby in the neonatal unit. Noise and light levels can be high and care often necessitates much handling. Severe hearing loss occurs with frequent or continuous exposure to sound over 90 dB and the mean noise inside an incubator should not exceed 60 dB.
- High light levels increase the risk of the preterm baby developing retinopathy of prematurity. The harmful effect of light can be reduced by establishing a day/night pattern of lighting. When noise and light stimulus was reduced at night babies slept on average 2 h in 24 more and increased their weight gain more rapidly than babies who did not undergo the day/night cycling.
- Prolonged nursing in the prone position results in externally rotated hips and everted feet which may delay standing and walking. A lack of careful positioning may result in developmental delay. Preterm babies often develop flattened, elongated and asymmetrical head shapes which can be avoided by frequent changes in the position of the baby's head.
- The immaturity of the preterm baby's immune system makes it easy for infectious organisms to enter his body. The most important aspect of infection prevention is careful washing of hands and forearms as these enter the incubator during care. Each baby should have his own equipment which can be stored in the cupboards under the incubator or cot. Disposable items are useful.
- Babies who are small for gestational age may be affected by asymmetrical growth retardation or symmetrical growth. Most of them are born after the 37th week of gestation and are neurologically mature. The fetal brain undergoes a growth spurt in the last trimester of pregnancy and is vulnerable to lack of oxygen and nutrients. These babies are at risk of hypoxia during labour and hypoglycaemia after delivery.
- SFGA babies may have long-term problems such as hypertension and cardiovascular disease and mature-onset diabetes mellitus. They should be delivered in a maternity hospital with a suitable neonatal unit where immediate care is available. Complications include perinatal asphyxia, meconium aspiration syndrome, hypothermia, hypoglycaemia, polycythaemia and pulmonary haemorrhage.
- The baby who has been growth retarded will have poor energy reserves of both fat and glycogen. These babies lack subcutaneous fat and lose heat rapidly. They are usually active, vigorous and alert, feed well and may not need admitting to a neonatal unit.
- Transitional care wards have been developed in many maternity units to allow mothers to care for neonates with minor problems. Mothers and babies are not separated and the mother is enabled to develop caring skills for her baby. Well babies may be transferred home as long as the surroundings are suitable.
- The early care of these babies in the first 48 h is aimed at prevention of the complications, especially hypoglycaemia. Energy-rich low birthweight formula milk is useful. There is a risk of the rare condition of transient neonatal diabetes mellitus. It is essential to offer follow-up care to ensure that these babies meet their growth and developmental milestones.

References

Barker DJP. 1992 Fetal and Infant Origins of Adult Disease. BMJ Books, London.

Bellefeuille-Reid D, Jakubek S. 1989 Adaptive positioning intervention for premature infants: issues for paediatric occupational therapy practice. British Journal of Occupational Therapy 52(3), 93–96.

Bottos M, Stefani D. 1982 Postural and motor care of the premature baby. Developmental Medicine and Child Neurology 24, 706–707.

Corff KE, Seideman R, Venkataraman PS et al. 1995 Facilitated tucking: a non-pharmacological comfort measure for pain in preterm infants. Journal of Obstetric, Gynaecologic and Neonatal Nursing 24(2), 143–147.

Crowley P. 1997 Corticosteroids prior to preterm delivery. In Neilson JP, Crowther CA, Hodnett ED, Hofmeyr GJ, Keirse MJNC (eds) Pregnancy and Childbirth module of The Cochrane Database of Systematic Reviews, The Cochrane Library. Update Software, Oxford.

Dubowitz LMS, Dubowitz V, Goldberg C. 1970 Clinical assessment of gestational age in the newborn infant. Journal of Paediatrics, 77(1):1–10.

Fetters L. 1986 Sensory-motor management of the high risk neonate. Physical and Occupational Therapy, Pediatrics 6, 217–229.

Gilady Y, Battino S, Reich D et al. 1996 Delivery of the very low birth weight breech: what is the best way for the baby? Israel Journal of Medical Sciences 32 (2), 116–120.

Grant A. 1997 Elective versus selective Caesarean delivery of the small baby. In Neilson JP, Crowther CA, Hodnett ED, Hofmeyr GJ, Keirse MJNC (eds) Pregnancy and Childbirth module of The Cochrane Database of Systematic Reviews, The Cochrane Library. Update Software, Oxford.

Greer F. 1991 Nutritional needs of the full-term and low-birth-weight infant. In Rudolph A (ed) Rudolph's Pediatrics. Appleton and Lange, New York.

Keeble S, Twaddle R. 1995 Assessing neonatal pain. Nursing Standard 10 (1), 16–17.

Kelnar CJH, Harvey D, Simpson C. 1995 The Sick Newborn Baby. Baillière Tindall, London.

Lacy JB, Ohlsson A. 1993 Behavioural outcomes of environmental or care-giving hospital-based interventions for preterm infants: a critical overview. Acta Paediatrica 82, 408–415.

Long GJ, Lucey JF, Philip AGS. 1980 Noise and hypoxaemia in the intensive care unit. Pediatrics 65, 143–145.

Lucas A, Morley R, Cole TJ et al. 1992 Breast milk and subsequent intelligence quotient in children born preterm. Lancet 339, 261–264.

Mann NP, Haddow R, Stokes L et al. 1986 Effect of night and day on preterm infants in a newborn nursery: randomised trial. British Medical Journal 293, 1265–1267.

Marieb EN. 1992 Human Anatomy and Physiology, 2nd edn. Benjamin/Cummings Publishing California

Parkin JM, Hey EN, Clowes JS. 1976 Rapid assessment of gestational age at birth. Archives of Disease in Childhood 51, 259.

Simpson C. 1997a The preterm baby. In Sweet BR with Tiran D (eds) Mayes Midwifery, 12th edn. Baillière Tindall, London, pp 833–851.

Simpson C. 1997b Neonatal surgery and pain. In Sweet BR with Tiran D (eds) Mayes Midwifery, 12th edn. Baillière Tindall, London, pp 921–926.

Stirling HF, Kelnar CJH 1995 Neonatal diabetes. In Kelnar CJH (ed) Childhood and Adolescent Diabetes. Chapman and Hall, London 419–426.

Sweet B. 1997 Mayes' Midwifery. Baillière Tindall, London.

Thomson E. 1996 Small and large babies. In Bennett VR, Brown LK (eds) Myles Textbook for Midwives, 12th edn. Churchill Livingstone, Edinburgh, pp 559–577.

Thomson E, Torley E. Intensive care of the newborn. In Bennett VR, Brown LK (eds) Myles Textbook for Midwives, 12th edn. Churchill Livingstone, Edinburgh, pp 578–560.

Recommended reading

Barker DJP. 1992 Fetal and Infant Origins of Adult Disease. BMJ Books, London.

Bellefeuille-Reid D, Jakubek S. 1989 Adaptive positioning intervention for premature infants: issues for paediatric occupational therapy practice. British Journal of Occupational Therapy 52(3), 93–96.

Corff KE, Seideman R, Venkataraman PS et al. 1995 Facilitated tucking: a non-pharmacological comfort measure for pain in preterm infants. Journal of Obstetric, Gynaecologic and Neonatal Nursing 24(2), 143–147.

Fetters L. 1986 Sensory-motor management of the high risk neonate. Physical and Occupational Therapy, Pediatrics 6, 217–229.

Gilady Y, Battino S, Reich D et al. 1996 Delivery of the very low birth weight breech: what is the best way for the baby? Israel Journal of Medical Sciences 32(2), 116–120.

Grant A. 1997 Elective versus selective Caesarean delivery of the small baby. In Neilson JP, Crowther CA, Hodnett ED, Hofmeyr GJ, Keirse MJNC (eds) Pregnancy and Childbirth module of The Cochrane Database of Systematic Reviews, The Cochrane Library. Update Software, Oxford.

Lucas A, Morley R, Cole TJ et al. 1992 Breast milk and subsequent intelligence quotient in children born preterm. Lancet 339, 261–264.

Mann NP, Haddow R, Stokes L et al. 1986 Effect of night and day on preterm infants in a newborn nursery: randomised trial. British Medical Journal 293, 1265–1267.

Chapter

51 Neonatal cardiovascular and respiratory disorders

In this chapter

INTRODUCTION

These next two chapters can only outline common problems to alert the practitioner to possible neonatal illness. Because of space limitation some conditions that the reader might have wished to read about have been omitted. The reader is referred to textbooks specialising in neonatology or paediatric pathology such as Behrman et al (1992), Hoffman (1991), Kelnar et al (1995) or McCance & Huether (1994).

Young babies can become ill very quickly and in some cases the speed of recognition that all is not well may save life. Any neonate who is causing anxiety should be referred to a medical practitioner, preferably a specialist in the care of the neonate. Some disorders are discussed elsewhere; for instance, haemorrhagic disease of the newborn (Chapter 48), rhesus isoimmunisation and ABO incompatibility (Chapter 14).

CARDIOVASCULAR PROBLEMS

Cardiac conditions

As discussed in Chapter 15, cardiac conditions are responsible for 30% of all congenital malformations, making up the largest group of abnormalities, with an incidence of eight per 1000 live births (Behrman et al 1992). Babies may have cyanotic or acyanotic heart disease and the disorders may lead to different problems of management. Babies may have severe cardiovascular lesions with complicated structural defects. Common abnormalities are divided by Kelnar et al (1995) into those leading to a right-to-left shunt in the heart, accompanied always by central cyanosis, a left-to-right shunt and obstructive disease. Any baby who develops heart failure will develop central and peripheral cyanosis.

Risk factors include:

- women with diabetes mellitus – ventricular septal defect, coarctation of the aorta, transposition of the great vessels;
- babies with Down's syndrome (in 40%) – atrioventricular defect, Fallot's tetralogy, ventricular septal defects, patent ductus arteriosus;
- babies whose siblings or a parent have a cardiac defect;
- rubella infection in pregnancy;
- part of a genetic syndrome.

Table 51.1 *Common cardiac defects and their relative percentage occurrence*

Right-to-left shunt	%	*Left-to-right shunt*	%	*Obstructive disease*	%
Transposition of the great arteries	4	Ventricular septal defect	33	Aortic stenosis	6
Fallot's tetralogy	5	Patent ductus arteriosus	10	Pulmonary stenosis	8
Total anomalous pulmonary venous drainage	1–2	Atrial septal defect	8	Coarctation of the aorta	6

Signs and symptoms in the neonate

One or more of the following features is usually present in babies with cardiac lesions although some are also suggestive of respiratory disorders.

- Tachypnoea
- Dyspnoea
- Cyanosis
- Tachycardia
- Heart murmurs
- Poor feeding ability
- Grunting
- Peripheral oedema
- Poor weight gain
- Cachexia

Any baby presenting with these symptoms must be examined by a paediatrician as soon as possible. Some disorders may not be diagnosed for several weeks as neonatal symptoms may at times be vague.

Investigations

Chest radiograph

Although difficult to achieve, a good film allows the size and position of the heart in relation to the lungs and the mediastinum to be seen. Some disorders have a characteristic heart shape.

Electrocardiogram (ECG)

ECG tracings change rapidly in the first 72 h of life but experienced practitioners may detect abnormalities.

Echocardiography

Echocardiography is a non-invasive technique involving ultrasound scanning that can be carried out at the mother's bedside (Fig. 51.1). Echoes from the heart chambers, valves, the large vessels associated with the heart and other structures can be identified (Simpson 1997a). Many anomalies can be identified in utero by 18 weeks of gestation. Surgical treatment may be initiated in some units solely on the echocardiography findings without undertaking cardiac catheterisation, depending on local expertise and the nature and severity of the cardiovascular lesion (Kelnar et al 1995).

Magnetic resonance imaging (MRI)

MRI scanning gives a clear picture of the anatomy of the heart and is becoming widely used in neonatal care.

Cardiac catheterisation and angiocardiography

These invasive investigations may be necessary in circumstances where cardiac defect(s) or related vascular defect(s) are complex. Cardiac catheterisation may also be used as a method for creating a life saving balloon atrial septostomy in lesions such as transposition of the great arteries. The procedure is carried

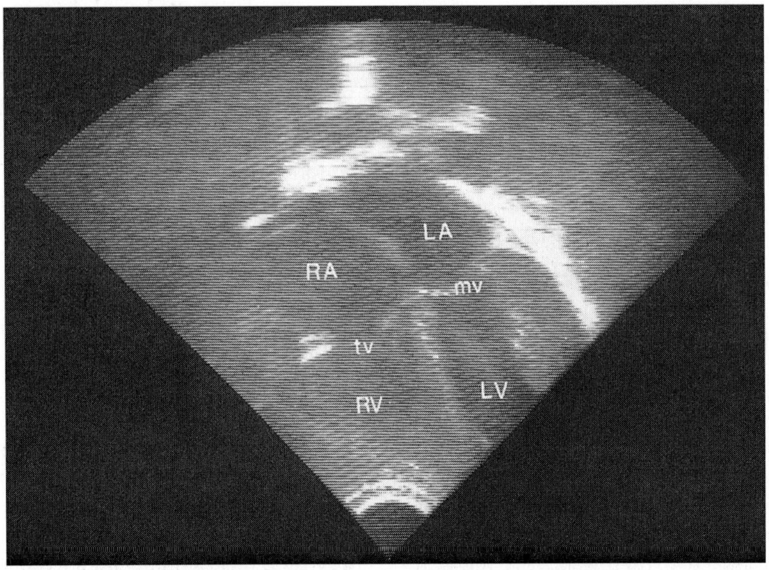

Figure 51.1 *A four chamber echo of the normal heart (LA, left atrium: LV, left ventricle; RA, right atrium; RV, right ventricle; TV, tricuspid valve; MV, mitral valve) (from Kelnar C, Harvey D, Simpson C, 1995, with permission).*

out under a general anaesthetic when a catheter is passed into the femoral vein then into the right side of the heart, and into the pulmonary artery and its branches. If there is a septal defect it may be possible to pass the catheter into the left side of the heart. Abnormal tracts can be identified and blood pressure and oxygen saturation within the heart and great vessels can be measured (Simpson 1997a).

Blood gases

Arterial blood gases from a baby breathing air followed by 100% oxygen can provide good evidence for a differential diagnosis of a right-to-left shunt in cyanotic heart disease. PO_2 seldom exceeds 25 kPa in a baby with cyanotic heart disease breathing 100% oxygen whilst a baby cyanotic because of a lung disorder will usually have a higher level of arterial oxygen. This test may provoke closure of the ductus arteriosus which may be disastrous in some babies who are dependent on ductal blood flow. Prostaglandin should be immediately available (Kelnar et al 1995), administered intravenously in order to induce the reopening of the ductus arteriosus for clinical reasons.

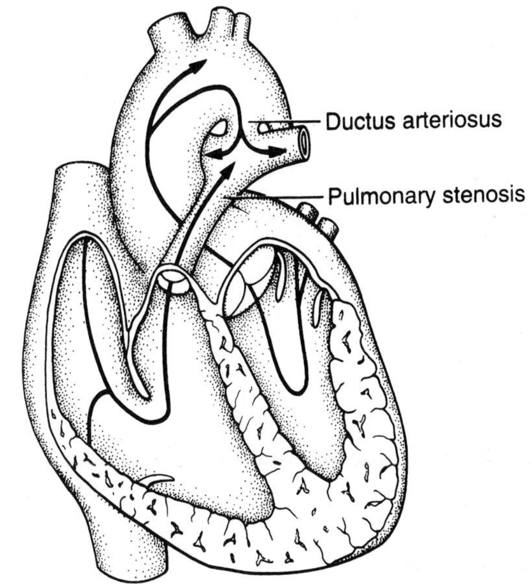

Figure 51.2 *Persistent ductus arteriosus in the presence of pulmonary stenosis (from Fitzgerald MJT, Fitzgerald M, 1994, with permission).*

Acyanotic lesions

Patent ductus arteriosus (PDA)

In a term infant the ductus arteriosus usually closes by 15 h following birth. Closure in the preterm infant may take up to 3 months when the specialised contractile tissue which enables the ductus to close develops. This usually occurs spontaneously. PDA is twice as common in baby girls as in boys. In circumstances where the ductus arteriosus remains open, pulmonary resistance is reduced at birth, blood flow is reversed and flows through a PDA from left to right, shunting oxygenated blood back into the pulmonary circulation. The ductus arteriosus may remain open when certain cardiac anomalies such as pulmonary stenosis are present (Fig. 51.2). Congestive cardiac failure, pulmonary hypertension and subacute bacterial endocarditis are complications most common in the preterm baby with respiratory distress syndrome.

Symptoms of PDA usually arise between the 3rd and 7th days following birth and the baby develops tachypnoea, dyspnoea and lethargy. Systolic and diastolic murmurs are almost always present. Treatment includes restriction of fluids and adequate oxygen administration. Indomethacin may be used to close the PDA in preterm babies but is not effective in the full-term baby (Kelnar et al 1995). Indomethacin is transported around the circulation by serum albumin and may displace bilirubin, leading to jaundice. Digoxin and diuretics may be necessary if congestive heart failure develops and surgical ligation may be tried if medical management fails (McCance & Huether 1994).

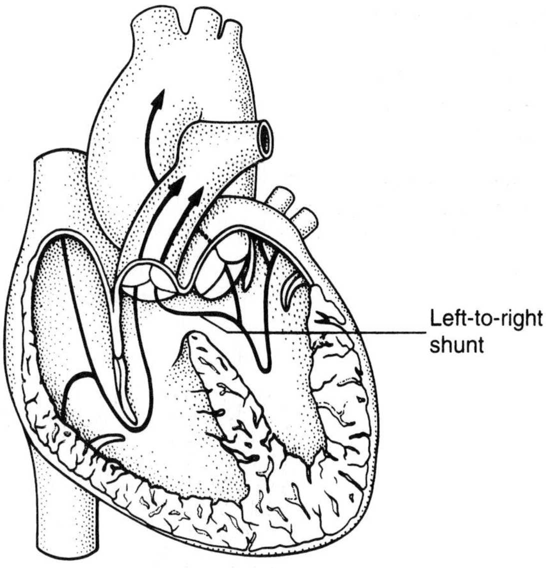

Figure 51.3 *Ventricular septal defect (from Fitzgerald MJT, Fitzgerald M, 1994, with permission).*

Ventricular septal defect (VSD)

A ventricular septal defect usually occurs as an isolated cardiac abnormality but it may be associated with other abnormalities in 50% of children with congenital heart lesions. The membranous septum is the most common site but a defect may occur anywhere in the interventricular septum (Fig. 51.3). Defects vary in size from minute openings to almost complete absence of the interventricular septum. Precise anatomical definition of the defect(s) is critical because some forms of ventricular septal defects have a high incidence of spontaneous closure whereas others do not and are consequently more likely to lead to complications such as congestive cardiac failure and failure to thrive. Small VSDs cause no symptoms and may close spontaneously in 80% of all babies with a VSD.

VSD is an acyanotic heart defect with increased pulmonary blood flow. Because pressure is higher in the left ventricle, the defect in the ventricular septum allows a left-to-right flow of blood through. In circumstances where there are multiple VSDs, a left-to-right shunt develops equalising pressure in both ventricles. The rise in right intraventricular pressure is almost entirely attributable to the ongoing shunting of oxygenated blood from the left ventricle directly to the right ventricle. This causes right ventricular volume overload.

In turn, the abnormal increase in the right ventricular volume gives rise to pulmonary plethora or increased blood flow to the lungs via the pulmonary artery. The persistent increase in pulmonary blood volume contributes to an increase in the pulmonary venous return to the left side of the heart. Not surprisingly, this unusual haemodynamic situation eventually contributes to left ventricular volume overload and exacerbation of the existing left-to-right shunt and to left ventricular hypertrophy. For a time the enlarged left ventricle pumps more efficiently but eventually heart failure occurs. Pulmonary hypertension also occurs. This is **Eisenmenger's syndrome** and cyanosis usually occurs. It is usually fatal but is almost never seen in neonates (McCance & Huether 1994).

If the VSD is large, there will be a loud murmur heard shortly after birth. Congestive cardiac failure will develop between 4 and 12 weeks after birth. Treatment with diuretics and digoxin is commenced until surgery can be performed. If possible, surgery is delayed until the infant is aged 1 year or more but the VSD which shows no sign of spontaneous closure must be closed surgically before permanent lung changes occur.

Atrial septal defect

Interference with the development of the future atrial septum may result in the formation of a variety of atrial septal defects. Atrial septal effects may be **simple**, with a hole in the septum, or **complex** with involvement of the tricuspid or mitral valve. Severe atrioventricular defects may involve the ventricular septum, mitral and tricuspid valves. The most common of these defects are as follows.

- **Septum primum with endocardial cushion defects** This form of lesion is generally associated with abnormalities of the mitral and tricuspid valves and atrioventricular canals (Fig. 51.4b). Although it may occur in isolation in otherwise normal infants, the most frequent occurrence of this defect is in infants born with trisomy 21 (Down's syndrome). The involvement of the endocardial cushions may contribute to the defective formation of the upper portion of the intraventricular septum.
- **Ostium secundum** A characteristic defect found in the central portion of the atrial septum. Because of its close anatomic association with the fossa ovalis, this defect may be appropriately known as the **fossa ovalis defect** (Fig. 51.4a).
- **Sinus venosus defect** This form of atrial septal defect is characteristically found in the superior portion of the atrial septum. The defect generally extends into the superior vena cava.

Simple defects cause few problems and repair can be carried out at about 5 years of age. The shunt is usually from left to right in a simple ASD and no cyanosis occurs. There is a poor prognosis for babies with atrioventricular defects (AVD), many of whom do not survive surgery. Babies with complex defects are usually diagnosed in the first few weeks when they develop dyspnoea, poor feeding and failure to thrive. Mild cyanosis occurs and abnormal heart sounds include a systolic murmur (Simpson 1997a). About 30% of babies with AVD have Down's syndrome.

Cyanotic lesions

Transposition of the great arteries (TGA)

A complete transposition of the great arteries is the most common cardiovascular cause of peripheral and central cyanosis in newborn infants. In this defect, the aorta arises from the right ventricle and the pulmonary artery arises from the left ventricle, a complete switch between the great vessels (Fig. 51.5). The transposition leads to the formation of two completely separate and closed circulatory systems so blood from the pulmonary system cannot enter the systemic system and vice versa. These babies survive long enough to be treated because of the patency of the right-to-left shunts of the ductus arteriosus and/or the foramen ovale. There is sometimes an accompanying VSD which also allows mixing of the oxygenated and deoxygenated

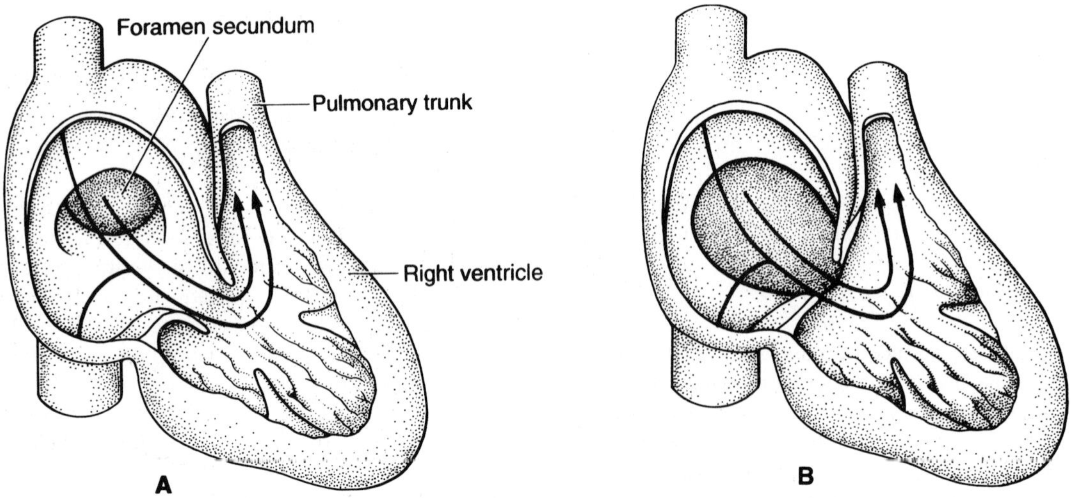

Figure 51.4 *(a) Ostium secundum lesion. (b) Ostium primum lesion (from Fitzgerald MJT, Fitzgerald M, 1994, with permission).*

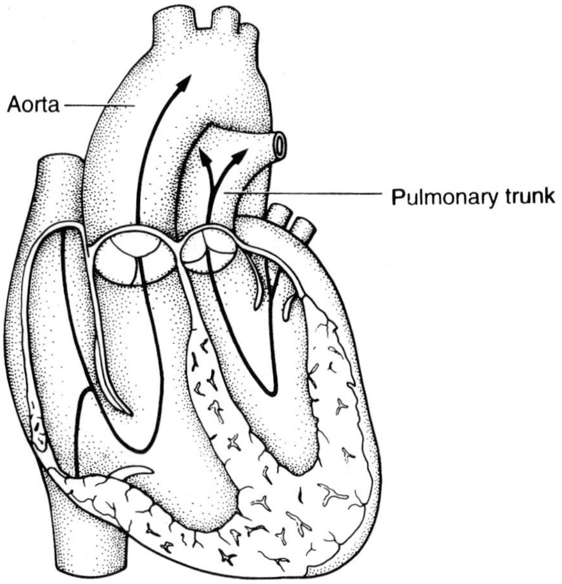

Figure 51.5 *Transposition of great arteries (from Fitzgerald MJT, Fitzgerald M, 1994, with permission).*

blood (Wolfe & Wiggins 1991). Boys are affected twice as often as girls.

Within 24 h of birth the baby who has a complete transposition and no VSD will become increasingly cyanotic as the ductus arteriosus begins to close. The cyanosis is not relieved by the administration of 100% oxygen and urgent treatment is needed to save life. Prostaglandin is given to maintain a PDA until the baby can be transferred for palliative or corrective surgery (Kelnar et al 1995). A **balloon septostomy** (e.g. Rashkind's) is carried out as an emergency treatment to enlarge the foramen ovale and surgical repair can begin as early as 2 weeks (Fig. 51.6). The **Jatene arterial switch**, where the arteries are physically reversed, has a survival rate of up to 90% (McCance & Huether 1994).

Total anomalous pulmonary venous drainage (TAPVD)

Total anomalous pulmonary venous connection is characterised by the absence of any direct connection between the pulmonary veins and the left atrium. The pulmonary veins are in this instance connected to the right atrium or various systemic veins which drain into the right atrium, such as the superior vena cava, the coronary sinus or the ductus venosus.

About 30% of this small group of babies with TAPVD have other cardiac anomalies. There is a right-to-left shunt of blood at atrial or ventricular level allowing mixed arterial and venous blood to circulate to the lungs and body. Central cyanosis, dyspnoea, tachypnoea and congestive cardiac failure occur and urgent surgical correction is necessary but mortality is between 15% and 50% (Kelnar et al 1995).

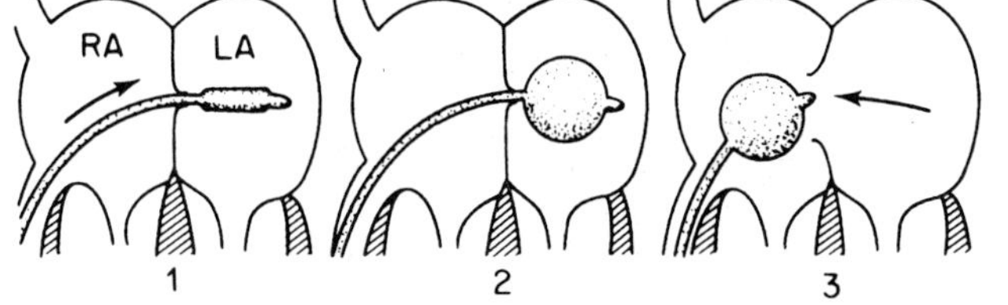

Figure 51.6 *Rashkind's atrial septostomy. 1. A catheter is passed into the right atrium (RA) and pushed through the foramen ovale into the left atrium (LA). 2. A balloon at the tip of the catheter is inflated. 3. The catheter is withdrawn sharply so that the inflated balloon tears the atrial septum, allowing oxygenated blood to reach the systemic circulation. (Reproduced with permission from Wallis & Harvey 1979.)*

Tetralogy of Fallot

The tetralogy of Fallot classically consists of four anatomic defects (Fig. 51.7).

1 A high, large ventricular septal defect.
2 An overriding aorta which straddles the VSD.
3 Pulmonary stenosis – a funnel-shaped opening at the entrance to the pulmonary artery. The pulmonary artery and valve may rarely be completely obliterated.
4 Right ventricular hypertrophy developing because of the obstruction to blood flow.

The defects are associated with Down's syndrome (trisomy 21), first-trimester rubella infection and Noonan's syndrome, similar to Turner's syndrome but in a male with short stature, low-set ears and webbing of the neck. Testicular function may be normal but fertility is decreased. Chromosomes appear normal and the cause is not yet known (Anderson et al 1994).

The clinical features of this defect reflect the magnitude of the neonate's pulmonary blood flow. This in turn depends on the severity of the right ventricular outflow tract obstruction, the relative resistance to ventricular outflow imposed by the systemic and pulmonary circulations and the presence of

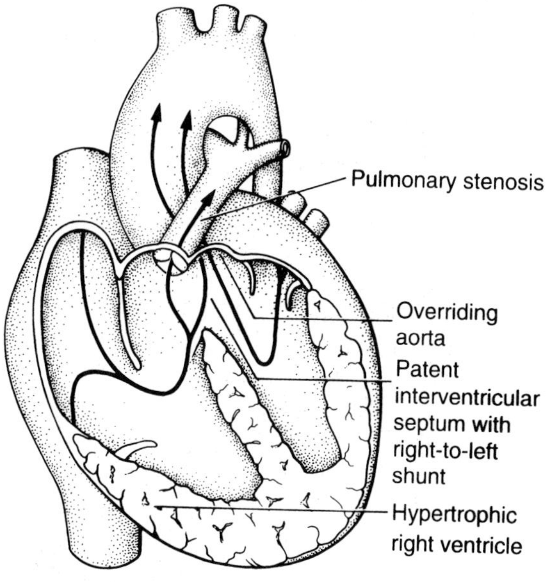

Figure 51.7 *Tetralogy of Fallot (from Fitzgerald MJT, Fitzgerald M, 1994, with permission).*

systemic-to-pulmonary collateral blood flow through the bronchial arteries or, rarely, a persistent ductus arteriosus.

The symptoms vary, depending mainly on the degree of pulmonary stenosis although the size of the VSD is important. Stenosis decreases the flow of blood to the lungs and the return of oxygenated blood to the left side of the heart. If there is a large VSD blood may shunt from right to left, causing a further reduction in oxygen content, and cyanosis may be present. However, giving oxygen causes the PDA to close which increases the degree of cyanosis. More red cells will be produced, resulting in polycythaemia. Older children are likely to have sudden spells of dyspnoea, cyanosis and restlessness and typically squat to alleviate these hypoxic episodes. Surgical correction is necessary.

Infants born with tetralogy of Fallot and pulmonary atresia usually require specialist surgical intervention of a corrective or palliative nature in the first few days or weeks of life. All infants born with tetralogy of Fallot manifesting in growth failure or history of congestive cardiac failure should be evaluated and treated in a specialist cardiac centre for children.

Obstructive lesions

Coarctation of the aorta

In this condition there is an abnormal narrowing of the aorta anywhere between the origin of the aortic arch and the bifurcation of the abdominal aorta at its lower end. Commonly, it occurs at the junction with the ductus arteriosus (Allen et al 1988) with 98% of cases being at this site (Behrman et al 1992). The narrowing may be before (**preductal**), as shown in Figure 51.8, at or after (**postductal**) the opening of the ductus arteriosus. Collateral arteries develop to bypass the obstruction.

In postductal coarctation, circulation to the upper body is from the ascending aorta via the subclavian arteries and blood pressure to the upper body is increased. Blood supply to the lower extremities via the descending aorta is decreased, resulting in decreased or absent femoral pulses and cyanosis of the lower extremities. Coarctation results in obstruction to the outflow from the left ventricle and possible development of left ventricular failure. Once heart failure has developed generalised cyanosis occurs.

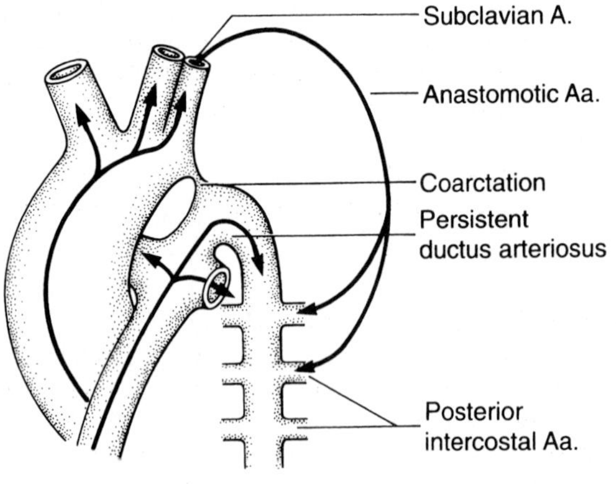

Figure 51.8 *Preductal coarctation of the aorta (from Fitzgerald MJT, Fitzgerald M, 1994, with permission).*

Preductal coarctation is associated with other anomalies and the ductus arteriosus may remain patent, creating a shunt where blood may flow in either direction depending on the pressure differences in the aorta and pulmonary artery. If blood flows from right to left, the right ventricle acts as a systemic pump and the blood pressure and pulse differences between the upper and lower extremities disappear. If the blood flow is left to right more than the normal amount of blood will be sent to the lungs, causing congestive heart failure with left ventricular hypertrophy.

Congestive heart failure is usually the first sign and must be treated. High oxygen levels must be avoided and prostaglandins may be given to maintain patency of the ductus arteriosus. Diuretics such as frusemide 1 mg/kg body weight are given to decrease fluid overload and oedema. Surgical resection is carried out when the child's condition is stable.

Pulmonary valve stenosis and aortic valve stenosis

Narrowing of the pulmonary valve occurs on its own in about 8% and aortic stenosis in 6% of congenital cardiac abnormalities. Mild cases of both valvular defects improve with age and even severe narrowing causes few symptoms in neonates. Surgical correction may be necessary in children who are experiencing low exercise tolerance or heart failure.

Congestive cardiac failure

Congestive cardiac failure is a syndrome in which the failing heart cannot sustain a normal cardiac output and consequently is unable to supply adequate volumes of oxygenated blood to the tissues. The major causes of congestive cardiac failure in the newborn infant are excessive volume overload, excessive pressure load and abnormal myocardial function.

Excessive volume overload

Large valve incompetence or left-to-right shunts are the most common causes of volume overload. In the newborn infant, the cause of the volume overload is likely to be attributed to a patent ductus arteriosus, large ventricular septal defects or endocardial cushion defects with gross valve incompetence. Less commonly, volume overload may be initiated by excessive placental transfusion at the time of birth.

Excessive pressure load

Severe forms of aortic stenosis and coarctation of the aorta, commonly referred to as **left ventricular outflow tract obstruction**, may cause severe forms of congestive cardiac failure within the first month following birth. Infants suffering with either of these lesions are likely to present with very poor pulses and a large left-to-right shunt at the atrial level. Consequently, in the initial period following birth the infant is likely to present with right-sided congestive cardiac failure which may be attributed to the moderately severe pulmonary hypertension. Once the intraatrial left-to-right shunt reverses or a large right-to-left shunt develops through the ductus arteriosus, the infant will present with moderately severe peripheral and central cyanosis.

Myocardial dysfunction

Hatch et al (1995) argue that the fetal and neonatal myocardium develops much less active tension during isometric contraction than the myocardium of an adult. Furthermore, in the adult, 60% of the myocardium is a contractile mass, whereas in the newborn infant or fetus the myocardium is much less compliant, resulting in a significant reduction in the myocardial contractile force. Myofibrils are sparse and randomly organised. It is therefore likely that the filling pressures in the heart of a newborn infant must be higher in comparison to the values seen in adults to optimise myofilament alignment.

At birth the morphology of the two ventricles is similar. However, as the infant's physiological pulmonary vascular resistance falls, the right ventricle gradually adapts, losing power as it pumps to a low resistance system that does not require as much muscular effort.

Normal myocardial function in the neonate

The myocardium of a neonate has less sarcoplasmic reticulum. Therefore it is more dependent on transsarcolemmal calcium influx than the mature, adult myocardium. This is because the mature myocardium stores calcium in its sarcoplasmic reticulum. This maturational phenomenon explains why there is a significant though shortlived increase in ventricular performance in infants given bolus doses of calcium.

Hatch et al (1995) hold that the neonatal myocardium is much less susceptible to hypoxia than the mature adult myocardium. This reflects a greater neonatal capacity for anaerobic metabolism. Similarly there is evidence to suggest that the neonatal myocardium displays a greater resistance to acidosis. This may be partly attributable to a greater buffering capacity of the immature myocytes which allow smaller changes in intracellular pH.

Causes of neonatal myocardial dysfunction

Reed et al (1995) and Rudolph (1996) maintain that the most likely causes of myocardial dysfunction in neonates may be attributed to myocardial ischaemia caused by an anomalous coronary artery. However, in neonates, the myocardium can also be severely depressed by metabolic abnormalities such as severe postpartum asphyxia or marked hypoglycaemia, hypocalcaemia and hypomagnesaemia. Arrhythmias such as congenital heart block or paroxysmal tachycardias can cause cardiac failure in both the fetus and neonate. However, as the tachycardias in neonates are often intermittent, difficulties may occur in diagnosing the condition.

All causes of congestive cardiac failure must be effectively diagnosed and treated to avoid permanent damage not only to the heart as a physiological pump but also to the entire cardiorespiratory system.

Common manifestations of congestive cardiac failure

According to Rudolph (1996), the most common manifestations of congestive cardiac failure in a newborn infant are tachypnoea, pulmonary oedema, cyanosis, diaphoresis, feeding difficulties and, occasionally, periorbital or peripheral oedema.

In the light of possible complexities of the causes of congestive cardiac failure, it is essential that the neonate is examined by a specialist neonatologist with experience in cardiovascular paediatric medicine. Effective diagnosis and efficient treatment of the congestive cardiac failure and its underlying causes are essential if the neonate's survival and quality of life are to be assured.

RESPIRATORY PROBLEMS

This section of the chapter is about lower respiratory tract problems in the neonate. Breathing difficulties make up the commonest problems of newborn babies and it is often difficult to make a clearcut diagnosis, even after examining a chest X-ray. A further problem which is difficult to rule out is that of infection and many babies are treated with antibiotics until the results of any specimens sent for culture are known. Time of onset is an important factor in confirming a diagnosis, as are the birth records. A major problem is the differential diagnosis of cyanosis which may be caused by respiratory disorders or congenital heart disease (Kelnar et al 1995). Babies with respiratory problems will usually need caring for in a neonatal intensive care unit (Fig. 51.9). Birth asphyxia is dealt with in Chapter 46.

Respiratory distress syndrome (RDS)

At birth the baby initiates breathing and the lungs, which have been filled with fluid in utero, are now inflated with air. There is a marked increase in pulmonary blood flow as the vascular tree expands and there is a 10-fold increase in pulmonary capillary blood. Surfactant is a collection of fatty substances called phospholipids including lecithin and sphingomyelin. It begins to be secreted into the lung alveoli from about 22 weeks with surges at 33 weeks and again at birth. It coats the inner aspect of the alveoli and reduces surface tension, so that the alveoli do not collapse at the end of expiration. Before 34 weeks the ratio of lecithin to sphingomyelin (L:S ratio) is 1:1 but the amount of lecithin increases until the ratio is 2:1 in the mature lung. Amniotic fluid contains these substances in their ratios and the L:S ratio can be tested to establish lung maturity.

Respiratory distress syndrome of the newborn is also referred to as **hyaline membrane disease** (HMD). This severe lung disorder is responsible for more neonatal deaths than any other condition, especially affecting between 5% and 10% of preterm infants when it is responsible for up to 70% of deaths. It is rarely seen after 37 weeks gestation (Kelnar et al 1995) but it is fairly common in term infants born to mothers suffering from diabetes mellitus.

Predisposing factors depend on lung maturation and most cases occur in babies born before term. Other important factors include:

- being male;
- birth by CS prior to the onset of labour;
- infants of diabetic mothers, regardless of gestational age, sex and mode of delivery, may have delayed lung maturity (Hollingsworth 1992);
- asphyxia neonatorum, because respiratory and metabolic acidosis interferes with the production of surfactant;
- hypovolaemia or hypervolaemia;
- maternal antepartum haemorrhage;

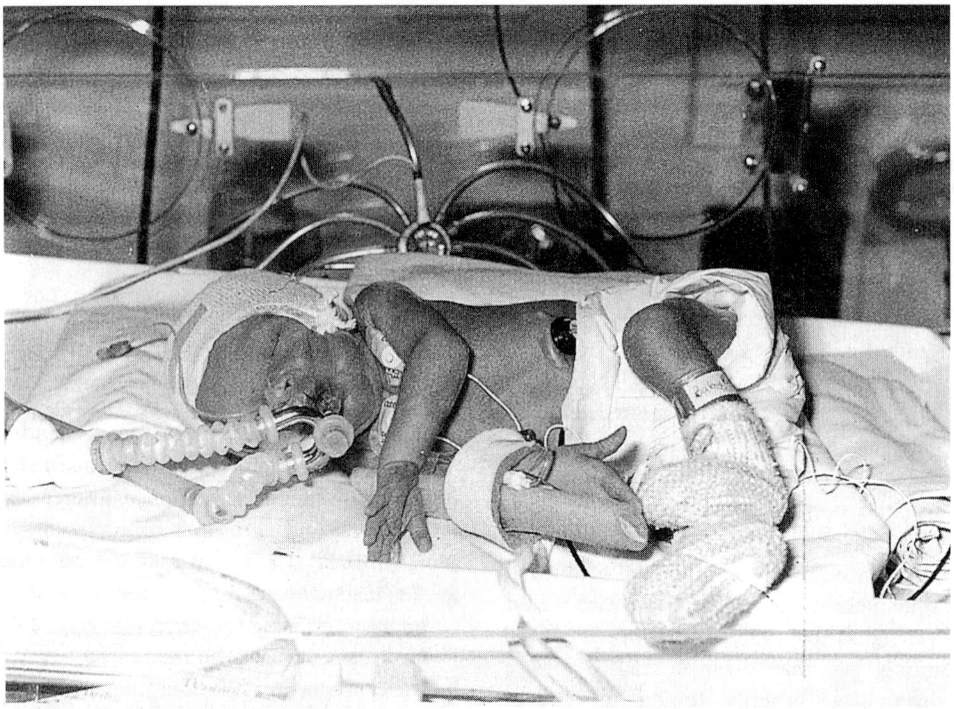

Figure 51.9 *A baby having assisted ventilation (from Sweet B, 1997, with permission).*

- shock;
- drug addiction.

Some maternal problems of pregnancy increase the amount of surfactant produced. Examples are hypertensive disorders and prolonged rupture of the membranes.

Pathophysiology

RDS is caused by a deficiency in surfactant production by the type II cells lining the lung alveoli which is associated with gestational age. Increasing inspiratory effort is needed to keep the alveoli open. The main problem in RDS is **atelectasis**, which is inadequate expansion or collapse of lung tissue, preventing respiratory gas exchange (Anderson et al 1994). Pressures in adjacent alveoli are unequal and some take longer to fill whilst others fill normally. The normal alveoli become overdistended and the smaller alveoli collapse, reducing functional residual capacity and creating dead space within the lungs (Blackburn & Loper 1992).

The resulting blood picture is one of hypoxia and hypercapnia which leads to vasoconstriction of the pulmonary artery. There is persistent fetal circulation with right-to-left shunting of blood through the foramen ovale and ductus arteriosus. Lung ischaemia exacerbates the damage to the epithelial surfaces of alveoli and capillaries. Metabolic and respiratory acidosis develop progressively and further decrease the production of surfactant (Simpson 1997b).

The increased alveolar surface tension combined with the low plasma protein levels present in the preterm baby lead to a shift of interstitial fluid towards the alveolar space. The exudate is rich in fibrinogen which is converted to fibrin which lines the alveoli. Blood products and cellular debris present within the alveoli are bound by the fibrin, resulting in the formation of hyaline membrane which further reduces lung surface area (Blackburn & Loper 1992). Recovery occurs if there is regeneration of alveolar tissue with increasing surfactant production.

Clinical symptoms

Affected babies do not present with symptoms at birth but gradually over the next few hours, typically about 4 h after birth, the neonate develops tachypnoea with increased respiratory effort and grunting on expiration. There is chest wall recession and cyanosis develops (Fig. 51.10). A chest X-ray will show a 'ground-glass' appearance with an air bronchogram (Fig. 51.11), where air is visible in the larger airways against the background opacity (Kelnar et al 1995).

Management

Prebirth maternal treatment with corticosteroids

Management of RDS includes prevention and treatment. It is possible to increase the production of surfactant in the fetal lung before delivery if time allows by treating the mother with a corticosteroid such as betamethasone for at least 24 h before birth. Indications for commencing corticosteroid administration may be finding a low L:S ratio or, if this invasive test is not possible, when there is an expectation of preterm birth. Crowley (1997) carried out a thorough review of the research, finding that this treatment reduces the risk of RDS in susceptible babies and also the morbidity and mortality.

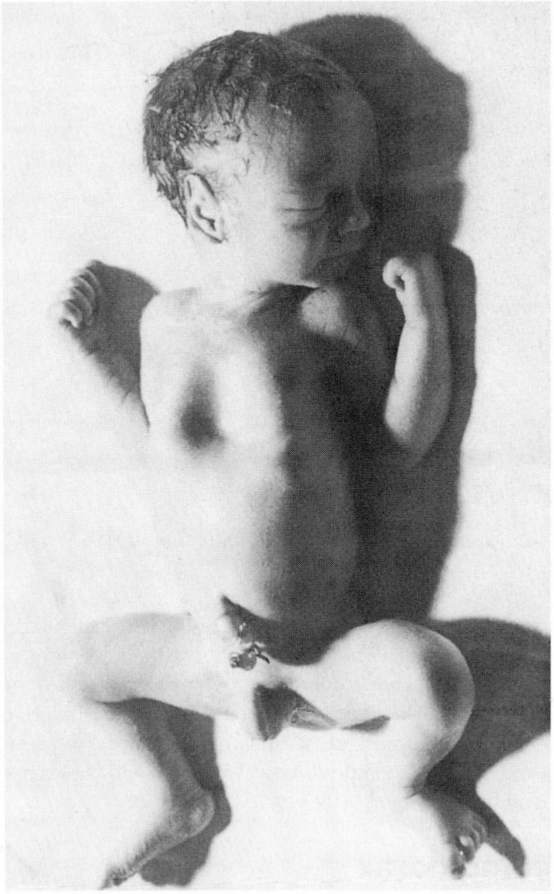

Figure 51.10 *A baby with respiratory distress syndrome (RDS). Note marked sternal recession (from Kelnar C, Harvey D, Simpson C, 1995, with permission).*

Surfactant therapy

The use of natural surfactant postdelivery has been widespread and artificial surfactant is also now available. Soll (1997a, b) has undertaken two substantive reviews of research into surfactant therapy, concerning the benefits or otherwise of natural versus synthetic surfactant and multiple versus single dose of natural surfactant. To summarise these two reviews, both natural and artificial surfactant were shown to be effective in the treatment of established RDS but there was earlier improvement in the need for ventilatory support with fewer cases of pneumothorax in those babies treated with natural surfactant extract. Multiple doses of natural surfactant extract resulted in greater improvements in oxygen and ventilatory needs and a decreased risk of pneumothorax. Multiple doses of natural surfactant extract therefore appears to be the most effective treatment.

Oxygen therapy

Oxygen therapy is necessary to prevent hypoxic brain damage. For some babies, introducing humidified oxygen into a headbox to provide oxygen-rich air is all that is needed. For others it is necessary to reduce the work of breathing by providing a **continuous positive airway pressure** (CPAP) of 5–10 cmH_2O within the alveoli at the end of expiration. Very small babies or those with severe RDS may require mechanical ventilation by intermittent positive pressure ventilation (IPPV) (Simpson 1997b).

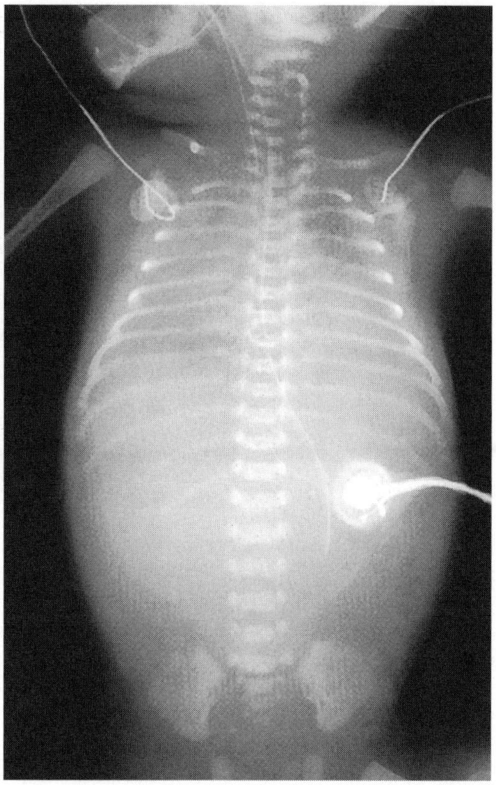

Figure 51.11 *Chest X-ray showing 'ground-glass' appearance of lungs in hyaline membrane disease (from Kelnar C, Harvey D, Simpson C, 1995, with permission).*

Complications of oxygen therapy include the following.

- Long-term IPPV may lead to pneumothorax or bronchopulmonary dysplasia, both of which may lead to periventricular haemorrhage.
- Infection and secondary pneumonia may follow intubation and the lavage and suction needed to keep the tube patent.
- Retinopathy of prematurity may follow the administration of high oxygen concentration.
- The treatment may cause stress with alterations in blood pressure and blood oxygen content.

It is essential to avoid hypothermia and hypoglycaemia, both of which increase oxygen requirements and energy expenditure.

Bronchopulmonary dysplasia

Bronchopulmonary dysplasia is a severe form of lung damage associated with prolonged assisted mechanical ventilation in the neonate. The disorder typically affects babies who weighed less than 1500 g at birth (Kelnar et al 1995). Infants remain oxygen dependent, have respiratory symptoms such as tachypnoea and intercostal recession and abnormal lung findings on radiography (Fig. 51.12) after 28 days (McCance & Huether 1994). There is scarring of the lung tissue with emphysema. Alveoli fail to multiply and there is inflammatory destruction of the ciliated epithelial surfaces in the lung and of the epithelial lining of lung

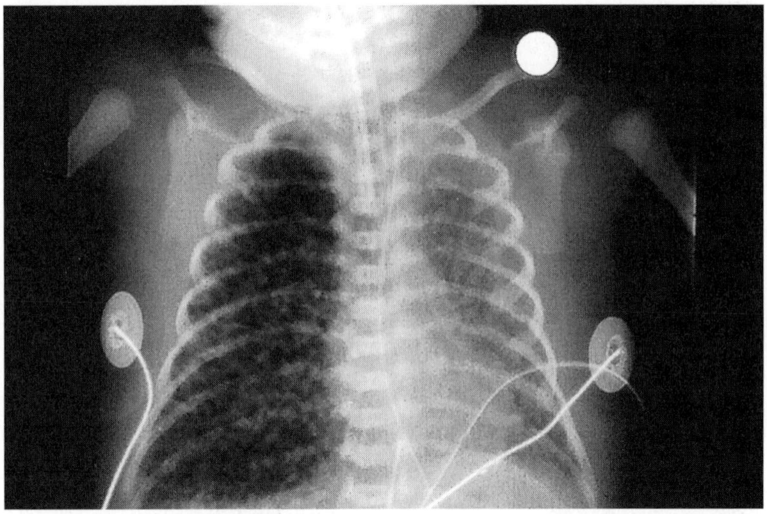

Figure 51.12 *Chest X-ray showing early stages of bronchopulmonary dysplasia (from Kelnar C, Harvey D, Simpson C, 1995, with permission).*

blood capillaries. Mucous plugs and debris clog the airways. The condition may last for months or years and whilst some babies go on to recover, others may die.

Treatment involves maintaining normal oxygen levels, preventing infection and ensuring adequate nutrition. The steroid dexamethasone may be used to reduce the inflammation and improve oxygenation without increasing the risk of infection (Ng 1993) and antibiotics are necessary to control infection. Once the baby's condition is stabilised and the parents know how to manage the oxygen therapy, the baby can be discharged home. A community specialist neonatal nurse will support the family.

Meconium aspiration syndrome (MAS)

If a baby suffers from intrapartum asphyxia he may pass meconium into the amniotic fluid and inhale it as he makes gasping movements. Prompt clearing of the mouth and upper airways at birth should be carried out if there is known to be a risk of inhalation of meconium. If there is thick meconium present on his body, the larynx and trachea should be cleared under direct vision.

Management

Meconium is a good culture base for the development of micro-organisms. Any baby suspected of having inhaled meconium should be observed for signs of respiratory distress manifesting as tachypnoea and cyanosis for the next 24 h. Oxygen therapy is needed and it is usual to use antibiotics to try and prevent the onset of pneumonia. There may be a right-to-left shunt through a persistent fetal circulation. Pneumothorax is a common complication (Kelnar et al 1995).

Surfactant treatment

Meconium in the lung may also inactivate surfactant and Findlay et al (1996) carried out a randomised controlled study of 40 babies. Twenty babies were given up to four doses of surfactant every 6 h to see whether high-dose surfactant therapy would reduce the morbidity of infants with meconium aspiration syndrome. They found that, compared to the control group of babies who received standard treatment, if surfactant therapy was commenced within 6 h of birth oxygenation improved, respiratory morbidity was reduced and babies needed to stay in hospital for shorter periods.

Pneumothorax

Pneumothorax is a condition where a collection of air in the pleural space, following rupture of alveoli, causes a lung to collapse (Anderson et al 1994). It may occasionally be spontaneous but it usually occurs following another respiratory complication. It may follow resuscitation attempts at birth, especially if high pressures have been used to achieve lung expansion. It may occur in babies with RDS or meconium aspiration who have been ventilated or given oxygen by CPAP. Significant reduction in the number of babies developing pneumothorax has followed the introduction of surfactant therapy.

Management

Pneumothorax does not present with the classic symptoms seen in the adult and therefore may be difficult to diagnose. The baby suddenly collapses and becomes cyanotic with bradycardia. There may be cardiac displacement. In small babies transillumination by shining a cold light onto them may demonstrate air around the lung (Kelnar et al 1995). A chest radiograph will confirm the diagnosis (Fig. 51.13). If the baby is in good clinical condition, draining the air is not necessary as it will be reabsorbed. If the baby is distressed and ill, underwater sealed drainage will allow the air to escape and the lung to reexpand.

Transient tachypnoea of the newborn

This condition is quite common and may occur in a term baby who would not be expected to develop RDS, especially if he has

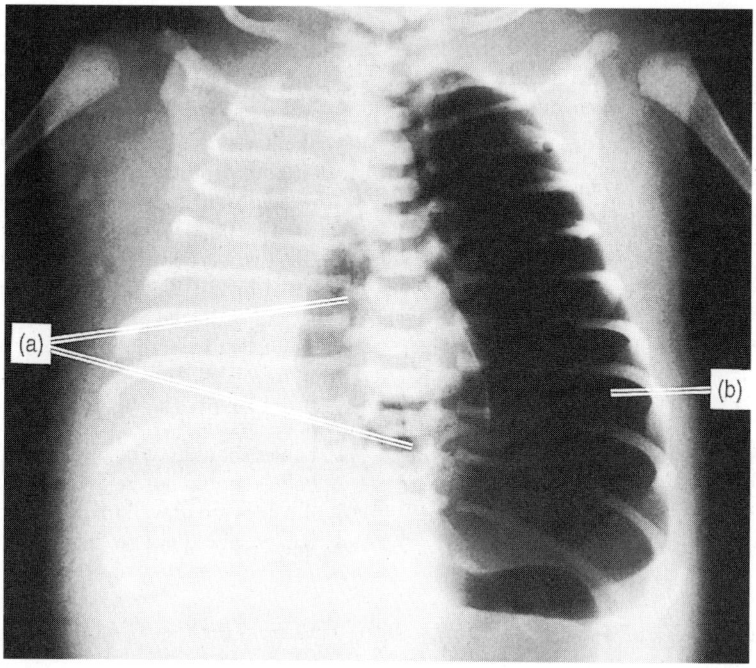

Figure 51.13 *Pneumopericardium (a) with a large left pneumothorax (b) (from Kelnar C, Harvey D, Simpson C, 1995, with permission).*

been delivered by CS. The baby develops a respiratory rate of 60 or more per minute. Rib recession, slight grunting and cyanosis may occur. A chest X-ray will show enlarged lymph vessels which appear as streaks and signs of oedema between the lobes of the lungs (Simpson 1997b). The illness lasts about 24 h. Possible causes include mild surfactant deficiency or failure to absorb lung fluid following delivery. Little treatment is necessary and oxygen should be given if needed. Some neonatologists would commence antibiotics until culture results are known.

Sudden infant death syndrome

A sudden infant death (SID) is one where an infant death is unexpected and remains unexplained by postmortem examination. The term sudden infant death should only be used when it is the only cause of death stated on the death certificate as SIDS, sudden infant death, sudden unexpected death in infancy or cot death (Simpson 1997b). Deaths almost always occur during sleep and the peak incidence of cot death is from 2 to 4 months and it occurs more commonly in winter. Fewer than 1% of the deaths occur in infants under the age of 2 months. Boys are more likely to die than girls and low birthweight babies are at higher risk. McCance & Huether (1994) wrote that 'The greatest single cause of death amongst infants between 1 week and 1 year of age is SIDS'.

The causes of SIDS

SIDS is a complex disorder and although key factors that place infants at risk have been identified, research is still ongoing. These key factors include sleeping position, co-sleeping with parents, overheating, illness and the effect of smoking. The common factor for all but smoking may be an increase in core body temperature.

Position of the larynx

An interesting evolutionary aspect is mentioned by Morgan (1994). Babies are born, as are all mammals, with the larynx in contact with the back of the palate. This facilitates their ability to breathe and swallow simultaneously. Early in infancy, from about the 3rd month, the larynx moves to a position below the back of the tongue, an arrangement necessary for human speech production. However, it results in the openings to the stomach and lungs being side by side low in the throat. Food and drink can now pass inadvertently into the trachea.

The possibility that the change in position may have some bearing on the development of SIDS was postulated by Crelin (1973), although seldom mentioned in medical and nursing books. The risk is highest in the transitional period and once the larynx has reached its new position at 6 months, the risk almost disappears. It is unlikely to be the sole cause but should be kept in mind by researchers. Morgan postulates that in prone position the uvula may enter the larynx and block the airway. If the infant is ill or weak and cannot change the position of its head and neck, suffocation could occur.

Sleeping position

The fashion for placing babies in the prone position for sleeping arose in The Netherlands in the 1970s. It was reasoned that babies were less likely to inhale regurgitated feeds if lying on their stomachs. However, the practice led to a threefold increase in SIDS. Interest in the effects of sleeping position and SIDS culminated in studies in the 1980s that indicated that rates were lowered if young infants were placed on their backs to sleep. Fleming et al (1990) found an eight-fold increase in risk if a baby was placed prone for sleeping rather than on its side or back. Even being placed on the side doubles the risk, possibly because babies can easily roll over onto their stomachs. The slogan 'Back to sleep' has been introduced to encourage mothers to place their babies on their backs to sleep.

Co-sleeping

There may be an increased risk when babies sleep with their parents. Tuffnell et al (1996) found that deep body temperature in infants who co-sleep with their parents was 0.1° higher than in infants who slept alone. Parents are advised to separate their bodies from the baby by making a separate 'nest' for the baby with pillows.

Overheating

Mothers tend to wrap up their babies in the winter months or during illness. The study by Fleming et al (1990) found that babies dying of SIDS tended to have been heavily wrapped, lain prone and to have had the heating on all night.

Smoking

Studies have shown that smoking in pregnancy increases the risk of SIDS ((Mitchell et al 1993, Schoendorf & Kiely 1992). Simpson (1997c) mentions that studies on the effect of passive smoking are not as easy to prove but there may be an increased risk if both parents smoke.

Because of a steady rise in SIDS in England and Wales, peaking at 2.3/1000 live births in 1988, campaigns aimed at reducing the deaths were introduced in 1991 by the Foundation for the Study of Infant Deaths and the Department of Health. Between 1991 and 1995 the SIDS rate in England and Wales, which had already fallen from the high point of 1988 mentioned above, fell 50% from 1.4 to 0.6/1000 live births (Office for National Statistics 1996). The recommendations were that:

1 babies should not be placed upon their fronts to sleep;
2 babies should not be overheated;
3 if babies are unwell medical help should be sought;
4 babies should not be exposed to cigarette smoke.

Summary of main points

- Cardiac conditions are responsible for 30% of all congenital malformations. Babies may have cyanotic or acyanotic heart disease and the disorders may lead to different problems of management. Common abnormalities are divided into those leading to a right-to-left shunt in the heart, accompanied always by central cyanosis, a left-to-right shunt and obstructive disease. Any baby who develops heart failure will become cyanotic.
- Risk factors for congenital heart disease include women with diabetes mellitus, babies with Down's syndrome, babies whose siblings or a parent have a cardiac defect, rubella infection in pregnancy and part of a genetic syndrome. The following features may be present in babies with cardiac lesions: tachypnoea, dyspnoea, cyanosis, tachycardia, heart murmurs, poor feeding, grunting and peripheral oedema.
- Closure of the ductus arteriosus in the preterm infant may take up to 3 months. Patent ductus arteriosus is more common in baby girls than in boys. Treatment includes restriction of fluids and adequate oxygen administration. Indomethacin may be used to close the PDA in preterm babies. Surgical ligation may be necessary if medical management fails.
- Ventricular septal defect may be present in conjunction with other defects in 50% of children with congenital heart lesions. Small VSDs cause no symptoms and may close. In a large defect volume overload leads to left ventricular hypertrophy, pulmonary hypertension and heart failure. Treatment with diuretics and digoxin is commenced. Surgery is delayed until the infant is 1 year old.
- Atrial septal effects may be simple, with a hole in the septum, or complex, with involvement of the mitral valve. Simple defects cause few problems and repair can be carried out at about 5 years of age. The shunt is usually from left to right in a simple ASD and no cyanosis occurs. There is a poor prognosis for babies with atrio-ventricular defects, many of whom do not survive surgery.
- Transposition of the great arteries leads to the formation of two completely separate and closed circulatory systems as blood from the pulmonary system cannot enter the systemic system and vice versa. These babies survive long enough to be treated because of the patency of the right-to-left shunts of the ductus arteriosus and the foramen ovale and the commonly associated VSD.
- Boys are affected twice as often as girls. Within 24 h of birth the baby who has a complete transposition and no VSD becomes increasingly cyanotic as the ductus arteriosus begins to close. Prostaglandin is given to maintain a PDA until the baby can be given surgery. An emergency balloon septostomy will enlarge the foramen ovale. Surgical repair begins as early as 2 weeks.
- In babies with total anomalous pulmonary venous drainage, there is a right-to-left shunt of blood at atrial or ventricular level allowing mixed arterial and venous blood to circulate to the lungs and body. Cyanosis, dyspnoea and tachypnoea occur and urgent surgical correction is necessary.
- The tetralogy of Fallot classically consists of four anatomic defects: a high, large ventricular septal defect, an overriding aorta which straddles the VSD, pulmonary stenosis and right ventricular hypertrophy. Symptoms vary depending on the degree of pulmonary stenosis although the size of the VSD is important. Surgical correction is necessary.
- Coarctation of the aorta commonly occurs at the junction with the ductus arteriosus. Collateral arteries develop to bypass the obstruction. Congestive heart failure is usually the first sign. High oxygen levels must be avoided and prostaglandins may be given to maintain patency of the ductus arteriosus. Diuretics will decrease fluid overload and oedema. Surgical resection is carried out when the child's condition is stable.
- The major causes of congestive cardiac failure in the newborn infant are excessive volume overload, excessive pressure load and abnormal myocardial function. In the newborn infant the cause of the volume overload may be patent ductus arteriosus, large ventricular septal defects or endocardial cushion defects with gross valve incompetence and, less commonly, excessive placental transfusion at the time of birth.
- In the initial period following birth the infant may present with right-sided congestive cardiac failure attributed to moderately severe pulmonary hypertension. Once the intraatrial left-to-right shunt reverses or a large right-to-left shunt develops through the ductus arteriosus, the infant will present with moderately severe peripheral and central cyanosis.
- The most common manifestations of congestive cardiac failure in a newborn infant are tachypnoea, pulmonary oedema, cyanosis, diaphoresis, feeding difficulties and, occasionally, periorbital or peripheral oedema. Effective diagnosis and efficient treatment of the congestive cardiac failure and its underlying causes are essential for survival and quality of life.

- Breathing difficulties make up the commonest problems of newborn babies. A problem is the differential diagnosis of cyanosis which may be caused by respiratory disorders or congenital heart disease. Respiratory distress syndrome is a severe lung disorder responsible for many neonatal deaths. It is caused by a deficiency in surfactant production.
- Increasing inspiratory effort is needed to keep the alveoli open. The main problem in RDS is atelectasis. Pressures in adjacent alveoli are unequal and some take longer to fill whilst others fill normally. Normal alveoli become overdistended and the smaller alveoli collapse, reducing functional residual capacity.
- Hypoxia and hypercapnia lead to vasoconstriction of the pulmonary artery. There is persistent fetal circulation with right-to-left shunting of blood through the foramen ovale and ductus arteriosus. An exudate rich in fibrinogen which is converted to fibrin lines the alveoli. Blood products and cellular debris bound by the fibrin result in the formation of hyaline membrane. Affected babies do not present with symptoms at birth but after about 4 h, the neonate develops tachypnoea with increased respiratory effort and grunting with expiration.
- The production of surfactant in the fetal lung can be increased before delivery by treating the mother with a corticosteroid for at least 24 h before birth. This treatment reduces the risk of RDS in susceptible babies and also the morbidity and mortality. The use of natural surfactant postdelivery has been widespread and artificial surfactant is also now available. Both natural and artificial surfactant are effective in the treatment of established RDS. Oxygen therapy is necessary to prevent hypoxic brain damage.
- Bronchopulmonary dysplasia is associated with prolonged ventilation in the neonate. Infants remain oxygen dependent. The condition may last for months or years and some babies may die. Treatment involves maintaining normal oxygen levels, preventing infection and ensuring adequate nutrition. Dexamethasone may be used to reduce the inflammation and improve oxygenation.
- Any baby suspected of inhaling meconium should be observed for signs of respiratory deterioration for the next 24 h. Oxygen therapy may be needed and it is usual to use antibiotics to prevent the onset of pneumonia. The presence of meconium in the lung may also inactivate surfactant. Surfactant therapy commenced within 6 h of birth improves prognosis and recovery.
- Pneumothorax may occasionally be spontaneous but it usually occurs following another respiratory complication. Significant reduction in the number of babies developing pneumothorax has followed the introduction of surfactant therapy. If the baby is in good condition, draining the air is not necessary as it will be reabsorbed. If the baby is ill, underwater sealed drainage will allow air to escape and the lung to reexpand.
- Transient tachypnoea of the newborn is quite common. The illness lasts about 24 h. Possible causes include mild surfactant deficiency or failure to absorb lung fluid at delivery. Little treatment is necessary and oxygen should be given if needed.
- Sudden infant death almost always occurs during sleep with a peak incidence from 2 to 4 months, commonly in winter. Boys and low birthweight babies are at higher risk. Causative factors include sleeping position, co-sleeping with parents, overheating, illness and parental smoking. The common factor, except for smoking, may be increased core body temperature.
- Babies are born with the larynx in contact with the back of the palate and it descends by 6 months to lie under the back of the tongue. The change in position of the larynx may have some bearing on the development of SIDS. Fleming et al (1990) found an eight fold increase in risk if a baby was placed prone for sleeping rather than on its side or back. Fleming et al (1990) also found that babies dying of SIDS tended to be heavily wrapped and to have had the heating on all night.
- Studies have shown that smoking in pregnancy increases the risk of SIDS. The effect of passive smoking is not as easy to prove but there may be an increased risk if both parents smoke. Because of a steady rise in SIDS in England and Wales, campaigns aimed at reducing the deaths were introduced in 1991.

References

Allen LD, Chita SK, Anderson RH et al. 1988 Coarctation of the aorta in prenatal life: an echocardiographic, anatomical and functional study. British Heart Journal 59, 356–360.

Anderson KN, Anderson LE, Glanze WD (eds), 1994 Mosby's Medical, Nursing and Allied Health Dictionary, 4th edn. Mosby, St Louis.

Behrman RE, Kleigman RM, Nelson WE, Vaughn VC. 1992 Nelson's Textbook of Paediatrics, 14th edn. WB Saunders, Philadelphia.

Blackburn ST, Loper DL. 1992 Maternal, Fetal and Neonatal Physiology, A Clinical Perspective. WB Saunders, Philadelphia.

Crelin E. 1973 Functional Anatomy of the Newborn. Yale University Press.

Crowley P. 1997 Corticosteroids prior to preterm delivery. In Neilson JP, Crowther CA, Hodnett ED, Hofmeyr GJ, Keirse MJNC (eds) Pregnancy and Childbirth module of The Cochrane Database of Systematic Reviews, The Cochrane Library. Update Software, Oxford.

Findlay RD, Taeusch HW, Walther FJ. 1996 Surfactant replacement therapy for meconium aspiration syndrome. Pediatrics 97, 48–52.

Fitzgerald MJT, Fitzgerald M. 1994 Human Embryology. Baillière Tindall, London.

Fleming PJ, Gilbert R, Azaz Y et al. 1990 Interaction between bedding and sleeping position in sudden infant death syndrome: a population based case-control study. British Medical Journal 301, 85–89.

Hatch D Somner E, Hellman J et al. 1995 The Surgical Neonate: Anaesthesia and Intensive Care. Edward Arnold, London.

Hoffman J. 1991 Congenital heart disease. In Rudolph A (ed) Rudolph's Pediatrics. Appleton and Lange, New York.

Hollingsworth DR. 1992 Pregnancy, Diabetes and Birth. Williams and Wilkins, Baltimore.

Kelnar CJH, Harvey D, Simpson C. 1995 The Sick Newborn Baby. Baillière Tindall, London.

McCance KL, Huether SE. 1994 Pathophysiology: The Biologic Basis for Disease in Adults and Children, 2nd edn. Mosby, St Louis.

Mitchell EA, Ford RPK, Stewart AW et al. 1993 Smoking and the sudden infant death syndrome. Pediatrics 91, 893–896.

Morgan E. 1994 The Descent of the Child. Souvenir Press, London.

Ng PC. 1993 The effectiveness and side effects of dexamethasone in preterm infants with bronchopulmonary dysplasia. Archives of Diseases in Childhood 68, 330–336.

Office for National Statistics 1996 Population and Health Monitor DH3 (Sudden Infant Deaths), 96/2. ONS, London.

Reed G, Claireaux A, Cockburn F et al. 1995 Diseases of the Fetus and the Newborn, Vol 1. Chapman and Hall Medical, London.

Rudolph A. 1996 Rudolph's Pediatrics. Prentice-Hall, New Jersey.

Schoendorf KC, Kiely JL. 1992 Relationship of sudden infant death syndrome to maternal smoking during and after pregnancy. Pediatrics 90, 905–908.

Simpson C. 1997a Cardiac and circulatory conditions in the newborn. In Sweet BR with Tiran D (eds) Mayes Midwifery, 12th edn. Baillière Tindall, London, pp 882–888.

Simpson C. 1997b Respiratory disorders of the neonate. In Sweet BR with Tiran D (eds) Mayes Midwifery, 12th edn. Baillière Tindall, London, pp 889–895.

Simpson C. 1997c Sudden infant death syndrome. In Sweet BR with Tiran D (eds) Mayes Midwifery, 12th edn. Baillière Tindall, London, pp 927–932.

Soll RF. 1997a Natural surfactant extract versus synthetic surfactant in the treatment of established respiratory distress syndrome. In Neilson JP, Crowther CA, Hodnett ED, Hofmeyr GJ, Keirse MJNC (eds) Pregnancy and Childbirth module of the Cochrane Database of Systematic Reviews, The Cochrane Library. Update Software, Oxford.

Soll RF. 1997b Multiple versus single dose natural surfactant for severe RDS. In Neilson JP, Crowther CA, Hodnett ED, Hofmeyr GJ, Keirse MJNC (eds) Pregnancy and Childbirth module of the Cochrane Database of Systematic Reviews, The Cochrane Library. Update Software, Oxford.

Sweet B. 1997 Mayes' Midwifery Baillière Tindall, London.
Tuffnell CS, Petersen SA, Wailoo MP. 1996 Higher rectal temperatures in co-sleeping infants. Archives of Diseases in Childhood 75 (3), 249–250.
Wallis S, Harvey D. 1979 Intensive Care of the Newborn 3. Disorders of the Newborn. Nursing Times, 75(31): 1319–1327.
Wolfe R, Wiggins J. 1991 Cardiovascular diseases. In Hathaway W, Groothuis J, Hay W et al (eds) Current Pediatric Diagnosis and Treatment, 10th edn. Appleton and Lange, Norwalk, pp 412–469.

Recommended reading

Crowley P. 1997 Corticosteroids prior to preterm delivery. In Neilson JP, Crowther CA, Hodnett ED, Hofmeyr GJ, Keirse MJNC (eds) Pregnancy and Childbirth module of The Cochrane Database of Systematic Reviews, The Cochrane Library. Update Software, Oxford.
Mitchell EA, Ford RPK, Stewart AW et al. 1993 Smoking and the sudden infant death syndrome. Pediatrics 91, 893–896.
Schoendorf KC, Kiely JL. 1992 Relationship of sudden infant death syndrome to maternal smoking during and after pregnancy. Pediatrics 90, 905–908.
Soll RF. 1997a Natural surfactant extract versus synthetic surfactant in the treatment of established respiratory distress syndrome. In Neilson JP, Crowther CA, Hodnett ED, Hofmeyr GJ, Keirse MJNC (eds) Pregnancy and Childbirth module of the Cochrane Database of Systematic Reviews, The Cochrane Library. Update Software, Oxford.
Soll RF. 1997b Multiple versus single dose natural surfactant for severe RDS. In Neilson JP, Crowther CA, Hodnett ED, Hofmeyr GJ, Keirse MJNC (eds) Pregnancy and Childbirth module of The Cochrane Database of Systematic Reviews, The Cochrane Library. Update Software, Oxford.
Tuffnell CS, Petersen SA, Wailoo MP. 1996 Higher rectal temperatures in co-sleeping infants. Archives of Diseases in Childhood 75(3), 249–250.

Chapter 52 Neonatal jaundice and metabolic disorders

In this chapter

NEONATAL JAUNDICE

Morphological issues

Because fetal growth is of an **ontogenetic** (developmental) nature with respect to the evolutionary process, transition to extrauterine life should ideally only occur when the fetus can survive outside the uterus. At birth those structures and critical functions which are fundamental to postgestational life must have achieved sufficient maturity to permit independent survival. This is true of a variety of vital organ functions, including the formation of bile.

Nevertheless, hepatic disease in neonates is not rare and at times is present as a unique clinical or physiological phenomenon characteristic of the newborn infant. Ontogenetic studies of bile synthesis, metabolism and its subsequent transport across the hepatic and intestinal epithelia have convincingly demonstrated that all the processes are immature in the newborn infant.

As in adults, the neonatal biliary apparatus consists of primary secreting units, the bile canaliculi and a system of collecting tubules delivering the product of hepatocellular secretion onto epithelial lined surfaces, the gallbladder and the duodenum. Bannister et al (1995) hold that the biliary canaliculus is a narrowly constructed tube of approximately 1 μm in diameter formed by the plasma membrane of two hepatocytes joined to each other by occluding junctions.

In functional terms these regions of cell-to-cell attachments represent a barrier to diffusion and bulk flow between plasma and bile. The lumen of the bile canaliculus contains numerous microvilli which increase the surface area of the canalicular membrane. Since only two hepatocytes form a canalicular lumen, most canaliculi communicate with each other and thereby form a complex anastomosing network suited to the continuous drainage of bile.

As with other biological structures, the biliary membranes are permeable to water. Consequently a continuous water exchange between plasma and bile will take place along the entire length of the biliary apparatus. In this respect, all cells, hepatocytes and the bile ductal cells lining the biliary network, can be assumed to be participating in bile synthesis. However, although bile is isotonic with respect to plasma, striking concentration differences exist between the two fluids with respect to a number of solutes such as bile acids. Current physiological concepts suggest that the actual flow of bile is an osmotic process deriving its energy from metabolic sources. Water transport would consequently be a secondary process to the translocation of osmotically active solutes from blood to the biliary tree.

Metabolism of bilirubin

Bilirubin is a catabolic byproduct of haemoglobin derived primarily through the breakdown of haem from haemolysed erythrocytes (Fig. 52.1). It appears that only a small proportion of bilirubin produced in the newborn infant is the direct consequence of ineffective erythropoiesis; most of the bilirubin is synthesised from the breakdown of circulating erythrocytes. Cashmore (1992) suggests that as the erythrocytes are

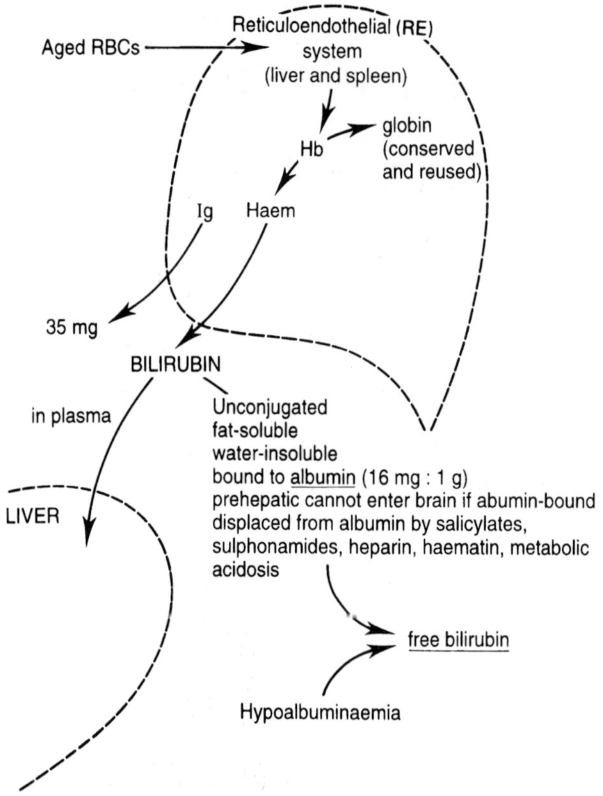

Figure 52.1 *The formation of bilirubin (from Kelnar C, Harvey D, Simpson C, 1995, with permission).*

destroyed, the globin chains are removed and the α double bond is catalysed.

The iron atom at the centre of the haem skeleton is reused while a molecule of carbon dioxide is removed from the haem ring and excreted in a reaction catalysed by the enzyme hepatic haem oxygenase. The degradation of 1 mole of haem to 1 mole of bilirubin releases 1 mole of carbon dioxide. It is therefore possible to estimate the rate of haem degradation from the rate of carboxyhaemaglobin production.

Once released into the bloodstream, molecules of **unconjugated** (sometimes called indirect or prehepatic) bilirubin are tightly bound to serum albumin and transported to the liver for conjugation and excretion (Fig. 52.2). The liver cells easily take up the unbound lipid-soluble bilirubin but need a carrier molecule to take up the bound complex. The unconjugated bilirubin is **conjugated** (joined together, fused) to form bilirubin diglucuronide in the presence of a catalytic enzyme called bilirubin uridine diphosphate (UDP) glucuronyl transferase (Storer 1996). Oxygen and glucose are necessary for this process and hypoxia or hypoglycaemia may slow conjugation (Kelnar et al 1995).

The conjugated (sometimes called direct or posthepatic) bilirubin, which is now water soluble, passes into the bile and enters the intestine. In the terminal ileum and colon some of the bilirubin is metabolised by bacterial activity to produce urobilinogen, known in this form as stercobilinogen, which gives faeces the typical brown colour. In its absence faeces are greyish white (Marieb 1992). Small quantities of urobilinogen enter the circulation and are reexcreted by the liver and kidney as urinary urobilinogen.

Bilirubin in the neonate

Before birth bilirubin clearance is handled by the placenta and maternal system. After birth the liver must take over bilirubin metabolism, a change as complex as the changes in the circulation at birth (Kelnar et al 1995). At birth the intestines contain up to 200 g of meconium, of which 175 g may be bilirubin, about half of which is conjugated. Delay in excretion of meconium may lead to the return of unconjugated bilirubin to the circulation.

Plasma bilirubin concentration

The plasma bilirubin concentration depends on the balance achieved by its production and elimination. In the adult the rates of hepatic uptake, conjugation and excretion of unconjugated bilirubin are highly efficient. In the newborn infant the physiological processes involved in bilirubin conjugation and excretion are considerably less efficient. This phenomenon may be partly attributed to the somewhat dormant behaviour of the fetal hepatic conjugating system and the bowel.

Consequently, newborn infants usually manifest a progressive rise in their plasma unconjugated bilirubin which peaks at 180 μmol/l on the 3rd or 4th day of life, resulting in the clinical condition known as **physiological jaundice**. The possible cause of this physiological jaundice may be attributed to the increase in load of bilirubin to the liver, a decrease in hepatic uptake and a transient deficiency of hepatic bilirubin glucuronyl transferase activity culminating in a reduced excretion of conjugated bilirubin.

The neonate produces about twice as much bilirubin as the adult but levels fall to normal by about 6 weeks. This results from destruction of the large pool of red cells that are not needed after birth, a decreased red blood cell life of 80 days rather than 120 days and increased numbers of immature or fragile cells.

The transport and conjugating mechanisms for unconjugated bilirubin are complex and not fully understood. Newly formed bilirubin is released from the reticuloendothelial system and is tightly bound to plasma albumin. Levels of unbound, unconjugated bilirubin are higher in the neonate because of lower plasma albumin concentrations, decreased albumin-binding capacity and decreased affinity of the albumin for bilirubin, possibly due to an immature albumin molecular structure (Blackburn & Loper 1992). The capacity of a term neonate to excrete bilirubin is only one-fiftieth that of an adult so that all babies have hyperbilirubinaemia by adult standards and jaundice is common (Kelnar et al 1995).

Kernicterus

It is now well established that unconjugated bilirubin is toxic to the central nervous system, even though the precise mechanism of bilirubin toxicity is still not fully understood. The most likely scenario involves the entry and deposition of unconjugated, unbound bilirubin in the central nervous system. This unconjugated, unbound bilirubin fraction appears to be the toxin which disrupts several neural cell functions.

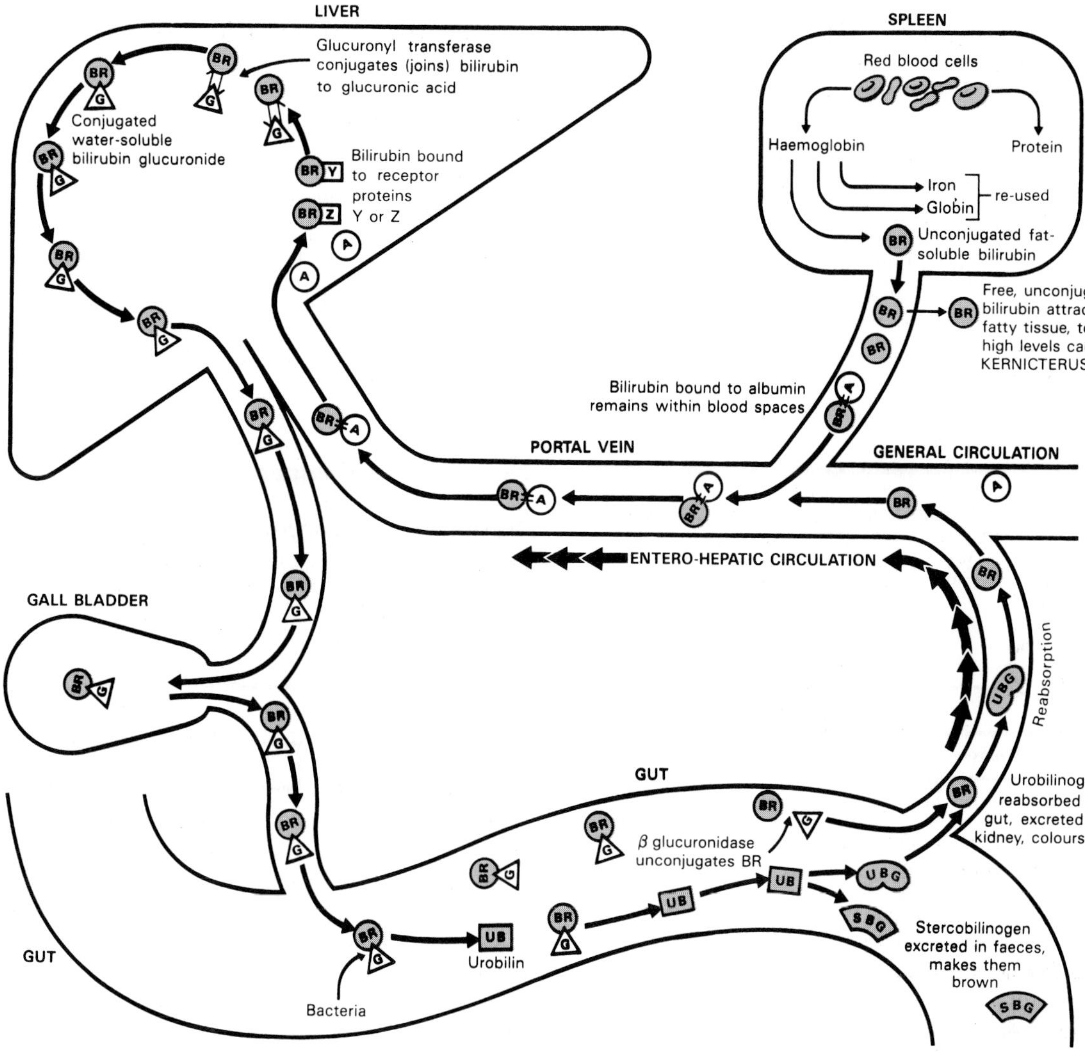

Figure 52.2 *Schematic diagram showing the conjugation of bilirubin. Key: BR bilirubin, = bound to, A albumin, G glucuronic acid, UB urobilin, UBG urobilinogen, SBG stercobilinogen (from Bennett VR, Brown L, 1993, with permission).*

Unconjugated bilirubin is fat soluble and cannot be eliminated. If it cannot be conjugated and there is an increase in free bilirubin, it is deposited in fatty tissue. Neural tissue, in particular the basal ganglia in the brain, contains a high proportion of fat. Molecular unconjugated bilirubin has a high affinity for several of the phospholipids present in the plasma membrane. It appears to form complexes with these phospholipids. Also, the inclusion of protein in membrane vesicles increases the binding of bilirubin to the plasma membranes.

Deposition of bilirubin causes irreversible tissue changes which lead to a condition known as kernicterus (yellow kernel, so-called because the basal ganglia are likened to the stone in the centre of a fruit). Strictly speaking, the word kernicterus refers to staining of the basal ganglia and cranial nerve nuclei. However, the term bilirubin encephalopathy is more appropriately applied in acute clinical findings where the newborn presents with a mild but reversible hyperbilirubinaemia.

However, deposition of unconjugated bilirubin in neural tissue may cause irreversible neural damage. The baby develops muscular twitching, hypertonicity of the limbs and neck retraction. There may be long-term sequelae of cerebral athetosis and mental retardation. This is most likely to happen if the serum bilirubin level rises above 350 μmol/l but paediatricians become anxious if the bilirubin level rises above 250. Kernicterus can be prevented in all but the very small, sick neonate where the blood–brain barrier may be inefficient so that even quite low levels of bilirubin may be damaging to the fragile tissues.

Conjugation of bilirubin

Conjugation may be delayed if there is excessive production of unconjugated bilirubin, so that there is a delay in its binding to serum albumin and deposition in fatty tissue, or if there is low serum albumin. Some of the binding sites may be occupied by other molecules such as the drugs salicylates, sulphonamides, heparin, diazepam and chloramphenicol (Sweet 1997). This could be likened to a large queue at a bus stop. A bus comes along but there is no room for all the passengers and some must wait for the next bus. Some of the bus seats may already be taken up by other passengers. Some people in the queue decide to sit down in the comfort of the bus station.

Jaundice

Jaundice is a common problem sign seen in the neonate and is the yellow colouration of the skin and sclera caused by deposits of bilirubin. It becomes visible when the serum bilirubin rises above 85 µmol/l. Bilirubin is a normal yellowish green bile pigment which, prior to its alteration by the liver, is a weak acid, very soluble in lipid and slightly soluble in water. About 75% of bilirubin is released along with biliverdin when red blood cells are broken down in the mononuclear phagocytic cells of the liver and spleen with the release of haem and globin to the body stores. The rest comes from tissue cytochromes and other haem products (Storer 1996). Excessive bilirubin may enter the bloodstream in three ways (McCance & Huether 1994), all three of which may affect the neonate:

1. during haemolysis of red blood cells;
2. liver disease, which affects the metabolism and excretion of bile;
3. conditions that obstruct the common bile duct.

Investigation and possibly treatment are needed if:

- the jaundice appears within the first 24 h after birth;
- jaundice persists for longer than 2 weeks;
- the total bilirubin level is over 250 µmol/l;
- there is conjugated hyperbilirubinaemia (above 30 µmol/l);
- jaundice appears in an ill baby (Kelnar et al 1995).

Causes of neonatal jaundice

Kelnar et al (1995) divide causes of jaundice into three groups: prehepatic, originating before bilirubin arrives at the liver; hepatic, with problems within the liver; and posthepatic, with obstruction or delay in the posthepatic pathways. A further consideration of importance is whether the free bilirubin is unconjugated or conjugated. Causes of neonatal jaundice, shown in Figure 52.3, include the following.

Prehepatic unconjugated bilirubin

- Physiological jaundice/jaundice of prematurity

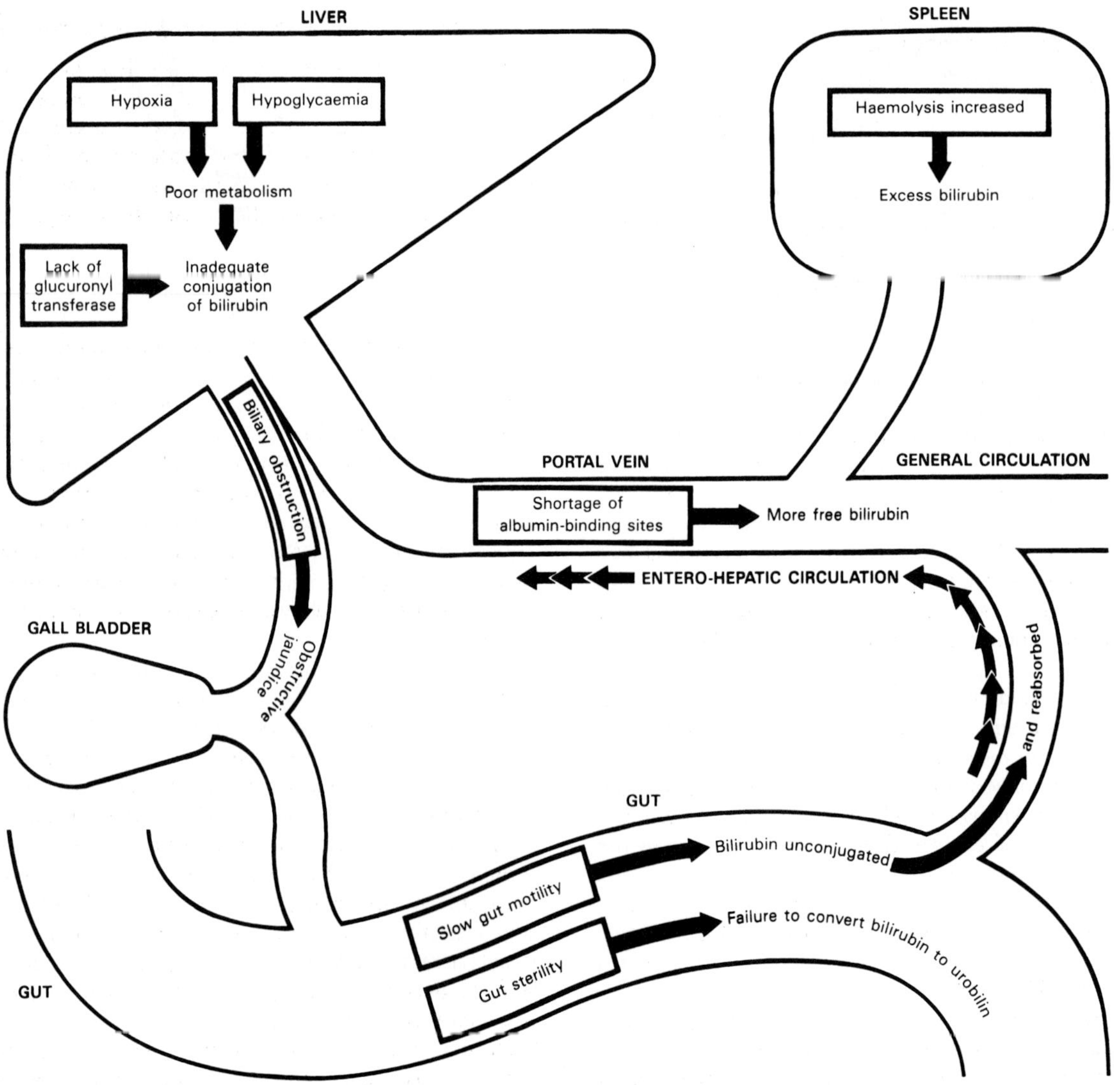

Figure 52.3 *Sites of events leading to jaundice (from Bennett VR, Brown L, 1993, with permission).*

- Haemolytic jaundice
- Bruising and haematoma
- Polycythaemia
- Postnatal infections

Hepatic unconjugated

- Breast milk jaundice
- Congenital hypothyroidism

Hepatic, mixed unconjugated and conjugated

- Inborn errors of metabolism
- Hepatitis, commonly due to transplacental infections (e.g. TORCH organisms)

Posthepatic mixed unconjugated and conjugated

- Congenital biliary atresia
- Bile plug syndrome

Posthepatic unconjugated

- Paralytic ileus
- High intestinal obstruction such as duodenal atresia

Prehepatic unconjugated bilirubin

Physiological jaundice usually appears on the 3rd day and has faded by the 8th day. The infant's general condition is good. It occurs because of the features of red cell and bilirubin metabolism discussed above. There is destruction of up to a third of the red cells present at birth, less efficient binding of unconjugated bilirubin to albumin and an immature liver. The bilirubin present in meconium may add to the unconjugated bilirubin load. Late clamping of the cord results in an increased blood volume and may exacerbate the problem. Treatment with phototherapy is occasionally necessary.

Jaundice of prematurity is a more serious form of the above and is caused by the same factors. In the preterm baby each feature is more exaggerated and jaundice begins earlier, lasts longer and is deeper. It is essential to prevent the onset of bilirubin encephalopathy and sometimes an exchange transfusion is necessary.

In **haemolytic jaundice**, the two main causes of red cell haemolysis are rhesus isoimmunisation, which is serious, and ABO incompatibility, which is rarely severe. These have been discussed fully in Chapter 12. Jaundice appears in the first 24 h of life.

Bruising and haematoma lead to extravasation of red cells, such as is found in a cephalhaematoma. Extra breakdown of red cells occurs during the resolution of the bruise.

Polycythaemia or the presence of excess red blood cells which must be broken down and their bilirubin metabolised occurs in twin transfusion syndrome, delayed cord clamping and infants of diabetic mothers.

Infection following birth, such as septicaemia, urinary tract infections and meningitis, may cause haemolysis and jaundice.

Hepatic unconjugated

Breast milk jaundice causes no ill effects and should not be a reason to discontinue breastfeeding but it creates anxiety in parents who see it as an illness or dysfunction. Breastfed babies are significantly more likely to develop hyperbilirubinaemia than bottlefed babies and it may occur early at 3–4 days or late from 4–10 days.

The absolute cause of breast milk jaundice is as yet not clear. It may involve:

1 inhibition of the glucuronyl transferase by substances found in breast milk such as the maternal hormone pregnanediol and unsaturated fatty acids;
2 the presence in breast milk of lipase which releases free fatty acids into the neonate's intestines;
3 the presence in breast milk of the enzyme β-glucuronidase that will split conjugated bilirubin (Kelnar et al 1995) and increase shunting of unconjugated bilirubin from intestine back to liver;
4 the delay in the passage of meconium seen in fully breastfed babies. Early breastfeeding with adequate colostrum intake will act as a laxative and prevent breast milk jaundice (Blackburn & Loper 1992, Salayira & Robertson 1993).

Congenital hypothyroidism causes mental retardation if undetected. It is one of the disorders screened for by the Guthrie test on the 7th day.

Hepatic, mixed unconjugated and conjugated

Some **inborn errors of metabolism**, such as cystic fibrosis and galactosaemia, may lead to neonatal jaundice. Inadequate metabolic pathways release toxins which damage the liver.

Hepatitis may be part of the syndrome which accompanies transplacental infection by organisms such as rubella, toxoplasmosis, cytomegalovirus, herpes simplex or hepatitis.

Posthepatic mixed unconjugated and conjugated

Congenital anomalies of the biliary ducts often interfere with normal bile flow which ultimately gives rise to cholestasis. The more common biliary malformations are extrahepatic biliary atresias, intrahepatic biliary hypoplasia and cystic dilatation of the major intrahepatic bile ducts. Differentiation between these dysmorphic lesions and parenchymal disorders associated with cholestasis in the newborn infant is important as surgical correction of biliary malformations may be life saving, whereas in infants with cholestasis caused by inflammatory response, infections or metabolic disorders, surgery is ineffective and may be life threatening.

Extrahepatic biliary atresia is by far the most common of the biliary malformations with an incidence of 5–10 infants in every 100 000 births. It tends to be more common in girls. The origins of the atretic lesions have not been clearly established. The main histological feature associated with extrahepatic biliary obstruction is proliferation of the hepatic interlobular bile ducts and periportal fibrosis. The baby may develop a deep bronze jaundice in the 2nd week of life, the stools are putty coloured and the urine contains bilirubin (Sweet 1997). The liver becomes firm and enlarged. Because the bilirubin is conjugated the baby is not at risk of kernicterus. Progressive destruction of tissue leads to biliary cirrhosis, portal hypertension and liver failure (McCance & Huether 1994).

Depending on the extent of the obliteration, surgical intervention is necessary but prognosis is generally poor, only those 10% with extrahepatic atresia being suitable for early surgery which needs to be carried out before liver damage is irreparable, i.e. before the age of 2 months (Kelnar et al 1995). The success rate is about 70%. Liver transplantation is a long-term therapy and about 35–50% of children receiving transplants have biliary atresia. If transplantation is not available, 80% of children will die before the age of 3 years (McCance & Huether 1994).

Management

Investigations

Depending on the history, signs and symptoms and gestational age of the baby, investigations may include serum bilirubin estimation, haemoglobin estimation, blood group, rhesus antibody estimation, infection screening, viral antibody screening, thyroxine and enzyme assays.

Phototherapy

If jaundice persists the first line of treatment to prevent the development of kernicterus is phototherapy. When a light of wavelength 400–500 nm is shone on the skin any unconjugated bilirubin is converted to a non-toxic water-soluble substance which can be excreted. Phototherapy has risks attached such as damage to the retina if the eyes are not covered and it is now considered safe to withhold treatment in a healthy term baby until the serum bilirubin reaches 320 μmol/l (Yau & Stevenson 1995). In preterm babies born around 28 weeks, treatment is commenced when the bilirubin level exceeds 150–180 μmol/l and in babies born about 34 weeks, at 200–240 μmol/l (Kelnar et al 1995). The baby's stools may become loose and extra fluids should be given and normal feeding continued to reduce the risk of dehydration.

Exchange blood transfusion

This procedure is mainly carried out in rhesus haemolytic disease of the newborn to remove excess bilirubin from the baby's blood or antibodies to prevent further haemolysis and a further rise in bilirubin levels, leading to the development of kernicterus.

COMMON METABOLIC DISORDERS

The scope of this book does not allow exploration of the mainly recessively inherited inborn errors of metabolism. Detailed accounts of conditions such as phenylketonuria, cystic fibrosis and galactosaemia can be found in McCance & Huether (1994). Preconception, antenatal and neonatal screening tests such as the Guthrie test for phenylketonuria are becoming more widely available. Disturbances in common substances such as glucose, calcium and sodium may lead to cerebral symptoms and permanent neurological damage. In most cases this is avoidable by prevention and prompt treatment. The main conditions are described briefly below.

Hypoglycaemia

In any given situation, a newborn infant's plasma glucose levels are the net result of glucose synthesis, release and utilisation. When the rate of glucose utilisation exceeds the rate of production, the plasma glucose concentration falls. Conversely, when glucose production exceeds utilisation, plasma glucose levels increase over the normal threshold.

Regulation of hepatic glucose production appears to be critical to the maintenance of glucose homeostasis. Although the kidneys are capable of glycogen synthesis, glycogenolysis and gluconeogenesis, the contribution of glucose in this instance is not of sufficient magnitude to maintain some degree of homeostatic balance except in prolonged starvation and metabolic acidosis.

Most neonates who develop hypoglycaemia in the first 24 h after birth have a history of:

- a mother who suffers from diabetes mellitus;
- a mother who developed pregnancy-induced hypertension;
- neonatal asphyxia;
- being large or small for gestational age.

Most infants who develop hypoglycaemia make a spontaneous recovery. However, recurrent or persistent hypoglycaemia may be caused by hepatic enzyme defects, endocrine deficiencies or hyperinsulinism.

Following much debate over what constitutes a normal value for blood glucose, it is now accepted that plasma glucose level of 2.6 mmol/l in symptomatic babies may lead to neurological dysfunction and later abnormalities. Hypoglycaemia is commoner in low birthweight babies and in babies of diabetic mothers. Other babies at risk are those with birth asphyxia or respiratory distress syndrome, hypothermia, cerebral damage, severe haemolytic disease or an inborn error of metabolism (Simpson 1997).

Signs

Hypoglycaemic babies have non-specific signs which can be associated with other conditions. These include lethargy, hypotonia, shallow respirations with periods of apnoea, cyanosis, muscle twitching, convulsions and coma.

Management

Prevention is the best form of management when the baby is known to be at risk. Early feeding and repeated blood screening by ward tests or laboratory tests are essential. In mild cases where the blood glucose level is 1.7 mmol/l or more an immediate milk feed should be given. If the level is below 1.7 mmol/l an intravenous infusion of 10% glucose solution may be necessary. If symptoms have been present for some time the baby should be given follow-up appointments to check for neurological damage.

Hypocalcaemia and hypomagnesaemia

In the last trimester of pregnancy there is active movement of calcium from mother to fetus. This significant shunting of calcium ensures that by term the infant's skeleton is well mineralised. A manifestation of this positive calcium movement in favour of the fetus is represented by the total and ionised calcium levels in fetal blood, which are usually 10% higher than maternal values.

This **fetal hypercalcaemic state** appears to suppress fetal parathyroid secretion and stimulates the release of calcitonin, a balance which favours mineral deposition in the fetal skeletal system. At birth the newborn infant's parathyroid functions are suppressed and this contributes to the onset of a **transient hypoparathyroid state** with a fall in plasma calcium levels. In the term infant plasma calcium levels decrease during the first 24–72 h after birth, reaching relatively low levels of 1.75–2.0 mmol/l. It would appear that the physiologically induced hypocalcaemia is of functional significance as it stimulates the parathyroid glands and suppresses calcitonin secretion.

Although plasma calcium levels increase to more acceptable levels within 5 days of birth, in circumstances where the transition to normal calcium metabolism fails to take place, symptomatic hypocalcaemia will develop. Hypocalcaemia with neonatal tetany occurs when the blood calcium level is less than 1.7 mmol/l. Hypocalcaemia can occur in the first 3 days of life in babies who are preterm, have suffered birth asphyxia, hypothermia or RDS. Late hypocalcaemia occurring between days 5 and 6 is usually associated with feeding a baby unmodified cow's milk. It is therefore rare in developed countries. Cow's milk is high in phosphorus and the increase in serum phosphate level causes the serum calcium level to fall. In some immigrant mothers and mothers in the lower socioeconomic groups, because of dietary habits, there may be a deficient intake in vitamin D and calcium, leading to hypocalcaemia in pregnancy. Their babies are at risk of developing tetany.

Signs

Neonatal tetany results in irritability followed by muscle twitching, apnoea and convulsions. The baby is generally alert between convulsions.

Management

Prevention can be aided by advising women about diet, encouraging breastfeeding and ensuring all cow's milk given to babies is modified. If the baby is convulsing treatment is by the administration of an infusion of 10% calcium gluconate diluted in a ratio of 1:4 with sterile water or 10% dextrose. It must be given slowly and attention must be paid to the heart rate and rhythm as bradycardia and arrhythmias may occur. In most cases and if babies are asymptomatic, oral calcium supplements can be given and are safer (Kelnar et al 1995).

Associated hypomagnesaemia

Failure of the plasma calcium concentration to respond to the administration of intravenous calcium salts should raise the suspicion of coexisting hypomagnesaemia. If hypocalcaemia persists there may be an associated hypomagnesaemia and an intramuscular injection of 0.2 mmol/kg 50% magnesium sulphate will correct both metabolic conditions (Simpson 1997). There may be a long-term hypoplasia of tooth enamel in the milk teeth. The normal serum magnesium range is 0.6–1.0 mmol/l. Hypomagnesaemia is often associated with hypocalcaemia and the serum magnesium level will be below 0.6 mmol/l.

Hypernatraemia

Campbell & McIntosh (1992) hold that hypernatraemia in neonates is almost invariably the consequence of water depletion. Hypernatraemia is present if the plasma sodium level is above 143 mmol/l. It may be provoked by excessive fluid loss, for instance during phototherapy or in vomiting and diarrhoea, or excessive sodium intake, sometimes in intravenous solutions such as bicarbonate. Any baby receiving intensive care should have plasma electrolytes checked at least once a day.

Inappropriate feeding of babies may lead to hypernatraemia. Extra packing of scoops during the mixing of formula feeds will increase the sodium content of the feed and mothers should be taught the principles of feed preparation and encouraged to breastfeed whenever possible. In hot weather babies perspire, become thirsty and cry. If mothers misinterpret the cry as a demand for food more sodium is added to the already high plasma levels. Babies cannot excrete a high solute load by concentrating their urine and water is lost in the dilute urine produced as water passively follows the excess sodium along the kidney tubules.

Signs

The baby appears fretful and thirsty at first, followed by dehydration and pyrexia. If the condition remains untreated convulsions occur, leading to death. The characteristic features of this clinical problem may be associated with failure to gain weight, evident irritability, hypertonicity and convulsions, especially in circumstances when plasma sodium levels exceed 150 mmol/l. Neonates presenting with hypernatraemic dehydration may manifest a full and pulsatile anterior fontanelle. As the osmotic gradient favours maintenance of extracellular fluid at the expense of intracellular fluid, it may be difficult at times to establish the true diagnosis.

Management

Management of persistent hypernatraemia in neonates may be difficult because of its association with cerebral haemorrhage and renal vein thrombosis. Overaggressive correction may cause cellular overhydration of brain tissue. The baby is slowly rehydrated with an infusion of an isotonic solution such as 0.9% saline. Sedation may be necessary to control the convulsions. Follow-up care is necessary to observe for signs of neurological damage.

Summary of main points

- Jaundice is a common problem of the neonate. Excessive bilirubin may enter the bloodstream during haemolysis of red blood cells, in liver disease affecting the metabolism and excretion of bile and in conditions that obstruct the common bile duct. Molecules of unconjugated bilirubin are transported to the liver to be conjugated.
- The neonate produces about twice as much bilirubin as the adult because of destruction of excess red cells but levels fall to normal by about 6 weeks. Levels of unbound, unconjugated bilirubin are also higher in the neonate. The capacity of a term neonate to excrete bilirubin is only one-fiftieth that of an adult so that all babies have hyperbilirubinaemia by adult standards and jaundice is common.
- Unconjugated bilirubin is fat soluble and the basal ganglia in the brain contain a high proportion of fat. Deposition of bilirubin causes irreversible tissue changes which lead to kernicterus. Long-term sequelae include cerebral athetosis and mental retardation. Kernicterus can be prevented in all but the very small, sick neonate.
- Prehepatic causes of neonatal jaundice with excess unconjugated bilirubin include physiological jaundice/jaundice of prematurity, haemolytic jaundice, bruising and haematoma, polycythaemia and some postnatal infections.
- Hepatic unconjugated causes of jaundice include breast milk jaundice and congenital hypothyroidism. Hepatic, mixed unconjugated and conjugated causes include inborn errors of metabolism and hepatitis, commonly due to transplacental infections (e.g. TORCH organisms).
- Posthepatic mixed unconjugated and conjugated causes include congenital biliary atresia and bile plug syndrome. Posthepatic unconjugated causes include paralytic ileus and high intestinal obstruction such as duodenal atresia.
- Physiological jaundice occurs because of destruction of up to a third of the red cells present at birth, less efficient binding of unconjugated bilirubin to albumin and an immature liver. Treatment with phototherapy is occasionally necessary. In the preterm baby jaundice begins earlier, lasts longer and is deeper. It is essential to prevent kernicterus and an exchange transfusion may be necessary.
- Bruising and haematoma lead to extravasation of red cells such as is found in a cephalhaematoma. Extra breakdown of red cells occurs during the resolution of the bruise. Polycythaemia occurs in twin transfusion syndrome, delayed cord clamping and infants of diabetic mothers.
- Breast milk jaundice causes no ill effects and should not be a reason to discontinue breastfeeding. Breastfed babies are significantly more likely to develop hyperbilirubinaemia than bottlefed babies and it may occur early at 3–4 days or late from 4–10 days.
- Congenital hypothyroidism may present with jaundice. Some inborn errors of metabolism such as cystic fibrosis and galactosaemia may lead to neonatal jaundice. Hepatitis may be part of the syndrome which accompanies transplacental infections. Infection following birth may cause haemolysis and jaundice.
- Biliary atresia presents with a deep bronze jaundice in the 2nd week of life, the stools are putty coloured and the urine contains bilirubin. The liver becomes firm and enlarged. Because the bilirubin is conjugated the baby is not at risk of kernicterus. Progressive destruction of tissue leads to biliary cirrhosis, portal hypertension and liver failure. Surgical intervention is necessary but prognosis is poor.
- Phototherapy and exchange blood transfusion may be carried out to remove excess bilirubin from the baby's blood. This will also remove antibodies to prevent further haemolysis and a further rise in bilirubin levels, leading to the development of kernicterus.
- Disturbances in common substances such as glucose, calcium and sodium may lead to cerebral symptoms and permanent neurological damage. Plasma glucose levels of 2.6 mmol/l in symptomatic babies may lead to neurological abnormalities.
- Hypoglycaemia is commoner in low birthweight babies and in babies of diabetic mothers. Early feeding and repeated blood screening by ward tests or laboratory tests is essential. In mild cases an immediate milk feed should be given. If the level is below 1.7 mmol/l an intravenous infusion of 10% glucose solution is necessary.
- Hypocalcaemia can occur early, in the first 3 days of life in babies who are preterm, have suffered birth asphyxia, hypothermia or RDS. Late hypocalcaemia occurs between days 5 and 6 and is usually associated with feeding a baby unmodified cow's milk. Mothers with a deficient intake in vitamin D and calcium may develop hypocalcaemia in pregnancy and their babies are at risk of developing tetany. In most cases oral calcium supplements can be given. If a baby is convulsing an infusion of 10% calcium gluconate diluted in a ratio of 1:4 with sterile water or 10% dextrose is given. Long-term hypoplasia of milk tooth enamel may follow.
- Hypernatraemia may be provoked by excessive fluid loss or excessive sodium intake. Babies cannot excrete a high solute load by concentrating urine and water is lost in their dilute urine. The baby is slowly rehydrated with an infusion of an isotonic solution such as 0.9% saline.

References

Bannister L, Berry M, Collins P et al. 1995 Gray's Anatomy. Churchill Livingstone, Edinburgh.

Bennett VR, Brown L. 1993 Myles Textbook for Midwives. Churchill Livingstone, Edinburgh.

Blackburn ST, Loper DL. 1992 Maternal, Fetal and Neonatal Physiology, A Clinical Perspective. WB Saunders, Philadelphia.

Cashmore W. 1992 Bilirubin metabolism and toxicity in the newborn. In Polin R, Fox W (eds) Fetal and Neonatal Physiology. WB Saunders, Philadelphia.

Campbell A, McIntosh A. 1992 Forfar and Arneil's Textbook of Paediatrics. Churchill Livingstone, Edinburgh.

Kelnar CJH, Harvey D, Simpson C. 1995 The Sick Newborn Baby. Baillière Tindall, London.

Marieb EN. 1992 Human Anatomy and Physiology, 2nd edn. Benjamin/Cummings Publishing, California.

McCance KL, Huether SE. 1994 Pathophysiology: The Biologic Basis for Disease in Adults and Children, 2nd edn. Mosby, St Louis.

Salayira EM, Robertson CM. 1993 Relationships between baby feeding types and patterns, gut transit time of meconium and the incidence of neonatal jaundice. Midwifery 9(4), 235–242.

Simpson C. 1997 Metabolic and endocrine disorders of the newborn. In Sweet BR with Tiran D (eds) Mayes Midwifery, 12th edn. Baillière Tindall, London, pp 889–895.

Storer J. 1996 The liver. In Hinchliff SM, Montague SE, Watson R (eds) Physiology for Nursing Practice, 2nd edn. Baillière Tindall, London.

Sweet BR. 1997 Neonatal jaundice. In Sweet BR with Tiran D (eds) Mayes Midwifery, 12th edn. Baillière Tindall, London, pp 872–881.

Yau TC, Stevenson DK. 1995 Advances in the diagnosis and treatment of neonatal hyperbilirubinaemia. Clinics in Perinatology 22(3), 741–758.

Recommended reading

Cashmore W. 1992 Bilirubin metabolism and toxicity in the newborn. In Polin R, Fox W (eds) Fetal and Neonatal Physiology. WB Saunders, Philadelphia.

Roberton NRC. (ed) 1992 Textbook of Neonatology. Churchill Livingstone, Edinburgh.

Rudolph A. 1991 Rudolph's Pediatrics. Appleton and Lange, Norwalk.

Salayira EM, Robertson CM. 1993 Relationships between baby feeding types and patterns, gut transit time of meconium and the incidence of neonatal jaundice. Midwifery 9(4), 235–242.

Sinclair JC, Bracken MB. (eds) 1992 Effective Care of the Newborn Infant. Oxford University Press, Oxford.

Yau TC, Stevenson DK. 1995 Advances in the diagnosis and treatment of neonatal hyperbilirubinaemia. Clinics in Perinatology 22(3), 741–758.

Chapter 53

Infections and trauma in the neonate

In this chapter

INTRODUCTION

Infections in the neonate may be acquired by the fetus in utero either transplacentally, such as the TORCH organisms, or during invasive investigations, such as amniocentesis when pneumonia is a likely consequence. Some infections are acquired perinatally by microorganisms that ascend the maternal reproductive tract, especially if the membranes are ruptured. These include streptococci, group B streptococcus, which is now one of the commonest causes of neonatal infection, *Escherichia coli* and *Listeria monocytogenes*. Others are acquired in labour, such as *Candida albicans*, *Neisseria gonorrhoeae*, *Chlamydia trachomatis*, *Listeria monocytogenes* and herpes infections and acquired immunodeficiency disease (AIDS). These last-named fetal infections are discussed in Chapter 14.

POSTNATAL INFECTIONS

Babies become colonised by commensal organisms during labour and after birth, during exposure to those living in the mother's vagina and rectum and on the perineal skin. Staphylococci colonise the skin, streptococci the upper respiratory tract and *Escherichia coli* the lower gut (Simpson 1997). Infection in the neonate is difficult to recognise and, like many neonatal problems, signs may be non-specific. The baby may be reluctant to feed, lethargic and fretful. He may vomit or have diarrhoea with weight loss. Temperature control is poor with either hyperpyrexia or hypothermia. There may be tachypnoea, apnoeic attacks, cyanosis and bradycardia. The baby's skin may be mottled, jaundiced, grey or pale. Sudden collapse may occur and differential diagnoses include metabolic disturbances, respiratory or cardiovascular problems or intracranial haemorrhage.

Any baby whose condition is healthy for 2 or 3 days and then deteriorates should be considered to have a systemic or topical infection until diagnosed. In the neonate there is an urgent need to diagnose infection and to commence treatment. Any delay in diagnosing a local infection may result in a spread to septicaemia. Following resuscitation if needed, a full infection screen is carried out including nasal, umbilical, throat and skin swabs, collection of urine and stool samples, a full white cell count, platelet count and blood culture and, if the baby is ill, a lumbar puncture.

Broad-spectrum antibiotics are commenced before the results of the screening test are known until the organism and its range of sensitivities are identified. Units usually have specific combinations of antibiotics, depending on the organisms commonly seen there, for instance amoxycillin and gentamicin (Kelnar et al 1995). Maintenance of correct body temperature and adequate food and fluid intake are necessary and systemic support such as ventilation is provided if needed.

Serious infections

Septicaemia may accompany any serious neonatal infection and can be confirmed by blood culture. Group B β-haemolytic streptococcus and *Staphylococcus epidermidis* have replaced *Escherichia coli* as the commonest causes. Septicaemia may lead to disseminated intravascular coagulation (DIC). Both the systemic sepsis and the abnormal clotting problems must be treated.

Meningitis is also more likely to be caused by the group B β-haemolytic streptococcus rather than the previously common *E. coli*. Other organisms include *Listeria monocytogenes*, pneumococci, staphylococci and *Candida albicans*. The typical vague symptoms are followed quite late in the illness by convulsions, a bulging fontanelle and head retraction and these neurological signs must be sought before suspecting meningitis. A lumbar puncture will aid diagnosis and identification of the causative organism. The mortality rate in meningitis is 25% and complications in babies that survive include mental retardation, deafness and nerve palsies (Kelnar et al 1995) and pneumonia, all of which may lead to death.

Pneumonia may be congenital, acquired by inhaling infected amniotic fluid. It then presents with respiratory distress within hours of birth. Aspiration pneumonia may follow inhalation of milk or fluids given by nasogastric tube. It occurs in preterm or ill infants whose swallowing and coughing reflexes are absent. Organisms acquired after birth cause pneumonia after the first few days of life. The baby develops respiratory symptoms and becomes cyanosed. He will require nursing in an incubator and humidified oxygen may be needed. Mechanical respiratory support may be required if the pneumonia is severe. Broad-spectrum antibiotics are commenced. Feeding is by nasogastric tube unless there is severe respiratory embarrassment when intravenous feeding is necessary.

Gastroenteritis is rare in the breastfed baby. Outbreaks are commonly caused by rotavirus and there is rapid spread from one baby to another and a high mortality. *Salmonella* and some strains of *Escherichia coli* may also cause an outbreak. There is rapid deterioration and dehydration. Vomiting occurs and the stools are watery and frequent. Segregation of an infected baby is essential and units may be closed if more than one baby is affected. Reopening follows total discharge of all mothers and babies and disinfecting of the unit. Fluids and electrolytes are administered in order to correct the existing haemodynamic disturbances and antibiotics commenced if required.

Skin and surface infections

Any rash on a baby's skin should be considered abnormal. Infection, especially staphylococci, may be spread from the ear, nose, mouth and skin of a carer or from another baby. **Pyoderma** is the appearance of small spots or pustules on the skin and may spread rapidly if the baby is preterm or ill. **Paronychia** is a localised staphylococcal infection of the nail bed. In both situations a doctor should be informed and antibiotics are occasionally necessary.

Pemphigus neonatorum is a much more serious skin infection which is caused by staphylococcal entry through a broken skin surface such as a scratch. It is highly contagious and may lead to epidemics resulting in the need to close a maternity unit. Any blister appearing on a baby's skin should be notified to the doctor. Blisters filled with pus appear on the skin. They break and leave a raw skin surface, mainly on the head and trunk. Large areas may be involved and the blisters run into each other, giving the typical 'scalded skin' appearance. The baby then becomes seriously ill. Fluid loss and the development of septicaemia may lead to shock. An affected baby is isolated and antibiotic treatment begun.

Omphalitis or infection of the umbilicus can be serious because of a possible spread through the umbilical vein to the liver (Fig. 53.1). Staphylococci are the common invading organism. Widespread erythema around the umbilicus or any discharge of pus indicates infection and should be treated with antibiotics.

Ophthalmia neonatorum means the presence of a purulent discharge from the eyes of the infant within 21 days of birth and should not be confused with the commonly occurring sticky eye. It became a notifiable disease in 1914 because at that time 50% of blindness was due to neonatal infection. It is now rare that a child's sight is threatened by this condition. In the past gonorrhoea was a problem and it is returning with the advent of penicillin-resistant strains of *Neisseria gonorrhoeae* but the most commonly identified organisms are now staphylococci, *Escherichia coli* and *Chlamydia trachomatis*. The baby should be nursed with the affected eye downwards and it is usual to treat both eyes with the appropriate local and systemic antibiotics.

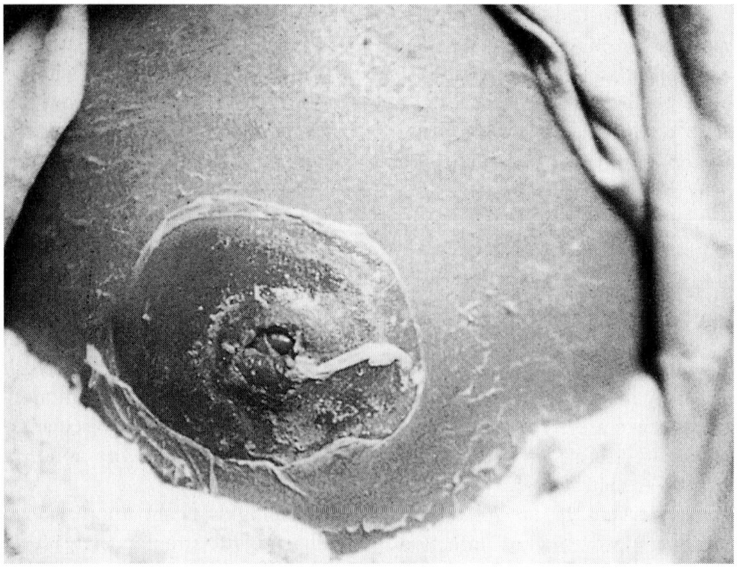

Figure 53.1 *Severe periumbilical infection (from Kelnar C, Harvey D, Simpson C, 1995, with permission).*

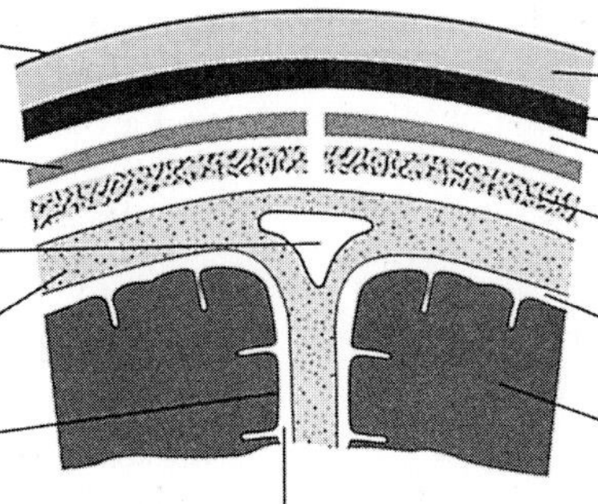

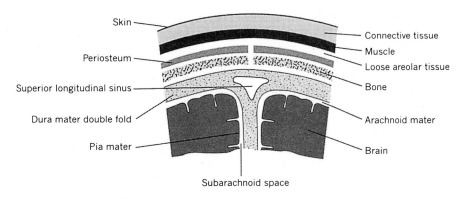

Figure 53.2 *A cross-section through the skull (from Sweet B, 1997, with permission).*

Necrotising enterocolitis

Necrotising enterocolitis (NEC) is an inflammatory disease of the bowel which is associated with septicaemia. No specific cause has yet been identified and several factors probably act together to result in bowel damage (Beeby & Jeffery 1992). Gut ischaemia resulting from a combination of hypoxaemia, hypoglycaemia and/or hypothermia may cause oedema, ulceration and haemorrhage in the wall of the bowel and perforation may occur. If the baby is not breastfed factors such as IgA and lymphocytes from colostrum are absent. This allows invasion of the bowel wall, portal system and bowel lymphatics by bacteria such as *Klebsiella*, *Clostridium*, *Bacteroides* and *Escherichia coli*. Endotoxin release leads to DIC, septicaemia and peritonitis. Failure of temperature control occurs and there is abdominal distension and melaena with bilestained vomiting (Kelnar et al 1995).

Treatment

Treatment is conservative at first. The baby is isolated, oral feeds are discontinued and intravenous fluids are commenced. The infant requires analgesia such as morphine. The stomach is kept empty by nasogastric tube on free drainage. Assisted ventilation and fentanyl may be necessary for the most severely affected babies. Blood and stools are sent to the laboratory for culture and sensitivity screening and a combination of broad-spectrum antibiotics is commenced. Surgery may be indicated if there are signs of bowel perforation, with the removal of the smallest amount of bowel possible to prevent later problems with absorption. There is a mortality rate of 40% so it is essential to prevent the onset or detect early signs so that treatment can be commenced (Simpson 1997).

Prevention

Lucas & Cole (1990), in a multicentre study of 926 preterm babies, found that NEC developed in 51 (5.5%) with a mortality rate of 26%. The disease was up to 10 times more common in exclusively formula-fed babies than those fed on breast milk alone and three times more common in those receiving a combination of formula and breast milk feeds. A link may be the prevention of pathogenic presence by the early colonisation of the gut by lactobacilli.

BIRTH TRAUMA

Normal labour rarely results in birth injuries. Severe birth trauma is now rare (Kelnar et al 1995) and should be considered avoidable (Lang 1996). Minor damage may occur during a complicated labour such as rotational forceps, ventouse extraction, shoulder dystocia or breech delivery. Preterm babies are at most risk, with head injury leading to intracranial haemorrhage at various levels of the protective structures around the brain (Fig. 53.2) still being a major cause of perinatal death. A tentorial tear involving a cerebral vein known as the great vein of Galen, a subaponeurotic haemorrhage or subdural haemorrhage (see below) may occur. Babies at risk are those who are large in relation to the mother's pelvis, those of low birth weight, those born by vaginal breech delivery and those who are members of a multiple pregnancy. Nerve injuries and fractures of the long bones of the arm or leg may follow a difficult vaginal delivery of the shoulders or aftercoming head of the breech.

Cephalhaematoma

A cephalhaematoma is a swelling on the head of a baby caused by an effusion of blood under the periosteum of the skull (Fig. 53.3). Friction between the baby's head and the hard maternal pelvis or forceps causes a tear in the periosteum which is confined in spread by the attachment of the periosteum to its bone. It is differentiated from the superficial oedema of the caput succedaneum as:

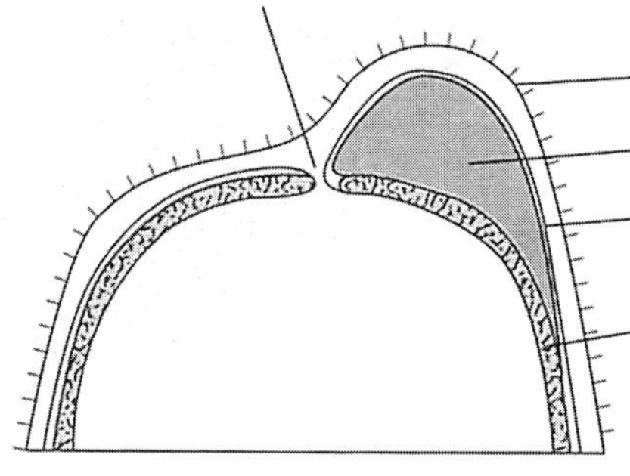

Figure 53.3 *Cross-section of a cephalhaematoma (from Sweet B, 1997, with permission).*

- it appears in the first 12 h after birth;
- it is clearly circumscribed and confined to one bone, never crossing a suture line;
- it does not pit;
- it tends to grow larger rather than disappear;
- it persists for 6–9 weeks and may ossify.

Late-onset jaundice may result as the blood cells are reabsorbed. No treatment is needed and the swelling usually disappears within 6–9 weeks.

Subaponeurotic haemorrhage

Subaponeurotic haemorrhage is a serious birth injury which is commonly associated with vacuum extraction (Lang 1996). Bleeding occurs from beneath the epicranial aponeurosis. Swelling can cross suture lines and the swelling may be confused with a caput succedaneum. It is present at birth and increases in size. Haemorrhage is extensive and may extend into the subcutaneous tissues of the neck or eyelids and may result in anaemia and jaundice. A blood transfusion may be necessary and the condition resolves in about 2–3 weeks.

Intracranial haemorrhage

Bleeding into brain tissue in the neonate may occur at different sites and differ in severity. The time of onset and duration of the bleeding are important when considering prognosis. Intracranial haemorrhage is most likely to occur in the preterm infant and may be caused by hypoxia or trauma, both often occurring together. Tears leading to haemorrhage usually occur in the falx cerebri or tentorium cerebelli (Fig. 53.4) as the fragile blood vessels of the preterm baby are easily torn. Types of haemorrhage according to the site of bleeding are (Lang 1996):

- subdural haemorrhage;
- subarachnoid haemorrhage;
- intraparenchymal haemorrhage;
- periventricular/intraventricular haemorrhage.

Subdural haemorrhage is almost exclusively traumatic. A tear occurs, most often in the tentorium cerebelli at its junction with the falx cerebri, causing rupture of the venous sinuses and the great vein of Galen. Signs include irritability, a highpitched cry and a bulging anterior fontanelle. Convulsions may occur and will require therapeutic interventions with anticonvulsant drugs and dexamethasone. Diagnosis can be confirmed by ultrasound scan. A subdural tap may be necessary to drain large collections of blood.

Subarachnoid haemorrhage is bleeding from small vessels into the subarachnoid space following mild trauma or asphyxia. It may be symptomless and be undetectable on ultrasound scan and therefore more common than is realised. Lumbar puncture will reveal bloodstained cerebrospinal fluid (CSF). Hydrocephalus may be a complication.

Intraparenchymal haemorrhage is bleeding into the cerebral tissue. It may occur due to birth asphyxia or be a complication of DIC. Cerebral irritation and convulsions may be present. Ultrasound scan or computed tomography (CT) scan may be useful to diagnose the problem. There may be destruction of cerebral tissue with formation of porencephalic cysts (Lang 1996).

Periventricular (PVH)/intraventricular haemorrhage (IVH) is the most common and most serious of the intracranial haemorrhages (Fig. 53.5). There may be direct damage to neurones due to pressure and inflammation and hydrocephalus may occur. Long-term outcomes include motor and sensory disabilities and cognitive delay (Blackburn & Loper 1992). It is a common cause of death in neonates of less than 32 weeks gestation. Most likely to be affected is the preterm baby with birth asphyxia and trauma who then develops respiratory distress syndrome.

The length of gestation and developmental stage of the brain are related to the site of the bleeding. The germinal matrix or subependymal layer which surrounds the ventricles of the brain in a preterm baby consists of actively dividing cells. From 24 to 32 weeks of gestation a large capillary bed of blood vessels supplies these actively dividing cells and holds a large proportion of the cerebral blood flow. These are very fragile and easily disrupted, especially when dilated by hypoxia and hypercapnia. From 32 weeks the matrix becomes less prominent and has almost completely disappeared by term.

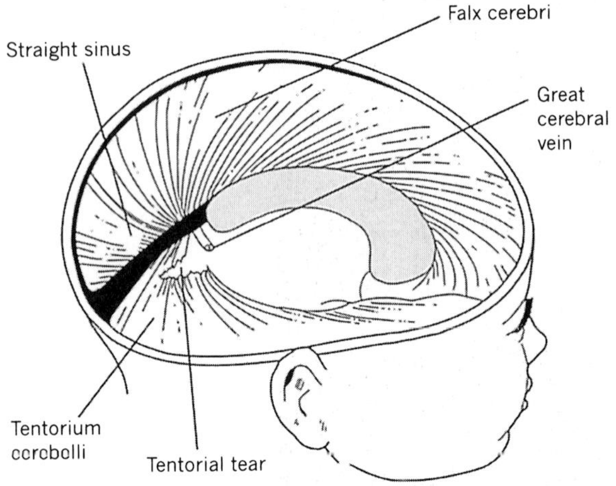

Figure 53.4 *A tentorial tear (from Sweet B, 1997, with permission).*

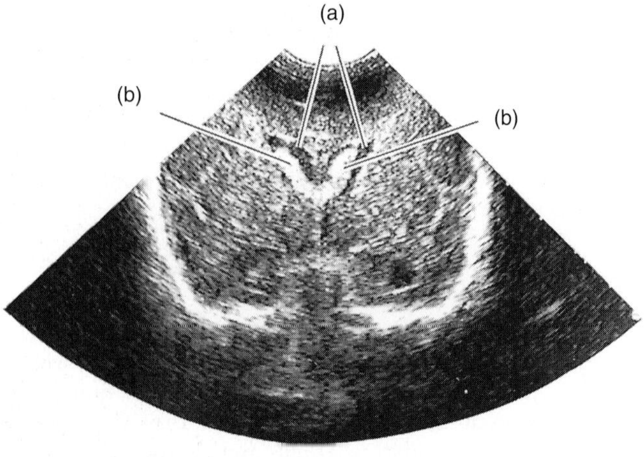

Figure 53.5 *Coronal cranial ultrasound scan showing intraventricular haemorrhages (b) in dilated lateral ventricles (a) (from Kelnar C, Harvey D, Simpson C, 1995, with permission).*

The more mature the fetal brain is, the less likely are PVH and IVH to occur. In term infants the haemorrhage is mainly in the choroid plexus and is due to trauma. In preterm infants the bleeding is more likely to occur in the capillaries supplying the subependymal germinal matrix located adjacent to the lateral ventricles. Other factors which may exacerbate the risk of haemorrhage in the preterm baby are handling, suctioning, erratic temperature control, pain and motor activity (Blackburn & Loper 1992). If the bleeding extends into the ventricle the thrombus may block the drainage of CSF and hydrocephalus may occur.

The neonate with a sudden, large PVH/IVH presents with apnoea and circulatory collapse with marked bradycardia (Kelnar et al 1995) which may lead rapidly to death. The anterior fontanelle may be enlarged and tense. Ultrasound scan will confirm the diagnosis. The baby will need active resuscitation and ventilation if he is to survive (Lang 1996). Fluids are given intravenously but may be restricted at first. Prognosis for babies with small haemorrhages is good. Babies with massive haemorrhages usually suffer from convulsions, cerebral atrophy and hydrocephalus.

Periventricular leucomalacia (PVL) is a condition in which ischaemia leads to necrotic changes in the white matter near to the brain ventricles. Blood flow is interrupted, usually by hypotension, and this area of the brain is vulnerable because it is a boundary zone between different areas of blood supply (Blackburn & Loper 1992, Kelnar et al 1995). Dubowitz et al (1985) remind us that PVL destroys tissue of the corticospinal motor pathways, resulting in spastic cerebral palsy (Fig. 53.6).

Nerve palsies

Facial palsy is caused by damage to the 7th cranial nerve by pressure applied to the facial nerve as it emerges near the angle of the jaw. The affected side shows no movement at all, the eye remains open and the corner of the mouth droops (Fig. 53.7). The baby almost always recovers facial movement completely.

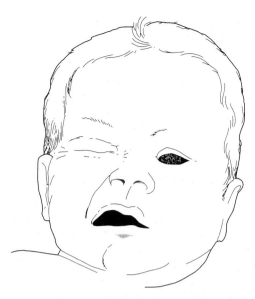

Figure 53.7 *Left-sided facial palsy. The right side is active when the baby cries but the left side is relaxed (from Sweet B, 1997, with permission).*

Erb's palsy results from damage to the 5th and 6th cervical nerves resulting in paralysis of the arm and the 'waiter's tip position' (Fig. 53.8). The arm is inwardly rotated and hangs limply at the side. The half-closed hand is turned outwards. It is caused by injury to the nerves of the upper brachial plexus due to dragging on the neck in a breech or difficult cephalic delivery. These nerves control the arm and some neck and chest muscles.

Klumpke's palsy is caused by traction on the arm with damage to the 8th cervical and first thoracic nerve roots which make up the lower brachial plexus. There is paralysis of the hand and wrist drop. The upper arm has normal movement. Klumpke's palsy is much less common.

Investigations to rule out fractures to the humerus and clavicle, which result in the baby not moving the affected arm, and to assess joint involvement are necessary. Recovery is slow,

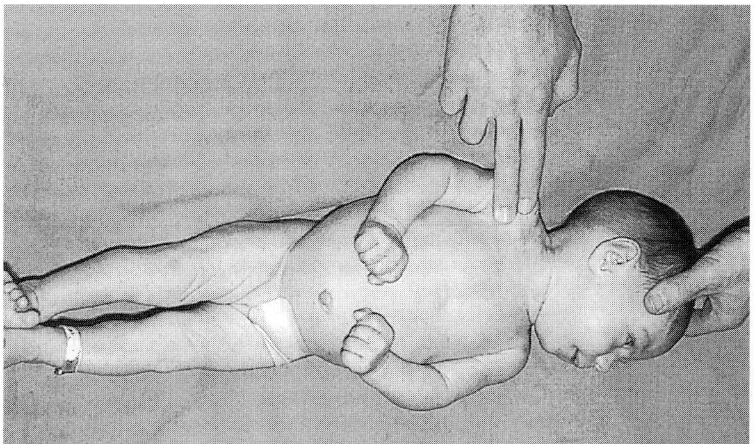

Figure 53.6 *Hypertonic baby with cerebral palsy (from Kelnar C, Harvey D, Simpson C, 1995, with permission).*

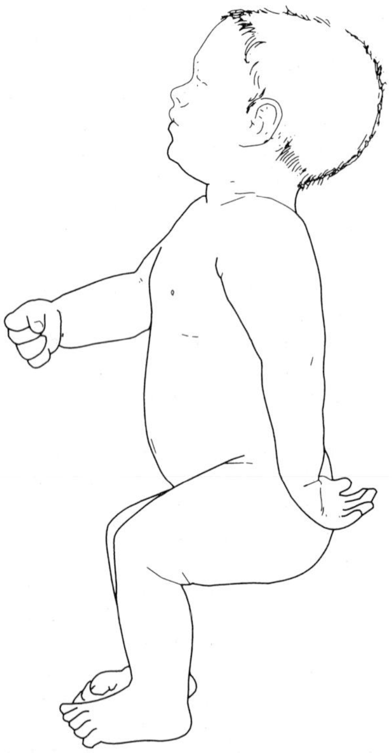

Figure 53.8 *Erb's palsy (from Sweet B, 1997, with permission).*

taking up to 2 years and more likely to be complete in Erb's palsy. Rest for the first week followed by physiotherapy to avoid contractures is of value. Cases not recovering spontaneously may benefit from surgical intervention with nerve graft or repair (Shenaq & Dinh 1990).

Soft tissue injuries

The most common cause of soft tissue injuries is vaginal delivery of the baby in the breech position. There may be:

- superficial bruising;
- injury to liver and spleen;
- injury to the kidneys, renal and adrenal glands;
- injury to the intestines.

Complications of bruising include hypovolaemia with circulatory collapse, consumptive coagulopathy and jaundice. Injury to internal organs may result in haemorrhage and anaemia. Diagnosis is by ultrasound scan and treatment is supportive with the possible need for blood transfusion. Surgical repair may be necessary.

Summary of main points

- Infections in the neonate may be acquired by the fetus in utero either transplacentally, such as the TORCH organisms, or during invasive investigations, such as amniocentesis. Some infections are acquired perinatally by microorganisms ascending the maternal reproductive tract, especially if the membranes are ruptured, and others are acquired in labour.
- Infection in the neonate is difficult to recognise and signs may be non-specific with lethargy, poor feeding, vomiting, diarrhoea and weight loss. There may be hyperpyrexia or hypothermia, tachypnoea, apnoeic attacks, cyanosis and bradycardia. The baby's skin may be mottled, jaundiced, grey or pale. Sudden collapse may occur.
- Any delay in diagnosing a local infection may result in a spread to septicaemia. Broad-spectrum antibiotics are commenced prior to the results of the screening test until the organism and its range of sensitivities are identified. Maintenance of correct body temperature and adequate food and fluid intake are necessary and systemic support such as ventilation is provided if needed.
- Septicaemia may accompany any serious neonatal infection and can be confirmed by blood culture. Group B β-haemolytic streptococcus and *Staphylococcus epidermidis* have replaced *E. coli* as the commonest causes. Septicaemia may lead to disseminated intravascular coagulation.
- Meningitis is more likely to be caused by the group B β-haemolytic streptococcus rather than the previously common *E. coli*. Mortality in meningitis is 25% and complications in babies that survive include mental retardation, deafness and nerve palsies and pneumonia.
- Pneumonia may be congenital and acquired by inhaling infected amniotic fluid. It then presents within hours of birth. Aspiration pneumonia may follow inhalation of milk or fluids given by nasogastric tube. Organisms acquired after birth cause pneumonia after the first few days of life. Mechanical ventilation may be required if it is severe. Broad-spectrum antibiotics are commenced.
- Gastroenteritis is rare in the breastfed baby. Outbreaks are commonly caused by rotavirus and there is a high mortality. *Salmonella* and some strains of *E. coli* may also cause an outbreak. Vomiting occurs and the stools are watery and frequent. Segregation of an infected baby is essential. Fluids and electrolytes are administered as needed and antibiotics commenced.
- Pemphigus neonatorum is a highly contagious serious staphylococcal skin infection which may lead to epidemics. Blisters filled with pus appear on the skin and break, leaving a raw skin surface. Fluid loss and the development of septicaemia may lead to shock. An affected baby is isolated and antibiotic treatment begun.
- Omphalitis can be serious because of a possible spread through the umbilical vein to the liver. Staphylococci are the common invading organism. Widespread erythema around the umbilicus or any discharge of pus should be treated with antibiotics.
- Gonorrhoea is a recurring problem with the advent of penicillin-resistant strains of *Neisseria gonorrhoeae* but the most commonly identified organisms in eye infections are staphylococci, *E. coli* and *Chlamydia trachomatis*. The baby with ophthalmia neonatorum should be nursed with the affected eye downwards and both eyes are treated with the appropriate antibiotics.
- Necrotising enterocolitis is an inflammatory disease of the bowel with invasion of the bowel wall, portal system and bowel lymphatics by pathogenic bacteria which may lead to oedema, ulceration and haemorrhage in the bowel wall. The disease is much less common in exclusively breastfed babies. Endotoxin release leads to disseminated intravascular coagulation, septicaemia and peritonitis. Treatment is conservative initially but surgery may be indicated if there is bowel perforation.
- Normal labour rarely results in birth injuries but minor damage may occur during a complicated labour such as rotational forceps, ventouse extraction, shoulder dystocia or breech delivery. Preterm

babies are at most risk, with head injury leading to intracranial haemorrhage, still a major cause of perinatal death.

- Friction between the baby's head and the hard maternal pelvis or forceps tears the periosteum and bleeding is confined by the attachment of the periosteum to its bone, forming a cephalhaematoma. No treatment is needed and the swelling usually disappears within 6 weeks. Jaundice may occur.
- Subaponeurotic haemorrhage is a serious birth injury commonly associated with vacuum extraction. Bleeding occurs from beneath the epicranial aponeurosis. Swelling can cross suture lines. Haemorrhage may extend into the subcutaneous tissues of the neck or eyelids resulting in anaemia and jaundice. A blood transfusion may be necessary.
- The time of onset and duration of the bleeding into neonatal brain tissue are important when considering prognosis. Intracranial haemorrhage is most likely to occur in the preterm infant and may be caused by hypoxia or trauma, both often occurring together. Tears leading to haemorrhage usually occur in the falx cerebri or tentorium cerebelli.
- Subdural haemorrhage is usually traumatic. A tear occurs, most often in the tentorium cerebelli at its junction with the falx cerebri, causing rupture of the venous sinuses. Signs include irritability and a bulging anterior fontanelle. Diagnosis can be confirmed by ultrasound scan. A subdural tap may be necessary to drain large collections of blood.
- Subarachnoid haemorrhage is bleeding into the subarachnoid space following mild trauma or asphyxia. It may be symptomless and more common than is realised. Lumbar puncture will reveal bloodstained cerebrospinal fluid. Hydrocephalus may be a complication.
- Intraparenchymal haemorrhage is bleeding into the cerebral tissue. It may occur due to birth asphyxia or be a complication of disseminated intravascular coagulation. Ultrasound scan or computed tomography scan may be useful to diagnose the problem. There may be destruction of cerebral tissue with formation of porencephalic cysts.
- Periventricular/intraventricular haemorrhage is the most common and most serious of the intracranial haemorrhages, occurring in the preterm baby. It is a common cause of death in neonates of less than 32 weeks gestation. Long-term outcomes include motor and sensory disabilities and cognitive delay.
- If the bleeding extends into the ventricle the thrombus may block the drainage of CSF and hydrocephalus may occur. Ultrasound scan will confirm the diagnosis. Prognosis for babies with small haemorrhages is good. Babies with massive haemorrhages usually suffer from convulsions, cerebral atrophy and hydrocephalus.
- In periventricular leucomalacia ischaemia leads to necrotic changes in the white matter near to the brain ventricles. Blood flow is interrupted usually by hypotension and this area of the brain is vulnerable because it is a boundary zone between different areas of blood. The corticospinal motor pathways are destroyed, resulting in spastic cerebral palsy.
- Facial palsy is caused by damage to the 7th cranial nerve by pressure applied to the facial nerve as it emerges near the angle of the jaw. The affected side shows no movement at all, the eye remains open and the corner of the mouth droops. The baby almost always recovers facial movement completely.
- Erb's palsy results from damage to the 5th and 6th cervical nerves resulting in paralysis of the arm and the 'waiter's tip position'. Klumpke's palsy is much less common and is caused by damage to the 8th cervical and first thoracic nerve roots which make up the lower brachial plexus. Recovery is slow, even with physiotherapy, and surgical intervention may be necessary.
- The most common cause of soft tissue injuries is vaginal delivery of the baby in the breech position. Complications of bruising include hypovolaemia with circulatory collapse, consumptive coagulopathy and jaundice. Injury to internal organs may result in haemorrhage and anaemia. Treatment is supportive but surgical repair may be necessary.

References

Beeby PJ, Jeffery H. 1992 Risk factors for necrotising enterocolitis: the influence of gestational age. Archives of Diseases in Childhood 67, 432–435.

Blackburn ST, Loper DL. 1992 Maternal, Fetal and Neonatal Physiology, A Clinical Perspective. WB Saunders, Philadelphia.

Dubowitz LMS, Bydder GM, Mushin J. 1985 Developmental sequence of periventricular leucomalacia. Correlation of ultrasound, clinical and nuclear magnetic resonance functions. Archives of Diseases in Childhood 60, 349–355.

Kelnar CJH, Harvey D, Simpson C. 1995 The Sick Newborn Baby. Baillière Tindall, London.

Lang MA. 1996 Trauma and haemorrhage. In Bennett VR, Brown LK (eds) Myles Textbook for Midwives, 12th edn. Churchill Livingstone, Edinburgh.

Shenaq SM, Dinh TA. 1990 Paediatric microsurgery. Clinics in Plastic Surgery 17(1), 79–83.

Simpson C. 1997 Infections of the newborn. In Sweet BR with Tiran D (eds) Mayes Midwifery, 12th edn. Baillière Tindall, London, pp 896–905.

Sweet B. 1997 Mayes' Midwifery. Baillière Tindall, London.

Recommended reading

Brock TD, Madigan MT. 1991 Biology of Micro-organisms, 6th edn. Prentice-Hall, New Jersey.

Gaffney G, Sellers S, Flavell V, Squier M, Johnson A. 1994 Case-control study of intrapartum care, cerebral palsy and perinatal death. British Medical Journal 308 (6931), 743–750.

Greenhough A, Oxborne J, Southerland S. (eds) 1991 Congenital, Perinatal and Neonatal Infections. Churchill Livingstone, Edinburgh.

Lucas A, Cole TJ 1990 Breast Milk and Necrotising Enterocolitis. Lancet, 336:1519–1523.

McCance KL, Huether SE. 1994 Pathophysiology: The Biologic Basis for Disease in Adults and Children, 2nd edn. Mosby, St Louis.

Remington JS, Klein JO. (eds) 1990 Infectious Diseases of the Fetus and Newborn Infant, 3rd edn. WB Saunders, Philadelphia.

Roberton NRC. (ed) 1992 Textbook of Neonatology. Churchill Livingstone Edinburgh.

Sinclair JC, Bracken MB. (eds) 1992 Effective Care of the Newborn Infant. Oxford University Press, Oxford.

Section

4B

PUERPERIUM – THE MOTHER

Section contents

Section 4B examines the physiology of the woman following childbirth and the parent-infant relationship. Breast anatomy and the physiology of lactation are discussed in chapter 54 and the following chapter is about infant feeding, both breast and by artificial milk. Chapter 56 is about the other physiological changes in the puerperium and the pathological conditions affecting the woman. Some common pathological conditions such as puerperal infection, not mentioned elsewhere in the book are discussed. The last chapter in the book considers the development of mother-infant relationships in terms of biobehavioural theories. Although these theories are highly biological in nature the student should not lose sight of the integration of biology, psychology and sociology in behavioural sciences.

Chapter 54 The breasts and lactation

In this chapter

INTRODUCTION

Lactation is the production of milk by specialised cutaneous organs called mammary glands (Mepham 1987). Animals such as humans that produce milk are called mammals and are distinguished from other vertebrates by that ability (Mepham 1987). It is probable that lactation was a key physiological feature that enabled the mammals to survive the climatic changes that led to the demise of the dinosaurs about 65 million years ago (Czerkas & Czerkas 1990).

The two advantages of lactation over other means of feeding the young (Mepham 1987) are:

1 the precursors of milk can be stored in maternal tissues so that milk can be produced on demand;
2 short-term variations in maternal diet have little impact on the nutrition of the young.

It is important to encourage mothers to breastfeed their babies and in order to achieve this practitioners should be knowledgeable about the anatomical and physiological aspects of lactation.

ANATOMY OF THE BREAST

Situation, shape and size

Breasts develop bilaterally on the ventral surface of the body and possibly originated from modified apocrine sweat glands. They are therefore part of the skin. In humans there are two hemispherically shaped breasts situated on the anterior chest wall on either side of the midline which vary in size depending on the amount of adipose tissue present. The mature breast lies over the pectoralis major muscle and extends from the 2nd to the 6th rib and from sternum to axilla (Fig. 54.1). The breasts are not completely circular in shape. There is a tail of breast tissue extending from the upper outer quadrant up into the axilla as far as the 3rd rib (Anderson 1992) – the axillary tail of Spence. Protruding from the centre of each breast, at the level of the 4th intercostal space, is the nipple surrounded by the areola.

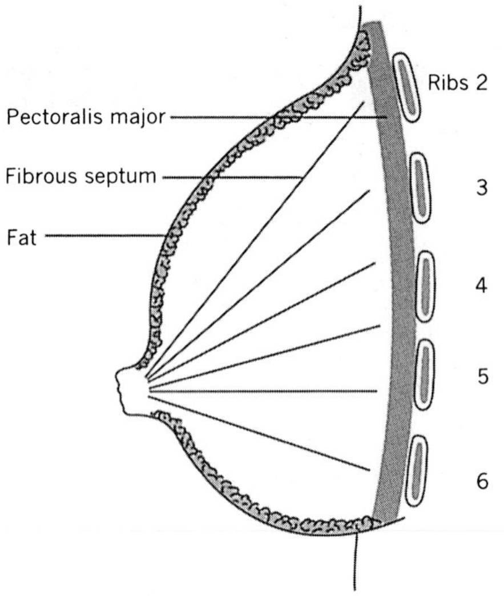

Figure 54.1 *The supporting structures of the breast (from Sweet B, 1997, with permission).*

Structure

Mammary tissue is divided into the **parenchyma** or the functional substance of the breast, which is a radiating compound **racemose** (bunch of grapes) gland, and the **stroma** which comprises the connective tissue, adipose tissue, blood and lymph vessels, nerve tissue and the surrounding skin. The parenchyma is arranged into about 15–20 lobes, shown in Figure 54.2, radiating out from the nipple like the spokes of a wheel (Herbert 1996). The lobes are separated from each other by fibrous connective tissue partitions so that they do not communicate and each functions independently.

The alveoli

As with all exocrine glands, the glandular tissue contains two types: secretory and ductal (Mepham 1987). Each lobe is divided into between 20 and 40 smaller **lobules** made up of the functional milk-producing units, the alveoli and their ductules known as the **lobuloalveolar system** (Fig. 54.3).

Each alveolus contains specialised milk-forming cells which surround a small duct. The cells are arranged in a single layer surrounding the hollow lumen. Milk is secreted into the lumen and drains via narrow ductules into the duct system. Some of the cells lining the ductules may also secrete milk.

The basal lamina

Each alveolus is surrounded by a **basement membrane** (basal lamina) made up of collagen, glycoprotein and glycosaminoglycans secreted by the epithelial cells where they are in contact with connective tissue. This provides a barrier between the epithelial and stromal components of breast tissue which cannot be crossed by cells other than leucocytes (Mepham 1987). Lymphocytes or monocytes are found wedged between the secretory cells of the alveoli and have migrated there. They play a role in local production of antibodies in the form of immunoglobulin A (IgA) for secretion into the breast milk.

The secretory cells

The secretory cells lining the alveoli are cuboidal and very polarised in structure (Fig. 54.4). The nucleus is situated at the base of the cell facing the circulation and facing the lumen is a well-developed Golgi apparatus with layers of flattened vesicles. Most of the cell is occupied by rough endoplasmic reticulum and there are a large number of mitochondria. There are large fat droplets and vesicles containing granules of protein. The basal surface of the cell has numerous infoldings for the uptake of substrate for milk production whilst the surface facing the lumen is covered with microvilli for secretion of milk.

The ducts

Groups of 10–100 alveoli drain into a small duct into which they pour their secretions. These small ducts join up to form larger ducts draining the lobules. The ducts from the lobules unite to form a central **lactiferous duct** for each lobe. Each lactiferous duct expands into a dilated sac as it passes beneath

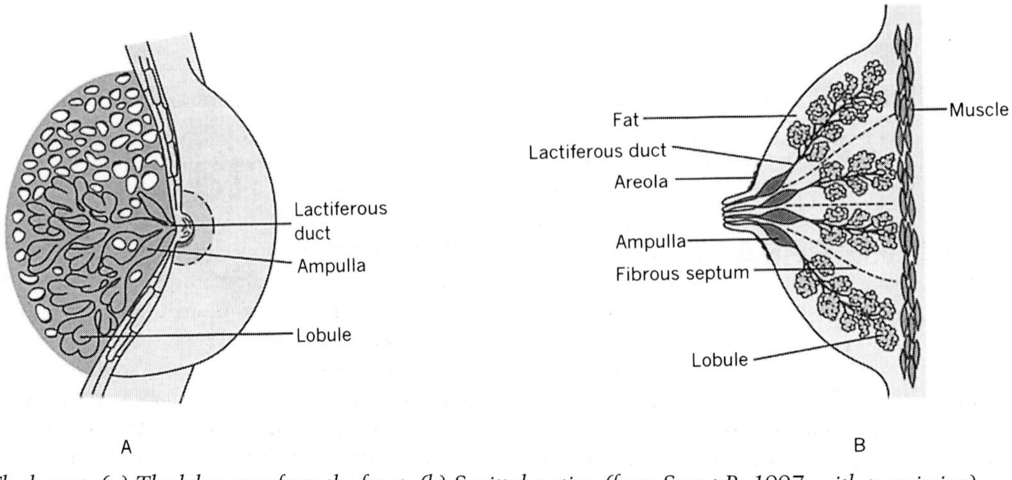

Figure 54.2 *The breast. (a) The lobes seen from the front. (b) Sagittal section (from Sweet B, 1997, with permission).*

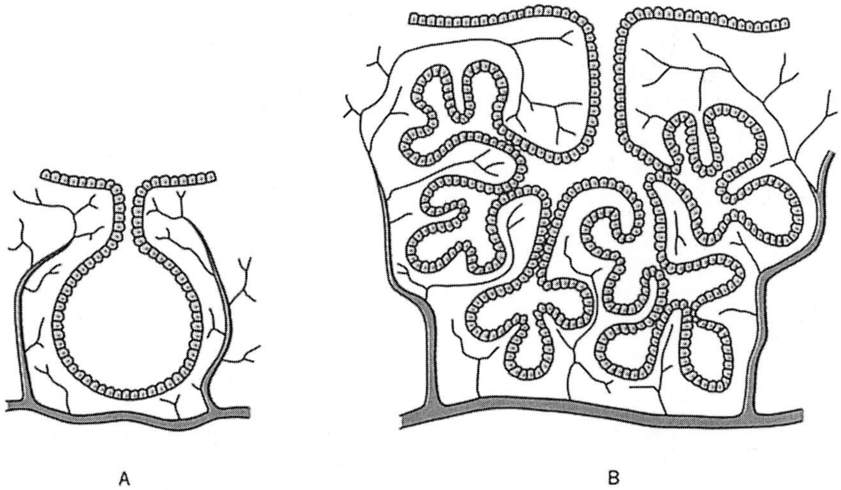

Figure 54.3 *The structure of the breast. (a) Single alveolus. (b) One lobule (from Sweet B, 1997, with permission).*

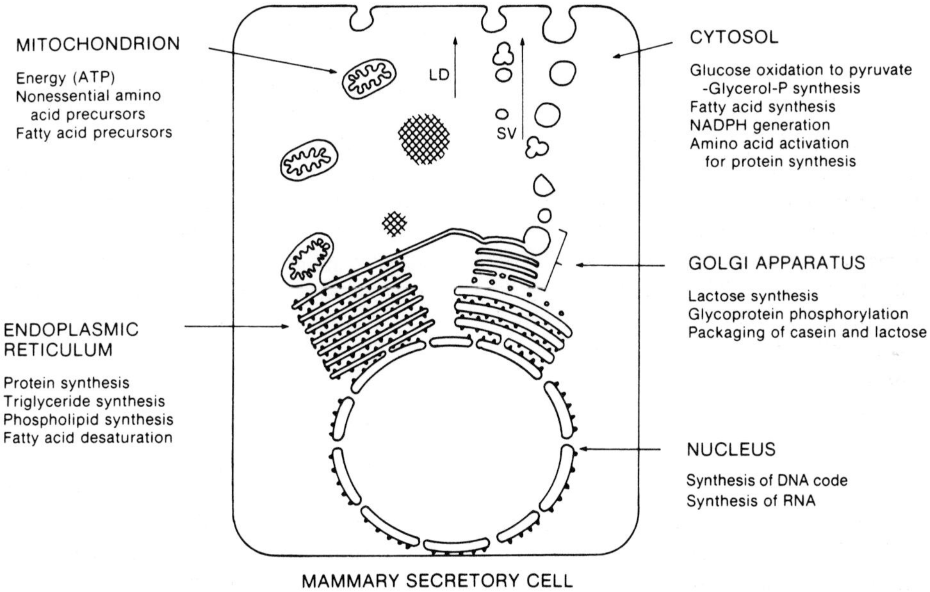

Figure 54.4 *Schematic representation of cytologic and biochemical interrelationships of secretory cell of mammary gland. LD, liquid droplet; SV, secretory vesicle. (Reproduced with permission from Lawrence 1985.)*

the areola to form an **ampulla** (lactiferous sinus) where milk can be stored prior to suckling. It then narrows to open out onto the nipple surface. The walls of the ducts are lined by a layer of cuboidal epithelial cells resting upon a basement membrane. Surrounding the alveoli and smaller ducts are the contractile branching myoepithelial cells. Smooth muscle surrounds the larger ducts near the nipple.

The stroma

The radiating lobes of glandular tissue are separated and supported by the connective and adipose tissue which forms the largest part of the mammary glands in the non-pregnant state (Sweet 1997). The breasts are held in position by the suspensory ligaments of Astley-Cooper which form from the interlobar connective tissue. These fibrous bands of tissue attach the breast to the underlying muscle fascia and to the overlying dermis (Marieb 1992).

Blood supply

The internal and external mammary arteries supplying the breasts are branches of the thoracic and pectoral arteries. The arterial blood supply terminates in networks of 5–12 capillaries surrounding each of the alveoli. Venous drainage is by venules into a circular vein behind the nipple and then into the mammary and axillary veins (Sweet 1997). There may be arteriovenous shunts that bypass the secretory tissue to drain deoxygenated blood from the breasts.

Lymphatic vessels

There is an extensive lymphatic drainage system forming a plexus beneath the areola and between the lobes of the breast with free communication between the two breasts. The smallest of these vessels are embedded in the lobuloalveolar tissue. Lymph glands drain into the axillary nodes of both axillae, glands in the anterior mediastinum and into glands in the portal fissure of the liver.

Nerve supply

Two types of nerves supply the breasts:

- somatic sensory nerves conveying impulses from skin receptors to the central nervous system;
- sympathetic motor (efferent) nerves which innervate blood vessels and the contractile muscles of the nipple.

The nipple and areola

The nipple is composed of connective tissue and smooth muscle fibres surrounding the lactiferous ducts which open onto the surface. It is covered by pigmented stratified squamous epithelium containing papillae which allow bundles of unmyelinated nerve endings to lie close to the skin surface. This makes the nipple one of the most sensitive areas of the body surface. Within the areola are about 18 sebaceous glands which enlarge during pregnancy and are known as **Montgomery's tubercles**. The red colour may be an important stimulus for the newborn baby to make the nipple easier to find. During suckling, the nipple becomes erect so that the baby can grasp and retain it in the mouth. This erection is a consequence of smooth muscle contraction and blood vessel engorgement in response to smooth muscle stimulation.

BREAST DEVELOPMENTAL CHANGES

In fetal life a line of immature breasts extends from the axilla to the inguinal region on each side. These disappear early to leave the normal number of two. Sometimes rudimentary breasts may persist and are known as **accessory breasts**, often mistaken by women for pigmented moles (Anderson 1992). They undergo pregnancy changes and lactation. Rudimentary mammary glands are present in both sexes but normally become functional only in females (Marieb 1992).

At puberty the breasts develop and enlarge under the influence of oestrogen from the growing ovarian Graafian follicles. Oestrogens develop the lactiferous tubules and ducts and cause a small amount of growth of the nipple and areola. Breasts may tingle and feel full during a menstrual period due to congestion stimulated by progesterone from the corpus luteum. However, the breasts are not mature until the woman undergoes pregnancy when new glandular tissue and ducts appear. Under the influence of prolactin, milk appears on about the 3rd day following delivery (see below).

Changes during pregnancy

Breasts begin to exhibit changes at about the 6th week of pregnancy and may be useful in confirming pregnancy (Anderson 1992, Blackburn & Loper 1992, Sweet 1997). The developmental changes are referred to as **mammogenesis** and are brought about by the increasing presence of oestrogen and progesterone from the fetoplacental unit (Fig. 54.5).

1 During the first trimester of pregnancy the structure of the breast changes and it feels nodular and lumpy due to the

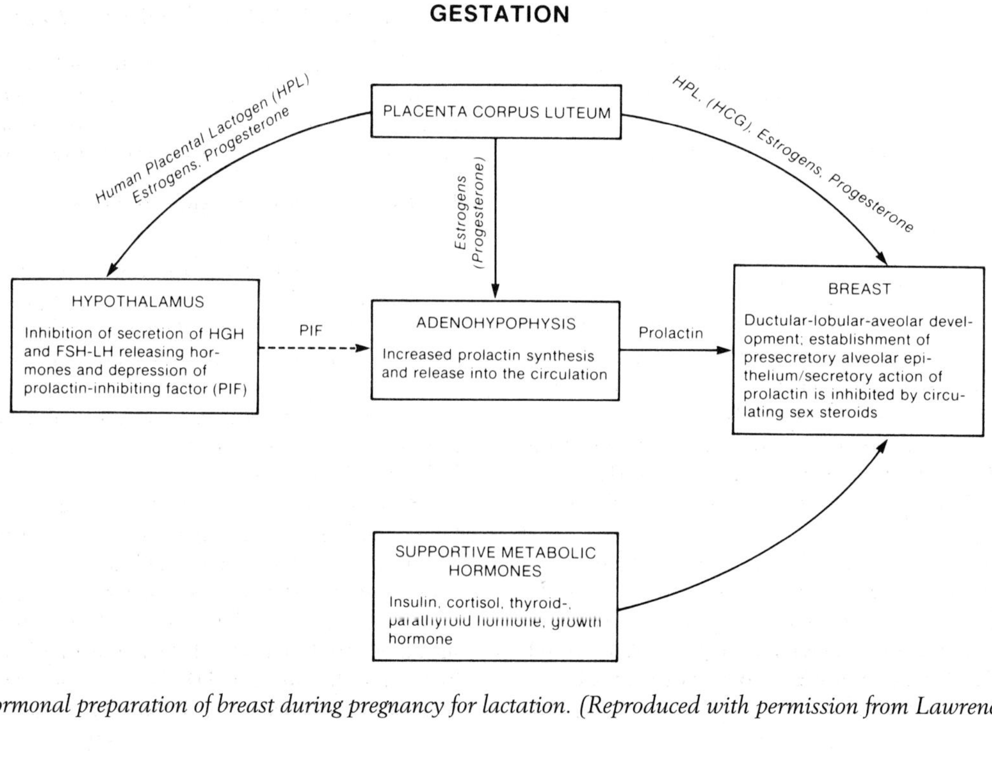

Figure 54.5 *Hormonal preparation of breast during pregnancy for lactation. (Reproduced with permission from Lawrence 1985.)*

growth and enlargement of the duct and alveolar systems. The duct systems develop under the influence of oestrogen and the alveolar systems enlarge under the influence of progesterone. The growth continues throughout pregnancy and the breasts increase in size.

2 During the 3rd trimester the epithelial cells of the alveoli differentiate into cells capable of secreting milk.
3 There is increased vascularity demonstrated by the appearance of a network of subcutaneous veins beneath the skin of the breasts. This network increases in size and complexity throughout pregnancy. By term the breasts have increased by 5 cm in size and 1400 g in weight (Sweet 1997).
4 By 12 weeks the nipples have become more prominent and the areola develops an increased fullness and brown pigmentation, the **primary areola** of pregnancy.
5 About 18 modified sebaceous glands develop in the primary areola. These are Montgomery's tubercles and are about 3 mm in diameter with a pinpoint orifice in their centres. They excrete a lubricating fluid to keep the nipple skin moist and protect it during suckling.
6 At about 16 weeks colostrum is present in the breasts and can be expressed if the breast is massaged from the periphery towards the nipple.
7 By the 24th week of pregnancy a secondary area of pigmentation called the **secondary areola** may occur, especially in dark-haired people.

Maternal nutrition and lactation

During pregnancy energy is stored in the form of body fat, mainly deposited on the woman's trunk and legs. In women with adequate nutrition this portion of the weight gain of pregnancy amounts to 4 kg, equivalent to an energy store of 35 000 kcal. This will provide for 4 months of lactation and 300 kcal per day for the baby, enough to ensure survival if the mother is deprived of food, as may happen in famine conditions (Ebrahim 1991). If a woman does not breastfeed these fat stores may be difficult to remove, leading to obesity as successive pregnancies deposit their stores. Women who breastfeed are much more likely to regain their figures.

There are two physiological aids to the accumulation of these fat stores:

1 the effect of progesterone and other hormones on the metabolism during pregnancy;
2 the slowing down of energy usage as pregnancy proceeds.

After delivery of the baby these extra stored calories are converted into milk and Ebrahim (1991) mentions a study carried out in Aberdeen where women were found to lose weight at about 0.28 kg per week whilst eating an average of 590 kcal more than those of the control group who were not lactating. Ebrahim recommended that an additional 500 kcal per day is needed by women whilst they are breastfeeding a baby.

The conversion of calorie intake to milk is very efficient. The enhanced ability to store energy in pregnancy coupled with the highly efficient conversion of food energy to breast milk enables women who suffer marginal nutrition (below 1800 kcal/day), such as those in developing countries, to breastfeed for at least 6 months or more (Ebrahim 1991).

THE PHYSIOLOGY OF LACTATION

The process of lactation can be divided into three stages.

1 The initiation of lactation, called **lactogenesis**
2 The production of milk, called **galactopoiesis**
3 The withdrawal of milk

Lactogenesis

Mepham (1987) commented that the 'switching on of milk secretion is a precipitous event'. Although small amounts of colostrum may be present in the breasts during pregnancy, following the birth of the baby a copious supply of milk must be established within the first 2 or 3 days. This must be seen as a major shift in the metabolic processes of the mother and occurs gradually with an increase in lactose content and a decrease in immunoglobulins.

Mepham also distinguishes two stages in lactogenesis.

- Stage I begins when milk components are first seen in breast tissue and colostrum can be expressed from the breast, about week 16 in humans. A specific milk protein called **α-lactalbumin** can be detected in maternal blood from midpregnancy. During this stage the physical changes in the breasts are accompanied by hormonal changes resulting from an interplay between the pituitary gland, the ovary and the placenta. These will culminate in the initiation of lactation following the birth of the baby.
- Stage II follows the birth when the flow of milk begins. There are rapid cardiovascular changes with an increase in breast blood supply, metabolic processes with the glandular tissue absorbing large amounts of milk substrates from the extra blood supply and secretory changes with the onset of milk production.

Hormonal control of lactogenesis

The four hormones involved in the initiation and maintenance of lactation are **oestrogen**, **progesterone, prolactin** and **oxytocin** (Fig. 54.6). The pituitary gland produces prolactin in increasing amounts under the stimulus of the hypothalamus.

Oestrogen and progesterone

It is highly likely that the onset and control of labour and the production of milk share the same endocrine trigger. Immediately prior to the onset of labour, during labour and following delivery of the placenta, there are abrupt changes in the hormonal content of maternal blood. Although the pathways have not been fully worked out in humans, it is possible that rising fetal cortisol levels may alter the balance of the placental hormones, increasing the level of oestrogen and decreasing the level of progesterone.

The drop in serum progesterone just before the onset of labour may be the lactogenic trigger, releasing the mammary secreting cells from their inhibitory state (Mepham 1987). The secretory cells can now respond to the circulating prolactin by producing milk. Following delivery, the pituitary gland produces low levels of follicle-stimulating hormone (FSH) and luteinising hormone (LH). The ovaries respond poorly to stimulation by FSH and LH and there is low level of oestrogen

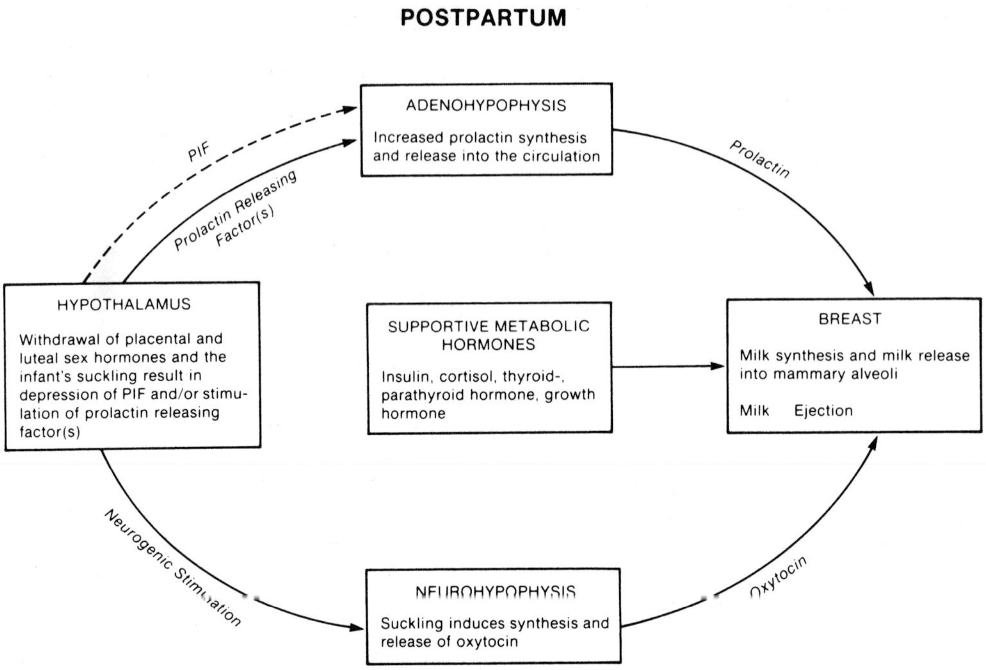

Figure 54.6 *Hormonal preparation of the breast postpartum for lactation. (Reproduced with permission from Lawrence 1985.)*

and progesterone production enhancing the production of prolactin.

Prolactin

During pregnancy plasma prolactin concentrations rise steadily to reach a concentration at term of up to 20 times that of the non-pregnant woman. The **lactotrophs** of the anterior pituitary produce increasing levels of prolactin under the influence of the rising fetoplacental production of oestrogens. This stimulatory effect may be inhibited by human placental lactogen (HPL) because of its similar biological structure and activity (Jacobs 1991). The effect of prolactin on breast tissue is inhibited during pregnancy by high levels of circulating progesterone (Mepham 1987).

The production of prolactin varies normally following a **circadian rhythm** (a rhythmic variation over 24 h). Rossmanith et al (1993) found sleep-related and diurnal variations in prolactin production. Prolactin secretion seems to be controlled by chemical factors, some inhibitory and some stimulatory (Fig. 54.7). The release of most anterior pituitary hormones is controlled by the stimulatory effect of hypothalamic releasing factors. In contrast, the release of prolactin under normal physiological circumstances is regulated in the non-lactating woman by an inhibitory factor – **prolactin inhibitory factor** (PIF) – thought to be the neuroregulatory substance dopamine (Chiocchio et al 1991). This factor is transported from the hypothalamus along the portal system to have its effect in the anterior pituitary.

Prolactin production is supported by growth hormone insulin and cortisol. Thyrotrophin-releasing hormone (TRH) may be the prolactin-releasing hormone (PRF). Administration of TRH has been shown to elevate blood prolactin levels as well as thyrotrophin. TRH also improves milk output in women whose lactation is declining (Ebrahim 1991) although Sweet (1997)

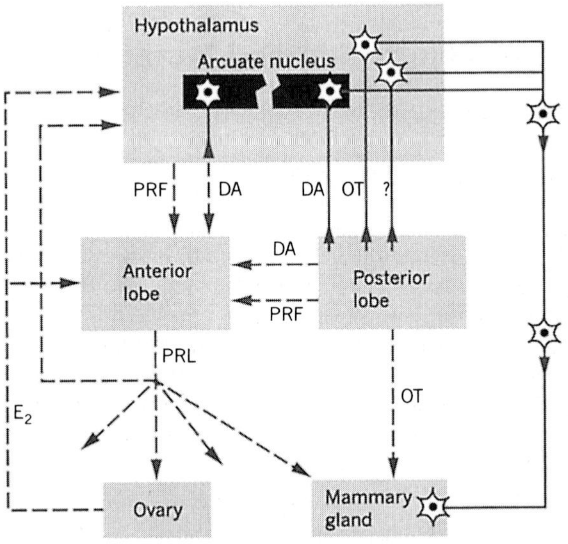

Figure 54.7 *A model depicting the neuroendocrine regulation of prolactin secretion. TH, tuberohypophyseal; T1, tuberoinfundibular; OT, oxytocin; E2, oestradiol; PRF, prolactin-releasing factor; PRL, prolactin; DA, dopamine. (Reproduced with permission from Ben-Jonathan et al 1991.)*

summarises research which suggests that TRH does not increase during suckling nor demonstrate any effect on milk production.

Another substance that has been investigated as a possible PRF is vasoactive intestinal peptide (VIP) (Mepham 1987). Recently the release of the neurotransmitter serotonin (5-hydroxytryptamine; 5-HT), β-endorphins and melanocyte-stimulating hormone induced by suckling and their reduction of dopamine inhibition of prolactin production have been studied (Sweet 1997).

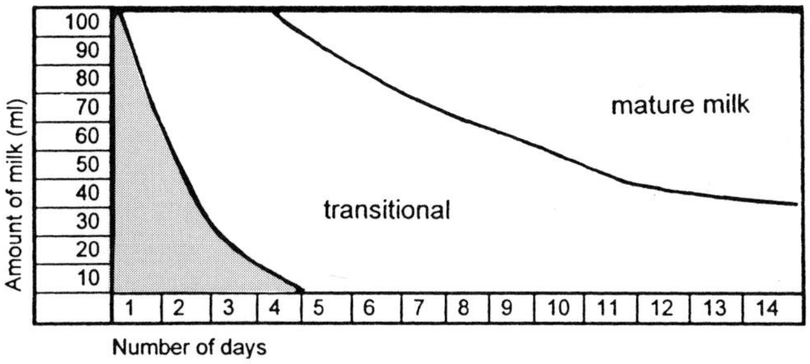

Figure 54.8 *The sequence of milk production (from Lang S, 1997, with permission).*

Galactopoiesis

After delivery plasma prolactin levels fall rapidly due to the reduction in oestrogen levels but still remain higher than in non-pregnant women. Prolactin is involved in galactopoiesis and suckling is the main stimulus for its release. Hypersecretion of prolactin follows suckling (Jacobs 1991). Plasma prolactin levels rise within 10 min of the onset of suckling and the amount of rise correlates with the length of suckling.

Prolactin levels peak 30 min after a feed and return to a baseline after 3–4 h (Sweet 1997). As might be expected of a system under the influence of circadian rhythm, suckling-induced prolactin production is minimal in the morning and greatest at night. However, no correlation has been found between the amount of milk produced and the concentration of prolactin (Diaz et al 1989, cited in Sweet 1997).

The production of milk

Colostrum is present from the 16th week of pregnancy and gradually changes into mature breast milk between the 3rd and 14th days following delivery (Fig. 54.8). It is high in density and low in volume, containing more protein, minerals and fat-soluble vitamins (A and K) than mature milk but less lactose, fats and water-soluble vitamins. It also contains more antiinfective agents such as IgA, lactoferrin, lysozymes and leucocytes than mature milk. It is eminently suited for the newborn baby (Sheridan 1997).

Mature breast milk is highly variable both within and between women. Its contents change from one feed to another, over the course of a specific feed and as the baby grows and develops. The milk obtained by the baby at the beginning of a feed is called the **foremilk** and differs from the **hindmilk** obtained towards the end of a feed (Fisher 1996).

THE CONTENTS OF BREAST MILK

The main contents of milk include proteins, carbohydrates, fats, electrolytes, minerals, vitamins, enzymes, hormones and antiinfective substances (Ebrahim 1991). All mammalian milks differ in the relative quantities of the above contents and have evolved specifically to maximise development of the newborn. Feeding one mammal's milk to another can only be second best although sophisticated modifications of cow's milk for human babies are achieved.

Protein

The **acinar** (milk-producing) cells are very efficient in removing breast milk precursors from maternal blood. Milk proteins are formed on the ribosomes bound to the rough endoplasmic reticulum from amino acids derived mainly from maternal blood. The protein molecules are then stored in the Golgi apparatus. Vesicles move the protein molecules to the apex of the cell where they are discharged into the lumen of the alveolus.

The main protein of human milk is α-lactalbumin (whey protein) and there are small amounts of caseinogen. A 3rd protein found in milk is β-lactoglobulin. There is over twice as much lactalbumin as caseinogen, with a ratio of 7:3. Besides their nutritional function, milk proteins have other specific functions (Ebrahim 1991). Casein is an important carrier of calcium and phosphate with which it forms micelles.

The amino acid composition of breast milk has developed to be perfect for the human baby and is totally different from that of other mammalian milk, for instance cow's milk. It is now apparent that not only the total protein content but the balance of amino acids present are essential for the maximum functioning of enzyme systems. For instance, the amino acids phenylalanine and tyrosine are present in much lower amounts than in cow's milk, modified or unmodified (Ebrahim 1991). The important amino acids glutamic acid and taurine are abundant in human milk but low in cow's milk. Taurine is necessary for the conjugation of bile salts and fat absorption in the first week of life. It is also essential for the myelination of the central nervous system (Sheridan 1997).

Carbohydrate

The main carbohydrate in human milk is lactose which is formed from glucose or galactose in the Golgi apparatus under the influence of the enzyme lactose synthetase. The enzyme has two components: an 'A' protein called galactosyl transferase and a 'B' protein which is α-lactalbumin. Thus the regulation of lactose is linked to the production of milk protein, in particular α-lactalbumin (Ebrahim 1991). Lactose in turn is linked to the water and mineral content of milk by exerting osmotic pressure, drawing water from the cytoplasm into the Golgi apparatus. Water makes up more than 80% of milk volume. The lactose content of milk varies between a high 7 g/100 ml in human milk to 4 g/100 ml in other mammals. Cow's milk is low in lactose.

Lactose is important for brain growth. It is also necessary for the growth of the microorganism *Lactobacillus bifidus* whose presence leads to increased acidity of the stool. Several important effects follow the increase in pH of the stools.

- Calcium salts are easier to absorb.
- Lactoferrin binds iron, making it more easily absorbed.
- The growth of pathogenic microbes is inhibited.

Fats

The lipids found in breast milk are mainly globules of triglycerides and are easy to digest and absorb. Long chain fatty acids are transported directly from maternal blood to the breast as **chylomicrons**. The acinar cells manufacture short and medium chain fatty acids. Although long chain fatty acids make up most of the fat content of milks, human milk contains more long chain (95% against 83%) than cow's milk. In both human milk and cow's milk, 5% of the remaining fatty acids are medium chain and cow's milk also contains 12% short chain fatty acids.

Arachidonic acid (AA) and docosahexaenoic acid (DHA) are two long chain fatty acids found in breast milk which are essential for the development of the brain and nervous system and for vascular tissue. The intake of biologically inappropriate fatty acids could have long-term effects on the growth of nervous tissue. In infants fed on cow's milk the unavailability of some fatty acids with a corresponding alteration in body tissue composition may be a long-term problem. In particular, the formation of the myelin sheaths may be permanently affected.

AA and another fatty acid, linoleic acid, are found in high quantities in human milk and enable prostaglandin synthesis which matures intestinal cells, aids digestion and adds to the antiinfective protective effect of breast milk. However, an illustration of the difficulty in achieving a balanced formula in modified milks was seen when linoleic acid was added to one infant formula to produce a milk rich in polyunsaturated fats. The infants fed on this formula developed a type of haemolytic anaemia. It was shown that the anaemia was caused by ingestion of large amounts of linoleic acid in the absence of vitamin E, which led to peroxide formation and haemolysis (Ebrahim 1991).

Variations in fat content of milk

The fatty acid content of breast milk varies according to the dietary source whilst the fat content varies with calorific intake (Ebrahim 1991). High quantities of free fatty acids and cholesterol are present in breast milk and act as an important energy source for the baby, providing more than 50% of the calorific requirements. The amount of fat present also undergoes diurnal variations, being lowest in the morning and highest in the afternoon. The fat content of the hindmilk is significantly increased, especially in late morning and early afternoon (Sheridan 1997). It increases during the course of a feed and may reach values of five times the initial level (Fisher 1996). As fat contains 9 kcal/g, the calorific content will vary significantly with the fat content.

Electrolytes

Lactose secretion is directly involved in the transfer of ions across the acinar cell membrane into the milk. The total content of mineral salts is less than a third of that present in cow's milk, with only 0.2% of the sodium, potassium and chloride content. The kidney of the neonate does not cope well with an increased sodium load.

Despite modification of the solute load in formula feeds, there is a risk of hypernatraemia with dehydration in bottle fed babies when the feeds are incorrectly reconstituted with too much milk powder over a period of time. High solute content leads to thirst and crying. This is generally interpreted by inexperienced parents as hunger and more feed is offered with a long-term effect of obesity. Irreversible brain damage may rarely occur in severe hypernatraemia. There may be a link between high solute loads and a predisposition to hypertension in later life. The breastfed baby is less likely to need additional fluid intake except in extreme temperatures (Sachev et al 1991).

Minerals

Calcium, phosphorus and magnesium are present in milk in concentrations higher than in plasma, suggesting active transportation. Absorption in the gut of the neonate depends on the availability of fats and vitamin D. Human milk contains 33 mg calcium and 15 mg phosphorus/100 ml, much less than cow's milk which contains 125 mg calcium and 96 mg phosphorus.

Despite these much higher levels infants fed on unmodified cow's milk are unable to absorb calcium and may suffer hypocalcaemia with tetany. Even if cow's milk is modified by replacing the cow's milk fat with a mixture of vegetable and animal fats and the addition of vitamin D, formula-fed infants tend to have lower serum calcium levels than breastfed infants (Ebrahim 1991). Low levels of magnesium may exacerbate neonatal tetany.

Trace elements

The levels of iron, copper and zinc are higher in colostrum than in mature milk (Ebrahim 1991). More zinc is present in cow's milk but is not as readily absorbed as that present in human milk. Other necessary trace elements such as copper, cobalt and selenium are present in optimal quantities (Sweet 1997). Small amounts of these elements are associated with the protein casein, large amounts with the whey proteins and moderate amounts with fats bound to specific carrier proteins (**ligands**). A small amount of zinc is necessary to ensure the baby's health.

Vitamins

The fat-soluble vitamins A, D, E and K are present in breast milk, with higher quantities of vitamin K than was previously realised being present in colostrum and hindmilk during the early days after delivery (Fisher 1996). The need to give vitamin K to neonates is discussed in Chapter 46. All B complex vitamins and vitamin C are also present in breast milk.

Enzymes

The function of many of the enzymes present in breast milk is unknown. The three following enzymes are important. **Lipase**, the fat-digesting enzyme, is present in breast milk in a form which becomes active in the baby's intestine, making fat digestion easier in breastfed babies (Fisher 1996). Also present is the starch-digesting enzyme **amylase**, the presence of which may compensate for low salivary and pancreatic amylase activity in neonates (Lonnerdal 1985). **Lysozyme** is an important bacteriolytic enzyme present in many body fluids.

Hormones

Hormones present in breast milk include prolactin, oxytocin, prostaglandins, insulin, thyroid-stimulating hormone, thyroxine and growth hormones – specifically epidermal growth factor which is important for the development of the gut lining Endocrine responses are different in breastfed babies from those who are artificially fed (Sweet 1997). Growth factor concentration is maximal in the colostrum produced on the first day of life.

Antiinfective factors

The following breast milk factors are present (Fisher 1996).

- There is a high level of **leucocytes** present in breast milk, especially in the first 10 days. These are mainly macrophages and neutrophils whose job is to surround and destroy pathogenic bacteria.
- Although **immunoglobulins** IgA, IgG, IgM and IgD are found in breast milk the most important is IgA which lines the intestinal mucosal surfaces to protect against pathogenic bacteria and viruses such as *E. coli*, salmonellae and shigellae species, streptococci, staphylococci, poliovirus and the rotaviruses.
- **Lysozyme** is a protein present in breast milk in concentrations thousands of times that of cow's milk. It is bacteriolytic and helps to break down the cell walls of pathogenic organisms.
- **Lactoferrin** is an iron-binding protein found in breast milk. It increases the absorption of enteric iron which prevents survival of pathogenic organisms such a *E. coli*, which depend on iron for their metabolism.
- The **bifidus factor** is present in human milk. This encourages the growth of the Gram-positive *Lactobacillus bifidus* which in turn discourages the growth of Gram-negative pathogenic organisms.

The transmission of viruses in milk

Babies can be infected with HIV during breastfeeding, especially if the infection is new during pregnancy and in the postnatal period (Black 1996). In developed countries it is usual to advise infected mothers not to breastfeed (Cutting 1994). However, in undeveloped countries where the alternatives to breastfeeding are poor and the risks of death due to disease or malnutrition are high, mothers should be encouraged to breastfeed. Lang (1997) suggests that mothers with HIV infection may protect their babies by breastfeeding but this is not accepted by most.

In other viral diseases such as cytomegalovirus, rubella and hepatitis B, the virus may be present in breast milk but no adverse effects on the baby occur.

Antiallergic properties

The newborn baby has an immature immune system and gut mucosa, allowing the absorption of large foreign proteins. The IgA and other factors present in breast milk encourage maturity of the gut mucosa to form a barrier against these large proteins. Sensitivity to certain allergens may be inherited and there may be a reduction in atopic diseases in childhood if mothers with known sensitivities breastfeed and avoid giving their babies cow's milk derivatives for the first few months. They may even be advised to avoid eating or drinking such allergens as cow's milk for the period of breastfeeding.

Researchers are divided as to the benefits of such advice. Gustafsson et al (1992) found no significant increase in atopic disease in children who had been fed cow's milk from their earliest days whilst Saarinen & Kajosaari (1995) found great benefit in reducing atopy in babies who were fully breastfed for 6 months. They also found that any form of breastfeeding was significant in reducing the incidence of food or respiratory allergy. Similarly, Burr et al (1993) found that children who had ever been breastfed had the lowest incidence of wheeze. Withholding cow's milk protein and replacing cow's milk with soya milk did not reduce the incidence of wheeze and allergy. It is likely that breastfeeding prevents the development of atopic diseases in children.

THE WITHDRAWAL OF MILK

There are two linked aspects of milk withdrawal. The first is the **let-down (milk ejection) reflex** and the role of the posterior pituitary hormone oxytocin. The second is the role played by infant suckling in the withdrawal of milk.

Oxytocin

Oxytocin is a peptide hormone produced in the hypothalamus and stored in the posterior pituitary gland (Blackburn & Loper 1992). The contractile tissue in the breasts, such as the myoepithelial cells surrounding the alveoli and the smooth muscle surrounding the larger ducts, have receptors for oxytocin on their cell walls. This allows them to respond to the presence of oxytocin by contracting.

The neuroendocrine mechanism or let-down reflex

Plasma oxytocin concentrations increase just prior to commencing a feed and the pattern of its release is pulsatile for the duration of the feed. The nipple and areola are provided with a rich sensory afferent supply terminating in the dorsal horn of the spinal cord where they synapse on ascending fibres which transmit the messages received from the suckling of the baby to the brainstem. The messages are then relayed to the midbrain and hypothalamus, resulting in oxytocin release. Milk is propelled out of the alveoli into the larger ducts by the contraction of the myoepithelial cells. The contraction of the smooth muscle results in shortening and widening of the ducts to allow milk to flow into the ampullae. Suckling and the subsequent emptying of the breast result in the release of prolactin (see above).

The effect of higher brain centres

The **neuroendocrine regulation** of oxytocin release and the resulting milk ejection is complex and can be inhibited or stimulated by neural influences projected by nerves synapsing on the hypothalamus from higher centres of the brain. These include those parts of the brain involved in emotion, such as the limbic system, and the cognitive interpretation of all aspects of the activity from the prefrontal cortex. These higher centre controls can be more powerful than the nipple–hypothalamic pathway. The let-down reflex can be stimulated by the sound, sight or smell of the baby and by anticipatory thoughts of suckling. It is known that anxiety, stress or embarrassment can inhibit milk ejection (Wakerley et al 1994).

Suckling

Although repeated emptying of the breast will stimulate milk secretion and flow, any factor which interferes with suckling will affect milk production (Ebrahim 1991). It is essential to put the baby to the breast as early as possible after delivery, ideally in the first hour, and allow suckling as frequently as the baby demands.

Several reflexes enable the baby to play his part in breastfeeding: the rooting, suckling, swallowing and breathing reflexes. Obstetric medication, particularly pethidine, may have negative effects on the ability of the newborn baby to respond with appropriate behaviour (Barrett 1982, Ebrahim 1991).

The **rooting reflex** is elicited when the baby's mouth is touched gently, such as by the nipple. He responds by turning his head towards the stimulus and opening his mouth wide. The wider he opens his mouth, the easier it will be for the mother to attach him to the breast.

The **suckling reflex** is complex. When the baby feels his mouth is full as far back as the hard palate and the back of his tongue, he will use jaws, tongue and cheek muscles to suckle (Ebrahim 1991). During suckling breast tissue is drawn into the baby's mouth so that an elongated teat is formed from the areola and nipple and the lactiferous sinuses are within the baby's mouth (Woolridge 1986). The lips are closed around the junction of the nipple and areola. The baby's gums are pressed against the areola and the tongue grasps the nipple and presses it against the hard palate, compressing the breast tissue beneath the areola to strip milk from the ducts (Fisher 1996). The muscles of the cheeks create suction and a negative pressure within the mouth.

The **swallowing reflex** is well developed in the term infant and the baby swallows about 0.6 ml at each mouthful. Oesophageal function is not as developed, with irregular peristalsis.

Breathing is coordinated with swallowing with an upper airways reflex to prevent aspiration (Ebrahim 1991). Under experimental conditions the introduction of water or milk from another species into the upper airway causes intermittent apnoea. Normal saline or same-species milk does not cause this. It has been observed that infants fed breast milk from a bottle suck intermittently but breathe continuously. If the infant is fed formula milk from the same bottle he sucks continuously and breathes intermittently. Breathing appears to be much more regular in babies fed breast milk. Neonates are nose breathers and cannot suckle adequately if their noses are blocked, for instance by breast tissue.

Summary of main points

- In humans two hemispherically shaped breasts are situated on the anterior chest wall on either side of the midline. There is a tail of breast tissue extending from the upper outer quadrant up into the axilla as far as the 3rd rib. Protruding from the centre of each breast, at the level of the 4th intercostal space, is the nipple surrounded by the areola.
- Mammary tissue is divided into parenchyma and stroma. The parenchyma is arranged into about 15–20 lobes. Each lobe is divided into the lobuloalveolar system. Each alveolus contains specialised milk-forming cells. Groups of 10–100 alveoli drain into small ducts which join up to form larger ducts draining the lobules. A central lactiferous duct from each lobe expands to form an ampulla where milk can be stored prior to suckling. It narrows to open onto the nipple surface.
- Lymphocytes or monocytes are found wedged between the secretory cells of the alveoli and have migrated there. They play a role in local production of antibodies in the form of IgA for secretion into the breast milk.
- The internal and external mammary arteries supply the breasts and venous drainage is into a circular vein behind the nipple and then into the mammary and axillary veins. There is an extensive lymphatic drainage with free communication between the two breasts. Two types of nerves supply the breasts: somatic sensory and sympathetic motor nerves.
- The nipple is composed of connective tissue and smooth muscle fibres surrounding the lactiferous ducts which open onto the surface. It is covered by pigmented stratified squamous epithelium. Within the areola are about 18 sebaceous glands which enlarge during pregnancy, known as Montgomery's tubercles.
- During pregnancy energy is stored in the form of body fat, mainly deposited on the woman's trunk and legs. After delivery of the baby these extra stored calories are converted into milk. An additional 500 kcal per day is needed by women whilst they are breastfeeding a baby.
- The process of lactation can be divided into three stages: the initiation of lactation, called lactogenesis, the production of milk, called galactopoiesis, and the withdrawal of milk. Although small amounts of colostrum may be present in the breasts during pregnancy, following the birth of the baby a copious supply of milk must be established within the first 2 or 3 days.
- The four hormones involved in the initiation and maintenance of lactation are oestrogen, progesterone, prolactin and oxytocin.
- It is likely that the onset of labour and the production of milk share the same endocrine trigger. The drop in serum progesterone occurring just before the onset of labour may be the lactogenic trigger, releasing the mammary secreting cells from their inhibitory state so that the secretory cells can respond to the circulating prolactin by producing milk.
- During pregnancy plasma prolactin concentrations rise steadily to reach a concentration at term of up to 20 times that of the non-pregnant woman. Prolactin secretion seems to be controlled by chemical factors, some inhibitory and some stimulatory. The prolactin inhibitory factor may be dopamine. Thyrotrophin-releasing hormone may be the prolactin-releasing hormone. Prolactin is involved in galactopoiesis and suckling is the main stimulus for its release.
- Colostrum is high in density and low in volume, containing more protein, minerals and fat-soluble vitamins than mature milk but less lactose, fats and water-soluble vitamins. It contains more anti-infective agents such as IgA, lactoferrin, lysozymes and leucocytes than mature milk. Mature breast milk is highly variable and changes from one feed to another, over the course of a specific feed and as the baby grows and develops.
- The main contents of milk include proteins, carbohydrates, fats, electrolytes, minerals, vitamins, enzymes, hormones and anti-infective substances. The main protein of human milk is α-lactalbumin and there are small amounts of caseinogen. A third protein found in milk is β-lactoglobulin. It is now apparent that not

only the total protein content but the balance of amino acids present is essential for the maximum functioning of neonatal enzyme systems.

- The main carbohydrate in human milk is lactose and its regulation is linked to the production of α-lactalbumin. Lactose in turn is linked to the water and mineral content of milk. Lactose is important for brain growth and for the growth of the microorganism *Lactobacillus bifidus* which leads to increased acidity of the stool, making calcium salts easier to absorb. Lactoferrin binds iron, making it easily absorbed, and inhibits the growth of pathogens.
- The lipids found in breast milk are mainly globules of triglycerides and are easy to digest and absorb. Long chain fatty acids are transported directly from maternal blood to the breast as chylomicrons. The acinar cells manufacture short and medium chain fatty acids, two of which – arachidonic acid and docosahexaenoic acid – are essential for the development of brain and nervous system and vascular tissue. Linoleic acid enables prostaglandin synthesis which matures intestinal cells, aids digestion and adds to the antiinfective protective effect of breast milk.
- Fats act as an important energy source for the baby, providing more than 50% of the calorific requirements. The amount of fat present undergoes diurnal variations, being lowest in the morning and highest in the afternoon. The fat content of the hindmilk is significantly increased. Lipase is present in breast milk, making fat digestion easier in breastfed babies.
- Lactose secretion is directly involved in the transfer of ions across the acinar cell membrane into the milk. The total content of mineral salts is less than a third of that present in cow's milk. Calcium, phosphorus and magnesium are present in milk in concentrations higher than in plasma, suggesting active transportation. Absorption in the gut of the neonate depends on the availability of fats and vitamin D.
- The levels of iron, copper and zinc are higher in colostrum than in mature milk. Other necessary trace elements such as copper, cobalt and selenium are present in optimal quantities. A small amount of zinc is necessary to ensure the baby's health.
- The fat-soluble vitamins A, D, E and K are present in breast milk with higher quantities of vitamin K than was previously realised being present in colostrum and hindmilk during the early days after delivery. All B complex vitamins and vitamin C are present in breast milk.
- Immunity factors present in breast milk include a high level of leucocytes, mainly macrophages and neutrophils to destroy pathogenic bacteria. The most important immunoglobulin is IgA which lines the intestinal mucosal surfaces to protect against pathogenic bacteria and viruses. Lysozyme, lactoferrin and the bifidus factor are other antiinfective agents.
- Babies can be infected with HIV during breastfeeding, especially if the infection is new during pregnancy and in the postnatal period. In other viral diseases such as cytomegalovirus, rubella and hepatitis B, the virus may be present in breast milk but no adverse effects on the baby occur.
- The newborn baby has an immature immune system and gut mucosa, allowing the absorption of large foreign proteins. Sensitivity to certain allergens may be inherited and there may be a reduction in atopic diseases in childhood if mothers with known sensitivities breastfeed and avoid giving their babies cow's milk derivatives for the first few months.
- There are two linked aspects of milk withdrawal: the let-down reflex and role of the posterior pituitary hormone oxytocin, and the role played by infant suckling. The myoepithelial cells surrounding the alveoli and the smooth muscle surrounding the larger ducts respond to the presence of oxytocin by contracting and propelling milk out of the alveoli into the larger ducts. Suckling and the subsequent emptying of the breast result in the release of prolactin.
- The neuroendocrine regulation of oxytocin release and milk ejection can be inhibited or stimulated by parts of the brain involved in emotion and cognitive interpretation. These higher centre controls can be more powerful than the nipple–hypothalamic pathway. The let-down reflex can be stimulated by the sound, sight or smell of the baby and by anticipatory thoughts of suckling. Anxiety, stress or embarrassment can inhibit milk ejection.
- Any factor which interferes with suckling will affect milk production. Several reflexes enable the baby to play his part in breastfeeding: the rooting, suckling, swallowing and breathing reflexes. Obstetric medication, particularly pethidine, may have negative effects on the ability of the newborn baby to respond with appropriate behaviour.

References

Anderson A. 1992 The Anatomy and Physiology of Obstetrics. Wolfe Publishing, London.

Barrett JHW. 1982 Prenatal influences on adaptation in the newborn. In Stratton P (ed) Psychobiology of the Human Newborn. John Wiley, Chichester, pp 267–296.

Ben-Jonathan et al. 1984 Novel aspects of posterior pituitary function: regulation of prolactin secretion. Frontiers of Endocrinology 12(3), 231–277.

Black RF. 1996 Transmission of HIV-1 in the breast feeding process. Journal of the American Dietetic Association 96(3), 267–274.

Blackburn ST, Loper DL. 1992 Maternal, Fetal and Neonatal Physiology, A Clinical Perspective. WB Saunders, Philadelphia.

Burr L, Limb ES, Maguire MJ et al. 1993 Infant feeding, wheezing and allergy: a prospective study. Archives of Diseases of Childhood 68, 724–728.

Chiocchio SR, de las Nieves Parisi M, Leisa Vitale M. 1991 Suckling-induced changes of vasoactive intestinal peptide concentrations in hypothalamic areas implicated in the control of prolactin release. Neuroendocrinology 54, 77–82.

Cutting WAM. 1994 Breast feeding and HIV – a balance of risks. Journal of Tropical Paediatrics 40(1), 6–11.

Czerkas SJ, Czerkas SA. 1990 Dinosaurs, A Global View, Dragon's World, London.

Diaz S, Seron-Ferre M, Cardenas H et al. 1989 Circadian variation of basal plasma prolactin, prolactin response to suckling and length of amenorrhoea in nursing women. Journal of Clinical Endocrinology and Metabolism 68(5), 946–955.

Ebrahim GJ. 1991 Breast-feeding: The Biological Option. Macmillan, Basingstoke.

Fisher C. 1996 Feeding. In Bennett VR, Brown LK (eds) 1996 Myles Textbook for Midwives 12th edn. Churchill Livingstone, Edinburgh, pp 519–538.

Gustafsson D, Lowhagen T, Anderson K. 1992 Risk of developing atopic disease after early feeding with cow's milk based formula. Archives of Diseases of Childhood 67, 1008–1010.

Herbert RA. 1996 Reproduction. In Hinchliff SM, Montague SE, Watson R (eds) Physiology for Nursing Practice, 2nd edn. Baillière Tindall, London, pp 679–734.

Jacobs HS. 1991 The hypothalamus and pituitary gland. In Hytten F, Chamberlain G (eds) Clinical Physiology in Obstetrics, 2nd edn. Blackwell Scientific, Oxford, pp 345–356.

Lang S. 1997 Breast milk may cut risk of HIV infection for babies. Nursing Times 93(20), 10.

Lawrence R. 1985 Breastfeeding: A Guide for the Medical Profession. Mosby, St Louis, p 57.

Lonnerdal B. 1985 Biochemistry and physiological function of human milk proteins. American Journal of Clinical Nutrition 42, 1299–1377.

Marieb EN. 1992 Human Anatomy and Physiology, 2nd edn. Benjamin/Cummings Publishing, California.

Mepham TB. 1987 Physiology of Lactation. Open University Press, Buckingham.

Rossmanith WG, Boscher S, Ulrich U et al. 1993 Chronobiology of prolactin secretion in women: diurnal and sleep related variations in pituitary lactotroph sensitivity. Neuroendocrinology 58, 589–593.

Saarinen UM, Kajosaari M. 1995 Breast feeding as prophylaxis against atopic disease: prospective follow up study until 17 years old. Lancet 346 (8982), 1065–1069.

Sachev HPS, Krishna J, Puri RK. 1991 Water supplementation in exclusively breast fed babes during the summer in the tropics. Lancet 337, 929–933.

Sheridan V. 1997 Breastfeeding. In Sweet BS with Tiran D (eds) Mayes Midwifery, 12th edn. Baillière Tindall, London, pp 801–812.

Sweet BR. 1997 The anatomy of the breast. In Sweet BR with Tiran D (eds) Mayes Midwifery, 12th edn. Baillière Tindall, London, pp 458–459.

Wakerley JB, Clarke G, Summerlee AJS, 1994 Milk ejection and its control. In Knobil E, Neill JD, Greenwald GS et al (eds) The Physiology of Reproduction. Raven Press, New York, pp 1131–1377.

Woolridge MW. 1986 The anatomy of sucking. Midwifery 2, 164–171.

Recommended reading

Black RF. 1996 Transmission of HIV-1 in the breast feeding process. Journal of the American Dietetic Association 96(3), 267–274.

Cutting WAM. 1994 Breast feeding and HIV – a balance of risks. Journal of Tropical Paediatrics 40(1), 6–11.

Ebrahim GJ. 1991 Breast-feeding: The Biological Option. Macmillan, Basingstoke.

Jelliffe DB and Jelliffe WEFP. 1979 Human Milk in the Modern World, Oxford University Press.

Rossmanith WG, Boscher S, Ulrich U et al. 1993 Chronobiology of prolactin secretion in women: diurnal and sleep related variations in pituitary lactotroph sensitivity. Neuroendocrinology 58, 589–593.

Saarinen UM, Kajosaari M. 1995 Breast feeding as prophylaxis against atopic disease: prospective follow up study until 17 years old. Lancet 346 (8982), 1065–1069.

Stables D, Hewitt G. 1995 The effect of lateral asymmetries on breast feeding skills: can midwives' holding interventions overcome unilateral breast feeding problems? Midwifery 11, 28–36.

Woolridge MW. 1986 The anatomy of sucking. Midwifery 2, 164–171.

Chapter 55

Breastfeeding practice and problems

In this chapter

INTRODUCTION

Breastfeeding is the optimal method of feeding babies, promoting closeness between mother and baby (Sheridan 1997). However, it cannot be discussed outside its social context and each nation has a rich folklore about the meaning and method of breastfeeding. One belief is that breast milk is not always adequate for the non-supplemented nourishment of babies. Jelliffe & Jelliffe (1979) suggested that successful lactation is a practical art depending on instinctive behaviour in the mother and neonate, encouraged by social support and promoted by knowledge and information given by lay and professional advisors.

Although many women in developed countries choose not to breastfeed their babies, it has been estimated that 97% of women are physiologically capable of breastfeeding. The information given in this chapter may allow practitioners involved in helping women to successfully establish breastfeeding.

PHYSIOLOGY APPLIED TO PRACTICE

In Western countries it is rare for a young woman to hold a newborn baby until she bears her own and even rarer for her to closely observe breastfeeding. A primipara is therefore faced with the need to rapidly acquire these two skills without the benefit of prior experience. The midwife must understand the above physiology and apply it to practice if mothers are to be helped to breastfeed. The baby must receive adequate nourishment at the breast and the mother must be enabled to develop the necessary skills to feed the baby herself (Fisher 1996).

Fisher (1996) demonstrates the false beliefs that interfere with the successful establishment of breastfeeding.

- The length of the feed during the first few days should be limited to avoid sore nipples.
- Both breasts must be used at each feed.
- The baby should be fed at regular intervals.
- The breast should be held away from the baby's nose during the feed. (This author has counselled many women who have been so enthusiastic to keep the breast away from the

baby's nose that they continuously pulled the nipple out of his mouth!)

There are many more misconceptions, including beliefs about the quality of colostrum and milk; for instance, that colostrum is poisonous or that the milk is too thin. This is now made more complex for the practitioner by the multicultural nature of society. As well as the physical help needed, the midwife needs to know what these beliefs are so that she can offer sensible explanations to a mother.

Practical help

Antenatal preparation

Fisher (1996) believes that most women know whether or not they wish to breastfeed before they become pregnant although a few do not make a definite decision until after the birth of their baby. Although in the past antenatal preparation of the breasts has been advocated, there is little evidence to show that it is successful other than promoting a normal standard of cleanliness and the wearing of a well-fitting supportive brassiere. Teaching pregnant women about breastfeeding physiology and skills may be more important. Women with nipple problems (see below) may find their nipple shape improves as pregnancy proceeds. The use of breast shells to help reshape the nipple and of Hoffman's exercises to free the nipple by manipulation are ineffective (Main Trial Collaborative Group 1994).

The first feed

Because of the nature of human experience in forming long-lasting beliefs, it is important that time is taken to achieve a successful first feed. Although it is preferable to feed the baby within the first hour, both mother and baby need to be suitably recovered from the birth and interested in the proceedings.

Positioning

The midwife needs to be flexible about her approach to the mother and baby. The mother may be lying down or sitting upright with her back at a right angle to her lap (Fisher 1996) but she must be comfortable. The baby should be held with his body turned towards the mother's body and his head slightly extended with his mouth opposite the nipple (Fig. 55.1). It is wise to offer the baby to the mother in a neutral position so that she can hold him on the arm she prefers for the first attempt.

Attachment of the baby's mouth to the breast

The mother should be taught to elicit the rooting reflex and shown how to offer the breast to the baby when his mouth is wide open. She should be helped to recognise when the baby has taken enough breast tissue into his mouth so that a teat is formed (Fig. 55.2) and to avoid letting him chew on the nipple. The midwife should explain that pausing is a normal part of feeding and that it will occur more frequently as the feed progresses.

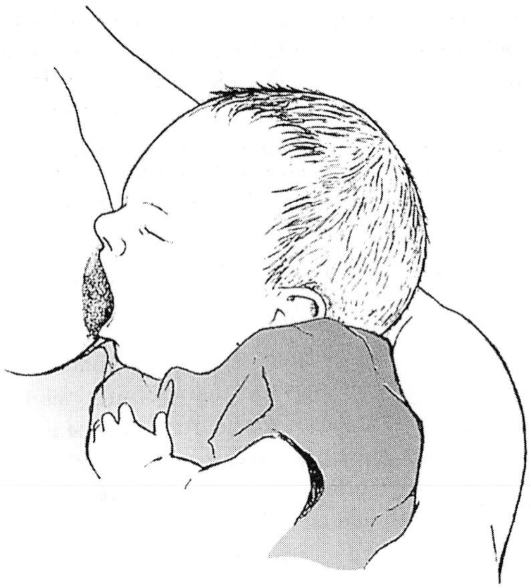

Figure 55.1 *The correct position for breastfeeding (from Sweet B, 1997, with permission).*

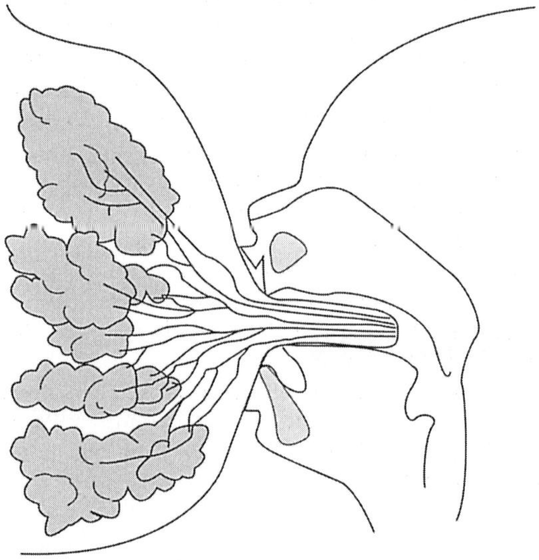

Figure 55.2 *Breast tissue formed into a teat in the baby's mouth (from Sweet B, 1997, with permission).*

Nutritional aspects

The baby must be allowed to obtain both the foremilk and hindmilk from one breast before he is offered the other to maximise his calorie intake. Changing breasts too early prevents him from obtaining the fat-laden hindmilk. If the next feed is commenced on the alternate breast, both breasts will continue to make milk.

Baby-led feeding (Fisher 1996)

Women should be assured that there is no need to know how much milk has been taken (one reason for wishing to bottlefeed). If the baby is satisfied and sleeps between feeds, he is well nourished. In particular, women need to understand that breast milk is not designed to last 4 full hours between each feed and that newborns do not differentiate night from day. At first, there may be a few problems for the mother as she may become tired with feeding too frequently. Also, it is often difficult to plan her day. However, the interval between feeds demanded will settle down as the baby develops his own circadian rhythms.

The role of lateral behavioural preferences

Human beings have at least three lateral preferences in behaviour that may influence the establishment of breastfeeding. The author carried out research into the effect of these lateral preferences (Stables & Hewitt 1995).

- The use of a dominant hand for skilled tasks, commonly the right hand.
- The use of a dominant arm to hold the baby, usually the left arm.
- A preference by the baby for turning his head to the right.

In essence, if a mother is right-handed and prefers to hold her baby in her left arm and the baby prefers to turn his head to the right, there may be a preference for feeding the baby on the left breast. This combination of events leads to the mother feeling comfortable with the baby held in her left arm which leaves her dominant right hand to manipulate the breast. The baby, who prefers to turn his head to the right, will automatically turn to face the left breast. The mother may perceive that feeding at the right breast is more difficult. These lateral preferences occasionally cause transient problems, usually overcome by the 3rd day as the mother and baby develop skills. However, some women who are ambivalent about breastfeeding may feel unable to continue.

Taking note of the lateral preferences of mother and baby, the baby may be held across his mother's lap or tucked under her arm (Fig. 55.3) if it is noticed that he consistently turns his head away from one breast (Stables & Hewitt 1995). The mother can be shown how to attach the baby to each breast using her skilful hand (Fisher 1996).

BREASTFEEDING PROBLEMS

The main problems reported by women are:

- insufficient milk;
- abnormal nipples;
- sore or cracked nipples;
- engorgement of the breasts;
- mastitis;
- breast abscess.

Other problems include:

- feeding after breast surgery;
- congenital abnormalities in the baby;
- prematurity in the baby.

Insufficient milk

This is the commonest reason given by mothers for dis-

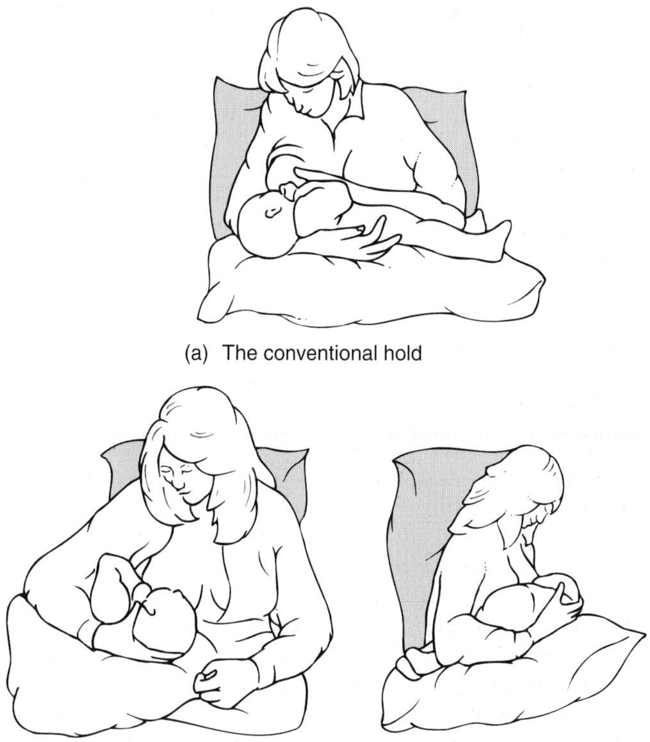

(a) The conventional hold

(b) Holding under one arm, dominant hand supports head

(c) Holding across the body, dominant hand supports head

Figure 55.3 *Ways of holding babies during breastfeeding.*

continuing breastfeeding (Graffy 1992). If breastfeeding is managed correctly with early and unrestricted feeding and no artificial milk, it should be a rare happening. **Complementary** feeding, given following a feed, and **supplementary** feeding, given instead of a feed, will eventually diminish the output of milk from the breasts as lactation is a supply-on-demand function. If the baby is not positioned correctly on the breast there may be inadequate emptying of the breast with reduction in milk supply. However, a new mother may need much support and help to overcome her beliefs. If the baby does not appear to be obtaining sufficient milk, putting him to the breast more frequently should increase milk production within a day or two (Sheridan 1997).

Abnormal nipples

Nipples may be too long so that the baby has difficulty drawing breast tissue into his mouth. Abnormally large nipples may cause difficulties for a small baby. However, probably more frequently seen are inverted (Fig. 55.4) or flat (Fig. 55.5) nipples. If the breast tissue is soft this should not cause too much of a problem as the baby will usually manage to attach to the breast, leading to an improvement in nipple shape, but difficulties arise when breast tissue is engorged. It may be necessary to express milk to give to the baby until the breast texture returns to normal.

Sore or cracked nipples

Nipples may be tender for the first few days but should not feel

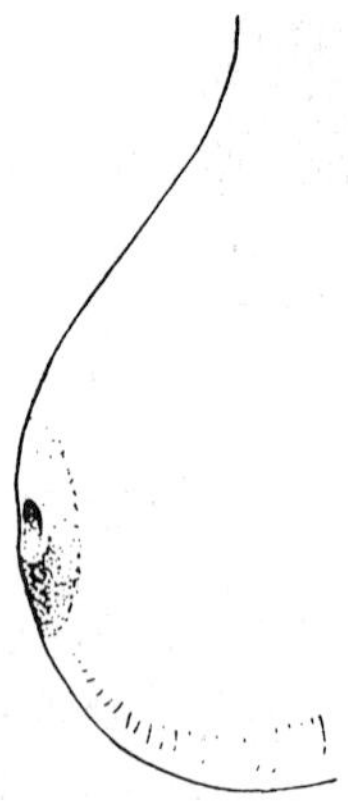

Figure 55.4 *An inverted nipple (from Lang S, 1997, with permission).*

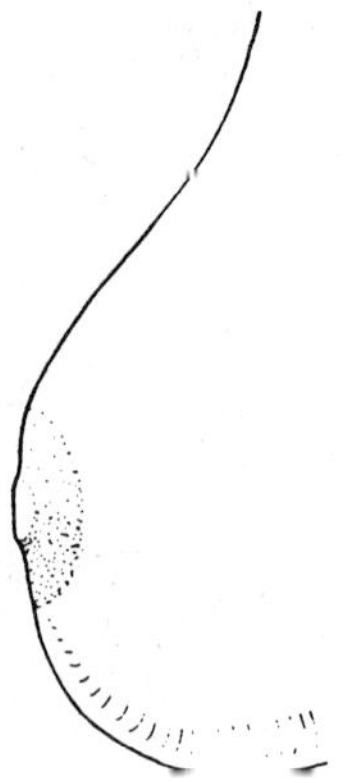

Figure 55.5 *A flat nipple (from Lang S, 1997, with permission).*

sore. If the baby has not been enabled to take sufficient breast tissue into his mouth he may have caused friction on the nipple, leading to soreness. This is more likely to occur in women with flat or inverted nipples. Depressing the breast away from the baby's face may alter the shape of the nipple and also lead to friction and abrasion. Repositioning the baby should be successful. If the nipple is too sore for the mother to continue feeding, she should rest that side and hand express, recommencing feeding when the lesion is healed.

Engorgement

Engorgment refers to the breast which becomes hard and painful. Vascular engorgement with oedema occurs between days 2 and 4 due to the increase in blood supply following delivery. The breasts appear flushed and the mother may have a slight rise in pulse and temperature. Milk production follows the increased blood supply, leading to milk engorgement if it is not removed from the breast. The breasts now become hard and painful and the alveoli are distended with milk. Suppression of milk manufacture may follow if the condition is not treated.

The midwife should ensure that the baby is positioned correctly and is attaching to the breast. Analgesia is offered and the breasts are well supported. The breasts need to be emptied of excess milk. It may help to express a little milk before the baby is put to the breast. The condition may be resolved more quickly if the baby is allowed to empty one breast at one feed and the other breast at the following feed. Illingworth & Stone (1952) demonstrated that early and unrestricted feeding helps to prevent the onset of engorgement.

Mastitis

Non-infective mastitis

Inflammation of the breast or mastitis is not always due to infection. In 50% of cases there is no infectious agent at first. Poor drainage of milk from the breast may lead to local inflammation. Signs and symptoms are rarely seen before the 8th postpartum day. The affected wedge-shaped segment of breast tissue is swollen, painful and the overlying skin is reddened. The woman complains of throbbing pain and tenderness. It is common for the woman to develop a raised temperature and pulse rate and rigors. Establishing correct breastfeeding techniques will help to prevent the development of mastitis. If it does develop, breastfeeding should be continued unless pus is present. Analgesics may be necessary and the breast should be well supported. Expression of breast milk at the end of the feed will ensure that the breasts are emptied. It is important to continue to breastfeed as milk stasis is an ideal culture for microorganisms. Prophylactic antibiotics may be commenced if it is not possible to closely observe the progress of the condition (Fisher 1996).

Infective mastitis

If bacteria enter the breast through a crack in the nipple, commonly *Staphylococcus aureus* from the baby, infective mastitis results and a breast abscess may develop. The axillary lymph glands will be enlarged. A specimen of breast milk will confirm whether or not infection is present and antibiotics may be necessary.

Breast abscess

If a breast abscess develops additional signs include pitting oedema of the overlying skin and a fluctuant swelling under the reddened area (Abbott 1997). Surgical incision and drainage is necessary. Although breastfeeding could be continued on the affected side pain usually precludes this until the incision has healed.

Feeding after breast surgery

Breast surgery may be performed to alter the shape and/or size of the breast for aesthetic purposes. These operations include the insertion of silicone breast implants and reduction mammoplasty. Surgery may also be carried out for pathological conditions and include biopsy and conservative surgery for cancer.

Breastfeeding with a silicone implant in situ may lead to risks for the baby of developing autoimmune disease such as scleroderma-like oesophageal disease in later childhood (Jordan & Blum 1996, Levine 1994). However, Williams (1994) argued that the benefits of breastfeeding outweighed the slight risk of scleroderma.

Milk production

Marshall et al (1995) found no difficulties in women who breastfed after reduction surgery. Neifert et al (1990) conducted a prospective study of the associations between biologic and surgical breast factors. Women who had had periareolar breast incisions were five times more likely to have lactational insufficiency as those without surgery. Widdice (1993) reviewed the literature over 10 years and found that women were likely to succeed in breastfeeding after breast augmentation surgery but, depending on the type of surgery, those who had undergone breast reduction ranged from 0% to 70%. Radiation following conservative surgery may interfere with breast milk production. Tralins (1995) found that following such treatment, only one in four women was able to successfully feed from the affected breast.

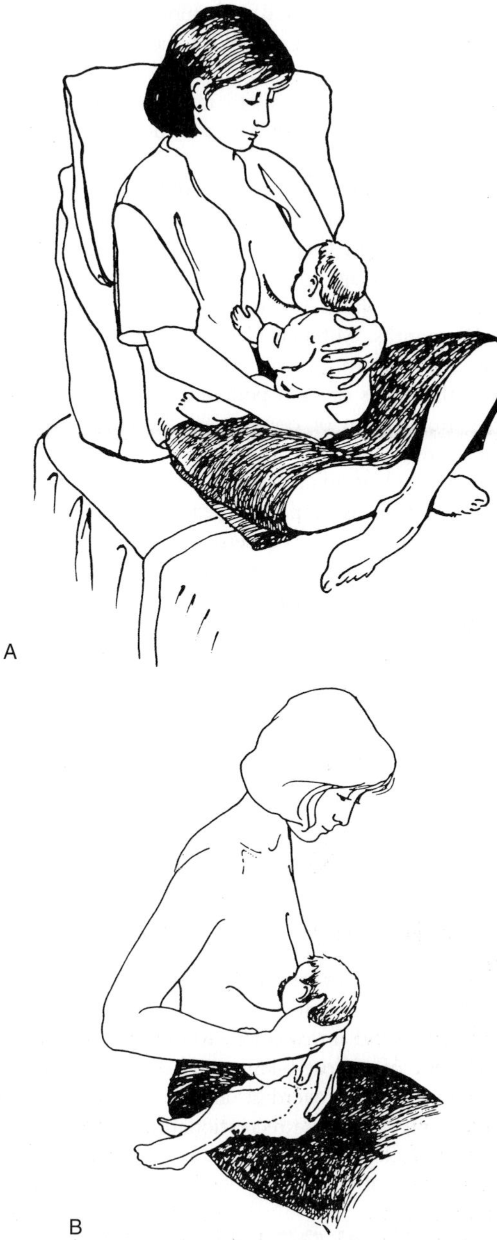

Figure 55.6 *Positions for feeding a baby with a cleft abnormality (from Lang S, 1997, with permission).*

Congenital abnormalities in the baby

Structural abnormalities of the lip and palate may make a mother feel she cannot breastfeed. In practice, if the cleft is in the lip only there should be no problem. A cleft palate will not allow the baby to obtain the suction necessary to withdraw milk as he will not be able to form a teat out of the mother's breast tissue. Some mothers have expressed their breast milk until the defect has been repaired and then achieved feeding success (Fisher 1996). Different positions for feeding (Fig. 55.6) may help a mother achieve success in breastfeeding her baby with a cleft abnormality (Lang 1997).

Prematurity in the baby

Once the baby has developed a sucking and swallowing reflex, breastfeeding is possible. If the baby tires quickly it may be necessary to complement his feeding by tube. The calorific needs of the small baby may also indicate complementary feeding.

CHEMICALS IN BREAST MILK

In recent years there has been much concern about the amount of environmental toxins that may be present in human breast milk (see Chapter 7). Also, most drugs are of a small enough molecular weight to pass into breast milk and so be ingested by the baby. Substances such as cocaine and nicotine taken as recreational drugs may also have adverse effects on the baby.

Medications

The British National Formulary (1996a,b) devotes a number of pages to the effects of prescribing in pregnancy and during breastfeeding. During the first trimester drugs may interfere with development of the fetus, resulting in congenital malformations, whilst in the 2nd and 3rd trimesters drugs may alter the growth and functional development of the fetus. Drugs given to the mother in labour may affect the neonate after delivery. Drugs given to breastfeeding mothers may inhibit lactation or may be toxic to the baby. The BNF states: 'For many drugs there is insufficient evidence available to provide guidance and it is advisable only to administer essential drugs to a mother during breast feeding'.

However, many drugs are bought over the counter and taken by lactating women. Some even take drugs prescribed for other family members. There is also the issue of women taking recreational drugs during breastfeeding. It is important that women of childbearing age should be advised to take care in the drugs that they use for minor symptoms and to seek advice from their family doctor for more severe illness.

Environmental toxins

Chemicals such as dioxin, organochlorine pesticides such as

polychlorinated biphenyls (PCB), dichlorodiphenyl dichloroethylene (DDE) (Dewailly et al 1996, Gladen & Rogan 1997, Huisman et al 1995, Hine 1997), methylmercury (Grandjean et al 1995) have provoked much research and discussion. Of concern is the ongoing motor and mental development of the growing child.

A consensus of opinion suggests that women who are anxious about pollution and breastfeeding should be reassured. There is no reason to avoid feeding their babies. Koopman-Essboom et al (1996) found that although there may be a small negative effect on breastfed babies of about 3–7 months this has disappeared by the age of 18 months. Mitchell (1997) concluded that whilst there is room for concern, breast milk is still best for the baby. Some believe the levels of such pollutants have now begun to fall following publication of popular articles and through the actions of pressure groups (DOH 1997).

Taking a wider look at infant feeding, phthalates, which act as environmental oestrogens, appear to leach out of plastics and there has recently been huge concern about their presence in formula milks. An effect on male reproductive development and function is the possible sequel to ingestion by babies (Cadbury 1997, Safe 1995).

Recreational drugs

Cigarette smoking and nicotine inhalation/ingestion in breast milk may be associated with sudden infant death (Klonoff-Cohen et al 1995), poor infant growth at 1 year (Little et al 1994), infant colic (Matheson 1995) and a reduction in breast milk quantity (Vio et al 1991). Women should be advised to stop or cut down their smoking if they are breastfeeding their baby.

Although the effect of recreational drugs on the fetus is known, there is less understanding about the effects of such drugs passed to the infant during breastfeeding. Cocaine use during breastfeeding may affect the brain of the young baby, causing convulsions and intoxication. Robinson (1996) reports the imprisonment of a drug-taking mother whose baby died through an amphetamine overdose and there are general discussions on the effect of some recreational drugs (Fulton 1990, Hansen & Moore 1990).

SUPPRESSION OF LACTATION

When women choose not to breastfeed, when there are absolute contraindications or following the loss of a baby, lactation needs to be suppressed (Fisher 1996). As breast milk is supplied on demand there is no need to provide treatment as the lactation will cease spontaneously. There may be discomfort for a day or two but it is rare to find extreme discomfort with engorgement. There is no need to restrict fluids and the woman should not be prescribed a diuretic drug.

Medication

If medication is required, bromocriptine, which acts to support dopamine's inhibition of prolactin production, can be given. It is well absorbed orally and reaches peak plasma concentrations 2 h after administration. It may cause nausea and vomiting but this risk can be minimised by taking the drug with meals. Other unwanted effects include dizziness, postural hypotension and constipation (Rang & Dale 1991). Bromocriptine should not be used in women with hypertension, coronary artery disease or present or past mental illness. A typical regime is 2.5 mg daily for 3 days followed by 2.5 mg twice daily for 14 days (British National Formulary 1996b). Although oestrogen preparations such as stilboestrol are effective there is a high risk of thrombosis with pulmonary embolism and death. Such drugs are no longer used.

LACTATION AND FERTILITY

The frequent pregnancies and births seen in developing nations are not typical of the normal human pattern. In hunter-gatherer societies babies are fed on demand, extremely frequently, day and night for up to 3 years. This intensive breastfeeding behaviour keeps the level of prolactin in the mother's blood high enough to block the development of ovarian follicles. Five children seems to be the norm and 50% of them may die before reproductive age. Thus the population would remain stable. The woman may only have a dozen or so periods throughout her life and ovulate equally as infrequently. Throughout the world prolonged breastfeeding prevents more pregnancies than all other forms of contraception added together (Short 1993).

In the human female, as in many species, regular suckling delays the resumption of fertility, probably by inhibition of the pituitary-ovarian hormonal cycle (Sweet 1997). McNeilly et al (1994) discuss the hormonal physiological mechanisms underlying lactational amenorrhoea, which may last from 2 to 4 years (Bender et al 1991). The pattern of feeding is important with frequent suckling being the most successful in reducing the risk of ovulation (Gray et al 1990).

Women who remain amenorrhoeic may be 98% protected against a further pregnancy for up to 6 months (Kennedy et al 1991). Once amenorrhoea extends beyond 6 months there is an increasing tendency for the first ovulation to precede the return of menstruation so the effect of breastfeeding as a method of contraception is reduced (Short 1993).

The use of the lactational amenorrhoea method (LAM) is of great value in spacing pregnancies in underdeveloped countries where access to scientific contraceptive methods is limited. However, the timing of returning ovulation varies widely between women and LAM is not totally reliable for women who do not wish a further pregnancy. Other contraceptive methods should be used by those women. The combined oral contraceptive has been shown to reduce breast milk output, an effect not seen in women who take the progestogen-only pill.

Breast cancer and amenorrhoea

Breast cancer is a complex disease with involvement of different tissue types. The last decade has seen a large rise in the incidence of cases and it is currently the most common cancer amongst women (Cooper 1992). About 5% of all breast cancers are familial, many involving the inheritance of the BRCA1 gene (Leutwyler 1994). Risk factors mainly involve the effect of hormones on breast tissue. Breast cancer risks are increased three times in women who have never had children or who have their first child after the age of 35. Menarche before the age of

12 or menopause after the age of 55 is associated with a twofold increase in risk (Cooper 1992). Davis & Bradlow (1995) postulate that the increased incidence in breast cancer is associated with the increase in environmental toxins.

Nesse & Williams (1995) discuss the incidence of breast, ovarian and uterine cancer and summarise findings suggesting that:

> The probability of a cancer of the female reproductive tract at any age increases directly in relation to the number of menstrual cycles a woman has experienced. The most likely victim of a cancer of reproductive tissues is an elderly woman who had an early menarche and late menopause and never had her cycling interrupted by pregnancy and lactation.

If this is so, it will involve repeated cyclical cellular responses of breast tissue to the changing hormonal environment of the female body. Nesse & Williams suggest that hormone manipulations may mimic the protective effects of repeated pregnancies and lactation divided by only one or two menstrual cycles. Currently there is evidence that oral contraception is protective against ovarian and uterine cancer but not breast cancer (Henderson et al 1993).

MODIFICATION OF COW'S MILK

Differences between human and cow's milk

In the previous chapter, reference was made to the many differences between cow's milk and human milk. All mammalian milks differ in the relative quantities of the contents and have evolved specifically to maximise development of the newborn. Feeding one mammal's milk to another can only be second best although sophisticated modifications of cow's milk for human babies are achieved. Relatively few women are absolutely unable to breastfeed their babies but many choose to bottlefeed for their own reasons. Therefore it is important that a safe alternative is available. Some of the differences in contents between human milk and cows milk are listed below, taken from Ebrahim (1991).

- The amino acids phenylalanine and tyrosine are present in human milk in much lower amounts than in cow's milk. The important amino acids glutamic acid and taurine are abundant in human milk but low in cow's milk.
- The lactose content of milks varies between a high 7 g/100 ml in human milk and 4 g/100 ml in other mammals. Cow's milk is low in lactose.
- Human milk contains more long chain fatty acids (95% against 83%) than cow's milk. In both human milk and cow's milk 5% of the remaining fatty acids are medium chain and cow's milk also contains 12% short chain fatty acids.
- The total content of mineral salts is less than a third of that present in cow's milk, with only 0.2% of the sodium, potassium and chloride content. The neonatal kidney does not cope well with an increased sodium load.
- Human milk contains 33 mg calcium and 15 mg phosphorus/100 ml, much less than cow's milk which contains 125 mg calcium and 96 mg phosphorus. Despite these higher levels, infants fed on unmodified cow's milk are unable to absorb sufficient calcium.
- More zinc is present in cow's milk but is not as readily absorbed as that present in human milk.
- Lipase, the fat-digesting enzyme, is present in breast milk in a form which becomes active in the baby's intestine, making fat digestion easier in breastfed babies (Fisher 1996).
- There is a high level of leucocytes in breast milk, especially in the first 10 days, mainly macrophages and neutrophils. The main immunoglobulin present is IgA which lines the intestinal mucosal surfaces to protect against pathogenic bacteria and viruses.
- Lysozyme is present in breast milk in concentrations thousands of times that of cow's milk.
- Lactoferrin increases the absorption of enteric iron which prevents survival of pathogenic organisms such as *E. coli*, which depend on iron for their metabolism.
- The bifidus factor present in human milk encourages the growth of the Gram-positive *Lactobacillus bifidus*, which discourages the growth of Gram-negative pathogenic organisms.
- If mothers with known allergies breastfeed, atopic disease in the child may be avoided.

The manufacture of infant formulae

Although manufacturers have achieved a high level of success in approximating cow's milk to human milk in food, electrolyte, vitamin, mineral and fluid content and calorific value, it is impossible to match the antiinfective and antiallergenic properties of human milk and breast milk will never be totally replaced. The essential composition of infant formulae so that they best approximate breast milk has been set down in statute and manufacturers must adhere closely to the guidelines.

Formula milk is modified from skimmed milk and whey milk (Fisher 1996). Much of the casein protein is removed and replaced by whey protein. There are some differences between milks and they can be divided mainly into two groups: casein dominant and whey dominant. Although whey-dominant formulae are recommended for the early weeks and casein-dominant formulae for the older baby, there is no evidence to show that one is superior to the other (Coates 1997). Lactose is added and some of the milk fat is replaced by vegetable fat. The solute load is reduced. Extra iron is added and the vitamin content is supplemented.

In order to reduce the worldwide movement towards artificial feeding, the World Health Organisation (WHO) and the United Nations Children's Fund (UNICEF) produced an international code of marketing for breast milk substitutes (WHO 1981). Most countries use this or a modified version. The recommendations for manufacturers of infant formulae include the following.

- No advertising or promotion directly to the public.
- No free samples given to mothers.
- No free gifts such as discount coupons or special offers.
- Accurate and scientific evidence provided by manufacturers to health-care workers.
- No financial or other gifts to health-care workers to promote products.
- Health workers should encourage and promote breastfeeding.

Summary of main points

- In Western countries it is rare for a young woman to hold a newborn baby until she bears her own or to closely observe breastfeeding. A primipara is faced with the need to acquire these two skills without the benefit of prior experience. The midwife must ensure that the baby is adequately nourished and that the mother is enabled to develop the necessary skills to feed the baby.
- There are many misconceptions, including beliefs about the quality of colostrum and milk; for instance, that colostrum is poisonous or that the milk is too thin. This is now made more complex for the practitioner by the multicultural nature of society. The midwife needs to understand these beliefs so that she can offer sensible explanations to a mother.
- Although in the past antenatal preparation of the breasts has been advocated there is little evidence to show that it is successful other than promoting a normal standard of cleanliness and the wearing of a well-fitting supportive brassiere. The use of breast shells to help reshape the nipple and of Hoffman's exercises to free the nipple by manipulation have been found to be ineffective.
- Because of the nature of human experience in forming long-lasting beliefs, it is important that time is taken to achieve a successful first feed. Both mother and baby need to be suitably recovered from the birth and interested. The mother may be lying down or sitting upright with her back at a right angle to her lap. The baby should be held with his body turned towards the mother's body, his head slightly extended and his mouth opposite the nipple. The baby should be offered to the mother in a neutral position so that she can hold him on the arm she prefers.
- The baby must be allowed to obtain both the foremilk and hindmilk from one breast before he is offered the other to maximise his calorie intake. Changing breasts too early prevents him from obtaining the fat-laden hindmilk.
- Human beings have three lateral preferences in behaviour that may influence the establishment of breastfeeding. These are the use of a dominant hand for skilled tasks, the use of a dominant arm to hold the baby and a preference by the baby for turning his head to one side. These preferences may cause transient problems during feeding, usually overcome by the 3rd day. However, some women may feel unable to continue. Taking note of individual lateral preferences, the baby may be held across his mother's lap or tucked under her arm if he consistently turns his head away from one breast. The mother can be shown how to attach the baby to each breast using her skilful hand.
- Insufficient milk is the commonest reason given by mothers for discontinuing breastfeeding. If breastfeeding is managed correctly with early and unrestricted feeding and no artificial milk, it should be a rare happening.
- Nipples that are too long or too large may make it difficult for the baby to draw breast tissue into his mouth. More frequently seen are flat or inverted nipples. If the baby has not been enabled to take sufficient breast tissue into his mouth he may have caused friction on the nipple, leading to soreness. If the nipple is too sore for the mother to continue feeding, she should rest that side and hand express, recommencing feeding when the lesion is healed.
- Vascular engorgement with oedema occurs between days 2 and 4 due to the increase in blood supply following delivery. Milk production follows the increased blood supply, leading to milk engorgement if it is not removed from the breast. Suppression of milk manufacture may follow if the condition is not treated. Early and unrestricted feeding helps to prevent its onset.
- Poor drainage of milk from the breast may lead to local inflammation. Establishing correct breastfeeding techniques will help to prevent the development of mastitis. If bacteria enter the breast through a crack in the nipple, infective mastitis results. A specimen of breast milk will confirm whether or not infection is present and antibiotics may be necessary. If a breast abscess develops surgical incision and drainage is necessary.
- Breast surgery may be performed for aesthetic purposes or for pathological conditions. Breastfeeding with a silicone implant in situ may lead to risks for the baby of developing autoimmune disease. Women may succeed in breastfeeding after breast augmentation surgery. Radiation therapy may interfere with breast milk production.
- A cleft palate will not allow the baby to obtain the suction necessary to withdraw milk as he will not be able to form a teat out of the mother's breast tissue. Some mothers have expressed their breast milk until the defect has been repaired and then achieved feeding success.
- Once the preterm baby has developed a sucking and swallowing reflex, breastfeeding is possible. If the baby tires quickly it may be necessary to complement his feeding by tube. The calorific needs of the small baby may also indicate complementary feeding.
- There has been much concern about the amount of environmental toxins that may be present in human breast milk. Most drugs are of a small enough molecular weight to pass into breast milk and so be ingested by the baby. Substances such as cocaine and nicotine taken as recreational drugs may also have adverse effects on the baby.
- When women choose not to breastfeed or cannot breastfeed, lactation needs to be suppressed. As breast milk is supplied on demand, lactation will cease spontaneously. There is no need to restrict fluids and the woman should not be prescribed diuretics. If medication is required, bromocriptine is well absorbed. Although oestrogen preparations are effective, there is a high risk of thrombosis, pulmonary embolism and death.
- The frequent pregnancies and births seen in developing nations are not typical of the normal human pattern. In hunter-gatherer societies babies are fed on demand, extremely frequently, for up to 3 years. Throughout the world prolonged breastfeeding prevents more pregnancies than all other forms of contraception. Lactational amenorrhoea may last from 2 to 4 years. The pattern of feeding is important, with frequent suckling being the most successful in reducing the risk of ovulation.
- About 5% of breast cancers are familial, many involving the inheritance of the BRCA1 gene. Breast cancer risks are increased in women who have never had children or who have their first child after the age of 35. Early menarche or late menopause is associated with a twofold increase in risk. Breast cancer may be associated with the increase in environmental toxins.
- Findings suggest that cancer of the female reproductive tract at any age increases directly in relation to the number of menstrual cycles a woman has experienced, especially if she has never had her cycling interrupted by pregnancy and lactation. Currently there is evidence that oral contraception is protective against ovarian and uterine cancer but not breast cancer.
- Formula milk is modified from skimmed cow's milk and whey milk. In order to reduce the worldwide movement towards artificial feeding, the World Health Organization and the United Nations Children's Fund produced an international code of marketing for breast milk substitutes.

References

Abbott H. 1997 Complications of the puerperium. In Sweet BS with Tiran D (eds) Mayes Midwifery, 12th edn. Baillière Tindall, London, pp 719–728.

Bender DE, McCann MF, Rodriguez S et al. 1994 The promotion of breast feeding as a method of child spacing in periurban Bolivia. International Journal of Health Sciences 5(4), 161–169.

British National Formulary 1996a Number 32 (September) Prescribing in Pregnancy, Appendix 4. BMA/RPSGB, London, pp 581–590.

British National Formulary 1996b Number 32 (September) Prescribing in Breast Feeding, Appendix 5. BMA/RPSGB, London, pp 591–597.

Cadbury SD. 1997 The Feminisation of Nature. Hamish Hamilton, London, pp 154–184.

Coates T. 1997 Artificial feeding. In Sweet BR with Tiran D (eds) Mayes Midwifery, 12th edn. Baillière Tindall, London, pp 813–818.

Cooper GM. 1992 Elements of Human Cancer. Jones and Bartlett, Boston.

Davis DL, Bradlow HL. 1995 Can environmental estrogens cause breast cancer? Scientific American 273(4), 144–149.

Dewailly E, Ayotte P, Laliberte C et al. 1996 Polychlorinated biphenyls (PCB) and dichlorodiphenyl dichloroethylene (DDE) concentrations in the breast milk of women in Quebec. American Journal of Public Health 86(9), 1241–1246.

Department of Health 1997 Department of Health statement (on the review by the Committee on Toxicity of Chemicals in Food, Consumer Products and the Environment of polychlorinated biphenyls and dioxins in food. DOH, London.

Ebrahim GJ. 1991 Breast-feeding: The Biological Option. Macmillan, Basingstoke.

Fisher C. 1996 Feeding. In Bennett VR, Brown LK (eds) Myles Textbook for Midwives, 12th edn. Churchill Livingstone, Edinburgh, pp 519–538.

Fulton B. 1990 Recreational drug use in the breast feeding mother. Part 2: Licit drugs. Journal of Human Lactation 6(1), 15–16.

Gladen BC, Rogan WJ. 1997 Effects of polychlorinated biphenyls and dichlorodiphenyl dichloroethylene on later development. Journal of Paediatrics 119(1) part 1, 58–63.

Graffy JP. 1992 Mothers' attitudes to and experience of breast feeding: a primary case study. British Journal of General Practice 42, 61–64.

Grandjean PP, Weihe P, White RF. 1995 Milestone development in infants exposed to methylmercury from human milk. Neurotoxicology 16(1), 27–34.

Gray RH, Campbell OM, Apelo R et al. 1990 Risk of Ovulation during lactation. Lancet 335 (8680), 25–29.

Hansen B, Moore L. 1990 Recreational drug use by the breast feeding woman. Part 1: Illicit drugs. Journal of Human Lactation 5(4), 178–180.

Henderson BE, Ross R, Pike MC et al. 1993 The reduction in uterine and ovarian cancer risk as a result of oral contraceptive use. Science 259, 633–638.

Hine D. 1997 Review of Dioxins and PCBs. Welsh Office, Cardiff.

Huisman M, Koopman-Essboom C, Lanting CI et al. 1995 Neurological condition in 18-month-old children perinatally exposed to polychlorinated biphenyls and dioxin. Early Human Development 43(2), 165–176.

Illingworth RS, Stone DGH, 1952 Self-demand feeding in a maternity unit. Lancet 1, 683–687.

Jelliffe DB, Jelliffe WEFP. 1979 Human Milk in the Modern World. Oxford University Press, Oxford.

Jordan ME, Blum RWM. 1996 Should breast-feeding by women with silicone implants be recommended? Archives of Pediatrics and Adolescent Medicine. 150(8) 880–881.

Kennedy KI, Parenteau-Carreau S, Flynn A et al. 1991 The natural family planning–lactational amenorrhoea interface: observations from a prospective study of breast feeding users of natural family planning. American Journal of Obstetrics and Gynecology 165(6), 2020–2026.

Klonoff-Cohen HS, Edelstein SL, Lefkowitz ES et al. 1995 The effect of passive smoking and tobacco exposure through breast milk on sudden infant death syndrome. JAMA 273(10), 795–798.

Koopman-Essboom C, Weisglas-Kuperus N, de Ridder MAJ et al. 1996 Effects of polychlorinated biphenyl/dioxin exposure and feeding type on infants' mental and psychomotor development. Pediatrics 97(5), 700–706.

Lang S. 1997 Breast milk may cut risk of HIV infection for babies. Nursing Times 93(20), 10.

Leutwyler K. 1994 Deciphering the breast cancer gene. Scientific American 271(6), 18–19.

Levine JJ, Ilowite NT 1994, Sclerodermalike esophageal disease in children breast-fed by mothers with silicone breast implants. Journal of American Medical Association, 271(3), 213–216.

Little RE, Lambert MD, Worthington-Roberts B et al. 1994 Maternal smoking during lactation, relation to infant size at one year of age. American Journal of Epidemiology 140(6), 544–554.

McNeilly AS, Tay CCK, Glasier A, 1994, Physiological mechanisms underlying lactational amenorrhoea. Annals of New York Academy of Sciences, 709: 145–155.

Main Trial Collaborative Group 1994 Preparing for breast feeding: treatment of inverted and non-protractile nipples in pregnancy. Midwifery 10, 200–213.

Marshall DR, Callan PP, Nicholson W. 1995 Breast feeding after reduction mammoplasty. British Journal of Plastic Surgery 47, 167–169.

Matheson I. 1995 The effect of smoking on lactation and infant colic. JAMA 261(1), 42–43.

Mitchell P. 1997 Pollutants in breast milk cause concern, but breast is still best. Lancet 349(9064), 1525.

Neifert M, DeMarzo S, Seacat J et al. 1990 The influence of breast surgery, breast appearance and pregnancy induced breast changes on lactational sufficiency as measured by infant weight gain. Birth 17(1), 31–38.

Nesse RM, Williams GC 1995 Evolution and Healing, Weidenfield and Nicolson, London.

Rang HP, Dale MM. (1991) Pharmacology, 2nd edn. Churchill Livingstone, Edinburgh.

Robinson J. 1996 Six years in jail – for breast feeding. MIDIRS, Midwifery Digest 6(2), 241–242.

Safe SH. 1995 Assessing the role of environmental oestrogens in human reproductive health. Health and Environment Digest 8, 79–81.

Sheridan V. Breastfeeding. In Sweet BR with Tiran D (eds) Mayes Midwifery, 12th edn. Baillière Tindall, London, pp 801–812.

Short RV. 1993 Lactational infertility in family planning. Annals of Medicine 25(2), 175–180.

Stables D, Hewitt G. 1995 The effect of lateral asymmetries on breast feeding skills: can midwives' holding interventions overcome unilateral breast feeding problems? Midwifery 11, 28–36.

Sweet BR. 1997 The physiology of lactation. In Sweet BR with Tiran D (eds) Mayes Midwifery, 12th edn. Baillière Tindall, London.

Tralins AH. 1995 Lactation after conservative breast surgery combined with radiation therapy. American Journal of Clinical Oncology 18(1) 40–43.

Vio F, Salazar G, Infante C. 1991 Smoking during pregnancy and lactation and its effects on breast-milk volume. American Journal of Clinical Nutrition 54(6), 1011–1016.

Widdice L. 1993 The effects of breast reduction and breast augmentation surgery on lactation: an annotated bibliography. Journal of Human Lactation 9(3), 161–167.

Williams AF, 1994, Silicone breast implants, breastfeeding and scleroderma. Lancet 343(8904), 1043–1044.

World Health Organization 1981 International Code of Marketing of Breast Milk Substitutes. WHO, Geneva.

Recommended reading

Bender DE, McCann MF, Rodriguez S et al. 1994 The promotion of breast feeding as a method of child spacing in periurban Bolivia. International Journal of Health Sciences 5(4), 161–169.

Cadbury SD. 1997 The Feminisation of Nature. Hamish Hamilton, London, pp 154–184.

Davis DL, Bradlow HL. 1995 Can environmental estrogens cause breast cancer? Scientific American 273(4) 144–149.

Diaz S, Seron-Ferre M, Cardenas H et al, 1989, Circadian variation of basal plasma prolactin, prolactin response to suckling and length of amenorrhoea in nursing women, Journal of Clinical Endocrinology and Metabolism, vol 68, no 5: 946–955 in Sweet BR, The Anatomy of the Breast, Chapter 35 in Sweet BR with Tiran D (eds.), Mayes Midwifery, Baillière Tindall, 1997: 458–459.

Graffy JP. 1992 Mothers' attitudes to and experience of breast feeding: a primary case study. British Journal of General Practice 42, 61–64.

Gray RH, Campbell OM, Apelo R et al. 1990 Risk of ovulation during lactation. Lancet 335(8680), 25–29.

Kennedy KI, Parenteau-Carreau S, Flynn A et al. 1991 The natural family planning–lactational amenorrhoea interface: observations from a prospective study of breast feeding users of natural family planning. American Journal of Obstetrics and Gynecology 165(6), 2020–2026.

Main Trial Collaborative Group 1994 Preparing for breast feeding: treatment of inverted and non-protractile nipples in pregnancy. Midwifery 10, 200–213.

Neifert M, DeMarzo S, Seacat J et al. 1990 The influence of breast surgery, breast appearance and pregnancy induced breast changes on lactational sufficiency as measured by infant weight gain. Birth 17(1), 31–38.

Short RV. 1993 Lactational infertility in family planning. Annals of Medicine 25(2), 175–180.

Stables D, Hewitt G. 1995 The effect of lateral asymmetries on breast feeding skills: can midwives' holding interventions overcome unilateral breast feeding problems? Midwifery 11, 28–36.

Chapter 56 The puerperium

In this chapter

INTRODUCTION

Anderson et al (1994) define the word puerperium as:

> The time after childbirth, lasting approximately six weeks, during which the anatomic and physiologic changes brought about by childbirth resolve and a woman adjusts to the new or expanded responsibilities of motherhood and non-pregnant life.

It commences immediately after completion of labour. The postnatal period is a social concept and, in the Midwives' Rules (UKCC 1993), it is defined as:

> A period of not less than 10 days and not more than 28 days after the end of labour during which time the continued attendance of a midwife on the mother and baby is requisite.

This chapter will address the physiology of the puerperium and the biological content of the multifactorial influences on emotional and cognitive reactions to childbirth and parenthood. Other aspects of postnatal care include family planning, which is considered in Chapter 5, and interactive aspects of parenting, which is the content of Chapter 57. The main maternal puerperal complications include postpartum haemorrhage, thromboembolic disorders, puerperal infections and psychiatric disorders. Postpartum haemorrhage can be found in Chapter 45, thromboembolic disorders, including thrombophlebitis, deep vein thrombosis and pulmonary embolism, are discussed in Chapter 33 and the other two problems are considered below.

PHYSIOLOGICAL CHANGES

During the puerperium the physiological changes can be divided into:

- involution of the uterus and genital tract;
- secretion of breast milk;
- other physiological changes.

The anatomy of the breast, initiation and maintenance of lactation and breastfeeding are so important that Chapter 55 has been devoted entirely to the topic.

Endocrine changes

Following delivery of the placenta, there is a profound fall in the serum level of placental hormones human placental lactogen, human chorionic gonadotrophin, oestrogen and progesterone. Removal of the placental hormones initiates the return of the body systems to their prepregnant state. The rate of removal of the hormones depends on their half-life, firstly and more rapidly in maternal blood and later in tissues. Within 24 h plasma oestradiol reaches levels of less than 2% of those seen at the end of pregnancy. Oestrogen levels return almost to prepregnant levels by 7 days. Progesterone levels return to those found in the luteal phase of the menstrual cycle by 48 h and to the follicular phase by 7 days (Fig. 56.1). The enlarged thyroid gland regresses and the basal metabolic rate returns to normal.

Resumption of menstruation and ovulation

Most women are relatively infertile during the postnatal period. This infertility may continue during the period of lactation. However, there is wide variation among women in the return to ovulation, regardless of whether the woman breastfeeds or not. The return of ovulation is preceded by an increase in plasma progesterone. In most cases the first menstrual cycle following delivery is anovulatory but in 25% of women ovulation may occur before menstruation and pregnancy may result. Anovulatory cycles are more common in lactating women (Blackburn & Loper 1992). Two maternal hormones involved in initiation and maintenance of lactation will be briefly mentioned here and are discussed more fully in Chapter 55. **Prolactin** is secreted by the anterior pituitary gland in increasing amounts during pregnancy but its effects are suppressed by oestrogen. **Oxytocin** is produced in the hypothalamus and stored in the posterior pituitary gland. This hormone stimulates electrical and contractile activity in the myometrium to aid involution and is critical for milk ejection during lactation (Blackburn & Loper 1992).

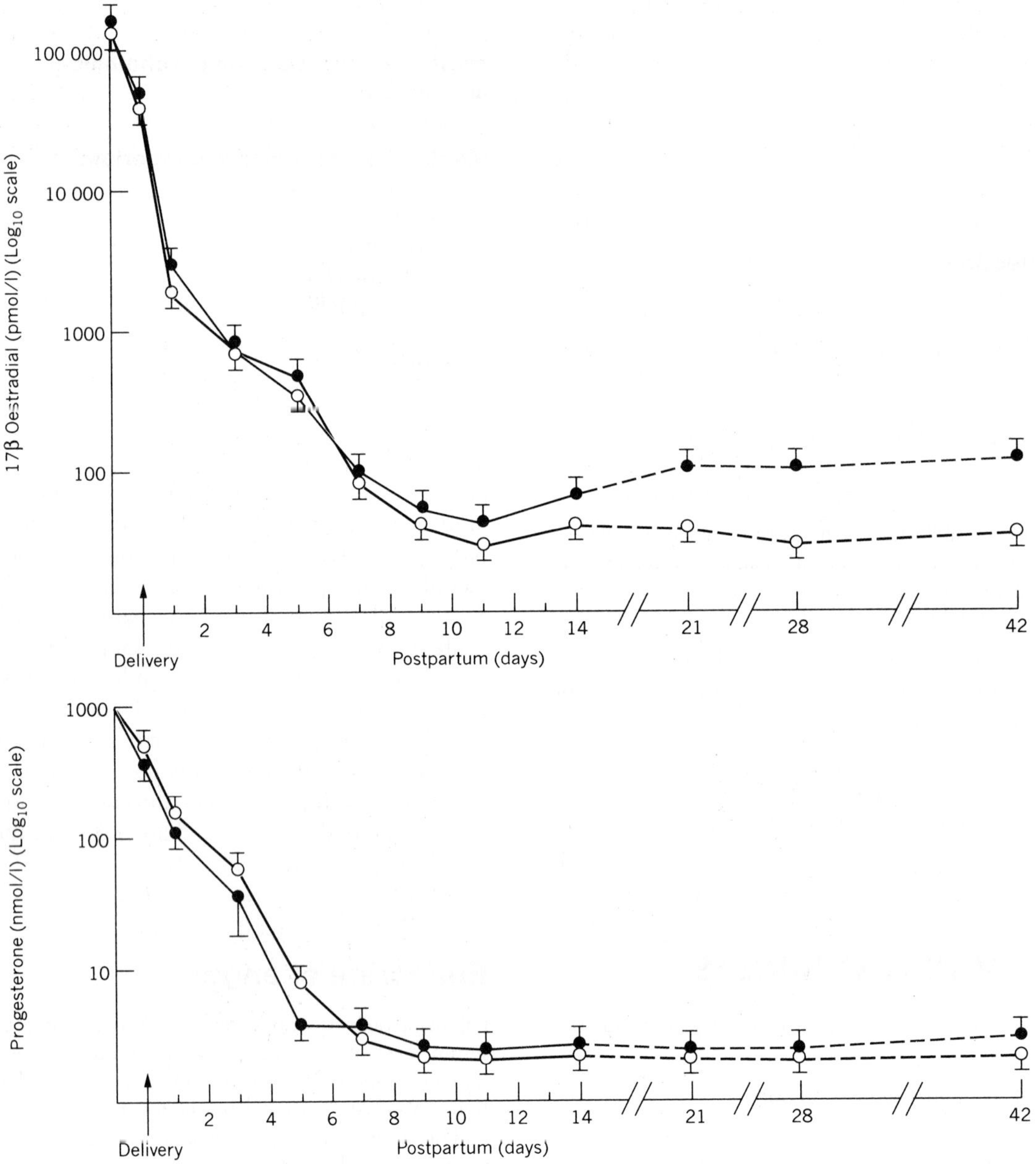

Figure 56.1 *Mean (± SEM) serum concentrations of 17β-oestradiol and progesterone in lactating and non-lactating subjects. Lactating subjects (n = 10) o-o; non-lactating subjects (n = 9) •-• (from Sweet B, 1997, with permission).*

Involution

Anderson et al (1994) define the word involution as 'A normal process characterised by a decrease in the size of an organ caused by a decrease in the size of its cells, such as postpartum involution of the uterus'. The uterus now returns to its normal size, tone and position and the vagina, uterine ligaments and muscles of the pelvic floor also return to their prepregnant state (Sweet 1997a). The pelvic floor and problems that can arise if the ligaments and muscles are permanently weakened have been discussed in Chapter 25.

Physiology

During involution there are changes to the myometrium and the decidua of the pregnant uterus (Fig. 56.2). The return of the muscle layer to normal thickness is brought about by the processes of ischaemia, autolysis and phagocytosis. The decidua is shed as the **lochia** and there is regeneration of the endometrium.

Ischaemia occurs when the muscles of the uterus retract at the end of the 3rd stage to constrict the blood vessels at the placental site, resulting in haemostasis. Blood circulating to the uterus is greatly reduced.

Autolysis is the process of removal of the redundant actin and myosin muscle fibres and cytoplasm by proteolytic enzymes and macrophages. Individual myometrial cells are reduced in size but there is no significant reduction in the numbers of cells (Blackburn & Loper 1992).

Phagocytosis removes the excess fibrous and elastic tissue. This process is incomplete and some elastic tissue remains so that a uterus that has held a pregnancy never quite returns to the nulliparous state (Sweet 1997a).

Positional changes

Immediately after delivery of the placenta the uterus weighs about 1000 g. It is situated with its anterior and posterior walls in close apposition in the midline of the body, with the fundus about midway between the umbilicus and symphysis pubis. The muscles are well contracted and the uterus feels hard and globular, like a cricket ball. Over the next 12 h the muscles relax slightly and the fundus returns to the level of the umbilicus, about 12 cm above the symphysis pubis.

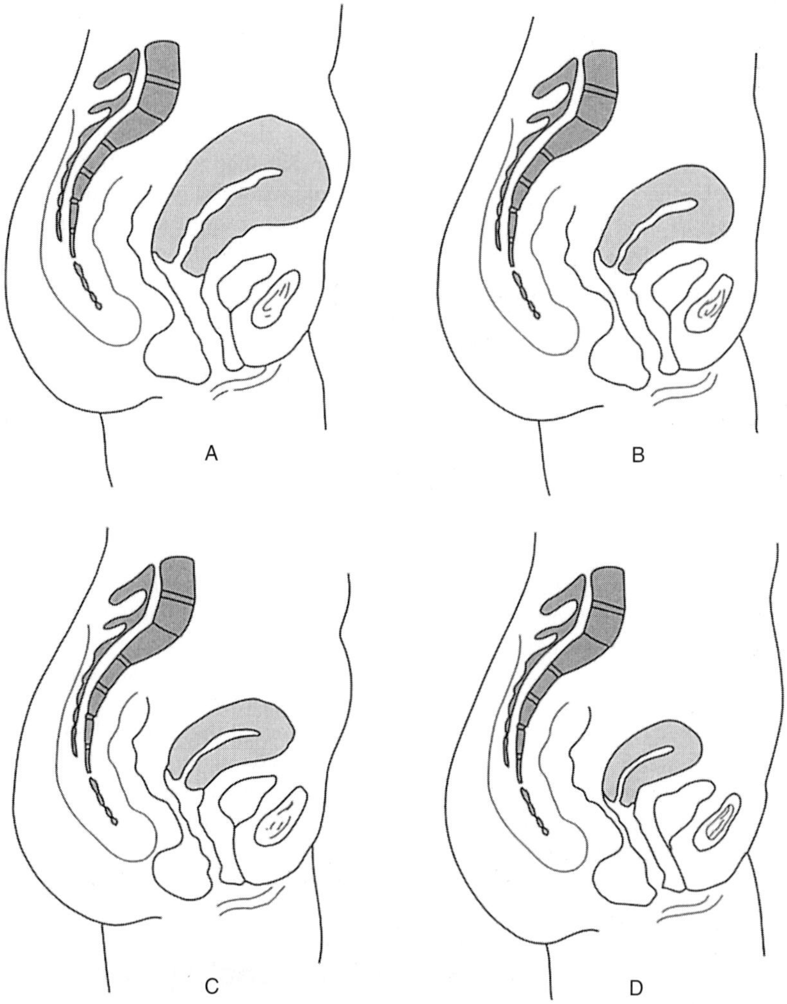

Figure 56.2 *Involution of the uterus. (a) At the end of labour. (b) One week after delivery. (c) Two weeks after delivery. (d) Six weeks after delivery (from Sweet B, 1997, with permission).*

The height of the fundus then decreases at a rate of 1 cm daily. At the end of the first week the uterus has lost 50% of its bulk and weighs about 500 g and is about 5 cm above the symphysis pubis. It has returned to the true pelvis by the 10th postnatal day. By the end of the 6th week after delivery the uterus should weigh between 60 and 80 g and have returned to its prepregnant position of anteversion and anteflexion.

This normal process is slower after a multiple pregnancy, after the birth of a large infant or after a pregnancy complicated by polyhydramnios. Although multiparous women have been thought to have a slower rate of involution, ultrasound studies of primiparous and multiparous women (Lavery & Shaw 1989) have shown a relationship between the size of the baby and the size of the uterus postnatally but there appeared to be no link between parity and the rate of involution, although the study did not state whether grand multiparous women were included (Sweet 1997a). Slow involution may be associated with retained placental tissue or blood clot, particularly if there is an associated infection (Sweet 1997a).

Uterine contractions

During the first 24 h after delivery oxytocin leads to uterine contractions which are quite strong with further retraction, often resulting in afterpains, especially in multiparous women. Oxytocin release is stimulated by suckling. These gradually diminish over the next 4–7 days and are relieved by paracetamol.

The decidua

The upper portion of the spongy endometrial layer is sloughed off when the placenta is delivered. The remaining decidua is organised into basal and superficial layers. The superficial layer consists of granulation tissue which is invaded by leucocytes to form a barrier to prevent microorganisms invading the remaining decidua. This layer becomes necrotic and is sloughed off as the lochia. The basal layer remains intact and is the source of regeneration of the endometrium which begins about 10 days after delivery and is completed, except at the placental site, by 2–3 weeks following delivery.

Healing of the placental site is completed by the end of 6 weeks. Immediately after delivery, the placental site is reduced to a raised roughened area about 12 cm in diameter. It contains many thrombosed sinusoids. The large blood vessels that had supplied the intervillous space are invaded by fibroblasts and their lumen is obscured. Some of the blood vessels later recanalise.

Lochia

The vaginal loss during the puerperium is known as the **lochia** (a plural word). Lochia vary in amount, content and colour as the excess tissue is lost. Women lose between 150 and 400 ml of lochia, averaging 225 ml. Women who breastfeed have less lochia, possibly due to more rapid involution and healing, although flow may increase temporarily during suckling (Blackburn & Loper 1992). Three forms of lochia are described: **rubra** (red), **serosa** (pink) and **alba** (white).

The lochia may remain red for 3 weeks or there may be a brief increase in blood content in the 2nd week. However, if the lochia remain heavily bloodstained or if there is a sudden return to profuse red lochia, there may be retained placental tissue. If the lochia are offensive and the woman becomes pyrexial uterine infection may be present. The woman must be seen and assessed by a doctor and appropriate treatment commenced (see below).

Table 56.1 *The characteristics of lochia*

Type	*Content*	*Average days*
Lochia rubra	blood, amnion and chorion, decidual cells, vernix, lanugo, meconium.	1 to 3
Lochia serosa	blood, wound exudate, erythrocytes, leucocytes, cervical mucus, microorganisms, shreds of degenerating decidua from the superficial layer	4–10
Lochia alba	leucocytes, decidual cells, mucus, bacteria, epithelial cells	11–21

Other parts of the genital tract

Immediately after delivery the **cervix** is soft and highly vascular but it rapidly loses its vascularity and returns to its normal consistency within 3 days of delivery. The cervical os reduces in size, measuring 1 cm wide 10 days after delivery. By the end of 6 weeks the external os is reduced to a slit. The **ovaries** and **fallopian tubes** return with the uterus to the pelvic cavity. The **vagina, vulva** and **pelvic floor** respond to the reduced amount of circulating progesterone by recovering normal muscle tone. Early ambulation and postnatal exercises can enhance this return to normal. Any oedema is reabsorbed within the first 3 or 4 days and bruising or tears to genital tissues heal rapidly.

The cardiovascular and respiratory systems

During pregnancy the increased circulatory volume and haemodilution were needed to ensure adequate blood supply to the uterus and placental bed. Following the withdrawal of oestrogen, a diuresis occurs for the first 48 h of the puerperium and the plasma volume and haematocrit rapidly return to normal. The reduction in circulating progesterone leads to removal of excess tissue fluid and a return to normal vascular tone (Ball 1996). Cardiac output and blood pressure return to non-pregnant levels.

Delivery of the baby and reduction in uterine size remove the compression of the lungs. Full inflation of the lungs, including the basal lobes, is again possible. With the reduction in cardiac work and circulatory volume and the decrease in metabolism, oxygen needs return to normal. The tendency to hyperventilation disappears and blood carbon dioxide levels return to normal, as does the slight alkalosis.

The renal system

The kidneys must cope with the excretion of excess fluids and an increase in the breakdown products of protein. The dilatation of the renal tract resolves with the removal of progesterone and the renal organs gradually return to their prepregnant state. During labour the bladder is displaced into the abdomen and the urethra is stretched. There may be loss of tone in the bladder and bruising of the urethra, leading to difficulty in micturition.

Because of these features and the diuresis the bladder may become overdistended and retention of urine may occur (Ball 1996). This may be missed if the carer fails to notice that frequent small amounts of urine are being passed but the bladder is becoming ever more distended. Early ambulation with frequent encouragement to pass urine and ensuring that the bladder is emptied will help to avoid this situation. Catheterisation may occasionally be necessary.

The alimentary tract

With the lower levels of circulating progesterone, smooth muscle tone throughout the body gradually returns to normal. The minor inconveniences of pregnancy affecting the alimentary tract, such as heartburn and constipation, resolve. Constipation may persist as a problem, possibly due to inactivity or a fear of pain on defaecation.

POSTNATAL INFECTION

Any woman developing a raised temperature and pulse rate should be screened for infection. Because of tissue trauma sustained in labour and the presence of the placental site, women are susceptible to invasion by pathogenic organisms in the postnatal period. Prior to the introduction of aseptic techniques and development of antibiotics, puerperal sepsis was an important cause of maternal mortality. Puerperal pyrexia was then a notifiable disease. Although this is no longer so, any woman developing a temperature in the puerperium should be examined by the medical team.

Other sites for infection are the breasts and the epithelial linings of the veins. Thromboembolic disorders are the leading cause of maternal death (DOH 1996). The possibility that the woman has developed an infection unrelated to pregnancy, such as an upper respiratory tract infection, should be kept in mind. Infection of surgical incisions is a significant cause of maternal morbidity.

Identification of site of infection

A raised temperature and pulse rate are only indicators that infection may be present. Other signs and symptoms present on clinical examination will help to identify the site of infection. The timing of the onset of pyrexia may also indicate the source of the problem. Swabs may be taken from all possible sites and specimens sent to the pathology laboratory for organism culture and antibiotic sensitivity. Depending on the signs and symptoms, these may include high vaginal, perineal, wound, ear, nose and throat swabs, breast milk, blood, urine and stool specimens. Antibiotic therapy should commence prior to the results of such investigations if the woman is ill.

Causative organisms

It takes time for invading organisms to multiply sufficiently to cause symptoms and postnatal infection occurs after the first 24 h from delivery. As in any infection, the severity depends on two factors: the virulence of the causative organism and the resistance of the host. Infecting organisms may originate from the commensal organisms normally present in the woman's own body. These are called **endogenous** organisms and cause problems if they invade susceptible sites. They may come from the vagina, bowel, skin, nose or throat of the woman and include *Escherichia coli*, *Clostridium welchii* and *Streptococcus faecalis*.

Other organisms are transmitted from sites other than the woman's body, commonly from an attendant. These are called **exogenous** organisms and are responsible for the more serious infections. The most dangerous organism is the **β-haemolytic streptococcus group A** (see below), which may be the organism found in people with a sore throat and is the cause of serious intrauterine infection. A common organism which causes spots, pustules and sticky eyes in babies and breast or wound infections in their mothers is *Staphylococcus aureus* (Abbott 1997) which can linger in dust. A strain of this organism, called methicillin-resistant *Staphylococcus aureus* (MRSA), is resistant to most antibiotics. Overuse and misuse of antibiotics in human disease and animal husbandry has been one of the causes of these mutations (Coughlan 1996).

β-haemolytic streptococcus Lancefield group A

The genus *Streptococcus* contains a wide variety of species of bacteria with many habitats. Some species are pathogenic to human beings. One group of related species are those which cause haemolysis when grown on blood agar, an action referred to as **β-haemolysis**. Streptococci are also subdivided depending on the presence of carbohydrate antigens on their surfaces and are named after Rebecca Lancefield who was a pioneer in the classification of streptococci. They are called **Lancefield groups** and are given the letters of the alphabet from A to O (Brock & Madigan 1991).

The danger of the β-haemolytic streptococcus Lancefield group A is its ability to gain access to the circulation via the placental site to cause septicaemia and haemolysis of red cells. This strain was responsible for deaths from childbirth fever and was virulent before the development of antibiotics, being responsible for the serious childhood illness scarlet fever, as well as sore throats. It was also an organism that damaged kidneys.

Garrett (1995) explains why this organism became much less of a problem until its resurgence recently. Streptococcus group A was found to be very vulnerable to penicillin and other common antibiotics and disappeared as a serious cause of illness from the war years until the 1980s. In the late 1980s new virulent strains emerged, with Lancefield group B being a problem with babies.

Group A streptococci began to attack people of all ages and became lethal despite vigorous treatment. In America, the inventor of the Muppets, Jim Henderson, died rapidly from a virulent strain of streptococcus group A that caused a syndrome similar to toxic shock syndrome (*Staphylococcus aureus*). Although there is hope on the horizon and scientists are developing new drugs that combat the ability of bacteria to resist antibiotics, it may be some years before these are readily available on the market (Chin 1996). Vigilance in preventive measures must be maintained if childbearing women are to be protected.

Genital tract infection

Infection of the genital tract may remain localised to the perineum, vagina or cervix or may ascend the genital tract to infect the uterine cavity (**endometritis**). Infection may then spread to the fallopian tubes to cause salpingitis and to the tissues of the pelvic cavity to cause cellulitis and peritonitis.

Postpartum endometritis

In the USA postpartum endometritis affects 1–3% of women delivering vaginally and 10–30% of those delivered by CS which is the most important risk factor (Arias 1993). Other predisposing factors are prolonged labour, prolonged rupture of the membranes, frequent vaginal examinations and traumatic delivery (Abbott 1997). Women who are anaemic are more at risk (Arias 1993). However, Newton et al (1990), in their multivariate analysis of predictive factors, found only caesarean section, lack of prophylactic antibiotics prior to caesarean delivery and the presence of particular organisms in the amniotic fluid during labour to be linked to endometritis. The more traditional explanations may facilitate rather than cause puerperal endometritis. Some authorities advise antibiotic treatment of women with vaginal vaginosis.

Signs and symptoms

- Pyrexia occurs about the 3rd postnatal day, rising to 39°C.
- There is a rise in pulse rate of about 10 bpm for every degree Celsius.
- Pain is present in the lower abdomen.
- The uterus is tender on palpation.
- Headache and rigors may occur.
- Localised infection is sometimes seen in the perineum.
- Lochia may be heavy and offensive if the invading organism is an anaerobe (Arias 1993).
- Blood cultures may be positive in up to 10% of women.

Spread of infection

If there is spread of the organism by bacteria such as *Clostridium welchii*, the mother's condition may deteriorate rapidly. In the last report into maternal deaths (DOH 1996), there were 15 deaths associated with genital sepsis with no improvement over the previous report.

Treatment

The woman is isolated and seen by the doctor. High vaginal and wound site swabs and urine and blood specimens are taken. Antibiotic therapy is commenced with a combination of drugs active against Gram-negative and Gram-positive organisms. Gentamicin and clindamycin therapy is commonly used (del Priore et al 1996, Maccato et al 1991). The drugs may need changing when the results of the culture and sensitivity tests are known. Care is provided to meet the woman's needs depending on the severity of the illness.

An intravenous infusion may be necessary if the woman is dehydrated. Analgesics will relieve pain. It is necessary to check the haemoglobin content of her blood as anaemia may precede or follow infection. A blood transfusion is sometimes necessary (Ball 1996). Any localised wound infections are treated. A light nourishing diet is provided if the woman is well enough to eat. It may be necessary to provide care for the baby.

Urinary tract infection

About 12% of women develop urinary tract infection (UTI) in the puerperium which may present as cystitis or pyelonephritis. Because of the delay in return to normal of the urinary tract changes of pregnancy, there is susceptibility to infection for the first 6 weeks. Women who had asymptomatic bacteriuria, antenatal urinary tract infections or were catheterised in labour or had retention of urine during labour or following delivery are more likely to develop a UTI. The most common organism cultured is *Escherichia coli*.

Signs and symptoms

In cystitis there is urinary frequency, dysuria and possibly a slight rise in temperature. In the more serious pyelonephritis the woman will have:

- pain radiating from loin to groin;
- pyrexia and rapid pulse;
- rigors;
- nausea and vomiting.

She will feel ill. The urine is acidic on ward testing, opalescent and offensive. Pus and blood may be found on microscopic examination.

Treatment

A midstream specimen of urine is sent for culture and sensitivity testing. The woman is requested to drink at least 3 litres of fluid daily and urinary output and fluid intake are recorded. If necessary drugs are given to relieve pain and nausea and to reduce temperature. A broad-spectrum antibiotic is commenced and changed if necessary when the culture and sensitivity results are known. Following completion of the antibiotic treatment, a further specimen of urine is sent to ensure the infection is defeated. Many midwives would add oral administration of potassium citrate to make the urine alkaline and inhibit the growth of *E. coli*.

At the end of the puerperium, when the urinary tract has returned to the prepregnancy state, any woman who has suffered recurrent urinary tract infections should have investigations of kidney function including intravenous pyelography.

Breast infections

These are discussed in Chapter 54.

HORMONAL INFLUENCES ON PSYCHOLOGICAL ADJUSTMENT

Behaviour is a complex function influenced by the interaction of biological factors, such as genes with their hormone and neurotransmitter products, and social, economic and cultural factors (Jessel & Moir 1995). If one accepts the influence of hormones on mood in the premenstruum, which affects 40% of women mildly and 2% of women seriously (Carlson 1991), and not everyone does, then it must be accepted that the fluctuating hormones in pregnancy and the puerperium must have an effect on mood. Behaviour in response to the childbearing process may also be influenced by obstetric factors (Cox & Holden 1994).

'Baby blues'

Emotional lability is common in the early puerperium with an early feeling of elation at delivery and during the first 3 days, often replaced by 'the blues' with mild depression, feelings of anxiety, tearfulness, irritability, forgetfulness, fatigue and inability to concentrate (Blackburn & Loper 1992), commonly on the 5th day (Sweet 1997a). It is so common as to be considered a normal reaction, occurring in 70–80% of all births (Ball 1994). Most women recover within a couple of days but a prolonged, serious episode may be predictive of the onset of postnatal depression (Cox et al 1982, cited in Sweet 1997b).

The cause of 'the blues' is unknown but, because it is almost universal, it is likely to be due mainly to the physiological changes occurring in the puerperium such as the decrease in oestrogen and progesterone, alterations in blood electrolytes and in the balance of the neurotransmitters serotonin (5-hydroxytryptamine; 5-HT) and dopamine, a close relative of adrenaline, while changes in body fluid content may affect brain function (Blackburn & Loper 1992). These factors may interact with minor anxieties, attitudes and beliefs about the birth of the child and sociocultural stress to influence maternal mood to a greater degree. This may result in the clinical depression that affects one in 10 women, reported by Cox et al (1982) and Kumar & Robson (1984).

MENTAL DISORDERS IN THE PUERPERIUM

In ethological terms, behaviour is complex and is caused by the influence of environmental factors upon the internal state of the organism (Bowlby 1987, Hinde 1982). The concept of nature or nurture is a redundant and simplistic one. There is an increased risk of mental disorders in childbearing, mainly in the postnatal period. Psychiatric disorders can be divided into two main groups: the **neuroses** and the **psychoses**.

In the neuroses the individual, though likely to be depressed, remains in touch with reality. In the much more severe psychoses, there is great impairment in the perception of external reality, often with delusions and hallucinations (Carlson 1991). In most cases the woman will suffer from the neurotic disorder of postnatal depression and only a few women, many of whom will have a history of prior severe mental illness, will suffer from a puerperal psychotic episode such as schizophrenia.

Postnatal depression

Postnatal depression is a non-psychotic depressive illness which usually commences within 2 weeks of delivery but may develop at any time in the first year following childbirth. Postnatal depression is thought to be a separate illness differing from other depressions and the cause is likely to be multifactorial, with contributions from physiological and psychosocial stresses (Cox et al 1993). The disorder is not always detected by professionals and usually recovery is complete. In some women the illness is protracted and may persist for over a year (Taylor et al 1994). The effect on the woman and her family is devastating and early recognition and treatment are essential.

Causes

Biological causes include hereditary factors, genetic make-up, hormonal changes in pregnancy and the puerperium, physical health problems related to childbearing such as anaemia, nausea and vomiting, obstetric factors such as type of labour and delivery, pain and the effect of the appearance and behaviour of the baby. Psychological factors include the mother's personality, especially obsessive or anxious women, quality of relationship with her own parents, previous experience of babies and her own expectations of motherhood. Social factors include stressful life events, low socioeconomic status and lack of support (Levy & Kline 1994, Stein et al 1989).

Recognition

It is only by close contact with women, observing their behaviour and reactions to events and encouraging them to discuss their feelings and anxieties that a midwife or doctor may recognise postnatal depression. The following symptoms may be present.

- A lowering of mood.
- Feelings that they cannot love their baby although the mother obviously cares for the baby.
- Feelings of inadequacy and inability to cope.
- Guilt about their mothering skills.
- Tearfulness and constant tiredness.
- Sleep disturbance with difficulty in achieving sleep and early morning waking.

Stamp et al (1995) utilised the Edinburgh Postnatal Depression Scale (EPDS) to detect postnatal depression. It is a simple self-rating 10-item scale which can be used at about 6 weeks after delivery (Sweet 1997b).

Management

The usual three methods of treating mental illness can be used in postnatal depression, namely: counselling, cognitive therapy or antidepressant drugs. An appropriate postnatal support group may also be helpful. Counselling seems to be satisfactory as it allows support to enable the woman to find her own solutions (Clement et al 1995). Women who do not respond to antidepressant drugs or who are suicidal must be referred to a psychiatrist. A few severely depressed women will need admission to a psychiatric hospital with a mother and baby unit. Support from the community psychiatric nurse (CPN) is available. Most women recover within 4–6 weeks.

Recently it has been thought that falling oestrogen levels after delivery of the placenta may provoke postnatal depression due to the effect on the dopaminergic system in susceptible women. Dopamine is a catecholamine related to epinephrine (adrenaline) and is an activating neurotransmitter in the central nervous system, linking the reticular activating system of the brainstem, with its attention to incoming information, with the emotional limbic system and the cognitive frontal lobes of the brain. Disturbances of this system may affect both emotional and thought content. This seems a likely explanation for a condition that affects up to 15% of women.

Treatment with transdermal oestrogen (skin patches) have been effective in some cases (Gregoire et al 1996, Henderson et al 1991). Dalton (1985) favours the postdelivery fall in progesterone levels and progesterone prophylaxis. Harris et al (1994) have found an association between postnatal blues and rapidly falling progesterone levels after delivery. It may be possible to treat the more severely affected mothers with progesterone.

Puerperal psychoses

Psychoses can be subdivided into two types of illness: an affective disturbance of mood that may be depressive or manic and the less commonly seen (in this group of people) schizophrenia. The incidence of puerperal psychosis is about two per 1000 births. The onset is quite often rapid, occurring on about day 3–14 of the puerperium. The woman may suffer from insomnia – a key symptom – is confused, frightened and distressed and may be disoriented in space and time.

Delusions and hallucinations often focus on the delivery or on the baby. The author can give two examples to support this statement. One woman with a diagnosis of schizophrenia thought her baby was Jesus reborn and none of us were allowed to touch him. A 2nd, seriously depressed lady believed that her baby must be killed as the earth was so evil he would be better off in heaven.

Causes

In keeping with recent thinking about psychotic disease, it is believed that these illnesses have a strong biological component due to imbalance of the relationship between pregnancy hormones and neurotransmitters, as discussed above. Many women have affected family members and may have known previous psychotic episodes themselves. In the latter case Cox & Holden (1994) recommend an antenatal referral to a psychiatrist so that early intervention can be made should their illness recur in the puerperium.

Management

Admission to a mother and baby psychiatric unit is usually necessary for these seriously disturbed women and their babies. Unfortunately these units are not available in many health districts. Separation of the baby from the mother may lead the woman to have increased delusions about the safety or even survival of the child. Initially sedation is useful to allow the mother to rest and take adequate food and fluid. Once the condition has been accurately diagnosed the appropriate treatment drug and supportive treatment can be commenced. Prognosis is good, most women recovering within 6 months. However, there may be a relapse in a subsequent pregnancy.

Summary of main points

- The puerperium lasts approximately 6 weeks after childbirth during which time anatomic and physiologic changes brought about by childbirth resolve and a woman adjusts to the new or expanded responsibilities of motherhood and non-pregnant life. The main maternal puerperal complications include postpartum haemorrhage, thromboembolic disorders, puerperal infections and psychiatric disorders.
- Following delivery of the placenta there is a profound fall in the serum level of the placental hormones human placental lactogen, human chorionic gonadotrophin, oestrogen and progesterone. Removal of the placental hormones initiates the return of the body systems to their prepregnant state.
- Involution is characterised by a decrease in the size of an organ caused by a decrease in the size of its cells. The uterus now returns to its normal size, tone and position. During involution, the return of the muscle layer to normal thickness is brought about by the processes of ischaemia, autolysis and phagocytosis. The decidua is shed and there is regeneration of the endometrium.
- Immediately after delivery of the placenta the uterus weighs about 1000 g and the fundus is about midway between the umbilicus and symphysis pubis. Over the next 12 h the fundus returns to the level of the umbilicus. The height of the fundus then decreases at a rate of 1 cm daily until after 6 weeks the uterus weighs between 60 and 80 g and has returned to its prepregnant position of anteversion and anteflexion. Slow involution may be associated with retained placental tissue or blood clot, particularly if there is an associated infection.
- Lochia vary in amount, content and colour. Women who breastfeed have less lochia, possibly due to more rapid involution and healing. If the lochia remain heavily blood stained or if there is a sudden return to profuse red lochia, there may be retained placental tissue. If the lochia are offensive and the woman becomes pyrexial uterine infection may be present.
- Immediately after delivery the cervix is soft and highly vascular but returns to its normal consistency within 3 days of delivery. The cervical os reduces in size, measuring 1 cm wide 10 days after delivery. The vagina, vulva and pelvic floor respond to the reduced amount of circulating progesterone by recovering normal muscle tone. Any oedema is reabsorbed within the first 3 or 4 days and bruising or tears to genital tissues heal rapidly.
- Following the withdrawal of oestrogen a diuresis occurs for the first 48 h of the puerperium and the plasma volume and haematocrit rapidly return to normal. The reduction in circulating progesterone leads to removal of excess tissue fluid and a return to normal vascular tone. Cardiac output and blood pressure return to non-pregnant levels. The kidneys must cope with the excretion of excess fluids and an increase in the breakdown products of protein.
- Delivery of the baby and reduction in uterine size remove the compression of the lungs. Oxygen needs return to normal and the tendency to hyperventilation disappears. Blood carbon dioxide levels return to normal, as does the slight alkalosis.
- There may be loss of tone in the bladder and bruising of the urethra, leading to difficulty in micturition. Retention of urine may occur but early ambulation with encouragement to pass urine and ensuring that the bladder is emptied will help to avoid this. With the lower levels of circulating progesterone, smooth muscle tone throughout

the body gradually returns to normal. Constipation may persist as a problem, possibly due to inactivity or a fear of pain on defaecation.

- Women are susceptible to invasion by pathogenic organisms in the postnatal period. Although puerperal pyrexia is no longer a notifiable disease, any woman developing a temperature in the puerperium should be examined by the medical team. Infection of surgical incisions is a significant cause of maternal morbidity.
- A raised temperature and pulse rate are only indicators that infection may be present. Other signs and symptoms help to identify the site of infection. The timing of the onset of pyrexia may also indicate the source of the problem and specimens are sent to the pathology laboratory for organism culture and antibiotic sensitivity. Antibiotic therapy should commence prior to the results of such investigations if the woman is ill.
- The most dangerous organism is the β-haemolytic streptococcus group A which is the cause of serious intrauterine infection. A common organism which causes spots, pustules and sticky eyes in babies and breast or wound infections in their mothers is *Staphylococcus aureus*. Methicillin-resistant *Staphylococcus aureus* (MRSA) is resistant to most antibiotics. In the late 1980s new virulent strains emerged, with Lancefield group B causing problems for babies.
- Predisposing factors for the development of postpartum endometritis include prolonged labour, prolonged rupture of the membranes, frequent vaginal examinations and traumatic delivery. Pyrexia and a rise in pulse rate occur about the 3rd postnatal day. Pain is present in the lower abdomen and the uterus is tender on palpation. Lochia may be heavy and offensive. Antibiotic therapy is commenced with a combination of drugs active against Gram-negative and Gram-positive organisms.
- About 12% of women develop urinary tract infection in the puerperium which may present as cystitis or pyelonephritis. Women who had asymptomatic bacteriuria or antenatal urinary tract infections or were catheterised in labour or had retention of urine during labour or following delivery are more at risk. A mid stream specimen of urine is sent for culture and sensitivity testing, the woman is requested to drink at least 3 litres of fluid daily and drugs are given to relieve pain and nausea and to reduce temperature. A broad-spectrum antibiotic is commenced. On completion of the treatment a further specimen of urine is sent to ensure the infection is defeated.
- Behaviour in childbearing may be influenced by obstetric as well as social factors. Emotional lability is common in the early puerperium. The 'baby blues' occurs in 70–80% of all births and most women recover within a couple of days but a prolonged, serious episode may herald the onset of postnatal depression.
- The cause of 'the blues' is likely to be due mainly to the physiological changes occurring in the puerperium such as the decrease in oestrogen and progesterone, alterations in blood electrolytes and in the balance of the neurotransmitters serotonin and dopamine. These factors may interact with minor anxieties, attitudes and beliefs about the birth of the child and sociocultural stress to influence maternal mood, resulting in clinical depression.
- Psychiatric disorders can be divided into the neuroses and the psychoses. Postnatal depression is a non-psychotic illness commencing within 2 weeks of childbirth. Close contact with women, observing their behaviour and reactions to events and encouraging them to discuss their feelings and anxieties enables a midwife to recognise postnatal depression.
- The usual methods of treating mental illness are counselling, cognitive therapy or antidepressant drugs. An appropriate postnatal support group may help. Women who do not respond to antidepressant drugs or who are suicidal must be referred to a psychiatrist. Severely depressed women will need admission to a psychiatric hospital with a mother and baby unit.
- Falling oestrogen levels after delivery of the placenta may provoke postnatal depression due to the effect on the dopaminergic system in susceptible women. Treatment with transdermal oestrogen has been effective in some cases. Others believe there is an association between postnatal blues and rapidly falling progesterone levels after delivery. It may be possible to treat the more severely affected mothers with progesterone.
- Psychoses can be subdivided into an affective disturbance of mood that may be depressive or manic and the less commonly seen schizophrenia. The woman may suffer from insomnia and is confused, frightened and distressed and may be disoriented in space and time. Delusions and hallucinations often focus on the delivery or on the baby. Admission to a mother and baby psychiatric unit is usually necessary for seriously disturbed women and their babies. Separation of the baby from the mother may lead the woman to have increased delusions about the safety or survival of the child.
- Sedation is useful to allow the mother to rest and take adequate food and fluid. Once the condition has been accurately diagnosed the appropriate treatment can be commenced. Most women recover within 6 months but there may be a relapse in a subsequent pregnancy.

References

Abbott H. 1997 Complications of the puerperium. In Sweet BR with Tiran D (eds) Mayes Midwifery, 12th edn. Baillière Tindall, London, pp 719–727.

Anderson KN, Anderson LE, Glanze WD. (eds) 1994 Mosby's Medical, Nursing and Allied Health Dictionary. Mosby, St Louis.

Arias F. 1993 Practical Guide to High Risk Pregnancy and Delivery, 2nd edn. Mosby Year Book, Chicago.

Ball JA. 1994 Reactions to Motherhood. The Role of Postnatal Care. Hale: Books for Midwives Press, London.

Ball JA. 1996 Physiology, psychology and management of the puerperium. In Bennett V R, Brown LK (eds) Myles Textbook for Midwives. Churchill Livingstone, Edinburgh, pp 233–250.

Blackburn ST, Loper DL. 1992 Maternal, Fetal and Neonatal Physiology, A Clinical perspective. WB Saunders, Philadelphia.

Bowlby J. 1987 Attachment and Loss: Volume 1, Attachment, Penguin. Harmondsworth.

Brock TD, Madigan MT. 1991 Biology of Micro-organisms, 6th edn. Prentice-Hall, New Jersey.

Carlson NR. 1991 Physiology of Behavior, 4th edn. Allyn and Bacon, New York, p 370.

Chin J. 1996 Resistance is useless. New Scientist 152(2054) 32–35.

Clement S 1995 'Listening visits' in pregnancy: a strategy for preventing postnatal depression, Midwifey, 11: 75–80.

Coughlan A. 1996 Animal antibiotics threaten hospital antibiotics. New Scientist 151(2043) 7.

Cox J, Holden J. (eds) 1994 Perinatal Psychiatry. Gaskell, London.

Cox J, Connor Y, Kendall RE. 1982 Prospective study of the psychiatric disorders of childbirth. British Journal of Psychiatry 140, 111–117.

Cox J, Murray D, Chapman G. 1993 A controlled study of the onset, duration and prevalence of postnatal depression. British Journal of Psychiatry 150, 27–31.

Dalton K. 1985 Progesterone prophylaxis used successfully in postnatal depression. Practitioner 229, 507–508.

Del Priore G, Jackson Stone M, Shim EK, Garfinkel J, Eichmann MA, Frederiksen MC. 1996 A comparison of once daily and 8-hour dosing in the treatment of postpartum endometritis. Obstetrics and Gynaecology 87, 994–1000.

Department of Health 1996 Report on Confidential Enquiries into Maternal Deaths in the United Kingdom, 1991 to 1993. HMSO, London.

Garrett L. 1995 The Coming Plague. Virago Press, London, chs 12 and 13.

Gregoire AJ, Kumar RD, Evritt B, Henderson AF, Studd JW. 1996 Transdermal oestrogen for treatment of severe postnatal depression. Lancet 347, 930–933.

Harris B, Lovett L, Newcombe RG, Read GF, Walker R, Riad-Fahmy D. 1994 Maternity blues and major endocrine changes: Cardiff puerperal mood and hormone study 11. British Medical Journal 308, 949–953.

Henderson AF, Gregoire AJ, Kumar RD, Studd JW. 1991 Treatment of severe postnatal depression with oestradiol skin patches. Lancet, 338: 816–817
Hinde RA. 1982 Ethology. Fontana, London.
Jessel D, Moir A. 1995 A Mind to Crime. Signet, London.
Kumar R, Robson K. 1984 A prospective study of emotional disorders in childbearing women. British Journal of Psychiatry 144, 35–47.
Lavery JP, Shaw LA. 1989 Sonography of the puerperal uterus. Journal of Ultrasound in Medicine 8, 481–486.
Levy V, Kline P. 1994 Perinatal depression: a factor analysis. British Journal of Midwifery 2(4) 154–159.
Maccato ML, Faro S, Martens MG, Hammill HA. 1991 Ciprofloxacin versus gentamycin/clindamycin for postpartum endometritis. Journal of Reproductive Medicine 36, 857–861.
Newton ER, Prihoda TJ, Gibbs RS. 1990 A clinical and microbiologic analysis of risk factors for puerperal endometritis. Obstetrics and Gynaecology 75, 402–406.
Stamp GE, Williams AS, Crowther CA. 1995 Evaluation of antenatal and postnatal support to overcome postnatal depression: a randomised controlled trial. Birth 22, 138–143.
Stein A, Cooper PJ, Campbell EA. 1989 Social adversity and perinatal complications: their relationship to postnatal depression. British Medical Journal 171, 1073–1074.
Sweet BR. 1997a Postnatal care. In Sweet BR with Tiran D (eds) Mayes Midwifery, 12th edn. Baillière Tindall, London, pp 472–495.
Sweet BR. 1997b Psychiatric disorders associated with childbirth. In Sweet BR with Tiran D (eds) Mayes Midwifery, 12th edn. Baillière Tindall, London, pp 728–737.
Taylor A, Adams D, Glover V. 1994 Postnatal depression: identification, risk factors and effects. British Journal of Midwifery 2, 1073–1074.
United Kingdom Central Council 1993 Midwives' Rules. UKCC, London.

Recommended reading

Ball JA. 1994 Reactions to Motherhood. The Role of Postnatal Care. Hale: Books for Midwives Press, London.
Bowlby J. 1987 Attachment and Loss: Volume 1, Attachment. Penguin, Harmondsworth.
Cox J, Holden J. (eds) 1994 Perinatal Psychiatry. Gaskell, London.
Cox J, Murray D, Chapman G. 1993 A controlled study of the onset, duration and prevalence of postnatal depression. British Journal of Psychiatry 150, 27–31.
Gregoire AJ, Kumar RD, Evritt B, Henderson AF, Studd JW. 1996 Transdermal oestrogen for treatment of severe postnatal depression. Lancet 347, 930–933.
Kumar R, Robson K. 1984 A prospective study of emotional disorders in childbearing women. British Journal of Psychiatry 144, 35–47.
Newton ER, Prihoda TJ, Gibbs RS. 1990 A clinical and microbiologic analysis of risk factors for puerperal endometritis. Obstetrics and Gynaecology 75, 402–406.

Chapter

57 Biobehavioural aspects of parenting

In this chapter

APPROACHES TO THE STUDY OF BEHAVIOUR

For thousands of years the brain and mind were seen as separate entities. The brain was the realm of scientists but the mind was studied by philosophers (Greenfield 1997). In the middle of the 19th century scientists began to realise that sensations such as sight and hearing were the result of nerve impulses and experiments began to be devised to explore these concepts. Wilhelm Wundt opened the first psychology laboratory at the University of Leipzig in 1879. Since then other disciplines have been developed to study behaviour, such as:

- **ethology**, which is the study of animal (including human) behaviour;
- **cognitive psychology**, which is the study of the way people process information;
- **physiological psychology**, which is the study of the physical substance and processes in the brain;
- **behaviourism**, which concentrates on observed behaviour, made famous by Pavlov and Skinner;
- **psychoanalysis**, stating that people's psychological history explains their current behaviour;
- **Gestalt psychology**, where the integrated brain is seen as greater than the sum of its parts;
- **evolutionary psychology**, which traces the development of behaviour.

This chapter draws on ethology and physiological psychology. The roots of physiological psychology involve concepts from philosophy and biology and have generated much discussion. In the past this has been referred to as the **mind-body question** (Carlson 1991).

Ethology

The study of animal behaviour was developed by scientists such Tinbergen and Lorenz in the 1950s and 1960s. Perhaps the most readable and accessible book is by Hinde (1982). He commented that:

> Ethologists follow a biological tradition in attempting to start their analyses from a secure base of description. And as biologists ... they are aware that ... the behaviour of each species (should) be seen in relation to the environmental context to which it has been adapted.

Ethologists ask four types of questions about behaviour.

1 What is its immediate causation?
2 How does it develop?
3 What is its function?
4 How did it evolve?

Other biological sciences related to ethology and the study of behaviour, which may help to answer the above four questions when related to the human species, are ecology, endocrinology and neuropsychology. Hinde discusses the relationship between ethology and human social sciences such as sociology, psychology and anthropology, believing that ethology alone cannot provide answers to human behaviour but that 'an amalgam of techniques, concepts and theories appropriate to the problem being tackled is essential'. An example is the influence that field primatology, such as Jane Goodall's (1986) studies on chimpanzee behaviour, has had on thinking about the evolutionary development of human behaviour, including parenting. Ethology has a contribution to make to the description and analysis of human behaviour.

Physiological psychology

Philosophical roots

One of the first people to discover that thoughts originated in the brain was Hippocrates who lived from 460 to 377 BC. He believed that the mind was in the brain and controlled the body. He postulated that mental illness was caused by disease and injuries to the head, not by demons (Greenfield 1997). Based on early thinking by Descartes in the 17th century, **dualists** consider the mind and body to be separate, with the body being constructed from chemical elements but the mind not. Arising from religious belief, the soul is thought to be located in the brain and to control the body. Descartes believed that only human beings have God-given souls.

Later philosophers have argued against this using logic. If the soul is not part of the physical world then it cannot move the physical body. If the soul does possess material properties, allowing it to interact with the body, then it too must be physical. This led to the concept of **monism** which is the belief that reality consists of a unified whole and that the mind is a product of the working body. If the function of the nervous system is known, human consciousness and the way we perceive, think, remember, act and are self-aware will be understood and the mind-body problem will be solved.

The nature of human consciousness produces a second major philosophical issue, that of **determinism** versus **free will**. Most of us feel that we are in control of our minds and believe that our mental abilities give us choice over our behaviour. The mind therefore cannot be constrained by the physiological body and the environment. However, this is related strongly to a belief in dualism and suggests that it is difficult, if not impossible, to search for physiological causes of behaviour. Greenfield (1997) reminds us that there is still no agreement as to whether monists or dualists are correct in their beliefs but that there is a middle course. Consciousness is a process of the whole brain, not individual brain cells.

Although physiological psychologists take a monistic approach to their study of human behaviour, they remain aware that it is complex and that a **reductionist** process will never predict behaviour in all circumstances (Greenfield 1997). This problem exists in other disciplines and is that of attempting to use general laws to predict the functioning of complex systems. This can be examined using the mathematical theory of **complexity** which is about the spontaneous emergence of order from the internal dynamics of complex systems.

Biological roots

The belief of monism led to the development of experimental physiology and the search by some scientists for specific causes of behaviour. Other biologists, including Charles Darwin, continued to base their theories on observation. Darwin developed his theory of **natural selection** which is at the centre of the discipline of evolution and revolutionised biological thinking, leading to the concept of **functionalism**; that all characteristics of a living organism perform useful functions for that organism.

Structural changes between animals of a species are brought about by genetic mutations. The effects of some changes are seen in the way the animal is **adapted** to its environment; that is, how it is formed and the way it behaves. Physiological psychologists ask questions about the selective advantage a particular behaviour may have for the species. Although they have not concerned themselves with evolution the principle of natural selection has been central to their theories. Recently, the discipline of evolutionary psychology has developed to examine the wider issue of the evolution of behaviour.

MOTHER–CHILD INTERACTION

Instinctive behaviour

Bowlby (1984) wrote:

> Behaviour of even the simplest animals is enormously complex. It varies in systematic ways from members of one species to another and in less systematic ways from individual to individual within a species . . . Yet there are many regularities of behaviour and certain of these regularities are so striking and play so important part in the survival of individual and species that they have earned the name instinctive.

He gives four main characteristics of instinctive behaviour.

1 It follows a recognisably similar and predictive pattern in almost all members of a species (or sex).
2 It is not a simple response to a stimulus but a sequence of behaviour that runs a predictable course.
3 Some of its usual consequences are of obvious value in contributing to the preservation of an individual or the continuity of a species.
4 Many examples of it develop even when all the ordinary opportunities for learning are absent.

In the past there was argument over which behaviours were **innate** (inborn, genetic, nature) and which were **acquired** (learned, environmental, nurture) but this is now known to be a meaningless division. Every biological character, physiological or behavioural, is a product of the interaction between genes and environment. Hinde (1982) introduced new terminology. If a biological character is little influenced by environmental variations, it is called **environmentally stable** and any characteristic that is much influenced by the environment is **environmentally labile**. Behaviour traditionally called instinctive is environmentally stable.

Can any human behaviour be said to be environmentally stable? Some believe that the immense variability of human behaviour proves that it is culturally driven and nothing is instinctive. Bowlby (1984) disagrees but accepts commonalities in the patterns of human behaviour (characteristic 1). In particular, he mentions mating, the care of infants and young children and the attachment of the young to their parents as having survival value for both individual and species (characteristic 3). In higher species instinctive behaviour is not stereotyped but follows a recognisable pattern (characteristic 1) and runs a predictable course (characteristic 2). Despite the immense variety of cultural norms in childbearing, some behaviours repeatedly emerge (characteristic 4).

Bowlby goes on to say that behavioural attributes contribute to survival and reproduction when they develop and operate within a prescribed environment. Environmentally stable behaviours are controlled by elements within the environment, **environments of adaptedness**, one for each body system; for instance, the range of environmental temperatures that the body can tolerate or the altitude at which the cardiovascular system can function. What is different about humans is how evolutionary and cultural change has led to the ability to survive in a wide range of environments.

The human environment of evolutionary adaptedness

Bowlby (1984) considered two main characteristics of humans to be versatility and the capacity for innovation. These have allowed an enormous extension of the natural environments in which humans live and procreate. Also, humans have built environments which has led to an incredible increase in the world population but with an increased risk of infection or pollution. Within these environments the environmentally stable components of behaviour related to childbearing can be found. Of interest is the stable environment of adaptedness in which human behaviour developed over the last 2 million years (Leakey & Lewin 1992). Only in the last 15 000 years has the rise in pastoralism and agriculture allowed the growth of cities and the environment in which most of us now live.

The social surroundings of the woman are part of the environment in which childbearing and childrearing take place (Morgan 1994). It is also important to take into consideration the environmental effects of relationships between the sexes. The basis of sexual difference is in **dimorphism** (size and structure difference between males and females) and investment in the gametes (Trevathen 1987). Humans are mammalian and not only does the female produce fewer large, energy-expensive ova compared to the millions of small, energy-inexpensive male sperms, she also has to provide energy to grow the fetus in utero and to supply milk during its infancy.

Fox (1967) believed that throughout human societies the tie between females and their young forms the basic social unit and it is the manner in which males are attached to the basic unit that creates differences in society. If this is so, it is very similar to our nearest living relatives, the great apes, and the role of the male within a small group would be to create a role model for young males to follow in a particular society.

Other writers such as Lovejoy (1981) believe that **pair bonding** (monogamy) is part of human ethology, typical of species who produce **altricial** (needing much care) infants rather than **precocial** infants (able to move about immediately at birth). Male parenting is necessary for the support of the woman and her children during the long growth to maturity of the human child (Trevathen 1987). It may be initiated by the continuity of female sexual receptiveness. There is no consensus on the nature of the family in human biological terms and it is risky to define evolutionary behaviour in terms of modern hunter-gatherers such as the !Kung. However, some conclusions can be drawn about human innate behaviour.

HUMAN CHILDBEARING BEHAVIOUR

Ethograms

An ethogram is a graphic way of depicting patterns of behaviour. Their use has arisen from 'painstaking descriptions of behaviour in the ecological and social setting where it has evolved and naturally occurs' (Klaus et al 1975). What are the stable interactive behaviours involving both mother and infant chosen by key authors (Bowlby 1984, Klaus & Kennell 1976, Morgan 1994, Papousek & Papousek 1982, Trevathen 1987) to fit into an ethogram of human maternal–infant behaviour? The main interest of the authors will first be presented.

Klaus and Kennell (1976)

This innovative book introduced the concept of a **sensitive period** lasting for a few minutes or hours after birth in which maternal–infant **bonding** or **attachment** (and paternal attachment) is ensured. They define attachment as 'a unique relationship between two people that is specific and endures through time'. Important to their theory is the idea of species-specific behaviour. The impetus for their work arose from concern about the effects of separating mothers and their babies for large periods of the day. Attachment is facilitated if the mother has social support during pregnancy and birth. Rooming in is a direct development of their work. The concept of a sensitive period is also known as **imprinting**.

Papousek and Papousek (1982)

Papousek & Papousek (1982) examine the evidence for importance of the first 28 days in the integration of the newborn into a social world. In particular, they are interested in the biological roots or 'fundamental behaviours of major adaptive significance' of social integration. They wrote that highly structured patterns are present in neonatal and parental behaviour but at the time of writing they thought there was a lack of systematic research. The Papouseks discuss but do not necessarily support the innateness of dyadic maternal–infant behaviour. They suggest that **social learning** may play a large part, building rapidly on the instinctive behaviours.

Bowlby (1984)

Bowlby chose a methodology distinct from Freudian psychoanalysis to achieve his ends. To quote him: 'The data drawn on are observations of the behaviour of young children in real-life situations'. His focus therefore is on the infant and child rather than on the parent. He distinguishes this from parental caregiving. He acknowledged the ethological nature of this work and his conceptualisation of instinctive behaviour and the environment of adaptedness have been discussed above.

Bowlby wrote: 'Because the human infant is born so very immature and is so slow to develop there is no species in which attachment behaviour takes so long to appear'. He discusses sensitive periods in humans and finds it hard to believe that they would not be present, particularly in the parents. He does not believe there is a neonatal sensitive period because of the slow development of attachment behaviour over the first 6 months of life. However, he does use the term imprinting, suggesting that the infant's focusing on a single figure, although slow to develop, is sufficiently like that of other mammalian species.

Maternal involvement in ensuring that infants remain close to them depends on the relative helplessness of the infant. Bowlby talks of an 'evolutionary shift in balance', from the infant taking all the responsibility for keeping contact to total maternal responsibility in human mothers because of the immaturity of the infant. However, every sensory function is present in the neonate from birth.

Trevathen (1987)

Trevathen has studied human birth from an evolutionary perspective. She has written about the process of birth and about the neonate and neonatal behaviour. She observed more than 200 midwife-assisted deliveries in a birthing centre and in women's homes in El Paso, Texas, and recorded intense observation over the first hour of maternal and neonatal behaviour. Trevathen writes: 'Although the process may not always be perfect behaviours of mammalian females have been selected to complement the needs and capabilities of their young'. Two categories of neonatal behaviours are described. The first is adaptation at birth (Chapters 48, 49) and the second includes behaviours that enhance mother–infant bonding.

The baby is described as **secondarily altricial** at birth, requiring a period of **exterogestation** (gestation outside the uterus) in order to complete maturation. A secondarily altricial baby has his eyes open and can use them extremely well to interpret his environment, unlike a primarily altricial animal such as a kitten. Evolution has selected for early onset of labour at 40 weeks when the fetus is still immature compared with most other mammals as a trade-off between the size and shape of the human pelvis, developed because of bipedal walking, and the complexity and size of the human brain (Chapter 24). Trevathen believes that a period of exterogestation, where babies are completely dependent on the mother, is a necessity because of the prolongation of infancy.

Scientists, including Gould (1977), have suggested that the human gestation period should be about 18 months if comparisons with the maturity of the infants of other species is made. In order to be delivered safely, both for the mother and the baby, human infants are born half way through this time and do not achieve equality of developmental status with other primates until they are at least 6 months old. In evolutionary terms this has been made possible by the high commitment to infant care shown by human mothers. This equates with Bowlby's observation that attachment with purposive clinging and distress behaviour, reaching the equivalent of a newborn gorilla infant, does not occur until the human infant is about 6 months old.

Stratton (1982) pointed out that:

> Over the last two decades we have amassed great quantities of data on the behaviour of newborn infants but . . . few psychologists and ethologists have paid much attention to what the human mother (or father) was doing in the immediate post-partum period.

Trevathen followed the example of Klaus & Kennell (1982) and developed an ethogram of mother–infant interactions. She concentrated on maternal behaviours, suggesting that the behaviours described were shown by nearly all human females delivering in normal circumstances. Her criteria were:

1 no medications used;
2 vertex presentation of a single healthy infant;
3 assistance from at least one other person;
4 the mother and infant are in contact with each other for the first hour after birth.

Morgan (1994)

Morgan discusses the following behaviours of a human baby.

- He can see and can distinguish faces and see what they are doing. From the first day of life, he can imitate facial expressions.
- The human baby is the only mammal to maintain eye contact whilst suckling. He signals social pleasure by smiling.
- The baby learns to root for a nipple within 48 h.
- Talking in a high voice accompanied by nodding head movements help to stimulate a new baby and keep him in an alert aware state.
- Unlike most mammalian young, human babies cry easily and are difficult to pacify. Morgan describes this as the 'on' button working more efficiently than the 'off' button. This may have evolved to remind a mother that she had put her baby down and not to forget to pick him up. Research has shown that babies who are carried by their mothers cry less than Western babies who are placed in cots and prams for much of the day.

IMPORTANT BEHAVIOURS

To those helping the mother at the birth of her baby, it is important to be aware of these behaviours as their presence helps create the relationship between the mother and baby. If there is an attempt to create an environment of evolutionary adaptedness, the experience will have maximum impact for the mother, father and their baby. Trevathen (1987) believes the birth attendants also benefit by being present and taking part.

The behaviours to be discussed are bonding, tactile behaviour, the senses – vision, hearing and olfaction – and lateral preferences.

Bonding

Bowlby, from the 1950s, was specifically interested in how the infant forms attachments with its parents. In contrast, Klaus & Kennell in the 1970s examined parental aspects of attachment. It is important to remember these differing viewpoints when considering the meaning of the word bonding. Klaus & Kennell (1976) open their book with the statement: 'Perhaps the mother's attachment to her child is the strongest bond in the human'. They believed that this mother–infant bond formed the basis on which the infant's future attachments are built and through which the child develops a sense of self.

Developing their theory from an ethological basis, they suggested that there was a sensitive period when maternal and paternal attachment to their newborn took place. Hinde (1982) describes a sensitive period as a time when 'a given event produces a stronger effect on development, or a given event can be produced more readily during a certain period than earlier or later'. This is less restrictive than the Lorenz concept where, if the behaviour does not occur within the critical period, the opportunity is lost. Attachment may be difficult if the early opportunity is missed but still develops. In ethological terms there is a balance between environmentally stable and environmentally labile species-specific behaviour allowing adjustments to occur in response to novel situations (Bowlby 1984).

The concept of a sensitive period for the infant is complex. Infant attachment develops over the first 6 months and Bowlby (1984) suggested that infant behaviour develops in phases from simple response to stimuli to a full **dyadic relationship** in response to parental behaviour. Parental behaviour depends on the presence of a sensitive period and if this is disrupted, the attachment behaviour of the infant may not develop normally. De Chateau (1976) found that when mothers were allowed an hour of skin-to-skin contact following birth, they demonstrated more hold-ing, encompassing and *en face* behaviour. Their infants cried less and smiled more than those of mothers separated from their infants in the first hour. Other studies reported similar findings (Anisfeld & Lipper 1983, Kontos 1978).

There has been much criticism of the bonding theory. Many studies lacked scientific methodology and have been difficult to replicate. Feminists objected to the studies because they believed that the theory was an attempt to keep mothers tied to their babies and in the home (Arney 1980.) Michael Lamb (1983) has been one of the most outspoken critics of bonding theory. He believes it is highly unlikely that a species as dependent on social learning as the human would exhibit such narrow behaviour as sensitive periods. However, even though the earlier studies may have been flawed, the events within the first few hours of birth are important.

Trevathen (1987) believes that there is a sensitive period in the first hour of birth but it is highly variable across time and between cultures. In support of the theory, she takes into consideration the intense physical and emotional experience of giving birth and the changes in hormonal status that accompany the process. She writes: 'It is a period of excitement for the parents that is valuable and meaningful in itself'.

Holding the infant close provides warmth, stimulation, eye contact and a chance for the mother to talk to the infant in the typical high-pitched voice. Also, by holding the baby on her left side, the rhythmic sounds of her heart beat may provide continuity for him from uterus to independent life. Licking and nuzzling the nipple stimulates the production of oxytocin and stimulates uterine contractions to expel the placenta. Colostrum is the infant's only source of vitamin K which acts to prevent haemorrhage at the umbilical cord. Trevathen concludes that there is scant evidence in today's world that contact between mothers and babies in the immediate postpartum period is necessary for survival or for bond formation.

The observed behaviours are probably 'relics from the past' and no longer have any significant function. Trevathen also says that we might not be able to survive if confronted with our past 'environment of evolutionary adaptedness'. At that time the only infants who survived were those whose bond with their mothers began at birth and continued until they could survive independently. In modern society even the basic aspect of nurture, feeding, can be undertaken by others if necessary.

In similar mode, Bowlby (1984) wrote: 'Almost from the first many children have more than one figure towards whom they can direct attachment behaviour'. Morgan (1994) introduced the concept of the extended family and repeated Bowlby's reminder that almost from the first day the infant is given the opportunity to form attachments to other family members, particularly the father. She makes the point that usually the mother does not have to accept the whole responsibility for childrearing. However, a child constantly surrounded by a succession of stranger caregivers may become withdrawn.

If the sensitive period is present in humans but plays little part in survival or eventual attachment, how should the professional interpret the first hour after birth? Ball (1994) refers to the hour as the 'fourth stage of labour'. Sweet (1997) advises midwives that they have a duty to ensure that all mothers have the opportunity to be with their new babies during this hour. Absence of this time may have an adverse effect on the way mothers perceive the birth, reducing their emotional satisfaction, and this is still evident 6 weeks after the delivery (Ball 1994). Although infant survival and maternal–infant attachment may not suffer if this behaviour is omitted, the mother may find birth less fulfilling.

Tactile behaviour

Attendants present at normal births report a specific maternal behaviour when first given the infant to handle. Klaus & Kennell (1976) quote Rubin (1963) who noted this orderly progression of behaviour. Rubin noticed that mothers took about 3 days to complete the behavioural sequence but they had limited access to their babies without clothing. Klaus et al (1970) saw the same sequence of behaviour occurring within minutes if mothers were given their nude babies to hold after birth. The mothers began with fingertip touching of their baby's extremities. Within 4–8 min they began to massage, stroke and place the palms of their hands around the baby's trunk. Klaus & Kennell (1976) report the findings of Lang (1972) who observed babies born in their own homes. The touching began with fingertips in a gentle stroking motion, face first. This occurred before the delivery of the placenta and before the first breastfeed. When the baby was offered the breast, the nipple was explored by the baby's tongue, licking continuously. Klaus & Kennell (1976) believe that this may be species-specific behaviour but has been modified by cultural behaviour at births. Papousek & Papousek (1982) stated: 'In the human the typical behaviours providing the newborn with comfort, protection and nourishment have been taken over by cultural institutions . . .'.

Trevathen (1987) places the tactile interaction between mother and baby in an evolutionary context. Many mammals lick their young to stimulate breathing and defaecation. Trevathan suggests that in humans, stroking has taken over from licking. Rubbing or massaging the infant is used by both mothers and birth attendants as a means to stimulate respirations. Trevathen (1981) observed 66 of the women in her study for the first 10 min of contact specifically to examine the possibility that tactile interaction was a species-specific behaviour.

Touching behaviours were recorded every 10 s and grouped into seven categories.

1 Holding the infant with both hands.
2 Holding with one hand.
3 Not holding or touching although the infant is with her.
4 Holding with one arm with fingertip stroking of the infant's face.
5 Holding with one arm with fingertip stroking of the infant's extremities.
6 Holding with one arm with fingertip stroking of the infant's trunk.
7 Holding with one arm with palmar massaging of the infant's extremities and trunk.

Although Trevathen noted fingertip and palmar touching, these behaviours reduced together over the 10 min when looked at in three time intervals each lasting 3 min 20 s. The percentage of the total time is given below. Most of the time was spent in passive holding (categories 1 and 2 above), a category not included in other studies.

Time interval	Fingertip touching	Palmar massage
1	18.7%	6%
2	18.2%	3.9%
3	17.8%	2.3%

Although the previously described tactile behaviours were observed in all the women, they varied widely from woman to woman. Trevathen could not accept the concept of invariant behaviour. She therefore looked for **endogenous** (from within) and **exogenous** (environmental) factors that might create the differences. She analysed the behaviour in:

1 'Hispanic' mothers and 'Anglo' mothers in her multicultural subjects;
2 mothers of boys and of girls;
3 primiparous and multiparous women.

The Anglo mothers spent less time holding their babies and changed state more often than the Hispanic women. Boys were less likely to be touched for longer periods but more likely to be actively explored than girls. Primiparous women spent more time not touching their infants than the multiparous women but they spent slightly longer exploring their babies. Based on the evidence from her study, Trevathen decided that there is a species-specific pattern of tactile interaction but the more typical pattern of mother–infant interaction is to 'cradle or encompass' the baby for the first few minutes after birth with occasional palmar massage to stimulate the baby's respirations. If the mother was not distracted, finger exploration of face, hands and extremities followed soon.

The role of the senses

The motor state of the newborn is rudimentary and babies can do little for themselves. However, in contrast, the neonate has functioning senses of vision, hearing and olfaction and appears capable of differentiating stimuli. From the early days neonates can take in information from the world around them. Their lack of motor response has made it difficult to determine how good their sensory abilities are and it would seem likely that their sense of smell and taste would be in advance of vision and hearing as feeding is so central to their well-being and they regulate their own feeding and drinking (Atkinson & Braddick 1982).

The method of studying sensory processes in the neonate relies on the ability of a stimulus to elicit a reflex response. One of the best used responses is that of high-amplitude sucking when infants are presented with visual and auditory stimuli (Siqueland & Delucia 1969). Other methods used include electrical measurement of the neonate's brain activity, examination of the organs with instruments such as an ophthalmoscope and observation of responses to stimuli such as head turning.

Vision

The commonest measure of vision is **visual acuity**, that is, what detail can be resolved. In infants this involves discrimination of simple black and white patterns. Newborn babies do not focus very well and the level of visual acuity is about 20–30 times lower than in the adult. Alternative black and white stripes can only be distinguished if they are 3 mm wide and held at a distance of 30 cm from the eyes (Oates 1988). Infants see with binocular vision and focus best at a distance of between 30 to 50 cm (Slater & Findlay 1975) which is approximately the distance between them and the adult face when cradled in adult arms and the distance at which the visual interest of the baby is captured.

Preferential looking (PL) studies have shown that infants prefer to look at some stimuli rather than others. All normal alert newborns will follow a moving object with their eyes and head and prefer to look at moving objects (Brazelton et al 1966). They prefer three-dimensional objects over two-dimensional and high-contrast to low-contrast patterns. They prefer curved contours rather than straight contours (Fantz & Miranda 1975) and novel objects more than familiar ones.

Of importance in the above findings are the *en face* position, the development of social smiles and left side holding which will all be discussed below. *En face* is part of attachment behaviour between mothers and their infants and fathers and their infants. Klaus et al (1975) noted that a mother's interest in her baby's eyes increased during the first 10 min following birth. This author has heard mothers saying to their babies 'Open *your* eyes so that *I* can see *you*'. It is also, marvellous evolutionary arrangement, the distance at which a mother holds her baby when she is breastfeeding, a time of optimal contact for the mother and her baby (Fig. 57.1).

Women hold their babies in the *en face* position which is defined as the position in which the mother's face is rotated so that her eyes and those of the infant meet fully in the same vertical plane of rotation (Klaus & Kennell 1976). Trevathen found that all mothers in her study spent some time in the first

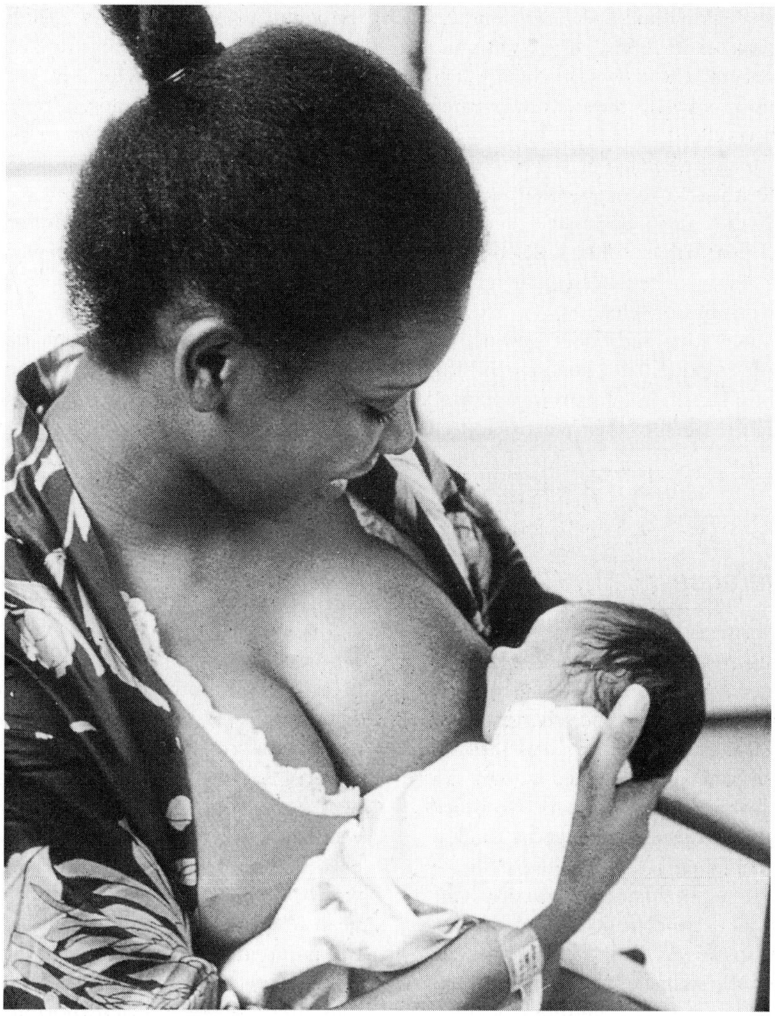

Figure 57.1 *Eye contact during breastfeeding (from Kelnar C, Harvey D, Simpson C, 1995, with permission).*

hour of birth looking at their infants *en face*. An additional fact is that women tend to cradle their newborn babies on their left arms regardless of their own handedness. The implications for this linked with the *en face* position for the monitoring of the emotional state of the baby will be discussed below.

Imitation of facial expressions suggests that the newborn has the ability to both recognise expressions and to copy them. This is a staggering feat as facial expressions utilise many muscles. The most famous expression is poking out the tongue. In a quiet moment with the baby, hold him in the *en face* position and poke out your tongue. If you persevere and the baby is quietly alert, he may poke out his tongue in imitation. Another expression that the baby will imitate is the open mouth. The earliest smiles shown by babies soon after birth tend to be one-sided, fleeting and do not involve the muscles around the eyes. As early as 14 days after delivery, some babies will begin to smile in response to social interaction.

Hearing

Neonates orientate to sound by turning their heads. They show interest in human speech and will suck more vigorously in response to the mother's voice as early as 3 days after birth (DeCasper & Fifer 1980). Many researchers (Brazelton 1963, Klaus & Kennell 1976, Lang 1972, Trevathen 1987) have recorded that women typically unconsciously speak to babies in a high-pitched voice. They even hold two conversations at once, reverting to normal speech when talking to an adult. The neonatal auditory system responds more readily to the higher frequencies of the human voice as demonstrated by orienting responses. Trevathen (1987) found all but two of her mothers changed their voice pitch to talk to their infants.

Speech is not one-sided. Entrainment is the rhythmic movement made by a baby in response to human speech. Condon & Sander (1974) demonstrated this interactional synchrony as early as 12 h after birth. Besides altering the pitch of their voices, adults tend to use repetitive, simplistic language when talking to infants (and pet animals). The baby moves its body and limbs in synchrony with the mother's voice and she responds by continuing to talk, thus prolonging the synchrony.

Olfaction

Bronson (1982) hypothesised that the older a brain function is in evolutionary terms, the earlier it will appear in the neonate. The olfactory centre is a very old brain centre and is the main mode of interaction with the environment for many animals. Macfarlane (1975) demonstrated that young babies recognise breast pads worn by their own mothers and preferentially turn towards them if offered a choice between those worn by their mothers and by other lactating mothers.

Fleming et al (1995) confirmed earlier findings (Porter et al 1983) that mothers quickly learned to recognise the odour of their own baby, especially if they have been given an early opportunity to hold and feed their babies. They recognised by smell T-shirts worn by their babies when allowed to choose between them and T-shirts worn by other babies. Vernix provides a source for bacterial colonisation and odour production. This recognition may have been important for bonding and this evidence for the importance of olfaction in humans is supported by studies of people preferring the smell of their partner to that of other adults.

Lateralities

Maternal holding preference

Salk (1973) discovered that women prefer to hold their babies on the left side of their bodies irrespective of handedness. This observation has been confirmed by many studies of people all over the world and in photographs, paintings and sculptures over the last 30 years although Dagenbach & Fitzgerald (1988) did find that maternal and parental handedness affected holding side preference in their study. However, the left-handed mothers showed the strong left-handed preference at birth and a handedness bias appeared only after some time.

Various hypotheses have been put forward to explain this left-sided holding preference, all derived from a belief that the baby elicits the behaviour in some way. Briefly, these include Salk (1973) who thought that the sound of the maternal heart beat if the baby was held on the left side of the thorax soothed the infant. Ginsburg et al (1979) found mothers' holding side preference was related to their baby's head-turning preference. Infants who preferred to turn their heads to the right, as 90% do, were preferentially carried on the left side of the body and vice versa. More recently, Manning & Chamberlain (1991) hypothesised that mothers carrying their babies on their left sides could monitor their emotions with the right side of the brain.

Neonatal head-turning preferences

More than 80% of newborn babies prefer to turn their heads to the right when lying supine (Gesell 1945, Turkewitz et al 1965). There is a probable link between this behaviour and eventual handedness which may develop out of a continued attention to the hand most often in their visual field (Michel 1981). Liederman & Kinsbourne (1980) found that there is evidence that head-turning behaviour is inherited and thus is genetically programmed.

They believed that the asymmetrical behaviour was linked to asymmetry in the motor development of the brain hemispheres. As the left hemisphere controls movements on the right side of the body, this could account for the right-sided turning preference and the later development of right handedness. Cornwell et al (1985) carried out an indepth study of infant head-turning preferences, observing spontaneous behaviour. They found that the strong right-sided preference at birth has disappeared by 3 months and babies then turn their heads to either side equally.

Implications of maternal and neonatal asymmetries

Mothers often report more difficulty feeding their babies on one breast than the other. Stables researched this phenomenon for an MSc dissertation (Stables & Hewitt 1995). The problem most often arose when the woman was right-handed, preferred to carry the baby on her left and the baby preferred to turn its head to the right. This set up a situation where the left breast was much easier to feed from. The woman enjoyed carrying the baby on her left arm and had her right dominant hand free with which to offer the baby the nipple. When the baby turned his head to the right he turned towards the breast. Unfortunately this group included most of the mothers!

Two aspects of this phenomenon can be discussed. The first is that after a few feeds most mothers and babies soon adapted to each other but some women gave up feeding because of the initial difficulty. Second, there is an opportunity for midwives to use their skills by varying the way the mother holds the baby to ensure that the early feeding efforts are successful. Basically, in women with the above problem, if the baby is moved across the mother's body and tucked under the right arm so that he can suckle at the right breast with his head turned towards the right, the mother is more likely to be successful. This is not a new strategy. Midwives have used it for decades but may not have known why. That is why research-based practice is so important to decide what care is of value.

Summary of main points

- For thousands of years the brain was the realm of scientists but the mind was studied by philosophers. Wilhelm Wundt opened the first psychology laboratory at the University of Leipzig in 1879. Since then other disciplines have been developed to study behaviour such as ethology and branches of psychology.
- Ethologists ask four types of questions about behaviour: what is its immediate causation, how does it develop, what is its function and how did it evolve? Other biological sciences related to ethology of the human species are ecology, endocrinology and neuropsychology. There is also a relationship between ethology and human social sciences.
- Physiological psychology has roots in both philosophy and biology. Physiological psychologists take a monistic approach to the study of human behaviour but remain aware that human behaviour is complex and that a reductionist process cannot predict behaviour in all circumstances. Recently the discipline of evolutionary psychology has developed to examine the evolution of behaviour.
- There are four main characteristics of instinctive behaviour. It is species specific, it is a sequence of behaviour that runs a predictable course, its consequences contribute to the preservation of an individual or the continuity of a species and many examples of it develop even though opportunities for learning are absent.

- The nature–nurture debate is now thought to be a meaningless division. Every biological characteristic is a product of the interaction between genes and environment. If a characteristic is little influenced by environmental variations it is environmentally stable and if it is much influenced by the environment it is environmentally labile. Instinctive behaviour is environmentally stable.
- Some believe that the variability of human behaviour proves that it is culturally driven and cannot be called instinctive. However, in higher species instinctive behaviour is not stereotyped but follows a recognisable pattern and runs a predictable course. Despite the immense variety of cultural norms in childbearing, some behaviours repeatedly emerge.
- Two main characteristics of humans are versatility and the capacity for innovation. These have allowed an enormous extension of the natural environments in which humans live and procreate. Within these multiple environments the environmentally stable components of behaviour related to childbearing can be found. The social surroundings of the woman are part of the environment in which childbearing and childrearing take place.
- Pair bonding may be part of human ethology, typical of species who produce altricial rather than precocial infants. Male parenting is necessary for the support of the woman and her children during the long growth to maturity of the human child and may have been initiated by the continuity of female sexual receptiveness. There is no consensus on the nature of the family in human biological terms.
- The use of ethograms in the study of people has arisen from painstaking descriptions of behaviour in the ecological and social setting where it has evolved and naturally occurs. Behaviours that could fit into an ethogram of human maternal–infant behaviour are interactive, involving both mother and infant.
- To those helping the mother at the birth of her baby, it is important to be aware of these behaviours as their presence helps create the relationship between the mother and baby. If there is an attempt to create an environment of evolutionary adaptedness, the experience will have maximum impact for the mother, father and their baby.
- Bonding concerns the mother's attachment to her child and may form the basis on which the infant's future attachments are created and through which the child develops a sense of self. There has been criticism of the bonding theory. Many studies lacked scientific methodology and have been difficult to replicate. Although the earlier studies appear to have been flawed, this does not mean that the events within the first few hours of birth are unimportant.
- Holding the infant close provides warmth, stimulation, eye contact and a chance for the mother to talk to the infant in the typical high-pitched voice. Holding the baby on her left side near the rhythmic sounds of her heart beat may provide continuity during his transition to independent life. Licking and nuzzling the nipple stimulates the production of oxytocin and stimulates uterine contractions to expel the placenta.
- Lack of time to be alone with her baby may have an adverse effect on the way a mother perceives the birth, reducing her emotional satisfaction and this is still evident 6 weeks after the delivery. Although infant survival and maternal–infant attachment may not suffer if this period of time is omitted, the mother may find it less fulfilling as a life experience.
- Attendants present at normal births where there is minimal medical interference report a specific maternal behaviour when first given the infant to handle. Mothers begin with fingertip touching of their baby's extremities. Within 4–8 min they begin to massage, stroke and place the palms of their hands around the baby's trunk.
- Although the motor state of the newborn is rudimentary, the neonate has functioning senses of vision, hearing and olfaction and appears capable of differentiating stimuli. From the early days neonates can take in information from the world around them. Studying sensory processes in the neonate relies on his ability to respond to a stimulus. One of the best responses is that of high-amplitude sucking when infants are presented with visual and auditory stimuli.
- Infants see with binocular vision and focus best at a distance of between 30 to 50 cm. This is also the distance at which the visual interest of the baby is captured. Infants prefer to look at three-dimensional objects over two-dimensional and high-contrast rather than low-contrast patterns. They prefer curved rather than straight contours and novel objects more than familiar ones.
- Women hold their babies in the *en face* position. Imitation of facial expressions suggests that the newborn has the ability not only to recognise expressions but to copy them. As early as 14 days after delivery some babies will begin to smile in response to social interaction.
- Neonates orientate to sound by turning their heads. They show interest in human speech and suck more vigorously in response to the mother's voice as early as 3 days after birth. Women typically speak to babies in a high-pitched voice and the neonatal auditory system responds more readily to the higher frequencies of the human voice. Entrainment is the rhythmic movement made by a baby in response to the mother's or other human voice. This interfactional synchrony is seen as early as 12 h after birth.
- Young babies recognise breast pads worn by their own mothers and preferentially turn towards them if offered a choice between those worn by their mothers and by other lactating mothers. Mothers quickly learn to recognise the odour of their own baby, especially if they have been given an early opportunity to hold and feed their babies.
- Women prefer to hold their babies on the left side of their bodies irrespective of handedness. Various hypotheses to explain this preference are derived from a belief that the baby elicits the behaviour. These include the sound of the maternal heart beat soothing the infant, mothers' holding side preference being related to their baby's head-turning preference and mothers carrying their babies on their left sides monitoring their emotions with the right side of the brain.
- Most newborn babies prefer to turn their heads to the right when lying supine. There is a probable link between this behaviour and eventual handedness so that head-turning behaviour is genetically programmed. The strong right-sided head-turning preference disappears by 3 months.
- Mothers often report more difficulty feeding their babies on one breast than the other. In one study the problem most often arose when the woman was right-handed, preferred to carry the baby on her left and the baby preferred to turn its head to the right. This set up a situation where the left breast was much easier to feed from.
- There is an opportunity for midwives to use their skills by varying the way the mother holds the baby to ensure that the early feeding efforts are successful. Basically, if the baby is moved across the mother's body and tucked under the right arm so that he can suckle at the right breast with his head turned towards the right, the mother is more likely to be successful.

References

Anisfeld E, Lipper E. 1983 Early contact, social support and mother-infant bonding. Pediatrics 72, 79–83.

Arney WR. 1980 Maternal-infant bonding: the politics of falling in love with your child. Feminist Studies 6, 547–570.

Atkinson J, Braddick O. 1982 Sensory and perceptual capacities of the neonate. In Stratton P (ed) 1982 Psychobiology of the Human Newborn. John Wiley, Chichester.

Ball JA. (ed) 1994 Reactions to Motherhood. Hale: Books for Midwives Press, London.

Bowlby J. 1984 Attachment and Loss: Vol 1 Attachment. Penguin, Harmondsworth.

Brazelton TB, 1963, The early mother-infant adjustment. Pediatrics, 32:931–938.

Brazelton TB, Scholl ML, Robey JS. 1966 Visual responses in the newborn. Pediatrics 37, 284–290.

Bronson GW. 1982 (Neonatal) capacities and characteristics. In Stratton P (ed) Psychobiology of the Human Newborn. John Wiley, Chichester.

Carlson NR. 1991 Physiology of Behavior, 4th edn. Allyn and Bacon, New York.

Condon WS, Sander LW. 1974 Neonate movement is synchronised with adult speech: interactional participation and language acquisition. Science 183, 99–101.

Cornwell KS, Barnes CL, Fitzgerald HE, Harris LJ. 1985 Neurobehavioral reorganisation in early infancy; patterns of head orientation following lateral and midline holds. Infant Mental Health Journal 6(3), 126–136.

Dagenbach D, Harris L J, Fitzgerald H E, 1988 A longitudinal study of lateral biases in parents' cradling and holding of infants. Infant Mental Health Journal, 9(3), 218–234.

De Chateau P, 1976, Neonatal care routines: influences on maternal and infant behaviour and on breast feeding (thesis) Umea, Sweden, Umea University medical dissertations, N S no. 20.

DeCasper AJ, Fifer WP. 1980 Of human bonding: newborns prefer their mothers' voices. Science 208, 1174–1176.

Fantz RL, Miranda S. 1975 Newborn infant attention to form and contour. Child Development 46, 224–228.

Fleming A, Corter C, Surbey M, Franks P, Steiner M. 1995 Postpartum factors related to mothers' recognition of newborn infant odours. Journal of Reproductive and Infant Psychology 13(3–4), 197–210.

Fox R, 1967, Kinship and Marriage. Penguin Books, Harmondsworth.

Gesell A, 1945, The Embryology of Behaviour, Harper, New York.

Ginsburg HJ, Fling S, Hope ML, Musgrove D, Andrews C. 1979 Maternal holding preferences: a consequence of newborn head turning behaviour. Child Development 50, 280–281.

Goodall J. 1986 The Chimpanzees of Gombe, Patterns of Behaviour. Belknap Press/Harvard University Press, Cambridge, Mass.

Gould SJ. 1977 Ontogeny and Phylogeny. Harvard University Press, Cambridge, Mass.

Greenfield SA. 1997 The Human Mind Explained. Cassell, London.

Hinde RA. 1982 Ethology. Fontana, London.

Kelnar C, Harvey D, Simpson C. 1995 The Sick Newborn Baby. Baillière Tindall, London.

Klaus MH, Kennell JH. 1982 Parent-Infant Bonding. CV Mosby, St Louis.

Klaus MH, Kennell JH, Plumb N, Zuehlke S. 1970 Human maternal behaviour at first contact with her young. Pediatrics 46, 187–192.

Klaus MH, Trause MA, Kennell JH. 1975 Does human maternal behaviour after birth show a characteristic pattern? Parent-Infant Interaction, Ciba Foundation Symposium Vol 33. Elsevier, Amsterdam.

Kontos D. 1978 A study of the effect of extended mother-infant contact on maternal behaviour at one and three months. Birth and the Family Journal 5, 133–140.

Lamb ME. 1983 Early mother-neonate contact and the mother-child relationship. Journal of Child Psychology and Psychiatry 24, 487–494.

Lang R. 1972 Birth Book. Genesis Press, Ben Lomond, California.

Leakey R, Lewin R. 1992 Origins Reconsidered: In Search of What Makes Us Human. Little, Brown, Boston.

Liederman J, Kinsbourne M. 1980 Rightward turning biases in neonates reflect a single neural asymmetry in motor planning. Infant Behaviour and Development 3, 245–251.

Lovejoy CO, 1980, Hominid Origins: The Role of Bipedalism, American Journal Of Physical Anthropology, Vol 52: 250. In Johanson D C, Edey M A, 1981, Lucy, the beginnings of mankind, William Clowes (Beccles) Ltd, Beccles and London.

Macfarlane A. 1975 Olfaction in the development of social preferences in the human neonate. Parent-Infant Interaction, Ciba Foundation Symposium Vol 33. Elsevier Amsterdam.

Manning JT, Chamberlain AT. 1991 Left-sided cradling and brain lateralisation. Ethology and Sociobiology 12, 237–244.

Michel G. 1981 Right-handedness: a consequence of infant supine head-orientation preference? Science 212, 685–687.

Morgan E. 1994 The Descent of the Child. Souvenir Press, London.

Oates J. 1988 Cognitive development in infancy. Block 1 of the Open University course Cognitive Development: Language and Thinking from Birth to Adolescence. Open University Press, Buckingham.

Papousek H, Papousek M. 1982 Integration into the social world: survey of research. In Stratton P (ed) 1982 Psychobiology of the Human Newborn. John Wiley, Chichester.

Porter RH, Cernock JM, McLaughlin FJ. 1983 Maternal recognition of neonates through olfactory clues. Physiology and Behavior 30, 151–154.

Rubin R. 1963 Maternal touch. Nursing Outlook 22, 828–831.

Salk L. 1973 The role of the heartbeat in relations between mother and infant. Scientific American 228, 24–29.

Siqueland ER, Delucia CA. 1969 Visual reinforcement of non-nutritive sucking in human infants. Science 165, 1144–1146.

Slater A, Findlay J. 1975 Binocular fixation in the newborn baby. Journal of Experimental Child Psychology 20, 248–273.

Stables D, Hewitt G. 1995 The effect of lateral asymmetries on breast feeding skills: can midwives' holding interventions overcome unilateral breast feeding problems? Midwifery 11, 28–36.

Stratton P. (Ed) 1982 Psychobiology of the Human Newborn. John Wiley, Chichester.

Sweet BR. 1997 The psychology of childbirth. In Sweet BR with Tiran D (eds) Mayes Midwifery, 12th edn. Baillière Tindall, London. pp 151–158.

Trevathen WR. 1981 Maternal touch at first contact with her newborn infant. Developmental Psychobiology 14, 549–558.

Trevathen WR. 1987 Human Birth: An Evolutionary Perspective. Aldine de Gruyter, New York.

Turkewitz G, Gordon EW, Birch HG. 1965 Head turning in the human neonate: spontaneous patterns. Journal of Comparative and Physiological Psychology 59, 189–192.

Recommended reading

Anisfeld E, Lipper E. 1983 Early contact, social support and mother-infant bonding. Pediatrics 72, 79–83.

Ball JA. (ed) 1994 Reactions to Motherhood. Hale: Books for Midwives Press, London.

Bowlby J. 1984 Attachment and Loss: Vol 1 Attachment. Penguin, Harmondsworth.

Fleming A, Corter C, Surbey M, Franks P, Steiner M. 1995 Postpartum factors related to mothers' recognition of newborn infant odours. Journal of Reproductive and Infant Psychology 13(3–4), 197–210.

Lamb ME. 1983 Early mother-neonate contact and the mother-child relationship. Journal of Child Psychology and Psychiatry 24, 487–494.

Klaus MH, Kennell JH. 1982 Parent-Infant Bonding. CV Mosby St Louis.

Manning JT, Chamberlain AT. 1991 Left-sided cradling and brain lateralisation. Ethology and Sociobiology 12, 237–244.

Trevathen WR. 1981 Maternal touch at first contact with her newborn infant. Developmental Psychobiology 14, 549–558.

Index

Note: page numbers in **bold** are to references in figures only; page numbers in *italic* are to references in tables only.